Realities in Childbearing
SECOND EDITION

Mary Lou Moore, R.N.C., M.A., A.C.C.E., F.A.A.N.

Nursing Consultant and Childbirth Educator
Formerly Nursing Coordinator and Instructor
North Carolina Perinatal-Neonatal Nursing Program
Bowman Gray School of Medicine
Winston-Salem, North Carolina

With a contribution by

Ora Strickland, R.N., Ph.D., F.A.A.N.

Associate Professor and
Doctoral Program Evaluator
School of Nursing
University of Maryland at Baltimore

W.B. SAUNDERS COMPANY
PHILADELPHIA   LONDON   TORONTO   MEXICO CITY   RIO DE JANEIRO   SYDNEY   TOKYO

W. B. Saunders Company: West Washington Square
                          Philadelphia, PA   19105

                          1 St. Anne's Road
                          Eastbourne, East Sussex BN21 3UN, England

                          1 Goldthorne Avenue
                          Toronto, Ontario M8Z 5T9, Canada

                          Apartado 26370—Cedro 512
                          Mexico 4, D.F., Mexico

                          Rua Coronel Cabrita, 8
                          Sao Cristovao Caixa Postal 21176
                          Rio de Janeiro, Brazil

                          9 Waltham Street
                          Artarmon, N.S.W. 2064, Australia

                          Ichibancho, Central Bldg., 22-1 Ichibancho
                          Chiyoda-Ku, Tokyo 102, Japan

Library of Congress Cataloging in Publication Data

Moore, Mary Lou.

Realities in childbearing.

Includes index.

1. Obstetrical nursing.   2. Pregnancy.   3. Infants (New-
born)—Care and hygiene.   I. Strickland, Ora.   II. Title.
[DNLM: 1. Family—Nursing texts.   2. Neonatology—
Nursing texts.   3. Obstetrical nursing.   4. Pregnancy—
Nursing texts. WY 157 M823r]

RG951.M66 1983   618.2'0024613   82–40188

ISBN 0–7216–6498–9

Cover photo by J. T. Chalmers

Realities in Childbearing   ISBN   0-7216-6498-9

Last digit is the print number: 9   8   7   6   5   4   3   2

To Our Parents
MARY BLACKWELL HANSON
and
HAROLD EPHRAIM HANSON

GLADYS HARTZ MOORE
and
RONALD ROBERTS MOORE

Nursing Care Plan Contributors

Hazel N. Brown, R.N., B.S.N., M.A.Ed., Ed.D.
Assistant Professor
School of Nursing
University of North Carolina at Greensboro

Elizabeth K. Dickson, C.N.M., M.S.N.
Director
Carolina Birth Center
High Point, North Carolina

Mona B. Ketner, R.N., M.S.N.
Clinical Educator, Labor and Delivery Room and Ob/Gyn Recovery Room
Forsyth Memorial Hospital
Winston-Salem, North Carolina

Preface

Perinatal nurses have a unique opportunity to share in one of the most significant times of their clients' lives, the period of childbearing. Nurses enhance that period through interaction with individual clients and families, through nursing research in which new and better approaches to care are developed and evaluated, and through advocacy of such principles as the rights of persons and family-centered care.

During the 1970's perinatal nursing changed in a number of ways. Family members, including other children, became more involved throughout the childbearing year. Birthing rooms and alternative birthing centers provided choices in childbearing. Education for childbirth and parenting became available for many more families. Perinatal mortality decreased and many of those infants who survived premature birth could anticipate normal growth and development.

The 1980's offer even greater challenges. Ever-increasing technological potential must be balanced by an equally increasing understanding of human needs. The benefits of family-centered care and increased knowledge must be available to clients regardless of socioeconomic status and ethnicity. With infant mortality rates of nonwhite persons nearly double those of white persons, perinatal nurses face a formidable task.

We are aware that perinatal nursing will not be the career emphasis of many student nurses who use this text. Yet we believe an understanding of the needs of childbearing women and their families will enhance any nursing practice. Nurses in emergency rooms, in operating rooms, in medical and surgical and psychiatric practice may at times have clients who are pregnant or who have problems related in some way to childbearing. Nurses, as citizens, have the opportunity to be advocates for programs and practices that, through the improvement of childbearing, will affect the quality of life for future generations.

This edition is intended for all nurses, student and professional, with the belief that each of us, through our contribution to the quality of life for childbearing families, will also contribute to the quality of life in our society.

MARY LOU MOORE

Acknowledgments

It is impossible to acknowledge all of the individuals who contributed to a book such as this one. The families for whom we have cared, the students and professional nurses we have taught, colleagues in nursing, medicine, nutrition, and the sciences—each has contributed and continues to contribute to the knowledge we share with you here.

A particular debt is due to several individuals: Susan Rumsey, R.N., M.P.H., and Mary Brodish, R.N., M.N., who critically and helpfully read portions of the manuscript and shared many good ideas with me; Charlene Miller, R.N., who shared here knowledge of adolescent pregnancy; individuals and families from my childbirth education classes and from the Continuing Education Program of the Winston-Salem-Forsyth County school system who allowed themselves to be photographed; Laura and Charles Kesler and Tim Chalmers, who shared the pictures of the birth of Laura and Charles' child; Martha Ogburn, R.N., M.A., and Sarah Jones, R.N., A.C.C.E., who helped to locate photographs; Patrick Lawson, who contributed a number of photographs; Dr. Keith Moore for permission to use many excellent illustrations from his book *The Developing Human,* second edition; Dr. Lewis Nelson for the ultrasound photographs; Dr. Elsie Broussard for permission to use the Broussard assessment; Drs. Ralph Traylor, Richard Trippie, and Rosita Pildes for photographs and charts; Ora Strickland, R.N., Ph.D., Hazel Brown, R.N., Ed.D., Elizabeth Dickson, R.N., M.S.N., C.N.M., and Mona Ketner, R.N., M.S.N., who contributed nursing care plans; Terri Welfare and Janet Somers, who turned manuscript into beautiful typescript; Betty Cobbs and Kathy Pitcoff of W. B. Saunders Company, who provided many excellent ideas as well as unlimited support; and all of those organizations, authors, and photographers who were so willing to share material with me.

Nursing Care Plans

Questionnaire

We are very interested in your comments concerning the second edition of *Realities in Childbearing* and your suggestions for its next edition. Your answers to any or all of the following questions and your comments will aid our evaluation and in this way, we believe, contribute to continually improving the ways in which nurses assist and care for families during childbearing.

1. What are the strongest features in *Realities in Childbearing*?

2. What parts of the book should be revised, expanded, shortened, etc., to make it more helpful to you?

3. What topics should be added?

4. What topics should be deleted?

Additional comments:

Please return to Mary Lou Moore, 701 Austin Lane, Winston-Salem, North Carolina, 27106.

Contents

Realities in Childbearing

The Context of
Childbearing

Childbearing in Today's World

All of us, student nurses and professional nurses, have accumulated many attitudes and feelings about childbearing long before we take a course or meet our first patient. These feelings and attitudes do make a difference in the meaning that a course in "maternity nursing" will have for us. This is the first reality each of us must consider.

Think back to the first time you were aware of pregnancy or of birth. What were the circumstances? How did you feel? Did you discuss your feelings with your family or your friends? Think about women you have known who were pregnant—their feelings and your reactions. Have you ever seen an infant during the process of birth or a film of the birth process? Have you ever seen a baby who was nursing at his mother's breast? What did you think? What did you feel?

Reality Versus "The Myth"

There is a popular myth in the United States, and probably in the rest of the world to a certain extent, that babies are born to couples who are married, who want them, and who are able to care for them, perhaps with a little help from those of us who provide health care. For some of the families we meet as we participate in maternity care, the myth appears to be close to the truth, although as we come to know these families more intimately we find that even for them there are adjustments to be made and stresses that they may not have anticipated that are not always readily apparent at first glance.

For many others, the myth bears little resemblance to the reality of their experience. There may be no husband or mate, only a mother alone. This does not mean that the baby is necessarily unwanted (just as marriage by no means guarantees a wanted baby), nor does it mean that there is not support from others (such as a grandmother). Poverty, poor health, inadequate nutrition, and family disorganization often coexist with pregnancy and birth. The disappointment of infertility or of the birth of a child who is less than normal may happen in any family.

The Pregnant Woman and Her Family

Throughout this text we will talk about the pregnant woman and her family. Who is her family? For some women, family means a husband and perhaps other children. But for many

pregnant women—more than half the women met in some agencies—there is no husband. The father may have a close, ongoing relationship with the mother, or he may have a very tentative relationship with her. The mother, or mother-to-be, may be living with her own mother and may have a close relationship with her, or she may be totally alienated from that family. The term *significant other(s)* is used by behavioral scientists to refer to the individual(s) who have a close, meaningful relationship with a particular person. Because significant other is a somewhat unwieldy term to use over and over throughout a text, we have used the words "father" or "family" frequently, while recognizing that for some women the significant person in her life may be neither of these.

The needs of each woman and the significant people in her life must be assessed and met on an individual basis. Families don't fit into neat boxes—husbands and wives in this one, unmarried mothers in a second, and the like—a theme that will be repeated throughout this text.

Care and Conflict in Contemporary Childbearing

Caring for childbearing families often places nurses in situations of conflict. This is one of the realities we must face each day. Three major areas of conflict, briefly discussed here, are recurrent themes, occurring in actual practice and referred to throughout this volume:

1. The conflict that may result between nurses and physicians because of their differing perspectives about care.
2. The conflict in values that may occur both among professionals and between professionals and patients over issues such as out-of-wedlock pregnancy and abortion.
3. The conflict between consumer desire and traditional practice.

Conflict: Nursing Support Versus Traditional Obstetric Care

Does obstetric care, which we will define as the *medical* care of the obstetric patient, differ from the nursing care of the childbearing family? Although there are obvious variations in individual practice settings, some specific, very important differences do exist.

Traditional obstetric care has focused on physiology and pathology. A focus on physiology has frequently meant that the social and emotional needs of women and their families were overlooked or considered less important than clearly physical needs. A focus on the search for the recognition of pathology has viewed mothers as "patients" rather than persons and pregnancy as a time of illness or potential illness rather than a period in which a natural biologic process is occurring.

Concepts from Maslow[2] (Chapter 2) suggest at least a part of the basis for this focus. Until well into the twentieth century many women and infants died during childbearing. Maslow suggested that needs for safety and security must be met before higher order needs, such as meaningfulness and individuality, can be satisfied. It is not too difficult to understand why health care professionals, both nurses and physicians, who began their practice at a time when childbirth was a major source of mortality, would place primary emphasis on physical safety.

While safety can never be ignored, childbirth is no longer a time of "death and mutilation," a phrase used by Breckenridge,[1] the founder of the Frontier Nursing Service. Nurses are able to provide not only safe and secure childbirth experiences, but experiences that meet needs for love and belongingness, self-esteem, and growth.

Recognition of the changes in both the mother and father as individuals and in the dynamics of family interaction at each stage of pregnancy is significant for nurses.

Closely related are those skills that offer support to the family in coping with these changes. The importance of understanding the physiologic aspects of the maternity cycle is not ignored; such understanding is, however, considered insufficient in itself.

In these areas, nurses function in an independent role. For example, nurses may teach classes in preparation for childbirth or postpartal classes. Supporting the family during labor, teaching the mother and father to care for their new baby, assessing the need for help from other professionals (a nutritionist or a social worker, for example), and referring the family to a professional are but a few examples of ways in which *nurses* care for childbearing families.

The difference in emphasis between traditional obstetrics and contemporary nursing may lead to conflict between professionals (particularly between nurses and physicians) or may result in combining the strengths of both professions to offer the best talents of both for the care of patients. The physician who sees the nurse's role as one of a "handmaiden" who is available to prepare supplies for him, but never to counsel *his* patient, does not under-

stand the role of nursing. The nurse who practices to meet this kind of expectation deprives her patient of comprehensive care.

Nurses who are knowledgeable about the total process of childbearing—its physiologic, emotional, and social components—have much to offer families that is unique and essential. It is toward this concept of care that this book is directed.

Conflicts in Values

Childbearing is important to every society; it is the means by which the society is perpetuated. So it should not be surprising that in every society there are strongly held values and beliefs about activities related to childbearing—sexual intercourse, abortion, and infanticide, for example.

Because we live in a society that is (1) pluralistic, i.e., with many cultural traditions, and (2) undergoing rapid social change, there are many conflicts about cultural beliefs.

Nurses who care for childbearing families are often caught in the conflict between their own values (marriage should occur before pregnancy; abortion is "murder"; or abortion is a woman's right, for example) and the values or beliefs of their patients or coworkers.

A basic issue is that of control. Who should make decisions about the circumstances surrounding birth—issues such as who shall be present, the position the mother may assume, the technology that shall be used? The desire of women and their families to have more control over events during pregnancy and childbirth is not isolated from the desire of persons to have more control in many aspects of their health and health care. Moreover, the opportunity to be an active participant in, rather than a passive recipient of, one's own care appears to be one factor in achieving a positive outcome.

During the same period in which family-centered values have become increasingly important, there has been a significant increase in the "technology of childbirth." Examples of this technology are the use of ultrasound and electronic fetal heart rate monitoring. Originally designed for mothers with complications during pregnancy, the use of such technology has increased in the care of all mothers and infants in many hospitals. Issues related to the causes and effects of technological intervention are discussed throughout this volume and are summarized in Chapter 30.

When nurses do not have opportunities to explore their own feelings about conflicts in values in a supportive environment, the woman or family who holds values that differ from those of the nurses who care for her may suffer. For example, the unmarried mother may, in some settings, receive less supportive care than the married couple. Nurses cannot ignore value conflicts; to do so is a source of stress to women and their families and to nurses themselves. (See Chapter 30, under Stress in Perinatal Nurses.)

Conflict: Traditional Practice, Consumer Desire, and Childbirth Technology

A growing number of families are searching for new and more meaningful experiences surrounding pregnancy and birth—experiences that do not separate families at one of the significant times of their lives and experiences that they feel are oriented in favor of human dignity.

The 1970's saw a rise in consumer activism in all areas of life, including the way in which maternity care is provided. Among the lay and lay-professional organizations that have been active (through conferences, publications, and the efforts of individuals) in bringing about changes in the care of childbearing families are the International Childbirth Education Association (ICEA), the American Society for Psychoprophylaxis in Obstetrics (ASPO), the American Academy of Husband Coached Childbirth, and the La Leche League. (The addresses of these and similar organizations are found in Appendix I.) These organizations, which we will term advocacy groups, have played a part in bringing about changes toward a more family-oriented system of maternity care in many areas of the United States.

Nurses may feel "caught" between two adversaries when advocacy groups and institutional policies conflict. On the one side are families who view nurses as implementers of institutional policy. On the other are administrators and physicians who are resistant to change and against whom nurses may feel quite powerless in effecting the changes that families desire. Student nurses at times feel very antagonistic toward staff nurses who fulfill traditional roles and who are not able to bring about changes.

Why should there be such conflict? Unlike most areas of practice, both outpatient and hospital, maternity nursing largely involves "patients" who are well rather than ill. The healthy mother, with no complications, does not really fit into a "medical model" designed primarily for individuals who are sick. Yet often she is treated within the framework of illness.

A major function of nurses who care for childbearing families is the examination of both traditional practices and the desires of families in relation to knowledge currently available to us—knowledge of both the biologic and the psychosocial needs of parents and infants—in order to chart the most appropriate course for contemporary maternity nursing.

Not every encounter between nurses and advocacy groups is helpful to either, especially in the beginning. Sometimes the clash is a matter of individual personalities. Often nurses feel that their professional competence is being attacked. If members of advocacy groups are demanding change, then they are obviously dissatisfied with current care.

Many nurses, of course, are a part of advocacy groups or maintain close associations with members of these groups. They have discovered that their nursing role as an advocate for families can often best be served by working along with families to bring about changes that both feel are desirable.

For example, in one community there was a strong desire on the part of a group of mothers, many of whom were members of the La Leche League, for "rooming-in" (i.e., allowing the baby to spend most of his day in his mother's room rather than in a central nursery). Over the period of a year, conversations between individual mothers and nurses resulted in a shared enthusiasm for a change in policy within the hospital. Nurses began to look at the practical aspects of the changes within the framework of safe and acceptable maternal and newborn care. Their professional expertise was essential before the desires of the families could become reality. Mothers and fathers were encouraged to communicate their feelings to the hospital administration, a factor also seen as significant to success. This feedback was continued after a trial period of rooming-in was established.

During the trial, data were collected from both mothers and staff to assess both good and bad aspects of the change. By the conclusion of a 3-month trial period, the change was firmly established, and within the year a similar change occurred in the community's other hospital.

Moreover, the bridges built between the La Leche group and the staff nurses have resulted in cooperation in other aspects of care. Money was raised by the group to purchase a breast pump for the hospital. There has been cooperation in the teaching of prenatal classes in the community. Hospital nurses more frequently refer mothers to La Leche leaders for help after they return home from the hospital. Undoubtedly, further enhancement of care will occur as a result of future cooperation.

Nurses can also become effective advocates of other aspects of care at local, state, and federal levels.

Problem: Fragmentation of Care

Who cares for, nurtures, and supports the family during pregnancy? At least part, and often a major part, of that support comes from people other than nurses, physicians, or other professionals. It is well that it does, for professional care is frequently fragmented, divided among many professional people.

Consider just the number of nurses the woman (and her family) meets. One or more are in the antepartal clinic or the physician's office. If the woman attends prenatal classes, she meets another. Still another nurse may teach a specific class in preparation for labor. Within the hospital there are often a variety of nurses in the labor room and nursery and on the postpartal unit. Upon discharge, the mother may be referred to a public health nurse and/or a family planning nurse and/or a follow-up clinic.

In addition, she must cope with a variety of physicians, nutritionists, social workers, and others. Even if she is the patient of a physician in private practice, the physician is probably in a group practice, and she may see a different member of the group at each visit.

If childbearing were a purely biologic occurrence, if all that were required were checks of hemoglobin and blood pressure and urine, such a fragmented approach to care might possibly suffice. But childbearing is a complex biologic psychosocial process that is best served by a continuous relationship between the woman, the family, and the provider of care. Nurses, of all the potential providers, are in the best position to supply that care.

In order to provide this kind of comprehensive care, nurses are developing new roles and expanding established ones (Chapter 30).

Problem: Perinatal Mortality

Perinatal mortality is the term used to describe the death of a fetus or infant between 20 weeks of gestational age (i.e., age since the mother's last menstrual period) and 28 days after birth (Chapter 10).

In the United States perinatal mortality is higher than it is in much of the rest of the industrialized world. This difference appears to be not merely a matter of the way in which statistics are kept, but an actual difference in the number of deaths.

Much of the technological development described above has been pursued in an effort to reduce this mortality. The problem is complex and is discussed more fully in the chapters on the high-risk infant.

Nursing Roles in Transition

The problems described above—the desires and needs of families for meaningful, humanistic, family-centered childbearing; the proliferation of technology at least in part to deal with the very real issue of high perinatal mortality with its own special demands, and fragmentation of care—have put diverse pressures on nurses.

Nurses have found the need to increase their skills in assessment, in communication, and in support of families, for example, and also to increase their skills in technical areas, such as vaginal examination of the woman in labor and the administration of intravenous fluids to preterm infants weighing 2 pounds or less.

What is the role of nurses who care for childbearing families? Some nurses suggest that the supportive, teaching roles are paramount for the professional nurse and that the purely technical tasks may best be performed by someone else. To us this seems a further fragmentation of care, and so we emphasize, both in our practice and in this text, a nursing role that to us combines the best of both worlds. For example the nurse most intimately concerned with the minute-by-minute care of a sick newborn infant, care that is in some aspects highly technical, has the best opportunity, we believe, to foster attachment of parents and baby, to help parents grieve (Chapter 22), and, in short, to give the comprehensive care that the family needs. Other professionals and paraprofessionals, such as physicians, social workers, nutritionists, and respiratory therapists, play a part in that care, but the nurse devises and implements the comprehensive nursing plan.

How Do Nurses Improve Care by Developing New or Expanded Roles?

If fragmentation of care and the desire of families for a human experience are major issues, what answers can nurses offer?

Many nurses are now practicing in settings that enable them to care for families throughout a childbearing cycle. They see women and families in the antenatal period, both individually and in classes that prepare them for childbearing. They may coach the mother or couple during labor, counsel both parents following delivery about self-care and care of their baby and family, and make one or more home visits. If the nurse is a certified nurse-midwife, she may also deliver the baby if the delivery is expected to be uncomplicated.

While there are barriers to this kind of care, it is a possibility in every community if nurses make a real commitment to achieving it.

What Must Nurses Know to Care for Childbearing Families?

How much and what must a nurse know to adequately care for childbearing families? Until fairly recently, much nursing knowledge was set in a medical model. The body of knowledge that might be described as pertaining purely to nursing was relatively small.

We view the knowledge needed for the nursing care of families as:

1. A body of basic knowledge derived from the physical and psychosocial sciences.

2. A body of knowledge specifically related to reproduction.

3. A body of concepts derived from the humanities, to assist in developing a philosophy that helps one cope with the value issues of childbearing, issues such as abortion and the care of a dying, malformed newborn.

4. Specific knowledge that is chiefly or entirely a part of nursing practice, including an understanding of the nursing process.

5. A knowledge of, and expertise in, specific skills utilized in the care of mothers and newborn infants.

From the biologic sciences we gain an understanding of the anatomy and physiology of the male and female reproductive tracts, of genetics, and of embryology, for example. From social science we must understand concepts such as individual and family developmental tasks, the dynamics of changing roles, and the way in which culture influences our lives.

Examples of knowledge of reproduction include the circumstances of conception; the body's reaction to pregnancy, labor, birth, and recovery; the meaning of pregnancy for men and women; and their reaction to it.

All of these types of knowledge serve as the basis from which nursing knowledge has developed—the specific ways in which we, as nurses, care for families and enable families to care for themselves and to cope physically, emotionally, and socially with childbearing.

Nurses who specialize in the care of child-bearing families frequently seek additional educational preparation. Some are nurse-midwives; others are obstetric, neonatal, family planning, or family nurse practitioners. Some participate in continuing education programs to enhance their knowledge. Some earn advanced degrees in maternal-child health care (Chapter 30).

For all nurses a basic course in the care of childbearing families is a foundation, a beginning, not the sum total of knowledge.

Nursing Research and Childbearing

In *The Logic of Scientific Discovery,* Karl Popper states:

. . . it is not in the *possession* of knowledge, of irrefutable truth, that makes the man of science, but his persistent and recklessly critical *quest* for truth. . . Science never pursues the illusory aim of making its answers final, or even probable. Its advance is, rather, towards the infinite yet attainable aim of ever discovering new, deeper and more general problems, and of subjecting its very tentative answers to ever renewed and ever more rigorous tests.[3]

Nursing is barely a generation away from rigid proscriptions about how care should be given. Many nurses practicing today were educated by rigid models. In our student years, mothers who had delivered not only were confined to bed for several days but were given bedpans only at specific intervals, the rationale being that this would help them to void regularly! (To our credit, we, as students, provided bedpans on request, an activity that required considerable stealth lest our unlawful activities be discovered.)

We know that there are always, as Popper suggests, better ways of doing what we do—better ways of helping families cope, better ways of facilitating care. Many of the suggestions in this book will be improved upon, through nursing research, by those of you now reading it as undergraduate students or as practicing nurses. Some of this research will be formal, supported perhaps by grants; other projects will be on a smaller scale but nevertheless valuable. Several nursing research projects that we feel have made significant contributions to care have been described in some detail in this volume (for example, study of the newborn's temperature under the warmer and on his mother's abdomen, in Chapter 15).

We hope that readers—both nursing students and professional nurses—will consider the ideas in this volume, use them as a springboard to develop new concepts and ideas, and share their new ideas with us and with nurses everywhere. In this way our nursing care of childbearing families will continue to grow and improve, to their benefit and to our own satisfaction in a nursing job well done.

REFERENCES

1. Breckinridge, M.: *Wide Neighborhoods*. New York, Harper, 1952.
2. Maslow, A.: *Motivation and Personality*. New York, Harper, 1954.
3. Popper, K.: *The Logic of Scientific Discovery*. New York, Basic Books, Inc., 1959.

2

Nursing and Childbearing Families: Theory and Practice

OBJECTIVES

1. Define:
   a. theory
   b. concept
   c. proposition
   d. variable
   e. adaptation
   f. focal stimulus
   g. contextual stimulus
   h. residual stimulus
   i. adaptive mode
   j. developmental task
   k. role
   l. symbolic interaction
   m. culture
   n. ethnocentrism
   o. culture conflict
   p. cultural imposition
   q. culture shock
   r. dissonance
2. Discuss the value of theory to nurses who care for childbearing families.
3. Describe ways in which the nursing theories of Abdellah, Orem, and Roy may be utilized in the care of childbearing families.
4. Explain the issues of nature/nurture and continuity/discontinuity and how nurses' perspectives on these issues can affect their practice.
5. Differentiate the perspectives of psychoanalytic theory, learning theory, and humanistic theory; identify ways in which these theories may contribute to the care of childbearing families.
6. Differentiate the perspectives of the following family theories: symbolic interaction, exchange, systems, conflict, developmental, functionalist. Consider the advantages and disadvantages of these theories in terms of their ability to assist nurses who care for childbearing families.
7. Describe the value of an understanding of the following anthropological concepts in the care of childbearing families: culture, culture conflict, ethnocentrism.
8. Identify ways in which an understanding of environmental stressors can be utilized within the nursing process.
9. Describe factors that influence cultural change.
10. Describe the nursing process. Discuss examples of the use of the nursing process in the care of childbearing families.

Theory is the basis of professional nursing practice. In the care of childbearing families, nurses utilize nursing theory and theories from other disciplines to better understand the needs of individuals and families. This chapter will explore selected theories from nursing and the behavioral sciences. It is not meant to be a comprehensive view of all the theoretical positions from which one might view the care of the childbearing family. Nor does it explore individual theories in depth.* The purpose is to demonstrate that one's theoretical perspective does influence the way in which one practices.

Theories, Concepts, and Propositions

The word *theory* has been variously defined. Multiple definitions include those that characterize a theory as a set of interrelated concepts, interrelated propositional statements, or a statement that characterizes. Theories may describe, or they may attempt to explain. *Concepts* are terms or words that represent some aspect of reality; family and marriage are examples of concepts. *Propositions* or propositional statements state (or attempt to state) a truth; frequently, propositions state a relationship between variables. For example, the following are examples of propositions related to family planning: (1) The greater the perceived satisfaction or rewards regarding pregnancy, the less the frequency of effective contraception; and (2) The greater the amount of communication with one's partner about contraceptive use, the greater the frequency of effective contraception.

Variables are concepts that vary along a dimension: size of family, marital status, number of pregnancies, and socioeconomic status are examples of variables. In the propositions given above, perceived satisfaction or rewards regarding pregnancy, communication between partners, and effective contraception are variables.

Some theories strive to be general, or global, attempting to answer major questions such as: What are nursing's unique functions? or What is nursing? or How do members of a family relate to one another? A number of theories described in this chapter are general theories. Other theories, such as crisis theory and attachment theory, are directed at specific issues.

There is not and probably will never be a single theory of nursing, or of the family, or of individual development that is the one right theory for all circumstances. The question one should raise as theories are evaluated is not Which one is best? but rather What theoretical perspective illuminates a particular problem in a way that helps me do what I need to do? The particular problem might be the organization of nursing in a prenatal facility, or it might be the development of a nursing plan to facilitate bonding or to provide care to grieving parents.

Theories are not static but are subject to modification and revision as a result of testing them through both research and practice. Nurses can provide valuable contributions to theory development by publishing in the nursing literature accounts of their experiences in utilizing various theoretical perspectives.

Nursing Theories

Three nursing theories have been selected to illustrate the application of nursing theories to childbearing clients. Abdellah focuses on nursing problems that were originally seen as problems of persons who were ill but that we see as relevant to healthy pregnant women and to newborn infants as well. Orem's focus is self-care and the role of nurses in educating individuals and families and facilitating self-care. Roy describes the role of adaptation to change, a constant process of the childbearing years.

Abdellah's Nursing Problems

Abdellah's (1960) identification of 21 nursing problems is strongly focused on the role of the nurse and is designed for persons who are ill.[1] However, the problems can be "translated" into concepts that apply to childbearing women and their families. We believe these "problems" are applicable throughout the childbearing period, although the focus will be different during different phases.

The first group of problems addresses activities of daily living such as:

1. To maintain good hygiene and physical comfort

2. To promote optimal activity—exercise, rest, and sleep

3. To promote safety through prevention of accident, injury, or other trauma and prevention of the spread of infection

4. To maintain good body mechanics and prevention and correction of deformities.

How do these concepts apply during each

---

*Stevens, 1979[69] and Nursing Theories Conference Group, 1980[46] are excellent introductions to nursing theory.

phase of childbearing? For example, how do hygienic needs change during pregnancy? Can we show gravidas more comfortable positions for resting, for sitting, for intercourse?

Do we counsel gravidas about exercise during pregnancy, demonstrate exercises that will provide comfort, improve her physical condition, prepare her body for labor and delivery, and enhance a rapid return of physical efficiency? Do we share information about rest and sleep needs?

Safety concerns include physical factors such as the shift in the woman's center of gravity as the fetus grows, safe use of drugs, and protection from environmental hazards. During pregnancy, concern is for the safety of both mother and fetus. Following delivery, the needs of the newborn for hygiene, rest, safety, and positioning are considered as well as those of the mother.

A second group of nursing problems stresses physiologic needs:

5. To facilitate the maintenance of a supply of oxygen to all body cells
6. To facilitate the maintenance of nutrition of all body cells
7. To facilitate the maintenance of elimination
8. To facilitate the maintenance of fluid and electrolyte balance
9. To recognize the physiologic responses of the body to disease conditions—pathologic, physiologic, and compensatory
10. To facilitate the maintenance of regulatory mechanisms and functions
11. To facilitate the maintenance of sensory function.

When one thinks of oxygen and nutrition, again one thinks of the fetus and newborn as well as the mother. Can we encourage the prospective mother, particularly in the last trimester, to maximize placental blood flow, thus aiding both fetal nutrition and fetal oxygenation?

Or, for another example, how can we help parents recognize and appreciate the unique sensory characteristics of their infant and care for him in a way that will enhance those characteristics?

Abdellah includes several nursing problems that focus on emotional reactions. A slight rewording of the statements (in parentheses) follows several of Abdellah's original statements as examples of their relevance to nursing care during childbearing. The others are, we believe, equally pertinent; the reader can interpret them in a manner similar to the examples.

12. To identify and accept positive and negative expressions, feelings and reactions (to

help the mother, father, and significant others accept positive and negative expressions, feelings, and reactions during each phase of childbearing)
13. To identify and accept the interrelatedness of emotions and organic illness (to help the childbearing family identify and accept the interrelatedness of emotions and childbearing)
14. To facilitate the maintenance of effective verbal and nonverbal communication (to help the childbearing family develop and maintain effective verbal and nonverbal communication)
15. To promote the development of productive interpersonal relationships
16. To facilitate progress toward achievement of personal and spiritual goals
17. To create or maintain a therapeutic environment
18. To facilitate awareness of self as an individual with varying physical, emotional, and developmental needs.

Of the three final goals, the last two are social in nature.

19. To accept the optimum possible goals in the light of limitations, physical and emotional
20. To use community resources as an aid in resolving problems arising from illness
21. To understand the role of social problems in causing illness.

As with the previous problems, one can phrase the statements in terms of childbearing rather than illness and visualize the nurse in the supportive-educative system describd by Orem. Even though most childbearing couples are not ill, there are community resources (classes in preparation for childbirth and parenting, for example) to which nurses can refer couples. For some families, a variety of other services in the community are appropriate (nutritional supper through WIC [Women, Infants and Children], for example).

While many families do not have "social problems" per se, all are experiencing the social changes that accompany the birth of a baby, as well as individual changes.

Orem's Premise of Self-Care

Dorothy Orem's concept of nursing focuses on the idea that persons are basically capable of and have a need for self-care, but because they are not totally self-sufficient, nursing can assist them by designing, providing, and managing systems of self-care.[47] These systems may be *wholly compensatory* (the person has no active role in her care as, for example, when she is totally incapacitated either physically or mentally) *partly compensatory* (the person has some role but requires some assistance); or *supportive-educative* (the person is able to perform the necessary care, given an appropriate environment and support, guidance, and teaching from the nurse).

Utilizing this approach, it is obvious that most of the care given to childbearing women and their families can be educative-supportive. A very small number of women may require wholly compensatory care (a mother who develops eclampsia or severe preeclampsia, for example), and a somewhat larger number may, for part of their pregnancy, need partly compensatory care. A mother who requires bed rest because of a rising blood pressure or heart disease would be an example.

The usefulness of Orem's theory in providing a new way of looking at an issue is evident if we look at the changes that have occurred in the care of childbearing families in the last decade. One way to conceptualize these changes is to see them as a move from a compensatory system to a supportive-educative system. The majority of mothers entering the labor-delivery suite in the 1960s left family and supportive friends at the door. Many knew little about what was to come, other than the old wives' tales of pain and suffering. Few women possessed knowledge of what was happening within their bodies or how they might work with labor. Medication frequently blotted out understanding and memory, making a woman a passive recipient of compensatory care. General anesthesia at the time of delivery meant that the woman required wholly compensatory care for a period of time.

By contrast, consider the couple of the eighties. The couple may be married or they may be a woman and another coach, such as a friend or sister or boy friend. Many will have participated in some form of childbirth education in which a nurse (or other childbirth educator) has provided guidance and teaching. The nurse works with the couple during labor and delivery to provide an environment that will enhance their childbirth experience. More and more frequently this environment will be designed to resemble a home setting rather than a hospital room. In this setting, a nurse supports a couple's own coping mechanisms, offering guidance and information. Even when the laboring mother has had no previous preparation, a nurse who practices within the supportive-educative system can guide the mother and her support person in a way that is very different from that of the nurse who sees her role and functions within a compensatory system.

Concepts of self-care during childbearing are not limited to the woman without complications. For instance, support and education from a nurse can help a gravida with diabetes mellitus enhance the well-being of herself and her fetus in specific ways, such as through consistent use of urinalysis for sugar and ketones, home blood-glucose determinations, and appropriate nutrition. The gravida with pregnancy-induced hypertension may be able, through bed rest in a side-lying position, both to keep her blood pressure within safe limits and to provide improved placental blood flow.

In a given situation, such as labor, care may be at any level depending on the needs of the individual woman. For example, a very few women may need wholly compensatory care because of serious maternal illness. A much larger group of women may need partly compensatory care, particularly toward the end of labor. They may need help with elimination, with hygiene, with the provision of comfort measures. Other women, either alone or working with a coach with whom they have prepared and practiced for labor, may need and desire only supportive and educative interaction with a nurse. During the course of an individual labor, the level of care may change. A complication, for example, may require more intervention and a compensatory level of care that was not originally planned.

Table 2–1 shows some examples of the use of Orem's theory during childbearing.

Roy's Adaptation Theory

Sister Callista Roy began the development of an adaptation framework of nursing in the 1960s.[57] Roy proposes the following ideas:

- Man is a biopsychosocial being
- Man is in constant interaction with a changing environment
- To cope with a changing world, man uses both innate and acquired mechanisms, which are biologic, psychologic, and social in origin
- Health and illness are one inevitable dimension of man's life
- To respond positively to environmental changes, man must adapt
- Man's adaptation is a function of the stimulus he is exposed to and his adaptation level
- Man's adaptation level is such that it comprises a zone that indicates the range of stimulation that will lead to a positive response. If the stimulus is within the zone, the person responds positively. If,

Table 2-1. EXAMPLES OF THE USE OF OREM'S MODEL DURING CHILDBEARING

	Mother	Father (or Other Family Member)	Newborn
Wholly compensatory	Provides care for seriously ill mother (e.g., mother with eclampsia). Supports mother in recipient role	Provides support when mother or child is ill	Provides care for seriously ill newborn. Supports parents when they are unable to care for infant
Partly compensatory	Provides care to mother in partial need of assistance (e.g., immediately following cesarean birth, or during labor)	Provides support and interprets change as mother or newborn require	Helps mother and father assume responsibility for caring for previously ill newborn
Supportive and educative	Provides parent education and support during each phase of childbearing to enhance self-care	Same as for mother	Provides education and support to mother or father to ensure care for newborn

however, the stimulus is outside the zone, the person cannot make a positive response

- Man has four modes of adaptation: physiologic needs, self-concept, role function, and interdependence relations[2]

One need only substitute the phrases "a pregnant woman" and "a newborn infant" to utilize this proposal as the basis for nursing interaction during childbearing. For example, both pregnant women and newborn infants are biopsychosocial beings. Therefore, it is not enough to plan only for the physiologic needs of a person; the psychologic and social needs must be planned as well. Similarly, concepts of the changing environment must include not only the external and internal environments (although the physical environment is important) but also psychosocial stimuli. To the degree that one is able to adapt to continual environmental change one is healthy. A healthy pregnancy would thus be one in which a woman is able to adapt or cope with physical, emotional, and social changes. A newborn's healthy transition to extrauterine life is also related to an ability to adapt to some momentous changes. One clear example of a physiologic failure to adapt in a newborn infant is called *persistent fetal circulation*, a condition in which the circulatory system of the newborn continues to function as it did in fetal life instead of making the transition necessary for postnatal life.

The term *adaptation level* is used to describe the person's state of coping. Adaptation level is determined by *focal, contextual* and *residual* stimuli. A *focal stimulus* is the environmental change in a given situation. A *contextual stimulus* is any other stimulus (external or internal) that affects the situation, can be measured, or is reported by the individual. A *residual stimulus* is any characteristic of the individual that is relevant to the specific situation.

For example, consider nausea, a condition that is found in many pregnant women during the first months of gestation. Nausea itself is the focal stimulus; nausea represents a change in the internal environment. Contextual stimuli include the conditions under which nausea occurs, such as only in the morning or throughout the day, the relationships to certain odors, and so on. Residual stimuli include cultural attitudes (as noted in Chapter 12, nausea during pregnancy does not appear to occur in all societies), and individual attitudes (research has been unable to establish any clear links between nausea and attitudes toward pregnancy). The attitudes of family and friends may also be relevant residual stimuli. If an individual is able to cope with all of the stimuli, adaptation occurs. In our example, the woman adapts to nausea; she uses measures such as dry carbohydrate foods, dietary changes, and perhaps medication to relieve symptoms, and she recognizes that this problem will probably improve within a few weeks. If the stimuli are greater than her capacity to cope, maladaptation occurs. Nausea may interfere with needed nutrition or disrupt family life.

Table 2–2. ROY'S ADAPTATION MODEL AND THE NURSING PROCESS: CARE OF A PREGNANT WOMAN DURING THE PRENATAL PERIOD IN AN AMBULATORY SETTING

	Examples of Areas to Be Assessed	Examples of Potential Nursing Diagnoses	Nursing Observations that Will Lead to Specific Diagnoses	Nursing Intervention
Physiologic mode	Physiologic adaptation to pregnancy Nutrition Modification of activities (e.g., elimination, exercise, rest)	Good or difficult adaptation Discomfort related to internal body sensations, restrictions, or diagnostic procedures Need for more rest, exercise, and so on Inadequate information about physiologic changes or needs during pregnancy	Physical examination (including evaluation of blood pressure, weight, fetal growth) Laboratory studies (e.g., urine, hemoglobin, VDRL, Pap smear) Evidence of favorable response to any therapy Evidence of good nutrition	Provides information about 1. normal physiologic changes in pregnancy 2. self-care during pregnancy 3. nutritional needs of pregnant women Teaches exercises (e.g., Kegel, pelvic rock, tailor sitting) Refers when assessment indicates special needs (e.g., extensive nutritional needs)
Self-concept mode	Effect of pregnancy on self-concept of mother or father, including moral-ethical self, self-ideal, self-consistency, self-esteem, physical self	Enhance or diminished self-concept related to "being pregnant" (or partner's pregnancy) Enhanced or diminished self-concept related to changing body (or partner's changing body) Sense of inadequacy	Statements by mother or father reflecting self-esteem (e.g., behavior, posture, dress) that suggest enhanced or diminished self-esteem	Counsels (and makes appropriate referral if necessary) when assessment indicates need Provides information about feelings common to expectant mothers, fathers

			Enhanced or diminished self-concept related to moral-ethical self
Role function mode	Progressive movement toward the parent role; evidence of prenatal attachment behaviors	Positive prenatal attachment behavior Absence of prenatal attachment behavior	Statements by mother or father reflecting role transition to parenthood Behavior indicating attachment (e.g., purchase of clothes for infant, other "nesting" behavior) (see Chapter 10)	Provides educational opportunities for expectant parents to learn knowledge and skills required in new roles Provides opportunities for individual counseling when assessment indicates need
Interdependence mode	Effects of pregnancy on relationship of mother and father or significant other persons Adequacy of support from significant other persons	Enhanced or diminished family relationships as a result of pregnancy Enhanced or diminished family relationships of single, teenage mother	Statements by mother or father indicating changes in relationship or feelings of support or lack of support Behavior by mother or father indicating changes in relationship or feelings of support or lack of support	Provides education about changing relationships during pregnancy Provides opportunities for individual counseling (and referral if assessment indicates need)

Two factors are significant in adaptation: the extent of the environmental change and the ability of the individual to cope. A pregnant woman, a new mother, an infant, may be able to cope with limited levels of change without exceeding their ability, but they may need a great deal of support when the change is major. Parents may be well prepared to care for a healthy newborn, for example, but few can initially adapt to a critically ill baby. The stimulus (critically ill baby) exceeds their ability to cope. With support from nurses, family, friends, and other health professionals, however, the ability of most parents to cope increases, and they are able to adapt to the changing environment and care for their baby.

Adaptation occurs in four areas or *modes*: physiologic needs, self-concept, role function, and interdependence relations. Adaptive modes are the intervening variable between basic needs and behavior. As the chapters that follow will indicate, each of these modes is highly relevant to individuals and families during childbearing. The *physiologic adaptive mode* includes the need for exercise, rest, nutrition, elimination, fluids and electrolytes, oxygen, and circulation, and the regulation of temperature, sensory activity, and the endocrine system. The changes that occur in pregnancy and the special requirements of newborn infants demand different consideration of each of these needs than at other times in life.

The *self-concept mode* is related to the need to maintain psychologic integrity. Every facet of reproduction is likely to affect self-concept. The person or couple who desire a child but remain infertile frequently have a diminished self-concept, as may parents who give birth to a child with a defect. A woman considering termination of pregnancy may experience a lack of adaptation in her moral-ethical self-concept if her previous values (contextual or residual stimuli) suggest to her that termination of pregnancy is wrong.

Role, in Roy's theory, involves holding a position in society and interacting with another individual who holds a position in society. The *role function mode* and the *interdependence mode* both address the need for social integrity. Whereas the role function mode addresses appropriate role behavior (the role of mother or father, for instance), the interdependence mode focuses on an individual's need for love and support. It is not unusual for expectant and new mothers and fathers to experience role conflict as they attempt to integrate new responsibilities with ongoing ones. Not is it unusual for individuals to experience increased needs for love and support

or to feel that they are receiving less. The new father, for example, may feel that he receives less attention from his wife (the focal stimulus) now that the new baby is here (contextual stimulus). If he understands that the baby's needs and his wife's depleted energy are transient, he will not feel overly threatened, or he may help with infant care and household tasks and thus enable his wife to spend more time with him. Both of these responses are adaptive. Maladaption and thus serious problems in interdependence may occur if he is unable to cope with his feelings of lack of love and support or to provide love and support to his wife.

The four modes form the basis of the use of nursing process. Table 2–2 is an example of the use of the adaptation model in healthy, ambulatory women and their families. The model does not include all possible factors but suggests how Roy's adaptation model can lead nurses to provide care that is both holistic and individualized. Evaluation, an essential part of the nursing process, is not included in Table 2–2 (see Nursing Process at the conclusion of this chapter).

Theories from Other Disciplines

In addition to nursing theory, nurses may adapt theories from other disciplines or utilize those theories to better understand some aspect of their practice. Throughout this book, biologic, chemical, and physical bases for practice are noted. For example, although the specific cause of the onset of labor is unknown, a theoretical explanation of what may occur is offered.

In this chapter the focus is on behavioral theories. Psychologic theories address inner states, whereas social-psychologic and sociologic theories are more concerned with interactions between persons and group behavior, including behavior in families. Anthropologic theory is interested in the relationships between aspects of societies and the behavior of persons in those societies. As in the discussion of nursing theories, the ideas described here are examples of ways in which the theories may be utilized rather than a comprehensive review.

Theories of Individual Development

Although childbearing is certainly a family affair, it is also a time of individual development for women and frequently for men as well. Important theories of individual development are psychoanalytic theory, social learning theory, cognitive theory, and humanistic perspectives. Each of these perspectives addresses basic issues that must be considered by nurses who interact with childbearing families. Two of the most important are described here.

Nature vs. Nurture. How much of what an individual does is due to innate qualities (e.g., nature, heredity) and how much is learned behavior (e.g., nurture, environment)? This issue has been debated in various forms over many centuries. Today the nature vs. nurture or heredity vs. environment issue is not usually stated in terms of the source of behavior but rather the manner of interaction between these two inseparable (but distinct) concepts. (For a more detailed discussion, see Lerner, 1976.[39]) Consider mothering and fathering behavior. If we assume that mothering, for example, is instinctive, then we will expect mothers to behave immediately in "motherly ways." The fact that "motherly ways" vary from culture to culture (an anthropologic observation) suggests that perhaps some learning is involved—not formal, planned learning, in most instances, but learning from one's family and neighbors and peers. If we believe that mothering (or fathering) is learned, then it becomes our responsibility to assess the need for learning and to provide or suggest opportunities for learning. We would recognize that certain environmental factors (economic constraints or the availability of support persons, for example) and certain hereditary factors (physical or mental disabilities such as blindness or diminished intellectual capacity, for example) would also affect learning.

Continuity vs. Discontinuity. Do the same "laws" apply to all species and to persons at different stages of their lifespan? This issue has been termed one of continuity vs. discontinuity.

Continuity and discontinuity appear to exist in both the biologic and behavioral sciences. For example, animal models are used to help us understand more about the effect of drugs on the fetus (the assumption is one of continuity), yet a major drug affecting the human fetus, thalidomide, caused birth defects in humans but not in animals (see Chapter 8 for further discussion). Some of our ideas about attachment behavior and relationships between infants and parents have been derived from studies of animal behavior.

A continuity perspective suggests that behavior such as learning occurs in the same way at different stages of life, whereas a perspective of discontinuity suggests that people learn in different ways at different times in their lives. Since a major role of nurses in interaction with childbearing families is that of educator, our understanding of how adolescents and adults learn will affect that interaction. Although early learning theorists favored a perspective of continuity, discontinuity, that is, the perspective that persons learn most things in ways that differ from other species and in different ways at different stages of life, is accepted widely today.

The theories discussed in this chapter have attempted to integrate a great many concepts into a comprehensive entity. Some theories deal with more specific issues. Attachment theory, described in several chapters throughout this book as it applies to prenatal, birth, and postnatal phases of pregnancy, is an example. Crisis intervention theory, described in Chapter 25, is another example of a theory that, while it is useful in many circumstances (and by no means only in interaction with childbearing families), deals with specific rather than general issues.

Humanistic Perspectives

Humanistic perspectives are also described by the term *phenomenologic* because they emphasize the systematic investigation of conscious experiences (phenomena), or by the term the *third force,* because they are a third alternative to older and more dominant psychoanalytic and behaviorist perspectives. Humanistic ideas, particularly those of Abraham Maslow, have been important and helpful to many nurses and are consistent with the concepts of many nursing theorists.

For the humanistic psychologist, people are seen as far more autonomous and self-governed than a learning theorist such as Skinner would accept. People need not be victims of either inner drives or their environments; they have the potential to become their best selves or, in Maslow's terms, to become self-actualized. Emphasis is also placed on persons as a whole, integrating biologic, intellectual, and emotional components.

The basic needs of all persons as described by Maslow (1954)[43] are:
1. Physiological needs (air, water, food, shelter, sleep, sex)
2. Safety and security
3. Love and belongingness
4. Self-esteem and esteem by others
5. Growth needs (e.g., meaningfulness, self-sufficiency, justice, order, individuality).

When all these needs are met, an individual achieves self-actualization, a state of being in which one is able to make full use of one's talents and potential.

It is not difficult to consider how Maslow's hierarchy of needs can be utilized in interaction with women during pregnancy and with newborn infants. Physiologic needs and needs for safety and security are met through education and facilitation for most mothers, although more active intervention is sometimes necessary (see the discussion of Orem's theories above), such as encouraging active rather than passive participation by parents in all phases of pregnancy. This theme recurs throughout this book.

Some pregnant women exhibit very low self-esteem; some single mothers, most mothers who are drug addicts, as well as women with no apparent reason for a low self-image will be in this group. Pregnancy may have brought them into contact with a professional nurse for the first time since their childhood. If nurses are able to accept them and make them feel cared for, they are more likely to develop a caring attitude about themselves. Humanistic psychologists use the term *unconditional positive regard* to describe the kind of acceptance from a professional that will help a client develop positive self-esteem. The hierarchical nature of Maslow's needs suggests that the first needs must be met before other needs can be addressed. The practical evidence of this is abundant. For example, the newly delivered mother who is ill or physically uncomfortable herself (unmet physiologic and perhaps safety or security needs) will experience difficulty in developing a close relationship (bonding) with her baby (need for love and belongingness). If her baby's basic physiologic needs for warmth and nutrition and oxygen are unmet, he will not provide the positive behavior—the gazing into his parents' eyes, for example—that establishes and reinforces love and belonging ness between parents and their infant. When childbearing is a positive experience, self-esteem and self-confidence are enhanced.[48, 49] As nurses we can facilitate that self-esteem.

If other needs are met, the period of childbearing can become a period of growth of both the individual and the family. Many couples do describe childbirth in words similar to those used by humanistic psychologists to define a *peak experience*—an experience that provides a deep sense of inner satisfaction and joy and that enables the couple to see themselves as changed in many ways, with enhanced potential for further development. One of the great satisfactions in nursing interaction with childbearing families is the experience of seeing a somewhat anxious, unsure couple early in pregnancy bloom into a confident mother and father a few weeks after the birth of their baby.

Psychoanalytic Theory

Classic psychoanalytic perspectives, derived from the insights of Sigmund Freud, focus on the inner, mental life rather than on social life. For Freud the unconscious was the largest and most important part of the mind. The period of external influence on the personality is brief, completed by the time the child is 6 years old and entering the period Freud labels as latency. From that time onward the focus is on the individual's reworking or reconstruction of events of the early years.

In psychoanalytic tradition, motherhood is the mechanism that enables a woman to rework childhood conflicts and thus become a mature adult. Freud (along with many other nineteenth century writers) saw women as weak, immature, and innately inferior. Only by becoming a mother could a woman achieve mature femininity. Benedek states, "Motherliness as a normal characteristic of femininity, of women's psychosexual maturity, and as a part and parcel of motherhood belongs to those enigmatic features of a woman's psychology that have eluded investigation."[4] This concept, sometimes termed "anatomy is destiny," is unacceptable to many people today.

Determinism is another concept in the psychoanalytic tradition. In relation to maternal roles, women who suffered excessive maternal deprivation as children are expected to experience major difficulty both in reworking childhood conflicts and in parental role performance. While research does not support the deterministic position,[19] the psychoanalytic notion that *remembrance* of one's childhood is part of one's conception of oneself, and that remembrances are awakened and reinterpreted during pregnancy, has been supported by research.[56] Remembrance is not of actual past events but of "fantasies expressing unconscious infantile wishes."[66] In a series of intensive interviews with 15 sets of parents, the Rosenbergs found that a mother's image of her own upbringing and the mothering she experienced "was probably the most pervasive element in the mother's development of a parental identity.... Some of the parents in the study struggled to become like their parents and thus relive their childhoods. Still others sought to fulfill perceived parental expectations and thus earn love and approval.... No type of encounter between mother and young child seemed to transpire without there being some sense of actual or potential repetition from the mother's own construction of her childhood."[56] This finding suggests that in our assessment of maternal history it is the mother's perception of her own childhood that should be a focus of our attention, and that how she thinks that perception affects (or will affect) her ideas about mothering is a theme to be explored with her.

Birth is a significant event in psychoanalytic thought. The Freudian view of birth as a shock in which overwhelming environmental stimulation impinges upon the newborn is, in some ways, similar to that of Leboyer, who in the 1970s stressed the need for "gentle birth" (Chapter 17). For Freudians, birth trauma results in intense fear and is the prototype for subsequent fear-producing situations. A more gentle birth would result in less fear in the unconscious of the growing child and subsequently lead to greater emotional control in later life.[71]

More influential to many nurses than the ideas of Freud are the concepts of Erikson, who is a "neo-Freudian," a theorist who has been influenced by psychoanalytic thought but has gone far beyond the original concepts. Erikson defines eight psychosocial stages of development that he considers to occur throughout history and in all societies.[15] In contrast to Freud, who saw development as limited to the first years of life, Erikson believes that human development occurs throughout the life cycle. The developmental tasks of each stage and the result of failure in the development of that task are summarized in Table 2–3. A developmental task is a problem in social development that must be dealt with at that time. Although each stage is necessary to the development of individuals and thus to childbearing mothers and to infants, the particular concerns

at this time in a person's life are those stages marked with an asterisk (*).

In considering psychosocial stages related to childbearing, adolescence seems a logical starting point. The adolescent's task is to answer the question, "Who am I?" The answer lies, for Erikson, in finding a role for oneself in society and thus establishing a sense of personal *identity*. A sense of identity is normally unconscious, "a feeling of being at home in one's body, a sense of 'knowing where one is going,' and an inner assuredness of anticipated recognition from those who count."[15] For Erikson, a sense of identity is necessary before one can move on to the tasks of adulthood (intimacy) and parenthood (generativity). This perspective suggests that one of the tragedies of adolescent parenthood is the movement into a new set of roles before a sense of one's own identity has developed. A person may then suffer identity diffusion, resulting in inability to adopt a role.

Intimacy is the ability to give of oneself totally to another person—to share not only in a physical sense but also feelings, ideas, values, and goals. If one cannot share and accept sharing, isolation is the inevitable result. *Generativity* has been defined for women in past generations as the generation of children, although men have been able to achieve generativity through their business and professional activities. Erikson, however, departs from psychoanalytic tradition in this regard; he feels that society must come to view women's generational fulfillment as possible in many ways, not through mothering alone.

Trust, the developmental task of the first year, is related to consistency in the care the baby receives during the first year. Here Erikson's concepts are similar to those of other psychoanalysts, who stress the importance of care in the first year. Erikson believes that a child who receives maternal nurturance and care will develop a sense of trust and, as a parent, provide the same care to his or her own children. Conversely, inadequate mothering leads to a deep *mistrust* and, according to the theory, an inability to develop subsequent developmental tasks.

Table 2–3. ERIKSON'S PSYCHOSOCIAL STAGES

Appropriate Chronologic Age (Years)	Developmental Task: Development of a Sense of:	Result When Developmental Task Not Achieved
0–1	*Trust	Mistrust
1–3	Autonomy	Shame, doubt
3–6	Initiative	Guilt
6–Adolescence	Industry	Inferiority
Adolescence	*Identity	Identity diffusion
Adulthood	*Intimacy	Isolation
	*Generativity	Stagnation
	Integrity	Despair

*Especially important to childbearing mothers and their infants.

Learning Theory

Learning "is a relatively permanent change in behavior potentiality which occurs as a result of reinforced practice."[39] Major contemporary learning theorists include Skinner, Bandura, and Walters, the last two men being associated with *social learning* theory.

Skinner focuses on conditioning as the basis

of learning; he maintains that the laws of learning, whether they involve classic conditioning or operant conditioning, are continuously applicable to the behavior of all organisms. Thus, for Skinner, a rat or a pigeon learns behavior in the same way that humans learn.

One way in which principles of conditioning are utilized in the care of childbearing families is in the use of techniques to help mothers cope with contractions during labor. The contractions of labor are stimuli that may produce commonly observed responses such as crying and twisting and turning in bed. In classes preparing them for labor, mothers learn how to use a different set of responses, which include focusing, relaxation, and breathing techniques. The success of their response reinforces the response to the next contraction (see Chapter 11 for a more complete discussion of these techniques).

Two concepts from social learning theory that can be helpful in nursing interaction with childbearing couples are modeling and the influence of rewards and punishments on behavior.

The concept of modeling suggests that much learning is derived from observation and modeling of what others do. Thus, a major part of learning to be a parent is derived from the observation of other parents. Models include one's own parents, originally imitated in doll play, as well as relatives and friends. One of the problems for couples today is that because there are so many small families, many persons approach parenthood with relatively few models and must find other resources to learn about parenthood.

Rewards and punishments are important influences in learning theory as it addresses the issue of sex differences between men and women, a subject important to couples as they develop their own maternal and paternal roles and as they consider how they plan to behave as parents to their own children.

In psychoanalytic theory, gender differences are believed to be innate, but in learning theory differences are attributed to differential reinforcement of the behavior of boys and girls. Girls and boys are rewarded for certain behaviors and punished for different behaviors; for example, girls may be praised for "feminine" behavior such as doll play and punished for "masculine" behavior such as getting dirty or being loud and boisterous. In addition, the models in books, on television, at home, and in the community convey a certain image of what is appropriate for each sex, thus (according to social learning theory) helping to develop a gender identity.

Research supports the idea that parents do perceive and treat their male and female infants differently. In one study, Rubin, Provenzano, and Luria (1974)[58] asked 30 pairs of primiparous parents, 15 with sons and 15 with daughters, to describe their baby as they would "to a close friend or relative" and then to rate their baby on 18 11-point, bipolar adjective scales such as firm-soft, relaxed-nervous, noisy-quiet, and hardy-delicate. There were no significant differences in the male and female infants in birth weight or length or in Apgar scores at 5 and 10 minutes.

Fathers rated their infants almost immediately after delivery; they were not allowed to be present during delivery and had seen their infants only through the nursery window. Mothers rated their infants during the first 24 hours; they had delivered under general anesthesia but had handled and fed their infants.

Both mothers and fathers labeled their infants differently according to gender. Daughters were rated as softer, finer featured, littler, and more inattentive. When the relationship between the sex of the parent and the sex of the infant was analyzed, it was found that fathers were more extreme in their ratings of both sons and daughters than were mothers. On one variable (cuddly-not cuddly), mothers rated the sons as more cuddly, whereas fathers saw their daughters as more cuddly.

In a series of studies, Lewis and colleagues[10, 25, 40] found that boys received more contact with their parents in the first 6 months and girls more contact after 6 months. Other studies of differential treatment include Moss (1967),[45] Rebelsky and Hanks (1971),[53] and Thoman, Leiderman, and Olson (1972).[70] Some studies do not reveal early differences. (See Maccoby and Jacklin, 1974,[42] for a review of studies.)

One criticism of social learning theory as an explanation is that differential treatment of infants may be a response to the infant's behavior; male and female infants develop at different rates, and this may account at least partially for differences in parental treatment. However, other studies with older infants and children elicited stereotypical behavior from both parents and nonparents when the sex of the same infant was described as a boy or girl to different observers.[13, 23, 65, 67]

Expectant parents often express concern about mothering and fathering in terms of gender roles. A common feeling in childbirth classes was stated by one father, "Mothers are just naturally better at taking care of babies." His wife felt that statement was an excuse to avoid certain aspects of child care. Learning theory suggests that mothers become more proficient because they have more opportunities to practice and probably because they have more models as well. Even in hospitals it is the mother who most often has opportunities for caregiving, although this need not necessarily be so.

Gender role is also important in the care of the baby. Not many parents buy toy trains for their infant daughters and even less often dolls for infant sons. Other behaviors considered inappropriate by one parent because of the baby's gender (e.g., "treating *him* like a sissy") can be a source of conflict.

Theories About Families

A fundamental belief about nursing care of childbearing families is that care is family-centered, focused not only on the mother or the infant but on other members of the family as well. Family theorists approach the study of the family from several perspectives. Major approaches are interactionist theory, exchange theory, and systems theory. Other theories include conflict theory, developmental theory, and structural fundamentalism.[34] Each of these theories has been or can be utilized by nurses who interact with childbearing families.

Symbolic Interaction

The symbolic interaction perspective encompasses a number of subtheories, including role theory, perceptual theory, reference group theory, and self theory. The interaction of family members with one another and the way in which others (e.g., a reference group) and one's own perceptions affect that interaction is a focus. Symbolic interaction emphasizes the *meaning* of actions for actors rather than behavior per se.

Role is a basic concept in the interactional perspective. Role is also an important concept for functionalists (see below), but the meaning of role is different in these two perspectives (Table 2–5). For the interactionist role is a dynamic concept in which "there is usually considerable room for individual differences in roles, and there is no clear-cut normative script for much of what persons do in a role."[9] Turner (1962)[72] uses the term *role playing* to describe the way in which individuals improvise, explore, and judge what is appropriate in a particular situation rather than acting on the basis of previously learned scripts or expectations. Burr and associates (1979) write, "It is indefensible to urge that roles are a static aspect of structure, because roles are dynamic and processual. . . . Even those parts of roles

that are the most clearly and precisely defined by social expectations are ongoing, dynamic processes rather than static events."[9]

The period of childbearing is a time in which new roles develop; the roles of father and mother are added to other roles—husband, wife, student, daughter, and so on. New roles are developed through *socialization*, a process that in recent years has come to be recognized as a reciprocal process in which the socialized individual both influences the process and is influenced by it. Socialization involves both knowledge of what is expected in a role and acquisition of the skills needed to fulfill that expectation. As nurses interact with women and their families in each phase of childbearing, they function as one agent in the socialization process, and they can be very influential agents. We must remember, however, that socialization for childbirth and parenting has been occurring since the expectant parent's own infancy. The stories she hears about pregnancy and childbirth from her reference group, the way in which her own parents acted toward her, and the role models of women who are pregnant or of friends and relatives who are mothers and fathers are all significant to socialization.

The *quality of role enactment*[59] or *quality of role performance*[6] describes how well a person performs a role relative to the expectations for that role. It is a concept that is part of the basic nursing assessment of parents. For example, "alterations in parenting" is one of the accepted nursing diagnoses identified by the National Group for the Classification of Nursing Diagnosis,[22] indicating a role performance that is expected by nurses as professionals. Depending on nurses' expectations, this diagnosis may or may not be appropriate.

Parents, too, have expectations for themselves, for each other, and for others. These expectations may be discussed between individuals (e.g., mother and father), but frequently they may be understood or thought to be understood but not expressed. For example, a prospective father may expect his baby to breast-feed because that is traditional in his family, or a grandmother may expect the baby's mother to give up her job and remain at home once the baby is born. In a given situation there may be a high level of *consensus of role expectations* or little or no consensus. Some authors use the term *role conflict* to describe a low level of consensus or lack of consensus, but others feel this term is too ambiguous.

The concept of *role strain*, originally developed by Goode (1960),[26] a functionalist, is defined as "felt difficulty in fulfilling role obligations." Role strain can be thought of as a continuous variable that can range from absence to a very high level. As role strain increases along the continuum, i.e., as individuals become increasingly uncomfortable in complying with the expectations of a role, anxiety, stress, and loss of self-esteem may occur. Labeling this concept role strain is less valuable than identifying the behaviors that produce stress, but because the term is widely accepted, it is used here.

Nursing intervention that can facilitate the development of new roles is described in Chapter 7.

Exchange Theory

The basic assumption of an exchange perspective is that persons (and groups) behave as they do to gain rewards and avoid costs. Whereas some exchange theorists approach rewards and costs from an individualistic perspective (e.g., Nye), others focus on interaction between individuals or groups (e.g., Scanzoni).

Childbearing can certainly be examined in a reward/cost framework. Perceived rewards may include being recognized by the community as an adult member of society, having a sense of personal achievement, achieving survival of family name, and receiving affection.[63] Other perceived rewards of childbearing may include saving a relationship, pleasing others, escaping from an undesirable situation, replacing a lost child, affirming masculinity or femininity, or acting out rebellion. Hoffman and Mannis (1979)[32] found that the rewards of childbearing included love and companionship, stimulation and fun, and expansion of self.

Childbearing also involves costs, even under the most ideal circumstances. A new baby requires a tremendous amount of attention; most new parents experience fatigue, disruption in routine, reduced social life, and diminished time for other activities.[62] Husbands may feel that the baby is more important to their wives than they are; wives at times have similar feelings of jealousy. There are financial costs as well, both in expenditures and, for some couples, in reduced earnings of the mother.

One concept important to exchange theorists is *resources*. Resources may be either tangible (e.g., money, job status, education) or intangible (e.g., self-esteem). The possession of resources is a principal source of *power*, which is defined as the ability to achieve intended effects, although other factors such as preferences, goals, and prevailing social values may also influence power.[54]

Issues such as power and resources have not

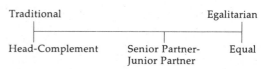

Figure 2–1. Three styles of marital interaction. (Derived from Scanzoni *In* Levinger and Moles: Divorce and Separation. New York, Basic Books, 1979.)

traditionally been a part of the conceptual framework of maternity nursing. Contemporary family theorists, however, are turning their attention to this facet of childbearing.

What does happen to couples when a child arrives? Let us assume that this is a first child and that the couple is either married or committed to one another over a period without marriage. The changes that childbearing brings will depend on the current pattern of interaction in the relationship.

Three styles of marital interaction, described by Scanzoni (1979),[61] may be thought of as a continuum from traditional to egalitarian (Fig. 2–1). Some couples interact in the traditional way described by the functionalists (see below). Scanzoni has called this type of marriage "head complement," in that the man, as head of the family, continues to hold greater power than the woman over areas such as family finance. The wife is his complement.

In the senior-junior partner relationship, the woman possesses resources that give her increased power in the relationship, although her power is not equal to that of her mate. Her power may be derived from a job that gives her increased economic resources, for example.

The equal partner marriage is similar to the dual-career marriage described by Rapoport and Rapoport (1976),[51a] in which men and women are coproviders in the economic sphere (possessing resources that are close to being equal) and in which no issues are non-negotiable. There are relatively few marriages at this time that approach this degree of equality, but as women's educational levels and job opportunities increase, it can be expected that equal-partner marriages will also increase.

If we accept the existence of various family patterns, the question becomes, Does childbearing affect each pattern equally? Lamb suggests that as childbirth approaches, the relationship between couples becomes more traditional. He cites as an example the wife's withdrawal from work, which "may facilitate a change from the more egalitarian values and role demands of dual-career couples to the more stereotyped role set of traditional nuclear families."[37a] Exchange theory suggests that if she does indeed withdraw from work, she will have fewer resources (such as her own source of income) and thus be more dependent, less equal, and less powerful than her husband.

This change in relationship may be stressful to at least some women, particularly young women in the 1980s who place a high value on equality. This process may explain reports of decreased marital satisfaction following childbirth. For some women, the costs of the altered relationship may be perceived as outweighing the rewards, and the woman may begin to negotiate with her partner for what she perceives as a more equitable solution. For example, she may negotiate to return to work, which could help to restore the balance of power. Such a move would probably require increased participation of the father in child care and house care.

Luker (1975)[41] uses a cost/reward framework to examine decision-making in relation to contraception and abortion. A sexually active woman (single or married) balances the costs and rewards of pregnancy against the costs and rewards of contraception. For example, a mother of four children with limited resources might consider another pregnancy very costly and minimally rewarding. However, contraception may also be costly. If she is past 40, the health risk (a cost) of oral contraception may be very high. If she is not able to use an intrauterine device (IUD) and her partner is uncooperative in the use of other contraceptives such as a diaphragm or condom, she must then decide whether the cost of contraception exceeds the cost of pregnancy. She may reason "I probably am too old to get pregnant," or "if I get pregnant, we'll manage somehow," or "if I get pregnant, I'll have an abortion." She concludes that the risk of unprotected intercourse is less costly than the risk of pregnancy. Other women, or couples, arrive at markedly different decisions.

Exchange theory provides insights that can be useful at each stage of the nursing process. What is the couple's current style of interaction? Is the relationship traditional, senior partner-junior partner, or egalitarian? Are both partners satisfied with their current life style? How do they expect the birth of the baby to change their lifestyle and how do they feel about that? What are the rewards of childbearing for them? What costs do they perceive?

Such questions might be raised in an individual assessment, but they could also be raised in a childbirth education group discussion or in a class for new parents after delivery. These and similar questions could also be the basis of research into the needs of childbearing couples.

A better understanding of an individual couple's needs and resources enables the nurse to plan teaching and support to meet their needs and utilize their resources. If the father is to have a major responsibility for child care, how can the nurse help him, as well as the mother, gain skill and confidence? If the mother who wants to breast-feed for just a few weeks before she returns to her job asks, "Will that be worthwhile?," can the nurse help her identify costs and rewards for herself, her baby, and her family?

Exchange perspectives can also serve as a conceptual framework for other childbearing clients. Hoffman and Mannis (1979)[32] suggest that in a teenage pregnancy, identifying the perceived rewards of parenthood for teenagers (e.g., the desire for adult status) and providing alternate sources of satisfaction may be helpful. Alternatively, indifference to or lack of awareness of costs may be a more important factor in a decision.

Systems Theory

Family systems theory, one of the major approaches to understanding families, is derived from general systems theory. Thus, systems theory focuses on the interaction of various parts of a system rather than on the function of those parts. The most frequently quoted definition of a system is "a set of objects together with relationships between the objects and between their attributes."[28]

The family is considered a living social system—organized, interdependent, interrelated, and having specific goals.[18] Because the family interacts with its environment (cultural and social as well as physical), it is considered an open system. This concept is important because it means that the family unit is different from and more comprehensive than the sum of the individual members. *Feedback*, the process by which output from the system is subsequently processed as input, is a necessary part of a system.

In systems theory, families are further organized into subsystems. A couple is a subsystem; the birth (or adoption) of a child creates a new subsystem. As additional children join the family, a sibling subsystem is created.

Many concepts of systems theory have yet to be developed (see Broderick and Smith, 1979[8] and Friedman, 1981,[18] for an expanded discussion). Nevertheless, in caring for childbearing clients, certain ideas in systems theory seem useful.

Each childbearing family can be considered an open unit interacting with the environ-

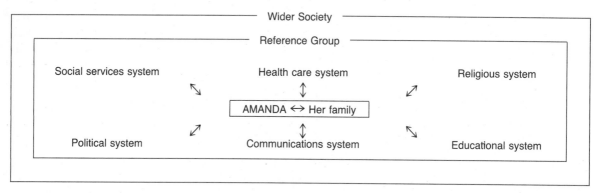

*Adapted from Friedman: *Family Nursing: Theory and Assessment.* New York, Appleton-Century-Crofts, 1981.
Figure 2–2. Influences on decision-making.

ment. Part of that environment is the health care system. At times health care providers behave as if they were the major source of input into the system, but this will rarely be true. It is incumbent upon nurses to be aware of other environmental interactions with the family if they are to provide the best possible care. Consider, for example, Amanda, 17 years old, single, and sexually active. The health care system advises her to utilize some form of contraception and provides input in the form of both information and matter (the specific contraceptive technology), an action supported by her family. Society at large supports contraception for persons who are sexually active (although many would object to sexual activity in a single 17-year-old).

Figure 2–2 suggests that other facets of the environment will also influence Amanda's decision. She and her family may be influenced by religious values. The political system can influence the availability of contraceptives, particularly for adolescents, and also the information she may be able to receive from the educational system (a comprehensive family-life education curriculum in her school, for example). The communications system, including the media, may provide information or support values gained from other systems. The effect of each of these systems will be mediated by Amanda and her family's reference group, both explicitly and implicitly. Amanda may "check out" her ideas with her peers; Amanda's parents may not directly discuss Amanda's use of contraception, but they may be aware of more general discussions within their own group of friends and relatives. Encompassing all of these influences are the values of the wider society. In some societies, adolescent sexuality is both expected and accepted and contraception may not even be an issue; in others, adolescent sexuality, at least for females, may be unthinkable.

A systems approach to the family is im-

mensely valuable in helping us as nurses to realize that our influence is only one of many on a family or individual. We should not be devastated when we are unable to accomplish *our* goals but should recognize that we are part of many systems that influence a family's goals. Systems theory also suggests that any attempt at major change, such as a reduction in the incidence of adolescent pregnancy, must involve many systems. No one system will accomplish change by itself, although all too frequently the health care system has endeavored to do just that. (See Chapter 29 for a description of a coalition of multiple systems that addresses the issue of adolescent pregnancy.

Conflict Perspectives

A conflict approach to marriage does not imply that couples are continually in conflict (i.e., fighting), but it does assume that a certain amount of confrontation is inevitable "over scarce resources, controversial means, and incompatible goals."[68] Although this idea may seem harsh, LaRossa (1977)[38] stated that the belief that marriage and the transition to parenthood could be free of conflict could, "more than anything else, be at the root of dissatisfaction and breakdown in marriage and family systems." LaRossa, who interviewed four times each of 16 couples expecting their first baby, identified shifts in marital organization that occurred even before the birth of the baby as well as areas of disagreement between couples. In my own practice I have encouraged couples to answer individually true/false questions about the roles of husband/father and wife/mother and then to discuss their ideas with one another. (Examples of such questions are: the mother should realize that a mother's greatest reward and satisfaction come through her children; the father should spend as much time as the mother looking after the daily

Table 2–4. THE FAMILY LIFE CYCLE

State	Status	Time Span
1	Beginning family	Prior to the birth of the first child
2	Early childbearing	Oldest child is 2.5 years old or less
3	Preschool children	Oldest child is 2.5 to 5 years old
4	School children	Oldest child is 6 to 13 years old
5	Teenage children	Oldest child is 13 to 20 years old
6	Launching	Period during which all children leave home
7	Middle years	From "empty nest" to retirement
8	Retirement, old age	From retirement until death of both spouses

needs of his children. See Scanzoni, 1980, for a complete list.[62]) In this way areas of conflict can be verbalized, and couples can be helped to understand that disagreement and subsequent exploration of feelings is a helpful rather than a harmful process. Particularly during pregnancy many couples seem afraid of disagreement (although conflict is escalated in others to the point of wife abuse—see Chapter 13). Reassurance that it is normal to disagree over such important issues as those involving childbearing can be helpful.

Developmental Perspectives

The developmental approach to family proposes an eight-stage family cycle (Table 2–4). Developmental tasks are associated not only with individual development but with families as well. Developmental tasks associated with pregnancy are discussed in Chapter 9.

Although many developmental perspectives are useful to nurses interacting with childbearing families, this perspective, like functionalism, assumes a very traditional, nuclear family–oriented lifestyle that does not reflect the life experience of many childbearing families today.

Functionalist Perspectives

Functionalism, or structure-function, was the predominant theory of family sociology in the 1940s, 1950s, and early 1960s. Parsons, Pitts, and Spiegel are major functionalist theorists; Parsons derived some of his ideas from Freud's concepts.

For functionalists, the family is nuclear, with the father playing an instrumental leadership role and the mother playing a subordinate expressive role; this division of labor is seen as not only true but necessary. Roles are fixed; they represent the way families *ought* to function (Table 2–5). Variations are seen as both deviant and a threat to the social order.

Functionalists espouse male superiority. "A generalized male superiority is a basic theme of the structure of the nuclear family in all known societies."[50] Women are accorded little prestige. "In relation to prestige, the first observation is that housekeeping is universally an activity of low status. . . . It is repetitious,

Table 2–5. TWO PERSPECTIVES ON SOCIAL INTERACTION*

Functionalist View	Symbolic Interactionist View
1. Objects and persons are stimuli which act on an individual.	An individual constructs objects on the basis of his ongoing activity. He gives meaning *to* objects and makes decisions on the basis of his judgments.
2. Action is a release or response to what the situational norms demand.	The individual decides what he wishes to do and how he will do it. He takes account of external and internal cues, interpreting their significance for his action.
3. Environmental forces act to "produce" behavior.	By a process of self-indication, an individual accepts, rejects, or transforms the meaning (impact) of such forces.
4. Prescriptions for action, or norms, dictate appropriate behaviors. They are social facts.	Others' attitudes are the basis for individual lines of action.
5. An act is a unitary, bounded phenomenon; i.e., it starts and stops.	An act is disclosed over time and what the end of the act will be cannot be foretold at the start.
6. The act (of an actor) will be followed by the response of an other with or without any interpretation taking place on the part of the other.	An act is validated by the response of an other.
7. Persons act on the basis of a generally objective reality; i.e., learned responses.	Reality is defined by each actor; one defines a situation as he "sees it" and acts on this perception.
8. Group action is the expression of societal demands and shared social values.	Group action is the expression of individuals confronting their life situations.

*From Hardy and Conway: *Role Therapy: Perspectives for Health Professionals.* New York, Appleton-Century-Crofts, 1978.

monotonous . . . [it] remains essentially a low-skill activity which requires for successful discharge a high sense of responsibility rather than complex training. The same is true of parenthood, especially care of the prepubertal child."[50]

Functionalism is no longer a viable theory for most family theorists. In a recent major textbook of family theory[9] there is no chapter on functionalism. The functionalist perspective almost never appears in a contemporary family journal. However, it is still a popular theoretical framework in some nursing literature[18] and in maternity texts (see quotes from Clark, 1979,[12] and Jensen et al., 1977,[36] below).

What is wrong with the functionalist approach? More important, does using a functionalist conceptual framework limit nursing practice? For the functionalist each role demands specific role behavior. The mother has her role and appropriate behavior as does the father. These roles are predetermined. Pitts (1964)[50] notes Parsons' "cogent case for the importance of this type of division of labor for the socialization of the child in any society." Clark (1979)[12] states that "the many practical attitudes necessary to take care of infants and guide learning are facilitated by characteristic qualities of a woman's personality." As for fathers, "fatherliness consists of instinctive responses of empathy for the children as the man fulfills his ultimate goal as protector and provides for his family."

Nursing approaches toward the new family, based on these concepts, would emphasize adaptation to the prescribed roles. But what if the mother is the major provider for the family, either by choice or by necessity? For functionalists, this pattern represents deviance.

A nurse practicing from a functionalist perspective will assume that particular tasks, such as bathing and feeding the baby, are a mother's responsibility. Baby bath classes will be held for mothers in the mornings rather than at a time that may be more convenient for fathers as well. The question has been raised in nursing literature and practice whether grandmothers who are the primary caregivers should be a focus of teaching (e.g., when the mother is a younger teenager); rarely are fathers thought of in this situation. Feeding help is generally given to the mother; how often does a nurse help a father with feeding? The nurse may assume that a mother will instinctively know how to feed her infant. Community health nursing and nursing clinics have also focused largely on the mother as the primary caregiver because contacts have been made during the day when many fathers are working.

What about the parents who ask about maternal employment after childbearing? From what perspective can nurses answer if they view this behavior as "deviant"?

In some hospitals, support persons other than husbands are not allowed in the labor/delivery areas. Again, the assumption seems to be that any relationship other than the nuclear family relationship represents deviance.

Aside from its clinical implications, functionalism is not a particularly useful theory for the researcher. If roles and functions are fixed, the researcher is limited in measuring adjustment or deviance. In a society in which the behavior of men and women within the family is changing markedly, a researcher's commitment to fixed roles and functions is not only nonproductive for research but potentially destructive for families that may be influenced by the results of such research.

Summary: Family Theories

Each of the family perspectives described here is helpful in the different ways that have been discussed. Interactionist theory has been very popular in nursing practice related to childbearing because of the usefulness of the concepts related to roles. In my practice and thinking, I find exchange perspectives of particular value. The rigidity of functionalist theories, from my point of view, makes functionalist concepts less valuable, although many nurses continue to use them.

Anthropologic Perspectives

In no society is childbearing ever considered a solely physiologic event. Every society, no matter how small or isolated or traditional, has social norms that prescribe where birth will occur, who will be present, how pregnant women and new mothers and infants will be cared for, whether pregnancy is seen as a time of health or illness, the kind of health care chosen during pregnancy, the kinds of food the mother will eat during pregnancy, whether the newborn infant will be breast- or bottle-fed, and so on. Examples of these practices will be found throughout this book.

Culture—the knowledge, beliefs, customs, laws, attitudes, values, and behavior of a society—is the focus of anthropologists. Concepts from the field of anthropology are increasingly recognized as important in nursing practice. A nursing subspecialty, transcultural nursing, has been developed. There is a nursing section within the Society for Medical Anthropology. For nurses caring for childbearing families it is the concepts of anthropology that provide an understanding of the customs, behaviors, values, attitudes, and beliefs of individuals and families.

Cross-cultural Perspectives and Childbearing

In a general sense, the physiology of pregnancy and birth is similar in all societies. It is cultural factors that make the experience of childbirth so different. A limited but growing number of cross-cultural comparisons of pregnancy and birth experiences can help us to understand better the extent of variation from culture to culture, something that is difficult to appreciate from the perspective of a single culture (see Jordan, 1980[37], and Clark, 1978,[11] for examples). For example, there appear to be some societies in which pregnancy-induced hypertension does not occur (Chapter 13). Could the reason be cultural? The discomfort of labor and birth seems to vary between cultures. Why? This question led an English obstetrician, Grantly Dick-Read,[14a] to suggest that anxiety and tension were important contributors to the pain of labor, an idea that has markedly changed the care of childbearing women in many societies.

It would be a mistake to believe that all traditional societies (i.e., societies in which the process of cultural change is very gradual) have the "right" answers to our questions and that we need only to emulate their practices to improve our own. There are traditional societies that see pregnancy as a time of illness (e.g., the Cuna Indians of Panama), and there are those who see pregnancy as a time of health. In many traditional societies the presence of the baby's father at childbirth would be unthinkable, yet this is important to many couples in our own society.

In addition to enhancing our understanding of human variability, a cultural perspective is essential in providing high quality care to individual women and their families. As noted throughout this book, the care-provider must understand the values, behaviors, and beliefs of the care-receiver. Table 2–6 suggests the basic components of a cultural assessment that will help nurses to individualize care to families when cultural values differ from their own.

Of course, within any society, persons do not act identically, regardless of similar cultural backgrounds. Individual differences, determined by both heredity and environment, are always important factors in behavior. Yet culture does exert its influence; the middle-class American mother would not be likely to pin a charm on her baby's dress to protect him from the "evil eye," nor would she use a cradle board

rather than a carriage to transport him. A nurse who does not consider cultural preferences in food will not be able to help a mother plan a diet that meets the nutritional needs of pregnancy.

The United States is a nation of many subsocieties, each with its own distinct cultural heritage. When the beliefs of these groups come in conflict with those of nurses and doctors, misunderstandings can and do arise, creating barriers that interfere with care.

Ethnocentrism is the belief that our own values and lifestyle are superior to the lifestyle of other groups of people. Thus an herb tied around the neck of a baby may seem only a dirty bag to the nurse or physician (after all, they "know" it has no value); to the mother, however, it is a symbol of her caring for her baby.

Because of ethnocentrism, *culture conflict* may result. Both nurse and patient may be critical of one another. The nurse may be more overt in her criticism and may attempt to impose her views on the patient *(cultural imposition)*. The patient may appear acquiescent in the presence of the nurse but may ignore the nurse's advice once she returns home.

Culture conflict is often subtle and unrecognized. For example, if the patient's culture emphasizes close family relationships during illness, but the nurse values quiet and sees kinship ties as relatively unimportant, there is culture conflict. If the nurse values stoicism in the face of pain, but the patient has been socialized in a culture where expressions of pain are encouraged, there is culture conflict.

Not only health-related behavior but also "everyday" behavior may lead to culture conflict between nurse and patient. To illustrate: middle-class Americans value direct eye contact between persons; continually looking down is taken to mean either lack of interest or "having something to hide." But to the man or woman from the Appalachian mountains, direct eye contact is "staring" and highly improper; the Appalachian will avert his eyes when looked at directly. Differences may be so overwhelming that *culture shock* results.

Culture Shock

Culture shock is a term anthropologists use to describe a reaction that occurs to persons in unfamiliar situations as a result of multiple environmental stresses. A traditional example of culture shock is the person from a western society who goes to live in a traditional society, such as that of an African village or an Indian tribe along the Amazon river. The language, technology, customs, values, and beliefs are all

Table 2–6. CULTURAL ASSESSMENT*

Area Assessed	Significance
Family	

Birthplace of parents-to-be
   Birthplace of grandparents-to-be
   (maternal and paternal)
	Younger generation may have different ideas of family tradition and culture, particularly if older generation was born in "home" country and younger generation was born in United States

Residence in culturally identifiable
    neighborhood (e.g., Indian reservation,
    Chinatown)
	Residents of identifiable neighborhood may have more traditional values

Nuclear or extended family
    Grandparents living in home
    Role of grandparents in decision making
	It is essential to understand family influence on young parents when teaching and counseling

Family support
    Companion or coach during labor
    Assistance during postpartal period at home
	In some societies a male labor coach is unusual; males may not expect to help in infant care

Diet: Traditional foods
   General
   During and following pregnancy
	Nutritional counseling must utilize foods acceptable to individual clients; appropriate foods must be provided to the mother during hospitalization

For infant	Understanding cultural beliefs about infant diet (e.g., delayed breast-feeding) must precede infant care and teaching
Pica	Pica is frequently deleterious
Traditional health care practices	Understanding traditional values of health and child care must precede both care and teaching

Use of herbs
    Herbs used
    Western medicines used
    Beliefs about value of herbs
	In assessing drug use (Chapter 3), traditional herbs must not be overlooked

Ritual practices Beliefs related to health and illness (e.g., *el mal ojo*)	
Utilization of traditional healers (e.g., faith healer, curandero, medicine man)	When advice is being received from other healers, knowledge of that advice is essential (Scott[64])

Child care practices
   Feeding
   Circumcision
	Understanding traditional values of health and child care must precede both care and teaching

Bathing, dressing, sleeping, etc. (e.g., is a
    belly band believed to be necessary; does
    baby sleep alone or with parents?)
   Special protection for infant
   Rituals or customs (e.g., cradle boards)	

*Adapted from Rose: *In* Clark, A. (ed.): *Culture, Childbearing, Health Professionals.* Philadelphia, F. A. Davis, 1978.

strange to the westerner. He sees unaccustomed sights, hears unaccustomed sounds, smells strange odors, is presented with unfamiliar food. Previous coping strategies may be of little value. At the very least, the situation may be frightening. The same situation exists, of course, when a person from another culture interacts with the dominant culture in our own society. That person may be Mexican-American, American Indian, Vietnamese, or someone from any of the many cultural groups within our society.

The health care system may be viewed as a subsociety within the larger society, with its own language, customs, and values, and even

sights, sounds, and smells that distinguish it from society as a whole. For many persons, interaction with the health care system is a cultural shock in that the situation is unfamiliar and there are multiple stressors in the environment. The degree of stress may be minimal in the prenatal care of a woman with no complications; it is intensified in the traditional hospital labor/delivery experience, even for the woman with no complications, and it is maximum in the experience of a high-risk mother or high-risk infant.

When the values, beliefs, and behavior of one group do not fit with those of another, *dissonance* is said to exist. Dissonance is thus a characteristic of cultures in conflict. Those cultures may very well be the culture of a childbearing family and the culture of the health care provider. Festinger (1957)[16] states that:

1. Dissonance is psychologically uncomfortable and therefore an individual experiencing it will try to reduce dissonance and achieve consonance.

2. When dissonance is present, an individual will actively seek to avoid situations and information that will increase it.

Brink (1976)[7] has identified five environmental stressors in hospital experience; we suggest that these stressors may also be present in ambulatory settings, although they may be less intense. Each of these stressors may result from dissonance.

Communication is always a potential stressor when individuals from two cultures interact. The subculture of health care providers uses a vast number of words (fundus, gestation, cervix) and abbreviations (pit, OCT, NST) that are often meaningless, at least initially, even to persons with a high level of general education. Student nurses in their first days in maternal-child health clinical experiences may be able to appreciate somewhat the confusion of childbearing women caused by our specialized use of language.

Mechanical differences, the ever-increasing, high-technology care of mothers (e.g., fetal monitors, amniocentesis) and sick newborn infants (e.g., equipment for respiratory assistance, monitors of respiratory and heart rates) are unfamiliar and thus can be stressful.

Customs include clinic, office, or hospital routines. As simple a matter (from the provider's perspective) as knowing where to go in a large clinic or hospital is stressful. Consider a mother who has been receiving prenatal care in an office or clinic in her rural community and who is referred to her regional center for further care. She may be so overwhelmed by the idea of a large medical center that she just doesn't go. (Remember that, according to dissonance theory, persons avoid situations that are likely to increase dissonance.) Absolutely clear instructions about how to proceed or, better, someone to go with her may help her to overcome this stress. For all mothers, the opportunity to tour the site where they will give birth as well as very specific information about routines and expectations will help reduce the stress of an unfamiliar experience.

Isolation from family or friends is always stressful. One of the best changes occurring in the care of childbearing families over the past decade has been the decrease in isolation of the mother from others in both ambulatory and hospital settings. "Rooming-in" has permitted parents and new infants to spend far more time together following birth, and high-risk and intensive care nurseries have become increasingly open to parents on a 24-hour basis. Periods of separation that are stressful still exist, however.

The *attitudes, values and beliefs* of health care providers frequently clash with the attitudes, values, and beliefs of the childbearing family. Women and families have an image of what they hope childbearing will be—a warm, loving, family-centered experience, with loved ones and perhaps their other children present. Health care providers also have an image of childbearing; it may include, for example, fetal monitoring for all women, intravenous fluids, and a delivery site that looks like an operating room (because it is). The dissonance in these two views is so great that in many instances a woman and her family may choose to leave the traditional system, opting for home birth even without a qualified birth attendant rather than endure a situation that conflicts so intensely with their values.[3]

Table 2–7 suggests some ways in which nurses may utilize the concepts of environmental stressors in caring for childbearing families. After assessing the relationship between a particular environmental stressor and an individual, nurses can use that knowledge to diagnose nursing problems and then to develop appropriate intervention.

Cultural Change

Another focus of anthropologic theory is *cultural change*. In nursing practice we may desire to change one individual's behavior or the behavior of a group of people. Graham (1973)[27] has suggested several factors that influence the success of proposed cultural change.

1. Does the proposed change add or eliminate a behavior? Changes that add behavior appear to be more successful than those that seek to eliminate behavior. For example, in trying to improve a pregnant woman's diet, the addition of a missing nutrient (milk, perhaps) will probably be achieved more readily than the elimination of a long-standing practice (e.g., cooking vegetables with "fat-back" or "streaky-lean").

2. How overt and simple are the advantages of the proposed change? Changes that are overt and simple with easily communicated advantages are more likely to be successful. Cigarette smoking is a cultural practice we would like to eliminate during pregnancy; there are

Table 2–7. ENVIRONMENTAL STRESSORS AND CHILDBEARING FAMILIES

Environmental Stressors	Assessment (initial and continuing evaluation)	Nursing Diagnosis	Intervention
Communication	Do the clients understand the words we are using?	Need of the client for clear definition of terms	Clearly define terms in language client can understand
Mechanical differences	Is the purpose of any equipment clearly explained, along with the effects or possible effects on mother or fetus?	Need of the client for clear explanation of all equipment	Clearly explain the use, effects, and need of all equipment
Customs	Do the clients know what is expected of them? Do they understand the routines and customs of the care setting?	Need of the client for clear explanation of customs, routines, role behavior, in each setting	Provide information about routines, role behavior. Encourage prenatal couple to visit delivery site prior to time of labor (Chapter 11)
Isolation	Is the woman isolated from significant persons during prenatal examinations, in labor, delivery, postpartum? Are parents, infants separated?	Need of client for contact with significant persons. Need of parents and infant for contact	May require changes in health care setting to reduce or eliminate isolation
Attitudes and beliefs	What is important to the woman or family at each period of childbearing? Are her values incorporated into the plan of care?	Need of woman or family to participate in developing plan of care	Involvement of woman or family in decision-making. May require changes in health care setting to allow incorporation of woman's values

abundant data indicating that the infant of mothers who smoke are smaller and thereby at greater risk than the infants of mothers who do not smoke (Chapter 8). This information can be clearly communicated and, although the change requires an elimination of a behavior, the required change is straightforward. Pratt (1971)[51] suggests that concentration on concrete behavior patterns rather than large amounts of *complex* information is helpful.

3. How easy and inexpensive will a trial of the proposed change be? If we hope to convince a pregnant woman with limited financial resources to add more protein to her diet, we must be able to suggest ways that are both easy and inexpensive as well as compatible with her culture's dietary practices. The facilities she has available for preparing meals are just as important as her resources for purchasing food. A family that doesn't own a pitcher or jar and has no means of refrigerating food is not helped by a demonstration of making a quart of powdered milk.

4. Is the decision to accept or reject the proposed change reversible? As Harrison et al. (1978)[30] suggested, oral contraceptives, which can be terminated at any time, are much more likely to be accepted as a method of birth control than is permanent sterilization by tubal ligation or vasectomy.

5. How many decisions are required to bring about the proposed change? Changes that require repeated decisions, such as a contraceptive that must be used prior to each act of intercourse, are more difficult to introduce than a change that requires a single decision, such as the insertion of an IUD.

Nursing Process and the Care of Childbearing Families

Nursing interaction with individual members of childbearing families utilizes the nursing process. Both nursing theories and theories from other disciplines suggest areas that should be integrated into the nursing process as we plan care. Some examples have been given earlier in this chapter.

Assessment: Assessment involves the development of a data base that includes information provided by a woman and other family members as well as data derived from physical examination and laboratory tests. All of the theories suggest the importance of a holistic approach that recognizes the importance of cultural, social, and individual psychologic aspects of a person's life as well as the physiologic changes that are so readily apparent during pregnancy.

Because pregnancy is a time of change, continuing assessment is mandatory at each opportunity for interaction. Feelings, attitudes, and behavior as well as physical status can change from week to week during the prenatal period; they may change from hour to hour during the time of labor. Rapid changes in status are characteristic of newborn infants.

Assessment is of limited value if the data are not systematically recorded. In planning care and evaluating the effects of that care, we must be able to look back at earlier assessments. Physiologically, for example, patterns of blood pressure, weight gain, and anemia are evaluated over the months of gestation. Often graphic recording is useful. The status of a mother's feelings about her changing body, her preparations for the baby (one type of attachment behavior), her relationship with the baby's father and other family members are other examples of data that are assessed on a continuing basis and recorded so that changes can be noted.

Nursing Diagnosis

An American Nurses Association resolution (1976) states that "nursing diagnosis describes actual or potential health problems which nurses are capable (of treating) and licensed to treat."[9a]

A number of nursing diagnoses have been noted earlier in this chapter. Some examples are listed in Tables 2–8 and 2–9. The diagnoses listed are by no means the only ones a nurse might utilize in the care of childbearing women and infants.

By definition, a nursing diagnosis identifies a *problem* or *potential problem*. For the majority of mothers who are healthy during their pregnancy, few problems may exist. In this instance, the nursing judgment is that "no problem exists and the client's state of wellness is affirmed."[73]

The nursing diagnosis may identify a potential problem. For example, a pregnant woman with two previous infants weighing 9 pounds, 8 ounces and 10 pounds, 13 ounces may be at risk of developing gestational diabetes with this pregnancy. Because she is at increased risk, her plan of care will vary from the plan developed for the woman in whom no problem

has been identifed. Figure 2–3 shows a sample decision tree for nursing diagnosis and action in the prenatal period.

If a problem has been identified during a previous assessment, the nursing diagnosis may indicate that the woman (or her husband or their infant) is coping well with the problem. For example, back pain is a frequent problem in the last trimester of pregnancy. A nurse may teach the mother to do an exercise called pelvic rock (Chapter 11); a subsequent assessment may indicate that the exercise has helped the mother cope with back discomfort to her satisfaction.

At times the nursing diagnosis indicates that progress has been made in solving the problem but that the problem is not yet resolved. Inadequate weight gain may have been identified as a problem; the mother's weight gain may have improved, but further improvement may be necessary to ensure the well-being of her fetus. A mother who has had difficulty accepting her pregnancy may show beginning signs of acceptance and attachment to her infant, but further counseling may be indicated.

Some problems will continue throughout pregnancy and into the postpregnancy period. A mother with hypertension or diabetes mellitus prior to pregnancy will require specialized care throughout pregnancy and afterward. If hypertension or diabetes mellitus develops during pregnancy, the plan of care will vary. A mother who is not married may have problems or potential problems during pregnancy that will continue following her child's birth.

Unexpected complications may occur with great rapidity during the course of pregnancy, threatening the life or well-being of the fetus or mother. Examples are bleeding early in pregnancy, indicating a threatened abortion (i.e., a possible miscarriage; see Chapter 13), a prolapse of the umbilical cord during labor (Chapter 19), or sudden respiratory distress in the newborn infant. Rapid diagnosis is essential so that a plan of care can be initiated immediately.

Developing a Plan of Care

Once nursing diagnoses have been made, a plan of care is developed, directed toward the goal of solving the problems or potential problems identified. Goals may be long-term, intermediate, or immediate, and are usually stated as specific client behaviors. For example, education provided during pregnancy may have

Table 2–8. EXAMPLES OF POSSIBLE NURSING DIAGNOSES RELATED TO CHILDBEARING*

Prenatal Period

Physiologic
Discomfort, pain, or physiologic distress related to changes of pregnancy
Discomfort, pain, or physiologic distress related to diagnostic procedures
Inadequate nutrition, potential malnutrition, or malnutrition
Intake of potential teratogens or harmful substances (alcohol, drugs, nicotine)
Nausea
Constipation
Backache
False labor

Social-Emotional
Self-dissatisfaction related to changing body
Diminished self-esteem
Emotional distress related to changes of pregnancy
Emotional distress related to diagnostic procedures
Difficult adaptation to role changes
Difficult adaptation to crisis situations
Difficult adaptation to lifestyle interruptions
Inadequate adaptation to lifestyle interruptions

Educational
Need for information about changes of pregnancy
Need for preparation for childbirth

General
Need for nursing supervision of normal pregnancy

Intrapartal Period

Physiologic
Discomfort, pain, or physiologic distress related to process of labor or birth
Inability to relax, breathe with contractions

Social-Emotional
Feeling of inadequacy in coping with labor
Inadequate emotional support
Diminishing ability to cope with labor as labor progresses
Distress related to intervention (e.g., fetal monitor)

Educational
Need for information about the process of labor
Need for specific instruction (e.g., effective pushing during second stage)

General
Need for nursing supervision during labor and birth

Postpartum Period (Mother)

Physiologic
Breast enlargement
Lactation suppression
Excessive lactation
Nipple pain
Breast tenderness
Perineal discomfort
Constipation
Subinvolution
Potential for thrombosis

Social-Emotional
Inadequate parent-infant bonding
Sense of inadequacy
Distress related to family reorganization
Difficult adaptation to new role

Educational
Need for information about infant care
Need for information about breast or bottle feeding
Need for information about self-care in hospital and at home
Need for information about family planning

General
Need for nursing supervision of mother, infant, or family

Neonatal Period (Infant)

Physiologic
Hypothermia
Hypoglycemia
Feeding difficulty
Need for circumcision care

Social-Emotional
Infant characteristics affecting bonding (e.g., irritable infant, sleepy infant)
(See also Postpartum Period, [Mother])

Educational
(See Postpartum Period, [Mother])

General
Need for nursing supervision of infant

*Many of these diagnoses are from Campbell, C.: *Nursing Diagnoses and Intervention in Nursing Practice*. New York, John Wiley and Sons, 1978.

as a goal a change in eating pattern within the next week (immediate behavior), preparation for labor and birth (intermediate behavior), or the development of ideas about parenting roles (long-term behavior).

Some actions will have a higher priority than others. As far as possible, the woman and the members of her family should be involved in the setting of priorities. The time span of the prenatal period frequently allows nurses and women some flexibility in the setting of priorities; obviously, the time frame is compressed during the time of labor and birth, and even further compressed when emergency sit-

uations arise (when a newborn must be resuscitated, for example). Maslow's hierarchy of needs, discussed earlier in this chapter, is one conceptual model that some nurses use to establish priorities. Top priority is given to meeting physiologic needs so that needs for safety and security can be met, and then the need for love can be met, and so on. During labor, for example, the need for physiologic comfort must be met before the goal of labor as a meaningful experience can be achieved.

Nurses and clients frequently do not share priorities. This is particularly likely when cultural and socioeconomic backgrounds vary, but

Table 2–9. EXAMPLES OF POSSIBLE NURSING DIAGNOSES RELATED TO CHILDBEARING IN MOTHERS OR INFANTS AT RISK FOR SPECIAL PROBLEMS

Prenatal Period
All of the diagnoses in Table 2–8

Physiologic
Obesity
Additional rest requirement
Predisposition to bleeding or hemorrhage (e.g., gravida with placenta previa)

Social-Emotional
Anger because of high-risk status
Conflict related to diagnostic or therapeutic intervention (e.g., amniocentesis, ultrasound)
Anxiety or potential anxiety about self or infant related to high-risk status

Educational
Need for information related to specific high-risk problem (e.g., pregnancy-induced hypertension, diabetes)

General
Need for nursing supervision of high-risk pregnancy

Intrapartal Period
All of the diagnoses in Table 2–8

Physiologic
Maternal exhaustion
Hypotonic uterine contrctions
Hypertonic uterine contractions
Potential for hemorrhage
Uterine relaxation, fourth stage of labor

Social-Emotional
Conflict related to diagnostic or therapeutic intervention (e.g., amniotomy, cesarean birth)
Anxiety or potential anxiety about safety of self or infant
Doubt about capacity to cope in face of complication

Educational
Need for information about variations from expected labor
Need for information when cesarean birth is necessary

General
Need for nursing supervision of a high-risk mother during the intrapartal period.

Postpartum Period
All of the diagnoses in Table 2–8

Physiologic
Elevated body temperature
Susceptibility to infection (e.g., prolonged labor, cesarean delivery, traumatic vaginal delivery)
"Boggy" uterus

Social-Emotional
Diminished self-esteem related to high-risk condition of self or infant
Guilt related to defect of infant
Delayed bonding due to illness in mother or infant
Need for interaction with infant

Educational
Need for information about self-care relevant to specific health problems (e.g., diabetes)
Need for information about course of future pregnancies (e.g., repeat cesarean delivery)

General
Need for nursing supervision of puerperium for high-risk mother

Neonatal Period (High-Risk Infant)
All of the diagnoses in Table 2–8

Physiologic
Hypotension
Hypoxia
Inadequate urine output
Potential vision loss related to oxygen therapy
Susceptibility to infection
Urinary obstruction
Dependence on endotracheal tube management
Predisposition to acidosis
Sucking difficulty
Potential inadequate pulmonary ventilation

Social-Emotional (Parents)
Denial of severity of infant illness
Guilt related to preterm birth or birth of infant with anomaly
Inability of parent(s) to grieve
Difficult adaptation to crisis changes

Social-Emotional (Infant)
Need for sensory stimulation
Need for interaction with parents

General
Need for nursing supervision of high-risk infant and family

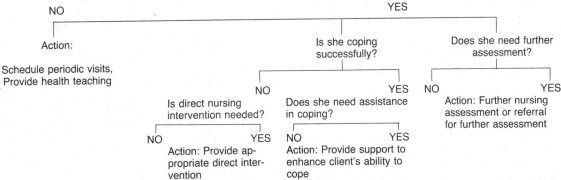

Figure 2–3. Nursing diagnoses and action in the prenatal period.

the professional values of the nurse (and of other health professionals) may in themselves lead to widely varying priorities. Clients who perceive pregnancy as a time of health may be very resistant to intervention during any phase of childbearing that may seem both appropriate and important to nurses. Examples of these interventions are the use of ultrasound, antenatal fetal heart rate testing, and fetal heart monitoring during labor. This difference in priorities results in cultural dissonance, described earlier. Negotiation may lead to a mutually satisfactory list of priorities; if priorities are not satisfactory to both nurse and client, the plan of care is not likely to be effective.

The plan of care will identify the action or intervention that will be primarily or completely the responsibility of the nurse, those actions for which the woman or her family will assume primary responsibility, and those that will be the responsibility of other professionals or agencies.

The plan must be written if there is to be continuity in the care a woman (or infant) receives. The written record of problems, diagnoses, and proposed actions forms the basis for subsequent interaction.

During some phases of childbearing, the prenatal period, for example, the development and modification of a plan of care over the course of prenatal visits is less difficult than in a more acute period, such as the time of labor and birth, in which assessment and nursing diagnoses must frequently be made very quickly. When nurses who care for women during labor have access to the prenatal care plan, care is greatly enhanced.

For the majority of women who receive prenatal care in a private physician's office, there may be no nursing care plan during the prenatal phase of childbearing. A prenatal medical history may or may not be available to the nurse. We believe this lack of knowledge of what has happened in the previous months hinders both physical and social-emotional nursing care during labor. A nursing assessment and diagnosis in early labor are certainly of value, but frequently women are not seen until the active phase of labor when contractions lasting as long as 60 seconds are occurring every 3 to 5 minutes. At this stage assessment and diagnosis are frequently limited to physical factors, and a great deal of important information that would facilitate a mother's care may not be obtained.

Although each woman or infant needs an individualized care plan, in emergency situations nurses should have a preliminary plan of management available. For example, if the nursing diagnosis is prolapse of the umbilical cord, the nurse should be aware of the plan of care for a prolapsed cord in her setting so that immediate intervention is possible.

Nursing Action and Interaction: Implementing the Plan of Care

Nurses use a variety of skills in implementing a plan of care for childbearing families. Yura and Walsh identify three types of skills: intellectual (using problem solving and critical thinking, making judgments), interpersonal (communication skills, sensitivity to nonverbal as well as verbal language, for example), and technical (involving specific procedures and the use of equipment, for example).[73] Although certain skills may be of more importance during specific nurse–client interactions, all are highly significant during the childbearing year.

For example, during the prenatal phase of healthy childbearing, much of the interaction with a woman and her family may involve interpersonal skills such as listening and providing information and reassurance. Technical skills will be used in assessment (assessing maternal blood pressure and fundal height, for example), but there may be little technical intervention. Critical thinking is involved in evaluating communication and deciding whether further nursing action is required. For example, a nurse may judge that a mother needs more extended nutritional counseling than she is able to provide in the time available and refer the mother to the nutritionist. Other frequent nursing referrals are to social workers, childbirth educators, and physicians.

When the assessment indicates that the mother is at risk during the prenatal phase, all types of nursing skills are utilized more intensely in both ambulatory and hospital settings. Nursing action and interaction during labor and birth are also intense, involving support and communication (interpersonal skills), a variety of technical skills, and, of course, constant use of problem-solving and decision-making skills.

Evaluation

Evaluation is a continuing aspect of nurse–client interaction within the framework of the nursing process. Evaluation asks such questions as: What was the effect of the planned intervention? Were the goals established in the planning stage met? Evaluation enables a nurse to modify the plan of care for an individual client and also to evaluate her approach to similar problems of other clients. Evaluation leads to a new nursing diagnosis, that is, a resolved problem, adequate coping, and so on. When evaluation indicates that problems are solved or goals attained, priorities involving other problems (if any) can be reevaluated.

Evaluation includes the client and her family when this is possible. For example, an evaluation of the experience of labor should include the mother's perception and the evaluation of her husband or other family members as well as the evaluation of the nurse.

Because of fragmentation of care of childbearing families, evaluation of intermediate and long-term goals is often difficult. A nurse who works closely with the family during the prenatal phase may not have the opportunity to evaluate the effects of her teaching about labor and birth or parenting. A nurse participating in newborn resuscitation in a community hospital may not see the infant again if he is transported to a regional center, and she will be unable to evaluate the care given the baby. Nurses who care for preterm infants in an intensive care nursery frequently are unable to evaluate the long-term results of their care. Aside from the personal frustration involved, the absence of evaluation prevents nurses from modifying their general approach. In a number of settings improved evaluation has been instituted. Nurses who teach childbirth education classes utilize a variety of mechanisms for evaluation—written reports from parents, reunions, and telephone calls. Some intensive care nurseries regularly inform community hospitals of the status of transported infants. Further development of mechanisms for evaluation will enhance nursing care.

Nursing Process: A Cycle

The nursing process is cyclical; nurses continually assess, diagnose, plan, act, evaluate, and modify their actions on the basis of evaluation. Particularly within the context of a developmental, continually changing stage in the life of a woman who is pregnant and her infant, recognition of the ongoing nature of the nursing process is essential.

Summary

Nursing theory, theories from other disciplines, and the nursing process are the core of understanding the nursing care of childbearing families. In the chapters that follow, specific information about childbearing from physiologic, psychologic, social, and cultural perspectives will enable us to augment that core to a fully developed understanding of childbearing families.

REFERENCES

1. Abdellah, F.: *Patient-Centered Approaches to Nursing.* New York, The Macmillan Company, 1960.
2. Aspinall, M., Jambruno, N., and Phoenix, B.: The Why and How of Nursing Diagnosis. *MCN,* 2(6), 354, 1977.
3. Bauwens, E., and Anderson, S.: Home Births: A Reaction to Hospital Environmental Stressors. *In* Bauwens, E. *The Anthropology of Health.* St. Louis, C. V. Mosby Co., 1978.
4. Benedek, T.: Motherhood and Nurturing. *In* Anthony, E., and Benedek, T. (eds.): *Parenthood: Its Psychology and Psychopathology.* Boston, Little, Brown & Co., 1970.
5. Bettman, S., and Zalk, S.: *Expectant Fathers.* New York, Hawthorn Books, 1978.
6. Biddle, B., and Thomas, E.: *Role Theory: Concepts and Research.* New York, John Wiley & Sons, 1966.
7. Brink, P.: *Transcultural Nursing.* Englewood Cliffs, N.J., Prentice-Hall, 1976.
8. Broderick, C., and Smith, J.: The General Systems Approach to the Family. *In* Burr, W., Hill, R., Nye, F., and Reiss, I. (eds.): *Contemporary Theories About the Family,* Vol. 2. New York, The Free Press, 1979.
9. Burr, W., Leigh, G., Day, R., and Constantine, J.: Symbolic Interaction and the Family. *In* Burr, W., Hill, R., Nye, F., and Reiss, I. (eds.): *Contemporary Theories About the Family,* Vol. 2. New York, The Free Press, 1979.
9a. Campbell, C.: *Nursing Diagnosis and Intervention in Nursing Practice.* New York, John Wiley, 1978.
10. Cherry, L., and Lewis, M.: Mothers and Two Year Olds: A Study of Sex-Differentiated Aspects of Verbal Interaction. *Developmental Psychology,* 12:278, 1976.
11. Clark, A.: *Culture, Childbearing, Health Professionals.* Philadelphia, F.A. Davis Co. 1978.
12. Clark, A., and Affonso, D.: *Childbearing: A Nursing Perspective.* 2nd Edition. Philadelphia, F.A. Davis Co., 1979.
13. Condry, J., and Condry, S.: Sex Differences: A Study of the Eye of the Beholder. *Child Development,* 47:812, 1976.
14. Conway, M.: Theoretical Approaches to the Study of Roles. *In* Hardy, M., and Conway, M. (eds.): *Role Theory: Perspectives for Health Professionals.* New York, Appleton-Century-Crofts, 1978.
14a. Dick-Read, G.: *Child birth Without Fear.* New York, Harper and Row, 1959.
15. Erikson, E.: Identity and the Life Cycle. *In* Klein, G. S. (ed.): *Psychological Issues.* New York, International University Press, 1959.
16. Festinger, L.: *A Theory of Cognitive Dissonance.* Evanston, Ill., Row, Peterson, & Co., 1957.

17. Foster, P., and Janssens, N.: Dorothy E. Orem. *In* Nursing Theories Conference Group: *Nursing Theories: The Base for Professional Nursing Practice.* Englewood Cliffs, N.J., Prentice-Hall, 1980.

18. Friedman, M.: *Family Nursing: Theory and Assessment.* New York, Appleton-Century-Crofts, 1981.

19. Fries, M.: Longitudinal Study: Prenatal Period to Parenthood, *Journal of the American Psychoanalytic Association, 25*:132, 1977.

20. Galbreath, J.: Sister Callista Roy. *In* Nursing Theories Conference Group: *Nursing Theories: The Base for Professional Nursing Practice.* Englewood Cliffs, N.J., Prentice-Hall, 1980.

21. Galligan, A.: Using Roy's Concept of Adaptation to Care for Young Children, *MCN, 4*(1):24, 1979.

22. Gebbie, K. (*ed.*): *Classification of Nursing Diagnoses.* Summary of the Second National Conference. St. Louis, Clearinghouse for The National Group for Classification of Nursing Diagnoses, 1976.

23. Gerwitz, S., and Dodge, K.: Adults' Evaluation of a Child as a Function of Sex of Adult and Sex of Child, *Journal of Personality and Social Psychology, 32*:822, 1975.

24. Gladieux, J.: Pregnancy—the Transition to Parenthood: Satisfaction with the Pregnancy as a Function of Sex-Role Conceptions, Marital Relationship and Social Network. *In* Miller, W., and Newman, L. F. (eds.): *The First Child and Family Formation.* Chapel Hill, N.C., Carolina Population Center, 1978.

25. Goldberg, S., and Lewis, M.: Play Behavior in the Year Old Infant: Early Sex Differences, *Child Development, 40*:21, 1969.

26. Goode, W.: A Theory of Role Strain, *American Sociological Review, 25*:488, 1960.

27. Graham, S.: Studies of Behavior Change to Enhance Public Health, *American Journal of Public Health, 63*:327, 1973.

28. Hall, A., and Fagan, R.: Definition of Systems, *General Systems, 1*:18, 1956.

29. Hardy, M., and Conway, M. (eds.): *Role Theory: Perspectives for Health Professionals.* New York, Appleton-Century-Crofts, 1978.

30. Harrison, G., Tymrak, M., and Friedman, G.: The Riverside School Heart Project: A Laboratory in Applied Medical Anthropology. *In* Bauwens, E. (ed.): *The Anthropology of Health.* St. Louis, C.V. Mosby Co., 1978.

31. Hennenborn, W., and Cogan, R.: The Effect of Husband Participation on Reported Pain and the Probability of Medication During Labor and Birth, *Journal of Psychosomatic Research, 19*:215, 1975.

32. Hoffman, L., and Manis, J.: The Value of Children in the United States: A New Approach to the Study of Fertility, *Journal of Marriage and the Family, 41*:583, 1979.

33. Hogan, R.: *Personality Theory: The Personalogical Tradition.* Englewood Cliffs, N.J., Prentice-Hall, 1976.

34. Holman, T., and Burr, W.: Beyond the Beyond: The Growth of Family Theories in the 1970's, *Journal of Marriage and the Family, 42*:7, 1980.

35. Hurley, B.: Socialization for Roles. *In* Hardy, M., and Conway, M. (eds.): *Role Theory: Perspectives for Health Professionals.* New York, Appleton-Century-Crofts, 1978.

36. Jensen, M., Benson, R., and Bobak, J.: *Maternity Care: The Nurse and The Family.* St. Louis, C.V. Mosby Co., 1977.

37. Jordan, B.: *Birth in Four Cultures.* Montreal, Eden Press, 1980.

37a. Lamb, M.: Influence of the Child on Marital Quality and Family Interaction during the Prenatal, Perinatal and Infancy period. In Lerner, R., and Spanier, G. (eds.): *Child Influences on Marital and Family Interaction,* New York, Academic Press, 1978.

38. LaRossa, R.: *Conflict and Power in Marriage: Expecting the First Child.* Beverly Hills, Calif., Sage Publications, 1977.

39. Lerner, R.: *Concepts and Theories of Human Development.* Reading, Mass, Addison-Wesley, 1976.

40. Lewis, M.: Parents and Children: Sex-Role Development, *School Review, 80*(2):229, 1972.

41. Luker, K.: *Taking Chances: Abortion and the Decision Not to Contracept.* Berkeley, University of California Press, 1975.

42. Maccoby, E., and Jacklen, C.: *The Psychology of Sex Differences.* Stanford, Calif., Stanford University Press, 1974.

43. Maslow, A.: *Motivation and Personality.* New York, Harper & Bros., 1954.

44. Miller, G., and Buckhout, R.: *Psychology: The Science of Mental Life.* 2nd Edition. New York, Harper & Row, 1973.

45. Moss, H.: Sex, Age and State as Determinants of Mother-Infant Interaction, *Merrill-Palmer Quarterly, 13*:19, 1967.

46. Nursing Theories Conference Group: *Nursing Theories: The Base for Professional Nursing Practice.* Englewood Cliffs, N.J., Prentice-Hall, 1980.

47. Orem, D.: *Nursing: Concepts of Practice.* New York, McGraw-Hill Book Co., 1971.

48. Peterson, G., and Mehl, L.: Some Determinants of Maternal Attachment, *American Journal of Psychiatry, 135*, 10, 1978.

49. Peterson, G., and Mehl, L.: *The Effects of Childbirth on the Self-Esteem of Women* (Publication no. 24). Berkeley, Calif., Psychophysiological Associates, 1980.

50. Pitts, J.: The Structural-Functional Approach. *In* Christensen, H. (ed.): *Marriage and the Family.* Chicago, Rand McNally, 1964.

51. Pratt, L.: The Relationship of Socio-Economic Status to Health, *American Journal of Public Health, 61*:281, 1971.

51a. Rapoport, R., and Rapoport, R.: *Dual Career Families Re-examined.* New York, Harper and Row, 1976.

52. Rausch, H., Barry, W., Hertel, R., and Swain, M.: *Communication, Conflict and Marriage.* San Francisco, Jossey Bass, 1974.

53. Rebelsky, F., and Hanks, C.: Fathers' Verbal Interaction with Infants in the First Three Months of Life. *Child Development, 42*:63, 1971.

54. Rodman, H.: Marital Power and the Theory of Resources in Cultural Context, *Journal of Comparative Family Studies, 3*:50, 1972.

55. Rose, P.: The Chinese American. *In* Clark, A. (ed.): *Culture, Childbearing, Health Professionals.* Philadelphia, F.A. Davis Co., 1978.

56. Rosenberg, S., and Rosenberg, H.: Identity Concerns in Early Motherhood. *In* Getty, C., and Humphreys, W. (eds.): *Understanding the Family: Stress and Change in American Family Life.* New York Appleton-Century-Crofts, 1981.

57. Roy, C.: *Introduction to Nursing: An Adaptation Model.* Englewood Cliffs, N.J., Prentice-Hall, 1976.

58. Rubin, J., Provenzano, F., and Luria, Z.: The Eye of the Beholder: Parents' Views on Sex of Newborns, *American Journal of Orthopsychiatry, 44*:512, 1974.

59. Sarbin, R., and Allen, V.: Role Enactment, Audience

Feedback, and Attitude Change, *Sociometry,* 27:183, 1964.

60. Scanzoni, J.: *Sex Roles, Life-Styles, and Childbearing: Changing Patterns in Marriage and Family.* New York, Free Press, 1975.

61. Scanzoni, J.: A Historical Perspective on Husband-Wife Bargaining Power and Marital Dissolution. *In* Levinger, G., and Moles D. (eds.): *Divorce and Separation.* New York, Basic Books, 1979.

62. Scanzoni, J., and Szinovacz, M.: *Family Decision-Making: A Developmental Sex Role Model.* Beverly Hills, Calif., Sage Publications, 1980.

63. Scanzoni, L., and Scanzoni, J.: *Men, Women and Change: A Sociology of Marriage and the Family.* New York, McGraw-Hill Book Co., 1976.

64. Scott, C.: Health and Healing Practices Among Five Ethnic Groups in Miami, Florida, *Public Health Reports,* 89:524, 1974.

65. Seavey, C., Katz, P., and Zalk, S.: Baby X: The Effect of Gender Labels on Adult Responses to Infants, *Sex Roles, 1*:103, 1975.

66. Shimek, J.: The Interpretations of the Past: Childhood Trauma, Physical Reality and Historical Truth, *Journal of the American Psychoanalytic Association, 23*:845, 1975.

67. Sidorowicz, L., and Lunney, G.: Baby X Revisited, *Sex Roles, 6*:67, 1980.

68. Spry, J.: Conflict Theory and the Study of Marriage and the Family. *In* Burr, W., Hill, R., Nye, F., and Reiss, I. (eds.): *Contemporary Theories About the Family.* Vol. 2. New York, The Free Press, 1979.

69. Stevens, B.: *Nursing Theory: Analysis, Application, Evaluation.* Boston, Little, Brown & Co., 1979.

70. Thoman, E., Leiderman, P., and Olson, J.: Neonate-Mother Interaction During Breast-Feeding, *Developmental Psychology,* 6:110, 1972.

71. Thomas, R.: *Comparing Theories of Child Development.* Belmont, Calif., Wadsworth Publishing Co., 1979.

72. Turner, R.: Role-Taking: Process Versus Conformity. *In* Rose, A. (ed.): *Human Behavior and Social Processes.* Boston, Houghton Mifflin, 1962.

73. Yura, H., and Walsh, M.: *The Nursing Process.* 2nd Edition. New York, Appleton-Century-Crofts, 1973.

Biologic Potential: The Genetic Basis of Reproduction

The links between parents (represented biologically by a single egg and a single sperm) and their child are hundreds of thousands of genes. Located on the chromosomes, genes are the blueprint for the developing human being.

An understanding of the basic principles of genetics is essential for any nurse who cares for persons during their childbearing years. Some of these men and women will be met in obstetric practice—as visitors to family planning clinics, as expectant mothers and fathers, or as parents following the birth of a child with an anomaly. Others may be parents of a child with a genetic disorder, such as cystic fibrosis; a teenager with hemophilia; or a young wife who has been found to have sickle cell trait following a visit to a screening clinic.

Some nurses are part of genetic counseling teams, while others recognize the need for counseling in their practice and know how to make appropriate referrals. Because genetic problems are so far reaching, all of us, at one time or another, are likely to be involved with people whose lives are affected by such problems. Genetic counseling is discussed in this chapter. The support of a family who give birth to an infant with a genetic disorder is discussed in Chapter 28.

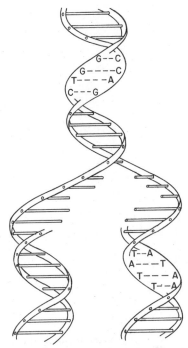

Figure 3–1. Replication of DNA. Note that the original molecule (top) unwinds, and the halves separate. The new half molecules of DNA are formed on the old halves by adenine *(A)* pairing with thymine *(T)* and by guanine *(G)* pairing with cytosine *(C)*.

The Genetic Basis of Development

The genetic potential of all organisms is encoded in genes. Genes are made up of nucleoproteins that are, in turn, composed of nucleic acid and protein. The principal substance in nucleic acid is deoxyribonucleic acid (DNA), with the exception of some of the simplest viruses in which DNA is replaced by ribonucleic acid (RNA).

Molecules of DNA are double helices of polynucleotide chains (Fig. 3–1). Each single segment of the helical strand, called a *nucleotide*, consists of a phosphate, deoxyribose (a special kind of sugar), one of two purines (adenine or guanine), and one of two pyrimidines (thymine or cytosine). The purines and the pyrimidines serve as bases.

The chains of the helix are held together by hydrogen bonds between the bases. Each chain is the exact complement of the other. An adenine base in one chain is always linked to a thymine base in the other; guanine is always bonded to cytosine. Thus, when the double helix separates into two single threads, each is able to re-form an exact copy of the original by coupling the proper bases. *It is this ability to re-form exact copies that makes replication (self-reproduction) possible.*

Since from 200 to 2000 nucleotides make up a single gene and as many as 3000 genes make up a single chromosome, in man each cell division involves more than 27 million nucleotide replications, an estimate that is probably conservative. When one considers the number of cell divisions that take place each day from conception to death, the intricacies of our biologic heritage are truly overwhelming.

It is in the arrangement of the bases (adenine, guanine, cytosine, and thymine) that genes differ from one another. The DNA molecule is the "blueprint" that directs all of development. If the DNA arrangement in a part of a particular gene varies, the wrong message may be delivered to the developing cell and a variation in development may occur. For example, sickle cell anemia is produced by a single gene, one that is probably different in one or a few nucleotides. This variation in the gene molecule causes a different message to be sent to the developing hemoglobin molecule. The red blood cell develops differently than it normally would, and the cell then behaves abnormally.

Ovum and Sperm

The genetic potential of an individual is present in every cell of his body, but it is transferred from generation to generation through specialized cells, the female ovum (egg) and the male sperm. Understanding the development of these cells and their division is essential background for understanding the action of genes and chromosomes.

Oogonia and *spermatogonia*, the forerunners of mature ova and sperm, originate as large, spherical *primordial germ cells* during the fourth week of intrauterine life. The processes by which they develop into mature ova and sperm *(oogenesis* and spermatogenesis) are described below and are summarized in Table 3–1.

Oogenesis

Ova develop from oogonia located in the cortical tissue of the ovary. During early fetal development, oogonia divide by *mitosis* (see below) to form additional oogonia. By the fifth to sixth month of fetal life, all of the oogonia for a woman's lifetime have been produced; many will degenerate before sexual maturity is reached.

The differentiation of the oogonium into a *primary oocyte* also occurs during fetal life, as does the first *meiotic division* (see below) of the primary oocyte. Then development ceases until after puberty, when a second meiotic division occurs for certain ova at some time in the years that follow. It will be 40 years or more before some of the primary oocytes resume meiotic division; many never will. The completion of the development of a mature ovum is described below in the discussion of meiosis.

Spermatogenesis

In contrast to the oogonia, in which the process of development of the mature ova begins during fetal life, the spermatogonia present in the newborn's testes at birth disappear until puberty. From that time, spermatogenesis continues throughout life.

Spermatogenesis begins as the germ cells lining the seminiferous tubules of the testes (Chapter 4) divide by mitosis to form spermatogonia, which in turn grow into primary spermatocytes. Two meiotic divisions result first in two secondary spermatocytes and, shortly afterward, in four spermatids (Fig. 3–2). Spermatogenesis occurs simultaneously in hundreds of thousands of spermatogonia in order to produce the millions of sperm that are constantly present in the adult male reproductive tract. Before the spermatid can become a functioning sperm, still other changes, described in Chapter 4, must occur.

Cell Division: Mitosis and Meiosis

In order to understand the way in which chromosomes affect inheritance, it is necessary to review the two processes of cell division—*mitosis* and *meiosis*.

Mitosis is the process by which all cells divide, except those that produce the ovum and sperm after the stage of the primary oocyte and primary spermatocyte. The stages of mitosis are diagrammed in Figure 3–3. Observe that when all the chromosomes are aligned in the equatorial plane of the cell (Fig. 3–3*C*), the nuclear membrane is no longer present. It is at this point that the *centromere* of the chromosome (i.e., the point at which the strands, called *chromatids*, are joined) splits to complete the chromosome separation. The chromosomes are pulled to the opposite ends

Table 3–1. PROCESS OF OOGENESIS AND SPERMATOGENESIS

Oogenesis	Spermatogenesis
Germ cell	Germ cell
(Mitosis)	(Mitosis)
Oogonium	Spermatogonium
(Develops)	(Develops)
Primary oocyte	Primary spermatocyte
(First meiotic division)	(First meiotic division)
Secondary oocyte First polar body	Secondary spermatocyte Secondary spermatocyte
(Second meiotic division)	(Second meiotic division)
Ovum Second polar body Polar bodies	Spermatid Spermatid Spermatid Spermatid

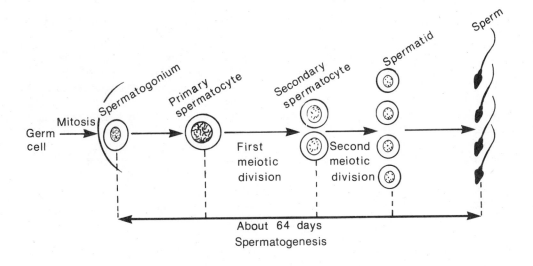

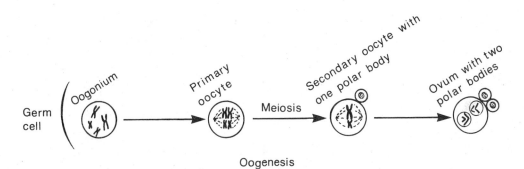

Oogenesis

Figure 3–2. Spermatogenesis.

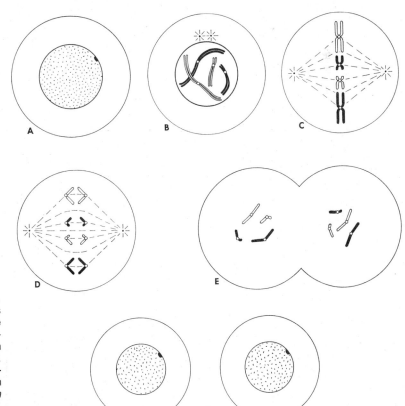

Figure 3–3. The stages of mitosis. Only two of the 23 chromosome pairs are shown. Chromosomes from one parent are shown in outline; chromosomes from the other parent are in black. *A,* Interphase; *B,* prophase; *C,* metaphase; *D,* anaphase; *E,* telophase; and *F,* interphase. (From Thompson and Thompson: *Genetics in Medicine.* 3rd Edition. Philadelphia, W. B. Saunders Co., 1980.)

(poles) of the cell with the centromeres leading (Fig. 3–3D). This gives each chromosome a special shape during anaphase that aids in the recognition of the different types of chromosomes. After the chromosomes arrive at the poles, they fade from sight, nuclear membranes form, and cell division is completed. *Two* cells now exist in place of one.

A second process of cell division, meiosis, is reserved for the *gametes* (i.e., sex cells). In meiosis the chromosomes split once, as in mitosis, but the cell divides *two times,* so that

four cells result, each with one-half the number of chromosomes of the parent cell.

Consider what would happen if this did not occur. At the end of mitosis, each cell in humans has 46 chromosomes, as did the original cell. (See section on Chromosomes, below). If the ovum and sperm were each to have 46 chromosomes, the resulting zygote would have 92 chromosomes. Meiosis gives the ovum and sperm 23 chromosomes each, so that the resulting zygote has 46 chromosomes, the correct number for humans.

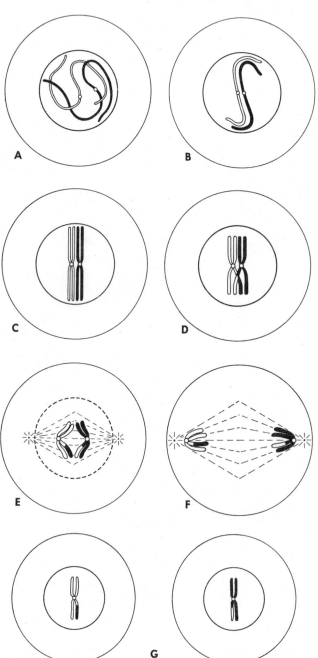

Figure 3–4.   The first meiotic division. One of the 23 chromosome pairs is depicted. Chromosome from one parent is shown in outline, chromosome from the other parent in black. *A,* Leptotene; *B,* zygotene; *C,* pachytene; *D,* diplotene, showing one chiasma (several may be present, and two, three, or all four strands may be involved); *E,* metaphase; *F,* anaphase; and *G,* telophase. (From Thompson and Thompson: *Genetics in Medicine.* Philadelphia, W. B. Saunders Co., 1966.)

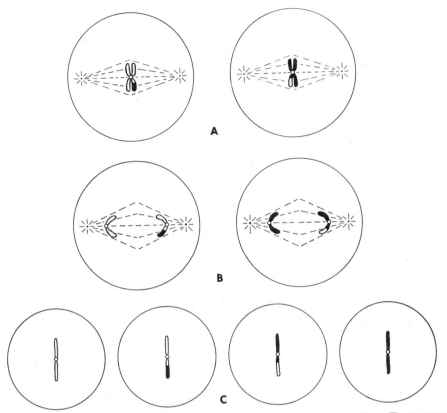

Figure 3–5. The second meiotic division. *A,* Metaphase; *B,* anaphase; and *C,* telophase. (From Thompson and Thompson: *Genetics in Medicine.* Philadelphia, W. B. Saunders Co., 1966.)

Figures 3–4 and 3–5 diagram meiotic division; compare them with Figure 3–3. Note first that the pairs of homologous chromosomes come together in the first phase (prophase). This process is called *synapse* (which means "coming together"). The chromosomes of each pair are aligned so that the loci for specific genes are next to each other and often touch. As in mitosis, the chromosomes are split, so that each of the 23 pairs consists of four strands, each two strands joined at the centromere. The centromere does not split during the first meiotic division; the daughter cells at the end of the first stage contain one of each of the homologous pairs. In the second meiotic division (Fig. 3–5), the centromere divides, and single strands go to opposite poles. As cell division completes, there are now four cells, each with 23 chromosomes.

Although both ovum and sperm undergo meiosis, there is a significant difference. In the male, the four resulting sperm are identical in size. In the female, however, the first meiotic division results in two cells that are identical as far as chromosomes are concerned but that differ greatly in size. Most of cellular material goes to one cell, the *secondary oocyte.* The other cell, the *first polar body,* contains the chromo-

somes but has only a very small amount of cellular material. The same process occurs at the second meiotic division, with the secondary oocyte producing the ovum and the *second polar body* (Figs. 3–6 and 3–7). The significance of this disparity in size is that should the ovum be fertilized, it contains all of the material of the original oocyte that will nourish the zygote prior to implantation in the uterine wall.

Chromosomes

The rod-shaped chromosomes exist in a variety of lengths and shapes. Not only the chromosomal number but also the size and shape of the chromosomes are specific for each species. Humans have 46 chromosomes, which are paired: 22 pairs of *autosomes* and one pair of *sex chromosomes.* Autosomes are alike in both sexes. Females have two X sex chromosomes; males have one X chromosome and one Y chromosome. Both autosomes and sex chromosomes carry genes that govern traits, with the possible exception of the Y chromosome.

Human chromosomes have been classified on the basis of size and the position of the

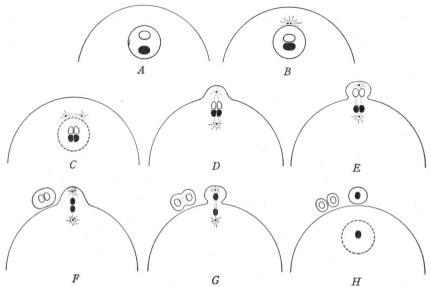

Figure 3–6. Diagrams of the maturation of the ovum in an animal with two chromosomes. *A-E,* Budding off of the first polar body. *F, G,* Formation of the second polar body and subdivision of the first. *H,* Mature egg with polar bodies. (From Arey: *Developmental Anatomy: A Textbook and Laboratory Manual of Embryology.* Revised 7th Edition. Philadelphia, W. B. Saunders Co., 1974.)

centromere. Since it is sometimes difficult to identify all 23 pairs of chromosomes in an individual sample, it has become an accepted practice to organize them into seven groups, identified by the letters A through G in order of decreasing length. A systematically arranged set of chromosomes is called a *karyotype* (Fig. 3–8). Cells used for karyotyping may be white blood cells (since red blood cells have no nucleus, they have no chromosomes) or tissue cells obtained during biopsy. Epithelial cells from the lining of the cheek are frequently used. Amniotic fluid is used to study fetal chromosomes. The cells are cultured and treated chemically, and slides are prepared for examination and photography. Individual chromosomes are then cut from the photograph, matched in pairs, and mounted according to the standard classification, called the Denver Classification because of its adoption at a meeting in Denver, Colorado, in 1960.

Figure 3–4; *D* through *G,* illustrates another facet of chromosomal inheritance, a process called "crossing-over," in which two chromosomes of a pair may exchange certain sections and thus certain genetic traits at the same *locus* (i.e., at the same location on the chromosome). Note in Figure 3–5 that in the four

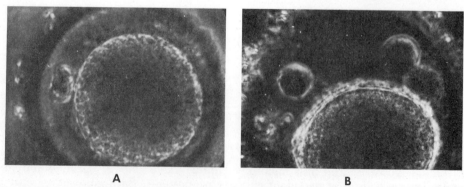

A **B**

Figure 3–7. Living human ova, shown as photomicrographs (Shettles). × 150. *A,* Secondary oocyte, with first polar body (beginning to subdivide), lying within the space bounded externally by the dark zona pellucida; at the left, spermatozoa lie on the zona. *B,* Ripe egg, said to be artificially fertilized and showing all three polar bodies; unsuccessful spermatozoa are embedded in the locally elevated zona pellucida. (From Arey: *Developmental Anatomy: A Textbook and Laboratory Manual of Embryology.* Revised 7th Edition. Philadelphia, W. B. Saunders Co., 1974.)

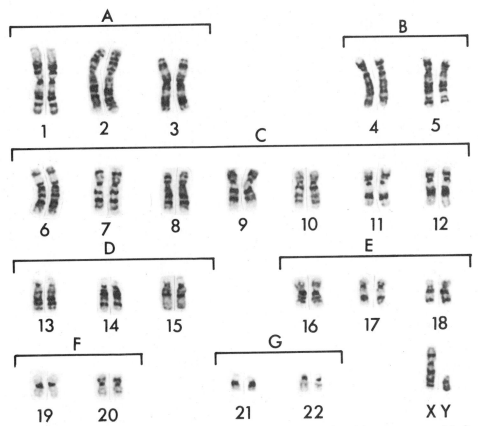

Figure 3–8. Normal male karyotype. The chromosomes are individually labeled, and the seven groups A to G are indicated. (From Thompson and Thompson: *Genetics in Medicine.* 3rd Edition. Philadelphia, W. B. Saunders Co., 1980. Photomicrograph courtesy of R. G. Worton.)

daughter cells one of the "white" chromosomes has exchanged sections with one of the "black" chromosomes.

Variations in Chromosomal Inheritance

Mitosis and meiosis do not always occur normally. As a result, chromosomal abnormalities occur in a small percentage of infants. Because of the large number of genes located on each chromosome, it might be expected that any chromosomal change would produce not just one but a constellation of changes. It appears that it is the total effect of the imbalance of genetic material that is responsible for the changes.

Several types of chromosomal abnormalities can occur, involving either the autosomes or the sex chromosomes. The most common is *nondisjunction* (Fig. 3–9). If during the meiotic process a chromosome pair fails to separate normally, one gamete will contain two of a

Figure 3–9. Nondisjunction occurring at the first and second meiotic divisions. Nondisjunction at meiosis produces gametes containing both members of the pair of homologous chromosomes concerned, or neither member. Gametes lacking a chromosome (other than X) are usually apparently unable to form a viable zygote. (From Thompson and Thompson: *Genetics in Medicine.* 3rd Edition. Philadelphia, W. B. Saunders Co., 1980.)

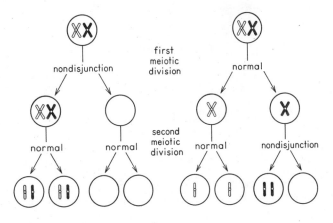

particular chromosome while the other will not have that chromosome at all. If the two-chromosome gamete then joins with a normal gamete to form a zygote, the zygote will have three of that particular chromosome, hence the term *trisomy* (Fig. 3–10). The gamete with no autosome does not seem to be able to form a viable zygote. Nondisjunction can also occur during mitosis, after the zygote has been formed.

Down's syndrome (Fig. 3–11), which is related to trisomy of chromosome 21, is usually the result of nondisjunction. Occasionally, Down's syndrome is due to a second type of abnormality, *translocation*, in which a piece of one chromosome breaks off and subsequently attaches itself to another chromosome. In translocation Down's syndrome, the long arm of the twenty-first chromosome breaks off and subsequently attaches itself to either a chromosome of the D group (chromosomes 13 to 15) or another chromosome of the G group (chromosomes 21 to 22) (Fig. 3–11). In this instance the child with Down's syndrome will have only two number 21 chromosomes (not three, as in trisomy 21). However, there is a chromosome that is a composite of number 14 and number 21 chromosomes and contains the genetic material of each, thus, the total amount of genetic material for the number 21 chromosome is equivalent to that of three chromosomes. The effect on the child is the same; the child has Down's syndrome.

When translocation occurs at the first meiotic division, four types of gametes are possible: (1) normal chromosomes and a normal gamete; (2) a normal number 14 chromosome and a fragment but no number 21 chromosome, so that if fertilized, the zygote would not be viable; (3) a composite of number 14 and number 21 chromosomes and a normal number 21 chromosome, which would result in a child with Down's syndrome although there are 46 chromosomes and (4) a composite of number 14 and number 21 chromosomes and a fragment; following fertilization the individual would have only 45 chromosomes but would have the normal amount of genetic material and would be a translocation carrier.

Of children with Down's syndrome born to mothers younger than 30, 8 to 10 per cent of the cases are due to translocation. Of these translocation Down's children, approximately two-thirds of the parent pairs have a normal karyotype, and the translocation occurred with the cell division at this pregnancy. In the remaining third one parent is a translocation carrier. For some reason not now apparent, the likelihood of a child being born with Down's syndrome is 10 per cent when the mother is the translocation carrier and only 2 per cent when the father is the translocation carrier.

Such differentiation has value in genetic counseling. When the basis of Down's syndrome in an individual child can be determined (by obtaining a family history related to Down's syndrome, by karyotyping the baby, and sometimes by karyotyping the parents as

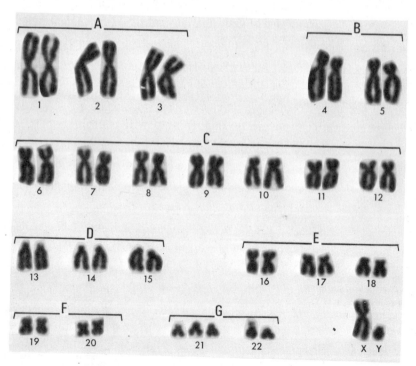

Figure 3–10. Trisomy 21 karyotype. Note the three number 21 chromosomes. Compare this karyotype with Figure 3–8. (From Walker et al.: *J. Mental Deficiency Research,* 7:150, 1963.)

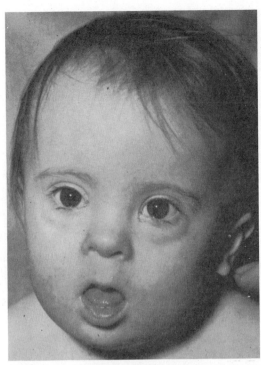

Figure 3–11. A child with trisomy 21 (Down's syndrome). (From Smith: *Recognizable Patterns of Human Malformation.* 3rd Edition. Philadelphia, W. B. Saunders Co., 1982.)

Table 3–2. RISK OF DOWN'S SYNDROME IN FETUSES AT AMNIOCENTESIS AND IN LIVE BIRTHS*

Maternal Age*	Frequency of Down's Syndrome	
	Fetuses	*Live Births*
–19	–	1/1550
20–24	–	1/1550
25–29	–	1/1050
30–34	–	1/700
35	1/350	1/350
36	1/260	1/300
37	1/200	1/225
38	1/160	1/175
39	1/125	1/150
40	1/70	1/100
41	1/35	1/85
42	1/30	1/65
43	1/20	1/50
44	1/13	1/40
45–	1/25	1/25

*Approximate (rounded) estimates from data of Hook and Chambers, 1977. Birth Defects: Orig. Art. Ser. 13(3A): 123–141; Trimble and Baird, 1978. Am. J. Med. Gen. 2:1–5; Hook, 1978. Lancet 1:1053–1054; and Spielman et al., 1978. Lancet 1:1306–1307. From Thompson and Thompson: *Genetics in Medicine.* 3rd Edition. Philadelphia, W. B. Saunders Co., 1980.

well), the likelihood that the syndrome may be repeated in future children can be evaluated more accurately. The risk of Down's syndrome in a second child is much greater if the mother is a translocation carrier than if the cause is nondisjunction. Only about 5 per cent of children have Down's syndrome due to translocation rather than to trisomy 21; about 2 per cent of these babies have inherited the translocation from a parent. The mother of a baby with Down's syndrome due to translocation is usually of normal childbearing age; the risk of trisomy increases markedly in older mothers (Table 3–2). The prenatal detection of Down's syndrome is discussed in Chapter 14.

In addition to trisomy 21, trisomy 18 (or trisomy E) and trisomy D also result from nondisjunction, the letters in both instances referring to the group of chromosomes involved. These babies usually have multiple and severe deformities and die in the first months after birth (Fig. 3–12).

Other chromosomal breaks include *deletion,* in which a piece of a chromosome breaks off and is lost; *duplication,* in which an extra piece of chromosome either is in the chromosome itself, is attached to another chromosome (translocation), or exists as a separate unit; the development of *isochromosomes* because of abnormal splitting; and chromosomal *mosai-*

cism in which an individual has at least two different groups of cells with different chromosome complements. Mosaicism always occurs after fertilization during the process of mitosis, leaving cells with two different types of chromosomes to develop. Mosaicism may involve the sex chromosomes or, less commonly, the autosomes. In rare instances, children with Down's syndrome may have mosaicism, with some cells having 46 chromosomes and others 47 chromosomes. Some of these children will have only a few symptoms of the syndrome, whereas others will have a full range of symptoms. Mosaicism is difficult to detect when tissue is taken from a single site for examination.

A number of anomalies are a result of sex chromosome alterations. Individuals may possess varying combinations of X and Y chromosomes. Klinefelter's syndrome (XXY), which occurs once in every 400 male births (Fig. 3–13), and Turner's syndrome (XO), which occurs once in every 3000 live births (Fig. 3–14), are two of the more common abnormal combinations.

In general, individuals with unusual combinations of chromosomes will be male if they have a Y chromosome (e.g., XXY) and female if they do not (e.g., XO). The higher the number of extra chromosomes, the greater the

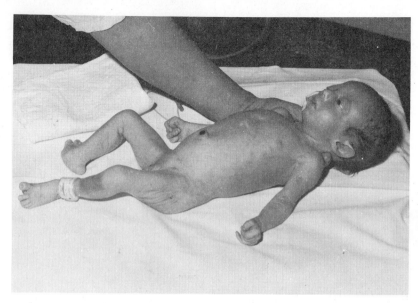

Figure 3–12. Infant with trisomy of a chromosome in group E, probably chromosome 18. Note the overlapping fingers, rocker-bottom feet, simplified patterns of the ears, and dorsiflexion of the big toe. (From Thompson and Thompson: *Genetics in Medicine.* 3rd Edition. Philadelphia, W. B. Saunders Co., 1980. Courtesy of D. H. Carr.)

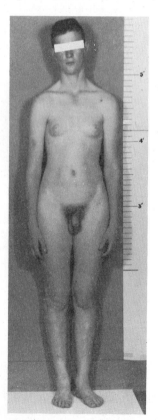

Figure 3–13. A young man with Klinefelter's syndrome, XXY karyotype. These men are usually tall, with small testes and sparse pubic hair. Approximately 20 per cent of the time they have gynecomastia (female development of the breasts), as this man does. Many affected males are mentally retarded. (From Thompson and Thompson: *Genetics in Medicine.* 3rd Edition. Philadelphia, W. B. Saunders Co., 1980. Courtesy of M. L. Barr.)

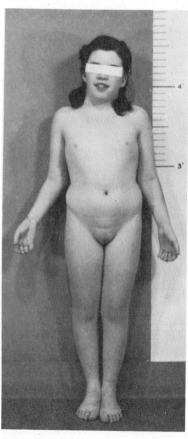

Figure 3–14. A girl with Turner's syndrome, XO karyotype. These girls are usually short and may have webbing of the neck, low set ears, poorly developed breasts with widely spaced nipples, and juvenile external genitalia. Note the absence of pubic hair. The ovary is usually only a streak of connective tissue. (From Barr: *American J. Human Genetics, 12*:118, 1960.)

likelihood of abnormality in the visible characteristics.

The following example of nondisjunction in a single ovum illustrates how some unusual combinations may arise. Nondisjunction may take place in the sperm as well.

XX
(First meiotic division)

XX   O
(Second meiotic division)
XX   XX   O   O

The potential combinations following fertilization with a normal sperm (XY) would then be:

	XX	O
X	XXX	XO
Y	XXY	YO

We have already noted that XO represents Turner's syndrome and XXY Klinefelter's syndrome. YO would be nonviable. Females with the XXX pattern have frequently been found in surveys of hospitals for the mentally retarded and among women in infertility clinics. They may be relatively common in the general population as well.

When ambiguity of the genitalia makes it difficult to assign a sex to an infant, chromosome analysis can be helpful. An additional evaluation is the examination for a *Barr body (sex chromatin body, chromatin-positive body)* (Fig. 3–15). The Barr body is a chromatin mass derived from one of the X chromosomes, therefore the number of Barr bodies is one less than the number of X chromosomes. A normal male (XY) or a female with Turner's syndrome (XO) would have no Barr body. Both a normal female (XX) and a male with Klinefelter's syndrome (XXY) would have one. An XXX female would have two Barr bodies.

Causes of Chromosomal Breakage

What causes chromosomal breakage, with resultant deletions, translocations, and other abnormalities? Like genetic mutations, some appear to arise spontaneously. Radiation is a factor in certain deletions and translocations. Maternal age correlates with nondisjunction. Since viruses can produce fragmentation of chromosomes, they may play a role in resultant abnormalities. LSD has been suspect in chromosomal breakage, but a final verdict awaits further research.

Genes

Genes exist in pairs because chromosomes are paired. The functions of genes at any specific point on each chromosome are the same for all chromosomes of that type. For example, a gene governing eye color is at a specific locus on a specific chromosome and at the same spot on every other chromosome that is identical to that chromosome. Geneticists are beginning to map the loci of some human genes; loci in some species, such as fruit flies, have already been mapped. In any pair of genes there are contrasting forms or states of the gene, known as *alleles.* Some genes have multiple alleles; there are three alleles for blood types A, B, and O. If an individual has the same alleles for a trait on each gene of a pair, he is said to be *homozygous* for that trait. A man with two alleles for A type blood, designated AA, is homozygous for A blood. When alleles differ, the individual is *heterozygous,* such as a man with AB blood. In heterozygous combinations one allele, the *dominant* allele, will manifest itself in the *phenotype* (visible characteristics). One cannot

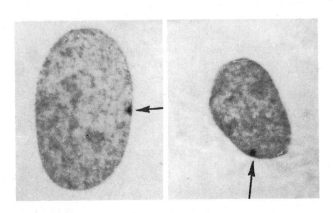

Figure 3–15. Sex chromatin or Barr bodies are indicated by the arrow. (Feulgen, magnification × 2200. Courtesy of Dr. Ursula Mittwoch, Galton Laboratory, University College, London. From Villee: *Biology.* 6th Edition. Philadelphia, W. B. Saunders Co., 1972.)

tell from the phenotype what the *genotype* (genetic characteristics) is, a matter of very practical concern in many instances.

Consider the father with blood that types Rh positive, who is married to an Rh negative mother. The capital letter D represents the positive allele, with a lower case d representing the negative allele. The positive father may be homozygous, with a genotype DD, or he may be heterozygous, with a genotype Dd. The only possible genotype for the negative mother is dd because recessive alleles are only expressed when no dominant alleles are present. Thus, recessive traits always represent a homozygous situation for that particular trait. The probability that this couple will have a child who is Rh positive will vary with the father's genotype. In the first example, the father is homozygous, i.e., DD (less frequently the case).

	D	D
d	Dd	Dd
d	Dd	Dd

As you can see, every child will have the genotype Dd, and the phenotype will be positive.

In the second example, the father has the genotype Dd.

	D	d
d	Dd	dd
d	Dd	dd

The probability is that 50 per cent of the children will have the genotype dd, and thus their phenotype will be negative.

It is very important to understand what this probability means. It does *not* mean that if this couple have two children with the genotype Dd the next child will be dd, nor does it mean the reverse. Because of the way in which genes segregate in meiosis and recombine at fertilization, each child born to a family has exactly the same probability of inheriting a specific condition as every other child of those two parents. (The obvious exception is the X-linked trait discussed below, in which the sex of the child is a factor.) The probability of a child's inheriting a specific trait is analogous to the toss of a coin. If a coin is tossed a great number of times, one expects an approximately equal number of heads and tails. But even if a

person happens to toss "heads" 50 times in a row, the chance of tossing either "heads" or "tails" is still even on the fifty-first toss. Chance alone determines which alleles will be present in a particular zygote. Thus, in the case of Rh incompatibility, even if the father's genotype is Dd, it is perfectly possible that all of the children will be Dd (with a positive phenotype), and it is also possible that all will be dd (with a negative phenotype).

Both normal and pathologic traits are inherited through alleles of a gene that may be dominant, recessive or X-linked. Many traits are controlled by more than one gene; this mode of inheritance is termed *polygenic*. Since genes are located on chromosomes and since each parent normally contributes 23 chromosomes to the zygote (see Chromosomes, above), inheritance from each parent is equal in terms of numbers. Genetically, there is no "chip off the old block" in the sense that no child can be just like either parent, nor is it likely that brothers and sisters (with the exception of monozygotic twins) will share identical genes. Two children of the same parents may resemble each other closely in genotype or in phenotype, or they may be very different, depending on the genes that they have received by chance and on the interaction of those genes with environment. The real surprise is not that some children fail to resemble either parent very closely but that, considering the almost infinite number of possible combinations of the thousands upon thousands of genes involved, strong similarities are seen fairly often between people who are only distantly related. We need no more than a very simple understanding of genetics to realize that each child is truly different from other children and from his parents, a unique individual in his own right.

Twins may or may not have the same genotype. Dizygotic (fraternal) twins result when two separate ova are fertilized by two separate sperm. The genotype, including sex, is no more likely to resemble that of the twin than is the genotype of any other brother or sister. Monozygotic (identical) twins result when one egg and one sperm unite to form a single zygote and then split at an early stage of zygote development. Monozygotic twins do have the same genotype and must be of the same sex.

The Genetic Inheritance of Characteristics

Dominant Characteristics

For a *dominant* allele to be manifest in the phenotype, only one gene from one parent is necessary. The illustration of the Rh factor above shows dominant inheritance. The dominant gene (in this case D) must be present in one parent (genotype DD or Dd) and must be present in the child for the trait to be inherited. The chance, or *probability*, of a dominant trait's being inherited is 50 per cent if the parent contributing the gene is heterozygous, which is usually the case. There are nearly 800 pathologic traits caused by dominant genes, in addition to the many, many normal traits governed by them. Examples of the former include hyperphalangy of the thumb; one type of achondroplastic dwarfism; and Huntington's chorea, a degenerative disease of the central nervous system that usually affects young adults. For the individual who knows he or she carries a dominant gene for a condition such as Huntington's chorea, or who suspects the possibility, feelings about marriage and childbearing may be strongly influenced by this knowledge.

While dominant traits are commonly expressed whenever the gene is present, the term *lack of penetrance* is used to describe an individual who carries and transmits a gene for a dominant trait but who does not express the trait in his own phenotype. Environmental interaction may be one factor accounting for lack of penetrance, but it is probably not the only factor. As genetic knowledge increases, it is likely that more specific reasons will be found to explain variability within individual genes.

Recessive Characteristics

Recessive genes are expressed in the phenotype only when one recessive allele is inherited from *each* parent. All of us carry many recessive genes, transmitted through generation after generation, but unexpressed until they find a "mate," i.e., a second identical allele. Approximately 800 recessive diseases are known, most of them rare.

Cystic fibrosis is a condition inherited through recessive genes. For purposes of illustration, the normal dominant gene is designated "F" and the recessive gene for cystic fibrosis "f." An individual with the genotype FF neither has the disease nor is a carrier of the recessive gene. The genotype Ff denotes a carrier (one recessive gene), while ff is the genotype of the person with cystic fibrosis. The following diagrams illustrate the inheritance of a recessive trait. We would suggest to nurses that it is much easier to construct this type of diagram than to try to remember probability figures. This can be done in an instant and clearly demonstrates possible combinations.

In this first example, neither parent has the disease nor is a carrier; thus, no child can have the condition or be a carrier.

	F	F
F	FF	FF
F	FF	FF

If only one parent is a carrier (Ff), there is a chance that 50 per cent of the children will be carriers (Ff), but no child will have cystic fibrosis. It is through such combinations that recessive genes may be carried for many generations yet never expressed.

	F	f
F	FF	Ff
F	FF	Ff

If both parents carry the recessive gene (Ff), the mathematical probability is that 25 per cent of the children will have cystic fibrosis (ff), 50 per cent will be carriers (Ff), and 25 per cent will be neither (FF).

	F	f
F	FF	Ff
f	Ff	ff

Again, remember just what probability means (page 50). If this seems to be unduly emphasized, it is only because so many misunderstandings are encountered, both in the literature describing the experiences of others and in life.

Now that children born with many recessive disorders are not only surviving infancy but growing to adulthood and possible childbearing, three other possibilities occur, which were rare until recent years. The first is the combination of an individual with the condition (ff) and an individual who is neither a carrier nor has the disease (FF). As you can see, all of the children would be carriers, but none would have cystic fibrosis.

	f	f
F	Ff	Ff
F	Ff	Ff

If, however, an individual with cystic fibrosis should mate with a carrier (who, in all likelihood, would not know he was a carrier), the chance is that half of their children would have cystic fibrosis and the other half would be carriers.

	f	f
F	Ff	Ff
f	ff	ff

In the event that two individuals with cystic fibrosis should mate, every child would also have cystic fibrosis; there is no alternative.

	f	f
f	ff	ff
f	ff	ff

Sickle cell disease is another condition caused by recessive alleles. Persons who are carriers (Ss) have sickle cell trait; individuals with two recessive genes (ss) have sickle cell anemia. Unlike most recessive traits whose presence is detected only after an affected child is born (such as the child with cystic fibrosis), carriers of the sickle cell gene can be identified. Since approximately 10 per cent of American blacks carry the sickle cell gene, sickle cell screening becomes an important factor for couples considering childbearing (see genetic counseling in Chapter 5). The prevalence of sickle cell trait is much higher in parts of Africa, where it apparently gives the individual an increased resistance to malaria.

X-linked Characteristics

The dominant and recessive genes discussed above are located on the 22 pairs of autosomal chromosomes. The remaining pair of chromosomes are sex chromosomes. Normal females have two X chromosomes; normal males have one X chromosome and one Y chromosome. For traits that are inherited through genes located on the autosomal chromosomes, it makes no difference whether a gene comes from the mother or the father. Virtually all of the characteristics known to be carried by the sex chromosones, however, are located on the X chromosomes. They are recessive traits, expressed only when they are not masked by a normal X chromosome. Thus, females who have two X chromosomes may carry an X-

linked trait, but it will not be expressed because of the presence of a normal X chromosome. Only if a female carries two affected chromosomes would the trait be expressed, a mathematical possibility but a rare occurrence (see the third example below).

In males, however, the recessive X chromosome will always be expressed when it is present, because there is no dominant allele on the Y chromosome to match it. Thus, males can never be carriers of X-linked traits; either they must express the trait, or it will be totally absent.

Hemophilia is possibly the best known example of an x-linked trait. Let X represent the normal X chromosome (which is dominant) and x the recessive gene for hemophilia. There are three possible combinations:

If the mother carries the hemophiliac allele (Xx) but the father does not (XY), the probability is that half of the daughters will be carriers (Xx) and half of the sons will have hemophilia (xY). The remaining half of the sons and daughters will receive the normal allele.

	X	x
X	XX	Xx
Y	XY	xY

If the mother carries no gene for hemophilia (XX) but the father is a hemophiliac (xY), all of the daughters will be carriers (xX), but the sons will neither have the disease nor be carriers.

	X	X
x	xX	xX
Y	XY	XY

Should a woman who is a carrier (xX) marry a man with hemophilia (xY), their daughters would all be either carriers or have hemophilia (xX or xx) (because they could inherit two recessive genes), while half of the sons would have the chance of having hemophilia (xY).

	x	X
x	xx	xX
Y	xY	XY

Some traits that are suspected to be X-linked are dominant rather than recessive. For example, in one type of oral-facial-digital syndrome (a disorder with a number of characteristics, including unusual facial appearance, absence of certain teeth, and a digital malformation such as syndactyly), transmission is from affected females to their daughters. Sons are rare in these families, but those who are born are unaffected. It is thought that the gene may be lethal to the male fetus. Thus, the sons who receive the particular gene die in utero, while those who receive the normal allele survive but do not inherit the trait.

Polygenic Inheritance

Unfortunately, at least from the standpoint of unraveling genetic puzzles, not all traits are inherited in as straightforward a manner as the three modes described. Polygenic or multifactorial inheritance is due to the combined action of two or more genes. Variations in height, fingerprint ridges, and arterial blood pressure are examples of traits in which there is a polygenic component.[12] Neural tube defects, such as spina bifida and anencephaly (see Chapter 24) are examples of polygenic disorders in the newborn. Other conditions believed to be transmitted by polygenes include clubfoot, congenital dislocation of the hip, cleft lip and palate, and pyloric stenosis.

Potential risk for polygenic traits cannot be calculated in the same way as risk for single gene traits. Instead, risk factors are based on actual birth records. For example, when parents have one child with cleft lip, there is a 4 in 100 chance of recurrence. When one child has spina bifida or anencephaly, the chances of recurrence are 5 in 100. Notice that the risks in these polygenic conditions are much lower than the risks in single gene disorders. In general, the risks for polygenic traits are approximately 5 per cent (5 in 100).

Genetic Penetrance

Penetrance refers to the fact that at times a gene may produce an effect that is easily recognized and at other times no effect at all. When an effect is produced or *expressed*, penetrance is said to be *complete*. When the effect is not produced, penetrance is *partial* or *incomplete*. Incomplete penetrance may be due to the action of other genes or to environmental factors. For example, environmental factors such as maternal nutrition and maternal illness may affect the fetus's genetic potential for growth and thus modify birth weight. Birth injury may modify the genetic potential for the development of intelligence. The possibility of incomplete penetrance makes interpreting genetic probabilities more difficult.

Prenatal Detection of Genetic Disease

Fetal assessment to detect genetic disease may include amniocentesis, maternal blood screening for alpha-fetoprotein, and/or ultrasound. This topic is discussed in Chapter 10.

Genetic Counseling

The concept of genetic counseling is not new. The Babylonian *Talmud* noted many centuries ago that there were families in which blood did not clot. A case is described in which the sons of three sisters died during circumcision. A rabbi advised a fourth sister not to have her son circumcised.

Today, with nearly 1200 conditions identified as genetic in origin, it has been estimated that 25 per cent of medical problems in the United States can be traced in part to genetic factors. Genetic counseling has thus become an important medical specialty and a vital part of family planning counseling.

Goals

The birth of a child with a defect is one major circumstance that brings families for genetic counseling. A second is the knowledge that someone in the family—a cousin, a sister, or perhaps an uncle—has some abnormality. "Could the same thing happen to my child? Or could it happen to another of my children?" parents wonder. A young man, newly married, has just learned that his second sister has diabetes mellitus. "What are the chances that my children might have diabetes?" he asks. Thus one goal of counseling is to help determine the risks of occurrence of a particular trait.

For those conditions that are governed by a single gene, these risks are relatively easy to determine and explain. For disorders that are polygenic or appear to be influenced by familial factors, such as diabetes or cleft lip and palate, only empiric risk figures are available, i.e., calculations based on the occurrence of the particular disorder in a large number of births.

If a genetic condition already exists in one or more children in a family, an important goal of counseling is to help the family recognize their feelings about the child and accept those feelings. It is normal to feel sad about giving birth to a child with a serious mental or physical handicap. (See Chapter 28.)

In a number of conditions, genetic counseling can help to assure prompt medical attention for a child in utero who may have an inherited condition. For example, phenylketonuria (PKU) is an inborn error in metabolism that can be treated by a diet low in phenylalanine but if untreated leads to severe mental retardation. If one child in a family has PKU, counselors can alert both the family and the medical personnel who care for them to the need for prompt evaluation and early treatment at any subsequent delivery.

Other disorders can be diagnosed prenatally by amniocentesis and the cultivation and analysis of amniotic fluid cells (Chapter 10). At least one condition, adrenogenital syndrome, is currently being treated in utero.

The importance of genetic counseling in ultimately reducing the number of abnormal genes in the population is the goal of some counselors, although this is not as significant in everyday practice as are the other goals that basically aim at helping individual families. Abnormal genes will never be totally eliminated because new ones arise by mutation in each generation, in addition to those that are carried undiscovered as recessive genes through many generations. However, because improved medical care now allows individuals to reach maturity and therefore to reproduce when formerly they did not (children with cystic fibrosis, for example), there is concern that without attention to the population aspects of counseling the number of persons with genetic diseases will increase.

It is important to remember that every one of us carries recessive genes for three to eight "diseases" or conditions. The vast majority of these conditions will never be expressed in our own phenotype or in the phenotypes of our children, their children, or the children for many generations. For example, in the United States about 4 persons in every 100 are estimated to carry the gene for cystic fibrosis, yet only 4 in 10,000 suffer from the disease. One of 160 individuals carries the gene for galactosemia (an inborn error in metabolism), yet only 1 in 100,000 inherits the condition. Thus it is evident that most deleterious genes are carried, unrecognized, by apparently healthy people rather than by individuals with the disease. Even if someone with a particular condition marries a carrier, the odds of producing a child with the condition are two out of four, compared with one out of four if carriers marry.

The number of people with some genetically related traits is certainly increasing. For example, since the advent of insulin, individuals with juvenile diabetes mellitus no longer die at an early age. Many reproduce successfully. The possibility that their children will develop diabetes at some time in their lives is greater than for children who have no family history of diabetes. Yet diabetes is controllable and will probably be even more easily controlled in the future than it is today. Is the number of persons with diabetes a serious problem for society?

The Process of Genetic Counseling (See Nursing Care Plan 3–1)

A proper diagnosis is the foundation of genetic counseling. When a newborn shows signs of an abnormality (often first recognized by an observant nurse), possible causes are carefully evaluated (such as maternal rubella, kernicterus, and so on) before the disorder is accepted as genetic in origin.

Data from the extended family provide the basis for construction of a pedigree chart (Fig. 3–16). Possible kinship between family members, the ages and causes of death of as many members as possible, exact diagnoses of any apparent familial disease, and the occurrence of spontaneous abortion and/or stillbirth are significant parts of the family history that are incorporated in the pedigree chart. Chromosomal studies are made of family members, when this is appropriate, as well as laboratory evaluations for carriers, when such persons can be determined.

It is only at this point that a discussion of risks is feasible. Risks may be described in Mendelian terms for some specific dominant or recessive disorders. Often, however, such clearcut risk figures are not available and empirical risk figures based on observation of the recurrence of the condition in actual practice, are used.

Each couple must decide what use they will make of the information they receive in genetic counseling. It is not the role of the counselor to determine a course of action for them. The counselor will, of course, make the family aware of the possibility of prenatal diagnosis for a particular condition, but some couples may choose not to follow that course.

Couples will react differently to risk figures. In a condition for which the empirical risk figures are 1 in 20, or 5 per cent, one couple may focus on the 95 per cent chance that a problem will not occur while another will focus on the 5 per cent chance that it may and find that risk unacceptable. Differences in the ac·

Nursing Care Plan 3–1.   Genetic Testing and Counseling*

NURSING GOALS:

To provide families at risk of genetic disease with a specific diagnosis and with information about genetic inheritance that is applicable to them.

To provide families at risk of genetic disease with objective, nonjudgmental information about alternatives.

OBJECTIVES: Following counseling, the client(s) will:

1. Understand the purpose of genetic testing and counseling.
2. Have a specific diagnosis of the genetic condition of concern.
3. Understand physiological, emotional, social, and economic factors related to the specific genetic condition.
4. Know if antenatal diagnosis is possible.
5. Understand the alternatives available to them.
6. Begin to cope with the realities of their particular genetic condition in a way that is consistent with their psychological, social, and ethical values.

ASSESSMENT	POTENTIAL NURSING DIAGNOSIS	NURSING INTERVENTIONS	COMMENTS/ RATIONALE
1. Prior to counseling a. family history of genetic disease b. birth of a child with genetic disorder c. identification of potential genetic disorder in screening program (e.g., sickle cell trait, elevated serum alphafetoprotein)	Need for genetic testing/counseling Need for information about purpose and process of genetic testing/counseling	1. Explain purpose of genetic testing and counseling in positive, reassuring terms. 2. Make appropriate referral for genetic testing and/or counseling. 3. Provide information about a. process of testing and counseling b. time and place of appointment c. specific location of counseling center (if other than family physician)	

2. During the Testing/Counseling Process
 a. Assist in the collection of data:
  1. outcome in each pregnancy for couple
  2. pregnancy history in mother of each partner
  3. genetic disease in brothers or sisters of each partner (both living and dead)
  4. genetic disease in children of siblings of each partner
  5. genetic disease in parents, aunts, uncles, cousins and cousin's children of each partner
  6. relationship of couple other than by marriage (e.g., cousins)
 b. Assess client(s) understanding of information presented; need for further testing, etc. at each stage of testing/ counseling process.
 c. Assess client(s) feelings at each stage of testing/counseling process.
 	
 d. Assess client(s) coping skills at each stage of testing/counseling.
	b. Need for information about the process, purpose of additional tests, if necessary
	
	c. Self-dissatisfactory, diminished self-esteem; emotional distress related to diagnostic procedures; emotional distress related to genetic problem
	d. Difficult adaptation to genetic problem
		b. Provide information about process, purpose of additional tests. Ask client(s) to repeat information to you to assure understanding
		c. Allow client(s) to express feelings about all aspects of problem and counseling process; accept client(s) anger, frustration.
		
		d. Reinforce positive coping behavior; provide (or refer to) resources to facilitate or enhance coping	

3. Following a specific diagnosis
 a. Assess understanding of risk factors.
 b. Assess understanding of specific condition
  1. course of illness
  2. long-term prognosis
  3. available therapy
  4. costs of care
 c. Assess meaning of information for individual couple.
 d. Assess knowledge of alternatives.
	Knowledge deficit; need for information related to . . . (risk factors, specific condition, alternatives)
	
	Negative self-image; fear related to diagnosis of genetic disease; anger, etc.
		Provide information to enhance understanding of risks
		Provide information about the course of the particular condition: long term prognosis, extent of care, costs of care.
		
		Provide opportunity for expression of anger, fear, and other feelings; allow for questions.
		Provide information about alternatives consistent with clients' diagnosis, values.
		 a. future pregnancy antenatal testing and possible abortion of affected infant
		 b. future pregnancy with knowledge of risks
		 c. avoidance of future pregnancy
			The meaning of risk figures to a couple will vary.

4. Following the testing/counseling process a. assess need for further counseling	Need for additional information. Need for counseling in relation to coping	Provide (or refer to) resources for continuing care (physiologic, psychologic, and/or social). Provide a telephone number where client can reach you (or other appropriate resource) as questions arise.	

*Genetic counseling requires a team approach; the team includes nurses, physicians, geneticists and may include other professionals as well.

55

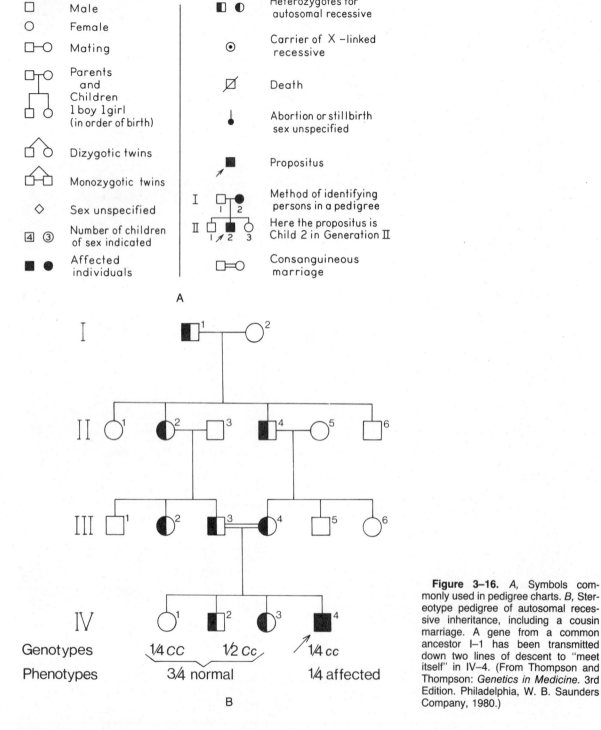

Figure 3–16. *A,* Symbols commonly used in pedigree charts. *B,* Stereotype pedigree of autosomal recessive inheritance, including a cousin marriage. A gene from a common ancestor I–1 has been transmitted down two lines of descent to "meet itself" in IV–4. (From Thompson and Thompson: *Genetics in Medicine.* 3rd Edition. Philadelphia, W. B. Saunders Company, 1980.)

ceptability of a risk will also vary with the condition in question. Some couples would risk a condition that is fatal in the neonatal period, as difficult as that situation would be at the time, but would be more hesitant to risk a condition that involves a long-term disease, such as Down's syndrome.

Counseling also attempts to help parents deal with the myriad of financial, medical, and social realities of their baby's condition. These questions are raised not just in relation to the affected baby but to the parents' considerations of future pregnancies.

What will the cost of care possibly be? What

alternatives for care should be considered (as, for example, in the case of a child with a severely handicapping condition)? Will special medical treatment be needed (such as for the child with cystic fibrosis)? What is the eventual prognosis? How able is the family to cope with the emotional and financial demands of the condition? What resources are available to help them cope? Many of these are not questions that counseling can answer, other than to inform families about what a particular community has to offer. But by raising questions, parents can be helped to consider these issues, particularly when they are trying to decide to have another child, which is so frequently why such counseling is sought.

Alternatives to future childbearing may also be considered in the genetic counseling process. Some families choose sterilization as a means of preventing future pregnancies. Others seek information about highly reliable contraception. Adoption is an alternative chosen by some of these couples.

Adoption, however, is by no means the right answer for every couple. For parents whose only child is defective, Macintyre[8] states, "there is a deep personal need to prove that they are capable of producing a normal child of their own." Macintyre uses the analogy of a baseball game to describe his perception of how parents feel when their infant, particularly a firstborn infant, is defective.

It's like being up to bat in a very important ball game where everything depends on you, and striking out; and the whole stadium boos, the whole of society boos, or you think it does. . . . For the individual who has struck out in that important ball game, there is a real need to offset society's criticism by hitting a home run the next time at bat. Adopting a child is like getting to first base on a "walk." It is no proof of your batting ability.[8]

Every couple will not feel this way, but the possibility that some will is certainly worth considering.

When the disorder in question is caused by a dominant gene carried by the father, artificial insemination may be an alternative for some families. With other conditions, pregnancy may be attempted with subsequent diagnosis in utero by the use of amniocentesis (Chapter 14) and possible therapeutic abortion. For example, when the disorder is X-linked recessive, thus affecting only male children, the knowledge that the fetus is a girl can make pregnancy far less stressful for both mother and father.

Cultured cells from amniotic fluid are also being used to detect the presence or absence of some enzymes that lead to the diagnosis of certain biochemical disorders, such as galactosemia.

A single example of prenatal monitoring for detection of an inherited defect may illustrate its value.

A three and a half year old child was referred to us for chromosomal analysis. The youngster had several external congenital malformations and was suffering from bilateral renal dysplasia, severe growth retardation (she weighed only 8 pounds), and severe mental retardation. She has two phenotypically normal sisters. Results of the chromosome analysis indicated that the defective child's karyotype was genetically unbalanced, and analyses were performed on both parents. The father's karyotype was normal, but that of the mother indicated that she is a carrier of a balanced reciprocal translocation....

The mother was pregnant at the time she was ascertained as having the genetic problem, and when she and her husband were informed that the risk of producing a second badly defective child might be as high as 50% both parents requested that the pregnancy be interrupted. They both desired more children, but neither could tolerate the thought of having another deformed one. We discussed the possibility of performing a prenatal chromosomal analysis on the developing fetus, and it was agreed that an attempt at such an analysis should be made. Amniocentesis was performed in the sixteenth week following the last menstrual period, and cultures were established from fetal cells in the amniotic fluid. By the eighteenth week the analysis was complete, and the fetal chromosome karyotype was obtained. It was obvious that the fetus carried the same translocation as the mother. . . . Since the karyotype represented that of a balanced carrier, we were able to predict that the child would develop normally. Furthermore, the parents were hoping for a boy and we were able to predict that their desires would be fulfilled in this regard also. In due time, at full term, the mother was delivered of a beautiful eight and a half pound, healthy son. The parents were ecstatic. . . .

Our ability to perform the prenatal chromosome analysis in this case literally saved the life of that youngster, for he would have been destroyed by therapeutic abortion on the basis of the high genetic risk involved, had we not been able to perform the prenatal evaluation.[8]

Genetic counseling is becoming one additional resource for families in their childbearing years. Like all counseling, it must never press solutions on families but rather should inform them of alternatives from which they can choose the best possible course for themselves.

REFERENCES

1. Arey, L.: *Developmental Anatomy: A Textbook and Laboratory Manual of Embryology.* Revised 7th Edition. Philadelphia, W. B. Saunders Co., 1974.
2. Asimov, I.: *The Genetic Code.* New York, The Orion Press, 1962.
3. Borek, E.: *The Code of Life.* New York, Columbia University Press, 1965.
4. Dobzhansky, T.: *Mankind Evolving.* New Haven, Yale University Press, 1962.
5. Eppink, H.: Genetic Causes of Abnormal Fetal Development and Inherited Disease. *JOGN Nursing 6(5):*14, 1977.
6. Hendin, D., and Marks, J.: *The Genetic Connection.* New York, New American Library, 1979.
7. Horan, M.: Genetic Counseling: Helping the Family. *JOGN Nursing 6(5):*25, 1977.
8. Macintyre, M.: Prenatal Chromosome Analysis—A Lifesaving Procedure. *Southern Medical Journal, 64*(Suppl. #1): 85, February, 1971.
9. Mellman, W.G.: The Genetic Basis for the Variability of Hereditable Disease. *Journal of Pediatrics.* 72:727, May 1968.
10. Page, E., Villee, C. A., and Villee, D. B.: *Human Reproduction: The Core Content of Obstetrics, Gy-necology and Perinatal Medicine.* 3rd Edition. Philadelphia, W. B. Saunders, Co., 1980.
11. Papazian, H. P.: *Modern Genetics.* New York, W. W. Norton and Co., Inc., 1967.
12. Roberts, J., Pembry, M.: *An Introduction to Medical Genetics.* 7th Edition. Oxford, Oxford University Press, 1978.
13. Smith, D. W.: Genetic Basis for Clinical Disorders. *Southern Medical Journal. 64:* Supplement #1, 4, Feb. 1971.
14. Thompson, C.: Legal Aspects of Genetic Screening. *JOGN Nursing 6(5):*34, 1977.
15. Thompson, J., and Thompson, M.: *Genetics in Medicine.* 2nd Edition. Philadelphia, W. B. Saunders Co., 1973.
16. Ursprung, H.: Developmental Genetics. In Cooke, R. E. (ed.): *The Biological Basis of Pediatric Practice.* New York, McGraw-Hill Book Co., 1968.
17. Wright, S. W.: Chromosomal Abnormalities in Man: The Autosomes. *In* Nelson, W. E., Vaughan, V. C., and McKay, R. J. (eds.): *Textbook of Pediatrics.* 9th Edition. Philadelphia, W. B. Saunders Co., 1969.

Biologic Readiness for Childbearing

1. Define:
   - a. penis
   - b. scrotum
   - c. testes
   - d. glans penis
   - e. prepuce
   - f. spermatic cord
   - g. vas deferens
   - h. epididymis
   - i. ejaculatory duct
   - j. seminal fluid
   - k. prostaglandins
   - l. capacitation
   - m. vulva
   - n. mons pubis
   - o. labia majora
   - p. labia minora
   - q. clitoris
   - r. hymen
   - s. bulbocavernous muscle
   - t. vaginismus
   - u. Bartholin's glands
   - v. Skene's ducts
   - w. infundibulum
   - x. ampulla
   - y. isthmus
   - z. Rubin test
   - aa. myometrium
   - bb. endometrium
   - cc. fornix (fornices)
   - dd. hypogastric plexus
   - ee. gonadotropin-releasing hormone
   - ff. follicle-stimulating hormone
   - gg. luteinizing hormone
   - hh. estrogen
   - ii. progesterone
   - jj. testosterone
   - kk. oocyte
   - ll. graafian follicle
   - mm. corpus luteum
   - nn. corpus albicans
   - oo. endometriosis
   - pp. spinnbarkeit
   - qq. ferning
   - rr. climacteric
   - ss. orgasmic platform
   - tt. refractory period

2. Identify the structures of the male and female reproductive tracts.
3. Describe the bony pelvis—the bones, the differentiation of the true and false pelves, and the types of pelves. Identify the terms pelvic inclination and pelvic axis.
4. Describe the muscles and fasciae of the pelvic floor.

Objectives continued on following page

5. Identify the major ligaments supporting pelvic organs and describe their location.
6. Describe pelvic circulation, including the major vessels and unique characteristics.
7. Explain the relationship between the central nervous system and the endocrine system.
8. Identify the following breast structures:
   a. alveolus
   b. ductule
   c. duct
   d. lactiferous duct
   e. lactiferous sinus
   f. ampulla
   g. nipple pore
   h. areola
   i. tubercles of Montgomery
9. Explain the relationship between the cerebral cortex, the hypothalamus, and the endocrine system.
10. Identify the gonadotropic hormones and their function in males and females.
11. Describe the production and action of testosterone, estrogens, and progesterone.
12. Compare the ovarian cycle and the endometrial cycle; describe the relationship between each phase of the two cycles.
13. Identify the role of prostaglandins in the reproductive cycle.
14. Identify possible causes of dysmenorrhea. Describe the factor considered primary and the process by which that factor causes dysmenorrhea.
15. Identify factors that should be included in a nursing assessment of a woman with dysmenorrhea.
16. Identify both nonpharmacologic and pharmacologic treatments for dysmenorrhea and describe the rationale for the use of each.
17. In relation to toxic shock syndrome, describe the proposed etiology, the criteria defining the syndrome, and treatment.
18. Cite important facts to be included in educating women about toxic shock syndrome.
19. Identify the physiologic basis of symptoms of the climacteric.
20. Describe physiologic reactions to sexual stimuli.
21. Describe the four phases of the cycle of sexual response.
22. Identify physiologic factors that facilitate or impede fertilization.

The biologic functioning of the male and female reproductive systems is a complex and fascinating process. While this might be said of each body system, it is only in the reproductive systems that two distinct individuals must function in concert to achieve their biologic purpose.

Consider, for example, that the character of the mucus of the female cervix changes in consistency to facilitate the passage of sperm into the female reproductive tract at precisely the time that the ovum is ready for fertilization. Or consider that the zona pellucida, the area surrounding the cytoplasm of the ovary, admits a single sperm and then repels others.

In this chapter, we will examine the reproductive tracts from a biologic point of view; in the chapters that follow, we will consider more closely how social and psychologic factors interface with reproductive biology.

The reproductive system serves three functions, all closely interrelated. Satisfying sexual desires is the first; without a strong sexual drive the human race might never have survived the long course of history. The production of some very potent hormones is a second function. The third is procreation, beginning with the production of the ovum and sperm and continuing for several weeks following an infant's birth.

Anatomy of the Reproductive System

In both males and females the reproductive system is divided into external and internal components. The major structures will be described here, and their functions will be discussed in greater detail later in the chapter.

Male Genitalia

The *penis* and *scrotum* are the external organs of the male reproductive system. Although the *testes* are found within the scrotum, they are generally considered internal structures.

Within the penis are three cylinders of spongy tissue: two *corpora cavernosa* and the *corpus spongiosum*. The urethra runs through the corpus spongiosum. A network of blood vessels and nerve endings crisscrosses the spongy tissue of each of these cavities; during sexual excitement they are engorged with blood, and the penis becomes characteristically stiff. The smooth, round head of the penis is the *glans penis,* a highly sensitive structure

with many nerve endings. In an uncircumcised male, a retractable foreskin *(prepuce)* covers part of the glans; circumcision totally exposes the glans (Fig. 4–1).

The scrotal sac (Fig. 4–2) contains a testis and its *spermatic cord* in each of two separate compartments. Within the spermatic cord, from which the testis is suspended, are blood vessels, nerves, muscle fibers, and the *vas deferens* through which spermatozoa leave the testes. The spermatic cord enters the abdomen through the inguinal canal.

Internal reproductive organs in the male are the testes and the duct system. In the latter, spermatozoa are both stored and transported.

Within each testis are many seminiferous tubules in which spermatozoa are produced. The combined length of the seminiferous tubules of both testes measures several hundred yards, which allows the production and storage of hundreds of millions of sperm.

Each testis is enclosed in a tight fibrous sheath *(tunica albuginea).* If mumps occurs in an adult male, the virus may infect the testes. They will swell, but because the tunica albuginea is unyielding, the seminiferous tubules may be destroyed, and the man will then become sterile.

From the seminiferous tubules, sperm enters the *epididymis* and then the vas deferens. They pass from the vas through the *ejaculatory duct* into the urethra.

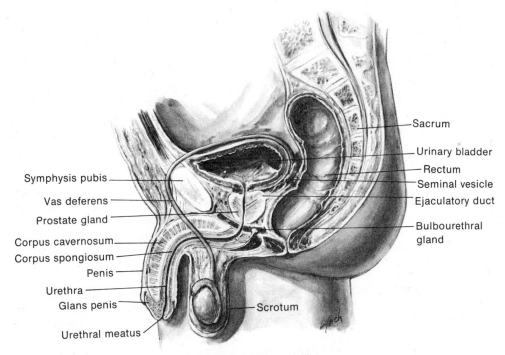

Figure 4–1. Male genitalia.

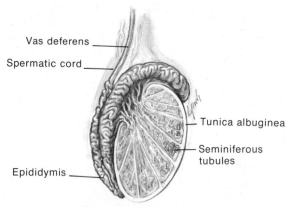

Vas deferens

Spermatic cord

Tunica albuginea

Seminiferous tubules

Epididymis

Figure 4–2. Testis and epididymis.

Seminal Fluid

Seminal fluid, or semen, is produced by several glands, including the *prostate* and the *bulbourethral glands;* the epididymis; the vas deferens; and the *seminal vesicles.* In addition to containing spermatozoa, semen includes amino acids, certain amines that give it a characteristic odor, fructose, and *prostaglandins.* Prostaglandins are fatty acid derivatives secreted by the seminal vesicles that affect uterine muscle (page 77).

Fluid from the seminal vesicles is believed to have a part in initiating sperm motility. The alkaline secretions of the bulbourethral gland may help to neutralize the acidic vaginal secretions that harm sperm. Some of this sticky fluid is secreted prior to ejaculation; because it may contain a few spermatozoa, pregnancy can result even when ejaculation does not occur.

The Completion of Spermatogenesis

The initial development of an individual sperm during the process of mitosis has been described in Chapter 3. Before a sperm can become functional, i.e., capable of fertilization, it must complete its development. The nucleus shrinks, becoming the head of the sperm, and most of the cytoplasm is shed. A pointed acrosome forms at the front of the sperm, while a tail forms behind (see Figure 3–2, page 41).

Biochemically, the sperm's energy is directed toward motility. Only motile sperm are capable of fertilization; sperm motility is one major factor evaluated during an infertility examination (Chapter 6). In the female reproductive tract, sperm may remain motile for as long as a week, although they are considered capable of fertilizing an ovum for only 48 to 72 hours.

The final step in sperm maturation is called *capacitation.* Probably because of some enzymatic difference, capacitation takes place only in the female reproductive tract; if a sperm is returned to the seminal fluid, the process is reversed *(decapacitation).* Just exactly what occurs during capacitation is unclear; probably the acrosome is detached.

Before mature sperm can be produced, there must be adequate production of follicle-stimulating hormone (FSH) and of other hormones, particularly thyroid hormone. Because a temperature lower than body temperature is necessary for the production of mature spermatozoa, they cannot be produced when the testes are undescended.

External Female Genitalia

The female reproductive tract is also divided into external and internal structures. The external genitalia, collectively termed the *vulva* (covering), are the mons pubis (mons veneris), the labia majora, the labia minora, the clitoris, and the vaginal opening.

The *mons pubis* is composed of fatty tissue; it covers the bony pubic symphysis (page 67). Following puberty, it is covered with hair (Fig. 4–3).

The *labia majora* (singular, labium majus) are also composed of fatty tissue and contain nerves, blood vessels, and smooth muscle fibers. The covering skin of the labia majora contains hair follicles and sebaceous glands, but the inner surface is smooth and hairless. The labia majora are usually close together; the area between them, visible only when the lips are parted, is the *pudendal cleft.*

The *labia minora* are thin, pink, and hairless. Posteriorly, the major lips merge with the minor lips. Anteriorly, the major and minor lips divide, with the upper portions forming the *prepuce* of the clitoris and the lower portions meeting beneath the clitoris to form the *frenulum.* The prepuce completely covers the clitoris in most women.

Between the labia minora is an area, the *vestibule* of the vagina, that contains the clitoris and the opening of the urethra and the vagina. The *clitoris* is homologous to the male penis; it consists of two *corpora cavernosa,* the tips of which are attached to the pubic bone. In function it is more like the glans of the penis in that it contains many nerve endings and is highly sensitive. Like the penis, the clitoris becomes engorged with blood during sexual excitement. However, because of its attachment, it does not become erect as the penis does.

The introitus (or opening) of the vagina is

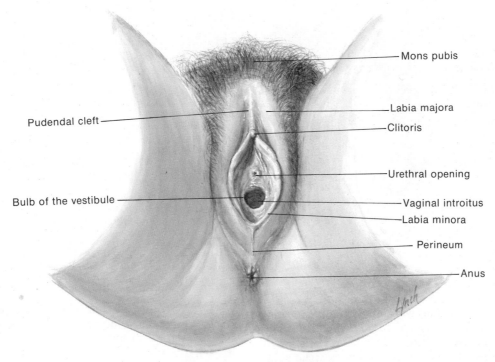

Mons pubis

Labia majora

Clitoris

Pudendal cleft

Urethral opening

Bulb of the vestibule

Vaginal introitus

Labia minora

Perineum

Anus

Figure 4–3. Female genitalia.

an area highly sensitive both to pain and to sexual stimulation. The appearance of the opening tends to vary with the shape, or the absence, of the *hymen,* a pinkish membrane composed of elastic and collagenous tissue.

Traditionally, great social importance has been attached to the intact hymen as proof of virginity, but it is a very unreliable sort of evidence. Not only may the hymen be torn accidentally, but it may sometimes remain intact following intercourse. The rare imperforate hymen (i.e., the hymen with no opening at all) is corrected by surgical incision (hymenotomy).

Usually the virginal hymen will admit one fingertip, sometimes two, or a tampon. If the hymenal orifice is small, self-dilatation, either with the fingers or with a dilator, for 2 to 3 weeks prior to initial intercourse not only will make intercourse less difficult but may prevent a tearing of the hymen that predisposes to bladder infection, often called "honeymoon cystitis."

Provision of good preventive care would suggest that this information should be more widely disseminated. The anticipation and prevention of such problems are considered one value of a premarital examination. However, considering that many, probably most, women never have such an examination and that many women have initial sexual intercourse

prior to marriage, some other way of educating both women and men should be found.

Alongside the vaginal opening are masses of erectile tissue, the *bulb of the vestibule,* and the muscular ring of the *bulbocavernous* muscle. These muscles allow for a certain amount of voluntary control over the size of the vaginal opening. Like the anal sphincter, the vaginal opening can be relaxed or tightened. The muscles can also be tightened through exercise. Such exercise should always be taught to mothers, preferably in the prenatal period (Chapter 11).

General body tenseness, anxiety, or physical pain communicates tenseness to the vaginal muscles. Such tenseness can make a vaginal examination much more difficult for a woman. It is a cycle in which anxiety and tenseness lead to pain, which, in turn, makes the woman more tense. The more a woman is able to relax, the less uncomfortable she will be, and the more she will relax.

The same cycle of tenseness—pain—tenseness may be a problem in sexual intercourse. *Vaginismus* is the term that describes such intense spasm of the muscles surrounding the vagina that the vagina itself cannot be penetrated.

Behind the vestibular bulbs are two small *Bartholin's glands* (greater vestibular glands), with ducts opening between the edge of the

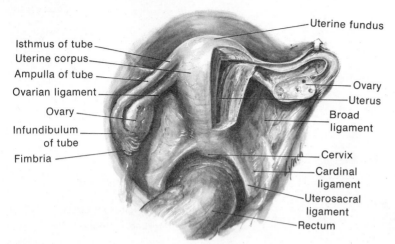

Isthmus of tube
Uterine corpus
Ampulla of tube
Ovarian ligament
Ovary
Infundibulum of tube
Fimbria
Uterine fundus
Ovary
Uterus
Broad ligament
Cervix
Cardinal ligament
Uterosacral ligament
Rectum

Figure 4–4. Female pelvis, posterior view.

hymen and the labia minora. Bartholin's glands, homologous to the bulbourethral glands in the male, were once thought to play a major role in vaginal lubrication. Now that the vaginal walls themselves have been shown to be the chief source of lubrication, the function of these glands is unclear. Bartholin's glands may be infected by the gonococcus or by other organisms, with resultant abscesses or cysts. *Skene's ducts* (paraurethral ducts), which are found on each side of the urethral meatus, are also subject to infection. Between the vulva and the anus is the perineum, made up of skin, muscle, and fascia.

Internal Female Genitalia

The internal organs of the female tract are a pair of ovaries and uterine (fallopian) tubes, the uterus, and the vagina (Figs. 4–4 and 4–5).

The Ovaries

Flanking the uterus and attached to it by the ovarian ligaments are the almond-shaped ovaries. Each ovary is approximately 1½ inches × 1 inch × ¾ inch (3.8 cm. × 2.5 cm. × 1.9 cm.) and weighs ½ ounce (15 grams). The periphery (cortex) of the ovary contains

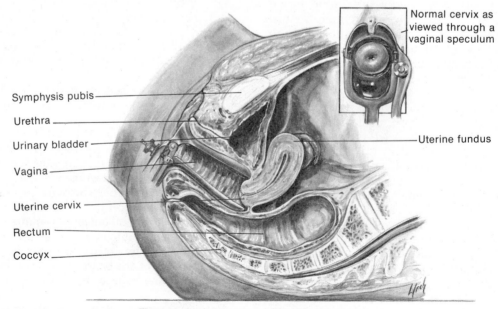

Symphysis pubis
Urethra
Urinary bladder
Vagina
Uterine cervix
Rectum
Coccyx
Normal cervix as viewed through a vaginal speculum
Uterine fundus

Figure 4–5. Internal female reproductive organs.

follicles in all stages of development (page 78), while the central medulla has many convoluted blood vessels. Each follicle contains one ovum (egg.).

Unlike the testes, which deliver sperm through a duct system, there is no tube attached to the ovary through which the egg passes directly into the uterus. Instead, the follicle containing the egg must rupture, and the ovum must be "captured" by the end of the uterine tube. Thus, it is important that the ovarian capsule be thin.

Prior to puberty the ovary appears smooth and glistening, but as years go by, with a follicle rupturing each month, it becomes scarred.

The Uterine Tube

The uterine (fallopian) tube is about 4 inches (10.2 cm.) long. At the uterine end, it extends within the wall of the uterus and opens into it.

The tube itself contains four segments. Beginning at the ovarian end, they are:

1. The *infundibulum,* which is funnel-shaped (hence the name) and fringed by fingerlike projections, the *fimbria.*
2. The *ampulla,* which accounts for half the length of the tube and in which fertilization occurs.
3. The *isthmus,* a thin segment resembling a cord.
4. The *interstitial* segment, which passes through the myometrium of the uterus. The diameter of the tube becomes progressively smaller and is very small in this segment.

The motions of the fimbria that occur at the time of ovulation may attract the ovum into the tube in some way, probably by ciliary action, for if the fimbria are diseased or cut off, the result is relative infertility.

The tubes are lined with hairlike *cilia.* The sweeping action of these cilia, along with the peristalsis of the muscular tubal wall, propels the ovum through the tube. Unlike the motile sperm, the ovum has no innate mobility.

Patency of the tubes is very important. Surgical ligation of the uterine tubes is an effective means of sterilization. Gonorrhea can cause sterility because the purulent exudate that is produced fastens the mucosal surfaces of the lining of the tubes together, and often seals off the infundibulum as well. In countries where abortion by vacuum aspiration has been practiced for a number of years, subsequent sterility from collapse of the tubes has occurred in some women who have had repeated aspiration procedures.

Two methods for determining the patency of the tubes are:

1. The Rubin test, in which carbon dioxide gas is introduced into the uterus and the pressures measured.
2. Serial x-ray studies following the injection of a radiopaque fluid.

(See discussion of infertility in Chapter 6.)

The Uterus

The hollow, pear-shaped uterus is moored to the pelvis by eight ligaments (page 69) and attached to the pelvic floor through the vagina. Prior to any pregnancy, the uterus is approximately 3 to 3½ inches long (7 to 9 cm.) and 2 inches (5 cm.) wide at the top. Following the tremendous expansion of pregnancy, it returns almost, but not quite, to this original size. Normally, the uterus is tilted forward (anteverted, anteflexed) (Fig. 4–6).

The uterus consists of two parts, the corpus (body) and the cervix, but four areas may be described:

1. The fundus, which lies above the openings of the uterine tubes and is the uppermost part of the corpus.
2. The corpus.
3. The narrow isthmus where the corpus joins the cervix.
4. The cervix, or neck, which projects into the vagina.

The fundus is a landmark for obstetric care in every phase of pregnancy. For example, the height of the fundus is one indicator of the age of the normally developing fetus. The prolongation of the uterus into which the uterine tube spins is termed the *cornu* (horn).

During pregnancy, the isthmus forms the *lower uterine segment,* with the remainder of the corpus and fundus forming the *upper uterine segment.*

About half of the inch-long (2.5 to 3 cm.) cervix protrudes into the vagina (Fig. 4–5) and is visible on vaginal examination with a speculum. The cervical canal expands somewhat between the *internal os,* where the cervix enters the isthmus, and the *external os,* which opens into the vagina. The external os, which is visible through the speculum, appears round prior to first childbirth; subsequently, it is transverse with an *anterior lip* and a *posterior lip.*

Prior to pregnancy, the walls of the uterus are approximately 8 mm. thick and consist of three layers:

1. The perimetrium, a serous outer layer.
2. The myometrium, layers of intertwined smooth muscle.

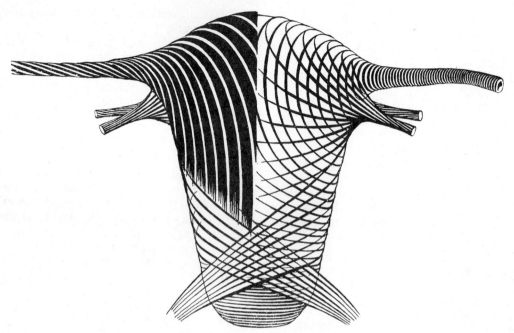

Figure 4–6. Highly schematized representation of the complex interlacing of the myometrial fibers, showing external longitudinal bands and internal circular arrangement. (From Bumm: *Grundriss zum Studium der Geburtschülfe.* 13th Edition. Wiesbaden, J. F. Bergmann, 1921.)

3. The endometrium, a mucous membrane covered with ciliated columnar epithelium.

The perimetrium covers all of the uterus except the lower part of the anterior wall; at this point it turns upward to cover the bladder.

About 90 per cent of the upper uterus, including the fundus, consists of myometrium. By contrast, 10 per cent or less of the cervix is composed of myometrium, the cervix consisting chiefly of fibrous connective tissue. The transition area occurs in the lower 1 cm. of the isthmus. A change in muscle fibers during pregnancy allows for growth of the uterus.

The glands and blood vessels of the endometrium change constantly with the menstrual cycle. These changes are discussed in detail later in this chapter.

The Vagina

Above the hymen, the vagina serves as a repository for semen, a duct for uterine discharges (menstrual flow, for example), and a birth canal. The vagina tilts posteriorly from the vulva to the place at which it joins the cervix. Because of the angle of attachment to the cervix (almost a right angle), the anterior wall of the vagina is shorter than the posterior wall by about an inch. (The anterior wall is approximately 2.4 to 2.8 inches or 6 to 7 cm. in length; the posterior wall 3.2 to 3.6 inches or 8 to 9 cm.)

The projection of the cervix into the upper one-third of the vagina creates a blind vaginal pouch surrounding the cervix. Four fornices describe the upper segment of the vagina in relation to the cervix:

1. The posterior fornix, which lies behind the cervix.

2. The anterior fornix, which lies in front of the cervix.

3. Two lateral fornices, one on each side of the cervix.

Ordinarily a collapsed tube, the vagina is soft and so highly distensible that it will accommodate an infant's head at the time of delivery. Unlike the vaginal introitus, the walls of the vagina above the hymen are largely insensitive.

The vagina has a mucosal inner layer and a fibromuscular layer. Prior to a first delivery, the thick mucous membrane of the vagina appears in folds, called *rugae,* which are stretched to give the vagina a smooth appearance during delivery. Within the mucosa are layers of several types of cells: flat cells closest to the surface; parabasal and intermediate cells; and small, round basal cells. Beneath the vaginal mucosa is a fibromuscular layer that consists of predominantly smooth muscle in the upper layer and connective tissue cells at the deeper levels. This fibromuscular layer may become stretched or torn during childbirth.

Other Pelvic Organs

Because of their proximity, both the rectum and anus and the urethra and its meatus must be considered in relation to the genitalia. As Figure 4–5 demonstrates, the bladder is anterior to the uterus and the rectum posterior. This pelvic "geography" explains many of the minor problems of pregnancy and the postpartal period that are discussed throughout the text.

Supporting Structures of Female Genitalia

A variety of systems support the genital organs and structures. They include the bony pelvis, muscles, ligaments, and segments of the circulatory and nervous systems.

The Bony Pelvis

The pelvis consists of four bones; two innominate bones, the sacrum, and the coccyx. The innominate bone is divided into three areas that in childhood were distinct bones; the ilium, the ischium, and the pubis. Pelvic bones articulate at the two sacroiliac joints, the sacrococcygeal joint, and the symphysis pubis (Fig. 4–7). The fibrocartilage lining these joints becomes soft during pregnancy. This softening allows mobility of the pelvis during labor but does not result in any change in pelvic size.

The size and shape of the bony pelvis are significant in determining whether a woman will be able to deliver her infant vaginally or whether a cesarean section may be necessary. Measurement of the pelvis is a part of the prenatal examination and is discussed in Chapter 10.

The *linea terminalis* divides the pelvis into two sections. The upper or *false* pelvis is of little obstetric interest; it does provide the general direction for the entry of the fetus into the true pelvis.

The lower or *true* pelvis determines the shape and direction of the birth canal and supports the muscles of the pelvic floor. The shape and size of the false pelvis give no indication of the shape and size of the true pelvis. The true pelvis has a basically cylindrical shape, which curves anteriorly much like a bent stovepipe (Fig. 4–8). Because of this curve, the canal is slightly less than 2 inches (4.5 cm.) anteriorly but is 5 inches (12.5 cm.) posteriorly.

Both the entrance and the outlet of the true pelvis are smaller than the middle portion. The entrance is termed the *superior strait,* or plane of the inlet, and the outlet is the *inferior strait,* or plane of the outlet (Fig. 4–9). It is the shape of the superior strait that determines the type of pelvis. Figure 4–10 illustrates the four pelvic types:

1. Gynecoid, rounded and "roomy."
2. Android, heart-shaped and funnel-shaped, narrowing from top to bottom.
3. Anthropoid, an ellipse, elongated from front to back.
4. Platypelloid, a flattened ellipse.

In most women the shape of the pelvis is somewhere between these four types. When there is doubt, the shape of the anterior segment is the guide. Approximately 50 per cent of childbearing women have a gynecoid pelvis, considered the most favorable for normal delivery. The anthropoid pelvis is the next most common. Because the funnel-shaped android pelvis narrows from top to bottom, vaginal delivery is difficult. The flat platypelloid pelvis is relatively rare. Disease in early life that has caused contraction and distortion of the pelvic bones may present obstetric complications.

Pelvic inclination refers to the angle that the inlet makes with the horizon. When a woman is standing erect, pelvic inclination is about 55 to 60 degrees.

The *axis* of the pelvis is formed by drawing a line perpendicular to each of the pelvic planes (Fig. 4–8). In the gynecoid pelvis, the

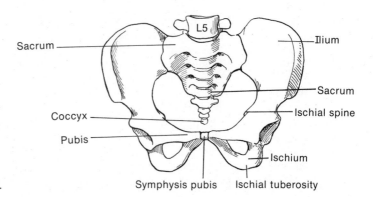

Figure 4–7. Female bony pelvis.

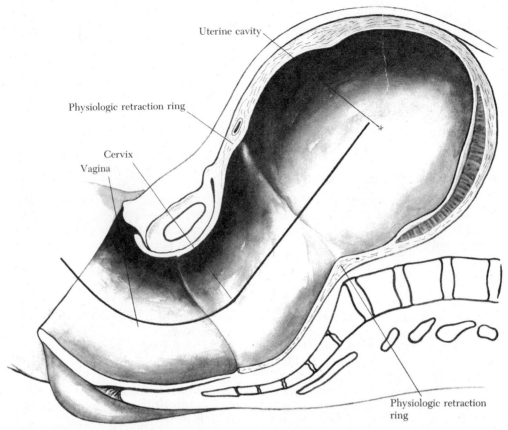

Uterine cavity

Physiologic retraction ring

Cervix

Vagina

Physiologic retraction ring

Figure 4–8. The pelvis curves anteriorly, much like a bent stovepipe. The uterus, cervix, and vagina are diagrammed as if all the component parts were distended at one time. The axis is the central curved line. (From Greenhill and Friedman: *Biological Principles and Modern Practice of Obstetrics.* Philadelphia, W. B. Saunders Co., 1974.)

curve begins at about the level of the spine. The pelvic axis is another important consideration in delivery.

Muscles and Fascia of the Pelvic Floor

The pelvic floor, or pelvic diaphragm (Fig. 4–11), is made up of two identifiable muscular diaphragms: (1) the deeper, stronger muscles and (2) the superficial muscle structures that close and control the urethral, anal, and vaginal orifices. Internally, the pelvic diaphragm forms the base of the abdominal cavity and is covered with peritoneum. It serves to anchor the cervix, vagina, rectum, and bladder. The muscle layers are surrounded by connective tissue, fascia, adipose tissue, and skin.

The deeper levator ani muscles are composed of the pubococcygeal, the iliococcygeal, and the puborectal muscles. The vagina, rectum, and urethra actually pass through this muscular diaphragm, which forms a slinglike support for the birth canal. Each pelvic organ has a fascial sheath surrounding or embracing it that supports it and assists in maintaining its

anatomic relationship to the other pelvic organs and the bony pelvis.

Four fascial layers arise from the deeper fascial covering of the levator ani muscles: (1) one layer extends in the front to the bladder and continues on to the pubic bone to form the pubovesical ligament; (2) another, the retrorectal layer, travels to the sacrum to form the uterosacral ligament; (3) two other layers, between the bladder and vagina and between the vagina and rectum, branch to each side to form the base of the broad ligament that attaches to the pelvic side wall and to each side of the uterus. It is the fascial layers surrounding the vagina with the bladder in front and the rectum in back that are most subject to tearing during the course of delivery. Persistent bowel and bladder problems may result from a weakening or tearing of these tissues.

The superficial layer of the pelvic floor is composed of the urogenital diaphragm, the perineal body, the vulva, and the glands of the vulva. The *urogenital diaphragm* is formed by the bulbocavernous muscle, the ischiocavernous muscle, and the superficial transverse per-

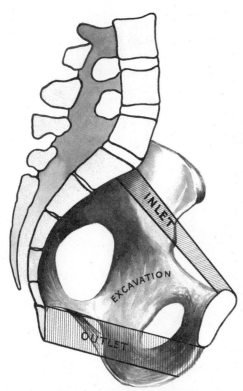

Figure 4–9. The pelvic inlet and outlet. (From Greenhill: *Obstetrics.* 13th Edition. Philadelphia, W. B. Saunders Co., 1965.)

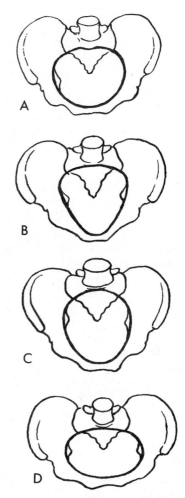

Figure 4–10. Caldwell-Moloy classification of pelves. *A,* Gynecoid; *B,* android; *C,* anthropoid; and *D,* platypelloid.

ineal muscles. It surrounds the upper part of the urethra and the lower part of the vagina, which supports the upper portion of the urethra. When there is an increase in intra-abdominal pressure, the pressure is transmitted to the upper urethra as well as to the bladder, and urine does not escape. However, if the urogenital diaphragm has been torn or stretched during childbirth, the bladder neck and urethra may sag downward, allowing urine to escape when intra-abdominal pressure increases. This is called *stress incontinence.* Often nurses are the first to hear of the symptoms of stress incontinence; a woman may feel it is too small a problem to mention to a physician, even though it is very aggravating to her.

The pelvic floor muscles and fascia differ in strength and tonus from one mother to another. They tend to be weaker in the mother who has delivered babies previously than in the mother who is delivering for the first time. The quality of pelvic floor support and the integrity of these tissues can be maintained or enhanced by an attentive birth attendant and by a knowledgeable care-agent during postdelivery recovery and adjustment.

Pelvic Ligaments

Four significant ligaments serve to bind the pelvic bones together and add strength to the pelvic structure: (1) the interpubic ligaments between the pubic bones strengthen the symphysis pubis, (2) the sacrotuberous ligaments between the sacrum and the ischial tuberosity, (3) the sacrospinous ligaments between the sacrum and the ischial spines, and (4) the sacroiliac ligaments between the sacroiliac joints and the inguinal ligaments between the anterior superior iliac spine and the pubic bone. The sacroiliac ligaments are probably the strongest in the entire body. The sacrotuberous and sacrospinous ligaments form the back portion of the pelvic outlet.

Other major ligaments supporting the pelvic organs are summarized in Table 4–1. Figure 4–4 illustrates several major ligaments.

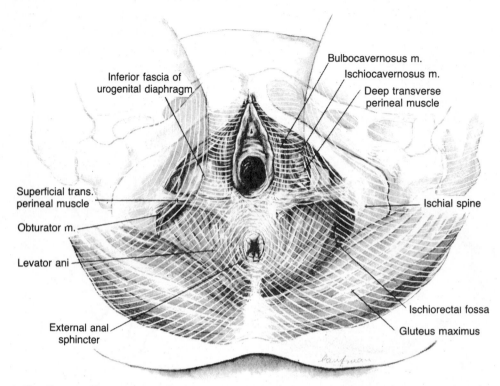

Inferior fascia of
urogenital diaphragm

Bulbocavernosus m.

Ischiocavernosus m.

Deep transverse
perineal muscle

Superficial trans.
perineal muscle

Ischial spine

Obturator m.

Levator ani

Ischiorectal fossa

Gluteus maximus

External anal
sphincter

Figure 4–11. Topographic anatomy of the important perineal structures showing the interrelationships between bony, muscular, and visceral structures. (From Greenhill and Friedman: *Biological Principles and Modern Practice of Obstetrics.* Philadelphia, W. B. Saunders Co., 1974.)

Circulation

Three paired vessels form the main arterial blood supply of the uterus (Fig. 4–12). They are: (1) the uterine arteries, branches of the hypogastric arteries; (2) the ovarian arteries, branches of the aorta; and (3) the funicular arteries (not shown), branches from the vesical arteries that join the ovarian arteries at the fundus. As Figure 4–12 shows, all of these vessels are highly convoluted with frequent anastomoses.

Veins follow the same paths as the arteries. The uterine veins empty into plexuses in the broad ligaments. The blood then flows through veins in the broad ligaments to the hypogastric vein and then to the common iliac vein. The ovarian veins empty into the renal vein on the left and the vena cava on the right. Veins penetrate all the layers of the uterus and are especially plentiful in the myometrium. Like the arteries, they anastomose frequently.

The arteries and veins of the uterine wall are unique in that they have no outer coat and so lie directly on the muscular bundles, where they form large blood spaces called sinuses. Because of this, the ovarian and pelvic veins are able to dilate as blood volume increases during pregnancy. It is estimated that their capacity is increased by more than 60 times by the thirty-sixth week of pregnancy. A second apparent advantage of this property of the ovarian and pelvic veins is the neutralization of changes in systemic pressure that is afforded, such as the sudden high central pressure that occurs during acute straining.

The pelvic organs are also richly supplied by lymphatic vessels and lymph nodes. The lymphatic system follows the overall pattern of the major blood vessels.

Nerve Supply

Both motor and sensory fibers from the autonomic and central nervous systems supply the genitalia (Fig. 4–13). Parasympathetic motor fibers stimulate vasodilatation and cause the inhibition of muscular contraction; sympathetic motor fibers affect vasoconstriction and muscular contraction. The *hypogastric plexus* is a large plexus of motor fibers formed above the promontory of sacrum near the bifurcation of the aorta. Sensory fibers arise from the spinal cord through the sacral nerves.

A basic knowledge of neural function is valuable in understanding a number of clinical phenomena that will be discussed in greater

Table 4–1. LIGAMENTS SUPPORTING THE PELVIC ORGANS

Ligament	Location	Comments
Broad	From the lateral walls of the uterus to the lateral pelvic wall.	Upper two-thirds: two thin layers of peritoneum. Divides pelvic cavity into anterior and posterior segments. Folds contain uterine tubes, ovaries, round and cardinal ligaments, blood vessels, lymphatics, and nerves.
Cardinal	Lower one-third of broad ligament, from cervix to lateral pelvic wall.	Dense connective tissue. Main supporting structure of uterus (along with muscles of pelvic diaphragm and perineum). Contains uterine artery and vein.
Round	From the uterus, just anterior to the insertion of the uterine tubes, upward and outward through the inguinal canal to the labia majora.	Forms the upper margin of the broad ligaments.
Uterosacral	From the posterior upper cervix backward to the fascia of the second and third sacral vertebrae.	Exerts traction, which keeps the uterus in normal position.
Anterior	A peritoneal fold between the bladder and the uterus.	
Posterior	A peritoneal fold between the uterus and the rectum.	
Ovarian	Suspends ovary.	Short.
Infundibulopelvic	Ovarian hilum to the lateral pelvic wall.	Contains ovarian vein and artery.

detail in the chapters that follow. For example, because sympathetic motor fibers that stimulate muscular contraction originate in the ganglia at the level of the T5 to T10 vertebrae, spinal anesthesia to the level of T5 will tend to abolish contractions of the uterine fundus. However, a transection of the spinal cord above the level of T5 will not necessarily prevent labor and delivery.

The stimulus for pain in hollow viscera such as the uterus and tubes is either stretching or ischemia. Thus, a cervical biopsy is only mildly uncomfortable but dilatation (as for a dilatation and curettage) requires anesthesia. A

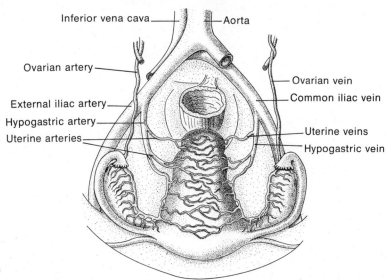

Figure 4–12. Blood supply of uterus and ovary.

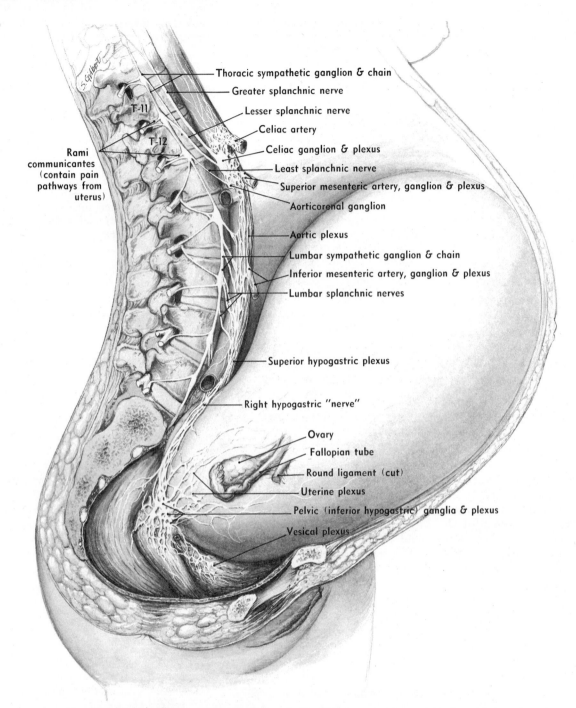

Figure 4–13. Schematic representation of uterine nerve supply showing nerve routes arising from the thoracic and lumbar spinal nerves and traversing the lumbar sympathetic chain to the aortic plexus, superior hypogastric plexus, and pelvic plexus. (From Bonica: *Principles and Practice of Obstetrical Analgesia and Anesthesia.* Philadelphia, F. A. Davis Co., 1967.)

twisting of the tube that interferes with blood supply will cause severe pain.

Breasts

While the breasts are not genitalia, they are influenced by the same hormones and play an important role in both sexual and reproductive functions. Externally, the nipples and the darkened areolae are the most obvious areas of the breasts. The nipples contain many nerve fibers, which make them highly sensitive. While nipples normally protrude, they may be flat or inverted. Occasionally, a woman may have one or more accessory nipples or breasts. These are usually found along a "milk line"

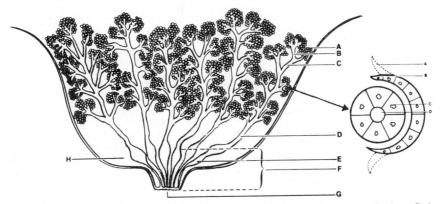

Figure 4–14. *Left,* Diagram of the breast as a "forest of trees." *A,* Alveolus; *B,* ductule; *C,* duct; *D,* lactiferous duct; *E,* lactiferous sinus; *F,* ampulla; *G,* nipple pore; *H,* areolar margin. With full development of the uterine-menstrual cycle, groups of gland secreting cells (alveoli) bud from the small ducts (ductules). The alveoli secrete milk under the influence of prolactin, a hormone of the pituitary gland. *Right,* Diagram of an alveolus. *A,* Uncontracted myoepithelial cell; *B,* contracted myoepithelial cell; *C,* gland secreting cell; *D,* ductule opening. Gland secreting cells are arranged in a circle about the ductule opening. About the alveolus is a contractile cell. When sucking begins, this cell, under the influence of oxytocin from the pituitary gland, contracts and squeezes the milk into the duct system. This reflex is called "let-down." (From Applebaum: *Pediatric Clinics of N. America,* 17:205, 1970.)

extending from the normally located nipple to the groin, as are multiple nipples in other species. The small papillae that appear on the surface of the nipples and the areolae are the *tubercles of Montgomery,* glands that secrete a lipoid substance that lubricates the nipples.

Internally, the breast is arranged in *lobes,* composed of about 15 to 20 *lobules* and *lactiferous ducts* (Fig. 4–14). Lactiferous ducts from each lobe join to form the *ampulla* or *lactiferous sinus.* From each ampulla a milk duct opens into the nipple. Connective and fatty tissue support the lobes.

Breast changes during pregnancy are discussed in Chapter 7 and those of lactation in Chapter 24.

The Endocrine System and Reproduction

Even during the embryonic and fetal period, hormones are necessary for the proper development of the reproductive organs. Hormonal influence continues to be significant throughout life, both in normal physiologic functioning and in pharmacologic intervention in a variety of circumstances.

The endocrine secretions that affect the reproductive system come from two reproductive sources: the anterior lobe of the pituitary gland and the ovaries or testes. These hormones are, in turn, affected by the hypothalamus and the central nervous system.

Endocrine function involves both positive and negative feedback. For example, a steroid hormone such as estrogen can stimulate the release of a gonadotropin such as luteinizing hormone. This is positive feedback. Negative feedback occurs when a hormone, such as a large amount of progesterone, prevents the release of a gonadotropin. The concentration of a particular hormone in the blood determines whether the feedback will be positive or negative. Examples of both positive and negative feedback can be found in the discussion of hormonal action that follows.

Neural Control of Endocrine System

At one time the anterior pituitary gland (the adenohypophysis) was considered the "master" of the endocrine system. It is known now that the "master" is itself influenced by the hypothalamus, which in turn can be stimulated by still higher nerve centers (Fig. 4–15).

A single releasing hormone secreted by the hypothalamus, gonadotropin-releasing hormone (GnRH), induces the release of both follicle-stimulating hormone (FSH) and luteinizing hormone (LH) from the anterior pituitary. At one time the releasing substance was termed luteinizing-hormone–releasing substance and it was believed that a second substance, not yet discovered but termed follicle-stimulating hormone–releasing factor, was responsible for the release of FSH. It is now known that a single factor is responsible for both actions; some texts refer to that factor as luteinizing-hormone–releasing factor (LHRH), and others now use the term GnRH.

GnRH is secreted by neurons with nuclei in

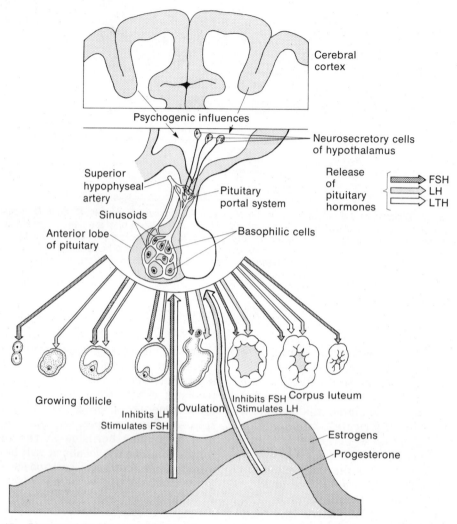

Figure 4–15. Diagram of the interaction between the nervous system, the endocrine system, and the ovarian cycle.

two areas. Nuclei in the suprachiasmatic area behave in a cyclic fashion and are responsible for the surge in LH that occurs at the midmenstrual cycle (see below). Secretions from arcuate nuclei maintain a basal level of gonadotropins in response to negative feedback from the steroid hormones (i.e., when levels of the steroid hormones drop, the arcuate nuclei produce more GnRH to stimulate production of steroid hormones).

The gonadotropin-releasing factors are carried to the anterior pituitary by way of the hypothalamic-hypophyseal portal system (Fig. 4–16).

Several brain centers modify the action of the gonadotropin-releasing factors. These centers are located mainly in the limbic system, a group of brain structures surrounding the hypothalamus and including the hypothalamus as one of its central elements. The centers are influenced by positive and negative feed-

back levels of steroid hormones (estrogen, progesterone, and testosterone) and probably by anterior pituitary hormones (FSH, LH, and luteotropic hormone [LTH]). The limbic centers are also sensitive to emotional stimuli, such as stress, and to factors external to the individual, such as light.

Examples of central nervous system influence on gonadotropin excretion can be found in animals and in humans. In sheep, goats, and deer, for instance, changes in the weather and in the amount of light during the day elicit responses in the nervous system that, in turn, increase the quanity of gonadotropins during the mating season. This, in turn, allows birth during a season of the year when the chances of survival are greatest.

Although there is no directly analogous behavior in humans, stress, mediated through the central nervous system to the endocrine system, certainly affects fertility. Rose[22] found

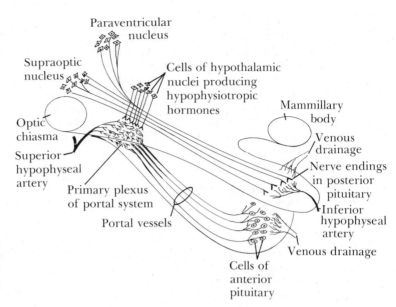

Figure 4–16. Diagram of hypothalamus and pituitary gland showing the portal system of the vasculature. (From Villee: *Human Endocrinology*. Philadelphia, W. B. Saunders Co., 1975.)

that levels of testosterone rose and fell in combat soldiers in response to the degrees of stress to which the men were exposed. A stressful emotional problem may suppress GnRH in a woman so that luteinizing hormone is not released, ovulation does not occur, and amenorrhea results. The emotional correlates of infertility are discussed in more detail in Chapter 6.

The Anterior Pituitary and the Reproductive System

The anterior pituitary secretes three gonadotropic hormones, i.e., hormones that act upon the gonads. These hormones are: (1) FSH, (2) LH, usually called interstitial cell-stimulating hormone (ICSH) in the male; and (3) LTH, also called lactogenic hormone or prolactin.

Follicle-Stimulating Hormone in the Male. FSH is essential for initiating the conversion of spermatogonia into sperm. In addition, it potentiates the effects of LH in promoting the production of testosterone.

Follicle-Stimulating Hormone in the Female. At the time of puberty, FSH stimulates the growth of the ovaries. From that time onward its primary function appears to be the initiation of the growth of the follicles. During each monthly cycle, 20 or more primordial follicles begin to develop under the influence of FSH. Ordinarily, one will outgrow the others and expel its ovum, i.e., ovulate. All the others degenerate completely.

FSH is not secreted continuously; FSH output follows a cyclic pattern that is related to the output of estrogen. As estrogen production

rises, the level of FSH falls (an example of negative feedback). Figure 4–15 shows this relationship during the menstrual cycle, discussed below. The level of FSH is high on day 1, drops to its lowest point on day 14 when estrogen levels are peaking, and begins to rise again on about day 25 in preparation for the beginning of the next cycle.

Luteinizing Hormone (Interstitial Cell-Stimulating Hormone) in the Male. LH (ICSH) stimulates the production of testosterone by the interstitial cells of Leydig in the testes.

Luteinizing Hormone in the Female. Whereas FSH initiates follicular growth, LH, acting along with FSH synergistically, is necessary for final growth and for ovulation. Together they cause rapid swelling of the follicle shortly before ovulation, which probably contributes to the rupture of the follicle. LH may also have a direct effect upon the breaking open of the follicle. It is known that an especially large amount of LH is secreted on the day immediately prior to ovulation, a condition termed the *ovulatory surge* (Fig. 4–15). Note also in Figure 4–15 that LH appears to be stimulated by estrogen (positive feedback).

LH is also responsible for the change of follicular cells into lutein cells following ovulation. (See discussion of the ovarian cycle, below.)

Luteotropic Hormone in the Male. At this time the role of LTH in the male is not considered significant.

Luteotropic Hormone in the Female. On the basis of animal experiments it is believed that LTH is responsible for the maturing of the corpus luteum and its secretion (see below). In animals LTH also stimulates the development of the mammary glands and milk production, hence the name prolactin. The name used for this hormone generally depends upon the function being described; remember that LTH and prolactin are one hormone with more than one action. LTH has not been proved to exist in humans.

Hormones Produced by the Reproductive System

Testosterone, secreted by the interstitial cells of the testes; estrogens, produced by the cells of the ovarian follicle and the corpus luteum; and progesterone, secreted by the corpus luteum, are the principal hormones produced by the male and female reproductive systems. During pregnancy the placenta also secretes estrogens, progesterone, and several other hormones (Chapter 7). (Small amounts of both estrogens and testosterone are also secreted by the adrenal cortex in both men and women.)

Testosterone

The production of testosterone begins in the second month of embryonic life. Testosterone is essential for the development of the penis, scrotum, prostate gland, seminal vesicles, and genital ducts. It is also essential for the descent of the testes. A deficiency of testosterone during this period of development may lead to male hermaphrodism, i.e., a male with ambiguous external genitalia.

The major production of testosterone begins between the ages of 11 and 13, dwindles after the age of 40, and by the age of 80 is only 20 per cent of the amount of peak years. It is testosterone production during adolescence that is responsible for the development of the distinguishing characteristics of the male body:

1. The penis, scrotum, and testes enlarge.

2. Male hair distribution is achieved.

3. Because of hypertrophy of the laryngeal mucosa and enlargement of the larynx, the voice changes; at first there is hoarseness, later a deepening of the voice.

4. Protein is increased in the body; muscles become stronger.

5. The quantity of the bone matrix increases; bones become thicker and have increased deposits of calcium salts.

6. The basic metabolic rate increases from 5 to 15 per cent.

7. Red blood cells are increased by 15 per cent.

8. There is slightly increased reabsorption of sodium in the distal renal tubules.

Testosterone is also necessary for the completion of spermatogenesis, i.e., the conversion of spermatogonia into sperm, a process begun by FSH (page 62). If the hypothalamus is functioning normally, testosterone acts as a feedback control system that inhibits the secretion of the gonadotropins (FSH, LH, and LTH). It is believed that testosterone does this by inhibiting the gonadotropin-releasing factors of the hypothalamus.

The Estrogens

There is no single substance, estrogen, but rather a group of estrogens. However, only two, β-*estradiol* and *estrone,* are secreted in quantities large enough to be considered significant. Of these two, estradiol is considered the major compound. The singular word estrogen is commonly used for these substances.

Estriol is the oxidized end-product of estradiol and estrone; it is formed in the liver shortly after the estrogens are secreted, from that part of the estrogens that has not entered cells. Other substances conjugated from estrogens in the liver are glucuronides, sulfates, and estroproteins.

Small quantities of estrogens are secreted even in childhood, but it is at puberty that the production of estrogens, now 20 times greater, becomes such a major factor in female life. The estrogens:

1. Are responsible for the development of primary and secondary sexual characteristics.

2. Are essential to the hypothalamic-pituitary-ovarian cycle.

3. Influence the thickening of the uterine endometrium during the proliferative and secretory phase of the endometrial cycle.

4. Diversely affect reproductive function.

5. Appear to influence numerous body processes.

Estrogens in the Development of Female Characteristics. Just as testosterone is responsible for the distinguishing characteristics of males, the estrogens govern female traits. During puberty:

1. The uterus, vagina, uterine tubes, and external genitalia increase in size. Fat is deposited in the mons pubis and labia majora.

2. The cells of the vaginal epithelium change from cuboidal to stratified, which enhances their resistance to trauma and infection.

3. The cells and glands of the uterine endometrium increase in number, a preparation for

possible pregnancies in the future. Similar changes occur in the lining of the tubes, where the increased number of ciliated cells aids the ovum in traveling toward the uterus.

4. Breasts grow and the milk-producing system begins to develop (to be completed under the influence of other hormones, progesterone and prolactin).

5. Bone growth is accelerated for several years. Because estrogens cause the epiphyses to unite with the shafts of long bones at an earlier age than does testosterone, the average woman does not become as tall as the average man.

6. Fat is deposited in the subcutaneous tissues, particularly in the breasts, buttocks, and thighs.

7. The basic metabolic rate is increased but not to the extent of the increase caused by testosterone.

8. Female hair distribution occurs.

Estrogens stimulate motility in the uterine tubes, which brings the fimbriated end of the tube into contact with the ovum, aiding in its capture and propelling it into the end of the tube.

The effects of estrogens alone and of estrogens and progesterone combined on the ovarian and endometrial cycles are discussed more fully below. Following implantation, estrogens stimulate the development of both the myometrium of the uterus and the ductile system of the breasts.

Progesterone

In the woman who is not pregnant, progesterone, produced by the corpus luteum, governs all of the morphologic and biochemical changes of the endometrium during the second half of the menstrual cycle (see below) (Fig. 4–15). These changes prepare the body for pregnancy or gestation (thus they are progestational). Progesterone also maintains the endometrium during pregnancy, making continuation of pregnancy possible (Chapter 7).

Before progesterone can be effective, tissues must first be exposed to estrogens. This has practical value in diagnosis. If, for example, in the absence of pregnancy the endometrium fails to bleed after the administration of progesterone, a low level of estrogen is being secreted by the ovary.

Progesterone has a number of other functions, some of which will be discussed in greater detail later. Under the influence of progesterone, the endocervical glands secrete a thick mucus that will not form fern patterns and that impedes sperm migration, a factor important in the contraceptive effects of progestins (Chapter 6).

Progesterone reduces the excitability of the myometrium; contractions that normally recur in uterine muscle are reduced and become sustained and tetanic rather than clonic.

Alveolar development of the breasts and the preparation of the breasts for lactation require progesterone. Progesterone exerts a feedback mechanism on the releasing factors of the hypothalamus, which is demonstrated elsewhere in this chapter. The effect of progesterone on the elevation of basal body temperature is important in understanding basal temperature in relation to both contraception and infertility (Chapter 6). Progesterone also stimulates respiration, so that the CO_2 tension of the blood is decreased during the last half of the menstrual cycle and during pregnancy.

Prostaglandins: Role in Reproduction

Prostaglandins (PG) are fatty acids derived from arachidonic acids (eicosatetraenoic acid). Arachidonic acid is present in essentially all tissues bound in intracellular phospholipid stores; release of arachidonic acid is governed by an enzyme, phospholipase A_2. Although prostaglandins are produced constantly, different tissues vary in their concentration of prostaglandin E (PGE) and prostaglandin F (PGF). Males produce significantly more prostaglandins than females because large quantities are produced by the seminal vesicles. It was in human seminal fluid that prostaglandins were first identified.

Metabolism of prostaglandins is rapid; 99% of prostaglandins in blood is cleared during a single circulatory passage through the lungs and liver, where enzymes convert prostaglandins to metabolites that are excreted in the urine. Of the many prostaglandin compounds, PGE_2 and $PGF_{2\alpha}$ are the most important in reproduction. (The subscript 2 denotes two double bonds in the chemical structure; PGE_1 and PGF_1 both have a single bond.)

Prostaglandin activity in relation to the reproductive cycle includes the following:

1. LH induces increased concentration of $PGF_{2\alpha}$ in the ripening ovarian follicle. If prostaglandin concentration does not rise, the ovum remains trapped within the follicle.

2. Prostaglandins may have a role in regulating steroid production by the corpus luteum.[21]

3. Prostaglandins in seminal fluid may stimulate uterine mobility at the time of intercourse, thus facilitating the passage of sperm through the uterus and uterine tubes to the

side of the egg (see Fertilization, below). High concentrations of prostaglandins in seminal fluid appear to be essential for normal fertility.

4. Because of the effect of prostaglandins on uterine motility, PGE_2 and $PGF_{2\alpha}$ have been used to induce abortion (Chapter 30).

5. Prostaglandins are elevated prior to and during the onset of labor and have been used in some instances to induce labor (Chapter 15).

6. Prostaglandins have been tested as a contraceptive, with a single monthly dose administered in suppository form. Possible mechanisms of action include regression of the corpus luteum, increased uterine motility, or direct effects on the endometrium.

7. Prostaglandins appear to be associated with dysmenorrhea (see below).

The Menstrual Cycle

The interaction of the hypothalamic, pituitary, and gonadotropic hormones controls the cyclic changes that occur in a woman's body from the time of *menarche* (first menstruation) until *menopause* (the cessation of menstruation). These changes include the ovarian and endometrial cycles as well as variations in basal body temperature and changes in other areas of the genital tract. Although each cycle is closely interrelated with the others, each will be discussed separately.

Each cycle is discussed on the basis of an "idealized" 28-day cycle, in which the first day of the menstrual period is day 1. Such numbering is convenient because the onset of menstruation is readily identified. Many normal cycles are either shorter or longer than 28 days; it is merely convenient in a textbook to discuss a 28-day period in which ovulation is presumed to occur on day 14.

The Ovarian Cycle

Because the cyclic changes of the endometrium are dependent upon the cyclic changes in the ovary, the ovarian cycle must be understood first.

At the twentieth week of fetal life there are about 7 million *oogonia* (immature ova) in the human ovary, the largest number that there will ever be. By the time an infant girl is born, the oogonia have been reduced to approximately 1 million, have begun their first meiotic division (Chapter 3), and are called *primary oocytes*. They do not undergo further change until ovulation occurs. Their number at pu-

berty is about 0.5 million. Approximately 450 primary oocytes will ovulate; consider how few will eventually be fertilized.

The Follicular Phase

In the 2 weeks prior to ovulation, the primary oocyte undergoes the changes that prepare it for fertilization under the influence of follicle-stimulating hormone (FSH). FSH output is very high at the beginning of the cycle (Fig. 4–15). The oocyte, along with the follicular (or granulosa) cells that surround it, is now called a follicle and is found in the periphery of the ovarian cortex (Fig. 4–17). The follicular cells are at first flattened, but they enlarge, become cuboidal in shape, and multiply in number. Follicular fluid, containing estrogen, develops between the follicular cells, accumulating in the center of the follicle to form a vesicle. Two layers of cells develop around the follicle, the outer *theca externa* and the inner *theca interna*. Theca interna cells play a part both in estrogen production and in the formation of the corpus luteum (see below). A mucoid membrane, the *zona pellucida*, develops between the primary oocyte and the follicular cells.

Thus developed, the immature primary follicle is now a *vesicular* or *graafian* follicle (it was first described by the anatomist de Graaf). During a normal cycle, several follicles will begin to develop, but usually only one will mature to the graafian follicle stage. The others degenerate and disappear. Should more than one follicle mature, rupture, and subsequently be fertilized, fraternal twins will develop. Identical twins, in contrast, develop from a single ovum.

As the graafian follicle matures, it moves to the surface of the ovary. Shortly before the follicle ruptures, it is approximately ½ inch in diameter (10 to 15 mm.) and could easily be observed if the ovary were to be removed for some reason.

Within the follicle the oocyte is also enlarging. Yolk granules are deposited in the cytoplasm for nourishment, should fertilization occur. Before the follicle ruptures, the first meiotic division is completed.

Changes continue to take place in the graafian follicle. At a late stage the ovum and the follicular cells bordering it (called the *corona radiata* because they appear as a radiating crown) may become detached from the wall of the follicle. Finally, on about the fourteenth day of the cycle, under the influence of FSH and LH, the follicle ruptures, and both the

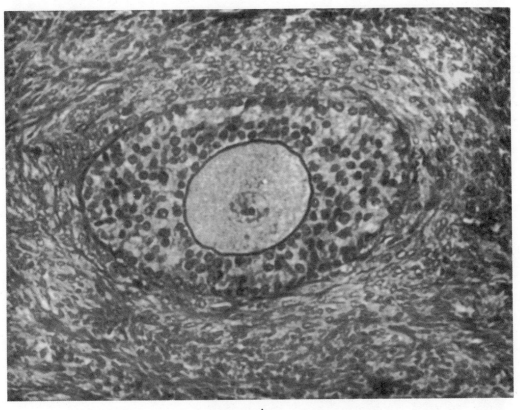

A

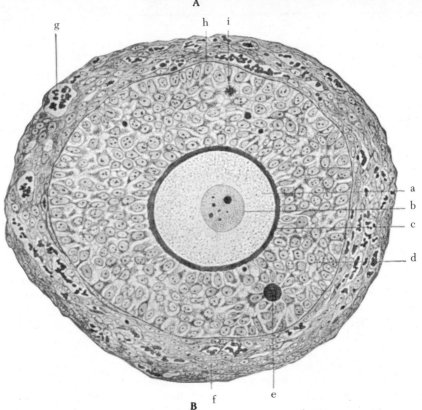

B

Figure 4–17. *A,* Follicle with early formation of oolemma or zona pellucida. (From Shettles: *Ovum Humanum.* New York, Hafner Publishing Co., 1960.) *B,* Follicle of a slightly later stage at the 18th day of the cycle showing *a,* ovum; *b,* oocyte nucleus; *c,* oolemma or zona pellucida; *d,* follicular epithelium with mitochondria; *e,* Call-Exner body or vacuole; *f,* theca folliculi with internal and external layers not yet differentiated; *g,* blood vessels containing erythrocytes; *h,* basement membrane; *i,* mitosis in follicular cell. (Magnification ×345.) (From Bloom and Fawcett: *A Textbook of Histology.* 10th Edition. Philadelphia, W. B. Saunders Co., 1975.)

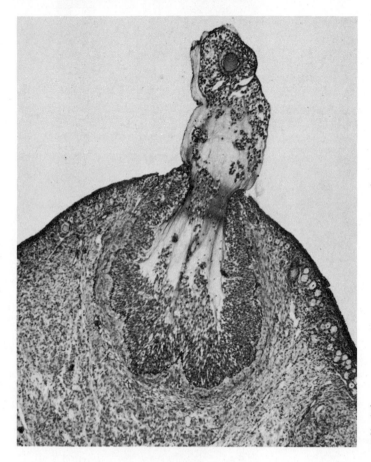

Figure 4–18. Photograph of a rabbit follicle taken at the moment of ovulation. (From Page, Villee, and Villee: *Human Reproduction: Essentials of Reproductive and Perinatal Medicine.* 3rd Edition. Philadelphia, W. B. Saunders Co., 1981.)

fluid (*liquor folliculi*) and the ovum and corona radiata are discharged from the ovary (Fig. 4–18).

The exact mechanism of ovulation itself is not well understood, but experimental evidence suggests that it is a slow process of extrusion, involving a gradual opening and oozing rather than an explosive event.

Variations in the overall number of days in the total cycle are usually variations in the length of the follicular phase.

The Luteal Phase

Following ovulation, the extruded ovum makes its way into the uterine tube. It may be fertilized in the outer one-third of the tube and subsequently makes it way to the uterus. Beginning shortly before ovulation and during the first 3 days following this (about days 14 to 17 of the cycle), capillaries invade the granulosa of the follicle, and both the granulosa and the theca interna become filled with a yellow material, hence the name *corpus luteum* (yellow body).

The corpus luteum produces progesterone and estrogen. Observe in Figure 4–15 that

there is a slight dip in estrogen production following ovulation. This occurs because estrogen secretion by the graafian follicle has ceased, but the corpus luteum is as yet not fully formed and producing estrogen at peak level. Note, in Figure 4–15, that the rise in progesterone level begins before ovulation; this is because the cells of the corpus luteum are beginning to mature in the graafian follicle.

Peak development of the corpus luteum comes about a week after ovulation, or about day 21 of the cycle, the time at which implantation will occur if the ovum is fertilized. From that point in time its development depends upon fertilization. If there is no fertilization, degeneration of the corpus luteum (now called the corpus luteum of menstruation) occurs rapidly. It ceases to secrete progesterone and estrogen, and the level of these hormones falls abruptly. Toward the end of the regressive phase, the corpus luteum is whitish in color and is called the *corpus albicans*. Following degeneration, it is replaced by connective tissue. The drop in hormone production leads to menstruation about a week later (see below).

Should the ovum be fertilized, the life of the corpus luteum (now termed the corpus luteum

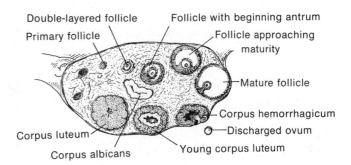

Figure 4–19. Schematic diagram of ovary, showing the sequence of events in origin, growth, and rupture of the ovarian follicle and the formation of retrogression of the corpus luteum. Follow clockwise around the ovary, beginning at the primary follicle.

of pregnancy) is extended by chorionic gonadotropin, which is produced by the trophoblast that developed from the fertilized ovum (Chapter 7). It will then continue to enlarge and be active throughout the first 3 months of pregnancy, with peak production of hormones during the first 60 days. The placenta gradually replaces the corpus luteum as the producer of estrogens and progesterone during pregnancy.

The luteal phase lasts from 13 to 15 days, regardless of the overall duration of the menstrual cycle. A luteal phase of less than 12 days is considered abnormal; a luteal phase of more than 16 days is suggestive of pregnancy. The presence of pregnanediol, a breakdown product of progesterone, in the urine indicates that luteinization has taken place.

The complete ovarian cycle is diagrammed in Figure 4–19 and summarized in calendar form in Figure 4–20.

The Endometrial Cycle

A second cycle, concurrent with and influenced by the ovarian cycle, prepares the endometrium for the implantation of the ovum should fertilization occur. The ovarian cycle involves the ovary; the endometrial cycle involves the uterus.

Before describing the phases of the endometrial cycle, the endometrium itself should be considered in somewhat more detail. Although the line of demarcation between the three layers of the endometrium is not sharp, they are the (1) zona basalis, (2) zona spongiosa, and (3) zona compacta.

The thin zona basalis, which lies next to the myometrium, responds very little to hormonal changes. Portions of the zona spongiosa, in which the endometrial glands are located, respond to ovarian steroids and are shed during menstruation. The zona compacta forms about one-third of the endometrium during the fourteenth to twenty-eighth days of the menstrual cycle. It is totally shed during menstruation.

Like the ovarian cycle, the endometrial cycle is divided into phases. The major phases are the proliferative, which precedes ovulation, and the secretory, which follows it. The first 4 days of the idealized cycle are the menstrual phase; some authors consider the menstrual phase as an early part of the proliferative phase. Terminology varies somewhat from one text to another. Although the menstrual phase

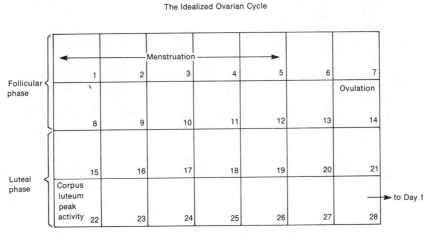

Figure 4–20. Calendar of ovarian cycle.

begins on day 1 of the cycle, in function it is a terminal activity and so will be discussed after the other phases.

The Proliferative Phase

The proliferative phase of the endometrial cycle corresponds to the follicular phase of the ovarian cycle. Estrogens produced by the developing follicles cause the initially thin endometrial epithelium to thicken; the epithelial cells increase in number through mitosis and become taller and columnar. The glands of the zona spongiosa hypertrophy and become more convoluted; blood vessels also grow. At the time of ovulation the endometrium is approx-

imately 2 to 3 mm. thick (0.08 to 0.12 inch) (Fig. 4–21).

The Secretory Phase

Following ovulation, the endometrium continues to thicken in preparation for the fertilized ovum. The secretory phase of the endometrial cycle corresponds to the luteal phase of the ovarian cycle. Glands and blood vessels coil (Fig. 4–21). Progesterone, produced by the corpus luteum, is the principal hormone that influences the changes of the secretory phase. At full development, about a week after ovulation when the endometrium is prepared to receive the embryo, it contains thousands of

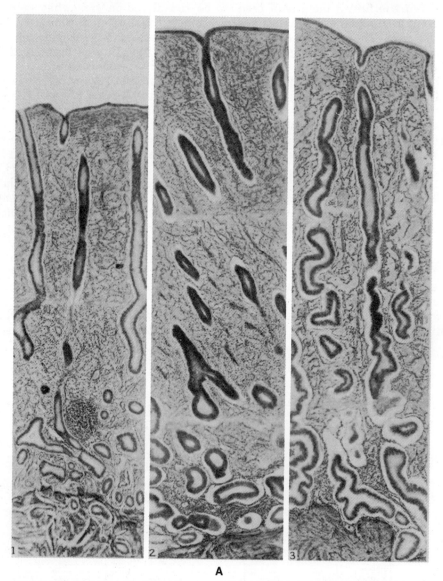

A

Figure 4–21.   Appearance of the human endometrium at various phases of the menstrual cycle. *A,* (1) Midfollicular phase; (2) late follicular phase, and (3) early luteal stage.

Illustration continued on opposite page

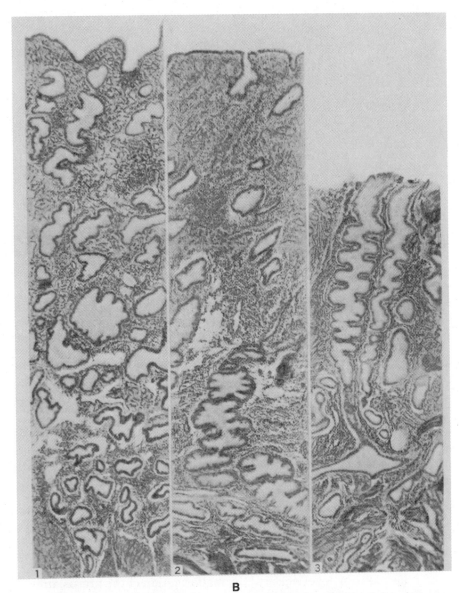

B

Figure 4–21 *Continued. B,* (1) Midluteal stage; (2) late or premenstrual phase; and (3) menstrual phase. (From Papanicolaou, Traut, and Marchetti: *The Epithelia of Woman's Reproductive Organs.* Commonwealth Fund, 1948.)

microscopic blood vessels surrounded by soft, spongy tissue. At this time also (about day 21 of the cycle), the biochemical activities of the endometrium (oxygen consumption, lipid storage, glycogen storage, and so on) are at their maximum, again in readiness for the implantation of the fertilized egg.

As in the ovarian cycle, what happens next depends upon whether or not fertilization occurs. If within 24 to 48 hours of ovulation (days 14 to 16) fertilization does take place, the changes of the secretory phase will continue and intensify under the influence of progesterone from the corpus luteum. If there has been no conception, the corpus luteum regresses, as

described previously, and levels of estrogen and progesterone drop. The endometrium becomes infiltrated by polymorphonuclear leukocytes. The last days of the secretory phase may be called the *ischemic phase* or phase of regression, as the endometrium prepares for menstruation (Fig. 4–22).

The Menstrual Phase

Spiral arteries in the endometrium are the key to the occurrence of menstruation. These arteries are very sensitive to fluctuations in the ovarian steroids. The fall of estrogen and progesterone levels causes the constriction of

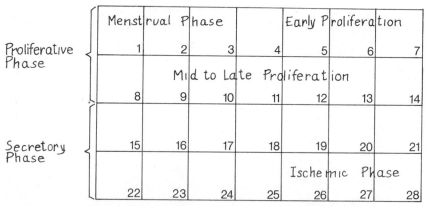

Figure 4–22. Calendar of idealized endometrial cycle.

intermittent segments of the spiral arteries in the endometrium, cutting off the supply of blood to the zona compacta and part of the zona spongiosa.

The combination of vasospasm and loss of hormonal stimulation leads to necrosis in the endometrium, particularly necrosis of the blood vessels. During the 24 to 36 hours preceding the onset of menstruation, blood seeps into the deeper layers of the endometrium, forming hemorrhagic areas. It is at these hemorrhagic sites that the separation of the necrotic outer layers of the endometrium occurs. The desquamated tissue and the blood in the uterine cavity initiate uterine contractions that expel the uterine contents. About 30 to 50 ml. of blood and an additional ounce of serous fluid are expelled during menstruation. When blood loss exceeds 80 ml., iron supplementation is required to prevent anemia. Women who report consistently heavy menstrual periods should have their hemoglobin level checked. *Menorrhagia* is the term for an abnormally heavy menstrual flow.

Physical Symptoms During the Menstrual Phase. Understanding the hormonal and physiologic basis of menstruation is only a part of understanding menstruation as it occurs in the lives of women. Menstruation can be viewed in two interrelated aspects: the physical symptoms encountered and the meaning of menstruation for an individual woman.

Symptoms related to the menstrual cycle fall into the general classifications of premenstrual tension and edema and of dysmenorrhea (painful menstruation).

Premenstrual Tension and Edema. Premenstrual tension is an "umbrella" term that describes a variety of symptoms some women experience for 1 or 2 days, or longer, during the second half of the endometrial cycle. Be-

cause of the timing of premenstrual tension and because the symptoms usually do not occur during anovulatory cycles (although menstruation does), the symptoms are thought to be associated with the corpus luteum. Among the symptoms reported fairly commonly are irritability and nervousness, less purposeful activity, and increased appetite.

Edema is also fairly common in the days prior to menstruation. Edema may be associated with premenstrual tension in some manner. However, successful treatment of the edema has not been shown to relieve the symptoms of premenstrual tension with any more frequency than would treatment with a placebo.

Dysmenorrhea. Dysmenorrhea is classified as primary or secondary. Secondary dysmenorrhea is that condition in which a specific pathologic reason can be demonstrated as the basis for pain. For example, there may be a malformation of the uterus, inflammation, and so on. In primary dysmenorrhea, no specific pathologic cause is discernible.

It is now believed that primary dysmenorrhea is due to contractions of the myometrium induced by prostaglandins, particularly $PGF_{2\alpha}$. Page[21] summarizes the evidence for this theory:

1. Endometrial concentrations of prostaglandins is highest during the menstrual phase.

2. Women with dysmenorrhea have significantly higher concentrations of prostaglandins in the menstrual discharge than do women without dysmenorrhea.

3. When $PGF_{2\alpha}$ is given to women from an exogenous source (i.e., outside their own bodies), symptoms of dysmenorrhea are duplicated.

4. Inhibitors of prostaglandin synthesis such

as aspirin, mefenamic acid (Ponstel), ibuprofen (Motrin), and naprosin (Naproxin) provide significant relief.

The pathogenesis of dysmenorrhea according to this theory is given below.

Shedding of the secretory endometrium
↓
Release of $PGF_{2\alpha}$
↓
myometrial contractions
↓
ischemia
↓
dysmenorrhea

Primary dysmenorrhea occurs only in ovulatory cycles; there is no increase of prostaglandins in proliferative endometrium. In the early months of menstruation following menarche, when cycles are usually anovulatory, primary dysmenorrhea should not occur. When ovulation is inhibited by oral contraceptives (Chapter 6), dysmenorrhea is also relieved.

There is little doubt that dysmenorrhea is a medical problem for a significant number of women in American society. Fay,[10] in a study of 701 girls in grades seven through twelve in Minnesota, found that 279 students (42.5 per cent) reported some pain during their menstrual cycles and that 196 students (27.7 per cent) lost time from school. In the group that reported pain, 76.3 per cent said they required bed rest for relief, 32.2 per cent had consulted a physician, and 66.6 per cent curtailed some favorite activity. Almost all of the students reporting pain said that they took some type of medication for it, including aspirin, aspirin with codeine, sleeping pills, and tranquilizers.

In another study, Doster[9] found that 38 per cent of a group of 1410 senior high school girls reported dysmenorrhea. Two-thirds of the girls with dysmenorrhea reported that they sometimes missed school because of it, and nearly half (45 per cent) reported that they missed school during every menstrual period. Eighty per cent said that they needed some degree of bed rest, and 73 per cent felt that their pain required medication. Doster used the same questionnaire to study 720 women employees in the Denver school system and summarized his data with women classified into two groups—one of teachers and clerical workers (white collar workers) and the other of lunchroom workers. While a higher percentage of white collar workers reported having had dysmenorrhea at some time, more lunchroom workers said they had dysmenorrhea regularly. Other studies of the frequency of dysmenorrhea have been done by Golub and Goldenwasser.

Table 4–2 summarizes Mead's findings concerning menstrual pain in a group of 25 adolescent girls in three villages in Samoa.[19] Future studies that try to differentiate women who have dysmenorrhea regularly from those who rarely do would seem very important, as this is a physical problem that involves so many women.

NURSING ASSESSMENT AND INTERVENTION. The nursing assessment of dysmenorrhea is summarized in Nursing Care Plan 4–1. Pharmacologic treatment of dysmenorrhea is now directed either at prostaglandin inhibition, using the medications mentioned above, or at prevention of ovulation in sexually active women through the use of oral contraceptives. Primary dysmenorrhea frequently improves following pregnancy, possibly because the increased uterine blood flow developed during pregnancy reduces the likelihood of ischemia.

Not every woman with dysmenorrhea requires pharmacologic intervention. Heat, applied either locally (e.g., with a heating pad) or from a warm bath or shower, leads to muscle relaxation and vasodilation (and thus to reduced ischemia and increased elimination of menstrual fluid). Regular exercise also reduces muscle tension and improves circulation. Several techniques taught in childbirth education classes, including relaxation, effleurage (light massage of the abdomen), slow chest breath-

Table 4–2. MENSTRUAL PAIN AMONG 25 SAMOAN GIRLS*

Amount of Discomfort	Number	Per Cent
None	2	8
Abdominal only	3	12
Back only	10	40
Abdominal and back	4	16
Extreme discomfort†	6	24

*From Mead, M.: *Coming of Age in Samoa.* New York, New American Library, 1949.
†Extreme discomfort was so characterized by the girls; in no instance were the girls so ill that they could not work.

Nursing Care Plan 4–1.   Caring for Women with Dysmenorrhea

NURSING GOALS: To assist women with dysmenorrhea in coping with periodic discomfort.

OBJECTIVES: The woman with dysmenorrhea will:
1. Be aware of physiologic, psychological and socio-cultured factors which contribute to dysmenorrhea.
2. Be able to utilize a variety of strategies to cope with dysmenorrhea.

ASSESSMENT	POTENTIAL DIAGNOSIS	NURSING INTERVENTION	RATIONALE/ COMMENTS
1. Knowledge and attitudes a. knowledge of menstruation. b. attitude of mother and significant others. c. cultural attitudes and beliefs about menstruation.	Need for information about menstruation, dysmenorrhea. Need for referral to evaluate possible underlying pathology.	Provide information about physiology of menstruation, dysmenorrhea (see text). Help woman to recognize influence of significant others, cultural beliefs. Referral if indicated.	Prior knowledge may influence expectation of dysmenorrhea. Attitudes of others may predispose toward expectation of dysmenorrhea.

2. Menstrual history
a. date of menarche
b. characteristics of cycle:
    duration (2–5 days)
    amount of flow (30–100 ml. average)
    character of flow (dark red; usually without clots)
    interval (may vary from 18 to 40 days; mean 30 days)
			First periods are anovulatory; primary dysmenorrhea should not occur.
			
			Characteristics outside of a range of normal may indicate underlying pathology.

3. Use of contraceptives a. oral contraceptives b. intrauterine device			Oral contraceptives alleviate dysmenorrhea. Intrauterine device may increase dysmenorrhea.
4. Reproductive history a. Pregnancies. b. Obstetric or gynecologic trauma.			Pregnancies may relieve primary dysmenorrhea. Trauma (gynecologic or obstetric) may lead to secondary dysmenorrhea.

5. Methods now used for relief of discomfort.
a. Non-pharmacologic.
b. Pharmacologic.
	Need for information about effective coping methods.	A. Provide information about non-pharmacologic method:
		1. heat
		2. regular exercise
		3. relaxation techniques
		4. effleurage
		5. dietary modifications
		    a. Decreased sodium intake 7 days prior to onset of menses.
		
		    b. Use of foods containing natural diuretics, such as coffee, tea, asparagus.
		    c. Increase intake of B-complex vitamins (meats, esp. pork, liver, poultry; peanut butter, dried beans and peas, milk, fish).
		    d. Increased protein.
		
		B. Medication inhibits prostaglandin synthesis (aspirin, mefenamic acid, ibuprofen, naprosin)
			
			Decrease fluid retention.
			
			Decrease fluid retention.
			
			Inactivation of excess estrogen by liver.
			Increase in use of protein.
			Decrease in fatigue, depression, tension.
			
			Altered carbohydrate metabolism may lead to hypoglycemia.
			May be helpful in inactivation of excess estrogen by liver.

ing, and exercises such as pelvic rock have been found valuable in treating dysmenorrhea (see Chapter 11). The physiologic contractions of orgasm, which facilitate menstrual flow and relieve pelvic congestion, are helpful to some women.[11] Dietary modifications that have been effective in some women are described in Table 4–3.

As nurses, we can suggest these techniques, recognizing that what is effective for one woman may not be the most helpful regimen for another. Dysmenorrhea may have socio-logic components (a cultural expectation of discomfort) and emotional as well as physio-logic components for an individual woman. All of these factors must be evaluated in helping women become more comfortable during men-struation.

In addition to pain from ischemia, dysmen-orrhea may also be accompanied by systemic symptoms including nausea or vomiting, diar-rhea (due to side effects of prostaglandins that increase gastrointestinal motility), backache, fatigue, vertigo, and syncope.

Menstruation and Toxic Shock Syndrome. The first description of toxic shock syndrome was published by Todd.[23] Todd's study included seven children aged 8 to 17 years and did not relate toxic shock syndrome to menstruation. In 1980, however, a series of reports by the Center for Disease Control[3, 4, 5]

Table 4–3. DIETARY MODIFICATIONS AND DYSMENORRHEA

Dietary Modification	Rationale
Decreased sodium intake 7 days prior to onset of menses	Decrease fluid retention
Use of foods containing natural diuretics, such as coffee, tea, asparagus	Decrease fluid retention
Increase intake of B-complex vitamins (meats, especially pork, liver, and poultry; peanut butter, dried beans and peas, milk, fish)	Inactivation of excess estrogen by liver Increase in use of protein Decrease in fatigue, depression, tension
Increased protein	Altered carbohydrate metabolism may lead to hypoglycemia May be helpful in inactivation of excess estrogen by liver

linked toxic shock syndrome to the use of tampons during menstruation. The problem does not appear to be the tampon per se but tampon use in susceptible individuals. The following chain of events have been proposed:

Susceptible woman colonized
with Staphylococcus aureus
↓
Uses tampon during menstruation
↓
Tampon causes microabrasions of vaginal mucosa
↓
Exotoxin enters circulation

Since *Staphylococcus aureus* is not an un-common organism and tampons have been widely used for a number of years, why has a new syndrome appeared? One possibility is a change in tampon composition. Prior to 1977 tampons were made of rayon or rayon and cotton blends. After 1977 more absorbent syn-thetic materials were utilized; some of these materials, like the carboxymethyl cellulose used in Rely tampons, are an excellent culture medium in the presence of moisture. All types of tampons have been associated with toxic shock syndrome, but Rely tampons, a "super-absorbent variety," was the brand most fre-quently implicated. Rely tampons were vol-untarily withdrawn from the market in 1980 following reports from the Center for Disease Control.

Toxic shock syndrome is a total body, mul-tiorgan disease. The case definition is sum-marized in Table 4–4. A case definition speci-fies the criteria by which a syndrome is defined.

Much of the treatment is supportive. Large volumes of intravenous fluids plus albumin and dopamine are used to treat the hypoten-sion that is frequently severe and difficult to control. Penicillinase-resistant penicillin is used against *Staphylococcus aureus*. Many women arrive at hospital unconscious; the ad-mitting nurse should always check for a tam-pon (or tampons) in the vagina. Treatment will be ineffective if the tampon remains. Most patients will begin to improve in 2 to 3 days. Approximately 1 to 2 weeks following the onset of the syndrome, there will be desquamation of the palms of the hands or soles of the feet and sometimes of other areas of the body as well. Mortality is approximately 10%. In some survivors, there are apparent long-term seque-lae, including abnormal electroencephalogram and changes in short-term memory.[25] There does seem to be a spectrum of disease, however, with some individuals displaying milder symp-

Table 4–4. CASE DEFINITION: TOXIC SHOCK SYNDROME

1. Fever — T 38.9° C. (102° F)
2. Rash — Diffuse macular erythroderma
3. Desquamation — 1 to 2 weeks after onset of illness, particularly of palms and soles
4. Hypotension — Systolic blood pressure 90 mm. Hg for adults or 5th percentile by age for children 16 years of age or orthostatic syncope
5. Involvement of three or more of the following organ systems:
   a. Gastrointestinal — vomiting or diarrhea at onset of illness
   b. Muscular — severe myalgia or creatine phosphokinase 2 times upper limit of normal
   c. Mucous membrane — vaginal, oropharyngeal, or conjunctival hyperemia
   d. Renal — BUN or creatinine values 2 times upper limit normal or 5 white blood cells per high power field, in the absence of urinary tract infection
   e. Hepatic — total bilirubin, SGOT, or SGPT 2 times upper limit normal
   f. Hematologic — platelets 100,000
   g. Central nervous system — disorientation or alterations in consciousness without focal neurologic signs when fever and hypotension are absent
6. Negative results on the following tests, if obtained:
   a. Blood, throat, or cerebrospinal fluid cultures
   b. Serologic tests for Rocky Mountain spotted fever, leptospirosis, or measles

toms. The disease can recur, emphasizing the importance of educating individuals who have had toxic shock syndrome.

Nurses can help to prevent instances of toxic shock syndrome through education of all menstruating women about tampon use (Table 4–4) and education of women who have had toxic shock syndrome about the prevention of recurrence. Recognition of milder forms of the disease symptoms during a menstrual period in a woman using tampons *may* prevent a subsequent, more serious form; this idea is unconfirmed but seems logical. Persons with toxic shock syndrome require the meticulous nursing care given to all critically ill patients.

Cyclic Changes in the Endometrium

Endometrial Hyperplasia and the Endometrial Cycle. When ovulation does not occur, the endometrium continues to proliferate under the influence of estrogen. Eventually there will be marked endometrial hyperplasia (i.e., cell proliferation). When estrogen levels do fall, the endometrium will often be shed in a patchy fashion, with excessive and prolonged bleeding.

Endometriosis and the Endometrial Cycle. Endometriosis occurs when patches of endometrium are found outside the uterus, most often in the cul-de-sac, the uterine ligaments, the ovaries, or the serosa of the uterus and bowel. The mechanism causing this is

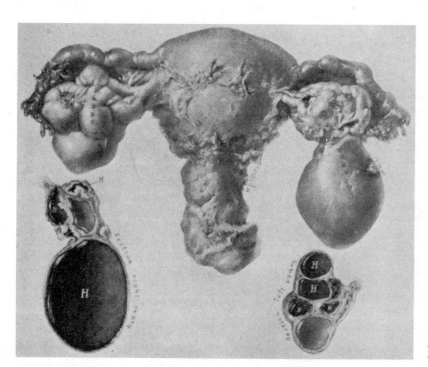

Figure 4–23. The gross appearance of endometriosis of the ovaries. Cross sections of ovaries show the hematomas (chocolate cysts). (From Sampson: *American J. Obstetrics and Gynecology,* 4:489, 1922.)

believed to be the regurgitation of menstrual blood through the uterine tubes. When endometriosis occurs in the ovaries, cysts filled with old blood (chocolate cysts) are a classic finding (Fig. 4–23).

Endometriosis most commonly occurs in white women who have never been pregnant; many have long-term infertility. Typically many are unmarried career women. This *may* be related to the production of progestins that occurs during pregnancy; progestins do cause endometriosis to regress and are one form of therapy. Surgery is also used in the treatment of some women.

Endometriosis may be quite painful, particularly during the menstrual phase (the endometrium outside the uterus responds to the hormonal cycle in the same way that the uterine lining does). On the other hand, some women have few symptoms.

Other Cyclic Changes in the Endometrium. As Figure 4–24 indicates, there are many additional changes in the endometrium that can be used to "date" the cells taken

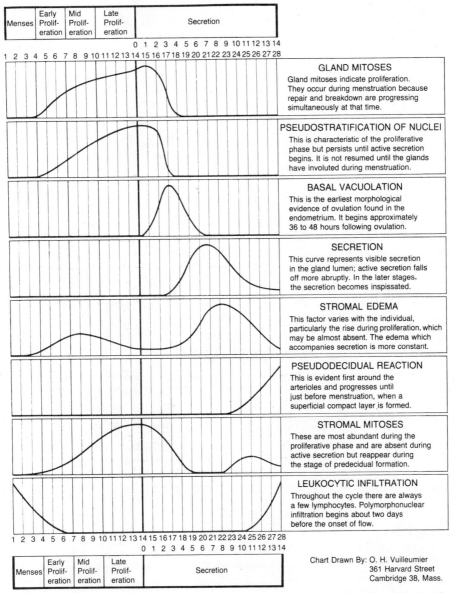

DATING THE ENDOMETRIUM
APPROXIMATE RELATIONSHIP OF USEFUL MORPHOLOGICAL FACTORS

GLAND MITOSES
Gland mitoses indicate proliferation. They occur during menstruation because repair and breakdown are progressing simultaneously at that time.

PSEUDOSTRATIFICATION OF NUCLEI
This is characteristic of the proliferative phase but persists until active secretion begins. It is not resumed until the glands have involuted during menstruation.

BASAL VACUOLATION
This is the earliest morphological evidence of ovulation found in the endometrium. It begins approximately 36 to 48 hours following ovulation.

SECRETION
This curve represents visible secretion in the gland lumen; active secretion falls off more abruptly. In the later stages, the secretion becomes inspissated.

STROMAL EDEMA
This factor varies with the individual, particularly the rise during proliferation, which may be almost absent. The edema which accompanies secretion is more constant.

PSEUDODECIDUAL REACTION
This is evident first around the arterioles and progresses until just before menstruation, when a superficial compact layer is formed.

STROMAL MITOSES
These are most abundant during the proliferative phase and are absent during active secretion but reappear during the stage of predecidual formation.

LEUKOCYTIC INFILTRATION
Throughout the cycle there are always a few lymphocytes. Polymorphonuclear infiltration begins about two days before the onset of flow.

Chart Drawn By: O. H. Vuilleumier
361 Harvard Street
Cambridge 38, Mass.

Figure 4–24. Criteria for dating the endometrium. Each curve represents the approximate quantitative change in each of eight factors considered most helpful. (From Noyes, Hertig, and Rock: *Fertility and Sterility, 1*:3, 1950.)

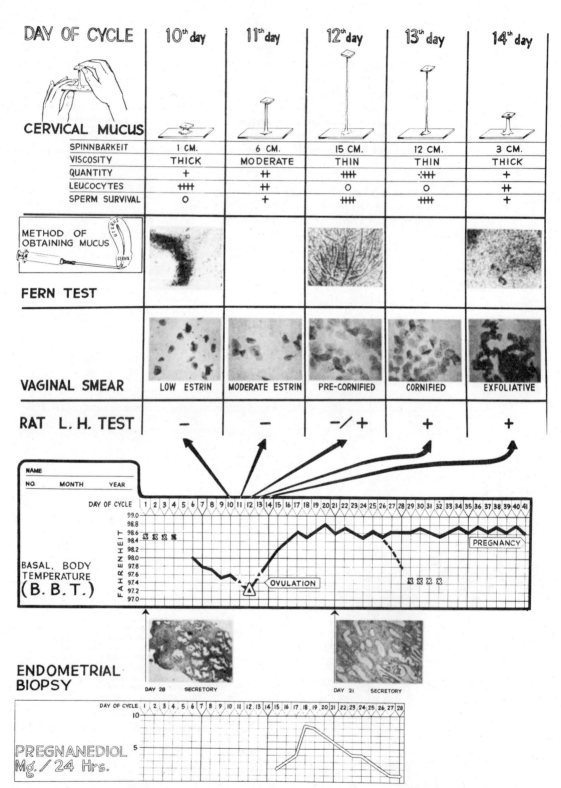

DAY OF CYCLE	10th day	11th day	12th day	13th day	14th day
CERVICAL MUCUS					
SPINNBARKEIT	1 CM.	6 CM.	15 CM.	12 CM.	3 CM.
VISCOSITY	THICK	MODERATE	THIN	THIN	THICK
QUANTITY	+	++	+++	+++	+
LEUCOCYTES	+++	++	O	O	++
SPERM SURVIVAL	O	+	+++	+++	+

METHOD OF OBTAINING MUCUS

FERN TEST

VAGINAL SMEAR	LOW ESTRIN	MODERATE ESTRIN	PRE-CORNIFIED	CORNIFIED	EXFOLIATIVE

| **RAT L. H. TEST** | − | − | −/+ | + | + |

BASAL, BODY TEMPERATURE (B.B.T.)

OVULATION

PREGNANCY

ENDOMETRIAL BIOPSY

DAY 28   SECRETORY   DAY 21   SECRETORY

PREGNANEDIOL Mg./24 Hrs.

Figure 4–25.   Clinical and laboratory changes at the time of ovulation. (From Cohen: Lying-in. *J. of Reproductive Medicine, 1*:182, 1968.)

during an endometrial biopsy to determine what is happening during the cycle. Such studies are helpful in the evaluation of various gynecologic problems, particularly infertility.

Changes in the Cervical Mucus

The mucus secreted by the endocervical glands also changes with the levels of estrogen and progesterone. Immediately following menstruation, when the level of both hormones is low, secretion of mucus is slight and the mucus is quite sticky. As the level of estrogen rises, secretion of mucus increases, and the mucus becomes more and more elastic. By day 13 of the idealized cycle, cervical mucus exhibits *spinnbarkeit* and *ferning*.

Spinnbarkeit (literally the ability to spin) refers to the property of cervical mucus to make a thread when it is placed between two glass slides. The length of the spinnbarkeit varies over a period of several days. It is longest immediately prior to ovulation (Fig. 4–25); at this time the cervical mucus resembles fresh egg white, both in appearance and viscosity.

Ferning describes the branching pattern that cervical mucus exhibits just prior to ovulation when it is allowed to dry on a glass slide. Ferning is caused by the increased sodium and water content of the mucus at this time. The disappearance of spinnbarkeit and

ferning indicates that ovulation has occurred (see discussion of infertility, Chapter 6).

As progesterone secretion rises during the second half of the cycle, endocervical glands secrete a thick mucus that impedes sperm migration. This property is an important factor in the contraceptive effect of progestins. As progesterone levels fall toward the end of the cycle, mucus again becomes scant.

Changes in the Vagina

Both the epithelial cells of the vagina and vaginal pH are influenced by the hormonal cycle. Cells exhibit different characteristics at different stages that may be identified by laboratory examination. The pH of the vagina is acid through much of the cycle (pH about 4.0 to 5.0). This is probably because of the activity of vaginal tract bacilli, which break down glycogen, producing lactic acid. The pH rises shortly before and during the menstrual phase because of alkaline cervical secretions and menstrual flow.

Changes in Basal Body Temperature

At approximately the time of ovulation or shortly afterward, basal body temperature (BBT), the temperature of the body at rest, rises. The increase is usually from 0.4 to 1.0 degree (Fig. 4–26). The rise is believed to be

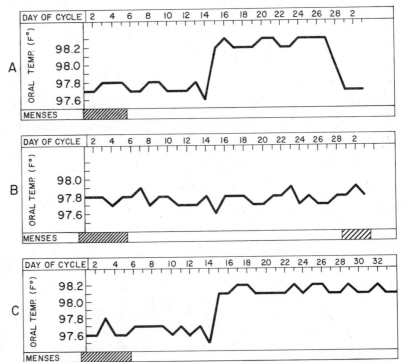

Figure 4–26. Typical oral basal body temperature curves in *A*, a normal cycle; *B*, an anovulatory cycle; and *C*, early pregnancy. (From Page, Villee, and Villee: *Human Reproduction: Essentials of Reproductive and Perinatal Medicine.* 3rd Edition. Philadelphia, W. B. Saunders Co., 1981.)

influenced by progesterone. Immediately prior to the temperature rise, there is often a marked drop, also illustrated by Figure 4–26.

A record of basal body temperature may be kept by a woman who is using the temperature-calendar method of contraception (Chapter 6) or by a woman with an infertility problem (Chapter 6). Special graphs are available for recording BBT. It is very important that any woman who is recording BBT, for whatever reason, understand that she must take her temperature each morning before she gets out of bed. The thermometer should be kept at the bedside and should even be shaken down the night before. If she rises to get the thermometer or to go to the bathroom before she takes her temperature, the BBT will not be valid.

Note in Figure 4–26 the temperature variations during an anovulatory cycle and when pregnancy occurs. If pregnancy does occur, the BBT remains high because progesterone continues to be secreted.

The Climacteric

The *climacteric* is that period of time, usually several years, during which ovarian function becomes less and less responsive to the stimulation of the gonadotropic hormones. Ovulation eventually ceases, and estrogen production slowly declines.

Menopause is the specific point in time at which menstruation ceases. (The word is often used incorrectly to refer to the climacteric.) The date of a woman's menopause can be determined only in retrospect. When she has not menstruated for a period of 6 months, the date of her last menstrual period is considered to mark her menopause.

While the body is in this process of disengagement from its cyclic preparation for pregnancy, pregnancy is possible and does occur during the climacteric. Since mothers of this age (commonly 45 to 55) are felt to be obstetrically at risk and the risk of a defective baby is greatly increased, contraception is usually advised for a year following the menopause.

The majority of the physiologic changes and symptoms of the climacteric (summarized in Table 4–5) are related to the decrease in estrogen production. No woman exhibits all of the symptoms noted; most will exhibit one or two, a few several. The difference is due in part to the fact that the amount of estrogen decrease varies from one woman to another. Estrogen is produced by the adrenal cortex as well as by the ovaries. In some women, estrogen production may be sufficiently adequate so that few

or no symptoms occur. The cells of the vagina may continue to show the effects of estrogen for more than 10 years after the cessation of menstruation. Possibly emotional factors, such as a woman's feelings about her life and about her femininity also influence the severity of some symptoms of the climacteric (Chapter 5).

Although estrogen production declines, the gonadotropic hormones not only continue to be produced but are produced in excess. (Remember the feedback mechanism; as estrogen and progesterone levels rise, the levels of the gonadotropic hormones decrease. During the climacteric, estrogen does not respond to the secretion of FSH and so more FSH is secreted.) Thus, the level of gonadotropins in the urine of the postmenopausal woman is high; this urine is the source of human gonadotropins used therapeutically to stimulate follicular growth.

Estrogen Replacement Therapy

It is readily apparent from scanning Table 4–5 that most of the changes that occur during the climacteric and in postmenopausal women are related to the decreased production of estrogen. Many physicians feel that this represents an endocrine deficiency and therefore feel that estrogen should be replaced for the remainder of life, just as other hormones are replaced when they are deficient. Other physicians use estrogen replacement only in specific individual instances. It is virtually always prescribed for women whose ovaries are diseased or removed before the age of 45. The dosage given to postmenopausal women is usually lower than that given to younger women for various gynecologic reasons.

There are certain disadvantages and contraindications to estrogen therapy, probably the chief reason why there is not universal agreement about its value. Episodes of uterine bleeding may occur, although this is often caused by a dose that is larger than necessary. Because estrogen appears to accelerate the growth of endometrial and breast cancers, it is contraindicated in women who have had any history of these malignancies within the preceding 5 years. Mainly as a precaution against the development of these malignancies, a regimen of 21 days of medication followed by 7 days of no medication is usually suggested.

Since the purpose of hormonal therapy prior to menopause is often to stimulate normal ovarian function, both estrogen and a progestin may be given. Following menopause or total hysterectomy, only estrogen is used.

Estrogen therapy, once started, should not be discontinued abruptly. Estrogen can be

Table 4–5. PHYSIOLOGIC CHANGES IN PERIMENOPAUSAL AND POSTMENOPAUSAL WOMEN

	Symptoms	Physiologic Basis
SYSTEMIC CHANGES	Hot flashes: sudden sensations of heat. Night sweats. Flushes: sudden reddening of face. Cold hands and feet (decreased blood supply). Dizziness (episodic decreased blood supply to brain).	Withdrawal of estrogen after many years of exposure *may* cause instability in hypothalamic vasomotor centers. Blood vessels do not dilate and constrict as formerly. These are probably the most widely discussed symptoms of the climacteric, but occur in only 20 per cent of women.
MUSCLE CHANGES	Decline in general muscle tone: Supporting muscles of uterus, bladder, and rectum lose tone and strength; muscle strength declines in arms and legs; decline in smooth muscles of bladder wall.	Estrogens function in protein storage, needed for muscle development.
REPRODUCTIVE CHANGES	Menstrual irregularity. Atrophic changes in vagina: vagina shortens, becomes more narrow, less elastic, and more susceptible to inflammation, infection, irritation, itching, discharge. Lining of vagina becomes pale and thin; may be painful during intercourse (dyspareunia). Shrinking of uterus.	Withdrawal of estrogen.
SKELETAL CHANGES	Osteoporosis leads to: loss of body height increased incidence of fractures slow healing of bone weakening of spinal vertebrae with low back pain, bowed posture, "dowager hump." Changes in joint cartilage may lead to aching joints.	Estrogen aids bone to utilize calcium; in the absence of estrogen, bone demineralization is significantly accelerated.
SKIN CHANGES	Fat pads beneath skin absorbed. Elastic material within skin absorbed; wrinkling. Brown spots on skin. Loss of firmness of breasts.	
CORONARY ATHEROSCLEROSIS	Thickening of arteries appears to be hastened.	Estrogen deficiency appears to correlate with the development of arteriosclerosis; conclusive evidence lacking.
MISCELLANEOUS CHANGES	Burning on urination following intercourse.	Thinning of vaginal lining between vagina and bladder and urethra.

gradually discontinued, but sudden withdrawal may result in endocrine imbalance and serious mental distress. Arras[2] reports evaluating a patient who became withdrawn, confused, and semicomatose following a mitral commissurotomy. When several weeks of studies failed to reveal a reason for her mental symptoms, she was to be transferred to a mental institution. A nurse during a clinical conference asked why her estrogens had never been restarted (she had had a total hysterectomy 2 years before). In less than 24 hours after estrogen therapy was resumed, the patient began to communicate; within 8 days she was planning her discharge from the hospital and her return to work.

Sexual Intercourse

The reproductive organs function not only in the production of hormones and of ova and spermatogonia, but also as the means of sexual intercourse. Intercourse is very much more than a physiologic phenomenon. Katchadourian states, "There is no denying the importance of knowing where the nerve centers are, but the current that feeds those centers is emotion."[16] In subsequent chapters we will look at the social and emotional factors in human sexuality during particular stages of life. Our purpose here is to examine the physiologic aspects of sexual intercourse as a foundation for understanding some of the concerns of couples during pregnancy and in the postpartum period and the interrelation between intercourse and fertilization, contraception, and infertility.

Physiologic Reactions to Sexual Stimuli

Sexual stimulation, whatever its source, activates the parasympathetic nervous system and inhibits the sympathetic system. An almost immediate reaction to parasympathetic stimulation is the relaxation of the arterial walls, which leads to *vasocongestion,* as more blood flows into an area than can be handled quickly by the veins. The most dramatic example of vasocongestion is the erection of the penis. Arterial blood under high pressure flows into the corpora cavernosa and spongiosum, the erectile tissue of the penis (see Fig. 4–1). Because venous flow is partially occluded and because the erectile tissue is surrounded by a strong fibrous coat, the pressure causes ballooning of the erectile tissue, and the penis becomes long and hard. The testes also increase in size because of vasocongestion.

Vasocongestion also occurs in the vaginal walls, which become darker in color. The congested walls of the lower vagina are called the *orgasmic platform* (Fig. 4–27). The clitoris, like its homologue the penis, also becomes erect from vasocongestion, although more slowly. The labia, uterus, and breasts are also affected and increase in size as well as change in color. In both men and women a flushing response of the skin, temperature change, and perspiration accompany sexual activity, again related to vasodilation and congestion. Skin reactions are somewhat more common in women.

A second physiologic response is increased muscle tension. Muscle tone increases in both smooth and skeletal muscles; part of the increase is voluntary, such as the flexing of muscles, and part involuntary, such as the muscular contractions of orgasm. The myometrium of the uterus also contracts, a consideration in planning care for some women who are pregnant.

Other physiologic responses include elevation of heart rate, blood pressure, and respiratory rate; hyperventilation; and increased secretion of saliva.

Secretion in the genital area (as well as of the sweat and salivary glands) is another correlate of sexual arousal. In males the genital secretion is limited. The bulbourethral (Cowper's) glands may secrete a small amount of alkaline mucus, which may neutralize the urethra (through which acidic urine has passed) and make it "safer" for sperm survival.

The vagina secretes a clear, alkaline fluid that may also neutralize the normally acid vaginal tract. The mechanism of vaginal secre-

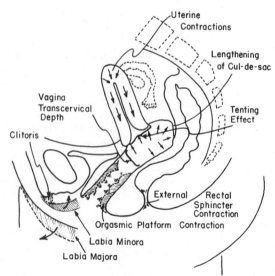

Figure 4–27. The female pelvis, orgasmic phase. (From Masters and Johnson: *Human Sexual Response.* Boston, Little, Brown & Co., 1966.)

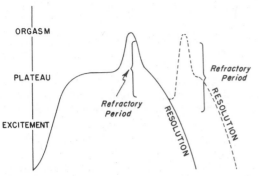

Figure 4–28. The male sexual response cycle. (From Masters and Johnson: *Human Sexual Response.* Boston, Little, Brown & Co., 1966.)

tion is unclear; it may be related to vasocongestion. The female bulbourethral (Bartholin's) glands and the cervix contribute limited secretions.

The Cycle of Sexual Response

In both men and women sexual response occurs in four phases: (1) the excitement phase, (2) the plateau phase, (3) the orgasmic phase, and (4) the resolution phase.

The *excitement* phase is the time of arousal. The couple become more aware of sexual excitement and less aware of other factors in their environment. Strong distractions, either internal or external, may inhibit sexual desire during the early part of the excitement phase. For example, a parent's concern about a new baby (internal) or the baby's cry (external) may be a barrier to sexual arousal.

The *plateau* phase precedes orgasm and is characterized by intense muscle tone throughout the body. Sensory perception of other stimuli is poor and becomes even less acute as *orgasm* is approached. Other changes already described—flushed skin, pounding heart, heavy breathing, and so on—also mark the plateau phase.

At the moment of orgasm, voluntary control is lost; the response not only is genital but also involves the entire body. Women are physiologically capable of multiple orgasms in rapid succession; men are not (see refractory period, below).

During the *resolution* phase, which follows orgasm, both genital organs and other body areas return to a prearousal state. Many persons feel pleasantly weary and go to sleep. Others may feel exhilarated, relaxed, hungry, or thirsty or may experience one of a wide variety of other possibilities.

While there is considerable individual variation, sexual responses are basically similar in both men and women. However, certain important differences do exist. Figure 4–28 diagrams male sexual response, based on the research of Masters and Johnson; Figure 4–29 illustrates female response.[18] Note the presence of a refractory period in the male cycle. (The term *refractory period* refers to the time that must elapse, following stimulation, before a cell, tissue, or organ can respond again.) During the refractory period, a male cannot respond to sexual stimulation, no matter how intense it is. No such refractory period occurs in females, hence the potential for multiple orgasms. Note also in comparing Figures 4–28 and 4–29 that while there is one basic pattern for male response, several variations in response are possible for females.

There is a great deal more that might be said about the physiology of sexual intercourse. Particularly helpful sources of information are Masters and Johnson[18] and Katchadourian and Lunde.[17]

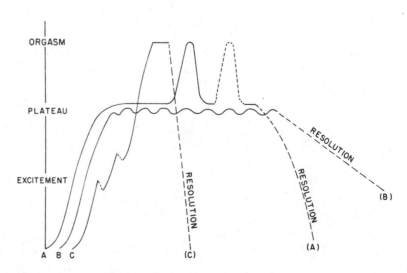

Figure 4–29. The female sexual response cycle. (From Masters and Johnson: *Human Sexual Response.* Boston, Little, Brown & Co., 1966.)

Fertilization as Result of Sexual Intercourse

When sexual stimulus becomes intense, the reflex centers of the spinal cord send out rhythmic sympathetic impulses to initiate *emission,* the forerunner of ejaculation. Peristaltic contractions begin in the ducts of each testis, the epididymis, and the vas deferens, and spermatozoa enter the internal urethra.

Ejaculation follows when impulses sent from the spinal cord to the skeletal muscles encasing the base of the erectile tissue of the penis cause rhythmic increases in the pressure of the erectile tissue. Semen is thus expressed from the urethra to the exterior. The average ejaculation contains approximately 100 million spermatozoa, some of which will be either immature or "senescent." Although only a single sperm will fertilize the ovum, the number of sperm is a significant factor in fertility (Chapter 6).

Spermatozoa are deposited at the mouth (os) of the cervix. Pregnancies have been reported from semen deposited on or near the vulva without intromission, a factor that is an important consideration in evaluating certain contraceptive practices, such as coitus interruptus (Chapter 6).

Throughout most of the cycle, viscid cervical mucus is a barrier to the ascent of the sperm from the cervix through the uterus to the uterine tube, where fertilization normally occurs. Sperm appear in the cervical mucus almost immediately after coitus; many never pass further. It has already been noted in the discussion of estrogen that at the time of ovulation the mucus increases in amount and becomes less viscid, making it more favorable for sperm penetration than at other times. Progesterone, on the other hand, makes the mucus unfavorable for sperm migration, so that very few reach the endometrial cavity either during the luteal phase of the menstrual cycle or when a woman is taking an oral contraceptive containing progestin.

Spermatozoa probably pass through the cervix by the movement of their tails. Upon reaching the uterus, they are apparently assisted in their passage to the tube by uterine contractions rather than by their own motility. Prostaglandins *may* be the agents that initiated the uterine contractions following coitus.

Probably only a few hundred to a few thousand of the original millions of sperm ever reach the ovum in the distal uterine tube. Those that do, however, do so in a few minutes. These few are likely the healthiest and the most vigorous sperm. Other sperm remain in the cervix, in the junction between the uterus and the tube, and in the isthmus of the tube. Some pass out of the body; others enter the endometrium of the uterus or the peritoneal cavity.

Additional Factors in Biologic Readiness

Development of the reproductive tract is the most obvious factor in biologic readiness for pregnancy. However, a number of additional biologic factors interact to affect the body's readiness. Such factors should be a part of educational programs for young people prior to the time of first sexual intercourse and also for women during and after childbirth. They include: (1) parental age, (2) maternal nutrition, (3) maternal health (chronic conditions, infectious processes, and use of medication), (4) hereditary disorders, and (5) Rh incompatibility.

Each of these areas is discussed more fully in the chapters that follow.

REFERENCES

1. Applebaum, R. M.: The Modern Management of Successful Breast Feeding. *Pediatric Clinics of North America,* 17:203, 1970.
2. Arras, B.: Don't Underrate Those Clinical Conferences. *RN, 38*(7):41, 1975.
3. Center for Disease Control: Toxic shock syndrome—United States. *Morbidity and Mortality Weekly Report, 29,* 229, May 23, 1980.
4. Center for Disease Control: Follow-up on toxic shock syndrome—United States. *Morbidity and Mortality Weekly Report, 29,* 297, June 27, 1980.
5. Center for Disease Control: Follow-up on toxic shock syndrome. *Morbidity and Mortality Weekly Report, 29,* 441, September 19, 1980.
6. Davis, M. E.: *Menopause and Estrogens.* Chicago, Budlong Press, 1969.
7. Diekelmann, N., and Gallaway, K.: A Time of Change. *American Journal of Nursing, 75*:994, 1975.
8. Dienhart, C. M.: *Basic Human Anatomy and Physiology.* 2nd Edition. Philadelphia, W. B. Saunders Co., 1973.
9. Doster, M. E., McNuff, A., Lampe, J., and Corliss, L.: A Survey of Menstrual Function Among 1668 Secondary School Girls and 720 Women Employees of the Denver Public Schools. *American Journal of Public Health, 51*:1841, 1961.
10. Fay, A.: Dysmenorrhea, A School Nurse's Findings. *American Journal of Nursing, 63*:77, 1963.
11. Fogel, C., and Woods, N. (eds.): The Gynecologic Triad: Discharge, Pain, and Bleeding. *In:* Fogel, C., and Woods, N. (eds.): *Health Care of Women: A Nursing Perspective.* St. Louis, C. V. Mosby, Co., 1981.

12. Greenhill, J. P.: *Obstetrics*. 13th Edition. Philadelphia, W. B. Saunders Co., 1965.
13. Greenhill, J. P., and Friedman, E. A.: *Biologic Principles and Modern Practice of Obstetrics*. Philadelphia, W. B. Saunders Co., 1974.
14. Guyton, A. C.: *Basic Human Physiology*. 2nd Edition. Philadelphia, W. B. Saunders Co., 1977.
15. *Introduction to Endocrinology*. Prepared by Educational Design, Inc. for Merrell-National Laboratories. Cincinnati, 1966.
16. Katchadourian, H. A., and Lunde, D. T.: *Fundamentals of Human Sexuality*. New York, Holt, Rinehart & Winston, 1972.
17. Lovesky, J.: Menstruation: Alternatives to Pharmacologic Therapy for Menstrual Distress. *Journal of Nurse Midwifery, 23*:34, 1978.
18. Masters, W. H., and Johnson, V. E.: *Human Sexual Response*. Boston, Little, Brown & Co., 1966.
19. Mead, M.: *Coming of Age in Samoa*. New York, New American Library, 1949.
20. Moore, K. L.: *The Developing Human*. 2nd Edition. Philadelphia, W. B. Saunders Co., 1977.
21. Page, E., Villee, C. A., and Villee, D. B.: *Human Reproduction*. 3rd Edition. Philadelphia, W. B. Saunders Co., 1981.
22. Rose, R. M.: Androgen Excretion in Stress. *In* Bourne, P. G. (ed.): *The Psychology and Physiology of Stress*. New York, Academic Press, 1969.
23. Todd, J., Fishnaualt, M., Kaprol, F., and Welch T.: Toxic shock syndrome associated with phage-group-I staphylococci. *Lancet, 2*:111b, 1978.
24. Tulchinsky, D., and Ryan, K.: *Maternal-Fetal Endocrinology*. Philadelphia, W. B. Saunders Co., 1980.
25. Wager, G.: Toxic shock syndrome. Presentation at Conference of Obstetrical-Gynecological Emergencies. Cook County Graduate School of Medicine, October 6, 1981.
26. Ziegel, E., and Van Blarcom, C. C.: *Obstetric Nursing,* 6th Edition. New York, The Macmillan Co., 1972.

5

The Social and Cultural Context of Childbearing Objectives

If the bearing and rearing of children were solely biologic, human lives would be far less complex—and far less satisfying and interesting. The word "culture" has been used by so many people in so many different ways that it seems important to define it in the way in which it is used here. An early anthropologist, Edward Tylor, described culture as ". . . that complex whole which includes knowledge, belief, art, morals, law, custom or any other capabilities and habits acquired by man as a member of society."[77] All of our behavior that is not instinctive (and very little human behavior is governed by instinct), all that we have learned, and all of our customary ways of doing things are a part of our culture.

Recognizing the influence of culture on childbearing is important for two fundamental reasons:

1. Culture influences how every man and woman experiences and deals with childbearing in his or her own life.

2. Culture affects the way in which *we* as nurses deal with and are affected by childbearing.

Individuals learn many of the values of a society from the families in which they grow to adulthood. These values are supplemented and modified by educational institutions, mass media, and a number of other forces in a technologic society such as our own. Nevertheless, families remain important, and in order to care for childbearing families in the best possible manner, we need to be aware of family characteristics and the ways in which we interact with families of varying lifestyles.

One way of looking at family lifestyles is in terms of social class. Over the past decades a number of similar but slightly varying class groupings have been developed, based on criteria such as income, education, and occupation. These classes have also been divided into subgroups, such as lower-middle, middle-middle, and upper-middle. The semantics of social class designation seem unfortunate. They appear to infer that upper is good and lower is bad. We intend no such judgment here; it is our belief that in each group there are strengths and weaknesses.

Another influence on family lifestyles is ethnicity. The forebears of American families have come from nearly every part of the world. For some families, America has been a "melting pot," and over several generations many cultures have blended. Other families have more distinctive ways of living, either because of their own choosing or because of barriers that have been raised to their entry into the "mainstream" of American life.

Some individuals and families have deliberately chosen alternate lifestyles. Families who participate in the counterculture are an example.

As we examine family lifestyles, even briefly, it is important to recognize other social factors that influence family life. Two interrelated factors that seem particularly relevant to childbearing families at this time are the women's movement and maternal employment.

The discussion in this chapter is necessarily brief. Just as we must continually increase our knowledge of other aspects of nursing practice, we must also grow in our understanding of the significance of culture as it influences families in every aspect of their lives.

Social Class

Families of the Affluent Society

Sociologists divide relatively or absolutely affluent families into three distinct social groups:

1. An upper-middle class of successful professional people, such as physicians, lawyers, and executives of large businesses.

2. A lower-upper class of families with considerable wealth, but wealth that is relatively recently acquired (the newly rich).

3. An upper-upper class, with both great wealth and a certain social prestige that no amount of money can purchase.

Because the number of sociologically defined upper class families is small (in a great many communities there are no people who would be considered upper class by these definitions) and because these families seem to share many characteristics in relation to childbearing, we are grouping them together here.

Both husbands and wives in affluent families are likely to be well educated. Some exceptions occur in the families of professional men who marry before their education is completed, with wives dropping out of school to support the family in the interim.

These families are aware of contraception and probably use it effectively, although other factors besides lack of knowledge (Chapter 6) may certainly influence the occurrence of conception. On the whole, these families are likely to have approximately the number of children they desire when they wish to have them.

Affluent mothers will usually seek good medical care early in pregnancy. Often the doctor will be a personal friend or a neighbor or a member of the same clubs (with the possible exception of families in very large cities). The doctor-patient relationship may be very different from that of the physician treating a blue collar mother, even if the latter is his private patient, or caring for a lower class mother in the outpatient department. Nevertheless, even upper class mothers may be subject to feelings of awe or fear toward their physician. Socialization to respond to the doctor as if he were on a pedestal is not always neutralized by social status or education.

Nurses and student nurses, who are usually from middle class families, sometimes feel threatened by mothers from families more affluent than their own. They may even keep their contacts to a minimum because of such feelings. In our own experience, when students have selected a mother for care and study throughout pregnancy, they have avoided these mothers, saying, "There's nothing I can teach her" or "She already knows everything I can tell her." We believe that such an appraisal is as unfair as assuming that our efforts will be wasted on a lower class mother.

Mothers and fathers in these affluent social groups have a certain amount of flexibility in the extent of involvement that they have with their infants because helpers can be hired. Fathers may be less likely to be participants in routine care, such as diapering, feeding, and bathing the baby, partly because of the press of "business" and partly because it is not customary. For men in the upper levels of corporate business (and perhaps even more for the young, middle class man aspiring to those levels), family relationships are part of a triangle that involves the corporation rather than "another woman" as the third angle. "Success here," said one official, "are guys who eat and sleep the company. If a man's first interest is his wife and family, more power to him—but we don't want him."[85] While such attitudes may have modified somewhat since that statement was made in 1951, partly because such a philosophy is less acceptable to many of today's young families, there is little question that similar attitudes are still present.

We caution against automatically interpreting this difference between upper and middle class norms of father participation, and our own expectations of a father's role, as a lack of caring. In our assessment of parental attitudes toward their baby (a significant part of nursing observation), social class differences should be borne in mind.

Mothers from affluent families may choose to delegate other responsibilities, such as house care, to hired helpers and thus have more time to spend with their babies, or they may allow helpers to assume most or all of their infant's care. The total abdication of responsibilities for baby care—all of the feeding, bathing, and even holding—suggests a rejection of the baby, although it may also indicate a severe lack of self-confidence, fear of harming the baby, anxiety about not being a good mother, or some other factor. How such a lifestyle may affect the baby will be influenced, as least in part, by the relationship that the baby has with other important people in his life—caretakers, grandparents, and the like.

Because most upper and upper-middle class mothers and fathers are reasonably well educated, some may tend to super-intellectualize the experiences of childbirth and the care they plan for their babies. Such trust may be placed in "experts" and books that their own feelings and reactions may be ignored and denied. This is particularly true of first babies, when parents have had no experence of their own with which to temper the advice of "experts." Variations in this experience, or in their baby's characteristics or appearance, may be difficult to cope with. We wish we could say to them, "Relax. Enjoy your baby. He's fine." We may be able to help them accept the concept of "range of normal" behavior that will make them more comfortable with these variations.

Middle Class Families

Middle class families have been grouped in various ways. For our purpose of looking at families in relation to childbearing, we have included the upper-middle class as a category of the affluent family groups. Two large groups remain, which appear to differ in a number of ways: a lower-middle class and a middle-middle class.

LeMasters,[49] calls the lower-middle class the "most rapidly growing group of parents in the United States." At least one factor is the mobility of blue collar workers, as the number of blue collar jobs shrinks and as greater numbers of blue collar children complete high school and at least some additional education.

Lower-middle class parents are usually high school graduates. They may have some college education and may even have graduated from one of the smaller colleges. By occupation they may be salesclerks in small businesses (shoe shops or hardware stores, for example), lower-paid municipal employees, and so on.

Incomes are often less than those of the best-paid blue collar workers, and often wife-mothers work to supplement earnings. While the mother's income is not usually necessary to provide basics such as food and clothing, as it often is in lower class families, her earnings can mean a home in a nicer neighborhood (which, in turn, can mean that her children go to a nicer school), better furniture, a vacation, and so on, all of which are important to these families who identify themselves more closely with the more affluent white collar workers. Credit is often used extensively, and indebtedness may be a chronic state, as the family tries to pattern their standard of living after that of the television family shows and the slick magazines.

Lower-middle class families are often caught in a "crunch" in relation to medical care, including, of course, obstetric care. Economically, they find it increasingly difficult to afford good private care. They may lack the comprehensive hospitalization insurance that gives security to the unionized blue collar worker. Yet they may be ineligible for free care or for care of reduced cost through clinics because their incomes are too high. Moreover, even if they were eligible, their close identification with the middle class may make such care difficult for them to accept. They may be embarrassed when the public health nurse comes to the door, associating her visit with that of the "welfare department." Medical costs can become a real burden if, for example, the mother has a longer period of hospitalization than was expected, or if their baby requires the very expensive care of an intensive care nursery (averaging $200 a day or more). These expenses are not covered by many hospitalization insurance policies, if the family is fortunate enough to have insurance at all.

Lower-middle class marriages tend to have more companionship and less sex-role segregation than do those of blue collar families. Both husband and wife share an interest in their home and in a hope for a better life for their children. Because these families are often upwardly mobile (both husband and wife may have grown up in blue collar families), there is less reliance on other family members (i.e., the extended family of parents, brothers and sisters, aunts and uncles) and more on one another (i.e., the nuclear family). This may limit the kind of support the young couple can count on in caring for the new baby and other young children.

Companionship and cooperation are the expectations of most husbands and wives in *middle class* marriages, even if these are not always found. Indeed, lack of companionship may be seen as a valid reason for divorce. Such cooperation involves not only the sharing of the work to be done, but also the sharing of

ideas and experiences. Much of the impetus for husband-father participation in childbirth comes from this group—in part because of the value given to sharing and also because of an openness to new ideas and a lifestyle that includes participation in groups in which individuals and couples exchange ideas and feelings.

These couples fulfill the expectations that many nurses have of what parents "should" be like. They accept our advice and are interested in the emotional as well as the physical aspects of pregnancy and infant care, a value that we share. Many of our breast-feeding mothers come from these middle class families. In short, our cultural model of the "good mother" and the "good family" is closely related to their behavior. However, we need to be very careful that we don't judge other families by this middle class model, labeling them as less than adequate when they behave in a different way.

The high ideals that middle class parents have for their children can be disadvantageous when both parents feel so overwhelmed by their idea that the total responsibility for producing "the perfect infant" is theirs alone. As a result, they may feel anxious and inadequate.

We also find parents in this class who have a very clear vision (although not always a realistic one) of how they plan to relate to their child in an intellectual and emotional sphere, but a less clear comprehension of day-to-day physical care. The college professor mother who was unsure about how long she should boil her baby's drinking water is an example. One reason for this uncertainty is probably that both fathers and mothers were reared in small, middle class nuclear families themselves and never had much experience with, or even exposure to, small children. David Steinberg writes:

> I knew nothing about babies when Dylan was born. I'm an only child and have never spent any time at all with babies. My confidence in myself as a father was very shaky. I felt deeply afraid of Dylan, always fighting an urge to close my eyes and shove responsibility for him over to Susan . . . I got very depressed at my lack of baby sense.[74]

We find that many middle class mothers share the same kinds of uncertainty, especially with their first babies.

Blue Collar Families

The term "blue collar family" encompasses a large but somewhat diminishing number of Americans, as automation and social change decrease the number of blue collar jobs. Traditionally, these jobs have included factory work, repair work, truck driving, bricklaying, carpentry, and many similar occupations. Many blue collar workers belong to strong labor unions.

There is a considerable range of both income and job security in blue collar families. Incomes may exceed those of many white collar workers, with fringe benefits and seniority within the union system offering a high level of security. Other blue collar workers have incomes that barely meet their basic needs, and jobs that are far less secure.

Segregation of sex roles seems to be a common characteristic of the relationship of many, but not all, blue collar husbands and wives. Some recent observations suggest that this kind of role segregation may be a little less rigid than formerly.

A corollary to segregated sex roles is the more limited communication between men and women, including husbands and wives, than is often found in many middle class families. Lines of communication are strongest between members of the same sex, and especially between family members of the same sex. A woman may turn to her mother or sister for advice; her husband will consult his brother. A nurse or other professional from a middle class environment may wrongly interpret such communication as evidence of a poor family relationship rather than as representative of a cultural pattern.

Families in Poverty

An estimated 12 million or more Americans, roughly 7 per cent of the population, have incomes that barely enable them to meet their daily needs. Sociologists call these families the lower-lower class.

The middle class stereotype of such families is one of unwed mother, nonwhites, and often of people who neither try nor care. Like most stereotypes, it describes some families and misses the mark many times.

For example, while the percentage of families headed by women is certainly higher among the poor (approximately 35 per cent as compared with approximately 14 per cent in the population as a whole), 65 per cent of lower class families are *not* headed by women. And although nonwhite families are overrepresented (only 12 per cent of all families but more than 30 per cent of poor families are nonwhite), it is obvious that the overwhelming number of poor families, nearly 70 per cent, are white.

A knowledge of families who live in poverty is crucially important to nurses who care for mothers and babies. Many will be high-risk mothers or have babies with special needs and problems. Prenatal care is often sporadic or nonexistent. Family planning is ineffective in many instances. Nutrition is usually poor.

Who are these families? They are Spanish-speaking and black families in urban ghettos and Anglo-Saxons in Appalachia. They are black or white farmers in the rural South—some tenants, some with their own small bits of land. They are the migrant families who follow the harvests along the Atlantic Coast from Florida to New England, or from Texas to the mountain states or the Midwest or across the deep South, or along the Pacific Coast. They are displaced farm workers who unsuccessfully sought jobs in the urban North. They are miners displaced by automation. They are American Indians. They are probably the most diverse group of families in the United States.

Not all of the poor are unemployed. Unskilled workers, day laborers, and domestics may work harder on a given day than a middle class man or woman. But income is low and work is often sporadic and inconsistent. A 2-week rainy spell can mean no income for an outdoor laborer. Nor do these jobs carry the fringe benefits—medical insurance, vacations, sick leave, and the like—that offer security to the unionized blue collar worker and the upper-middle class family.

Lower class families are often characterized as being improvident for not planning ahead. The mother who comes to the hospital to deliver with no money set aside to pay her bill, no clothes for the baby, and no bed for him at home is easily labeled a "poor mother" by middle class standards. After all, it is reasoned (and sometimes said) she had 9 months in which to get ready. It is worth considering that each day's needs in that 9 months may have seemed so pressing at the moment that they consumed the limited funds available.

Ethnicity

Black Families

For an increasing number of middle and working class black families, family organization is not unlike that of middle and working class white families. But for the poor black family, especially the family living in an inner city slum or at the end of a rural dirt road, family structure may vary considerably.

Many poor black families are headed by women, probably for a number of reasons. During the days of slavery, marriage between slaves was not recognized, and families were frequently broken up as members were sold to different masters. Black women, who could produce more slaves and who also often served as mistresses for their owners, were often accorded higher status than black men.

In the years that followed the abolition of slavery, job opportunities were often more available for women than for men, both in the rural South and in the North, where 10 million blacks migrated in the years between 1910 and 1960. Many fathers, unable to find employment, fled from their families.

Still another factor is our system of financial support for the poor in the United States (Aid to Families with Dependent Children—AFDC), which in many states does not allow payment if an unemployed father remains at home. Under such a system, families are financially better off if the father leaves than if he were to remain at home without a job. Since fathers with limited education and job skills are often the "last hired and the first fired" from their jobs, it is easy for a family to feel that consistent income from the government is more important than having a father at home.

Extended family organization is frequent in poor black families. In contrast to nuclear families that include only a father, mother, and their nonadult children, in an extended family other relatives live together. If we consider all of the world's families, the extended family system is far more prevalent than the nuclear family organization. There may be a grandmother living with her daughters, her granddaughters, and their children (her great-grandchildren). A teen-aged mother may turn her baby over to her own mother, or even to her grandmother, to care for while she continues her adolescent activities. Although this may seem an unusual pattern of infant care by American middle class standards, it is a common form of childrearing in many parts of the world.

Rainwater[63] observed that in Pruitt-Igoe, a low-cost housing project in St. Louis that he and his coworkers studied closely over a period of time, the babies seemed very secure in their homes. Quite a few people cared for them; they received considerable attention, being passed from mother to sister to grandmother and later toddling from person to person. Their care was regarded as routine. Normal development was greeted with neither anxiety nor undue interest.

If this description seems idyllic, remember that there are many problems as well. Incomes are low, with concomitant poor nutrition, inadequate housing, and marginal health care. Homes are adult-centered rather than child-centered; when children's needs conflict with adults' needs, those of the adults will often prevail. When new babies join the family, children of two years or older may easily be pushed into the background.

Understanding differences in behavior is specifically important for maintaining our relationship with patients from poor black families. For example, in conducting classes for mothers, a lack of interest on the part of the mothers in what a baby should be expected to do at a particular stage of development does not necessarily indicate a lack of interest in their babies, but merely that such indices are not as important to them as they are to us or to the middle class mother (who may be striving to have her baby compete with the baby next door).

In teaching a family about baby care, we need to try to discover just who is going to take care of the baby once he is home. If the mother is not to be the primary caretaker, some contact needs to be arranged with the person who will be.

Not only may the mother not be the primary caretaker, she may have limited authority as to what care is given. If her mother or grandmother believes that catnip is a constituent of baby formula (not an uncommon practice in the author's part of the country), it may be difficult for the mother to overrule the practice, even if we have convinced her that it is not such a good idea.

Much lower class black behavior seems to be in conflict with our middle class norms—views about the desirability of marriage, legitimacy of children, and sexual relations, for example. But Rainwater summarizes the norms of the 10,000 residents of Pruitt-Igoe as being the same as those shared by most Americans: "Lifelong marriage is the only really desirable way of living." "Children should be born only in marriage relationships; to procreate outside marriage is to fall short of the way things ought to be." "Any kind of sexual relationship outside marriage is dangerous, although it is attractive."[63]

It would appear, then, that it is not the norms that differ dramatically, but the ability to achieve those norms. As one father said, "I want my kids to be respectable and presentable wherever they go ... I got seven boys ... and I sure would like for one or two of them to be somethin'. I know they can't all make it, but if only one or two could be somethin'. . . ."[63]

Transracial Marriage: Black and White. Marriage between a black person and a white person has been illegal in some states and is socially unacceptable to many people. Nevertheless, transracial marriages are increasing, although the couples involved face many obstacles and will probably do so for years to come—obstacles such as finding a home and maintaining relationships with black and white families and friends.

Nurses who meet transracial couples during childbearing may be uncomfortable at first because they are dealing with an experience new to them. The couples may be alienated from their own families and from friends, although this will not necessarily be true, and therefore may be particularly in need of support. If we interact with them as people, as potential mothers and fathers, rather than as stereotypes, and if we examine the basis of our own feelings, we will find that transracial couples are no different from the other families we meet.

Spanish-American Families

Spanish-speaking Americans and Americans of Spanish heritage live in many areas of the United States. There are Mexican-Americans in Texas and California, Puerto Ricans in the Northeast, and Latin-Americans in Florida and Georgia. Some Spanish-American families have been in the United States for many generations; others are newcomers. Some of these families have adopted the lifestyle of "middle-America," but many others, because of language barriers, poverty, fear of or experience with discrimination, and loyalty to their own traditions have retained a cultural heritage that "Anglo" nurses and other professionals do not always understand.

Extended family relationships are very important to most Spanish-Americans. Although a young couple may live in a separate home, many relatives often live close by and will be seen very frequently. The advice and counsel of relatives is likely to be important in childbearing. There may be discussions among many family members before an important decision is made. The extended family, rather than the medical professional, may be regarded as the ultimate authority by the young couple (see below).

A second and equally important facet of Spanish-American life is the influence of *compadrazgo*. Compadres, or coparents, have social and economic obligations to one another beyond those that godparents have in most of American society. Compadres are expected to always be friends, no matter what happens; subsequently, there is a feeling of special obligation. The compadrazgo system offers each child a greater number of people upon whom he can depend for the necessities of life.

> . . . A woman will not hesitate to leave her husband and children to go to the aid of a compadre who needs help. When Paula's compadre, who lives in Hayward (about twenty-five miles from San Jose), was expecting her last baby, Paula left her own family for two weeks to care for her compadre during her confinement.[19]

Sex role division and a *double standard of sexual behavior* are characteristic of the relationship between men and women. It is not unusual for a husband to be several years older than his wife, who often marries between the ages of 16 and 19, a fact that enhances male dominance. There is limited dating prior to marriage, with very little acceptance of premarital sexual activity for girls. Women are categorized as "good women" and "bad women." One girl who became pregnant "out of wedlock" reported that "her family would throw her out" but added that she still wished to have the baby.

Childbearing is seen as a privilege and an obligation of married women; to be barren or to have only one or two children often elicits the sympathy of the community. Large families are still desired by many couples.

Many Spanish-speaking families have specific ideas about health care, about how they should act in situations of health and illness, and about the way in which the curer—nurse, physician, or *curandera* (folk-healer)—should behave. Many Spanish-speaking people are hesitant to seek care from someone who does not understand their beliefs.

Consider a pregnant mother who (in our view) needs hospitalization at some point in her pregnancy for diabetic control, perhaps, or for hypertension. There may be discussion among family members, relatives, and neighbors as to the proper course of action. We can become very distressed that our opinion about the necessity of the proposed hospitalization is not accepted as final, but it is the family group that has the ultimate authority to make such decisions. In the eyes of the Spanish community, the role of the curer is to advise, not to dictate. Authoritarianism is likely to drive patients away. The woman will rarely be openly defiant; she will smile and answer "si." But unless family consensus confirms medical opinion, medical advice may be ignored.

How is a nurse expected to behave? Clark

further describes the behavior of Paula, a curandera in California previously referred to, whose behavior typifies the expected role.

Paula's manner is as warm and friendly as her kitchen-dispensary.

She observes the requisite social amenities and always behaves in a manner which her clients regard as courteous. For example, she is always careful to wait for an invitation to enter the house before she goes in. She knows that she is expected to sit down with the family, drink a cup of coffee, and make small talk before getting down to the business at hand. . . . After a decent interval, the illness can be mentioned and the patient seen.

Families from Asian and Middle Eastern Societies

In the United States live many families from Asia—from China, Japan, India, Korea, Vietnam, the Pacific Islands, and many other Far and Middle Eastern nations. Some of these families have lived in the United States for several generations; others have only recently immigrated. Although families from Middle and Far Eastern cultures are not homogeneous, many share certain characteristics that are important for us to recognize if we are to help these families cope with and grow during childbearing.

The Importance of Family Support. When many of us think of family support during pregnancy, we think first of a nuclear family and the support that comes from the husband. For many Middle and Far Eastern women, however, the traditional support during pregnancy comes from women in the extended family—their mother, aunts, and sisters.

The Male Role. The traditional Asian husband will see pregnancy as "women's business"; his cultural values often tell him that it is not proper for him to be actively involved in his wife's pregnancy, labor, or delivery. To judge his degree of participation by our Anglo-Saxon standards and to thereby label him as being uninterested is, at the very least, unfair.

Because men are not expected to care for women, many Asian and Near Eastern women prefer a female physician or midwife and are very uncomfortable with a male physician. If they live in a community where there is no woman available for obstetric care, a nurse can help to some extent by protecting the mother's modesty with particular care and by reminding professional colleagues of this concern.

Traditional Practices. Traditional practices associated with childbearing will vary with the society and with the individual family. Check with the woman about concerns such as the:

1. Foods she believes are important for pregnant and newly delivered mothers.
2. Foods she customarily eats (see also Chapter 12).
3. Activities that are considered appropriate for mothers during pregnancy and the postpartum period.

A prolonged convalescence is customary for many societies, with special proscriptions about diet, bathing, and avoiding the "outside" or "unclean" world. Although these customs may seem unusual to us, from the viewpoint of ancient societies such practices probably served the new mother well by protecting both mother and baby from infection when there was no way to treat infection.

Similarly, the prohibition against the father's entering the room of the new mother and baby, common to many traditional societies, may have served to protect the new mother from intercourse and possible pregnancy too soon after birth during century after century when abstinence was the only sure means of contraception.

American Indian Families

Indian. The label is ours, not his. He has been an Indian for only 500 years. For as many as twenty-five thousand years, he has been Ottawa, Dakota, Shoshone, Cherokee—or one of several hundred distinct people who controlled this continent.[16]

Nearly 1,000,000 men, women, and children of American Indian tribes constitute approximately 1 per cent of the population of the United States. More than half live on or near reservations. Approximately 350,000 Indians live in urban areas in the Midwest and West (Fig. 5–1).

Most of the students and nurses who read this book may never care for Indian families. Yet because their health and human needs are so great, it seems important for anyone interested in people and in their care to become aware of the problems that Indians face, in order to serve, whenever possible, as an advocate for better opportunities for them.

Most of the Indians of the United States live in poverty; in general they are the poorest of the poor. Unemployment on the reservations is high.

Hunger, malnutrition, and poor health are constant facts of life. Even water, so taken for granted by most of us, must be hauled many miles on some reservations. Although neonatal

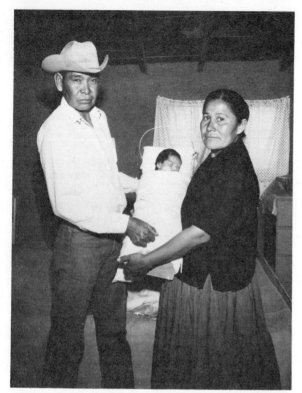

Figure 5–1. Navajo parents in Arizona with their new baby. Note the traditional cradle. (From the Office of Information Services, Indian Health Service, U.S. Public Health Service, Silver Spring, Md.)

mortality (death within the first 28 days of life) has declined as more Indian infants are born in hospitals, infant mortality (deaths in the first year) on reservations is higher than in any other group in our society.

Health care for Indians who live on reservations, other than the traditional care of the medicine man, is provided through the Division of Indian Health of the United States Public Health Service. Because of a shortage of personnel, it is largely crisis-oriented and overcrowded. An Indian may travel 90 miles to a clinic to find 200 to 300 persons ahead of him, with no hope of even being seen.

Transportation presents a major barrier to health care. Many families live miles from the nearest improved road. The *New York Times* (February 19, 1969) told of a Navajo woman who carried her sick baby 30 miles from her hogan (earth-covered dwelling) to the nearest traveled road. The *Times* noted that in the previous year 20 infants from the Pine Ridge Reservation in South Dakota were dead on arrival at medical stations. Eighteen of the deaths were attributed to delay in reaching medical aid.

Traditional beliefs about health care and the interrelatedness of health and other aspects of life, such as religion, are important in Indian

culture. Today most medicine men and Indian families recognize that some conditions (appendicitis, for example) are best treated by the "white man's medicine" while others are more appropriately treated in traditional ways (such as the Navajo "sing" or through a combination of Western and Indian medicine).

For Indians living on reservations, much of life in general is dictated by the Bureau of Indian Affairs, and matters of health are controlled by the Public Health Service. Both of these services are agencies of the United States government. The history of governmental intervention in Indian affairs has not always been one of which we can be proud, nor is it ideal today—a discussion well beyond the scope of this book. But nurses with an understanding of and an appreciation for Indian cultural values can make a difference in Indian care.

Rural Families

Approximately 57 million people live in rural America; of this number about 47 million are nonfarm families, living in small towns and villages scattered throughout the country.

Does life in rural areas differ from that in urban areas? In a time of mass media the differences are less distinct than formerly, but they remain. Recognizing some of these differences can be helpful as we care for childbearing families.

In contrast to the many impersonal relationships of people in urban areas, most relationships in rural communities are between people who know each other. The grocer is known by name and, in turn, knows his (or her) customers. Nurses and physicians will usually know the majority of their patients, unless they are serving unusually wide geographic areas. Families accustomed to this lifestyle can be tremendously overwhelmed by the apparent impersonality of a major medical center, where they must deal with a vast number of strangers in a single day. (The environment also intimidates the average urban resident, but he may have some skills for coping with impersonality.) Just knowing the name of their nurse, or their baby's nurse, and the name of their physician means a great deal to families.

Because "everyone knows everyone else" in a rural community, there is a great deal of pressure to conform to the community's norms and limited tolerance of those who deviate from these norms. For example, a single mother who wished to keep and raise her baby was forced to move to an urban community from her small hometown. "The people in my hometown would never accept me or my baby," she told us. "I was not even welcome in my church. My parents were suffering too."

The significance of family ties, such as she expressed, is far more important in rural areas. The family is the central group for a rural man or woman; for urban dwellers the family may be but one of many groups with which an individual is associated. An urban woman may, for example, belong to a club or professional group for many years with little or no involvement by the rest of her family.

Still another difference is the attitude toward change. In rural communities life changes less from day to day and from year to year than in large cities where change may be an inevitable part of daily life. Social attitudes change more slowly, and one may expect conservative attitudes toward issues such as male and female roles, single parenthood, and abortion, for example.

One easily overlooked aspect of rural life is the frequency of poverty. While one person in fifteen in suburbia and one person in eight in the city lives in poverty, one of every four persons in rural areas is poor. Among nonwhites living in rural communities, three of every five persons is poor. Poverty looms large in part of Appalachia, at the end of dirt roads throughout the South, on the Indian reservations already described, and along the paths that migrant workers follow year after year.

Rural poverty is not just a rural problem. Families who can find no way to support themselves in small towns or on farms migrate to inner city ghettos where they are ill-prepared for urban life. Although this migration has slowed in recent years, as it has become obvious that cities are no longer the promised land, the effects will be felt for many years.

Medical care in many rural areas, including care for mothers and infants, is often limited. Hospitals with limited facilities, particularly for high risk care; a limited number of physicians, many of them on the verge of retirement; and an inadequate number of professional nurses contribute to high infant mortality and morbidity in many rural communities. A concentrated effort toward the regionalization of perinatal care in many states is being initiated in an attempt to overcome these difficulties (Chapter 31).

Appalachian Mountain People

More than 24 million people live in Appalachia (Fig. 5–2); another 3.5 million Appalachians live in urban areas including Cleve-

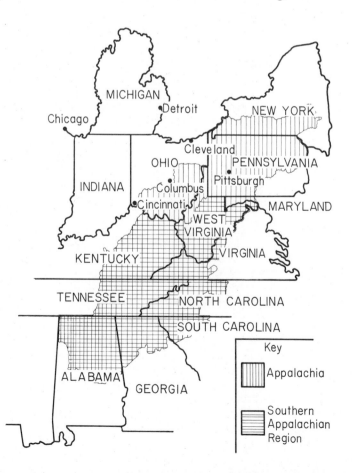

Figure 5–2. Appalachia and Southern Appalachia. (From Tripp-Reimer and Friedl: *Nursing Clinics of N. America*, 12:41, 1977.)

land, Detroit, and Pittsburgh, where they have migrated in search of employment, in many instances with minimum success. The poor and working class people of Appalachia tend to share values that may not always be understood and may therefore be misinterpreted by health care professionals with middle class values. A few examples are cited below.[76]

Time Orientation. Middle class Americans are largely *future oriented;* they plan today for events that are going to happen at some future time. Appalachians, like many of the world's peoples, are frequently *present oriented.* Prenatal care, which involves seeking medical care *now* to prepare for a *future* event may have low priority. Another aspect of their time orientation—a flexible attitude toward schedules—may lead to broken appointments. An appointment at 8:00 A.M. today may be kept "sometime today" or "sometime this week."

Relationship of Man and Nature. While middle class Americans tend to believe that man controls his own destiny to a large extent, Appalachians (again, like many of the world's peoples) believe that man has very limited control, if any, over the forces of nature. If one has no control over events—if "what will be will be"—then preventive health care such as prenatal and well baby care makes very little sense to that individual.

Importance of the Extended Family. The most important group influencing the Appalachian woman are her kinspeople, the members of her extended family. Their advice, especially about age-old matters such as pregnancy and birth, will often take precedence over the advice of professional strangers.

The Counterculture: Alternative Lifestyles

Any family, any commune, is like a Rorschach test. What you see when you come here says more about who you are than what it is. Visitors . . . completely miss what's really going on because they don't see what these things mean to us. (Melville,[52] quoting a member of an Oregon commune.)

Our knowledge of the counterculture, those young men and women who have chosen to live in a style different from that considered "mainstream American," is important not only so that we may give care to those young people but also because some facets of their alternative lifestyles may be advance signals of changes that will later become a part of the society as a whole. This is already evident in matters such as hairstyle and dress, and I think we are seeing examples in facets of childbearing as well.

The decision to live apart from the mainstream is hardly unique to the twentieth century. The Old Testament Jews saw themselves as a people set apart; so did the early Christians. Convents and monasteries offered medieval women and men the opportunity for communal living. Nineteenth century America saw both successful communities (Shakers, Oneida, the Harmony Society, for example) and many brief, less successful attempts at communal life (Brook Farm, Oberlin, Utopia, and a long list of others). Nathaniel Hawthorne lived at Brook Farm for a time. Bronson Alcott, the father of Louisa May Alcott, was one of the founders of a small, short-lived group called Fruitlands.

What of the people who choose alternative lifestyles today? It is estimated that there are more than 2000 communal groups in the United States at present, and in addition many couples and individuals reside outside of the communes with similar ways of life. Many communes are rural, but they exist in urban apartments and homes as well. Communities are scattered throughout almost every region of the country, although they are rare in the Southeast and Midwest. California, northern New Mexico, Southern Colorado, Washington, Oregon, Vermont, and the Hudson River Valley are popular areas. Some communities are small, with eight to ten members; the larger groups usually number 20 to 40. Despite regional and individual differences, there are also similarities because there is migration from one communal group to another.

Philosophically, communal groups appear to be of two basic types: those whose members are, in a sense, retreating from contemporary lifestyles and those formed with a specific mission in mind. Examples of the former are Twin Oaks in Virginia and Morningstar Ranch in California. Personal fulfillment and a more viable lifestyle are major foci of the individuals who live in these groups.

Koinonia, founded near Americus, Georgia, in 1943 is a well-known example of a community with a mission. Koinonia is an transracial community (consider what that meant in rural Georgia in the 1940s) formed for the purposes of demonstrating Christian ideals of community life and assisting local farmers by introducing scientific farming.

Observers have noted with some interest that in many communal groups there is little talk of "women's liberation." In those communities that succeed, everyone works hard, with heavy field work done by the men and cooking, sewing, and childcare mainly done by the women. A major difference from the life of women in suburbia, however, is that these tasks are not done in isolation but in the company of other adults. Moreover, the entire community, fathers as well as mothers, sees childcare as important.

"Unmarried" married couples may live in communities or as individual couples. Their commitment to one another is usually long-standing, although it may not last, just as the commitment of the "legally" married may not. It is the *idea* that a document from the government makes the difference between being married and being single that is rejected. In much the same way, birth certificates may be scorned as "the fatal beginnings of an official assembly line which leads to compulsory public education, military conscription, social security and taxation."[52]

A single mother who is part of the counterculture is more likely to be from a middle or upper class background and often is college educated. Unlike single mothers in the past, she may not share the guilt about an "out of wedlock" pregnancy, probably due in part to changing attitudes in mainstream society. These single mothers lead a life somewhat different from that of the lower class single mother, who often lives with her own mother or relatives in an extended family. The single mother of the counterculture is more likely to live in a community, with a group of other single mothers, or alone.

A detailed examination of the counterculture is obviously beyond the scope of this book. Our suggestions for further reading include the works of Kanter,[43] Melville,[52] and Hedgepeth[35] listed in the chapter references.

Childbearing and the Counterculture

Many of the expressed values of the counterculture concerning childbearing and childrearing are not very different from the ideals expressed in this and other nursing texts. For example, there is emphasis on the role of the father during pregnancy, at the time of delivery, and in childrearing. Natural childbirth is common, although many of us would find it more difficult to accept delivery within the community with nonprofessionals serving as midwives. Breast-feeding is almost universal, as is close, intimate contact between mother and baby during infancy. In some groups the child is rarely left with anyone but the mother and father, while in others childrearing tasks

may be shared, even to the point of exchanging breast-feeding infants among several lactating mothers.

There is considerable interest in nutrition, particularly in organic foods and herbs. One potential problem during pregnancy is that protein intake may be low. Diets with adequate protein can be planned within the framework of the dietary desires of most mothers, but some education and care in menu planning are necessary. For some mothers, the expense may be prohibitive.

The emphasis on naturalness and intimacy may put couples in conflict with the traditional medical world of hospitals and clinics—a world in which technology and bureaucracy often seem to be more important than people and relationships from the couples' point of view.

Bell* talks of this conflict and his reaction to it in describing the birth of Stephen Benson.[10] At the time he wrote the book, Dr. Bell was a pediatric house officer in an intensive care unit of a medical center—practicing medicine in a way as foreign to life in the commune as the bloodletting of the eighteenth century is to cardiac pacemakers. Stephen's parents, Kristin and Peter, lived on a farm with 13 other people. Kristin had received prenatal care from an obstetrician who was unwilling to participate in a home delivery. She said of him, "I don't think he likes us very much," and added, "We want to do everything possible for our baby. We don't want it to be unsafe, but we feel that it would be better for the child to be born at home." The couple agreed that should complications occur, they would immediately go to the hospital, a 15-minute drive.

In describing the labor, Bell comments, "We were witnessing something we had never seen in a hospital, a child being born in an atmosphere of love and caring. I wondered if the baby would somehow recognize this and, as Kristin and Peter believed, be a better, happier person because of it." A friend sang quiet songs during the long hours of labor. Kristin ate ice chips and sipped tea. At the time of Stephen's delivery, Bell records:

Finally, the vagina had stretched enough, and with a push the infant's head came out. Peter held the head and slowly guided out the shoulders and body of his son. The wet, warm, slippery body began to move, and after a cough, he began to cry . . . Peter and Kristin began crying, sobbing with joy as

---

*Dr. Bell's book, *A Time to be Born,* one that we highly recommend to all nurses who care for mothers and babies, describes in very readable fashion the first days of four infants: three sick babies in a medical center hospital and Stephen Benson.

their son moved about, flexing his arms, opening his eyes, looking around for the first time.

... The door opened and the other house members came in, everyone laughing, crying, hugging each other, rejoicing, and welcoming the new child ... Still overcome with joy, he (Peter) dried the baby, handing him carefully to Kristin, and they cried together for the joy of the new life they had produced. Their son was not crying but moving about, carefully studying this strange new world in the arms of his loving parents.[10]

What kind of persons will Stephen and his contemporaries, the children of the counterculture, be as adults? Melville[52] quotes a father in Taos Pueblo: "The test of this whole thing ... will be the next generation ... the kids who grow up here, they're going to be really high people, absolutely out of sight."

Veysey,[79] in looking at the children of earlier generations who sought alternative lifestyles, found that most of the children "slipped back into more conventional beliefs and styles of living" and that at least some "were soon enthusiastically playing baseball." He comments, "In America it seems little easier for radicals to hold on to their children than it is for any other parents."

Nursing and the Counterculture

We have chosen to stress some of the positive aspects of the counterculture, recognizing that there are problems as well. Misuse of drugs, venereal disease, and other health and social problems of our general society can hardly bypass those who choose to live differently.

As with everyone whose values differ from our own, it is important to listen to his or her ideas attentively and seriously. Bancroft,[8] in describing her nursing practice with the counterculture, concludes that there was "no need for us to participate in the life style of our clients ... As long as we did not try to impose our values on them, they did not impose theirs on us. ... " But, she adds, "It mattered a great deal that the staff were willing to work with hip clients."

Assessment of Cultural Factors

Incorporation of cultural factors into the nursing assessment is discussed in Chapter 10.

The Single Parent Family

It is customary, and comfortable, for us to think of childbearing in terms of a husband-

father and a wife-mother, married to one another. Much of our effort during the past decade has been devoted to breaking down barriers that have separated a husband from his wife and newborn child during significant phases of the birth of the child. While this continues to be an extremely important focus of our nursing practice, we must be just as interested in the needs of single parents.

The exact number of single mothers bearing children is difficult to compute because a number of states do not record marital status of the mother on birth certificates (a practice with much to commend it). Moreover, because of this, the poor, the black, and the very young mother are probably overrepresented in statistics. The mother with a higher income, frequently a white mother, may be able to travel to a state that will not record illegitimacy on her baby's birth certificate, and thus is probably underrepresented. Also unrepresented in statistics is the mother who is single at the time of conception and marries during, and perhaps largely because of, her pregnancy. For many couples, marriage under these circumstances may be short-lived, and the mother becomes a single parent at some future time.

Recognizing all of these limitations to the statistical data, we can still find some useful information about single mothers in the reported figures. Statistics are reported in terms of the total number of illegitimate births, the number of illicit births per 1000 live births, the number of illicit births per 1000 unmarried females, and the number of births to mothers who are white or nonwhite.

If we look at trends over a 40-year period (1938 to 1978) the number of births to single mothers has increased markedly (Table 5–1). Almost five times as many babies were born to unmarried mothers in 1978 as in 1938.

In looking at the age of the mothers (Table 5–2), the greatest number of babies are born to single mothers between the ages of 15 and 19. This was true in 1938 as well as in 1978. Two of every 100 unmarried girls in this age group and 3 of every 100 unmarried women between 20 and 29 years of age bear children, but absolute numbers are lower in the older age groups because so many women over 20 years of age are married.

In 1974, of all babies born to mothers between the ages of 15 and 19, approximately 20 per cent were born to single mothers. By 1978, over 44 per cent were born to single mothers. Of babies born to mothers under 15 years of age, 65 per cent of the mothers were unmarried at the time of birth in 1974 and over 87 per cent in 1978. Because of this, much of the

Table 5-1. BIRTHS TO SINGLE MOTHERS IN 1938, 1957, 1968, 1974, AND 1978, BY RACE OF THE MOTHER

	White		Nonwhite		
Year	*Number*	*Per Cent*	*Number*	*Per Cent*	**Total**
1938	41,200	47	46,700	53	87,900
1957	70,800	35	130,900	65	201,700
1968	155,200	46	183,900	54	339,100
1974	168,500	40	249,600	60	418,100
1978	233,600	43	310,200	57	543,900

emphasis, both in terms of care during and the prevention of the single pregnancy, has been directed toward the adolescent single mother. Special needs of adolescent mothers are discussed in Chapter 29.

Apart from the particular needs of the adolescent mother, what can we say about single mothers?

1. Single mothers represent a diverse group of people—diverse in terms of age, race, socioeconomic status, and individual characteristics. Reasons for pregnancy outside of marriage vary; they may be related to personality characteristics of the mother, such as low self-esteem; to cultural patterns in which successive generations of women in the same family have become single mothers; to ignorance of

the physiology of conception or effective contraception; to the desire for a child; and to a variety of other reasons important to a particular mother.

2. Not every pregnancy is unwanted by an unmarried mother, nor is every pregnancy seen by the mother as a problem (any more than every pregnancy to a married mother is wanted, planned, or without problems). Nurses and other professional workers tend to view single mothers from the perspective of their own values, values that are not necessarily shared, or shared with the same level of intensity, by the mother herself. A part of our role is to assess what the pregnancy means to an individual mother.

3. Pregnancies outside of marriage may fall

Table 5-2. NUMBER, RATIO, AND RATE OF BIRTHS TO SINGLE MOTHERS IN 1938, 1957, 1968, 1974, AND 1978, BY AGE OF THE MOTHER*

			Age of Mother				
Year	Under 15	15–19	20–24	25–29	30–34	35–39	40 and Over
Number of Births to Single Mothers							
1938	2,000	40,400	26,400	10,000	5,000	3,100	1,000
1957	4,600	76,400	60,500	29,800	18,000	9,400	2,800
1968	7,700	158,000	107,900	35,200	17,200	9,700	3,300
1974	10,600	210,800	122,700	44,900	18,600	8,200	2,300
1978	9,400	239,700	186,500	70,000	26,500	9,400	2,300
Illegitimacy Ratio *(Illicit Births per 1000 Live Births)*							
1938	608.5	135.5	36.6	16.4	13.2	15.3	14.2
1957	660.9	138.9	44.4	26.1	24.9	25.7	29.1
1968	810.2	267.2	82.6	38.9	41.0	47.1	51.4
1974	653.1	202.3	110.7	48.6	49.9	69.4	77.7
1978	872.6	441.1	163.7	69.0	55.9	74.5	96.3
Rate of Illegitimacy *(Births per 1000 Unmarried Females)*							
1938	0.3	7.5	9.2	6.8	4.8	3.4	1.1
1957	0.6	15.6	36.5	37.6	26.1	12.7	3.3
1968	0.0	19.8	37.3	38.6	28.2	14.9	3.8
1974	0.0	23.2	30.9	28.4	18.6	10.0	2.6
1978	—	25.4	36.1	29.4	17.3	8.1	2.2

*Adapted from the following sources: (1) Schacter, J. and McCarthy, M.: Illegitimate Births: United States, 1938–57. In *Vital Statistics—Special Reports, Selected Studies*, Vol. 47, No. 8. (Washington, D.C.: U.S. Government Printing Office, 1960); (2) *Trends in Illegitimacy: United States, 1940–1965.* (Washington, D.C.: U.S. Government Printing Office, 1968); (3) mimeographed reports for 1968 data from National Center for Health Statistics; (4) *Monthly Vital Statistics Report*, Vol. 24, No. 11, Feb. 13, 1976; and (5) *Monthly Vital Statistics Report*, Vol. 29, No. 1 (supplement), April 28, 1980.

into one of several categories. The couple may have no intention or desire to marry one another. Or one partner may desire marriage but the other may feel uninterested or unready. Contrary to the popular myth, it is not always the woman who desires marriage. Fairly frequently we see instances in which the man is very willing to marry, but the woman states that she "is not ready to settle down." These couples may continue their relationship during their pregnancy and after the birth of the baby. Some couples, as noted in the discussion of the counterculture, may choose to live together without a legal ceremony but may have a real commitment to one another and to their children. Pregnancy may occur to a couple already planning marriage, or to a woman following divorce. Or pregnancy may be the result of rape or incest. Pregnancy due to extramarital intercourse may result in a situation in which the mother is married but her husband is not the father of the conceptus.

Unmarried Fathers

Hundreds of studies, articles, and books have examined unwed mothers; very few have looked at the fathers of their babies. Why?

One reason is the double standard for sexual behavior in our society. Not only are men not condemned for sexual intercourse, but the adolescent boy receives many subtle (and some not so subtle) messages that sexual intercourse is expected. Society at large, and the medical world as well, places little blame on him when pregnancy occurs. Consider the following statements, part of a discussion following the presentation of a paper on the "Unwed Teenage Mother" at the Pacific Coast Obstetrical and Gynecological Society:

There is no question of the increased frequency of this aberrant behavior of young women in our culture . . . If we are to discover the least common denominator of illegitimate pregnancy we must investigate wherein the unwed mother's own mother failed in programming her daughter with enough basic emotional control to restrain her instinctive procreative drive until she meets the conditions required by the cultural mores.[46]

. . . I will tell them, and in many instances I sense that they know it to be true, that if they indulge in teen-age sexual intercourse and pre-marital intercourse most of the time their sexual partner has no respect for them whatsoever, and if he ever did, he usually loses it very rapidly.[7]

A second reason for little emphasis on the unmarried father is that he is, in a sense, invisible, while the mother is not only highly visible but in many instances a problem to a society that must support her and her child.

Traditionally, we have not expected much from the father involved in an unwed pregnancy. Our laws, which require only the consent of the mother for such actions as adoption and abortion, do, in fact, discourage the father's participation. And certainly there are some fathers who choose not to be involved.

However, when mothers and the professional people working with them have included the father in planning, they have found that many fathers were far more interested than they expected. Many chose to act responsibly when they were given the opportunity.

Auerbach describes two different paternal reactions to out-of-wedlock pregnancy.

The first woman had conceived due to contraceptive failure. The relationship with the father was shaky before the pregnancy and rapidly deteriorated after the announcement of expectant motherhood. Throughout her pregnancy her baby's father made no effort to help her in any way. She subsisted on a welfare check in an apartment house for singles only. After the baby was born she continued to live there with minimum financial support from her parents at the sufferance of the apartment house superintendent.

The second woman chose to conceive. While the father served a brief prison term, she decorated their rented house with care and devotion to the needs of their baby. They attended childbirth preparation classes together and he accompanied her to the obstetrician's office for prenatal visits. The physician treated them as he did married couples. Six months after the delivery of their daughter, they were hoping to have another child within two years.[5]

Pannor and his associates report that "the relationships between unwed mothers and fathers are much more meaningful than popularly supposed, and that unwed fathers have more concern for their offspring than is generally realized."[61] They describe a sense of isolation, alienation, and feelings of being cut off and denied meaningful human contact as some of the fathers' emotions.

In some clinics and hospitals, male partners are included in planning and support to the extent that they and the mother wish them to be. Part of our nursing role is to accept and support these fathers.

Decisions the Single Mother and Father Must Face

Unmarried parents must make one of four decisions: marriage, raising the child by a single parent, releasing the child for adoption, or abortion.

Marriage

Couples who are considering marriage because of pregnancy need to face their motives realistically. Does one, or both, of them feel guilty, if not for the act of coitus itself, for the pregnancy? Are sympathy or pity factors in their decision? In the months that follow such a decision, a bride may wonder, "Would he have married me if I were not pregnant?"

"Did she trick me into this?" may cross the mind of the groom. Such thoughts may be less important now than they will be in later years. Several of our patients have found that this kind of question becomes an issue during a subsequent pregnancy, when old feelings are rekindled.

Vincent[80] suggests that couples must face the reality that the question "Would he have married me if . . . ?" is unanswerable and is one form of a very universal problem. All couples, at some time during their marriages, drag events of the past into arguments, whether the issue be premarital pregnancy or some other circumstance of courting or early marriage. Thus, premarital pregnancy in itself does not constitute an absolute contraindication to marriage.

If marriage is chosen as the desired course, a wedding such as the couple would have had if there were no pregnancy may be a good idea. A hurried, secretive ceremony may be remembered longer by the couple themselves than the fact of a premature conception.

Often marriage, or at least marriage during the course of the pregnancy, is not desirable. No one can make this decision but the couple themselves, but the alternative of waiting until after the baby is born and perhaps placing the infant for temporary foster care before a marriage decision is made, might be suggested.

Keeping the Child Without Marriage: The Mother as a Single Parent

A mother's decision to keep her baby although she remains single is influenced by cultural norms and by individual circumstances. Women of lower socioeconomic classes are far more likely to feel that they should keep their babies than are middle class mothers. Quite a few of these lower class mothers are themselves products of single parent families; perhaps their own survival makes the idea of bringing up a child alone less threatening or strange.

Support for her chosen course from her parents is another positive factor that increases the likelihood that a mother may keep her baby. Older women who are already maintaining their own households, women who continue to have a relationship with the putative father (and who may consider future marriage a possibility), and women who have had prior pregnancies that were not carried to term have also been found to be more ready to keep their child.[50]

A mother who is a single parent faces some pressing issues concerning her lifestyle, both before and after the baby is born. She must decide where she will live; how she will meet increasing financial needs; how she will obtain medical care, both for herself and later for the baby as well; and how she will begin or continue a job or further education.

Where Will She Live?   The options available to her include: (1) living with her parents or other relatives, (2) living with her partner, (3) living with a friend, (4) living alone, (5) living in a maternity home, or (6) living in a foster home provided by some communities if she is under 18.

Each of these alternatives presents both advantages and problems that are highly individual. Living at home with genuinely supportive parents who accept their daughter and her pregnancy may be the best of all possible alternatives. However, in other instances constant friction between a young woman and her parents may make such a situation impossible. Still other parents totally reject an unmarried daughter. One of our patients, formerly married but now divorced and living at home, told us that her father would banish her when he discovered that she was pregnant. She was quite positive about this because he had already disowned her sister for the same reason.

Both in the past and somewhat more openly today, a woman may choose to live with her sexual partner, although marriage is not desired by one or both at the present time. Many nurses find this arrangement hard to accept; our feelings may affect our nursing relationship with this woman and this couple if we do not recognize and deal with them.

From a purely financial standpoint, living with a friend or living alone can present problems. At some point, income may cease; what will the woman do then? The problem is not unsolvable but needs realistic planning (see below).

Maternity homes, such as the Florence Crittenton homes, at one time played a significant role in the care of unmarried women during pregnancy. They are used far less today. A number have closed after many years of operation; others remain open but operate below capacity. The combination of legal therapeutic

Table 5–3. MEDIAN FAMILY INCOME, 1979

	All Races	White	Black
Male head of household	$21,703	$22,045	$17,248
Female head of household	$10,689	$11,849	$ 7,761

abortion and wider public acceptance of pregnancy outside of marriage is probably responsible for this decreased use. Those homes that do remain open offer the advantages of privacy and a protected environment, and often counseling and the chance for continued education are provided. Good medical care is usually assured. No good maternity home pressures the mother into placing the baby for adoption as some mothers seem to fear.

A foster home is an individual home licensed by the state. Foster homes are more commonly used for infant and child care, including the care of an infant awaiting adoption, but a young pregnant girl may also qualify for placement.

How Will Financial Needs Be Met? Most single mothers who deliver and keep their infants will have financial problems, regardless of socioeconomic status. The median family income for families headed by women was $10,689 in 1979, compared with a median income of $21,703 for husband-wife families. In our society even well-educated women rarely command the salaries of men with similar levels of education. With a high proportion of single mothers being teenagers and coming from nonwhite families, earning opportunities are even further restricted. (See Table 4–3.)

Each mother needs someone who will realistically help her balance the expenses of pregnancy and childrearing with the funds available to her. The economically poorest of patients may have a social caseworker who can help her assess her finances. For women with somewhat higher incomes, financial counsel may be more difficult to find. In some communities, home economists who are employed by the city or county government will help with budgeting.

Nurses can provide information about the costs of medical services and the resources available for meeting these and other needs. To those who would wonder if this is truly *nursing* care, we wonder how we can say it is not. How, for example, can we encourage a diet adequate for good prenatal care and remain oblivious to the fact that the mother can afford only pinto beans and fatback?

Many hospitals and clinics have departments or social workers to whom mothers can be referred for financial advice and assistance, and this should be done whenever it is possible.

Referral, for many mothers, means not merely telling them to go to Room 31-C if they need help but describing to them the service that is available and assisting them in whatever way seems individually appropriate. Although it is important for each mother to assume as much responsibility as possible in seeking help, women will vary in the amount of initiative they will be able to command, particularly when much of their coping strength is already channeled into dealing with the pregnancy itself.

Sources of financial assistance that may be available to an individual mother include: (1) employment, for at least part of the pregnancy, (2) help from the father of the child, (3) Medicaid, (4) food stamps, and (5) resources particular to the individual community.

Individual community resources may be services offered by an agency related to the National Foundation–March of Dimes, individual churches or groups of churches, women's clubs, Jay-cettes, and the like. When there is a definite gap in community services, nurses may be able to persuade such local groups to undertake unmet needs as projects. Such groups are not only helpful in securing clothes and food for mothers but in equipping hospital nurseries when a definite need is brought to their attention.

Support payments for the baby from the putative father that are ordered by the court may be a source of financial assistance *after* the infant is born, as may be public aid through Aid to Families with Dependent Children (AFDC). If the unmarried mother already has a child, she may be eligible for AFDC payments before delivery. Such eligibility is determined by the Department of Social Services of the AFDC. For some mothers the thought of any type of government assistance (which they translate as "welfare") is totally unacceptable. A nurse may be someone with whom they can share their feelings, explore alternatives, and eventually arrive at the best decision for themselves.

How Will She Obtain Medical Care? In the United States obtaining medical care is closely related to finances. At this point we would say that each nurse should be aware of the options for maternity care available in her own and neighboring communities and their relative costs in relation to other advantages and disadvantages, such as availability of transportation; length of waiting time; and most important, the quality of care given.

Placing the Baby for Adoption

Mothers should know that the decision to place the baby for adoption is not final and irrevocable until after the infant is born. The length of time following birth in which a mother may change her mind varies with the laws of each state. Counsel and support should be available to each mother not only at the time that she struggles to make her initial decision but during the weeks and months that follow. She will need reassurance that a good home will be found for her baby as she questions, to herself and to others, "Am I really doing the right thing?"

Adoption may be handled directly or through a licensed agency. In direct adoption the baby is placed in a specific adoptive home by the mother or couple. Usually this is less desirable than placement through a licensed agency, which preserves the anonymity of both natural and adoptive parents and has experience in selecting an adoptive home and dealing with the legal requirements.

While it is common to think that the adoptive decision is made near the time of birth, a mother may initially decide to keep her baby and then find, as the infant becomes a toddler or a preschool child, that caring for him is more than she can manage. A door should be left open for a change of plans at any time.*

Abortion

Since the Supreme Court ruling of January 22, 1973, a woman may legally choose abortion of any fetus before the seventh month of pregnancy, the time defined as the legal age of viability. The wording of that ruling (Roe vs. Wade, Texas—41 LW 4213) declared that since physicians, philosophers, and theologians are unable to reach a consensus on the issue of when life begins, it was not appropriate for the courts to speculate about it. For the purposes of constitutional protection, the unborn child was not to be considered a person. This issue, however, is again being debated in 1982, with the eventual outcome uncertain.

Almost all of the existing laws that limited abortion were declared unconstitutional because they were considered to invade the privacy of the pregnant woman. In the first trimester, abortion was judged to be strictly a medical decision between a woman and her doctor. From the beginning of the second trimester until the seventh month, individual states were allowed to enact laws to protect the health of the mother. But only after viability of the fetus was attained was the state permitted to limit abortion decisions to those instances in which the life or health of the mother was jeopardized.

In a second significant decision (Doe vs. Bolton, Georgia—41 LW 4233), a number of related laws were also declared invalid because they, too, were considered to violate the privacy of the pregnant woman. No longer could abortions be done only in accredited hospitals, only for residents of the state in which they were performed, or only when approved by a hospital abortion committee or the consensus of consulting physicians.

Abortion is discussed in Chapter 30.

The Women's Movement

The women's movement is not a recent phenomenon. Because the status of women is so closely related to our nursing practice, we would urge nurses to broaden their own knowledge of the movement by reading the works of authors such as Friedan, de Beauvoir, Sanger, Rossi, and others.

How does the women's movement relate to health care for childbearing families? First, because the majority of professional nurses are women, nurses have traditionally had less power to affect care than physicians and hospital administrators, the majority of whom are men. Ashley[4] points out that "nurses were not the equals of physicians in political and economic spheres, and so nursing's continuing subjection to male dominance resulted . . . They sought approval from men, not liberation. As a result, from the first decade of the century onward, physicians and hospital administrators have remained in positions of dominance and control over nursing and health care."

As recently as 1976, the president of the American Medical Association, Dr. Max Parrott, characterized nursing as ancillary to medicine and dependent upon it.[70]

As women become stronger, politically and economically, nurses will also practice from a position of greater strength. We may become more outspoken concerning issues that deal with health care for childbearing families,

*This later change of plans is dramatized well in the film "I'm Seventeen, Pregnant, and I Don't Know What to Do." (Appendix I.)

rather than deferring to others. We may seek to align public opinion on both national issues and problems within our own community, such as family life education in the school system, birth control information for all sexually active women (regardless of age or marital status), and family-centered care in maternity units, to name but three of many possible examples.

The status of women has also affected women's power in relation to their own health care, a large measure of which is obstetric and gynecologic care. As recently as the 1960s, obstetrician-gynecologists made decisions for women such as withholding birth control devices from unmarried women and deciding when a woman could be sterilized. The formula for sterilization (the woman's age times the number of children she had delivered had to equal or be greater than 120) was not dropped by the American College of Obstetrics and Gynecology (ACOG) until 1969, and is still a "rule of thumb" in many hospitals. By this formula, a woman of 25 would have had to have delivered five children before she could elect to be sterilized; a woman with four children would have to wait until she was 30. Pity the poor family that chose to have only two children; nature would solve the mother's fertility problems before the age of 60, at which time the ACOG formula would permit sterilization! Even if overpopulation were not one of the most pressing of the world's problems, the failure to allow women to make such decisions seems almost unbelievable.

The foregoing is one illustration why many women have felt that they have been unfairly treated by male physicians who have had so much control over their lives. In response, the women's movement has inspired a number of activities.

Learning to understand their own bodies and sharing their knowledge with other women has been one focus of the movement. *Our Bodies, Ourselves* is the result of such a study by one group, the Boston Women's Health Book Collective.[13] Originally published by the New England Free Press on newsprint and distributed to women's groups, the book is now available commercially. In a very frank and readable way, this volume discusses anatomy and physiology, female sexuality, venereal disease, birth control, abortion, and the many facets of pregnancy. *Vaginal Politics* by Ellen Frankfort[25] and *Free and Female* by Barbara Seaman[72] have similar goals. Frankfort warns (appropriately, we believe) that one danger of the health movement is that young women may become totally anti-doctor, as have some young couples at the time of pregnancy. The message is not total mistrust of physicians, she emphasizes, but understanding that doctors have areas of specialized information that can be utilized—"but not blindly."

The concerns of the women's movement for women's health parallel those of maternity nursing, although individual points of view certainly will differ. In relation to pregnancy, the emphasis is on making childbearing a fulfilling experience rather than a stressful one. Counseling for pregnant women who are

Some Relationships between the Status of Women and the Health Needs of Women

Low Status of Women

Women lack power to affect their own health and social needs

Nurses (because most nurses are women) lack power to affect health care of women

Male dominance of health care for women, including childbearing

↓

Health care structured to suit male professionals

↓

Desires and needs of women often ignored

↓

Entire family (mother, father, children) shortchanged from generation to generation experiencing difficulties, establishing pregnant couples groups, and placing heightened emphasis on dealing with the feelings as well as the physiologic facts of pregnancy are some suggested goals. The increased use of nurse-midwives for normal pregnancies, similar to the English model, is proposed, as well as the formation of organizations of visiting lay-women who would help with postnatal concerns. Maternity leave, not only for mothers but for fathers, so that the family can be together during the days following birth is already policy in Sweden. Providing daycare at every place of employment to enable the mother to return to work and to continue to breast-feed is a goal of some feminist groups.

Another area of concern to the women's movement has been the status of abortion in American society. Abortion is viewed by many women in "the movement" as a part of the right of a woman to control her own body. Obstruction to abortion, whether in the form of laws, hospital policy, high prices, physicians, adverse public opinion, or poor communication that keeps a woman from knowing what services are available, is a target for concern and for action of many women's groups (Chapter 30).

The Women's Movement and Changing Sex Roles

A second focus of the women's movement that seems particularly relevant to nursing care for childbearing families is the attempt to free both men and women from the stereotyping of sex roles. It has become obvious that the roles of women as wives and mothers cannot change to any great extent without changes in the roles of men as husbands and fathers.

What defines masculinity and femininity? Is it behavior such as bathing and diapering a baby or repairing an automobile engine? Is it a feeling, such as tenderness or sympathy? Is it a personality trait, such as aggressiveness or passivity? As people become parents, some are asking, "Can we raise children who will be free of sex stereotypes?"

To a large extent, sex roles are defined by cultural norms. There are societies in which sewing is the work of men rather than women, and even in our own country fine tailoring is frequently a man's occupation. In segments of our society the male dancer has been considered unmasculine (many little girls but few little boys go to dancing school); in other groups dancing is a male prerogative.

So, too, with the characteristics of personality. Mead[51] points out that among the Arapesh of New Guinea both men and women display traits that in our limited cultural perspective we might call maternal and feminine. They are "co-operative, unaggressive, responsive to the needs and demands of others." In another tribe, the Mundugumor, in marked contrast, both men and women are ruthless, aggressive individuals with little that we would call maternal or feminine in their personalities. In a third group, the Tchambuli, women are the dominant, impersonal, managing persons while men are "less responsible" and emotionally dependent.

Mead concludes:

If those temperamental attitudes which we have traditionally regarded as feminine—such as passivity, responsiveness, and a willingness to cherish children—can so easily be set up as the masculine pattern in one tribe, and in another be outlawed for the majority of women as well as for the majority of men, we no longer have any basis for regarding such aspects of behavior as sex-linked. And this conclusion becomes even stronger when we consider the actual reversal in Tchambuli of the position of dominance of the two sexes, in spite of the existence of formal partrilineal institutions.[51] (Author's note—patrilineal institutions might be expected to support male dominance.)

There seems little doubt that sex roles are changing in our own society. Can anyone imagine, if television had existed in Victorian days, that Victorian fathers (or the actors portraying them) would have appeared discussing the relative merits of two brands of diapers. Even a few years ago, fathers were rare in prenatal classes and labor rooms and nurseries. It was an unusual father who had the opportunity to touch his baby before the day of discharge. While this kind of situation still exists in some hospitals, it is rapidly changing.

Now society has, in a sense, given its permission. "It's all right to help at home and care for your baby. It doesn't make you a sissy. You may even like it" is the nonverbal message of television and magazines and even cocktail party conversations. A few men have experimented with being "househusbands" while their wives are employed.

As nurses, our practice changes too. More and more we find ourselves relating to couples, rather than to mothers, two people instead of one.

Changes in sex roles are by no means evenly distributed throughout our society. Most social change begins in urban areas and among middle class families, and sex role changes follow similar patterns. As we have already noted in the discussion of social class, sex role differentiation is still characteristic of many blue collar families and upper class families.

In single parent families one parent cannot and should not attempt to assume both male and female roles, although some mothers may feel, and may even be told, that they must do so. Nurses can assure the single mother that she is only expected to fulfill a mother's role. Male role models may be assumed by relatives or friends or other males in the community.

Families in Which the Mother is Employed Outside the Home

In spite of a popular myth that American families consist of fathers who are breadwinners and mothers who are homemakers (which the early sections of this chapter should have dispelled), a great number of American mothers have been employed outside the home for many years. In 1979, 43 per cent of married mothers, 53 per cent of separated mothers, and 69 per cent of divorced mothers with children under 6 were employed.

What is the effect of maternal employment on our society, and particularly on our families? In the general press and in popular discussion, mothers who are employed outside of their homes have often been treated as one homogeneous group. No real understanding of maternal employment is possible, however, without looking at the varied reasons why women seek employment.

Many mothers have no choice. They furnish all or most of the financial support for themselves and their children. In approximately 10 per cent of American households, a woman is the head of the family. Some of these women have never been married. Others are widowed, divorced, or separated from their husbands.

A second group of mothers work to supplement a family income that is, or seems to be, inadequate. Their husband may be unable to work because of physical or mental disability; even if he receives compensation of some sort, it is often insufficient for the family's financial needs. Unexpected expenses (frequently major medical expenses) may have overtaxed family resources. Two incomes may be necessary to meet basic needs or to provide the standard of living that would not be possible on one income.

For still other women, work offers emotional satisfactions that are as compelling as, or even more important than, economic considerations. This group includes many educated professional women who have spent time and money preparing for a career. Mothers who find themselves lonely at home with little adult companionship may also choose to work for social and emotional rather than for monetary reasons. Being a mother does not, unfortunately, bring much prestige in American society.

These categories are by no means mutually exclusive. For many women the decision to seek employment outside of their homes is influenced by social, emotional, *and* monetary considerations.

Societal Attitudes Toward Employed Mothers

Americans have some very contradictory attitudes about working mothers. The mother who works because she loves what she does or to provide income for "extras" (as opposed to basics such as food and shelter) is still largely regarded with ambivalence at best, and not infrequently with disapproval.

However, the lower class mother who accepts public assistance is often criticized for not putting her baby in a daycare nursery and going to work to support herself and her child. Thus, we offer one standard to one group of mothers and a second to another group.

The effect of criticism on an individual working mother varies. In a neighborhood in which necessity dictates that all mothers be employed away from home or when a mother's friends are equally career-oriented, the problem of criticism from her peers may be minimal. It is the mother who is "bucking the trend" of behavior in her own neighborhood who may feel guilty because of the attitudes of her contemporaries. As some of the studies reviewed below indicate, this guilt, rather than her working per se, may in turn affect her family.

Family Attitudes Toward Employed Mothers

A second source of comment and potential criticism comes from within the woman's own family. The mother's parents and relatives, or her husband's, may also create tension and anxiety by their comments. "When you (or your husband) were little, I stayed home and took care of you (him)," implies that the mother should do the same. The amount of stress that such comments can cause will depend on many factors; the support that a husband gives his wife's desire for employment and the couple's overall relationship with their parents are two such factors.

A major consideration in terms of family dynamics is the effect of the mother's employment on her relationship with her husband. If the mother gives her limited time at home to housework and baby care and if the father does not participate in these activities, when do the parents find time for one another? How resentful does the mother feel about the apparent unfairness of such a situation? On the other hand, if the father fully supports the mother's need or desire for employment and if homemaking and childcare tasks are shared, this is not only less likely to be a problem but can become a positive factor in the children's development, as they see both mother and father in more than one role.

A father's refusal to help his employed wife with tasks at home may be due to his own enculturation (men don't do women's work), or it may be a way of showing his unhappiness with his wife's employment. Lancaster[48] points out that it is not the husband who is unalterably opposed to his wife's job who creates the most difficult situation. Rather it is the huband who says, "It's O.K.," but then refuses to share in the other tasks or expects everything to be done as if the wife were home all day.

Howell[38] estimates that it takes 105 hours a week (that's 15 hours a day, 7 days a week) for a woman to hold a fulltime job and care for a home and family without help. Since some domestic chores are inevitable (cooking and dishwashing are hard to avoid, for example) it is easy to see that some important aspects of infant and child care, such as holding and singing and playing peek-a-boo, might be difficult to find time for, or that a mother with such a schedule might be too tired to play or even to talk if she must carry dual responsibilities alone.

One might hypothesize that if the mother's income is important to the family economically, the father would willingly share other tasks or, at the very least, be grateful for his wife's contribution. In some families, however, a wife's economic contribution may serve to make her husband feel that he has failed as a provider and thus as a man, and thereby may increase family tension. Douvan[22] reports that in homes in which the mother's working suggests the father's inadequacy, sons chose the father as a role model less frequently, were generally less active, and often showed a rebellious response to adult authority.

New studies of mother and infant interaction that show that importance of parenting for attachment and development during the early months (Chapter 26) raise questions about what happens when the mother is employed during this time.

Studies of babies receiving care by someone other than their mother have shown these babies to behave somewhat differently. This difference could be related to having received care from other people, or it could be related to a difference in the personality of their own mother (and thus the mothering they receive from her).

Moore[55] found that children receiving daycare before 1 year of age showed more fears and more dependent attachments to their parents than those who were not in daycare until after they were 3 years old. Infants who had a succession of child care arrangements during the first year demonstrated marked attention seeking and dependent behavior. When Moore compared "home-reared" children with those receiving any other kind of care, the home-reared infants appeared less aggressive, more obedient, and more concerned with approval. Schwarz and associates report similar findings.[71]

Murray[57] also found differences in babies who received care from their own mother as opposed to those who received care from multiple sources but suggests that the difference may be more related to the mother's personality. He found that the mothers who had sole responsibility for their baby's care (other than the care given by the father) when the baby was 6 months old were more self-confident and more personally involved with their baby than the mothers who shared care with one or more caretakers. At one year the babies who had been cared for by their mother alone had a more positive interaction with their mother, who, in turn, interacted more with her baby. We are impressed by the similarity of these findings with those of Klaus and associates[47] and Kennel and associates,[45] who found that mothers with early contact with their babies appeared more confident and interacted more frequently with them. Greenberg[31] reports similar findings for fathers (Chapter 26).

Long-term studies will be necessary to determine if the differences in mother-child interaction and infant personality during the first year are important as the child grows older. It seems obvious that such studies are vitally important to our society.

The effect of mothers' employment on older children has been investigated. Burchinal[15] found no apparent effect on personality, school-related characteristics, or social development in the school-aged children of 1100 families. The study included families in which the mother was employed during the first three years of the child's life, the second three years, and the first six years, as well as children of mothers who had never been employed. Some of the children who were tested were in the seventh grade; the remainder were eleventh graders.

Siegel reports similar findings.[74] She matched children for such factors as family size, age of siblings, and family income level so that she could more closely estimate if the differences she found were related to the fact that the mother was employed. The matched pairs of children, one of an employed mother and one of a mother who was not employed, were observed during free play period in kindergarten for self-reliance, conformity, and aggression. Siegel found no major differences in the two groups of children.

In the case of mothers of adolescents, there is some evidence that part-time employment may have a positive effect by helping adolescents become more independent. This may be because the part-time job helps the mother make the transition from the nurturing, protecting role of the mother of young children to the "letting go" that is important in allowing adolescents to mature.

The Mother's Feelings About Employment

How a mother feels about employment may be as important as employment itself in its effect on her children. Because of the proscriptions of our society about a mother's job, guilt is probably the emotion most commonly shared by employed mothers. Guilt is intensified if the baby has an accident while his mother is at work, if an older child is doing poorly in school, or if an adolescent commits some act of delinquency. A mother who feels guilty forgets that children whose mothers are not employed also have accidents and school problems and have trouble with the law.

Guilt can lead to efforts to compensate for being away part of the day by giving children attention and affection when their mother is home (not necessarily bad) or to overcompensate by being unable to say "no," buying too many toys and "things," and so on (obviously harmful).

Employment may either enhance or lower a mother's self-esteem, and this, in turn, affects her children. If a mother feels good about herself because of success in her job, her positive feelings can be contagious. On the other hand, if her self-esteem is lowered by employment ("If I had married a different man who could care for me and my children more adequately, I would not have to work"), her negative feelings may affect her children. The effect of her employment on the father's feelings about himself is also significant (see above).

Career or Job

One variable that has not been examined closely in formal studies is the effect of a "career" versus the effect of a "job" on infants and children. We use the term career to describe work that is not limited to hours at a place of employment but that makes many additional demands on time if one is to be reasonably effective—time for continuing education, traveling to attend professional meetings, reading, and even preoccupation with a challenging problem during the time a parent is at home. We consider nursing practice to be a career in this sense. Women who are lawyers, physicians, business executives, artists, writers, and teachers are other examples. A "job," by contrast, demand's one's time and energy only during the hours actually worked; assembly line work in a factory is an example.

In past generations, the number of mothers of infants and young children with careers was rather limited. But the number increases each year, as women seek and find new opportunities.

It has been suggested that a career is one's own favorite child. This is an issue to be considered not only by mothers, but by fathers as well. The demands of a man's career can shortchange his family, if he allows them to, just as much as the demands of a career on a woman. Although problems are not inevitable, career-oriented familes, both fathers and mothers, must consider what is important to them as they plan their families. Successful parenting cannot be fit into odd moments of leftover time.

Infant and Childcare for the Employed Mother

One of the biggest problems for mothers who must, or choose to, work is finding childcare—care that is not merely safe but that will be a positive factor in their infant's and child's development. For the mother who knows she must return to work within a few weeks after her baby's birth, this can be a major concern during pregnancy.

Potential caretakers commonly include another family member, such as a grandmother living in the home or nearby; someone who is hired to come into the home; or an individual or daycare center to which the baby is taken. In some families the husband and wife may arrange their employment so that one of them will always be with the baby. In a few families the husband may care for the baby while his wife is employed away from home, but this is still the exception in most American households. Communal living arrangements provide caretakers for a limited number of couples.

Although individual circumstances affect the decisions that a mother makes, social factors also appear important. Traditionally, few middle class mothers have chosen group care for small babies. This has been due, at least in the past, to the paucity of daycare centers in middle class neighborhoods, but it also seems to be related to a reluctance to use such centers even if they were present. Taking their baby to someone, either an older woman or perhaps a young mother with children of her own, is more acceptable to these mothers. An often preferred but more expensive alternative is hiring someone to come into the family's home to care for the child. Aside from the expense, finding a suitable person is difficult in many areas.

For other mothers daycare may be the alternative, unless they are living in an extended family. Currently there is a shortage of licensed daycare facilities. And only a small percentage of these facilities provide truly comprehensive services. Much daycare is custodial, providing safety but little more. Some is neglectful.

What should parents look for in choosing a caretaker? For small infants and children, a one-to-one relationship between caretaker and child would appear to be best. Murray[57] wonders whether a caretaker with four infants can provide sufficient responsiveness and stimulation.

The individual should be a warm, stimulating, nonrejecting person. Continuity is also important. A baby will need to form an attachment to his caretaker, just as he must to his parents, if he is to develop in an emotionally healthy way.

The caretaker's philosophy and rules of care must be similar to those of the parents; few small children can live by two sets of rules. Consider the confusion, for example, if parents encourage their 8 month old baby to try to feed himself and to experiment with the textures in his food, but his caretaker slaps his hand if he puts it in his plate and roughly scrubs his face with a washcloth, frowning all the while, when food misses his mouth.

For the adolescent mother, married or unmarried, the caretaker is often her own mother, an aunt, or even a grandmother. Under these circumstances it is often difficult for the young mother to make suggestions about how she feels the baby should be cared for. Young mothers tell of their distress over some of their own mothers' practices (dressing the baby too warmly on a hot day, for instance), yet they feel unable to change the situation.

Moreover, they may be unable, economically or emotionally, to care for the baby without that parent's help.

Unanswered Questions

The mother who is employed is an integral part of American life. Many of our childbearing women will return to work within a few weeks following delivery. It is necessary for us to be knowledgeable about the effect of maternal employment on children, both in order to help these women integrate their roles of wife, mother, and worker and to make a contribution to public planning for infant and child care for those families in which the mother is away from home.

There are no clear answers for the employed mother who is concerned about depriving her child, and almost all are concerned about this. Many more questions need to be explored. Does the age or sex or social class of the child make a difference? Is an unhappy mother at home better than a cheerful, hired caretaker? Is the effect of full-time work different from that of part-time work? Are fathers as effective as mothers in caring for infants and small children? The answers to these and similar questions are highly important to our society.

Cultural Norms of Nurses Who Care for Childbearing Families

It is important that we recognize the cultural factors that influence the behavior of childbearing families. It may even be more important for us to understand how cultural factors influence our professional lives. In essence, nurses and other professional workers are influenced by two sets of norms—those of their own cultural heritage and those acquired in the process of becoming a professional person.

Norms of the Nurse as a Person

Cultural factors that influence families also influence nurses. We bring to nursing the norms of our social class, our religion, the community in which we live, and the many other facets of our own cultural heritage. In the preceding pages, we have already illustrated some of the ways in which our values may differ from those of our patients—in relation to families in poverty and to American Indian families, for example. Many additional illustrations will be found throughout this book.

The "middle class" values of many nurses and other professionals can be a major barrier to providing health care for those who do not share them, if we do not consider these values in our planning. For instance, for many years the middle class assumption about unwed pregnant women has been that the pregnancy was an "accident" and the solution has been a hurried marriage or adoption. We now know that neither our assumption nor our solutions are necessarily correct, either for women who are not middle class or even for those who are.

Religious beliefs are another of our cultural norms that may conflict with patient values in many areas of nursing, and particularly in issues surrounding childbearing, such as family planning and abortion. The cardinal principle is that professionals, such as nurses, have no right to impose personal convictions or feelings on patients.

Norms of the Nurse as a Nurse

Values and norms of nurses can enhance good perinatal care, or they can be barriers to good care. Examples may be seen throughout this text and on any day on virtually every clinical unit.

One of the most pervasive cultural influences upon us is the "medical model" of childbearing. In sharp contrast is the view that for most mothers childbearing is a normal physiologic process. A basic question might be phrased. "Who runs the show?" Is childbearing a family function, supported and assisted by nurses and physicians? Or is childbearing within the purview of professionals, with compliance expected from families and those families who do not follow "orders" labeled as "bad"?

Although there have been some changes in recent years, the medical model of childbearing predominates in the United States. The medical model has even been upheld in the courtroom (Fitzgerald vs. Porter Memorial Hospital, No. 75–1203). The issue: could physicians and administrators bar fathers from the delivery room? In a ruling of the Seventh Circuit Court of Appeals, written by Justice John Paul Stevens (now a Justice of the United States Supreme Court), it was stated that an obstetric procedure "is comparable to other serious hospital procedures" and thus maternity patients had no greater right to determine hospital procedure than did other hospital patients.

Is the medical model essential to good perinatal care? Is it a barrier? Or does it really matter? Many nurses question this view of childbearing; others support it in whole or in part. Practices that evolve from the medical model and are a part of the cultural context of childbearing include labor in bed, usually in a recumbent position; elective induction of labor when there is no clear medical indication for this; separation of the family during the majority of the intrapartum period; frequent use of anesthesia, forceps, and episiotomy, and so on.

A physiologic, family-centered "culture of childbearing" does not need to be antimedical, although frustration with the prevailing system has led some couples to reject the system altogether for varying reasons. Physiologic care will work in rhythm with the woman's body, often making many of the procedures described above unnecessary during normal labor and delivery. Family-centered care makes parents informed partners in decisions and allows them to be together throughout as much of childbearing as they choose to be.

Beds that permit labor and delivery without a hurried rush down the hall and rooms that allow the same (and do not necessarily resemble operating rooms) are examples of environmental changes related to the idea that childbearing is a physiologic, family-centered process. Experiments with early discharge, which may return the mother and her infant who have no complications to their home 12 hours following delivery, along with modifications in hospital care following delivery are additional examples of changes in our norms that will be discussed, along with other options, in appropriate sections of this book.

Few of us wish to return to nineteenth century obstetrics, but the opposite extreme, that of seeing childbearing totally in terms of a medical model that is a part of nursing subculture as well, seems no more desirable.

When the Values of Families Differ from the Values of Nurses

Families come to childbearing with many and varying cultural values. Nurses, too, meet these patients with their own set of values. How can nurses give the best of care to patients whose life experiences and values differ from their own? A number of suggestions have already been made in this chapter. They are summarized below, along with some additional principles.

1. Every family can be treated with dignity, as individuals rather than as cases, regardless of whatever makes them seem "different."

2. We can talk with every family using terms that are familiar to them. This may mean the use of another language, such as

Spanish, or the use of idiomatic English. Often it will mean learning what terms a family or group uses that differ from those the nurse will ordinarily use.

3. We must understand the social organization of the families with whom we work, so that we will see why in some families the mother must defer decisions to the father and others in the extended family group, whereas in other situations the woman alone may make decisions about her plans.

4. We can involve the family in the planning of their care, so that plans are made in accordance with their priorities and needs.

5. We must understand the role expected of nurses by families with different cultural her-

itages and must work within these expectations as far as possible. This may involve slowing our pace (not an easy accomplishment) and observing social amenities that may seem time-wasting to us but are important to the families.

6. We can be willing to learn things that may differ from what we have previously experienced.

7. We must avoid making promises we cannot keep.

Knowing and working with families from a variety of cultural backgrounds add richness and depth to our nursing practice when we appreciate the significance of culture in the life of every individual.

REFERENCES

1. Abernethy, V.: Illegitimate Conception Among Teenagers. *Nursing Digest, IV*(3):8, 1976.
2. Adair, J., and Deuschle, K.: *The People's Health: Anthropology and Medicine in a Navajo Community.* New York, Appleton-Century Crofts, 1970.
3. Aichlmayr, R. H.: Cultural Understanding: A Key to Acceptance. *Nursing Outlook, 17*:20, 1969.
4. Ashley, J.: Nursing and Early Feminism. *American Journal of Nursing, 75*:1465, 1975.
5. Auerbach, K. G.: Behavior During Pregnancy: A Sociological Analysis. Unpublished doctoral dissertation, University of Minnesota, 1976.
6. Baldwin, B.: Problem Pregnancy Counseling: General Principles. *In* Wilson, R. (ed.): *Problem Pregnancy and Abortion Counseling.* Saluda, N.C., Family Life Publications, Inc., 1973.
7. Baldwin, G.: Discussion to paper by Von der Ahe. *American Journal of Obstetrics and Gynecology, 104*:286, 1969.
8. Bancroft, A.: Pregnancy and the Counterculture. *Nursing Clinics of North America, 8*:67, 1973.
9. Beauvoir, de, S.: *The Second Sex.* New York, Alfred A. Knopf, Inc., 1957.
10. Bell, D.: *A Time to Be Born.* New York, William Morrow and Co., Inc., 1975.
11. Bell, R. R.: *Marriage and Family Interaction.* Homewood, Ill., The Dorsey Press, 1971.
12. Benson, L.: *Fatherhood: A Sociological Perspective.* New York, Random House, Inc., 1968.
13. Boston Women's Health Book Collective: *Our Bodies, Ourselves.* New York, Simon & Schuster, Inc., 1973.
14. Brill, G.: *Indian and Free: A Contemporary Portrait of Life on a Chippewa Reservation.* Minneapolis, University of Minnesota Press, 1971.
15. Burchinal, L., and Rossman, J.: Personality Characteristics of Children. *Marriage and Family Living, 23*:334, 1961.
16. Cach, E., and Hearne, D. (eds.): *Our Brother's Keeper: The Indian in White America.* New York, New American Library, 1969.
17. Chesterman, H.: The Pubic Health Nurse and Family Planning. *Nursing Outlook, 12*:32 (September), 1964.
18. Chung, H.: Understanding the Oriental Maternity Patient. *Nursing Clinics of North America, 12*:67, 1977.
19. Clark, M.: *Health in the Mexican-American Culture.*
   Berkeley, Ca., University of California Press, 1959.
20. Curtis, G.: Retreat from Liberation. *Texas Monthly,* June, 1975, p. 58.
21. Deloria, V.: Custer Died For Your Sins: An Indian Manifesto. New York, The Macmillan Co., 1969.
22. Douvan, E.: Employment and the Adolescent. *In* Nye, F., and Hoffman, L. (eds.): *The Employed Mother in America.* Chicago, Rand McNally and Co., 1963.
23. Eiduson, B., Cohen, J., and Alexander, J.: Alternatives in Child Rearing in the 1970's. *American Journal of Orthopsychiatry, 43*:720, 1973.
24. Francoeur, R. T.: *Utopian Motherhood: New Trends in Human Reproduction.* New York, Doubleday & Co., Inc., 1970.
25. Frankfort, E.: *Vaginal Politics.* New York, Quadrangle Books, 1972.
26. Friedan, B.: *The Feminine Mystique.* New York, W. W. Norton & Co., Inc., 1963.
27. Gano, H. J.: *The Urban Villagers.* New York, The Free Press, 1962.
28. Gans, H. T.: *The Levittowners.* New York, Pantheon Books, 1967.
29. Goodwin, L.: Middle-Class Misperceptions of the High Life Aspirations and Strong Work Ethic Held by the Welfare Poor. *American Journal of Orthopsychiatry, 43*:554, 1973.
30. Gottlieb, D., and Heinsohn, A. L.: *America's Other Youth: Growing Up Poor.* Englewood Cliffs, N.J., Prentice-Hall, Inc., 1971.
31. Greenberg, M., and Morris, N.: Engrossment: The Newborn's Impact Upon the Father. *American Journal of Orthopsychiatry, 44*:520, 1974.
32. Greenberg, M., Rosenberg, I., and Lind, J.: First Mothers Rooming-In with their Newborns: Its Impact upon the Mother. *American Journal of Orthopsychiatry, 43*:783, 1973.
33. Haire, D.: *The Cultural Warping of Childbirth.* Milwaukee, Wisc., International Childbirth Education Association, 1972.
34. Halpern, F.: *Survival: Black/White.* Elmsford, N.Y., Pergamon Press, 1973.
35. Hedgepeth, W.: *The Alternative: Communal Life in New America.* New York, The Macmillan Co., 1970.
36. Hill, R.: *Families Under Stress.* New York, Harper & Bros., 1949.

37. Hoffman, L., and Nye, F.: *Working Mothers.* San Francisco, Josey-Bass, Inc., Publishers, 1974.

38. Howell, M.: Employed Mothers and Their Families: Part I. *Pediatrics, 52:*256, 1973.

39. *Indian Health Trends and Services.* Washington, D.C., U.S. Department of Health, Education and Welfare; Public Health Service, 1974.

40. Jorgensen, V.: The Gynecologist and the Sexually Liberated Woman. *Obstetrics and Gynecology, 42:*607, 1973.

41. Judd, J.: Nursing Implications. Comment on an article by Greenberg and Morris: Engrossment. *Nursing Digest IV*(1):22, 1976.

42. Kaiser, B., and Kaiser, I.: The Challenge of the Women's Movement to American Gynecology. *American Journal of Obstetrics and Gynecology, 120:*652, 1974.

43. Kanter, R.: *Commitment and Community: Communes and Utopias in Sociological Perspective.* Cambridge, Harvard University Press, 1972.

44. Keyerling, M.: Our Children Are Our Future: Early Childhood Development and the Need for Services. *American Journal of Orthopsychiatry, 43:*4, 1973.

45. Kennell, J., et al.: Maternal Behavior One Year After Early and Extended Post Partum Contact. *Developmental Medicine and Child Neurology, 16:*172, 1974.

46. Kimball, C.: Discussion to paper by Von der Ahe. *American Journal of Obstetrics and Gynecology, 104:*285, 1969.

47. Klaus, M., et al.: Maternal Attachment: Importance of the First Post-partum Days. *New England Journal of Medicine, 286:*440, 1972.

48. Lancaster, J.: Coping Mechanisms for the Working Mother. *American Journal of Nursing, 75:*1332, 1975.

49. LeMasters, E.: *Parents in Modern America: a Sociological Analysis.* Homewood, Ill., Dorsey Press, 1970.

50. McCoy, G., and Muth, F.: The Alternatives in Continuing the Pregnancy. *In* Wilson, R. (ed.): *Problem Pregnancy and Abortion Counseling.* Saluda, N.C., Family Life Publications, Inc., 1973.

51. Mead, M.: *Sex and Temperament in Three Primitive Societies.* New York, Dell Publishing Co., 1963.

52. Melville, K.: *Communes in the Counter Culture: Origins, Theories, Styles of Life.* New York, William Morrow and Co., Inc., 1972.

53. *Monthly Vital Statistics Report.* Vol. 24, No. II, February 13, 1976, Table 11, page 11.

54. *Monthly Vital Statistics Report,* Vol. 29, No. II (supplement), April 28, 1980.

55. Moore, T.: Children of Working Mothers. *In* Yudkin, S., and Holme, W. (eds.): *Working Mothers and Their Children.* London, Sphere Books, 1969.

56. Moustafa, A., and Weiss, G.: Health Status and Practices of Mexican Americans. Los Angeles, School of Public Health, University of California, 1968.

57. Murray, A.: Maternal Employment Reconsidered: Effects on Infants. *American Journal of Orthopsychiatry, 45:*773, 1975.

58. Newson, J., and Newson, E.: *Infant Care in an Urban Community.* New York, International Universities Press, 1963.

59. Nye, F., and Hoffman, L.: *The Employed Mother in America.* Chicago, Rand McNally & Co., 1963.

60. Pannor, R.: The Unmarried Father—the Forgotten Man. *Nursing Outlook, 18:*36, (November), 1970.

61. Pannor, R., Massarek, F., and Evans, B.: *The Unmarried Father.* New York, Springer Publishing Co., Inc., 1971.

62. Primeaux, M.: American Indian Health Care Practices: A Cross-Cultural Perspective. *Nursing Clinics of North America, 12:*55, 1977.

63. Rainwater, L.: *Behind Ghetto Walls; Black Families in a Federal Slum.* Chicago, Aldine Publishing Co., 1970.

64. Ringler, N. M., et al.: Mother to Child Speech at 2 Years: Effects of Early Postnatal Contact. *Journal of Pediatrics, 86:*141, 1975.

65. Rossi, A.: Family Development in a Changing World. *American Journal of Psychiatry, 128:*47, 1972.

66. Rossi, A. (ed.): *The Feminist Papers: from Adams to de Beauvoir.* New York, Columbia University Press, 1973.

67. Roszak, B., and Roszak, T. (eds.): *Masculine/Feminine.* New York, Harper and Row, Publishers, 1969.

68. Sanger, M.: *My Fight for Birth Control.* New York, Farrar Rinehart, 1931.

69. Schacter, J., and McCarthy, M.: Illegitimate Births: United States, 1938–57. *Vital Statistics—Special Reports, Selected Studies.* Vol. 47, No. 8. Washington D.C., U.S. Government Printing Office, 1960.

70. Schorr, T.: Current Shock. *American Journal of Nursing, 76:*911, 1976.

71. Schwarz, J., Strickland, R., and Krolick, G.: Infant Day Care: Behavioral Effects at Preschool Age. *Developmental Psychology, 10:*502, 1974.

72. Seaman, B.: *Free and Female.* New York, Coward, McCann and Geoghegan, Inc., 1972.

73. Siegel, A., et al.: Dependence and Independence in Children. *In* Nye, F., and Hoffman, L. (eds.): *The Employed Mother in America.* Chicago, Rand McNally & Co., 1963.

74. Steinberg, D.: Redefining Fatherhood: Notes After Six Months. *In* Howe, L. (ed.): *The Future of the Family.* New York, Simon & Schuster, Inc., 1972.

75. *Trends in Illegitimacy: United States, 1940–1965.* Washington, D.C., U.S. Government Printing Office, 1968.

76. Tripp-Reimer, T., and Friedl, M.: Appalachians: A Neglected Minority. *Nursing Clinics of North America, 12:*41, 1977.

77. Tylor, E.: *Primitive Culture.* New York, Henry Holt and Co., 1883.

78. U.S. Bureau of the Census: *Statistical Abstract of the United States: 1980* (101st Edition). Washington, D.C., U.S. Government Printing Office, 1980.

79. Veysey, L.: *The Communal Experience: Anarchist and Mystical Counter-Cultures in America.* New York, Harper and Row Publishers, Inc., 1973.

80. Vincent, C.: *Unmarried Mothers.* New York, The Free Press, 1961.

81. Vincent, C., Haney, C., and Cochrane, C.: Familial and Generational Patterns of Illegitimacy. *Journal of Marriage and the Family, 31:*659, November, 1969.

82. Von der Ahe, C.: The Unwed Teen-age Mother. *American Journal of Obstetrics and Gynecology, 104:*279, 1969.

83. Washburn, W.: The American Indian. *The Americana: 1974 Annual.* New York, Grolier, Inc., 1974, p. 63.

84. Weissman, M., et al.: The Educated Housewife: Mild Depression and the Search for Work. *American Journal of Orthopsychiatry, 43:*565, 1973.

85. Whyte, W. H.: "The Corporation and the Wife." *Fortune,* November, 1951, p. 109.

Family Planning

6

OBJECTIVES

1. Define:
    a. crude birth rate
    b. general fertility rate
    c. total fertility rate
2. Identify motives for childbearing.
3. Describe trends in population growth in the world and in the United States, and the major factors responsible for those trends.
4. Describe the relationship between family planning and family health.
5. Describe the mechanism of action and the advantages and disadvantages of the following methods of family planning:
    a. oral contraceptives
    b. intrauterine devices
    c. spermicidal preparations
    d. diaphragm
    e. natural family planning
    f. condoms
    g. coitus interruptus
    h. breast feeding
    i. surgical sterilization
6. Differentiate theoretical effectiveness and use effectiveness of contraceptives. Compare the effectiveness of contraceptive measures.
7. Explain potential reasons for family planning failure.
8. Describe the process of family planning counseling. Identify incentives and barriers.
9. Identify causes of infertility. Describe how fertility is evaluated in men and women and strategies for improving fertility.
10. Describe the process of artificial insemination.
    a. when husband provides semen
    b. when donor semen is used

In our society the term family planning has often been used as a synonym for contraception, which is unfortunate. Although family planning without the means of controlling birth would be virtually impossible, the mechanics of such control is a beginning, not an end in itself.

Family planning means advice to the apparently infertile couple, genetic counseling for the family of a baby with a genetically transmitted defect, or help for the woman who feels she cannot cope with pregnancy. It means education to help individuals and couples determine when, and if, they are ready to be parents, and then assistance to help them achieve their goal. Family planning may include adoption or artificial insemination.

Although nurses think of family planning primarily in terms of individual women and couples, we cannot escape the implications of our work for groups of people. For example, in an area where infant morbidity and mortality are high, can we improve the health of mothers and infants and even of older children through excellent family counsel? If we believe we can, how can we reach out to these families?

As a beginning, we need to be aware of the reasons why people choose to limit (or not to limit) their families, their motives for pregnancy, and their fears, as well as the advantages and disadvantages of various contraceptive devices. A special facility in communication is important, because family planning involves human sexuality, a topic some people find difficult to discuss.

Motivation for Childbearing

Every minute of the day, in every part of the world, children are born. Some are greatly desired; some are accepted as "God's will," with little understanding of the biologic principles of procreation; still others are viewed as "accidents" and are scarcely welcomed.

The motivations for pregnancy are many. Because the motivation for having a child may affect the child's development and the total family, it is an important consideration. Often the motivation is not apparent to the parent.

To create a new human being and to guide that infant, then child, then adolescent in a way that allows him to develop his own best self are deeply satisfying experiences, and rightly so. However, some of the motives discussed below have negative connotations. The pregnancy and the child may meet a need in the lives of the parents that is not necessarily in the best interests of the child.

Childbearing as a Source of Joy. In spite of the demands they inevitably make, one's children also bring occasions of pure joy that are difficult to match with any other experience. Few can resist eliciting a baby's smile, or the warm comfort of a baby sleeping on one's shoulder. Couples perceive these rewards in others and anticipate similar rewards for themselves.

Childbearing as a Manifestation of Their Love for One Another. For many couples a newborn baby is a tangible manifestation of their love for one another, a gift each gives to the other.

Childbearing to Create a Loved and Loving Family. Parents anticipate a child they will love and who will, in return, love them. No matter how difficult the rest of the world may become, even if one's partner is lost through death or divorce, a loving relationship with one's children provides a sense of belonging and mutual caring. Some parents are able to express affectionate feelings toward children that they cannot express to adults, even to their partners.

For most parents the desire to love and be loved creates a warm environment in which children grow and prosper. However, *overwhelming* needs to be loved, with expectations that are far beyond the capacity of the infant or young child, may lead to problems of child abuse when the infant is unable to satisfy the parents' needs.

Childbearing as a Bridge to the Future. Children offer parents a chance to achieve a kind of immortality. In the nineteenth century Thomas Campbell wrote, in the poem *Hallowed Ground,* "To live in hearts we leave behind/Is not to die." Some parents envision a life for their children that will be better than their own and, consequently, will be a source of satisfaction for them. Other parents believe that through their children they share themselves with the world of the future.

Childbearing as a Sacred Duty. For some couples the Biblical teaching to "be fruitful and multiply" is a divine command, and children are a sign of God's blessing on the marriage. The bearing of children is a part of the plan God has for their lives.

Childbearing as a Steppingstone into the Adult World. In many traditional societies, clearly defined "rites of passage" mark the transition to adulthood. There may be rituals, attended by the entire community; changes in the manner of dress; and so on.

There are fewer clear-cut indications of adulthood in our own society. Frequently both adolescents and young adults see pregnancy as an affirmation of their competency as adults. "We can do *something;* we can produce a child, therefore we are now a part of the adult world."

Childbearing to Save a Relationship. For some couples, childbearing is an attempt to "save" a faltering marriage or to stabilize a fragile relationship outside of marriage. This attempt may be the idea of one partner or of both.

One or both may feel that a child will give them a common experience that they can share, so that they will grow closer together. A woman may hope that a child will cause her mate to "settle down" and become more responsible and to care more about home and about her.

All of the odds are against the success of such an attempt. Pregnancy and the adaptation to a new member of a family add strain to even a firm, stable union; the stress on a fragile union may cause further disintegration.

Moreover, the child conceived for this purpose who fails in his appointed task is often rejected for that failure.

Childbearing as a Substitute for a Relationship. When the relationship between a man and a woman is poor, the woman, especially, may see in her child an opportunity for the satisfying relationship that is lacking with her partner. It is not difficult to imagine the tremendous burden such desires place on her relationship with a child who, in his early months and years, is very much a receiver of warmth and affection rather than a giver.

The unmarried girl or woman who feels she is unloved may also see a baby as an answer to her needs. She may have no special relationship with the baby's father but desires a baby as a love-object upon whom she can shower her love and who will love her in return. When the dependent, demanding baby fails to meet her needs, she is likely to feel highly ambivalent and frequently hostile toward the baby.

Childbearing to Please Others. "We had not planned to have children for several years, but the pressure from our parents, who wanted to become grandparents, was so intense that we decided to go ahead and start our family."

A variation on the theme quoted above is, "All of our friends were having children, and we felt left out, so we decided to have a baby too."

In a similar way, adolescents may experience *peer pressure,* which is not principally directed toward childbearing but toward sexual behavior that may result in childbearing. The more insecure an adolescent is, the more likely he is to feel the need to gain approval by competing with other adolescents in becoming sexually active or to copy the behavior of a sexually active peer. The fact that these experiences are frequently unhappy because the emphasis is on the sexual act itself and not on the relationship between the persons involved compounds the adolescent's insecurity and may lead to still more attempts.

Childbearing to Produce an Heir or a Child of a Specific Sex. "My husband wants a son," said the mother of two daughters, "and we are going to keep on having babies until there is a Quincy Gotrocks III."

"I've always wanted a little girl, to dress in pretty dresses and teach to sew and play the piano," said another woman.

But there are no guarantees that the child will be of the desired sex or even that the child of the desired sex will fulfill the parents' fantasy. Very likely, he or she will not. The baby may indeed be a little girl, but one who grows to love climbing trees and Little League baseball more than dresses and dolls.

Childbearing to Replace a Lost Child. When a sibling has died, some parents hope that another child may fill the void that they are experiencing. It seems important to discuss this issue as part of the counseling of parents after a child's death. Moreover, if the initial assessment during pregnancy reveals the death of a sibling, we need to be aware of this possibility and alert to any indications of this motive for pregnancy.

Childbearing to Affirm Femininity or Masculinity. For the woman who has doubts about her femininity or for the man who feels a need to prove his masculinity, the ability to become pregnant or to impregnate may be a way of affirming sexuality. The woman may seek a large family to confirm her womanliness; for the man fathering many children may represent "machismo" or maleness.

Childbearing as an Escape. Pregnancy may be viewed as a means of escaping from an undesirable situation. For the adolescent this may be an unhappy home life, with little realization that life in a forced marriage or as a single mother will often be no improvement. Older women also may see pregnancy as a chance for escape—from a job they don't like or as an excuse for avoiding other expected activities, for example.

Childbearing to Fill a Void. Women who express a feeling of "emptiness" may see in pregnancy a way to fill the psychic void within themselves. For such women, the desire may be not for the child but for pregnancy per se. One pregnancy may be followed by another.

Pseudocyesis, a condition that mimics the symptoms of pregnancy (often called false pregnancy), may occur in these women when the void is unfilled by an actual pregnancy.

Childbearing as Therapy for Physiologic Problems. Pregnancy may be undertaken as a cure for menstrual cramps, backache, migraine headache, and a variety of other ills. Here again it is the pregnancy that is desired; the child may almost be a byproduct.

Childbearing for the Emotional Satisfaction of Producing a Perfect Child. Every parent-to-be, and every parent, feels that his or her child is special. But some parents approach parenthood with the expectation of producing a "perfect child." They postpone pregnancy until the "perfect" time. Each detail is carefully planned. They expect to gain their satisfaction from their ability to produce a perfect child.

After the baby's birth the attempt to have everything "just so" continues. Here too there is a feeling of disappointment in the child who does not fit their plan. The scholar they fantasized is a nice but average child. Their athlete, in spite of all they do (and sometimes because of all they do), is on the second string.

Childbearing as an Act of Rebellion or Hostility. Adolescents, particularly, may choose sexual intercourse as a way of rejecting parental values. The more rigid they view their parents' values to be or the more uncomfortable their parents seem to be about sexual matters, the more valuable their sexual behavior becomes as a weapon.

Cohen and Friedman[18] quote one teen-aged girl, who had told her mother she was pregnant, as saying with great satisfaction, "Seeing the look of horror on my mother's face made the whole thing worthwhile."

The motives described here are mostly individual in nature. Social factors affecting high and low fertility are discussed in the section on population growth that follows. Some possible reasons for unplanned pregnancies are discussed later in this chapter.

Population Growth: The World in Which We Practice

Nurses have traditionally viewed population growth at the level of the individual family. The number of children born to particular parents has been more important to us than the fertility and reproductive rates of the nation and of the world. But population, as a national and as a worldwide issue, does affect us both as individuals and as nurses. As individuals, we are all a part of the problems of the world in which we live. As nurses, we find

that "official" attitudes toward reproduction can mean government funds for family planning clinics or, conversely, severe limitations on providing the family planning advice that we may feel is highly important to the physical and mental health of a particular family. Emphasis on zero population growth can mean that we fail to appreciate the concerns of an infertile couple.

Demographers have been concerned with population trends for many years, but population growth became an important social and political issue in the 1960's. Three terms are used by demographers to describe trends in births:

1. *Crude birth rate* (CBR) is the number of births per year per 1000 population.

2. *General fertility rate* (GFR) is the number of births per year per 1000 women aged 15 to 44 years.

3. *Total fertility rate* (TFR) is the sum of the fertility rates for women of different age groups in a given year.

Such distinctions may seem unimportant to the average person, but they assist demographers in more clearly understanding births. For example, if a large number of women between the ages of 20 and 30 were having babies, both the crude birth rate and the general fertility rate would rise; the total fertility rate would give an indication of the reason for the rise, i.e., an increase in the birth rate for women in a particular age group. Thus, although all three measures roughly follow the same pattern of ups and downs, each gives specific information that is valuable. In comparing birth rates of the world's nations, particularly the rates of underdeveloped nations, crude birth rate figures are often the most readily available.

Demographic Trends in the United States

Population in the United States, as well as in the rest of the world, began to grow not because birth rates increased but because death rates decreased. This growth was slow in the eighteenth century, accelerated in the nineteenth century, and became very, very rapid in the twentieth century (Fig. 6–1). Throughout this period of population growth, birth rates have been decreasing. In the United States there was a decrease in the white population from 7.0 births per woman in the year 1800 to 2.1 births per woman in 1936. Figures for nonwhite women have not been recorded over as long a period of time, but in general the downward trend has been the same, although the birth rate has been higher.

The fact that a level of 2.1 births per woman

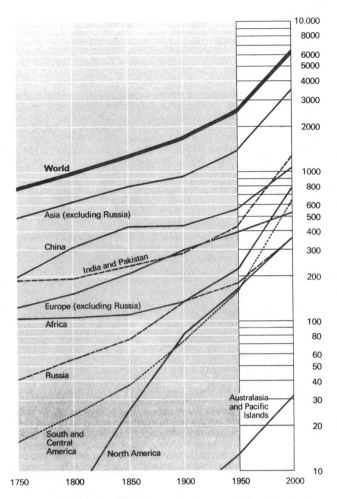

Figure 6–1. The growth of world population 1750–1950, with projections to 2000 (population in millions). (From Wrigley: *Population and History*. Copyright © 1969 McGraw-Hill Inc. Used by permission of McGraw-Hill Book Co.)

was achieved in the United States in 1936, considerably before the use of oral contraceptives and intrauterine devices (IUD's), suggests rather strongly that contraceptive technology is not the only factor in limiting births. Among the factors that apparently contributed to this low fertility rate were:

1. A higher proportion of women who never married.

2. A higher proportion of women who married at a later age.

3. A high level of unemployment and economic insecurity that motivated couples to postpone childbearing.

The downward trend of fertility in the United States reversed after World War II (the 1940's) with a tremendous rise occurring from 1946 through 1958. The "baby boom" came not from a rise in the number of large families but from a reduction in the number of childless couples and couples with only one child. The trends were the reverse of those of the depression years of the 1930's, as:

1. More women married.

2. Women married and had children at an earlier age.

3. Good job opportunities and opportunities

for homes in the suburbs made family living the lifestyle of many Americans. Pregnancy was "in"; childlessness was suspect.

Since the 1957 peak, birth rates in the United States have decreased steadily.

The crude birth rate (CBR) in the United States was 23.7 in 1960. By 1965 the CRB had dropped to 19.1; in both 1975 and 1976 a low of 14.8 was reached. The CBR rose slightly in 1977 (15.4), dropped slilghtly in 1978 (15.3), and rose again in 1979 (15.9). Comparable or slightly lower rates are found in other Western nations: Canada (15), United Kingdom (13), The Netherlands (13), France (14), Australia (15).

Although newer contraceptives have undoubtedly been a factor, again, as in the thirties, the decrease began before either the IUD or the oral contraceptives were being used widely enough to be a significant factor. Probably part of the reason for the drop is that couples in the peak years of the fifties achieved their desired family size rather quickly, and thus there were fewer births in the sixties.

A norm for smaller families is undoubtedly also important. Research studies in 1967 found an expected family size of 2.9 children; by 1972 similar studies found expected family size to be 2.1 children. Interrelated factors include a changing governmental policy toward family planning concepts (see below), an increase in the number of single women, the postponement of marriage and childbearing, and the desire or need of many women for jobs other than homemaking. The increased availability of abortion in the seventies has undoubtedly played some part. The rapidly rising cost of living may be related to postponement of marriage and childbearing and the need for women to work, much as economic factors in the depression years affected childbearing.

Government Policy and Family Planning in the United States

As early as the 1940's some political leaders had advocated federally supported family planning funds as part of maternal and child health programs for those states that wished them. But most Americans were not ready for such ideas, and there were many objections.

A major change in United States policy came in 1963, when Congress included the promotion of research on population growth in a foreign aid bill. Former President Eisenhower, who had previously blocked such legislation, now supported it as a means of helping nations keep fertility in check. But the program was slow in developing, and much of the hoped-for research into means of better fertility control was neither funded nor conducted.

In 1965 the Supreme Court of the United States ruled that laws prohibiting birth control were an invasion of "the right to privacy." Over the next 5 years congressional commitment to population problems grew, culminating in the Family Planning Services and Population Research Act of 1970, which encompassed support not only for research and family planning but also for manpower training and preparation of informational materials, and created an Office of Population Affairs in the Department of Health, Education and Welfare with full authority for family planning programs in the United States.

It was during these same years that biologist Paul Ehrlich wrote *The Population Bomb*,[24] which brought widespread public attention to population growth and advocated immediate and forceful action to control population. In the early years of the seventies, however, population growth in the United States dropped without the use of the strong measures suggested by Ehrlich.

Demographic Trends in the Rest of the World

In 1900 the world's population was roughly 1.5 billion. By mid-1975 there were 4 billion people living on earth. Currently the world's

Table 6–1. WORLD POPULATION DATA, 1979*

	Africa	Asia	North America	Latin America	Oceania	USSR	Europe	WORLD
Population, 1979 (in millions)	457	2498	244	352	23	264	483	4321
Growth rate (annual %)	2.9	1.8	0.7	2.7	1.3	0.8	0.4	1.7
No. years to double population	24	38	99	26	53	87	173	41
Birth rate (per 1000 population)	46	29	15	35	22	18	14	28
Death rate (per 1000 population)	17	11	9	8	9	10	10	11
Infant mortality rate (per 1000 live births)	143	99	14	86	43	30	20	95
Life expectancy at birth (in years)	47	57	73	62	69	70	72	60
% under age 15	44	38	24	42	31	26	24	36
Per capita gross national product (in U.S. dollars)	450	650	8620	1240	5560	3010	4910	1800

*From Page, Villee, and Villee: *Human Reproduction: Essentials of Reproductive and Perinatal Medicine,* 3rd Edition Philadelphia, W. B. Saunders Co., 1981.

population is increasing at the rate of approximately 2 per cent per year; in just 35 years, at this rate, the world will be expected to sustain twice the number of people as it does today.

As Table 6–1 indicates, population growth in Europe is lower than that of North America. The decline in fertility began in many European countries in the 1870's and 1880's, not only before modern contraception but largely without the use of any mechanical devices, such as the condom. Coitus interruptus was probably the most commonly used method. Gardner[32] uses the phrase "the collapse of fertility" to describe this phenomenon in Western Europe, a situation that the countries themselves (though obviously not individual families) view with mixed emotions. In some countries governments have attempted to increase fertility by various programs, such as free obstetric and child care and the payment of subsidies to mothers. At present rates of growth, it would take 175 years for the population of Western Europe to double.

The population of the Soviet Union is growing at a far faster rate than that of the other nations in Europe,[5] although the birth rate is declining. During the 1960's the Soviets opposed any international efforts toward family planning. Since that time, however, there has been an acknowledgement that excessive population growth can hinder economic development. In 1973 a demographic center was created at Moscow University to study both Soviet and world population problems.

Outside of the United States and Western Europe, Japan has led the way in slowing population growth, with a 50 per cent drop in births from 1948 to 1960, perhaps the most rapid decrease in reproduction in the world's history. Three factors are considered significant in this decline:

1. A strong interest in fertility reduction by a majority of Japanese families that caused a downward trend in fertility beginning in the 1920's.

2. The very energetic role of the Japanese government in birth control practices, probably the most active of any government ever.

3. Widespread, legal, induced abortion (about 1 in every 20 pregnancies in the peak year 1955).

Even though other Asian nations, such as India, are beginning to realize that overpopulation is a serious problem, and some (Taiwan, for example) are achieving a modest degree of success in family planning programs, some observers fear that these steps may already be too little and too late. For example, when compulsory vasectomy of men with three or

Table 6–2. PUERTO RICAN ADULTS' VIEWS OF IDEAL FAMILY SIZE*

Ideal Family Size	Men (Per Cent)	Women (Per Cent)
0	0.3	0.1
1	2.2	2.4
2	45.7	50.5
3	27.0	26.7
4	12.5	10.9
5	4.7	3.8
6–8	4.2	3.2
9 plus	1.0	0.6
As God wills	2.3	1.9

*From Hatt: *Background of Human Fertility in Puerto Rico.* Princeton, N.J., Princeton University Press, 1952.

more children was first under consideration in India, it was estimated that 100 surgeons or surgical technicians averaging 20 operations a day, 5 days a week, would take 8 years to cope with the existing candidates. In the meantime there would constantly be new candidates coming along. At today's rates the population of Asia will double in 30 years.

In the African nations, as death rates from diseases such as smallpox and malaria decline dramatically, governments vary in their feelings about population growth. Although some leaders are concerned about limiting fertility, others still consider their countries underpopulated and are suspicious of "outsiders" who advocate family planning. As Table 6–1 indicates, population increase is rapid in Africa; the population of Africa will double in 24 years at current rates of increase.

Population growth in Latin America is also rapid; continued growth at today's rates would mean a doubling of population in 26 years. Some governments support principles of family planning; in Venezuela the government appropriated a small amount of money for family planning programs in 1973 for the first time. Others are strongly opposed. There are approximately 80 million women of childbearing age in the Latin American nations; it is estimated that roughly 10 million middle class women use contraceptives. The remaining 70 million women average six children each, although surveys indicate that many of these women desire only three children. A study in Puerto Rico more than 20 years ago showed a preference for small family size (Table 6–2).

The Problems of World Population Growth

How many people can the earth sustain? We really don't know the answer. One question, of course, is "sustain at what level—in the lifestyle of an Asian or African farmer or of a Western European or middle class American?" A range of from 8 to 15 billion people is believed to be an absolute maximum at a very curtailed way of life. As we have already noted, the 8 billion mark will be reached within our own lifetime, just 35 years from now, if growth continues at current rates.

Some observers, such as Grant Cottam, a University of Wisconsin ecologist who was an official observer at the World Food Conference in Rome in 1974, feel that the world has possibly already reached its "carrying capacity" in terms of the number of people who can be fed using available resources. Only the food reserves of recent years have made survival possible, according to Cottam. Now that these reserves are gone to a large extent, he sees famine as inevitable *(Food and Population: Thinking the Unthinkable[29])*. In 1975 famine did occur in parts of central Africa and India and in Bangladesh.

Who is to feed the poor of the world is a major issue to be resolved throughout the remainder of this century. Not only will it probably become impossible to feed all of the world's hungry, but some people doubt the wisdom of even trying, feeling that food given to nations with no policy of population control will only lead to further population explosion and eventual disaster. Such ideas do not have universal acceptance. There are those who feel that technology, properly applied, can solve the world's food problems. Meanwhile the concept of triage, i.e., of cutting off food to groups of people who are starving, is unpleasant to everyone and unthinkable to a great many. Nevertheless, such triage already has occurred.

Starvation is not the only problem of unchecked population growth. The quality of life and economic standards of living are also adversely affected by rapid growth. For example, from 1945 to 1954 the gross domestic product of Latin America doubled, but rapid population growth kept the per capita increase far lower. Davis[19] says, "To put it in concrete terms, it is difficult to give a child the basic education he needs to become an engineer when he is one of eight children of an illiterate farmer who must support the family with the product of two acres of ground." Such problems are not limited to the developing nations. The cyclic dilemma of poverty leading to high fertility leading to poverty continues.

Another area sometimes overlooked in the concern for feeding the earth's people is the effect of high population density on life. Animal experiments (which can be applied to human populations only with great caution) indicate that when overcrowding exists, stress, rather than starvation, may be the major cause of death. Studies of chickens and of wild woodchucks have shown that caging too many animals together can cause a drastic increase in fatal heart attacks. Heart disease has also been found to increase in caged zoo animals (antelopes, deer, monkeys, and apes) when they are grouped together.

Calhoun[13] confined a population of Norwegian rats in a quarter acre enclosure and provided abundant food and protection from disease and predators. By the end of 27 months, the population could have expanded to 5000 animals, yet it stabilized at approximately 150. Although the adult rat mortality was unusually low, stress from the high level of social interaction led to such a disruption of maternal behavior that infant mortality was extremely high.

In other experiments Calhoun found that even moderate crowding affected rats by limiting their ability to carry pregnancy to term, to survive delivery, or to "mother" their litters. Males, too, showed behavioral disturbances.

Solutions: Family Planning Versus Population Policy

What is to be done about world population growth? Certain writers such as Kingsley Davis[19] and Bernard Berelson[6] draw a sharp distinction between "family planning" and "population policy."

A basic tenet of the family planning concept is voluntary contraception. The goal of family planning is to help parents have the number of children they want, when they desire them. It is not inconsistent with family planning principles for a couple to have four or six or more children if they so wish.

The aim of population control is to give society a feasible number of children. Although there are indications that many families, particularly poor families in many parts of the world, desire fewer children than they bear, just eliminating unwanted births would still leave a high birth rate in many societies.

No nation in the world has as yet developed what might be considered a population policy. Possible suggestions that might become part of such policy include:

1. Payments to people for allowing themselves to be sterilized.

2. Compulsory sterilization after a given number of pregnancies.

3. Free abortion.

4. Required abortion for illegitmate pregnancies.

5. A system of taxation that gives economic

advantages to single persons, such as taxation on marriage and on childbearing, elimination of tax exemptions for parents, and abandonment of tax policies that discriminate against couples when the wife works.

6. Creation of more opportunities for women to work outside the home, along with the assurance of equal education and equal pay for women.

7. Requiring a license to have children.

8. Temporary sterilization of all women by a technology not yet invented.

Although some of these suggestions are very much in conflict with our values (compulsory sterilization, for example), others, such as tax revision, may be politically unpopular but not totally unacceptable.

Family Planning and Family Health

Important as concerns about overpopulation are, they are not the only rationale for the planning of childbirth. Family health may also be affected in several ways:

1. The risk of stillbirth is relatively high for first births, low for second births, and increases thereafter, rising sharply after fifth and sixth births.[17]

2. The risk of infant and early childhood mortality increases steadily as the number of children in the family increases. (A second child has no advantage.) This has been found to be true in all social classes, although rates vary from one class to another.[2, 17, 33, 73]

3. Data on the relationship between family size and the frequency of specific diseases (respiratory infection, gastroenteritis, and so forth) are conflicting. Social class variation is probably one reason. The way in which data are gathered is important. If visits to a physician are the criteria for determining the frequency of illness, the mother of seven who is not overly concerned and does not seek treatment for a child's respiratory infection may appear to have a healthier family than the mother of two who does seek such assistance.

4. The risk of prematurity has been found to be higher when there is less than 12 months from the end of one pregnancy to the beginning of the next. Prematurity is the major cause of neonatal death (death within 28 days after birth) and a major cause of infant morbidity.

5. A number of studies show some decline in successful marital adjustment with increasing family size. One reason may be that success in controlling fertility may be a factor in marital satisfaction.[69]

6. Diminished maternal care has been found to be a correlate of some large families.[76] It is not difficult to understand the problems that a mother with several children under the age of 6 may have in meeting even the basic physical needs of each child individually.

7. Not only total family size but the spacing of pregnancy can affect family satisfaction. Before a subsequent child is born, a mother should feel both physically and emotionally ready. The father's feeling that he is ready is important too. When a previous child is 12 to 15 months old, he is still very demanding. It is hard for a mother to meet his still very strong needs for nurturing, as well as those of a new baby. By the time he is 3 years of age, the older child is less dependent. He is verbal enough to talk about the pregnancy and the new baby with his parents and to express his feelings about the baby.

A great volume of additional studies about the interrelation between family size and family health has been and is being conducted. One problem in studies of this type is determining what other variables are affecting the outcome. For example, malnutrition is often correlated with large family size, but is this because poor families are overrepresented in the large families of the study? One cannot compare the health of a middle class family with two children with that of a lower class family with six children. Future research should answer more of our questions.

Social Factors Affecting High Fertility

Family planning programs presuppose, in principle at least, that access to information about and materials of contraception will decrease birth rates. Although this is obviously true up to a point, we have already seen that fertility rates in many nations fell, often sharply, before the advent of modern contraceptives.

Obviously other factors are important in influencing high fertility. At certain times, and in certain societies, both industrialized and agrarian, large families brought status to both man and woman, often enhancing their position in the community. A woman's chief claim to fame might be the numbers of her children and grandchildren. Fertility has been thus extolled, even in our own country, until relatively recently. Moreover, a large family was insurance against both high infant mortality and loneliness and lack of care in old age.

Religious Factors

Religious beliefs are related to high levels of fertility in various ways. In some predominantly Roman Catholic countries, such as some nations of Latin America, church opposition

Table 6–3. THE TREND OF CATHOLIC BIRTH CONTROL PRACTICE BEFORE THE ENCYCLICAL*

	1955 (Per Cent)	1960 (Per Cent)	1965 (Per Cent)
Never used any method	43	30	22
Used rhythm only	27	31	25
Had used other methods	30	38	53

*From Westoff and Westoff: *From Now to Zero: Fertility, Contraception and Abortion in America.* Boston, Little, Brown & Co., 1971.

may influence governmental policy and may even make the use of birth control illegal, as it was in two states of the United States until the 1960's. Because of the large number of Roman Catholics and of families of other religions living in predominantly Roman Catholic countries, it is important for us to be aware of Catholic doctrine and practice in relation to birth control.

In July 1968 Pope Paul VI issued a 38-page encyclical *Humanae Vitae,* which defined Roman Catholic doctrine in relation to contraception, abortion, and sterilization. For contraception the rhythm method (and abstinence) is approved, and artificial means of birth control are rejected in these words:

If, then, there are serious motives to space out births, which derive from the physical or psychological conditions of husband and wife, or from external conditions, the church teaches that it is then licit to take into account the natural rhythms in the generative functions, for the use of marriage in the infecund [infertile] periods only, and this way to regulate birth without offending the moral principles. . . .

This encyclical was one more step in a long series of debates that have spanned the centuries of Christianity, influenced at various times by St. Augustine's condemnation of all contraception in the fourth century, Pope Gregory IX's decree in 1230 that contraception was to be considered the equivalent of murder, and St. Thomas Aquinas' views in the thir-

teenth century that the enjoyment of intercourse without the goal of procreation was not legitimate. By the mid-eighteenth century it was evident that in the Western world many couples, including Roman Catholic couples, were limiting their families. In 1930 Pope Pius XI issued *Casti Connubii,* reaffirming procreation as the primary goal of marriage and contraception as an "offense against the law of God and of nature, and those who indulge in such are branded with the guilt of a grave sin."

Not all Roman Catholics have agreed with these positions. One of the physicians chiefly responsible for the development of oral contraceptives, Dr. John Rock, a Roman Catholic, argues that the pill established a safe period similar to nature's safe period during pregnancy.

Following the encyclical of 1968, there was open disagreement in the Catholic press and among theologians about contraception. As Tables 6–3 and 6–4 indicate, women in the United States (and apparently in other parts of the world as well[78]) have been increasing their use of forms of contraception other than rhythm steadily over the last decades and have continued to do so following the *Humanae Vitae.*

In relation to our family planning practice, it seems evident that Roman Catholic families do not share a single set of beliefs about contraception. Individual wishes are our guide in counseling these families, as in any other family.

Table 6–4. METHODS OF CONTRACEPTION USED MOST RECENTLY BEFORE AND AFTER THE ENCYCLICAL BY CATHOLIC FERTILE WOMEN UNDER 44, MARRIED AT LEAST 4 YEARS*

	1965 (Per Cent)	1969 (Per Cent)
No method	7	4
Rhythm	35	32
Pill	14	37
Other methods	44	27

*From Westoff and Westoff: *From Now to Zero: Fertility, Contraception and Abortion in America.* Boston, Little, Brown & Co., 1971.

Black Fertility

When fertility statistics are tabulated by race, it is obvious that throughout the years black fertility rates are consistently higher. Further analysis of black fertility indicates that the reason lies in the higher number of blacks who are poor and who have had limited educations. Black women who are married to professional men or to men with college educations tend to have *lower* fertility rates than comparable groups of white women.

Black women interviewed in the 1965 National Fertility Study indicated a desire for the same number of fewer children (2.6 per woman) desired by the white women interviewed, but black women expected to have considerably more children (4.0 per woman). The chief difference between the black and the white women interviewed was therefore in the control of fertility rather than in the number of children desired. In this group of women only 8 per cent of the blacks and 28 per cent of the whites were completely successful both in achieving the number of children they desired and in timing the births as they desired. Although 58 per cent of the black couples and 60 per cent of the white couples were using some form of contraception, the methods of contraception used by black families were often the least effective methods. For example, among black couples 30 to 44 years old, 25 per cent used the douche, probably the least effective of any method.

Another reason for high rates of fertility among black women may be the meaning of pregnancy for the unmarried, lower class, black adolescent. Having a baby may be the "rite of passage" that signifies that she is no longer an adolescent, just as marriage or college is in other segments of our society.

Social Factors Affecting Low Fertility

In those nations in which fertility has been reduced, the principal factor appears to be industrialization, accompanied by increased job opportunities and education. Within nations, fertility is usually lowest among social classes in which women have the most education and opportunities for employment. The availability of skilled jobs lowers the economic value of children, makes it possible for more women to enter the work force, and raises the age of women at the time of marriage. No longer need the number of children she produces be the measure of a woman's status.

Postponement of marriage, coupled with social disapproval of premarital intercourse and out-of-wedlock pregnancy, was probably a factor in the longstanding low fertility rates of many European nations. Easily available abortion is also important; the very low fertility rates of the Eastern European nations and the sharp drop in the Japanese birth rate are undoubtedly related to the widespread availability of abortion in these nations.

Contraceptive Counseling

A major role of nurses in a total program of family planning is that of counseling individuals and couples about the use of contraceptives. In order to do this we need knowledge of:

1. The contraceptives available today—the way in which each prevents conception and the advantages and disadvantages of each.

2. Effective ways of introducing contraceptive information, both to women or couples who have never used contraceptives and to those who have been unsuccessful or dissatisfied with a method they had been using previously.

3. The reasons why people avoid contraceptives or fail to use them effectively.

Contraceptives in Current Use

Oral Contraceptives

Observation that the discharge of an egg from the ovary does not occur during pregnancy raised the initial questions about the possibility of using hormones to prevent pregnancy. Experiments followed that demonstrated the role of the corpus luteum, and in 1934 progesterone was isolated as the active chemical of the corpus luteum. But although the injection of progesterone prevented pregnancy, contraception by injection was not a practical solution.

As early as 1942 it had been discovered that oral estrogens would readily inhibit ovulation, but because long-term use of estrogen without progesterone often leads to endometrial hyperplasia with irregular bleeding and prolonged hypermenorrhea, estrogen was not considered as a possible contraceptive.

In 1954 synthetic progestin steroids were developed that had the properties of progesterone but were both more powerful and also active by the oral route. Human field trials followed in Puerto Rico in 1956, using a "pill" with a small amount of estrogen and one of the synthetic progestins. In May of 1960 oral contraceptives were first introduced for regular use; by 1965 they were the single most popular contraceptive in the United States.

Constituents of Oral Contraceptives.
All oral contraceptives currently available contain an estrogen and a progestogen, with the exception of the so-called "mini-pill," which contains no estrogen. The estrogen is either mestranol or ethinyl estradiol. Doses of mestranol range from 0.05 to 1.0 mg.; doses of ethinyl estradiol range from 0.02 to 0.05 mg. Both estrogens appear to be equally potent in protecting against pregnancy. However, because ethinyl estradiol appears to be more effective in protecting against "breakthrough bleeding" (i.e., bleeding during the time in which the pill is being taken rather than during the days in which it is not taken), low estrogen-dose contraceptives usually contain ethinyl estradiol.

There are five different progestogens utilized in oral contraceptives. They are listed in order of their potency with norgestrel being the most potent: norgestrel, ethynodiol diacetate, norethindrone acetate, norethindrone, and norethynodrel. No "pill" uses more than one type. Norgestrel is 30 times more potent than norethindrone and norethynodrel and twice as potent as ethynodiol diacetate.

Because the various products differ from one another in amount and type of estrogen and progestogen, some women are able to tolerate one preparation far better than another. It is important to reassure a woman that because she is having difficulty with one "pill" does not mean that she will be unable to use any form of oral contraception.

Action. The basic action of oral contraceptives is the prevention of ovulation. The hypothalamus is prevented from sending gonadotropin-releasing factor (GnRF) to the anterior pituitary, thus blocking the release of follicle-stimulating hormone (FSH) and luteinizing hormone (LH), which, in turn, are necessary for ovulation (see Chapter 4). Remember that the formation of the follicle and its subsequent rupture are determined by FSH and LH. The cells of the ruptured follicle form the corpus luteum, which secretes progesterone. A metabolite of progesterone, *pregnanediol,* is found in the urine, evidence of the level of progesterone in the body.

In women taking oral contraceptives, direct examination of the ovaries does not reveal any newly formed corpora lutea. In addition, urinary levels of pregnanediol are about one-tenth the usual level during the postovulatory period (0.5 mg. rather than the usual 5.0 mg.).

Progestins have additional antifertility actions. Under ordinary circumstances, as stated previously, the mucus of the cervix becomes thin and watery midway during the menstrual cycle, making it less difficult for sperm to ascend into the cervical canal (Chapter 4).

However, under the influence of oral contraceptives the mucus remains thick and sticky throughout the cycle and thus is hostile to sperm. Also, the endometrium matures more rapidly and thus becomes out of phase with the ovulatory cycle, making implantation less likely if fertilization should occur.

Regimens. An oral contraceptive is taken for 20 days of each 28-day cycle. The first pill is taken on the fifth day of the menstrual period, regardless of the length of the period (and thus it is important when teaching a woman to always say fifth day and not last day). If there is no menstrual period, the second cycle of pill-taking begins on the seventh day after the completion of the 20-day course.

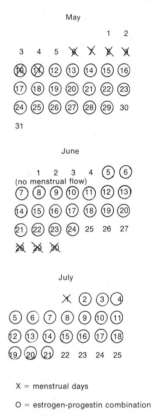

X = menstrual days

O = estrogen-progestin combination

When oral contraceptives fail, it is frequently because the user forgets to take her pill. Because of this, two regimens have been introduced to simplify pill-taking. In the 28-day regimen seven of the pills are placebos. The woman begins the pill on the *first* day of her menstrual period and takes one each day for 28 days. The active hormone is in the pills taken on days 5 through 26. She begins another package of pills immediately upon finishing the first package.

In the 21-day regimen pills are taken during a complete 3-week period of the cycle; no pills are taken during the fourth week. However, the pill-taking cycle always begins on the same day of the week, again, an aid to remembering.

Table 6–5. SIDE EFFECTS OF ORAL CONTRACEPTIVES

System	High Estrogen	Low Estrogen	High Progestin	Low Progestin
Reproductive System				
Hypomenorrhea		+	+	
Hypermenorrhea (heavy flow, clots)	+			+
Breakthrough bleeding, spotting				
cycle day 1–14		+		
cycle day 15–28				+
Amenorrhea			+	
Dysmenorrhea	+			+
Delayed withdrawal bleeding				+
Mucorrhea (clear vaginal discharge)	+			
Uterine enlargement	+			
Fibroid growth	+			
Cervical exstrophy	+			
Atrophic vaginitis; dyspareunia		+		
Pelvic relaxation (cystocele, rectocele)		+		
Small uterus		+		
Cardiovascular System				
Hypertension	+			
Vascular headache	+			
Venous relaxation, dilation of veins,				
venous stasis			+	
Edema	+			
Thrombus formation (increase in				
Factors III, IX, X, and platelets)	+			
Pulmonary embolus	+			
Skin				
Oily skin and scalp			+	
Acne			+	
Hirsutism			+	
Rash			+	
Pruritus			+	
Chloasma	+			
Hyperpigmentation	+			
Telangiectasia (dark red areas				
composed of dilated capillaries)	+			
Gastrointestinal System				
Nausea, vomiting	+			
Bloating	+			
Increased appetite			+	
Cholestatic jaundice			+	
Gallbladder disease	?		?	
Breast Tenderness				
Cystic breast changes	+		+	
Increase in ductal and fatty tissues	+			
Increase in alveolar tissue			+	
Decreased breast size				+
Decreased quantity of breast milk	+			
Altered composition of breast milk			+	
Weight				
Cyclic weight gain	+			
Increased fat deposition	+			
Noncyclic weight gain			+	
Weight loss				+
Emotions				
Irritability	+			
Fatigability			+	
Depression			+	
Change in libido			+	
Other				
Visual changes	+			
Leg cramps	+			
Vasomotor symptoms		+		

Side Effects. Among the most common of the side effects of oral contraceptives are those resembling some of the symptoms of pregnancy, such as nausea, weight gain, chloasma (yellowish-brown skin discoloration), headache, leg cramps, and breast enlargement and tenderness. These side effects are more often a nuisance than a serious medical problem, but they are of great importance to the individual woman. Some women find that nausea is lessened if they take their pill in the evening rather than in the morning, a change that does not affect the effectiveness of the contraceptive. After the first or second cycle of pill-taking, these side effects disappear in the large majority of women. If not, changing to a product with a lower estrogen content may help.

Acne may become worse; here a product with increased estrogen may help. Vaginal infections are more common in women using the pill; preexisting conditions may become more difficult to treat when oral contraception is started.

Depression has been reported in about 5 to 10 per cent of women using oral contraceptives. Approximately the same number of women become depressed following tubal ligation or the insertion of an intrauterine device, suggesting at least the possibility that psychologic rather than hormonal factors may be responsible. Possible emotional factors might be religious conflicts about the avoidance of pregnancy, a subconscious desire for children, or ambivalent feelings about the woman's own sexuality.

Considerable attention has been focused on the increase of thromboembolism in women who use oral contraceptives. Laboratory data show an increase in certain coagulation accelerator factors (Factors VII, VIII, IX, and X) both in the pill user and in women who are pregnant. The mortality rate from thromboembolitic disease has been found to be as much as eight times as great among women using the pill, and the risk of thromboembolism is from five to ten times higher. Statistics on both counts vary from one study to another.

The rate of thromboembolism is considered to be related to the quantity of estrogen contained in the product used. Those combined preparations containing 0.1 mg. of estrogen are associated with a risk of embolism that is two to three times greater than that of preparations containing only 0.05 mg. Products with still lower doses of estrogen and preparations containing only progestin are currently being evaluated. Theoretically, the absence of estrogen should reduce the incidence of blood-clotting, but this has not yet been demonstrated in studies.

As already mentioned, the possibility of pregnancy appears to increase very slightly with low estrogen products. Although the exact mechanism of progestin contraception is unknown, cervical mucus thickening (which affects the passage of sperm) and endometrial changes (which affect implantation) are two possibilities. Breakthrough bleeding, which at times is heavy, and failure of menstruation may also occur in some women and may account for the higher drop-out rates among women using contraceptives with low estrogen.

Two British studies, one of 63 women and the other of 153 women, have found the risk of heart attack to be more than four times greater among women who use oral contraceptives than among nonusers. The risk is compounded if the woman has other risk factors known to be associated with heart disease: cigarette smoking, diabetes, high blood pressure, obesity, or high serum cholesterol levels. The effect is suspected to be synergistic (i.e., the action of one factor potentiates the action of another). A 4.2 per cent increase in the risk of heart attack was found with one other risk factor being present; a 10.5 per cent increase with two other factors; and a 78.4 per cent increased risk with three or more additional factors.[72]

Still another area of concern has been the possible effect of oral contraceptives on subsequent pregnancy. When Peterson[65] compared 442 women who had become pregnant after they ceased to use the pill with 699 women who used other forms of contraception or none at all, he found that the incidence of abortion and infant death or illness within the first month after birth was similar in both groups. Premature births and congenital anomalies were less frequent in the group using oral contraceptives than in the control group. Peterson also found that long-term pill usage failed to result in either increased or decreased fertility.

For the breast-feeding mother, oral contraceptives appear to decrease milk production. In those parts of the world where infant nutrition is still highly dependent on successful breast-feeding, this is a major factor to be considered in family planning programs.

Sometimes the side effects that women report come from improper usage. For example, women will tell us that they take their pills "every once in a while" and that they tend to have irregular episodes of bleeding. The bleeding makes them feel that the pill is harming them in some way, and so they discontinue its use. History-taking in family planning involves finding out not only what is used for contraception but how it is used.

Effect on Sexual Enjoyment. The real or perceived effect of any contraceptive on sexual enjoyment will be an important factor in its continued use. For many couples the pill enhances sexual pleasure because:

1. It is taken at a time other than the moment of intercourse, so that remembering to use a contraceptive does not intrude.

2. It is highly effective in preventing pregnancy, so that the fear of pregnancy is removed from intercourse. For many couples this fear interferes considerably with sexual enjoyment.

For a woman who is experiencing some of the more unpleasant side effects of oral contraceptives, sexual intercourse may seem unpleasant while the other symptoms last.

Masters and Johnson[54] report an additional relationship between sexual desire and oral contraceptives in some women. These women begin to lose interest in sex after using the pill for from 18 months to 3 to 4 years. In about 90 per cent of affected women, 3 to 6 months of using some other form of contraception resulted in an improvement in sexual desire. To date no studies have examined this association, but it seems worth our awareness.

Contraindications to Oral Contraceptives. Because there are several physical conditions that are considered a definite contraindication to oral contraception, a thorough history and physical examination are mandatory before the pill is initially prescribed and at regular intervals during the entire course of its use. An annual check-up is a minimum precaution; many physicians prefer to see women once every 6 months.

Because of the increase of clotting factors discussed above, no woman with a *past history of thrombotic episodes* (pulmonary embolism or thrombophlebitis, for example) or with an *existing thrombotic condition* should use oral contraceptives at any time. The *development of migraine* after a regimen of oral contraceptives is started is also considered an indication for discontinuance because the incidence of cerebral thrombosis may be higher in these women. Postoperative thromboembolic complications also appear to be higher in women who use oral contraceptives. If surgery is anticipated in which an extended period of immobilization is expected or in which there is a risk of thromboembolism, oral contraceptives should be discontinued 4 weeks in advance (Federal Register, 1978).

Any woman with a *history of liver disease* or with *existing liver disease* (such as hepatitis or cirrhosis) should not take oral contraceptives, as they have been shown to produce subclinical changes in liver function tests. These changes are not felt to be significant for women with a normal liver and no past history of liver disease.

Malignancies of the breast or reproductive tract, either past or presently existing, are also contraindications. Although estrogen has never been shown to cause such malignancies, it may cause exacerbations.

Vaginal bleeding for which a cause cannot be ascertained is a definite contraindication.

Since glucose tolerance is decreased, women with *diabetes* or with a *strong family history of diabetes* are advised to use other forms of contraception.

Oral contraceptives (as well as pregnancy) may lead to sickle cell crisis in women with *sickle cell disease.* There is no contraindication in women with sickle cell trait.

Women with hypertension (blood pressure greater than 140/90) risk both cerebral vascular accidents and myocardial infarction because estrogen tends to further increase blood pressure.

Cigarette smoking, as noted above, appears to act synergistically with oral contraceptives in substantially increasing the risk of heart attack (Table 6–6). This means that the risk is higher for women who both smoke and use oral contraceptives than the total risk for either smoking or oral contraceptive use (Jain, 1976). Package inserts on all oral contracep-

Table 6–6. RISK OF FATAL HEART ATTACK* (PER 100,000 WOMEN)

Age	Nonsmoker, Non–pill user	Nonsmoker Pill user	Smoker, Non–pill user	Smoker, Pill user
40–44	7	10	16	All smokers 59
				Heavy smoker 83
35–39	4			Heavy smoker 24
30–34	2			Heavy smoker 16

*From data of Jain: Cigarette Smoking, Use of Oral Contraceptives, and Myocardial Infarction, American Journal of Obstetrics and Gynecology, *126:*301, 1976.

tives now must include the following statement: "Cigarette smoking increases the risk of serious adverse effects on the heart and blood vessels from oral contraceptive use. This risk increases with age and with heavy smoking (15 or more cigarettes per day) and is quite marked in women over 35 years of age. Women who use oral contraceptives should not smoke."

Risks Versus Benefits in Oral Contraception. After becoming aware of the possible risks of oral contraception, it is not unusual to wonder if this is a safe means of prevention. One does not have to practice very long to discover that some women, and their husbands, are afraid of the pill. Some of these fearful women have limited educations and are strongly influenced by "granny tales," but well-educated women are also sometimes hesitant.

Current medical consensus recognizes that although there is some risk, there is also a risk factor in pregnancy. It is felt that if the appropriate contraindications are observed, the advantages of oral contraception in terms of effectiveness (page 148), ease of administration, and acceptability by the woman and her mate far outweigh the risks. The ideal contraceptive, 100 per cent effective with no risks and no side effects, has yet to be discovered.

Intrauterine Devices

The idea that an object placed in the uterus could prevent conception is centuries old; Arab camel drivers placed stones in the uteri of their animals for that purpose many centuries ago. In modern times intrauterine devices (IUD's), usually of silkworm gut or gold or silver, were apparently first used to prevent pregnancy in Europe in the early twentieth century. However, IUD's came to be regarded as a possible cause of pelvic infection, and because of this and the occasional accompanying abnormal vaginal bleeding and/or perforation of the abdominal wall, their use fell into disrepute. It was not until new plastic materials became available that the potential of IUD's was again seriously considered.

The chief advantage of an intrauterine device is that, once inserted, very little thought need be given to contraception. This convenience is equally important to continued use and to sexual enjoyment. Once a week women are advised to make sure that the device is in place by checking for the presence of the thread that protrudes from the vagina. At the time of insertion we should be sure that each patient can "check for the string" effectively. She can do this by inserting her index finger in her vagina until the thread is felt. Obviously, if it

is not felt, she should contact her physician or clinic right away.

A second important advantage of the IUD is its comparatively low cost, an important factor in family planning programs, not only in underdeveloped nations but in our own country as well.

As a postpartal contraceptive, the IUD has one distinct advantage over the pill; it does not affect lactation. Although in the United States this may be a very important consideration for individual mothers, in those areas of the world where breast-feeding is still the only safe means of nourishing an infant, this is tremendously important.

Types of Intrauterine Devices. There are a number of different types of intrauterine devices; their advantages and disadvantages vary. Major characteristics of several IUD's are seen in Figure 6–2 and in Table 6–7. It is important to recognize that IUD's differ. Problems with one type of device do not necessarily mean that a woman will not be able to tolerate another type of IUD. Patient teaching also varies from one device to another. For example, women should be told that the copper Cu-7 should be removed 3 years after insertion. Because of the continuing changes in IUD's, nurses must constantly update their own information in order to answer women's questions correctly and to teach effectively.

Limitations and Side Effects. Intrauterine devices have seven basic limitations:

1. *They may be expelled by the uterus.*
2. *They often cause uterine bleeding and cramping,* the major reasons for discontinuance. The Lippes loop or Saf-T-Coil may double menstrual flow; the smaller Cu-7, Cu-T, and Progestasert cause less bleeding because they damage and distort the endometrium less. Damage to the endometrium from abrasion and necrosis is the major cause of increased bleeding. Bleeding is most severe in the first 3 months.
3. *The uterus may be perforated,* principally at the time of insertion. Most perforations can be avoided if the insertion is gentle and if a thorough pelvic examination is done prior to insertion to determine the position of the uterus (anteflexed or retroflexed) and the length of the uterine cavity (measured by a thin ruler called a uterine sound).
4. *They may fail to prevent pregnancy* (see section on Contraceptive Effectiveness later in this chapter).
5. *They may cause infections.* The risk of pelvic infection is three to five times higher for IUD users than for nonusers.[84] Approximately 2 to 3 per cent of IUD users will have a pelvic infection, which may range from rel-

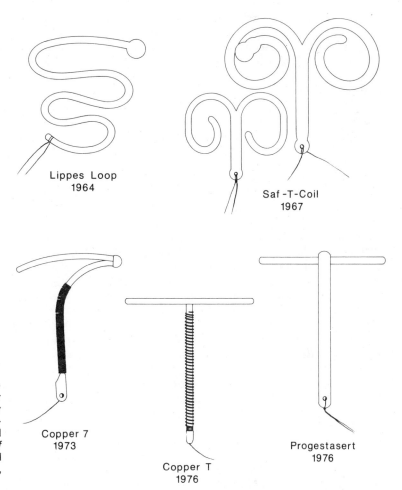

Figure 6–2. Five commonly used intrauterine devices. (Redrawn from Hatcher and Stewart: *Contraceptive Technology 1980–81*. 10th Edition. New York, Irvington Publishers, 1980 *in* Page, Villee, and Villee: *Human Reproduction: Essentials of Reproductive and Perinatal Medicine*, 3rd Edition. Philadelphia, W. B. Saunders. Co., 1981.)

Table 6–7. INTRAUTERINE DEVICES

Device	Advantages	Disadvantages	Status, 1981
Lippes loop	Proved relatively safe following several years of use	Expulsion or bleeding sufficient to cause removal in approximately 25% of patients	In use
Saf-T-Coil	Proved relatively safe following several years of use	Expulsion or bleeding sufficient to cause removal in approximately 27% of patients	In use
Cu-7	Causes less bleeding than inert IUD's; smaller size; ease of insertion	Leaches small amount of copper into system. Should be removed after 3 years of use	In use
Cu-T	Slightly larger than Cu-7	As for Cu-7	
Dalkon shield	Lower rate of expulsion	Difficulties in insertion and removal; multifilament tail conveys bacteria to uterus	Original shield withdrawn from market
Ypsilon	Shape believed to lower rate of expulsion	Currently being tested	
Progestasert	Reduced uterine cramps and menstrual flow	Increased risk of ectopic pregnancy; must be changed yearly	In use

atively mild to severe and sometimes fatal septic shock. Every woman should know these symptoms to be reported to her health care provider: temperature above 99° F, foul-smelling vaginal discharge, chills, pain with intercourse, vague lower abdominal pain, and "flu-like" symptoms (aches, fatigue). If there is any suspicion that the IUD is the source, it should be removed and antibiotic treatment started. The removed IUD should be placed in a sterile container and examined in the laboratory for culture of the organism and sensitivity to antibiotics. Tubo-ovarian abscess, a rare but serious infection, may require surgical removal.

6. *The risks of ectopic pregnancy* and *miscarriage* are higher in IUD users than in other women should accidental pregnancy occur.[86] If pregnancy should occur, the IUD is removed because of the risk of septic abortion, regardless of whether the mother wishes to continue the pregnancy. Spontaneous abortion occurs in 30 per cent of women following IUD removal.[80] These increased risks do not appear to apply to women who discontinue the use of IUD's in order to become pregnant.[86]

7. *Male partners may experience discomfort during intercourse.* In the first days following IUD insertion, the strings of the tail are firm and may cause penile irritation. Usually the strings become softer as they are bathed in vaginal secretion.[71]

The extent of each of these limitations varies with the type of IUD (Table 6–7). Exact comparisons between various types are difficult because the number of each type that has been inserted is unknown. Moreover, because a product must be in circulation for approximately 2 years before data on side effects begin to accumulate, comparison between devices available for a number of years and newly marketed products is also difficult. Experience with the Dalkon shield illustrates the problem of ascertaining limitations.

The Dalkon shield was first introduced in 1970. It had the advantage of a lower rate of expulsion than the other devices then in use; by 1973 it was reported that approximately 40 per cent of all IUD users had the shield. Early in 1972, however, it became evident that there were some difficulties with the shield. Because of its shape and because it was the largest of all the IUD's, it was the most difficult to insert. It did not show up on x-ray. The tail sometimes came off during insertion. But most significant was the finding in 1974 that the multifilament tail, which differed from the tails of the other devices, could convey bacteria to the uterus. If the woman were to become pregnant, the chances of infection and septic abortion (Chapter 13) were high. In 1974 Dalkon shield-related infected abortions accounted for 88 per cent of all such infections in IUD wearers. Subsequently, the Dalkon shield was withdrawn from the market and has been redesigned. However, it is estimated that as many as 800,000 women in the United States are still wearing the Dalkon shield.[71] They should be informed of the risks and, if they elect to keep the device, should seek immediate health care if they become pregnant or have symptoms of infection. The Dalkon shield is sometimes difficult to remove because of its shape and in some instances may require removal in the hospital under anesthesia.

Continuing research into new shapes and materials is being conducted in an attempt to deal with the varying limitations of the different products. The design of the Majzlin spring, for example, was created in an effort to lower the rate of expulsion; however, this device was so difficult to remove that the Food and Drug Administration forced its withdrawal from the market in 1974. A small percentage of women are unable to retain any IUD currently available.

Cramping at the time of insertion and an unusually heavy menstrual flow in the period following insertion are almost universal. Cramping is usually less severe in multiparous women; in nulliparous women cramping may be so intense that the device must be removed immediately. During the insertion of the device some women experience vasovagal stimulation with resultant bradycardia, irregular heartbeat, fainting, and, rarely, seizures and cardiac arrest. This reaction, when it occurs, is primarily in nulliparous women who have never had dilation of the cervix. A paracervical block (see Chapter 17) reduces but does not eliminate the pain of insertion; atropine may be given to reduce the vasovagal response.

Other complaints include cramps and backache, spotting, and bleeding between periods, although these problems do not occur in all women. Anticipating these side effects and explaining that in most instances they last for only a few weeks may help many women tolerate them. The newer copper-containing devices appear to reduce the incidence of bleeding.

Contraindications to an IUD. Contraindications to the insertion of an IUD may be absolute (applicable under all circumstances) or relative (varying from one woman to another). Absolute contraindications include pelvic infection, pelvic inflammatory disease, malignancy or abnormal Pap smears, pregnancy or a history of ectopic pregnancy, septic abortion, postpartal endometritis, and abnormalities of the uterus. Relative contraindications are hypermenorrhea or abnormal uterine bleeding, dysmenorrhea, and a uterus that is small (less than 6 cm.) or is markedly antiflexed or retroflexed. Women with anemia may be further compromised by hypermenorrhea. The possibility of infection may be a risk to women with valvular heart disease. Other relative contraindications include acute cervicitis and endometriosis. It is more difficult and more painful to insert an IUD in a nulliparous woman.

Choice of an IUD for an Individual Woman. If the insertion of an IUD is not contraindicated, a careful history and examination including the reason for contraception (child spacing or total avoidance of pregnancy), reproductive and menstrual history, pelvic examination including measurement of uterine size, and general health history will help determine the particular IUD that will be helpful to the patient. Every woman should be thoroughly informed of the disadvantages as well as the advantages of an IUD. She must know how to check the strings to ascertain the continued presence of the IUD and the extreme importance of contacting her health care provider if she has any signs of infection or suspects she may be pregnant. Removal of an IUD must be done by her health care provider. Follow-up care, at least once a year, should include a check of the IUD, Pap smear, breast examination, and hematocrit. A culture for gonorrhea is frequently recommended.

Spermicidal Preparations

Spermicidal preparations come in various forms—jelly, foam, or cream. Foams are more recent innovations than jellies or creams; they are less messy and spread more readily over the cervix. Originally used in combination with a diaphragm (see below), these contraceptives are now also used alone. Although they are somewhat less effective alone, they are readily available at most drugstores without a prescription, and this can be a decided advantage.

The preparation itself consists of a chemical that immobilizes and kills sperm and a base that mechanically blocks the cervical os.

Many women who purchase spermicidal contraceptives receive no instruction in their use. But we can, if we have the opportunity, teach their most effective application. The preparation should be inserted into the vagina within an hour prior to coitus. The applicator is filled and inserted while the woman is lying on her back. If the applicator is inserted as far as possible into the vagina and then withdrawn one-half inch, it will be at the mouth of the

cervix, where its contents should be deposited. The movement of the penis during coitus will distribute the foam (cream, jelly) throughout the vagina and over the cervix. If the woman gets out of bed prior to intercourse, she should insert a second applicator of spermicide. Getting out of bed following intercourse is not contraindicated, however.

The immobilization and killing of sperm take place in the 6 to 8 hours following coitus. There should be no douching during that time, since douching will either remove the spermicide or dilute it to the point of being ineffective, although it will not remove all of the sperm. Should the couple desire intercourse within the 6- to 8-hour period, reapplication of the spermicide is necessary. This is because vaginal secretions will dilute the spermicide and also because a certain amount of the preparation will leak from the vagina during and following coitus.

One disadvantage, apart from the necessity of applying the preparation shortly prior to intercourse, is that some women experience chemical irritation from the preparation itself. This is a relatively rare occurrence that may be an allergic reaction.

Diaphragm Plus Spermicide

A diaphragm is a dome-shaped device made of rubber with a metal spring contained within the rim. The spring fits the diaphragm to the walls of the vagina.

Diaphragms are always used in conjunction with a spermicidal preparation (see above). The diaphragm gives the additional advantage of a second mechanical barrier.

Diaphragms must be fitted by a physician or a nurse with specialized training. They come in a variety of sizes, with diameters ranging from 60 to 90 mm., and with several types of springs. Both the size and contour of the vagina influence the type and size of diaphragm for an individual woman. A diaphragm that is too small may not cover the cervix adequately; too large a diaphragm would at best be uncomfortable.

Most physicians and clinics prefer not to fit a virgin with a diaphragm, for once intercourse has stretched the vagina, the device must be refitted. Fit must also be checked: (1) following childbirth; (2) following therapeutic abortion or miscarriage; (3) following any surgery; (4) any time there is a weight change of 10 or more pounds, either gain or loss; and (5) every 2 years.

Displacement of the uterus will influence the type of diaphragm that can be used. If displacement is severe or if adjacent organs

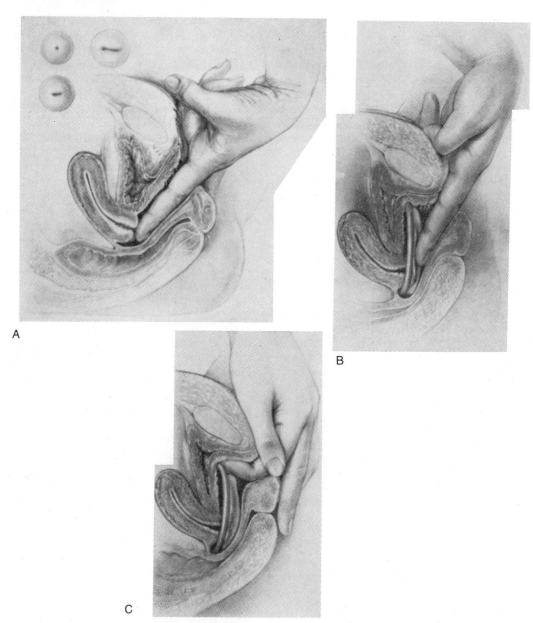

Figure 6–3. *A,* Finger recognizes cervix. Forms and sizes of cervix shown in upper left corner. *B,* Finger makes sure cervix is covered. *C,* "Front rim" test of fit. If finger cannot get by, neither can penis. (From Calderone: *Manual of Family Planning and Contraceptive Practice.* 2nd Edition. Baltimore, The Williams & Wilkins Co., 1970. Copyright © 1970 The Williams & Wilkins Co.)

are displaced (e.g., caused by a pronounced cystocele), use of a diaphragm may not be possible.

Once the diaphragm is fitted, the woman must learn how to position it properly. She needs the opportunity to practice insertion before she takes the device home with her.

The diaphragm is prepared for insertion by covering the dome and the rim with a spermicidal preparation.* With the woman lying

on her back, or squatting, or with one leg flexed (Fig. 6–3), she squeezes the opposite rims of the diaphragm together and inserts it deep into the vagina. She needs to be able to feel that it is over the cervix and behind the pubic bone. Some women may prefer to use plastic or metal inserters.

The diaphragm should be inserted no more than 2 hours prior to intercourse and should remain in place from 6 to 8 hours following coitus. As with spermicides used alone, there should be no douching during this period. If intercourse is desired again more than 2 hours after the initial coitus or if more than 2 hours

---

*Some recent reports have suggested that spermicide on the rim increases the possibility of dislodgment during coitus.

have elapsed after insertion but before coitus, additional spermicide should be inserted with an applicator, without disturbing the diaphragm. The diaphragm is removed by inserting a finger or the inserter over the front rim and pulling down and out. The device is then washed in soap and water, dried, and stored in a cool place. It should be checked for any holes each time it is used.

Disadvantages of diaphragms are mechanical and, for some women, personal. The mechanical difficulty is that even properly fitted diaphragms may slip out of place. Expansion of the vaginal canal during intercourse and frequent insertions of the penis are two common reasons for this. Dislodgment may be more likely when the female is above the male during coitus.

Use of a diaphragm will be difficult for a woman who feels she should not touch her genital area. She must be able to check the placement of the diaphragm, even if she uses an inserter to place it.

And, of course, the diaphragm, like the condom and spermicidal preparations used alone, requires forethought and action in the period immediately prior to intercourse.

Natural Family Planning

Nurses and physicians have in recent decades been less than enthusiastic about *natural family planning*, i.e., methods that are based on abstinence from intercourse during the time the woman is fertile. However, an increasing number of couples are indicating an interest in natural family planning. Some are concerned about the side effects of other methods of contraception. Some prefer "naturalness" in many aspects of their life (natural food, for example). Some have theological reasons.

In response to this interest, the Health Revenue Sharing and Health Services Bill of 1975 requires that agencies receiving federal funds for family planning provide information and counseling about natural family planning.

The Rhythm Method. The rhythm method is based on the concept of abstinence from intercourse during the period in which the woman is fertile (i.e., the period in which there is a recently expelled viable ovum capable of fertilization by a viable sperm in the upper portion of the reproductive tract). The ovum is capable of being fertilized no longer than 48 hours after ovulation (and probably only 12 to 24 hours), but since sperm remain viable for at least 48 hours and possibly for as long as 96 hours, intercourse must be avoided from 4 days prior to until 3 days following ovulation. Estimation of the time of the "fertile

period" may be done by means of a calendar method or by a calendar-temperature method.

The Calendar Method. The fertile period (and the corresponding safe period) is estimated in the following way by the calendar method. Consider a woman who has menstrual cycles that vary over a period of several months from 27 to 30 days in length.

1. Subtract 18 days from the shortest cycle duration (14 days for ovulation plus 4 days for sperm viability) to obtain the beginning of the period of abstinence:

$$27 - 18 = 9$$

Abstinence must begin on day 9 of the menstrual cycle.

2. Subtract 11 days from the longest cycle duration (14 days for ovulation minus 3 days for ovum viability) to obtain the day on which the period of abstinence may safely end:

$$30 - 11 = 19$$

Abstinence may end on day 19.

The best way to demonstrate this to a woman (and ideally to her mate) is by the use of a calendar. The example described above is shown on the following calendar:

```
              X  X  X  X  X   6
        7   8  ⑨ ⑩ ⑪ ⑫ ⑬
       ⑭ ⑮ ⑯ ⑰ ⑱ ⑲  20
       21  22  23  24  25  26  27
       28  29  30  X  X  X  X
```

X = menstrual period

O = fertile period

Note that the number of days in the menstrual period is not significant; the day is determined from the first day of the period.

Ovulation has been found to occur as early as day 8, meaning that the fertile period could begin as early as day 5 (and very rarely even earlier). The length of time between ovulation and menstruation appears to be more constant than the timing of the early part of the cycle, as we noted in Chapter 3.

The Calendar-Temperature Method. A method using the calendar alone is based on the presumption that in a 28-day cycle ovulation occurs on the fourteenth day. However, there is fairly wide variation in the day of the cycle on which ovulation occurs in an individual woman. Several physiologic criteria are useful in aiding the estimation of the exact time of ovulation: cervical mucus may be analyzed, an endometrial biopsy may be performed, and so on. The most practical method is by the determination of basal body temperature.

As discussed in Chapter 3, basal body temperature drops before ovulation and then, because of the influence of progesterone, rises from 1 to 3 days following ovulation and remains slightly elevated throughout the remainder of the cycle. The period during which the drop occurs is brief; the rise is considered the best indicator of ovulation. Because of ovum and sperm survival, pregnancy can occur within 72 hours following the rise in temperature. Thus the fertile period is considered to extend 3 days beyond the time at which the temperature rises.

The temperature rise does not indicate the beginning of the fertile period, only the end. Thus it is used in conjunction with the calendar method.

Consider now the woman described above with the same menstrual cycle of 27 to 30 days.

1. The beginning of the fertile period is estimated as in the calendar method, i.e., the shortest cycle duration minus 18 days:

$$27 - 18 = 9$$

2. The end of the fertile period is the day of the temperature rise plus 3 days. If the temperature rise occurs on day 15, day 18 would be considered the last day of the fertile period.

It seems obvious that the rhythm method requires a high level of motivation on the part of both the woman and her mate and a certain amount of intelligent understanding as well. Even if periods are always totally regular and of 28 days' duration, abstinence is necessary from day 10 to 17.

Rhythm will be ineffective for women who ovulate irregularly and thus have cycles of widely varying durations. Basal temperature can be helpful, but factors other than ovulation can cause a rise in temperature.

The Ovulation Method. Some of the disadvantages of the rhythm method are overcome by the ovulation method. In 1952 two Australian physicians, John and Evelyn Billings, began to work with couples who were "rhythm failures." They postulated that certain physiologic concepts that were being used to help couples achieve pregnancy might also be useful in avoiding pregnancy. Along with Professor James B. Brown of the Royal Women's Hospital in Melbourne, Australia, they developed a body of knowledge that has come to be known as the ovulation method of family planning.

Basic changes in cervical mucus prior to ovulation have been described in Chapter 4. Successful use of the ovulation method requires a woman's awareness of these changes in herself. As her awareness develops, she begins to perceive, during the days following ovulation, at first an absence of mucus. These are the "dry days." As the ovum begins to prepare for ovulation, a small amount of yellow or white mucus is present; it is opaque and sticky. As levels of blood estrogen reach a critical point, the fertile mucus appears. At first cloudy but not sticky, the mucus becomes clear and resembles raw egg white. The woman perceives a feeling of wetness. This slippery mucus usually appears about 3 days before ovulation.

Following ovulation, progesterone causes the abrupt cessation of the clear, fertile mucus. Mucus again becomes sticky.

It is possible for more than one estrogen peak to occur during the cycle. For example, if the woman has a high temperature, the growth of the ovum may be temporarily halted and then resume.

Women using the ovulation method keep a chart noting changes in the mucus; a system of colored stamps is frequently used. Red stamps are for the days of the menstrual period; white stamps (with the outline of a baby on them—thus white "baby stamps") are for the fertile or unsafe days. Unsafe days are those from the appearance of the slippery, fertile mucus until 72 hours after the change to progesterone mucus.

Following ovulation, light green "baby stamps" are used for 4 days. Green stamps designate safe days. The chart, stamps, and instructions are included in Billings' book *Natural Family Planning: The Ovulation Method.*[7]

The ovulation method requires awareness of one's body and a high level of motivation. In order to become acquainted with her own mucus pattern, the woman must abstain from intercourse for one complete cycle and thereafter every other day in subsequent cycles to detect fertile mucus. And, of course, she must abstain (or use some form of contraception) on the days in which she is fertile.

An advantage of the ovulation method, for women who choose it, is that it is effective for women with irregular cycles (for whom the rhythm method frequently is not satisfactory) and can be used by lactating and premenopausal women (in whom a menstrual period may not occur) to indicate fertility.

Billings suggests that the method be taught to each woman by a woman. Men have no personal experience with the feelings and sensations accompanying the changes in mucus and thus cannot communicate in the way that a woman can.

The Symptothermal Method. The symptothermal method utilizes observations of basal temperature, cervical mucus changes, and secondary signs such as increased libido and mittelschmerz to help couples recognize the period of fertility.

A lay group, the Couple to Couple League (CCL) (see Appendix I), suggests that the female partner identify the signs and symptoms and the male partner keep the records. Together the couple interprets the record, and thus each shares in the responsibility for pregnancy prevention. During the period of abstinence couples are encouraged to display affection through avenues other than intercourse, such as touch.

CCL also suggests that this method is best taught by one couple to another.

Condoms

Nearly one billion condoms are sold in the United States and Canada each year, making them the most widely used mechanical contraceptive in these countries. Most condoms are made of latex (hence the colloquial term "rubber") and may be purchased in lubricated or nonlubricated form. Condoms made from animal membranes are more expensive, but some men feel they interfere less with sensation.

Rarely does one see instructions about the use of a condom. It is assumed that all men are familiar with this technique, but experience gained from working in the kind of contraceptive clinics to which men feel free to come show that this is not necessarily so.

Condoms must be used throughout coitus, including foreplay if the penis is inserted into the vagina, since urethral secretions can also contain sperm. Most condoms come already rolled; if not, they should be rolled just before they are used. In either instance approximately one-half inch should remain unrolled at the tip to collect semen if the condom does not have a specialized ending for that purpose. As the condom is unrolled over the erect penis, this end space should be squeezed so that air does not collect in it. At the time that the penis is inserted in the vagina, it is important to avoid catching the extended end against the walls of the vagina, as the condom might break.

If the condom is not prelubricated, spermicidal jelly or surgical jelly makes insertion easier. Spermicidal jelly also gives additional protection, of course. The lubricant is applied to the outside of the condom after it is on the penis.

Condoms can be used more than one time if they are properly cared for. As they cost approximately 50 cents each, some men find reuse economically necessary, although condoms are available at considerably lower cost

through many family planning centers. If a condom is to be reused, it should be placed in a glass or jar filled with water immediately after removal from the penis. As soon as possible, it should be carefully washed in warm, soapy water, dried, and powdered with cornstarch. (Skin condoms are kept in a mild boric acid solution.) Condoms being reused should be tested for leaks before each use by filling them with water. Condoms are best stored in the containers in which they are sold. They will deteriorate from heat and moisture if carried in wallets or pockets or kept in other than a cool, dry place.

Disadvantages. One danger in the use of the condom is that it will slip off following ejaculation because of the loss of erection or that semen will leak from the open end. In withdrawing, the man should hold the upper part of the condom tightly against the base of the penis. If the condom has slipped off the penis, it should be removed from the vagina immediately, with the open end held tightly closed. Sperm deposited on the external genitalia can cause pregnancy.

Tearing or rupture of the condom is quite rare. If this should happen, the woman should insert an applicator of spermicidal jelly into her vagina, if a spermicide is available. Many physicians and clinics urge that condoms always be used along with spermicidal preparations and/or a diaphragm in case of condom failure.

The prevention of the spread of venereal disease is frequently cited as one advantage of condom contraception, and this is a real benefit. But because of this, some couples associate condoms with prostitution and other practices that they consider unacceptable and therefore find condoms undesirable as contraceptives for themselves.

Some couples feel that the condom itself is a barrier to sexual pleasure; both men and women may express this sentiment. But others, by incorporating the placing of the condom into sexual foreplay, find no such disadvantage.

Coitus Interruptus

Coitus interruptus is one of the oldest methods of conception control. It is believed to have been responsible for the drop in birth rates in Western Europe late in the eighteenth century. Also called *withdrawal,* the method consists of the withdrawal of the penis from the vagina prior to ejaculation. It is free of cost and always available.

However, there are a number of important disadvantages. Sperm not only must avoid the vagina but must not be deposited anywhere on the external genitalia because of the sperm's mobility. This is true even if the hymen is intact. Since sperm are present in urethral secretions as well as in the ejaculate, pregnancy can occur even if withdrawal is successful.

And successful withdrawal is not easily achieved. The time at which ejaculation occurs may be as early as 2 minutes after intercourse begins or as long as 20 minutes. Not every man is aware of the time at which ejaculation is imminent. Moreover, not every man has total ejaculation in a single emission; sometimes small amounts of semen are "leaked" prior to the ejaculation of which the man is aware. As the time of ejaculation approaches, coital movements become less voluntary, and withdrawal becomes more difficult.

Although there are no physical side effects, as once supposed, there are psychologic drawbacks for both men and women. The constant anxiety that withdrawal will not take place in time and that pregnancy will occur is a major disadvantage, as are ungratified sexual needs, particularly for the woman, who must often face interruption before orgasm.

So although withdrawal is probably better than nothing in an emergency situation, it is hardly a method of choice, considering the many other forms of contraception available today.

Contraceptive Effectiveness

How effective are the various types of contraceptives? *Theoretical effectiveness* describes how effectively a contraceptive prevents pregnancy under ideal conditions. Although there is no direct measure of theoretical effectiveness, it is estimated from the findings in the most successful groups of users.

Use effectiveness is determined by the actual number of pregnancies that occur in field trials when a method is offered to 100 women and is expressed in terms of pregnancies per 100 woman years.* There may be, and often is, a wide variation between the theoretical effectiveness of a product and its use effectiveness because of such factors as poor motivation on the part of the user and inconsistent usage. Studies of oral contraceptive failure demonstrate this principle quite well. Although the-

$$*R = \frac{\text{Total number of conceptions} \times 1200}{\text{Total months of exposure}}$$

R = rate of failure
1200 = 100 women × 12 months

From the denominator are subtracted 10 months for each pregnancy and 4 months for each abortion.

oretically there should be less than 1 pregnancy per 100 woman years with oral contraceptives, in reality some studies show failure rates as high as 25 pregnancies per 100 woman years.[86] As emphasized earlier, product improvement of oral contraceptives is directed not only toward achieving the optimum balance of estrogen and progestin but also toward trying to make the pill "unforgettable."

If no contraception is used at all, the pregnancy rate is approximately 80 to 85 per 100 woman years. With *any* type of contraception, even with relatively inadequate ones such as douching and withdrawal, pregnancy rates are more than halved. The two most effective methods are those that do not rely on some activity at the time of coitus, i.e., oral contraceptives and the IUD.

The theoretical failure rate of oral contraceptives is approximately 1.0 pregnancy per 100 woman years for sequential products and 0.5 pregnancy for combined products (for reasons already discussed), making both better than 99 per cent effective. The average use failure rate is about 5 pregnancies per 100 woman years, although it may be decidedly higher in some populations.

Pregnancy rates with the IUD average 2 to 3 per 100 woman years, making the method slightly more than 97 per cent effective. One reason for such a high rate of effectiveness is that the most common reason for the failure of many types of contraceptives is patient failure, i.e., the failure of the couple to use the method properly. The IUD is the only type of contraceptive that is virtually immune to patient failure. It requires only a single decision rather than sustained motivation.

When pregnancy does occur, it may be because the device has been expelled without the woman's knowledge; hence the need to check for the string. Spontaneous expulsion is more likely in women who have never been pregnant.

Approximately 1 per cent of women with IUD's become pregnant with the device in place. Should this occur, the device is left in the uterus and is delivered along with the baby. The device itself does not seem to present any problem to the developing embryo-fetus, but the spontaneous abortion rate is approximately 40 per cent, which is not really surprising in view of the suspected modes of action.

The theoretical effectiveness of the methods that necessitate some activity at the time of intercourse is lower than that of either the pill or the IUD, yet in several instances not much lower. Failure rates are approximately 2 to 3 pregnancies per 100 woman years for the diaphragm (about the same as for the IUD), 3 to 4 for the spermicidal preparations such as "foam," and 2 to 5 for the male condom. Use effectiveness, however, is not nearly as high. Failure to use these devices prior to every act of intercourse and improper insertion of the diaphragm or foam probably cause most failures from these methods. Failures from the condom method result most commonly from carelessness during removal after intercourse. The penis must be allowed to return to normal size before withdrawal, and the rim of the condom must be held during withdrawal, so that it will not slip off and spill its contents. If a fresh condom is used at each sexual act, breakage is quite rare.

The rhythm method averages 14 pregnancies per 100 woman years. Failure is most likely in women with irregular menstrual cycles, such as adolescents, postpartal women, and premenopausal women.

Coitus interruptus and douching are the least effective methods of contraception among those commonly practiced in the United States today. Even the theoretical effectiveness is about 15 to 20 pregnancies per 100 woman years; use effectiveness is estimated at approximately 30 to 35. Thus one woman in three using these methods will probably become pregnant.

Postcoital Contraception: Diethylstilbestrol

From time to time newspaper and magazine articles express an interest in the idea of a "morning-after" contraceptive. Diethylstilbestrol (DES), given within 72 hours after coitus, is such a medication. In one study of 100 women, no pregnancies resulted when 25 mg. of DES was given orally twice daily for 5 days, beginning within the 72-hour time frame.[48] It is believed that DES acts at the implantation site—thus the need to begin its use before the time of implantation. The medication may also increase the speed of ovum transport through the genital tract.

Currently, DES is most commonly given to rape victims. It may also be given after a known failure of contraception (rupture of a condom, for example) or when no contraceptive is used. But in all instances it is considered an emergency treatment only; good contraceptive counseling should be a part of follow-up care.

Nausea is the most frequently mentioned side effect, affecting 34 per cent of the patients in Kuchera's study.[48] About 16 per cent of the women experience both nausea and vomiting. Other side effects, all relatively rare, include headache, vaginal spotting, dizziness, diarrhea, and fluid retention. No serious side effects were noted, and 45 per cent of Kuchera's population reported no side effects at all.

A correlation between DES taken during the first trimester of pregnancy and vaginal cancer in the daughters of the mothers who had taken it has been reported. In each instance (all of which occurred in the 1940's and 1950's) DES was given to mothers with a history of miscarriages. The drug was often given throughout the first 3 months of pregnancy to prevent the possibility of another miscarriage.

Should DES fail as a contraceptive and pregnancy result, the question of the effect on the fetus would arise. There is no evidence, currently, that a 5-day dose of DES will cause these subsequent cancers. However, those few women who find themselves pregnant may elect abortion.

Natural Child Spacing: Is Breast-Feeding a Form of Contraception?

The term "natural child spacing" is heard with some frequency in these days when natural foods and natural cosmetics are very much in vogue. *Complete* breast-feeding, *without offering solids or supplements,* usually postpones the resumption of ovulation and menstruation for 7 to 15 months. Thus the minimum number of months between children, if all were to go according to schedule, would be about 16. Proponents suggest that this is the norm for the human species and is ideal for the child who is by this time a complete toddler.

However, breast-feeding carries *no* absolute *guarantees.* Although studies have shown that less than 1 per cent of women who completely breast-feed ovulate before their first menstrual period, it is fairly unusual for American women to offer neither solids nor supplements. Once menstruation has occurred, even though there is the possibility that the first period of a nursing mother is anovulatory, some other form of contraception should be used. Most of us would urge using other forms of contraception from the outset, although for the adamant believer in natural spacing our urging is likely to fall on deaf ears.

Granny Tales

The very fact that folk beliefs and "granny tales" abound with contraceptive advice shows a depth of concern that has been present in many different groups of people for a long time. Unfortunately, a large number of these beliefs are without foundation.

The idea that sperm can be washed away by douching seems the most pervasive of these beliefs about ineffective methods. Products advertised for feminine hygiene are frequent ingredients for those douching solutions. Shaking a cola beverage and then spraying it into the vagina is also popular.

Women have told us that pregnancy may be prevented by having intercourse while standing, jumping up and down following intercourse, and voiding or taking a hot bath afterward. Postpartum women have stated that the reproductive organs cannot function until 6 weeks after delivery, and thus they are "immune" during that time and need no contraception.

A list such as this could be very long. Our purpose here is to call attention to the existence of many erroneous beliefs and to raise the question, "How can we deal with them?" The answer is rather carefully, to say the least. Our objective is to substitute a more effective means of contraception without belittling the woman who has been using these other measures.

Surgical Sterilization

Twenty-nine per cent of couples in the United States who had reached their desired family size by 1973 had already undergone contraceptive sterilization, according to the National Survey of Family Growth in a study conducted for the National Center for Health Statistics. An additional 14 per cent said they intended to be sterilized. In 1970, 18 per cent of couples chose sterilization when they had completed their families; in 1965 the figure was 12 per cent. The same study found sterilizations to be almost evenly divided between male and female procedures.

Vasectomy is the operation for male sterilization. Perhaps the outstanding advantage of vasectomy is that it can be performed in a clinic or an office under local anesthesia. Small incisions are made on each side of the scrotum; the vas deferens is then cut and tied, blocking the passage of sperm (Fig. 6–4). Vasectomy does not diminish sexual drive or affect sexual performance. The man continues to have erection, orgasm, and ejaculation. Spermatozoa continue to be formed in the testes; they are absorbed by the body. Following vasectomy, the couple should continue to use some other form of contraception until examination of semen shows no sperm present, usually a period of 8 to 10 weeks.

Tubal ligation is the most common sterilization procedure for women. A segment of each uterine tube is tied with sutures and then cut to block the passage of the egg to the uterus.

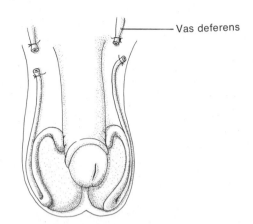

Figure 6–4. Vasectomy.

Tubal ligation in no way interferes with the menstrual cycle. The egg, however, does not reach the uterus; it is absorbed. Until the 1970's tubal ligations were most conveniently performed within 2 to 3 days following delivery, when the uterine tubes were more readily accessible. However, with the development of a procedure for tubal ligation using a laparoscope, the operation may be done quite easily at any time.

In a laparoscope tubal ligation, the laparoscope is inserted through a small incision in or just below the umbilicus, enabling the surgeon to visualize the abdominal cavity. Carbon dioxide gas is injected into the cavity so that the organs are separated and easily identified. An electric cautery is introduced through a second incision, about an inch long, below the first. The tubes are then severed and cauterized. Some surgeons perform the procedure through a single incision. Although some women report no discomfort afterward, others feel the need of rest for a day or two and/or experience abdominal pain that is the equivalent of menstrual cramps.

Since general anesthesia is used, the operation is usually performed in a hospital. However, a woman may be discharged once she recovers from the anesthesia or within a day after surgery. By contrast, 4 to 6 days of convalescence are usually required following traditional abdominal tubal ligation. A still simpler tubal ligation, which requires only local anesthesia and thus rarely an overnight stay in the hospital, is currently being tested at Johns Hopkins University and in some Asian countries. Through a small abdominal incision, the tubes are drawn into a loop that is then held by a silicone-rubber ring.

Neither men nor women should be sterilized with the hope of reversing the procedure. Although this is occasionally possible, it is never assured for a particular individual. However, research is currently being directed toward the development of a reversible vasectomy procedure. Many physicians and some state laws require that both husband and wife sign the permission form for sterilization. Both should understand the document they are signing.

When middle class couples seek sterilization, they have usually made a decision before they contact their doctor. With lower class families, it may be the professional personnel who first introduce the idea of sterilization. It is easy for us to see both medical and economic value in sterilization for low income families with many closely spaced children and to be eager for these families to share our views. But there is quite a difference between informing a patient about sterilization as an option that he or she may wish to consider and answering questions concerning the relationship of sterilization to sexuality and general health, on the one hand, and pressuring or coercing them to make a decision, on the other hand. Yet even in this area there is disagreement, as the example below indicates.

In 1974 the South Carolina Medical Association adopted a resolution declaring that a physician has a "moral and legal right to insist on sterilization permission before accepting a patient if it is done on the initial visit." The resolution was in support of a South Carolina physician who was being sued because of his policy that women on welfare with as many as three children *must* consent to sterilization before he would care for them. In response, a law professor at the University of South Carolina stated that such compelled sterilizations deprive women of their right to make personal decisions regarding their bodies, in violation of the First, Fourth, Fifth, Sixth, Eighth, Ninth, Thirteenth, and Fourteenth Amendments to the Constitution. In the trial, in which the American Civil Liberties Union sued the physician on behalf of two black women in 1975, the court found for the women, but awarded only token damages. The South Carolina Department of Social Services terminated the Medicaid contract of the physician.

Current Contraceptive Research

It should be obvious from the discussion in this chapter that a highly effective, coitus-independent, reversible, self-administered contraceptive with no side effects does not currently exist. Areas of current research address a variety of aspects of contraception.

Presently available methods of male contraception (condoms, withdrawal, vasectomy) are based on blocking the transport of sperm during intercourse. Research is focusing on methods that may arrest spermatogenesis. A chemical analog of GnRH (Chapter 3; also termed luteinizing hormone-releasing hormone) is in the process of clinical trials with male volunteers. Chinese scientists are using gossypol, a derivative of cottonseed oil, which they report as 99 per cent efficient in 4000 men.

GnRH analogs are also being investigated as a female contraceptive, both to prevent normal maturation of the egg during the follicular phase by interfering with the build-up of LH and FSH and by inducing luteolysis (premature decline in corpus luteum progesterone production) during the luteal phase.

The use of prostaglandin analogs in the form of vaginal tampons or injections appears to be at least 90 per cent effective in evacuating the uterus in the first 8 weeks of pregnancy and may be available within 2 to 3 years in the United States, even earlier in some other nations.

Currently, IUD's inserted immediately postpartum have an expulsion rate three times greater than later insertion. Researchers are investigating an IUD that could be inserted immediately after the placenta is delivered.

For more detail on the advantages and disadvantages of contraceptive methods under current investigation, as well as the social issues involved, see Atkinson et al., 1980[1] and Bendett, 1980.[5]

Unplanned Pregnancies: Why?

It is obvious that not every woman who becomes pregnant does so by choice. Many women who have not chosen pregnancy, however, accept it and welcome the baby by the time of birth. An unplanned child is not necessarily an unwanted child. Others choose abortion or adoption or resign themselves to an unwanted pregnancy and baby. A few, while denying that the pregnancy is desired, appear subconsciously to wish for the baby.

The immediate cause of unplanned pregnancies falls primarily into one of three categories: (1) failure to use any method of contraception, (2) irregular or improper use of effective methods, and (3) use of ineffective methods.

Since no contraceptive is even theoretically 100 per cent effective, *contraceptive failure* is another possible reason for an unplanned pregnancy.

Inadequate knowledge may be a factor in unplanned pregnancies, as suggested earlier in this chapter. At the most basic level, some patients do not appear to be aware of the biologic facts of conception. For others, including some women with a high level of formal education, such as college students, there is the obviously erroneous but rather prevalent belief that conception cannot occur from a single act of intercourse, or even from several acts. "I didn't do it very often; how could I be pregnant?" they ask. There may also be inadequate information about the efficacy of various contraceptive devices and practices, with reliance on inadequate practices such as withdrawal and douching.

For some unmarried patients, particularly girls still living at home with their parents, the *need to hide* pills or contraceptive devices in order to keep their coital activities secret makes use difficult.

And even in the "sexually liberated" eighties many women apparently feel that sexual activity outside marriage is permissible only if it is spontaneous, an "act of passion." The use of contraceptives makes the act "premeditated" and therefore unacceptable.

Introducing Contraceptive Information

Individual women and couples are motivated toward contraception for a variety of reasons. What seems to be an excellent rationale for limiting family size to one couple may have absolutely no appeal to another. Consider the concept of world population growth, discussed earlier in this chapter. To the family of a college professor—a sociologist or an ecologist, perhaps—world concerns may very well be the chief reason for a small family. But to the rural mother who cannot even see another house from her kitchen window, such an issue has no real or personal meaning. Providing for the children she already has or concern for her own health will probably be more valid for her. Stressing social issues to this mother may backfire. She may feel that we are more interested in the social issues than we are in her as a person. Or she may wonder if we want to limit the number of "her kind of people." Certain black leaders have expressed the feeling in recent years that whites want to control black power by limiting the birth of black infants.

Some of the patients who come to us are already highly motivated and basically desire specific information. Others have doubts, fears, and misconceptions that we may be able to resolve by facts.

There are other patients who never come to see us; we seek them out because *we* feel they need contraceptive advice for reasons that seem very valid to us—a number of closely spaced pregnancies, for example. Although many women in this last group may welcome our interest and advice, others are plainly hostile. Overenthusiasm about either specific birth control methods or about the subject of contraception itself can make these women less, rather than more, accepting of what we have to say. To cite one of my own experiences as an example:

A few years ago I was sitting in a clinic waiting-room with a friend who was a patient. There was no way in which anyone could identify me as a nurse. A public health nurse walked through and spoke to a woman nearby, saying, "I'll be out to see you next week." When she left, the woman said aloud to all of us sitting there, "I know what she wants. She don't want me to have no more babies. I really hate that woman!"

It nevertheless seems worthwhile to continue to try to reach out to such families. When 165 black urban mothers in Baltimore were asked if physicians or nurses should initiate family planning discussions or should wait until they were asked, 92 per cent said the nurse should not wait. The women said that many mothers were too shy or lacked adequate knowledge to ask. They added that teaching family planning was a medical and nursing responsibility.[23]

How, then, can we talk with these various patients? The initial statement during a contraceptive interview might be something like, "I'm glad to see you this morning. How can I help you today?"

After talking with the woman during these first few minutes, you can assess her feelings about contraception and her level of motivation. Is she there because someone told her to come—perhaps her social worker, or her mother, boyfriend, or husband? Is she doubtful? Curious? Does she really think you have something to offer her? (See Nursing Care Plan 6–1.)

What about her mate? If she is married, her husband's feelings about contraception are particularly important. If her sexual partner is constant, a single woman may also be strongly influenced by her mate's opinion. We need to give her the chance to talk about his feelings as well as her own. It would be even better if he were able to be present.

"Do you know how a woman gets pregnant?" may be the next logical question. Mitchell[56] suggests that for some women, anxious to discuss various methods, this question, which leads to a discussion of anatomy and physiology, gets in the way of her chief interest and is best deferred until later in the interview.

Nursing Care Plan 6–1.   Contraceptive Counseling

NURSING GOALS:

To provide an environment in which each client will be able to make decisions about the use of contraception to prevent unwanted pregnancy.

To provide knowledge and skills for each client that will enable the client to prevent unwanted pregnancy.

OBJECTIVES: Following counseling the client(s) will be able to:

1. Identify the relationship between sexual activity and possible pregnancy.
2. Identify a variety of possible methods of contraception.
3. Choose a method appropriate to the individual based on biological, psychological, and social parameters.
4. Utilize the chosen method correctly.
5. Identify the side-effects of the chosen method.
6. Recognize the need for continuing care appropriate to the chosen method.

ASSESSMENT	POTENTIAL NURSING DIAGNOSIS	NURSING INTERVENTION	COMMENTS/RATIONALE
1. General health history, physical, and laboratory assessment.		Provide for health care as indicated in assessment (e.g., treatment of infection, correction of anemia, etc.)	Health history, physical and laboratory exam, psychological and social needs provide the parameters within which contraceptive decisions are made. Client may have a general understanding of relationship of sexual intercourse and pregnancy, but still lack specific knowledge (e.g., likelihood of post-partum pregnancy).
2. Client's understanding of biological basis of human sexuality and sexual intercourse.	Need for information related to assessment (e.g., about human sexuality, sexual intercourse, etc.)	Correct misinformation, provide missing information as indicated in nursing assessment.	
3. Client's understanding of the psychological and social bases of human sexuality and sexual intercourse.			
4. Client's desire for contraception.		Provide information to assist client in deciding on need for contraception and in choosing appropriate method, based on total assessment.	
5. Client's need for contraception.			
6. Prior contraceptive experience.			
7. Client's knowledge of available contraceptives, possible side-effects, and limitations related to physical, psychological, social needs of individual and couple.		Provide information on side-effects, including the importance of reporting side-effects and methods of reporting.	
8. Client's skill in using chosen method.	Need for opportunity to practice necessary skills (e.g., insertion of diaphragm, checking IUD string).	Provide opportunity for practice of skills appropriate to chosen method.	
9. Client's knowledge of need for continuing care.		Provide information about continuing care appropriate to chosen method.	

For others, however, it may be the necessary door opener to an understanding of what contraception is all about. A pelvic model is very helpful in answering questions at this point. Lacking this, excellent illustrations are available in several pamphlets. Then, as various methods are discussed, they can be demonstrated in relation to the model or the drawings.

The woman or couple should decide what method is desired (and should feel free to reject any method if that is their wish). For a majority of patients, their own wishes can be the determinant of the methods they will use. For a few, there will be contraindications to specific methods, so it is always important to be sure that the woman understands that the final choice is dependent upon her physical examination and medical history. If an IUD is to be inserted or a diaphragm fitted, the process should be described to the woman before she sees the physician.

Once a method is chosen and, if necessary, approved by a physician, the woman must be taught very carefully and thoroughly the most effective use of the contraceptive of her choice. She needs ample time to tell us what she has learned in her own words and to practice the chosen method when that is appropriate, such as inserting a diaphragm or an applicator, or checking for the string or beads of an IUD.

There are also a number of practical questions that can be anticipated. "How much will I need? Where will I keep my supplies? How far in advance of intercourse should I use a particular product?" Estimated usage is aided if we can tell her how many applications are in a container of foam, for example. And although supplies should be kept out of the reach of small children, who have been known to eat oral contraceptives as well as nonoral products, coitally related supplies have to be convenient or they will not be used. The kitchen shelf isn't much help if the bedroom is on the second floor or at the back of the house.

Family Planning Programs: Incentives and Barriers

No family planning program ever achieves total success in the sense that it enables every family to eliminate all unwanted pregnancies (and enables families to have those children that they do desire). Some types of programs do seem particularly effective in helping "hard-to-reach" couples, however.

Stycos,[78] during field experiments in Puerto Rico, found that before a couple would use contraceptives effectively, they must first be made to see that family size was a salient issue for them, usually in terms of the pressure of children on the resources of the family. The experiments found that for families who had never used any form of birth control, pamphlets that made the issues relevant and offered information were more successful than group meetings when initiating contraceptive use. As many as 50 per cent of the nonusers became users in this way. However, when trying to help families who had already used birth control methods become more consistent and systematic users, group meetings were found superior to pamphlets because of the opportunity offered for reinforcement and commitment.

Another factor in helping the hard-to-reach family has been the use of "peer counselors," i.e., members of the couple's own community. One New York City program employed women from the communities served by the hospital who could relate to patients in their own language and at their own level. The women who became counselors were prepared by taking 7 weeks of specialized family planning classes, which included training in communication skills as well as in providing contraceptive information and facts about anatomy, physiology, and human behavior. One important outcome of this project was the finding that at first many professional nurses seemed to feel that the counselors were infringing on their practice.

Hardin cites the following as an example of the need for involving peer counselors in family planning:

I recall one instance where a Mexican woman had an unwanted pregnancy. She went to the Planned Parenthood group to find out if she could get an abortion, and the counselor told her that she could, but she would first have to see a psychiatrist. The Mexican woman interpreted this as an accusation that she was insane. Poor Mexicans in this community don't use psychiatrists just to pass an otherwise boring afternoon. To them, the psychiatrist is the last stop on the way to the insane asylum. The Mexican woman in this case was scared speechless, would not see the psychiatrist and tried to abort herself—all because of the frightening word "psychiatrist." Now, had the counselor been a Mexican, she would have known how to explain the situation to the patient, get her to a psychiatrist and a safe medical abortion. This kind of thing also is involved in making birth control services truly available.[37]

The importance of the feelings of each woman's sexual partner has already been mentioned. Yet traditionally, family planning clinics have been almost totally woman-centered, probably because they have been associated with equally woman-centered obstetric clinics. Men have felt very much out of place in these surroundings, which is unfortunate for both partners. Women report that one reason for contraceptive failure is the objection of their mate to their choice of contraceptive. Some males not only may object to contraceptives that might interfere with sexual pleasure because they must be used at the time of intercourse, but also may object to the pill and the IUD because of a belief that such use might encourage their partner to engage in sexual activity with other men.

One attempt to remedy this has been the availability of contraceptive centers staffed by nonmedical personnel, located in convenient neighborhoods, and open during evening hours on a walk-in, no appointment basis. Such a unit offers clients their choice of condoms, foam, or jelly and instructs them in the use of these methods, often on a free basis. Although all of these devices are available at the local drugstore (if one has the money and is motivated to spend it in that way), contraception education is not.

It has been a rather significant discovery that male clients in these walk-in units have been very responsive to the chance not only to learn more about contraception but to ask about conception and the development and birth of the baby as well. (In one such clinic more than 90 per cent of the new patients and 98 per cent of the returning patients were male.) Even when the counselors are female, because these women are seen as professionals, they do not appear to be a threat to masculinity. It has been found, however, that separate group discussions for males and females are more effective; in the presence of females of their own peer group young males do not like to show an ignorance of any subject related to sex.[34]

Questions about contraceptives asked by young men in these clinics cover such basics as how to put on a condom and how foam is used. When they are encouraged to use a combination of condom and foam for maximum effectiveness, many request both methods.

Other programs have been aimed at males visiting maternity wards and in clubs and prisons.

"Modesty" is sometimes a reason for women to avoid family planning programs. Contrary to middle class myths, women from lower income families are often more reluctant to undress for examinations than women from higher income groups. They may also be more reluctant to discuss subjects such as sexual intercourse. Modesty is an even greater barrier in some other areas of the world. Encouraging participation in family planning programs may therefore involve assurance that modesty is preserved and that a conscientious program to assure privacy and adequate protection in the clinic itself is maintained.

Many patients in family planning clinics have a low tolerance for barriers. Yet we continue to erect them: inconvenient locations and times, which necessitate long and/or costly travel, and long, frustrating waiting periods once the clinic is reached. Hardin describes one such program that is, unfortunately, not unique:

When the clinic was established with private funds it was located conveniently to where the poor lived; they could walk to the clinic and walk home. Finally, the county was persuaded that birth control was a legitimate public health function, and it took over the clinic. But after about a year the county supervisors decided that it was too expensive to maintain this separate medical facility. They decided to amalgamate it with the county hospital to save the tax-payers' money and to be more efficient. The only difficulty was that the hospital was 10 miles out of town. Now, California has been built on the assumption that man was born with an automobile between his legs. But many poor people either don't have automobiles or they have only one and the man of the house needs that to drive to work. How is his wife going to travel 10 miles to the birth control clinic? There is a bus which leaves every hour, but it sometimes skips. If she does get to the hospital, the woman will have to wait two or three hours for service because it is necessary to make "efficient" use of the doctor's time, and to hell with the patient. If she is lucky, a woman may leave her house at eight o'clock in the morning and get back home at two in the afternoon. For a poor woman who may already have several children to care for this can be a nearly impossible situation. So it has proved to be. Once afflicted by "efficiency," the whole system so discouraged patients that use dropped drastically. Thus, it isn't enough to establish birth control facilities; they must be located conveniently to where poor people live.

Similarly, to make birth control fully available to the poor we have to involve the poor in the delivery of services. There is a chain of people involved in any organized birth control effort, and direct communication must finally be with a staff person who can speak as a peer.[37]

What can we do about such problems? Relocation is one possible answer; a different way of scheduling appointments is another. While we attempt to unravel some of the red tape, we can at least acknowledge some of the frustration with comments such as "I know how hard waiting must be for you" or "You must be tired after your long trip. We will see you as soon as possible."

Family Planning Drop-outs

Once started, contraception is not necessarily continued. Table 6–8 summarizes some of the studies on the dropout rates of family planning clinics. Why this failure to continue? Major reasons cited in a variety of studies include:

1. Diminished need for contraception, including pregnancy.
2. Difficulty in getting to the clinic.
3. Poor service.
4. Feelings of sexual partner.
5. Side effects of the contraceptive method (physical and psychologic).

Individuals who are more likely to drop out include those who are not currently married, the teenager, the woman near the end of her childbearing years, and the woman with two children or less.

Table 6–8. DROP-OUTS FROM FAMILY PLANNING PROGRAMS*

Study	Country Studied	Observation Period	Definition of Drop-out	Contraceptive Method Used	Sample Size for New Admissions	Drop-out Rate (as % of New Admissions†)
Dubrow and Kuder	U.S.A. (New York City)	2 years	"Failure to return for further follow-up"	Jelly, cream, diaphragm	2046	44.5
Creedy and Polgar	U.S.A.	1 year	Did not return 3 months before due date or 6 months after it	All	21917	51.47
Population Council	Korea (Koyang)	1 year	Not actively registered at end of observation period	Diaphragm, condom, foam	490	About one-third
Population Council	Pakistan (Comilla)	2 years	Unspecified	Condom, foam	129	Fewer than 10%
Population Council	Pakistan (Lulliani)	1 year	IUD not in situ at end of observation period	IUD	134	36.5
Population Council	Taiwan	14 months	IUD not in situ at time of interview	IUD	2000	33.0
Population Council	Taiwan	6 months	Unspecified	Pill IUD	1017 Not applicable	"Almost 1 in 2" "About 1 of 4"
Population Council	India	1 year	IUD not in situ at end of observation period	IUD	20000	33.0
Hall	U.S.A. (Baltimore)	1 year	Pill would have run out if correctly used—did not return to clinic, IUD removed/expelled, accidentally pregnant	Pill IUD	12092	46.0· 37.0

Author	Location	Observation period	Definition	Method	N	Rate
Kanagaratnam and Kim	Singapore	1 year	Not using pill 4 months after end of observation period	Pill	2992	45.5
Beasely et al.	U.S.A. (New Orleans)	1 year	Failed to comply with revisit schedule during observation period	All	9210	13.6
Reynolds	Trinidad and Tobago	2 months	Patient not returned to clinic 3+ months since missing last scheduled appointment	All	680	19.1
Gordis et al.	U.S.A. (Baltimore)	1 year	"Terminated relation with program"	Pill	100 sexually active nulliparous adolescents	Nearly 50%
Takeshita et al.	West Malaysia	1 year	Not using given contraceptive at time of interview	Pill (91%)	2609	35.3
Keeny and Cernada	Taiwan	1 year	IUD not in situ at interview (after end of observation period), pill not being used at end of observation period	IUD Pill	4820 2217	33.3 68.0

*From Bracken: *American Journal of Public Health*, 63:262, 1973.

†In reviewing the literature it was sometimes necessary to calculate the clinic drop-out rates from other data presented in the paper. In all cases the drop-out rate reflects the magnitude of dropping out for all reasons.

Infertility: The Overlooked Side of Family Planning

In a society concerned with limiting population, with developing newer modes of contraception, and with the issues of abortion, it is easy to forget that more than 15 per cent of all married couples are not childless by their own choice. Some of these couples are unable to conceive; in other instances the woman is unable to carry the pregnancy to term.

A couple is considered infertile when conception does not occur within a year during which intercourse is frequent and contraception is not used. *Primary infertility* means that the couple has never achieved a pregnancy. If one or more pregnancies have been established at some time but the couple is now unable to achieve pregnancy, the term *secondary infertility* is used.

Determinants of Fertility

Basic factors affecting the fertility of any couple are the ages of both husband and wife, the frequency of intercourse, and the length of exposure.

Both male and female fertility are at their highest at approximately 24 to 25 years of age. About 75 per cent of couples in whom both partners are approaching their mid-20's will conceive within 9 months. Female fertility declines fairly rapidly after age 30. When the man is over 40, only 22 per cent of couples become pregnant.[52]

Frequency of intercourse enhances fertility not only because of the increased exposure but also because frequent ejaculation is a factor in sperm motility. Intercourse at least four times a week is advised for couples desiring pregnancy.

Length of exposure refers to the number of months of intercourse without the use of contraceptives. Eighty per cent of couples will conceive within a year; 90 per cent within 18 months. For those who do not, a fertility evaluation will attempt to pinpoint the reason. In all but 5 to 10 per cent of couples a cause may be found.

Physical Causes of Infertility

The reason for infertility in an individual couple may be physiologic or psychologic. In 30 to 40 per cent of couples the male partner is either completely or partially responsible.

Male infertility is usually due to sperm that are inadequate, either in number or in motility

(Chapter 4). Impotence can also be a reason. Social factors such as motorcycle riding (because of heat in the scrotal area) and working in an environment that is too hot may affect fertility.

Common causes of female infertility involve the uterine tubes, the endocrine system, and the cervix. Tubal causes account for the largest proportion of female infertility and have been found more often in women of lower socioeconomic groups. Pelvic inflammatory disease, of either gonococcal or enterococcal origin, and postabortal sepsis are major causes of tubal closure. Data from Eastern European countries, where abortion by suction curettage has been performed for a number of years, suggest that repeated suction abortion may affect tubal patency.

Failure of ovulation accounts for approximately 15 per cent of all infertility. Possible reasons why a woman may not ovulate include low levels of pituitary gonadotropin, absent or damaged ovaries, absence of ova, and endocrine system dysfunction.

Cervical and uterine causes of infertility result in inability to carry a pregnancy to term, rather than a failure to conceive.

Emotional Factors in Infertility

A number of the biologic changes that are causes of infertility may have a psychologic basis in an individual man or woman.

In women these conditions include tubal spasm, failure to ovulate, rapid expulsion of spermatic fluid, and vaginismus (painful vaginal spasm). An additional cause may be an unconscious avoidance of coitus at the time of ovulation.

Women with psychogenic infertility appear to share certain characteristics. Although they express, and appear to believe that they have, a strong desire to become pregnant, after counseling sessions such conflicting emotions as intense ambivalent feelings toward their own mothers and a variety of fears become apparent. These fears may be of the pregnancy itself (will it make me unattractive to my husband?), of labor (will I or my child die?), or of becoming a mother (can I possibly be a good mother?). Many women with psychogenic infertility find it difficult to express hostility and feel very guilty about their angry feelings. When therapy has helped them to express hostility without guilt, they become more free to develop warm relationships with others, including their own husbands, and in many instances conception occurs.

In men, erectile impotence (impotentia coeundi) and ejaculatory impotence (ejaculatio retardata) are the principal causes of psychogenic infertility. In addition, men, as well as women, may unconsciously avoid coitus. *Primary impotence* is used to describe the condition in which there has always been impotence. *Secondary impotence,* which occurs at some time after normal sexual potency has been established, may be a major problem or a very transitory one. Any normal male may experience periods of transitory impotence. There is agreement that a high percentage of male impotence is psychologic in origin. Not only is this felt to be true of younger men, but some investigators feel that it is an important factor in male impotence of old age.

Early psychic trauma, feeding problems, illness in childhood, and overprotection and overindulgence by their mothers are some of the characteristics seen in many men with the complex problem of psychogenic infertility. In general these men appear unaggressive and often view their sexual relationships with women as aggressive, hostile behavior. Since the sexual problem is a part of a more extensive personality disorder, particularly if it is long-standing, success in treatment may be limited. Psychologic care, combined with reeducation and retraining, is the principal treatment.

Evaluation of Fertility

The first step in helping an individual couple deal with infertility is to determine the reason. A thorough history is taken from both husband and wife. Significant information from the husband includes (see also Nursing Care Plan 6–2):

1. Occupation, past and present.
2. History of endocrine disorders.
3. Childhood diseases, especially if contracted during adulthood.
4. Genitourinary problems and/or surgery.
5. Excessive consumption of alcohol or use of tobacco.
6. Frequency of sexual activity.
7. Positions in coitus.
8. Impotence.

The wife will be asked about:

1. Occupation, past and present.
2. History of endocrine disorders.
3. Pelvic disease and treatment, and/or pelvic surgery.
4. Any previous pregnancies and their outcome.
5. Menstrual history.
6. Douching.
7. Coital technique.
8. Timing of coitus in relation to ovulation.

Occupation is important because hazards such as radiation and heavy metal poisoning affect fertility. Any disorder of the endocrine system, such as diabetes or thyroid disease, may be related to ovulatory failure. The contraction of a childhood disease during adult life, particularly of mumps, may lead to sterility (Chapter 4). Research has demonstrated that chronic alcoholism, nicotine intoxication, and habitual use of marijuana affect sperm production.

A complete physical examination follows the initial interviews. Specific fertility studies include the analysis of seminal fluid, the determination of ovulation, postcoital testing, and the determination of tubal patency.

Analysis of Seminal Fluid. Evaluation of seminal fluid for sperm count is a part of the initial evaluation of infertility. The specimen is obtained by masturbating directly into a clean bottle. The man should abstain from intercourse for 3 days before the sample is obtained. The specimen needs to be examined within 2 hours after collection.

In order to be considered "probably fertile" a specimen of seminal fluid should have greater than 20 million spermatozoa per ml., with more than 50 million sperm in the total specimen. The average ejaculation contains from 120 to 200 million sperm per ml. Counts between 20 million and 40 million may be considered subfertile, and some specific instructions may be given to the man about frequency of intercourse.

Sperm motility is also significant. Only motile sperm are able to reach the distal segment of the uterine tube, where fertilization takes place. Greater than 50 per cent of the sperm in a specimen of seminal fluid should be mobile, and more than 25 per cent should move forward. In addition, more than 70 per cent of the sperm in the sample should be of normal shape.

Failure to meet any of these five criteria in two or more samples suggests that male infertility is a very strong possibility, although only the total absence of motile sperm is considered absolute evidence of sterility.

Determination of Ovulation. The single most important tool in the determination of ovulation is the record of basal body temperature (Fig. 6–5). This is the same record that is kept by the woman who is employing the rhythm method of contraception. Again, we emphasize the importance of thorough patient teaching about the accurate taking and recording of basal body temperature. Ovulation is confirmed by endometrial biopsy.

Postcoital Testing. Cervical mucus undergoes characteristic changes a few days prior to ovulation (Chapter 4). The Sims-Huhner

Nursing Care Plan 6–2. Couples with a Fertility Problem*

NURSING GOALS:

To provide a couple with thorough evaluation of a fertility problem;

To assist a couple in coping with a fertility problem.

OBJECTIVES: At the completion of evaluation and counseling, the couple will have been provided with:

1. Physiologic and psychologic evaluation of fertility in both male and female.
2. Opportunity to openly discuss feelings related to fertility.
3. Treatment of conditions leading to infertility, when possible.
4. Information about alternatives to fertility when infertility cannot be resolved.

ASSESSMENT	POTENTIAL NURSING DIAGNOSIS	NURSING INTERVENTION	COMMENTS/RATIONALE

1. Health and sexual history
  a. Male
    (1) lifestyle (balance of work and leisure, stress)
    (2) nutrition
    (3) occupation, past and present
    (4) history of endocrine disorders
    (5) childhood diseases (esp. if contracted in adulthood)
    (6) genitourinary problems and/or surgery
    (7) excessive use of alcohol, tobacco, marijuana
    (8) medications used
    (9) personal habits (e.g., restrictive clothing, motorcycle rider, prolonged hot tubs, prolonged sitting)
    (10) coital history: frequency, positions, impotence
	Need for information about the relationship of assessment factors and infertility	Provision of information as indicated by assessment.	Excessive work, limited time for leisure may contribute to infertility in both women and men.
			
			Prolonged heat can interfere with male fertility.

b. Female
    (1) lifestyle (balance of work and leisure, stress)
    (2) nutrition
    (3) occupation, past and present
    (4) endocrine disorders
    (5) menstrual history (menarche, length and variability of cycles)
    (6) pelvic disease
    (7) previous pregnancy
    (8) previous contraceptives
    (9) douching; use of vaginal lubricants, perfumed tampons
    (10) coital history: frequency, positions, relationship to ovulation
		Provision of information as indicated by assessment.	Douching can change vaginal pH; vaginal lubricants can interfere with cervical mucus and thus sperm survival.
			
			Perfumed tampons, toilet paper may cause irritation which changes cervical and vaginal secretions.

ASSESSMENT	POTENTIAL NURSING DIAGNOSIS	NURSING INTERVENTION	COMMENTS/RATIONALE
(11) medications (esp. phenothiazines, psychotropic drug) (12) excessive use of alcohol, tobacco, marijuana			Limited intercourse at time of ovulation and frequency <4 times/week may be significant causes of infertility.
2. General physical examination (male and female)	Need for information about purpose and examination process.	Explain purpose and process of examination.	
3. Genitourinary examination (male) a. congenital anomalies b. discharges	Discomfort, pain or physiologic distress related to diagnostic procedures.		
4. Pelvic examination (female) a. congenital anomalies b. abnormal uterine position c. vaginal discharge d. pelvic pathology	Discomfort, pain or physiologic distress related to diagnostic procedures.	Explain purpose, process of examination; Assist with relaxation techniques.	
5. Laboratory evaluation a. complete blood count b. endocrine function studies c. endometrial biopsy d. analysis of seminal fluid	Need for information about collection of specimens, use of basal body temp. charts.	Explain purpose, process of examination.	
6. Special tests a. determination of ovulation (basal body temp. BBT); Billings method b. Sims-Huhner postcoital test c. determination of tubal potency		Explain purpose, process of each test; Explain purpose and use of BBT chart (text); Explain evaluation of cervical mucus (Billings method; text).	
7. Social and Psychological Assessment a. factors related to infertility 1. note if infertility is a shared concern (see also text) b. factors secondary to infertility and/or infertility testing c. assess desire for sexual counseling	Conflict in role, lifestyle Diminished self esteem; feelings of inadequancy; anxiety about results of examination; anger at self or partner; denial. Desire for sexual counseling.	Provide safe, nonjudgmental environment for expression of feelings; Remind that opportunity for new choices is available; Referral for more extensive counseling may be necessary. Explain that feelings are expressed are not unusual in infertile couples. Provide referral if needed or provide sexual counseling (if qualified).	Some couples seek infertility counseling in lieu of sexual counseling.
8. (following total assessment) Assess couple's understanding of information provided them.	Need for knowledge related to subfertility as it applies to them.	Review findings of all tests. If medical intervention required, review explanation of reasons. If no organic reason for subfertility identified, help couple to understand woman's cycle through BBT and mucus evaluation. Suggest fertility awareness classes, if available. Provide opportunity or refer for counseling if social or psychogenic causes identified. Provide information about adoption, if appropriate.	

*Fertility counseling requires a team approach; the team includes nurses, physicians, and may include other professionals as well.

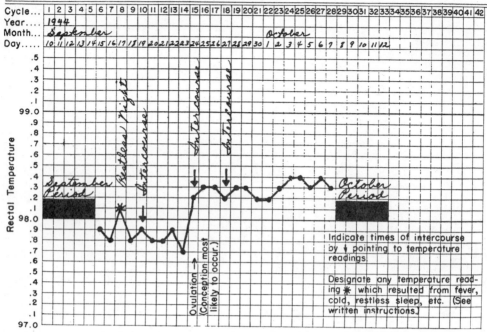

Figure 6–5. The use of a basal body temperature graph in infertility. (From Hamblen: *Southern Medical J., 38*:339, 1945.)

postcoital test examines both the quality of the cervical mucus and sperm survival. The woman is asked to anticipate ovulation from her record of basal body temperature and to have intercourse with her husband from 4 to 8 hours before the test.* In the clinic or the physician's office, a specimen of mucus is taken from the cervical area with forceps. The physical characteristics of the mucus are first examined. Near the time of ovulation the mucus resembles fresh egg white and "can be pulled from the slide in a long thread which will then retract to its original globule."[66] When placed on a slide at room temperature, the mucus forms a delicate fern pattern that is observable under a microscope (ferning). The number of viable and nonviable sperm and the motility and active forward progression of viable sperm are also noted under the microscope.

If the results of the Sims-Huhner test are less than optimal, the test is usually repeated, during either the same or the next cycle. Some clinics defer seminal fluid analysis until after examination of the sperm in a postcoital test.

Determination of Tubal Patency. When semen analysis indicates that the husband is probably fertile, a Rubin test determines the patency of the uterine tubes by means of the insufflation of carbon dioxide. Carbon dioxide flows through the tubes into the abdominal

cavity, irritates the subdiaphragmatic area as it rises when the patient sits erect, and causes a transient, referred pain in the shoulder.

Medications Used in the Treatment of Infertility

When the only apparent reason for infertility is failure to ovulate, clomiphene citrate (Clomid) may be a useful treatment. Clomiphene appears to stimulate the release of gonadotropins (FSH and LH) by the anterior pituitary, which, in turn, stimulates the growth of the follicle and subsequent ovulation (Chapter 4).

For clomiphene therapy to be successful, the pituitary must be capable of function and the ovary capable of response. Patients are screened to determine ovarian dysfunction (but not ovarian failure) and to rule out other types of reproductive tract problems, as well as untreated diabetes, or thyroid or adrenal disease that may be related to ovarian dysfunction. Any abnormal uterine bleeding must be evaluated. Patients with liver disease are not given clomiphene because it is metabolized in the liver. In women over 35 years old an endometrial biopsy to check for possible carcinoma is considered essential. The presence of some estrogen in the body, indicated by cervical mucus, biopsy of the endometrium, urine tests, or the administration of progestational agents, suggests that a woman may be a good candi-

---

*This length of time varies from one clinic to another. Page and associates suggest 4 to 18 hours.[66]

date for clomiphene therapy. Recognizing these constraints is important because of the widespread publicity given "fertility drugs" in the general press. Every infertile woman wonders, "Why can't I take these pills and solve my problem?"

A pelvic examination precedes each month's therapy. Following oral administration of clomiphene for 5 days, the woman is instructed to check basal body temperature to determine if ovulation has occurred. Endometrial biopsy and a rise in the urinary excretion of pregnanediol (a breakdown product of progesterone) are additional indications of ovulation.

Therapy is discontinued if:
1. The woman becomes pregnant.
2. The woman develops either visual symptoms (such as blurring of vision) or enlargement of an ovary.
3. After three cycles she has failed to ovulate.
4. After three ovulatory cycles she has failed to become pregnant.

The risk of multiple pregnancy is higher with clomiphene therapy (1:13) than in the general population (1:29), a fact that each couple should understand before the drug is given. Clomiphene has also been used experimentally to induce spermatogenesis, and in combination with human chorionic gonadotropin, given at midcycle, to enhance ovulation.[23]

Adoption

Adoption is one alternative for infertile couples who wish to become parents. Nurses who work chiefly with maternity patients are more likely to come to know mothers who give up their infants for adoption (Chapter 5) than couples who seek to become adoptive parents. Yet the same basic counsel is important for both groups: deal with a recognized adoption agency. In many communities departments of social services are an excellent source of information about recognized agencies.

Adoption is governed by state law (rather than by federal law), and thus regulations vary from one state to another. Although some privately arranged adoptions are probably successful, others have led to heartache. The mother who gives her infant for adoption, the adoptive couple, and the infant or child need the safeguards that recognized agencies afford.

The most frequently sought adoptive child is a white infant, newly born or a few weeks old. Relatively few such infants are available today. Most unwed mothers who feel they will not be able to care for a baby choose early

abortion. Many homes for unwed mothers, once crowded, have closed their doors. A shortage of adoptive infants has led to some questionable practices, including the buying and selling of babies (often couched in more subtle terms) in some instances. At the same time older children, nonwhite children, and children with anomalies (even such minor ones as missing fingers) are often overlooked as adoptive possibilities.

Adoption by a single parent has become a possibility in some areas of the country, but with infants in very short supply, single parent adoption represents only a tiny fraction of adoptions.

Couples considering adoption have a great many questions, most of which are best answered by specially trained counselors in adoption agencies. Ideas about adoption are changing. For example, there have been some questions in recent years about whether the identity of the biologic parents should always remain a secret, a tenet of adoption practice for many years. Nurses serve families best when these questions arise by referring couples to those who are qualified to answer their questions, usually the social workers and counselors of recognized agencies.

Artificial Insemination

As an alternative to adoption, artificial insemination was rather rarely suggested to infertile couples; it was usually considered only if the couple themselves pursued the subject. But as widespread elective abortion has diminished the number of infants available for adoption, more attention has turned to the possibility of artificial insemination as an alternative.

Although infertility is the most common reason for artificial insemination, it is not the only one. For example, when a mother has previously delivered an erythroblastotic infant, and when her husband is homozygous Rh positive (Chapter 3), the couple may choose artificial insemination from an Rh negative donor. Following genetic counseling (below) that indicates that the husband carries a serious genetic defect or that the husband and wife share a recessive gene for a major disease, a couple may again choose artificial insemination.

Either donor semen or the husband's own sperm may be used for artificial insemination, the choice being governed by individual circumstances.

Husband Insemination. Malformations

of the male or female reproductive tract that make it difficult or impossible to deposit semen in the posterior vaginal fornix are a major indication for insemination using the husband's semen. One of the earliest of all reasons for artificial insemination was penile hypospadias.

An adequate sperm count combined with low ejaculate volume or a low normal sperm count combined with a normal volume of ejaculate may suggest that the husband's semen be used for a number of inseminations before donor sperm is tried.

Donor Insemination. When the sperm count is very low or totally absent following medical therapy and when insemination using the husband's semen has not achieved pregnancy, donor semen may be used. Donor semen is also used when such factors as Rh incompatibility or genetic disease are the reasons for the insemination procedure.

Donors of semen often come from the university or medical community. They are paid for their semen, and they must agree both to the unrestricted use of their semen and to make no effort to discover the identity of the couples involved. Donors should not, to their knowledge, have any hereditary disease. Blood type, Rh factor, and serology are checked; ideally only compatible blood types are used. Matching the donor to the husband in relation to coloring and body type is not always possible, but physical characteristics serve as general guidelines. For example, semen from a tall, blond man would not be given to a Jewish or Italian couple who were short and olive-skinned.

Semen may be either fresh or frozen. Fresh semen must be delivered to the office or clinic shortly before the insemination procedure, which can be a disadvantage. On the other hand, freezing decreases sperm motility by about 40 per cent, and structural changes apparently take place in the individual sperm, lowering the conception rate.

The Insemination Procedure. Temperature charts for at least one cycle, and usually for several months, are reviewed. The initial day for insemination is then selected, about 1 to 2 days prior to basal temperature rise. Semen, obtained by masturbation into a clean cup (or a frozen specimen), is drawn into a syringe with a small length of polyethylene tubing attached. Or a metal cannula may be introduced into the cervix. A small amount (0.1 to 0.5 ml.) of semen is then inserted into the endocervical canal. The remainder of the semen is placed in a cervical cap—a small plastic cup that is held against the cervix by suction. After resting on the examining table for 15 minutes, the woman is ready to go home. She will remove the cervical cap about 6 hours later by pulling on the attached string.

Some physicians allow and encourage the husband to actively assist in the insemination procedure, believing that psychologically this is quite important. It is the husband who holds the syringe and deposits the semen. He is also instructed in the removal of the cervical cap. It is suggested that the couple have intercourse following the removal of the cap.

Two to three inseminations are done during each menstrual cycle, usually on alternate days, the last being performed on the day that the temperature drops just prior to ovulation.

When a woman's menstrual cycles are highly irregular, so that the time of ovulation is difficult to predict, she may be given clomiphene citrate, which is used to stimulate and control ovulation, or human chorionic gonadotropin, which will induce ovulation within 24 hours after administration if the follicle is ready.

Effectiveness of Artificial Insemination. An analysis of 630 couples who had artificial insemination with donor semen showed a success rate of from 55 to 78 per cent. Between 31 and 46 per cent of these successful couples achieved pregnancy in the first month. In 6 months 90 per cent of those who will become pregnant have already done so; rarely will there be success if pregnancy has not occurred within a year.[8]

Success with the husband's semen is as low as 15 per cent. The best results with frozen semen are no greater than 50 per cent.

REFERENCES

1. Atkinson, L., Schearer, S., Harkairy, O., and Lincoln, R.: Prospects for Improved Contraception, *Family Planning Perspectives, 12*:173, 1980.
2. Baird, D., Walker, J., and Thompson, A. M.: Causes and Prevention of Stillbirths and First Week Deaths, *Journal of Obstetrics and Gynaecology of the British Empire, 61*:433, 1954.
3. Beasley, J. D., Harter, C. L., and Fisher, A.: Attitudes and Knowledge Relevant to Family Planning Among New Orleans Negro Women, *American Journal of Public Health, 56*:1847, 1966.
4. Beasley, J. D., and Harter, C. L.: Introducing Family Planning Clinics to Louisiana, *Children, 14*:188, September-October, 1967.
5. Bendett, J.: Current Contraceptive Research, *Family Planning Perspectives, 12*:149, 1980.

6. Berelson, B.: Beyond Family Planning, *Science, 160*:533, 1969.

7. Billings, J.: *Natural Family Planning: The Ovulation Method.* 3rd Edition. Collegeville, Minn., The Liturgical Press, 1975.

8. Board, J. A.: Artificial Insemination in the Human, *MCV Quarterly, 8*:13, 1972.

9. Bracken, M. B.: Factors Associated with Dropping Out of Family Planning Clinics in Jamaica, *American Journal of Public Health, 63*:262, 1973.

10. Bradbury, B.: Preventing the "Diaphragm Baby Syndrome": A Matter of Technique, Teaching, and Time, *JOGN Nursing, 4*(2):24, 1975.

11. Britt, S.: Fertility Awareness: Four Methods of Natural Family Planning, *JOGN Nursing, 6*(2):9, 1977.

12. Calderone, M. (ed.): Manual of Family Planning and Contraceptive Practice. 2nd Edition. Baltimore, The Williams and Wilkins Co., 1970.

13. Calhoun, J. B.: Population Density and Social Pathology, *Scientific American, 206*:139, February, 1962.

14. Campbell, A. A.: Design and Scope of the 1960 Study of Growth of American Families. *In* Kiser, C. V. (ed.): *Research in Family Planning.* Princeton, Princeton University Press, 1962.

15. Campbell, A. A.: Family Planning and the Five Million, *Family Planning Perspectives, 1*:2, October, 1969.

16. Carrighar, S.: Nature's Balance, The Teetering See-Saw. *In* Young, L. B. (ed.): *Population in Perspective.* New York, Oxford University Press, 1968.

17. Chase, H. B.: *The Relationship of Certain Biologic and Socioeconomic Factors to Fetal, Infant and Early Childhood Mortality.* Albany, N.Y., State Dept. of Health, 1961 and 1962.

18. Cohen, M., and Friedman, S.: Nonsexual Motivation of Adolescent Sexuality, *Medical Aspects of Human Sexuality, 9*:9, 1975.

19. Davis, K.: Population, *Scientific American, 209*:62, September, 1963.

20. Davis, K.: Population Policy: Will Current Programs Succeed? *Science, 158*:730, 1967.

21. DiPalma, J.: The Pill, Pro and Con, *RN, 34*:61, January, 1971.

22. Edmands, E. M.: A Study of Contraceptive Practices in a Selected Group of Urban, Negro Mothers in Baltimore, *American Journal of Public Health, 58*:263, 1968.

23. Edwards, R. G.: Studies in Human Conception, *American Journal of Obstetrics & Gynecology, 117*:587, 1973.

24. Ehrlich, P.R.: *The Population Bomb,* New York, Ballantine Books, 1968.

25. *Federal Register:* Oral Contraceptives, Part II, January 31, 1978.

26. Finley, S. C.: Genetic Counseling, *Southern Medical Journal, 64* (Suppl. #1):101, 1971.

27. Flapan, M.: A Paradigm for the Analysis of Childbearing Motivations of Married Women Prior to Birth of the First Child, *American Journal of Orthopsychiatry, 39*:402, 1969.

28. Fogel, C.: Fertility Control. *In* Fogel, C., and Woods, N. (eds.): *Health Care of Women: A Nursing Perspective.* St. Louis, C. V. Mosby, 1981.

29. Food and Population: Thinking the Unthinkable, *Science News, 106*:340, November 30, 1974.

30. Frank, R., and Tietze, C.: Acceptance of an Oral Contraceptive Program in a Large Metropolitan Area, *American Journal of Obstetrics and Gynecology, 93*:122, September 1, 1965.

31. Freedman, R.: Norms for Family Size in Underdeveloped Areas, *Proceedings of the Royal Society,* B, *159*:220, 1963.

32. Gardner, R. N.: *The United Nations and the Population Problem: Planning for the 1974 World Population Conference.* Rensselaerville, N.Y., The Institute on Man and Science, 1973.

33. Gilson, J. R., and McKeown, T.: Observations on All Births (23,970) in Birmingham, 1947. Effect of Changing Family Size on Infant Mortality, *British Journal of Social Medicine, 6*:183, July, 1952.

34. Gobble, F. L., Vincent, C. E., Cochrane, C. M., et al.: A Nonmedical Approach to Fertility Reduction, *Obstetrics and Gynecology, 34*:888, 1969.

35. Greene, W.: Triage: Who Shall Be Fed? Who Shall Starve? *N.Y. Times Magazine,* January 5, 1975, 9.

36. Hamblen, E. C.: Minimal Standards for Sterility Surveys, *Southern Medical Journal, 38*:339, 1945.

37. Hardin, G.: Multiple Paths to Population Control, *Family Planning Perspectives, 2*:24, June, 1970.

38. Hatt, P. K.: *Background of Human Fertility in Puerto Rico.* Princeton, Princeton University Press, 1952.

39. Hellman, L. M.: Choices and Challenges for the Federal Family Planning Program, *American Journal of Obstetrics and Gynecology, 117*:782, 1973.

40. Hopkins, P., and Clyne, M.: Management of the Home Confinement. *In* Howells, J. (ed.): *Modern Perspectives in Psycho-Obstetrics.* New York, Brunner/Mazel, 1972.

41. Inman, W. H., and Vessey, M. P.: Investigation of Deaths from Pulmonary, Coronary, and Cerebral Thrombosis and Embolism in Women of Childbearing Age, *British Medical Journal, 2*:193, 1968.

42. Jaffe, F.: A Strategy for Implementing Family Planning Services in the United States, *American Journal of Public Health, 58*:713, 1968.

43. Jain, S.: Cigarette Smoking, Use of Oral Contraceptives, and Myocardial Infarction, *American Journal of Obstetrics and Gynecology, 126*:301, 1976.

44. Jekel, J., Klerman, L., and Bancroft, D.: Factors Associated with Rapid Subsequent Pregnancies Among School-Age Mothers, *American Journal of Public Health, 63*:770, 1973.

45. Kilby-Kelberg, S.: Why Some Won't Try the Diaphragm Method—Why Others Try and Fail, *JOGN Nursing, 4*(2):24, 1975.

46. Kippley, J., and Kippley, S.: *The Art of Natural Family Planning.* Cincinnati, The Couple to Couple League International, Inc., 1975.

47. Kistner, R. W.: The Infertile Woman, *American Journal of Nursing, 73*:1937, 1973.

48. Kuchera, L. K.: Postcoital Contraception with Diethylstilbestrol, *Journal of the American Medical Association, 218*:562, 1971.

49. Legans, J.: Artificial Insemination: Hope for Childless Couples, *JOGN Nursing, 3*(4):25, 1974.

50. Lynch, H. T., Krush, T. P., Krush, A. J., et al.: Psychodynamics of Early Hereditary Deaths, *American Journal of Diseases of Children, 108*:605, 1964.

51. Macintyre, M. N.: Prenatal Chromosome Analysis— A Lifesaving Procedure, *Southern Medical Journal, 64* (Suppl. #1):85, February, 1971.

52. MacLeon, J., and Gold, R. Z.: Male Factor in Fertility and Infertility, *Fertility Sterility, 4*:10, January-February, 1953.

53. Markash, R. E., and Seigel, D. G.: Oral Contraceptives and Mortality Trends in Thromboembolism in the United States, *American Journal of Public Health, 59*:418, 1969.

54. Masters, W. H., and Johnson, V. G.: Contraception and Sexual Pleasure, *Redbook,* May, 1975, 42.

55. McCalister, D., and Thiessen, V.: Prediction in Family Planning, *American Journal of Public Health, 60*:1372, 1970.

55a. McCusker, M. P.: The Subfertile Couple. *JOGN Nursing, 11*:157, 1982.

56. Mitchell, H. D.: How Do I Talk—Family Planning? *American Journal of Public Health, 56*:738, 1966.

57. Nadler, H. L.: Prenatal Detection of Inborn Errors of Metabolism, *Southern Medical Journal, 64* (Suppl. #1):92, February, 1971.

58. Notestein, F.: Zero Population Growth: What Is It? *Family Planning Perspectives, 2*:20, June, 1970.

59. Omran, A. R.: *The Health Theme in Family Planning.* Chapel Hill, N. C., Carolina Population Center, University of North Carolina, 1970.

60. Osborn, F.: Attitudes and Practices Affecting Fertility, *In* Young, L. B. (ed.): *Population in Perspective.* New York, Oxford University Press, 1968.

61. Page, E., Villee, C. A., and Villee, D. B.: *Human Reproduction.* 3rd Edition. Philadelphia, W. B. Saunders Co., 1981.

62. Peer-level Counselors Play Key Role in Success of N.Y.C. Family Planning, *Hospital Topics,* January, 1971, 85.

63. Pendleton, D.: IUD's: Intrauterine Danger? *Science News, 107*:226, April 5, 1975.

64. Perspectives in Genetic Counseling, *Pediatric Currents, 20*:9, February, 1971.

65. Peterson, W. F.: Pregnancy Following Oral Contraceptive Therapy, *Obstetrics and Gynecology, 34*:363, 1969.

66. Rainwater, L.: *And the Poor Get Children.* Chicago, Quadrangle Books, 1960.

67. Ratner, H.: Child Spacing II, Nature's Subtleties, *Child and Family, 9*:2, 1970.

68. Ratner, H.: Child Spacing III. Nature's Prescription, *Child and Family, 9*:99, 1970.

69. Reed, R. B.: Social and Psychological Factors Affecting Fertility: The Interrelationship of Marital Adjustment, Fertility Control, and Size of Family, *Milbank Memorial Fund Quarterly, 25*:383, 1947.

70. Scanzoni, L., and Scanzoni, J.: *Men, Women, and Change: A Sociology of Marriage and Family.* 2nd Edition. New York, McGraw Hill Book Co., 1981.

71. Shapiro, H.: The Birth Control Book. New York, Avon, 1978.

72. Shapiro, S.: Oral Contraceptives and Myocardial Infarction, *New England Journal of Medicine, 293*(4):195, July 24, 1975.

73. Siegel, E., Scurletis, T. D., Abernathy, J. R., et al.: Postneonatal Deaths in North Carolina, 1959–1963, *North Carolina Medical Journal, 27*:366, 1966.

74. Siegel, E., Thomas, D., Coulter, E., et al.: Continuation of Contraception by Low Income Women: A One Year Follow-Up, *American Journal of Public Health, 61*:1886, 1971.

75. Siegel, E., Thomas, D., and Coulter, E.: Family Planning—Changes in Attitudes and Practices Among Low Income Women Between 1967 and 1970– 1971, *American Journal of Public Health, 63*:256, 1973.

76. Spence, J., et al.: *A Thousand Families in Newcastle Upon Tyne: An Approach to the Study of Health and Illness in Children.* London, Oxford University Press, 1954.

77. Sterilization on the Rise, *Science News, 108*:58, July 26, 1975.

78. Stycos, J. M., and Back, K. W.: *The Family and Population Control.* Chapel Hill, N. C., The University of North Carolina Press, 1959.

79. Tabah, L., and Raul, S.: Preliminary Findings of a Survey on Fertility and Attitudes Toward Family Formation in Santiago, Chile, *In* Kiser, C. V. (ed.): *Research in Family Planning.* Princeton, Princeton University Press, 1962.

80. Tatum, H., and Schmidt, F.: Contraceptive and Sterilization Practices and Extrauterine Pregnancy: A Realistic Perspective, *Fertility Sterility, 28*:407, 1977.

81. Tietze, C., and Lewis, S.: The IUD and Pill: Extended Use—Effectiveness, *Family Planning Perspectives, 3*:53, 1971.

82. Timby, B.: Ovulation Method of Birth Control, *American Journal of Nursing, 76*:928, 1976.

83. Tips, R. L., Smith, G. S., Lynch, H. T., et al.: The "Whole Family" Concept in Clinical Genetics, *American Journal of Diseases of Children, 107*:67, 1964.

84. Tryer, L.: The Benefits and Risks of IUD Use. *International Journal of Gynecology and Obstetrics, 15*:150, 1977.

85. Tyler, C. W., Tillack, W. S., Smith, J. C., et al.: Assessment of a Family Planning Program: Contraceptive Services and Fertility in Atlanta, Georgia, *Family Planning Perspectives, 2*:25, March, 1970.

86. Vessey, M., Yeates, D., and Flavel, R.: Risk of Ectopic Pregnancy and duration of use of an intrauterine device, *Lancet, 2*:501, 1979.

87. Westoff, L. A., and Westoff, C. F.: *From Now to Zero: Fertility, Contraception and Abortion in America.* Boston, Little, Brown and Co., 1971.

88. Williams, J.: *Psychology of Women.* New York, Norton, 1977.

89. Wishik, S. M.: The Use of Client Characteristics as Predictors of Utilization of Family Planning Service, *American Journal of Public Health, 60*:1394, 1970.

90. Wolf, S. R., and Ferguson, E. L.: The Physician's Influence on the Nonacceptance of Birth Control, *American Journal of Obstetrics and Gynecology, 104*:752, 1969.

91. *The Womanly Art of Breastfeeding.* Franklin Park, Ill., La Leche League International, 1958.

92. Wrigley, E. A.: *Population and History.* New York, World University Library, 1969.

93. Wynne-Edwards, V. C.: Population Control in Animals, *Scientific American,* August, 1964.

94. Zatvchni, G. E.: *Post-partum Family Planning: A Report on the International Program.* New York, McGraw-Hill Book Co., 1970.

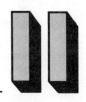

The Prenatal Period

7

Physiologic Change Following Conception: Mother and Conceptus

OBJECTIVES

1. Identify:
    zygote
    conceptus
    trimester
    embryo
    fetus
    embryologic age
    gestational age
    morphogenesis
    histogenesis
    induction
    competence
    agenesis
    hypoplasia
    cephalocaudal

    morula
    blastocyst
    decidua
    zona pellucida
    trophoblast
    ectoderm
    mesoderm
    entoderm
    lightening
    cotyledon
    septa
    ductus arteriosus
    ductus venosus
    foramen ovale

2. Estimate gestational age, using Nägele's rule.
3. Describe factors that may influence the accuracy of estimated gestational age.
4. Identify major developmental changes in the conceptus (embryo-fetus and supporting structures).
5. Identify major physiologic changes in the pregnant woman.
6. Describe in general the tissues that develop from each of the three germ layers: ectoderm, mesoderm, and entoderm.
7. Describe the major functions of the placenta.
8. Differentiate and describe Hegar's sign, Goodell's sign, Chadwick's sign.
9. Differentiate presumptive, probable, and positive signs of pregnancy; describe when they occur, their physiologic basis, and other possible causes.

From the moment an ovum is fertilized by a sperm, a pattern of development begins that will result, if all goes well, in the delivery of a healthy infant approximately 266 days later. From the fertilized ovum, or zygote, not only the infant but also the umbilical cord, the fetal membranes, the amniotic fluid, and the fetal portion of the placenta must develop. These products are jointly termed the *conceptus*. Concurrently, changes are taking place in the mother's body to accommodate and support this growing life.

Nurses who care for childbearing families must be aware of both embryologic development and maternal changes. Without an understanding of basic embryology, it is impossible to understand the capabilities and limitations of the term and preterm newborn, the reasons for many congenital malformations, and the rationale for certain practices in maternal care. A knowledge of the development of the conceptus in utero provides answers to questions such as, "I took an airplane trip when I was 6 months pregnant. Is this why my baby has a congenital heart defect?" We can understand why a viral disease such a rubella will have devastating effects in the first months of pregnancy but may cause only minor problems or no malformation at all late in pregnancy.

A knowledge of the basic concepts of embryologic development and maternal change is also important for nurses who choose other fields of practice—nurses who may be giving medications to women who are pregnant, nurses in venereal disease clinics, nurses who work with adolescent girls who have heart defects, industrial nurses and public health nurses with special concerns for environmental health, and nurses whose friends, neighbors, and relatives will be pregnant.

The period of time during which the baby develops in utero is divided into three divisions, called *trimesters*. The developing conceptus is called an *embryo* until the end of the seventh or eighth week (embryologists vary in their designation), and a *fetus* from that time until birth. Some embryologists designate the first 1 or 2 weeks following conception as the period of the ovum.

The mean length of human pregnancy is 266 days, or 38 weeks, from the time of conception. Approximately 70 per cent of all mothers deliver within 12 days of this period, plus or minus several days (i.e., from 254 to 278 days after conception). Because the exact date of conception usually is not known, the duration of pregnancy is usually calculated from the date of onset of the last menstrual period, the total period being considered as 280 days, or 40 weeks.

The *embryologic age* of the embryo-fetus is dated from the time of conception. *Gestational age* is dated from the time of onset of the last menstrual period. Thus 2 weeks after conception the embryo is 2 weeks old in terms of embryologic age, but the gestational age is 1 month. In the pages that follow the embryo is described in terms of embryologic age. After the period of viability, gestational age may be determined by adding 2 weeks to embryologic age. This aids in understanding the characteristics of the preterm newborn who is the same gestational age.

A common method for estimating the date of delivery, or estimated date of confinement (EDC), is Nägele's rule, in which one counts back 3 months from the *first* day of the last *regular* menstrual period and adds 1 year and 7 days. Thus if the last menstrual period (LMP) is March 10, the EDC will be December 17. In the review of the menstrual cycle in Chapter 4 it was noted that there is considerable variation in the length of the proliferative phase of the menstrual cycle, one major reason that the EDC is rarely exact.

Parents need to understand that the date they are given, based on Nägele's, rule is only approximate and may be revised during the course of the pregnancy; no predicted date is an absolute indication of the day their baby will be born. Revision is based on a variety of factors including uterine size, fundal height, the time fetal heart tones are first heard, and in some instances ultrasound evaluation of fetal biparietal diameters. All of these topics are discussed in Chapter 14.

Physiologic Adaptation in Pregnant Women

The changes that occur in a woman's body during pregnancy are far greater than those that are readily observable. As the mother's body grows and as the fetus makes demands upon the maternal system for nutrition, respiration, and excretion, physiologic adaptation must occur. Although it is necessary to consider physiologic adaptation in a system-by-system framework, we must remember that systems are interdependent. One change in one system may lead to a series of adaptations in other systems.

Cardiovascular Adaptation

Every aspect of the cardiovascular system undergoes adaptation during pregnancy— heart and blood vessels, cardiac output, blood volume and pressure, and the composition of the blood.

Heart size may increase, perhaps due to the hypertrophy of cardiac muscle. As the growing uterus elevates the diaphragm, the heart is displaced upward and to the left and rotated anteriorly. This change is evident on electro-cardiograms as a shift in the electrical axis. In assessment of the heart, a soft systolic murmur is heard in approximately 50 per cent of pregnant women.

The capacity of veins and venules is increased by more than a liter; should return blood flow be impeded or blood volume increase further, they will distend even more. It is believed that estrogen and progesterone are responsible for the changes in vessel walls. Estrogen and progesterone may also increase capillary permeability, which may in turn be a factor in the tissue edema frequently encountered in pregnancy. Estrogen may also affect arterial walls; the dilatation of the uterine artery occurs as a result of growth of the arterial wall and relaxation of the muscle coat.

Cardiac output increases from approximately 5.0 liters per minute in the nonpregnant woman to 6.7 liters per minute in late pregnancy. This represents an increase of approximately 35 per cent. During labor cardiac output is increased approximately 40 per cent; it remains elevated in the immediate postpartal period. (Table 7–1 compares cardiac output in several circumstances.)

Cardiac output is a function of stroke volume and heart rate. Resting heart rate is normally increased by 8 beats per minute by the end of the first trimester and by 15 beats per minute at term. Heart rate returns to prepregnancy rates 6 weeks following birth.

Increase in *blood volume* is slower than the increase in cardiac output, but it follows a similar curve. Blood volume begins to increase about 6 weeks after conception. At term the total increase is approximately 1700 ml.—

Table 7–1. CARDIAC OUTPUT IN WOMEN UNDER VARYING CIRCUMSTANCES*

Nonpregnant	
resting	5 liters/minute
walking 2 m.p.h.	15 liters/minute
walking 5 m.p.h.	20 liters/minute
running 7.5 m.p.h.	20 liters/minute
Pregnant	
resting	6.7 liters/minute

*Data from Bell et al., 1968.

1300 ml. in plasma and 400 to 450 ml. in red blood cells. About 1100 ml. is believed to be lost at the time of delivery, partly in bleeding (less than 500 ml.) and partly in blood in the delivered placenta. The remainder of the fluid is lost in urine and insensible water loss in the immediate postpartum period and over the next 2 to 6 weeks.

The relative difference in the increase in plasma volume and red blood cell (RBC) volume results in altered hemoglobin and hematocrit values. The increased RBC volume (400 to 450 ml.) contains approximately 500 mg. of iron, which is equal to or greater than the total body stores of iron in nonpregnant women.[9] The fetus contains 300 mg. of iron, further increasing total iron requirements; see Chapter 12.

Blood pressure changes are observed in mean arterial pressure and in systolic and diastolic pressures. Mean arterial pressure is derived by the formula:

$$\text{mean arterial pressure} = \text{diastolic pressure} + \frac{\text{pulse pressure}}{3}$$

in which pulse pressure is the difference between the systolic and diastolic pressures. For example, if blood pressure is $\frac{110}{70}$, pulse pressure is 40. Mean arterial pressure =

$$70 + \frac{40}{3} = 83.$$

It is possible to measure mean arterial pressure directly with the appropriate equipment. Mean arterial pressure remains unchanged or declines slightly in the first trimester, reaches a low point in the second trimester, and then rises until term (Fig. 7–1). In the past there has been considerable misunderstanding of blood pressure during pregnancy. This has been due in part to inaccuracies in blood pressure measurement because of failure to recognize the importance of factors such as maternal position and in part to a failure to appreciate the midtrimester drop in blood pressure as normal. The maximum fall in the second trimester is 8 mm. Hg for systolic pressure and 12 mm. Hg for diastolic pressure, resulting in an increase in pulse pressure.

If mean arterial pressure exceeds 90 mm. Hg in the second trimester or 105 mm. Hg in the third trimester, the risk of hypertension in the third trimester is increased (Fig. 7–2). Calculation of mean arterial pressure when blood pressure is assessed at $\frac{112}{80}$ will show

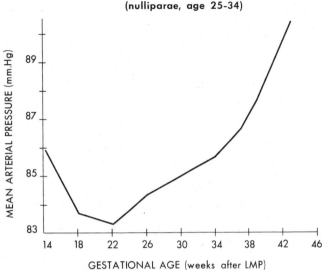

MEAN ARTERIAL PRESSURE BY GESTATIONAL AGE
FOR SINGLE WHITE TERM LIVE BIRTHS
(nulliparae, age 25-34)

Figure 7–1. Mean arterial pressure in pregnancy. (From Page, Villee, and Villee: *Human Reproduction: The Core Content of Obstetrics, Gynecology and Perinatal Medicine.* 3rd Edition. Philadelphia, W. B. Saunders Co., 1981.)

that, at midtrimester, the criterion of mean arterial pressure of 90 is exceeded and the patient is at risk. The assessment of blood pressure is discussed further in Chapter 10.

In the second half of pregnancy, inferior vena cava compression occurs to some degree in all women when they lie on their backs. The gravid uterus blocks part of the return flow of blood to the heart; venous pressure below the uterus may increase as much as 20 to 30 mm. Hg. About 8 per cent of women lying on their backs will experience a fall of 30 per cent or more in systolic blood pressure. After 4 or 5 minutes, reflex bradycardia occurs. The combination of hypotension and bradycardia (the *supine hypotensive syndrome*) can reduce cardiac output by half and may result in a feeling of faintness and symptoms of shock. Figure 7–3 illustrates cardiovascular changes in the supine and lateral positions. When the

mother is hypotensive, placental blood flow may be limited. The major changes in *regional blood flow* involve the kidneys, the uterus, and the extremities.

Renal blood flow increases during the first trimester by approximately 30 to 50 per cent or about 400 ml./minute and remains elevated until term.

Uterine blood flow supplies the endometrium and the myometrium early in pregnancy; by term 80 per cent of the uterine blood flow goes to the placenta. Total uterine blood flow is estimated at 50 ml./minute at 8 weeks, 75 ml./minute at 16 weeks, 150 ml./minute at 24 weeks, and 500 ml./minute near term.[3]

Capillary blood flow to the *skin* is increased, perhaps by as much as 400 to 500 ml. in the second trimester. Resting blood flow to the skin has been found to increase by as much as seven times in the hand and two to three times in

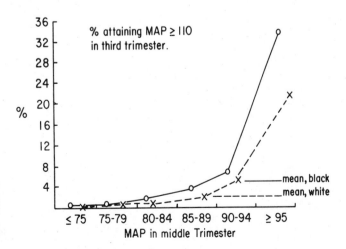

Figure 7–2. Relationship of middle trimester MAP to the percentage of blacks (circles) and whites (X's) that become hypertensive near term. (From data of Page, and Christianson: Am. J. Obstet. Gynecol. *125*:740, 1976.)

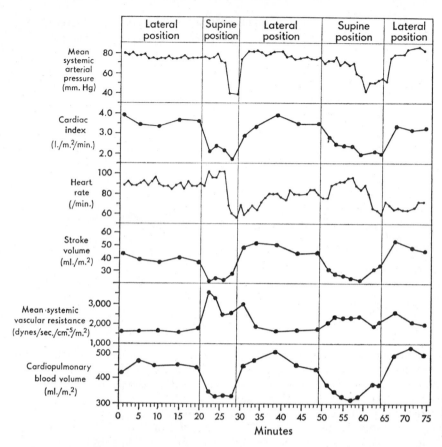

Figure 7–3. Cardiovascular changes induced by the supine position in late pregnancy. (From Kerri Br. Med. Bull., *24*:19, 1968.)

the foot[5] (Fig. 7–4). It is believed that the reason for increased blood flow to the skin is the elimination of heat generated by fetal metabolism.

Reports on blood flow to the *liver* are in disagreement. There is little information on increased *mammary* blood flow and on blood flow to the brain.

Hematologic Changes

The increase in *red blood cell (RBC) volume* has already been noted in relation to the increase in total blood volume. Increased RBC production is related to increased levels of erythropoietin and placental hormone hPL (see below). Reticulocytes account for 2 to 3 per

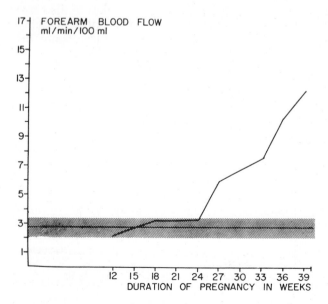

Figure 7–4. Blood flow through the forearm during pregnancy. Range of control values is within shaded area. (From Spetz: Acta Obstet. Gynecol. Scand., *43*:309, 1964.)

Table 7–2. CARDIOVASCULAR-HEMATOLOGIC ADAPTATIONS

Assessment	
Heart size and position	Recognize changes on x-ray and electrocardiogram

Heart rate	Expect increase:
	  8 beats/minute by 13 weeks
	  15 beats/minute by term

Blood pressure	Assess:
	  (1) absolute value
	  (2) relationship to stage of gestation
	  (3) relationship to previous values
	Consider effects of maternal position

Hemoglobin
Hematocrit
	Decreased from nonpregnant state
	  Hemoglobin should be greater than 11.0 to 11.5 g./100 ml.
	  Hematocrit should be greater than 35 per cent

RBC	Greater than 3,750,000/ml.
WBC	6000 to 12,000/cu. mm. 12,000/cu. mm. immediately before labor
Plasma proteins	May decrease to 6 g./100 ml. at term
Coagulation factors	Factors I, VI, VIII, IX, and X increase
Coagulation time	Reduced to 8 minutes

cent of red blood cells during pregnancy, compared with 1 per cent in nonpregnant women (Table 7–2).

White blood cell (WBC) counts are slightly increased during pregnancy; the increase involves neutrophils (rather than lymphocytes, T or B cells) and is believed to be related to estrogen. WBC counts may range between 6000 and 12,000/cu. mm. during pregnancy and exceed 20,000 immediately before or during labor. WBC changes increase the phagocytic and bacteriocidal properties of blood; resistance to viral infections, however, is decreased.

Plasma proteins fall from 7 g./100 ml. in the nonpregnant woman to 6 g./100 ml. at term. Most of the decrease occurs in the first trimester and is due to a fall in the concentration of albumin. This fall may be caused by suppression of albumin production by estrogen and progesterone, since decreased albumin concentration has been found in women taking oral contraceptives. Accompanying the decreased albumin concentration is a decrease in colloid osmotic pressure (from 37 cm. H_2O in nonpregnant women to 30 cm. H_2O in pregnant women). This *may* account for edema in the absence of hypertension and/or proteinuria, suggesting that in this instance generalized edema is part of the physiologic adjustment to pregnancy.[9]

In the *coagulation system* during pregnancy there are increases in Factor I (fibrinogen), Factor VII, Factor X, and , in some women, Factors VIII and IX. Factors XI and XIII are decreased, and there is no change in other factors. Platelet counts change little. The end result is an increase in blood coagulability, with coagulation time reduced from 12 minutes to 8 minutes. Thus the capacity for clotting is increased and the capacity for fibrin removal is decreased. Clinically, pregnant women are more subject to disseminated intravascular coagulation when complications such as infection, abruption of the placenta, amniotic fluid embolism, or eclampsia occur (see also Chapter 13).

Respiratory Adaptation

The major chemical control of respiration is the partial pressure of carbon dioxide (pCO_2) in the blood. In nonpregnant persons with no lung disease, pCO_2 is maintained at approximately 40 mm. Hg; if pCO_2 rises, the respiratory rate is increased to maintain homeostasis. Progesterone affects the respiratory center in the hypothalamus, reducing the threshold for pCO_2 from 40 mm. Hg. to 31 to 32 mm. Hg. and also increasing the sensitivity of the respiratory center to even small elevations in carbon dioxide concentration. These changes would result in a chronic respiratory alkalosis were it not for compensating adaptation in the renal buffering systems (see Urinary Tract Adaptation). This change has been noted during the luteal phase of the menstrual cycle when progesterone levels are high and in men who have been given progesterone; it is marked as progesterone production rises during pregnancy. Pregnant women thus tend to "overbreathe." Tidal volume (the amount of air exhaled during quiet expiration) increases by approximately 40 to 42 per cent, from 500 ml. in nonpregnant women to 700 ml. The respiratory rate remains essentially the same, but minute volume, the amount of gas exhaled per minute (minute volume = tidal volume × respiratory rate) increases from 8 to 11 liters/minute. Functional residual capacity (FRC), a combination of expiratory reserve (air exhaled with a maximum of effort) and residual volume (air remaining in the lungs no matter how great the effort), is decreased (Fig. 7–5). A decrease in FRC means increased alveolar ventilation and, therefore, more efficient gas exchange in the alveoli.

It is believed that lower levels of maternal pCO_2 make fetal elimination of carbon dioxide easier. As pCO_2 falls, the mother breathes more deeply, and oxygen tension rises from a mean of about 90 mm. Hg in nonpregnant women to 106 mm. Hg in pregnancy. Total oxygen consumption rises from 200 to 240 ml./minute, or about 15 per cent.

Anatomically, the lower ribs flare during pregnancy, resulting in an increased subcostal angle and an increase in the anterior/posterior diameter of the chest. The diaphragm rises earlier than might be expected from the growth of the fetus. These two changes offset one another so that there is no decrease in the size of the thoracic cavity nor are diaphragmatic movements limited.

In spite of the increase in pulmonary ventilation, many women report dyspnea (a conscious need to breathe) during pregnancy. Bruce (1981)[3] believes this may be due to the woman's feeling that she is breathing too rapidly, or it may be due to the change in the shape of the thoracic cavity combined with a decrease in functional residual capacity.

Capillary engorgement in the nasal passages causes symptoms of a "stuffy nose" in some mothers. Because of this, mothers may be

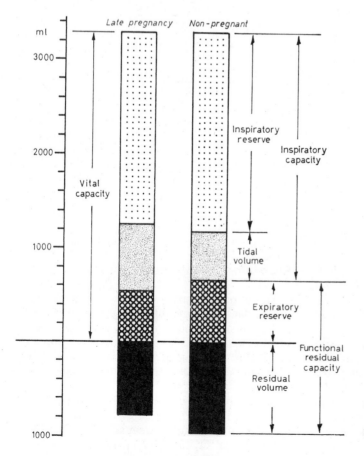

Figure 7–5. Respiratory changes in late pregnancy compared to the non-pregnant woman. (From Hytten and Leitch: *The Physiology of Human Pregnancy.* Oxford, Blackwell Scientific Publications, 1964.)

acutely uncomfortable if an upper respiratory infection or allergic rhinitis is superimposed.

Adaptation in the Urinary Tract

Because of the kidneys' important role in homeostasis, it is not surprising that there are a number of changes in the renal system during pregnancy. The metabolic, circulatory, and respiratory changes in the mother's body coupled with the need to excrete fetal waste products greatly increase the work to be done by the mother's kidneys.

Anatomically, there is dilation of the ureters and of the renal pelves and calyces. There are two theories about the reason for urinary tract dilation. The first suggests that the relaxing effect of progesterone on the smooth muscle of the uterus is primary. The second considers the primary cause to be mechanical obstruction to the flow of urine by the enlarging uterus.[6]

The fact that these changes begin as early as the tenth week suggests a hormonal role. The fact that dilation is greater on the right side later on (and that the uterus usually rotates to the right side) indicates mechanical factors may also be important.

Increased renal blood flow in pregnancy has already been noted (see Cardiovascular Adaptation, above). Glomerular filtration rate (GFR), the amount of plasma filtered by the glomeruli of both kidneys per minute, is also increased by 30 to 50 per cent in the first trimester and by 60 per cent by the third trimester (8 months). In nonpregnant women, GFR is 100 to 120 ml./minute/1.73 m.^{2}; by 4 to 8 months GFR is 150 to 180 ml./minute/1.73 m.^{2}.

Because of the dilation of the ureters, urine remains in the urinary tract longer in pregnant than in nonpregnant women. Urinary stasis increases the risk of urinary tract infection in pregnant women. Increased levels of glucose and other nutrients in the urine also favor the growth of bacteria and subsequent infection (Chapter 13).

Clearance tests of kidney function (such as creatinine clearance, frequently used in pregnancy) may be distorted because there is a time lag between the time the urine leaves the kidneys and the time it enters the bladder. An increase in fluid intake approximately 1 hour before the test, and asking the mother to lie in a lateral recumbent position (see below) will increase the accuracy of kidney function tests.

Creatinine clearance approximates the glomerular filtration rate and is commonly used as an index of glomerular filtration. Because the glomerular filtration rate increases more than the renal blood flow (50 to 60 per cent as compared with 30 to 50 per cent), the proportion of renal plasma flow filtered by the glomeruli is greater than in nonpregnant women. Also contributing to increased filtration is the lower plasma oncotic pressure that is due to lower serum protein levels. Simply stated, there are more waste products in the blood in pregnancy, and the system is designed to enhance the kidneys' opportunity to eliminate them. More effective clearance of substances like creatinine, urea, and uric acid with no increased production means that blood levels of these substances will be lower; they are approximately two-thirds of the levels in nonpregnant women, an important understanding in assessment. Because elevations in blood urea nitrogen (BUN) and creatinine are common indicators of impaired kidney function, it is essential to recognize that values that are normal for nonpregnant women represent an elevation in the pregnant women (Table 7–4).

Maternal posture is an important factor not only in maternal blood pressure but also in kidney function. In a standing or sitting position renal function may be decreased by as much as one-half compared with the lateral recumbent position. Recall the effect of position on blood pressure. When blood pools in the lower extremities and blood return to the heart are decreased, circulating blood volume and subsequently cardiac output are decreased as well. Renal vessels constrict when cardiac output decreases; decreased renal circulation leads to decreased glomerular filtration and thus to a decrease in the excretion of water and electrolytes. To improve renal function, the gravida should rest on her side. This becomes particularly important when kidney function is abnormal, as in pregnancy-induced hypertension. Postural effects also explain the changing pattern of urine excretion. In nonpregnant women urine excretion is increased during the daytime. The opposite is true during pregnancy; urine excretion increases at night when the mother is in bed, presumably because of her change in posture. Understanding the effects of posture on kidney function is particularly important in caring for women with kidney disease and pregnancy-induced hypertension (Chapter 13).

Sodium and water homeostasis is profoundly altered during pregnancy. Both sodium and water accumulate during the course of pregnancy in roughly proportional amounts. The total accumulation of sodium is about 400 to 900 mEq., distributed between the fetus, maternal extracellular tissues, and increased plasma volume. At term, the maternal body contains approximately 6 liters of extra water

Table 7–3. SODIUM EXCRETION DURING PREGNANCY

Factors Favoring Sodium Retention	Factors Favoring Sodium Excretion
Increase in renin and renin substrate → increase in angiotensin → increased aldosterone secretion	Increase in the glomerular filtration rate
Increase in estrogen	Increase in progesterone (antagonistic to aldosterone in the renal tubule)
Increase in free plasma cortisol	Increased renal blood flow
Posture	

in the fetus, placenta, uterus, breasts, and expanded blood volume. An additional 1.5 liters of water are found in the extracellular tissue of women with no evident edema; as much as 4 liters of extracellular water may be present in women who have generalized edema.

Changes in pregnancy that affect both the retention and the excretion of sodium are summarized in Table 7–3. Notice that estrogen and progesterone have opposite effects. One might wonder why increases in angiotensin do not, in most women, lead to increases in blood pressure. It appears that the blood pressure response to angiotensin is considerably reduced except in women who have pregnancy-induced hypertension.

Water retention also appears to be related to estrogen and progesterone, which may cause the receptors that respond to osmolality to be "reset." As previously noted in relation to plasma proteins, water retention in extracellular tissues may be partially related to the lower colloidal osmotic pressure of plasma; some edema, in the absence of hypertension, is now believed to be a normal part of pregnancy. Thompson (1967)[11] reported that 35 per cent of normotensive gravidas have clinically evident edema; these women had larger infants and a slightly lower mortality rate than women with no edema.

Glycosuria is increased during pregnancy. While nonpregnant women excrete an average of 100 mg. of glucose in urine every 24 hours, normal pregnant women may excrete from 100 to 2000 mg. per day, the amount varying widely not only from one woman to another but also from one sample to another taken from the same woman at time intervals of only a few hours. Moreover, glycosuria appears to bear little relationship to serum glucose levels. Because glucose is freely filtered across the glomerulus, the increased glomerular filtration rate is believed to be the major factor. A decline in the reabsorptive capacity of the proximal convoluted tubules may also contribute to glycosuria.[4]

The lower level of pCO_2 in pregnant women has been described in the section on respiratory adaptation. In nonpregnant persons, a pCO_2 of 31 to 32 mm. Hg would result in respiratory alkalosis with a high maternal serum pH. This does not happen in pregnancy because the kidneys maintain homeostasis through an increased renal excretion of bicarbonate. Although one does not ordinarily think of pregnant women in these terms, they may be described as being in a state of "chronic respiratory alkalosis fully compensated for by a chronic metabolic acidosis."[9]

In nonpregnant women, decreased pCO_2 would also cause the release of vasopressin, with subsequent diuresis. During pregnancy, however, there is a tendency to retain water (see below), suggesting that the osmoregulatory mechanisms are reset.[3]

Gastrointestinal Adaptation

Unlike changes in many of the systems that support the needs of the fetus, gastrointestinal changes seem largely to be side effects of hormonal changes. Although the cause of nausea remains unclear, rising estrogen levels may be one factor. The decreased tone of the gastrointestinal tract is probably due to the same hormonal effects that reduce tone in the veins

Table 7–4. ASSESSMENT OF KIDNEY FUNCTION AND URINE IN PREGNANT AND NONPREGNANT WOMEN

Parameter	Nonpregnant	Pregnant
Glomerular filtration rate	100–120 ml./min./1.73m^2	150–180 ml./min./1.73m^2
Blood urea nitrogen (BUN)	13 mg./100 ml. ± 3	8.7 mg./100 ml. ± 1.5
Serum creatinine	0.67 mg./ml. ± 0.14	0.46 mg./ml. ± 0.13
Glucose excretion (urine)	100 mg./day	100–2000 mg./day

and uterus. Both constipation and heartburn can be traced to the decrease in tone (Chapter 11). The swollen, frequently bleeding gums of pregnant women are also related to hormones. During the first two trimesters, there is reduced gastric secretion; one advantage of this is a reduced tendency for peptic ulcer during pregnancy.

Adaptation in Muscle and Connective Tissue

Connective tissue, under the influence of increasing levels of estrogen, relaxin (a hormone produced by the corpus luteum of pregnant women), and corticosteroids, becomes less supportive as pregnancy progresses, allowing increased relaxation and mobility in joints. This is particularly noticeable in the symphysis pubis, the sacroiliac and sacrococcygeal joints of the pelvis, the hip and knee joints, and the lower back.

As a result, body alignment and balance change during pregnancy. The center of gravity moves forward as the mother's abdomen enlarges, and she adapts by shifting her weight further back on her heels when she stands. An individual woman may unconsciously adopt any of a variety of postures. Back muscles bear much of the stress of these postural changes, resulting in low back pain for many pregnant women. Proper posture and prenatal exercise can alleviate much of the discomfort.

The loosening of the abdominal fasciae and reduced cohesion between collagen fibers in the skin allow the abdominal muscles and skin to stretch. As the collagen fibers pull apart, the skin may become thin in areas of maximum stretch, resulting in *striae gravidarium*, pinkish or bluish "stripes" (the color depends on the underlying vascular bed). Striae are seen not only in the abdomen but in the breasts and thighs as well because the skin is stretched over areas of accumulated subcutaneous fat. Mothers who were previously obese or who have inordinate amounts of weight gain or significant edema will have increased stretching.

Endocrine Adaptation

Endocrine changes involve hormones present in both nonpregnant and pregnant states

Table 7–5. PLACENTAL HORMONES

Polypeptide Hormones
  Human chorionic gonadotropin
  Human placental lactogen
  Human chorionic corticotropin
  Human chorionic thyrotropin
  Other placental proteins

Steroid Hormones
  Progesterone
  Estrogens
    Estradiol
    Estrone
    Estriol

(e.g., thyroid hormone and insulin) as well as hormones secreted by the placenta, some of which result in elevated levels of hormones that are also present in nonpregnant women (estrogen and progesterone, for example) and some of which are specific to pregnancy (or to the presence of trophoblastic tissue), such as human chorionic gonadotropin.

Placental Hormones

One of the major functions of the placenta is the synthesis of steroid and polypeptide hormones (Table 7–5). Nevertheless, the placenta is not an autonomous endocrine organ; precursors from the mother and the fetus are essential to placental hormone production.

Human Chorionic Gonadotropin (hCG). Human chorionic gonadotropin (hCG) is produced initially by the blastocyst (see below). Although some investigators report the detection of hCG prior to implantation of the ovum, others believe that detection is not possible until 8 to 10 days following conception. From that time concentration of hCG in serum doubles every 2 days (approximately), and serum levels therefore rise quickly (Fig. 7–6). In urine, hCG is found about 26 days after conception (approximately 6 weeks after the last menstrual period). Peak values are recorded at 60 to 70 days of pregnancy; after the tenth to eleventh week concentrations begin to decline. Following term pregnancy hCG disappears by the end of 2 weeks; it takes 4 weeks of hCG levels to disappear following therapeutic abortion.

The major function of hCG is diagrammed as follows:

hCG
↓
maintains the corpus luteum of pregnancy and thereby
↓
maintains progesterone production by the corpus luteum and thereby
↓
maintains the endometrium until there is sufficient progesterone production by the placenta.

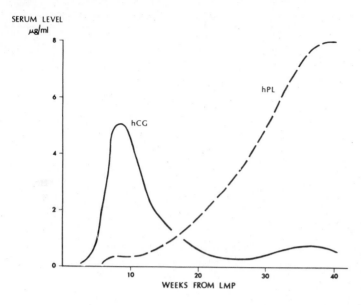

Figure 7–6. Maternal serum concentrations (μg/ml) of hCG (1 μg = 20 IU) and hPL. (From Tulchinsky and Ryan: *Maternal-Fetal Endocrinology.* Philadelphia, W. B. Saunders Co., 1980. Adapted from Dr. S. S. C. Yen, with permission.)

Thus hCG production is essential during the earliest weeks of pregnancy and but is less important after the development of the placenta.

In addition, hCG stimulates the fetal testicle to secrete testosterone during the period of gonadal differentiation (see below) and stimulates the fetal adrenal to secrete corticosteroids. The role of hCG in ovarian development, if any, is not clear at this time.

The presence of hCG is the basis of current pregnancy testing (Chapter 10) and is also used in the monitoring of women with gestational trophoblastic neoplasms (see Hydatidiform Mole in Chapter 13).

Human Placental Lactogen (hPL). Human placental lactogen (also called human chorionic somatomammotropin and chorionic growth hormone) is produced by the placental trophoblasts beginning about 12 to 18 days after the ovum is fertilized (5 to 10 days after implantation) and continues to rise, reaching a plateau at 34 to 36 weeks. Human placental lactogen appears to favor the growth of the fetus by mobilizing maternal free fatty acids to meet the mother's energy needs, thus sparing the mother's glucose for utilization by the fetus. The fetus is thereby assured of a constant glucose supply, which is its prime source of energy. By decreasing sensitivity to insulin and increasing the circulating levels of insulin in response to a glucose load, hPL affects carbohydrate metabolism. (Norms for the glucose tolerance test in pregnancy vary from those of the nonpregnant state; see discussion of diabetes in pregnancy, Chapter 13.) Thus, hPL contributes to the diabetogenic state of pregnancy. During fasting, both hypoglycemia and ketonemia (ketone bodies in the blood stream) develop more rapidly in pregnant women than in nonpregnant women.

Human placental lactogen may also affect protein metabolism by restricting the mother's use of amino acids, thereby making more

Table 7–6. FUNCTIONS OF HUMAN PLACENTAL LACTOGEN

Carbohydrate Metabolism	Fat Metabolism	Protein Metabolism	Preparation of Mammary Glands for Lactation
Decreased sensitivity to insulin + Increased circulating levels of insulin in presence of glucose ↓ Diabetogenic state of pregnancy + Increased availability of glucose to fetus	Mobilization of free fatty acids ↓ Fats as energy source for mother ↓ Decreased maternal utilization of glucose ↓ Decreased availability of glucose to fetus	Restriction of maternal utilization of protein ↓ Increased availability of amino acids to fetus	May directly, or, in combination with prolactin, prepare mammary glands for lactation

amino acids available to the fetus, and perhaps also by playing a part in the increased nitrogen retention found in pregnancy.

In addition, hPL may participate in the preparation of the breasts for lactation (the original source of the name lactogen), either directly or by interacting with prolactin. This action has been confirmed in animal studies.

The use of serum hPL levels as a test of placental function has been explored. Because the half-life of hPL is short, its presence in the blood reflects the rate at which it is produced and therefore, the functioning of the placenta on which the fetus is so dependent. There are varying reports of the success of hPL measurement as an indicator of placental function and fetal well-being. It does seem clear that hPL measurement is not of value in identifying fetal distress in mothers with pre-eclampsia, chronic hypertension, and intrauterine growth retardation (see Chapter 10); in addition, a low level of hPL does not necessarily indicate impaired function.

Other Polypeptide Hormones. The placenta also secretes an ACTH-like substance, human chorionic corticotropin, of which the physiologic role is unknown at present. Humanchorionic thyrotropin, also secreted by the placenta, is believed to be responsible for increased thyroid activity in women with gestational trophoblastic neoplasms (see Hydaditiform Mole in Chapter 13) but a role in normal pregnancy has not been identified.

Placental Secretion of Steroid Hormones

The corpus luteum, formed during the luteal phase of the ovarian cycle, secretes the steroid hormones estrogen and progesterone, as already noted (Chapter 4). Should conception occur, chorionic gonadotropin produced by the conceptus transforms the corpus luteum to the corpus luteum of pregnancy, which continues to secrete steroid hormones for at least 4 more weeks (until the eighth week of gestation or 6 weeks following conception), although by the seventh week of gestation placental production is sufficient to meet the needs of the pregnancy.

If for some reason the corpus luteum is removed before the seventh week of gestation, levels of both progesterone and estradiol (an estrogen) will drop markedly, and the fetus will be aborted. After the eighth week, removal of the corpus luteum does not affect the course of the pregnancy; blood levels of progesterone are affected briefly and slightly.

Progesterone. The placenta synthesizes progesterone from cholesterol, which is derived from the maternal circulation (see Placental Function, below). No substrate from the fetus appears to be required for progesterone production, since intrauterine fetal death does not affect production. Progesterone differs from estrogen in this regard (see below), and thus is not used in studies of fetal well-being.

Several of the effects of progesterone balance the effects of estrogen (Table 7–7). These include reduction of myometrial activity, constriction of blood vessels in the myometrium, decrease in the sensitivity of the respiratory center to carbon dioxide (see Respiratory Adaptation), and inhibition of prolactin secretion. Progesterone also leads to a decrease in muscle tone in other areas of the body. The effects of progesterone on the central nervous system result in feelings of sleepiness and listlessness for many women. Progesterone causes an increase in basal body temperature during the first half of pregnancy of approximately 0.4° to 0.6° C. Sodium and chloride excretion is increased in the presence of progesterone, but this effect is balanced by a compensatory rise in aldosterone, which works to prevent sodium loss.

Estrogens. The three major estrogens, estrone, estradiol, and estriol, have been described in Chapter 4. These three estrogens are synthesized in placental tissue. Of the three, estriol is the most highly sensitive to fetal well-being because 90 per cent of the precursor for estriol (16x-hydroxydehydro-epiandrosterone sulfate) is derived from the fetus. This process and the use of estriol in the assessment of fetal well-being are described in Chapter 14. In contrast, the precursors for the

Table 7–7. "BALANCING EFFECTS" OF ESTROGENS AND PROGESTERONE

Estrogens	Progesterone
Enhance myometrial activity	Reduces myometrial activity
Promote myometrial vasodilation	Constricts myometrial vessels
Increase sensitivity of respiratory center to CO_2	Decreases sensitivity of respiratory center to CO_2
Cause pituitary to secrete prolactin	Inhibits secretion or prolactin

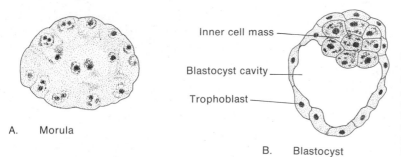

A.   Morula

B.   Blastocyst

Inner cell mass

Blastocyst cavity

Trophoblast

Figure 7–7 *A,* The morula is a mass of cells; it resembles a mulberry in shape and contains blastomeres and tropho-blast-producing cells. *B,* The blastocyst at approximately 5 days after conception, showing the inner cell mass (larger cells that will form the embryo) and prospective trophoblasts (smaller cells from with the fetal placenta, membranes, and cord will develop).

synthesis of estradiol and estrone (dehydro-epiandrosterone sulfate) are derived from both mother (40 per cent) and fetus (60 per cent).

Estrogens balance the action of progester-ones in many instances (Table 7–7). Other effects of estrogens include softening the fibers in collagen tissues of the cervix and increasing the sensitivity of the breasts to prolactin as well as a variety of hematologic changes, in-cluding an increase in the concentration of fibrinogen, an increase in serum binding pro-teins, and a fall in plasma proteins, particu-larly albumin. At the end of pregnancy estro-gens make the uterus more sensitive to prostaglandins.

Placental Development and Function

The role of placental hormones has been described in the previous section. Endocrine production is only one of several life-sustaining placental functions. "More than any other sin-gle factor, the welfare of the fetus is dependent upon an adequate perfusion by maternal blood of the effective exchange areas in the pla-centa."[9]

The placenta develops as the *trophoblast* (Fig. 7–7) invades the decidua. The maternal portion is derived from the *decidua basalis* (the maternal endometrium during pregnancy) and the arteries and venules that supply it; in the mature placenta the maternal surface is a "beefy" red. The fetal portion consists of *cho-rionic villi* (fingerlike projections from the cho-rion—see below) and multiple chorionic blood vessels covered by the amnion, giving the fetal aspect a shiny, gray appearance at term. Sep-arating the maternal and fetal circulations is a membrane, the syncytioendothelial mem-brane (or syncytium), which is derived partly from the chorion of the villi and partly from the endothelium of the blood vessels. The blood of the mother and the blood of the fetus do not mix under ordinary circumstances; fetal blood may enter the maternal circulation at the time

of placental delivery. For some mothers (e.g., mothers with Rh_D incompatibility) this may be a source of future difficulty (Chapter 13). The syncytium changes as pregnancy progresses and also varies with its position on a particular villus and the location of the villus. In general, the syncytium becomes more permeable as pregnancy progresses, allowing increased transport of nutrients, oxygen, and other sub-stances. In the last weeks of gestation, as the placenta begins to age and develop, infarctions (areas of tissue necrosis due to ischemia), permeability decreases. This explains why the infant of a prolonged pregnancy (more than 42 weeks) frequently exhibits signs of malnutri-tion and may have decreased oxygen reserves (see Chapter 23; post-term infant).

As the placenta develops, *septa* (partitions) derived from chorionic villi divide the placenta into segments called cotyledons. It is within the vascular system of the cotyledons that placental exchange occurs (Fig. 7–8). Cotyle-don formation begins about 40 to 50 days following ovulation. At 8 months, the time of maximum growth, there are approximately 10 to 12 large cotyledons, 40 to 50 small to me-dium cotyledons, and 150 rudimentary cotyle-dons. The sequential development of the pla-centa is described along with fetal and maternal development in this chapter.

Placental function includes the transport of nutrients, oxygen, potential toxins, antibodies, and fetal wastes through a variety of mecha-nisms (Table 7–8), and the synthesis of glyco-gen, cholesterol, and fatty acids for fetal nu-trition and as a substrate for the production of hormones. Placental function is summarized in Table 7–9.

The transport of substances across the pla-centa is of concern at every phase of pregnancy. Factors that appear important include placen-tal blood flow, the saturation of nutrients and gases in the blood, the molecular size, lipid solubility, and electrical charge of the sub-stances being transported, and the area of the placenta available for transport. Conditions that diminish blood flow (pre-eclampsia or se-vere maternal diabetes, for example) may re-

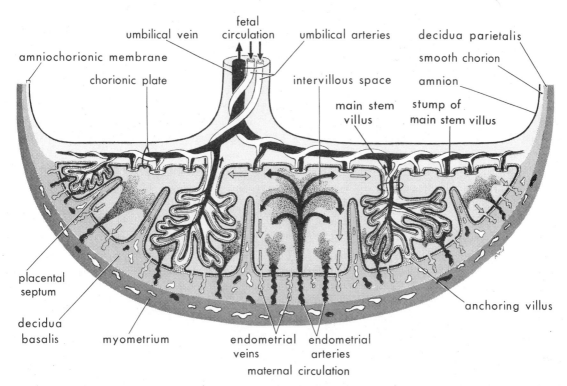

Figure 7–8. Schematic drawing of a section through a mature placenta, showing (1) the relation of the villous chorion (fetal placenta) to the decidua basalis (maternal placenta), (2) the fetal placental circulation and (3) the maternal placental circulation. Maternal blood is driven into the intervillous space in funnel-shaped spurts, and exchanges occur with the fetal blood as the maternal blood flows around the villi. The inflowing arterial blood pushes venous blood out into the endometrial veins, which are scattered over the entire surface of the decidua basalis. Note that the umbilical arteries carry deoxygenated fetal blood (shown in blue) to the placenta and the umbilical vein carries oxygenated blood (shown in red) to the fetus. (From Moore: *The Developing Human.* 2nd Edition. Philadelphia, W. B. Saunders Co., 1977. Based on Ramsey, 1965.)

sult in fetal growth retardation in the prenatal period and fetal distress during labor. If the maternal blood does not contain proper nutrients or adequate oxygen, the fetus will again be at risk of growth retardation or distress. Whether a drug or other substance will harm the fetus during the prenatal or labor phase will depend in part on the characteristics of that substance. Heparin, for example, is composed of large molecules that not cross the placenta. Some anesthetic drugs cross more rapidly than others. These concepts are thus important to a variety of maternal-fetal concerns.

Table 7–8. MECHANISMS OF PLACENTAL TRANSPORT

Mechanism	Action	Substances Involved
Simple diffusion	Molecules move from area of higher to lower concentration until equilibrium is established	Water, electrolytes, CO_2, O_2*
Facilitated diffusion	Transport through electrical charges (slow) carrier system, such as lipids (rapid)	Glucose, O_2*
Active transport	Transport against concentration gradient (i.e., moving from area of lower to higher concentration); requires energy and enzyme system	Calcium, iron, iodine, some vitamins, amino acids
Dinocytosis	Transport as plasma droplets	Large molecules (e.g., albumin, gamma globulins)
Other	Infection of placenta	Certain bacteria and protozoa
	Breaks in placental membrane	Fetal RBC's
	Unknown	Viruses, maternal leukocytes

*Simple diffusion has long been recognized as a mechanism of oxygen transport; facilitated diffusion may also play a role.

Table 7–9. SUMMARY OF PLACENTAL FUNCTION

Function	Substances Involved	Comment
I. Nutrition	Oxygen Glucose Protein Fat Water Vitamins and minerals Electrolytes	
II. Elimination of waste	Breakdown products of fetal metabolism → mother's kidneys and lungs	
III. Antibody transfer	Immunoglobulin-G (IgG) transferred from mother to fetus	Fetus immune only to IgG organisms to which mother is immune
IV. Hormone production	Human chorionic gonadotropin	Early maintenance of corpus luteum
	Estrogens and progestins	Placenta major source of estrogens and progestins after second month
	Human placental lactogen (human chorionic somatomammotropin)	Promotes growth
	Human chorionic thyrotropin	
V. Synthesis	Glycogen Cholesterol Fatty acids	Substrate for endocrine production Some fetal nutrition

The Umbilical Cord, Fetal Membranes, and Amniotic Fluid

The development and characteristics of the umbilical cord are described in the overview of development below (fifth through seventh weeks). Twisting of the cord occurs frequently because the umbilical vein is longer than the arteries and because all of the vessels are longer than the cord itself.

Two fetal membranes, the inner amnion and the outer chorion, are separated at first, but gradually the amniotic sac enlarges and eliminates the chorionic cavity (Fig. 7–9). The amnion also becomes the outer covering of the umbilical cord.

Amniotic fluid is produced within the amniotic sac; most of the amniotic fluid is derived from the maternal blood, but fetal urine is also important, especially late in pregnancy. At term there are approximately 1000 ml. of amniotic fluid. The fetus swallows up to 400 ml. of amniotic fluid each day and adds about 500 ml. of urine each day to the fluid.

Moore (1973)[7] describes several functions of amniotic fluid: (1) permits symmetrical growth and development of the embryo; (2) prevents adherence of the amnion to the jelly-like embryo; (3) cushions the embryo against jolts by distributing impacts the mother may receive;

(4) helps to control the embryo's body temperature by maintaining a relatively constant temperature; (5) enables the fetus to move freely, thus aiding musculoskeletal development.

In addition, amniotic fluid, aspirated through a procedure called amniocentesis, has proved valuable in a variety of types of fetal assessment (Chapter 14).

Principles of the Growth and Development of the Fetus

Growth and development follow very specific patterns in an orderly sequence. Both are part of a continuum that begins at the time of conception and continues for many years after birth.

The development of the embryo-fetus is dependent upon: (1) cell proliferation, (2) growth, (3) differentiation, and (4) integration.

The single fertilized ovum (zygote) divides by mitosis, as do the daughter cells, until trillions of cells are produced. The process of producing two cells from every one cell is so efficient that doubling the number of cells 45 times would result in all the cells needed for a complete individual.

Cell division per se does not result in growth.

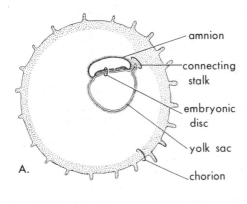

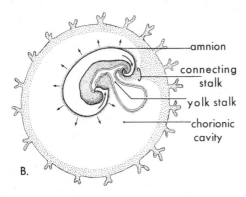

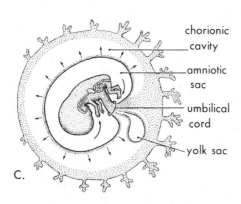

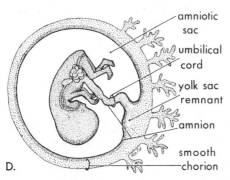

Figure 7–9. Drawing illustrating how the aminion becomes the outer covering of the umbilical cord and how the yolk sac is partially incorporated into the embryo as the primitive gut. *A,* 3 weeks. *B,* 4 weeks. *C,* 10 weeks. *D,* 20 weeks. (From Moore: *The Developing Human.* 2nd Edition. Philadelphia, W. B. Saunders Co., 1977.)

Growth is a result of: (1) the synthesis of protoplasm from amino acids, (2) the intake of water by the cells, and (3) the deposit of nonliving substances, such as fibers and parts of cartilage and bone.

Differentiation includes *morphogenesis,* by which the organs of the body and the body itself take shape, and *histogenesis,* by which the specification of tissue occurs. Changes in form are due to the fact that various regions of the body grow at different rates, both prenatally and postnatally. (See, for example, cephalocaudal development, below.) Different structures result as cells migrate to various areas of the body and aggregate, and the resultant tissues fuse, split, fold, and bend.

Induction is the process by which one tissue transmits a stimulus that leads to the development of neighboring tissues. *Competence* is the process by which the adjacent tissue responds to the stimulus. If induction fails, either because of inadequate stimulus or because the tissue to be acted upon does not react properly, an organ may fail to appear *(agenesis),* may be smaller than normal *(hypoplasia),* or may be incompletely differentiated. Irregularities in induction can also lead to organ duplication, such as a double kidney, or to abnormal positioning of an organ.

Cells first become specialized and later develop into specialized tissues. In the early stage of differentiation the suffix *-blast* often designates a developing cell (e.g., neuroblast) that will develop into a particular type of cell (such as a nerve cell).

The final stage of development is *integration,* during which organ systems become able to function in a coordinated way. The endocrine glands and the nervous system are the mechanisms for integration.

Developmental Trends

Both embryo-fetal development and development after birth are *cephalocaudal,* that is, they proceed from head to tail. The embryo's head develops more rapidly than the remainder of his body. Development of function, as well as of size, proceeds in a cephalocaudal direction. Thus a baby will raise his head and "reach out" with his eyes before he is able to use his arms and, still later, his legs.

Growth also proceeds from the *medial* aspect of the body to the *lateral* aspects. Thus the trunk develops before the arms and legs, which, in turn, precede the fingers and toes. As with cephalocaudal development, function following birth will also proceed in the same medial-lateral direction. Arms will be used before hands, and it will be many years before a child will be able to use his fingers for activities that require a high degree of precision.

General structures (i.e., arm buds and then arms) precede specific structures (i.e., hands and fingers). Postnatally, as noted, these general structures will be used before the more specific structures. Toys and activities for younger children should be planned with this principle in mind; a large soccer-sized ball is more appropriate for a preschool child than a baseball.

THE FIRST WEEK

Conceptus

Zygote undergoes cleavage as it traverses the uterine tube.

Forms morula, which reaches the uterine cavity in 3 to 4 days, undergoes further change to blastocyst stage.

Zona pellucida disappears about day 6 to 7.

Blastocyst attaches to endometrium (beginning of implantation), day 6 to 7.

Mother

Vascular changes influenced by progesterone prepare the endometrium for implantation.

Decidual reaction.

The First Week

The ovum is fertilized in the distal third of the uterine tube. During the next 3 to 4 days, it travels to the uterus, probably as a result of muscular peristaltic movement of the tube. The corona radiata disappears, so that the fertilized ovum can pass through the narrow infundibulum of the tube, but the zona pellucida remains until after the ovum reaches the uterine cavity.

During transport, cleavage (mitotic division) begins. The cells that result, called *blastomeres,* first form a ball called a *morula* (Fig. 7–7A). After reaching the uterine cavity, the morula begins to change its structure; a cavity filled with fluid forms in the center. The morula is now a *blastocyst* (Fig. 7–7B) with two types of cells: large cells (the inner cell mass) that will form the embryo and smaller *trophoblasts* from which will develop the fetal portion of the placenta, the amnion and the chorion and the umbilical cord.

Meanwhile, the endometrium, under the influence of progesterone from the corpus luteum, becomes highly vascular and stores glycogen in preparation for implantation.

On approximately the sixth day the zona pellucida disappears and implantation takes place, that is, the blastocyst attaches itself to the endometrium, commonly at the midposterior or midanterior portion of the fundus, and almost always close to a maternal capillary. Following the attachment of the blastocyst, the *decidual reaction* takes place, i.e., the endometrial stromal cells become large and pale. *Decidua* is the term used to describe the endometrium during pregnancy.

THE SECOND WEEK

Conceptus

Inner cell mass (embryo)—Embryo is a two-layered disc of ectoderm and entoderm, lying between a primitive amniotic cavity and the cavity of the yolk sac.

Trophoblast—Implantation continues; completed about day 12. Trophoblast differentiates into *syncytiotrophoblast* (outer layer) and *cytotrophoblast* (Langhans' cells).

Advancing Langhans' cells tap venules and capillaries of endometrium, forming *lacunae* filled with maternal blood, the predecessors of the intervillous spaces, at about 9 to 11 days.

Chorionic gonadotropin produced by syncytiotrophoblast.

Mesoblastic (mesodermal) cells, formed from the trophoblast at 11 days, give rise to the *amnion.*

The primary yolk sac develops.

Mother

Decidua engulfs blastocyst.

Chorionic gonadotropin acts on the corpus luteum of pregnancy to maintain production of estrogen and progesterone and thus prevents the changes that would lead to menstruation.

Human chorionic gonadotropin found in the mother's serum and urine at 10 days; basis of pregnancy tests 2 to 4 weeks after conception.

The Second Week

The endometrium erodes at the point at which the blastocyst has attached itself, and the point of entry is covered by maternal endometrial cells. The area beneath the implanting blastocyst is called the *decidua basalis;* the *decidua capsularis* covers the implanting blastocyst. *Decidua vera* is the term used to describe the remainder of the uterine lining. Once the decidua has engulfed the blastocyst, the blastocyst is no longer in the uterine cavity. The trophoblastic cells further differentiate and invade the decidua, as noted above and in Figure 7–10.

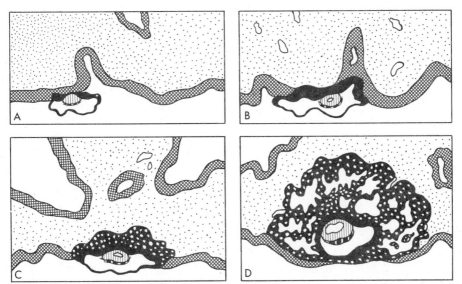

Figure 7–10. Stages of implantation. *A,* The blastocyst approaches the endometrium; *B,* begins to erode the epithelium; and *C* and *D,* is progressively buried within the decidua.

During the process of implantation, the future embryo has become a two-layered disc, consisting of ectoderm and entoderm. Table 7–10 indicates some of the major systems developing from each of these layers.

The *yolk sac,* which will further develop in the third week, does not store yolk in the human embryo, as it does in some species. Part of the digestive tract will develop from the entodermal roof of the yolk sac. A part of the sac, the proximal end of the yolk stalk, may persist to adulthood as an intestinal pouch (Meckel's diverticulum of the ileum). Some blood cells will be formed in the yolk sac during the third week.

The production of human chorionic gonadotropin by the syncytiotrophoblast is the basis of pregnancy testing.

THE THIRD WEEK

Embryo

Embryonic disc becomes pear-shaped and then slipper-shaped (Fig. 7–12).

Primitive streak and primitive node (head process) develop.

Mesoderm develops between ectoderm and entoderm.

Cloacal membrane formed at caudal end of primitive streak.

Neural plate, neural groove, and foregut develop.

Supporting structures:

Amnion continues to develop.

Body stalk connects caudal end of embryo with the chorion.

Table 7–10. THE GERM-LAYER ORIGIN OF HUMAN TISSUES*

Ectoderm	Mesoderm *(including mesenchyme)*	Entoderm
1. Epidermis, including: Cutaneous glands. Hair; nails; lens. 2. Epithelium of: Sense organs. Nasal cavity; sinuses. Mouth, including: Oral glands; enamel. Anal canal. 3. Nervous tissue, including: Hypophysis. Chromaffin tissue.	1. Muscle (all types). 2. Connective tissue; cartilage; bone; notochord. 3. Blood; bone marrow. 4. Lymphoid tissue. Epithelium of: 5. Blood vessels; lymphatics. 6. Body cavities. 7. Kidney; ureter. 8. Gonads; genital ducts. 9. Suprarenal cortex. 10. Joint cavities, etc.	Epithelium of: 1. Pharynx, including: Root of tongue. Auditory tube, etc. Tonsils; thyroid. Parathyroids; thymus. 2. Larynx; trachea; lungs. 3. Digestive tube, including: Associated glands. 4. Bladder. 5. Vagina (all?); vestibule. 6. Urethra, including: Associated glands.

*From Arey: *Developmental Anatomy.* Revised 7th Edition. Philadelphia, W. B. Saunders Co., 1974.

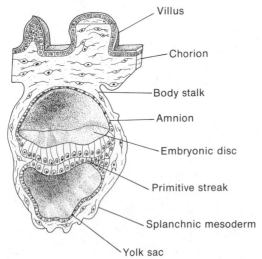

Figure 7–11. The right half of a human embryo of 14 days.

> Primary and secondary villi, and then tertiary villi, form.
> Umbilical vessels forming in body stalk; blood vessels in villi, chorion, and yolk sac.
> Circulation established between embryo and developing placenta.
>
> **Mother**
>
> Menstruation would have occurred during this week.

The Third Week

The embryo now has three layers of cells (ectoderm, entoderm, and mesoderm) and is divided precisely into right and left halves by the *primitive streak.* The ground work for the developing organ systems is thus established because from these three germ layers all of the systems will develop (Table 7–10). During the early stages of development, each germ layer has the potential for a variety of types of development. Cells differentiate first chem-

ically and then physically by means of induction and competence, as already described.

The chorionic villi begin to resemble branching trees. At the placental site the chorion is called the *chorion frondosum* (i.e., leafy) and becomes the fetal component of the placenta (Fig. 7–13). As the developing embryo grows, the remainder of the chorion, which becomes the outer layer of the fetal membranes, is pushed against the wall of the uterus, and its villi atrophy by the seventh week; it is then called the *chorion laeve* (smooth).

The missed menstrual period during this week is the sign that women most frequently associate with pregnancy. Because a single delayed or apparently missed menstrual period may be associated with a number of other circumstances, it is regarded as a presumptive factor. For example, amenorrhea may be caused by anemia, a debilitating disease such as tuberculosis, an endocrine disorder, strong emotional influences including a fear of pregnancy, and even by changes in climate or environment that a woman might encounter on vacation. Menstrual disturbances and other signs of pregnancy, such as breast changes, also occur in *pseudocyesis,* a condition in which a woman believes she is pregnant even though she is not. Pseudopregnancy is usually the result of either an intense desire to be pregnant or an intense fear of pregnancy. When pseudocyesis is diagnosed, the woman should receive emotional counseling as well as physical care.

Another reason that cessation of menstruation is not considered a positive sign of pregnancy is the fact that vaginal bleeding, difficult to distinguish from menstruation, may occur following conception. Three of the many possible causes are cervical erosion, polyps, and threatened abortion. One of the reasons for difficulty in establishing the EDC is postconception bleeding.

Pregnancy may also occur in a women with

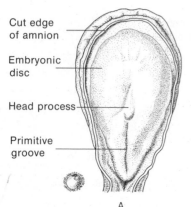

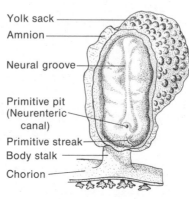

Figure 7–12. Human embryo viewed from above; *A,* at 18 days and *B,* at 19 days. (After Arey: *Development Anatomy: A Textbook and Laboratory Manual of Embryology.* Revised 7th Edition. Philadelphia, W. B. Saunders Co., 1974.)

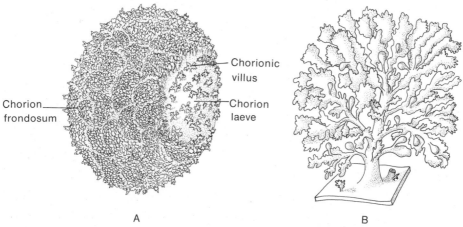

Figure 7–13. *A,* Human chorionic vesicle at 9 weeks, showing the chorion leave (smooth chorion) and the chorion frondosum, which will become the fetal component of the placenta. *B* shows a single chorionic villus. (After Arey: *Developmental Anatomy: A Textbook and Laboratory Manual of Embryology.* Revised 7th Edition. Philadelphia, W. B. Saunders Co., 1974.)

amenorrhea. The breast-feeding mother, for example, may conceive before she has her first menstrual period following delivery. Perimenopausal women may have amenorrhea for several months and therefore suspect that they have reached menopause—only to find themselves pregnant. Some healthy women have such irregular menstrual periods throughout their lives that it is difficult for them to know when a period is missed.

Mother

Early breast changes may be noticed.

The Fourth Week

The fourth week has been called the period of the embryo with *somites.* Somites are primitive segments that lie in pairs next to the spinal cord. The three somites that are present at 21 days become a total of 42 during the fourth week. A muscle mass, supplied by a spinal nerve, primitive kidney tubules, and blood vessels that arise from the aorta, develops in relation to each somite. Each pair of somites will collaborate to produce a vertebra. Somites first appear in the region of the head, consistent with the principle of cephalocaudal development.

The fourth week is tremendously significant in the embryo's development. During these 7 days he changes from a relatively simple disc to a complex organism (Fig. 7–14). The body becomes curved because the neural tube grows more rapidly than the ventral surface.

The potential for several anomalies dates to this week. If the anterior end of the neural tube fails to close, *anencephaly* (absence of cranial vault) results. If the posterior end fails to close, meningocele develops. Should the esophagotracheal septum fail to develop properly, the baby will have a *tracheoesophageal fistula.*

Aside from the missed menstrual period, the first physical changes that the mother may notice during the fourth week are in her breasts, which may be sensitive as they begin to enlarge. In subsequent weeks nipples also will enlarge and become erectile, and the ar-

---

THE FOURTH WEEK

Embryo

Grows from 2 mm. (0.08 inch) in length (crown to rump) at beginning of week to 5 mm. (0.2 inch) at end of week.

Body becomes cylindrical, flexed, and C-shaped.

Organs develop rapidly:

Heart tube fuses at 22 days and begins to beat at 24 days; blood circulates through fetus and chorionic villi.

Anterior end of neural tube closes to form brain; posterior end closes to form spinal cord.

Pronephros (forekidney) and mesonephros (midkidney) develop.

Esophagotracheal septum has begun to divide esophagus and trachea.

Sense organs indicated.

Limb buds present.

Primitive jaws present (as branchial arches).

Somites develop

Yolk sac begins to diminish in size.

Supporting structures:

Chorionic villi develop into an early placenta.

Chorionic sac is 20 mm. (0.8 inch) or slightly larger in diameter.

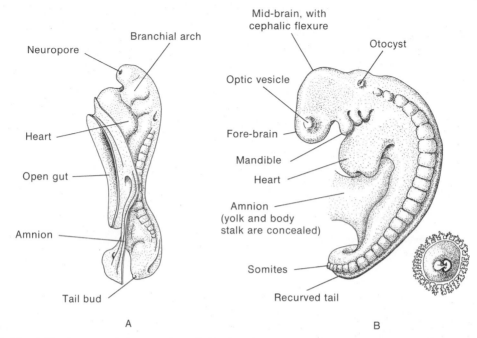

Figure 7–14. *A,* The human embryo at 24 days. *B,* The human embryo at 26 days. The heart begins beating on the 24th day. (After Arey: *Development Anatomy: A Textbook and Laboratory Manual of Embryology.* Revised 7th Edition. Philadelphia, W. B. Saunders Co., 1974.)

eolar area will darken. The sebaceous glands of the areola, called Montgomery's follicles, hypertrophy. Beneath the skin of the breasts, bluish veins may be traced. Breast changes are most obvious during first pregnancies.

FIFTH THROUGH SEVENTH WEEKS

Embryo

Crown-rump length 8 mm. (0.3 inch) at 5 weeks; 12 mm. (0.5 inch) at 6 weeks, 18 mm. (0.75 inch) at 7 weeks.

Five regions develop in brain.

Five main bronchi develop in lung.

Diaphragm separates abdominal and thoracic cavities.

Hepatic buds and ducts form.

Exterior heart formation essentially same as at birth; valves and septa form in the seventh week.

A portion of the intestinal loop enters the cavity of the umbilical cord.

Metanephros (hindkidney) begins to develop.

Wrist and elbow develop at 32 to 34 days.

Face develops: definite eye and nostril; pigment in eye at 34 to 36 days.

Palate developing; upper lip formed.

External genitalia appear, but sex cannot be determined from their appearance. Internal gonads begin to differentiate.

Supporting structures:

Umbilical cord organizes.

Trophoblast invades spiral arteries; cotyledons form; beginnings of maternal-placental circulation.

Human placental lactogen can be detected.

Mother

Hegar's sign.

Goodell's sign.

Nausea present in some women.

Mucous plug.

Corpus luteum may begin to regress.

Fifth Through Seventh Weeks

These weeks complete the period of the embryo. By the seventh week the beginnings of all the essential external and internal structures are present. Most major structural abnormalities will have occurred, although it is only 6 weeks after the first missed menstrual period (Fig. 7–15). Note that a portion of the intestines is outside the abdominal cavity, which is too small at this stage to contain the rapidly growing intestinal tract. Normally the intestines will return to the abdomen in the tenth week. Should they continue to remain outside, the baby may be born with an *oomphalocele* (a defect in the abdominal wall) or *gastroschisis* (a defect at the base of the umbilical stalk).

Deformities such as cleft lip and cleft palate occur during these weeks. Most congenital anomalies of the heart will have occurred before the end of the seventh week. If the diaphragm does not form correctly, the baby will have a *diaphragmatic hernia.*

The third and permanent kidney begins to develop early in the fifth week. Urine is first formed about the seventh to eighth week and is produced from that time on throughout fetal life. Urine mixes with amniotic fluid, which the fetus drinks. Thus in the absence of fetal kidneys (renal agenesis) or in certain other abnormalities of the fetal urinary tract, the mother may have a decreased amount of amniotic fluid (oligohydramnios). However, since the placenta assumes the function of the fetal kidney during pregnancy, it is only during the perinatal period that the baby with a kidney abnormality experiences difficulty.

Imperforate anus, related to abnormal development of the urorectal septum, dates to the sixth or seventh week.

During the sixth week, the placenta is developing to the stage at which maternal pla-cental circulation can take place. Each mainstem villus of the chorion develops into a lobule, called a *cotyledon,* divided from other cotyledons by *septa* (sheets of tissue) (Fig. 7–16). Within each cotyledon are blood vessels. At this time there are from 15 to 30 cotyledons; the mature placenta will contain about 200. The chorionic membrane in the placental area is called the *chorionic plate.* (See also page 180.)

Surrounding the cotyledons is the intervillous space, filled with maternal blood that comes from about 200 arterioles in the decidua basalis. The intervillous space is drained by collecting veins. Maternal blood flow at this stage is sluggish.

The umbilical cord is usually inserted near the middle of the fetal aspect of the placenta. The cord contains two umbilical arteries, which carry wastes from the fetus to the placenta, and one umbilical vein, which carries nourishment from the placenta to the fetus. When the cord is inspected at the time of birth,

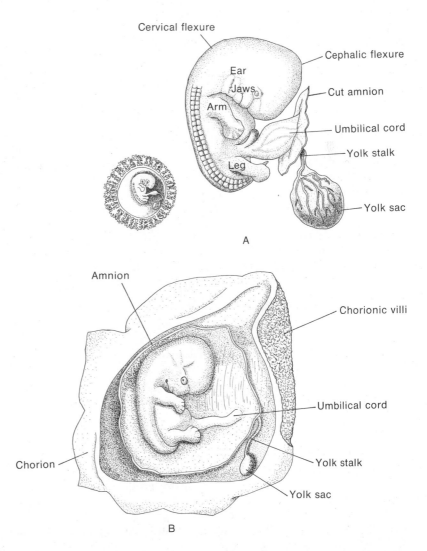

Figure 7–15. The human embryo. *A,* At 6 weeks and *B,* at 7 weeks. (After Arey: *Developmental Anatomy: A Textbook and Laboratory Manual of Embryology.* Revised 7th Edition. Philadelphia, W. B. Saunders Co., 1974.)

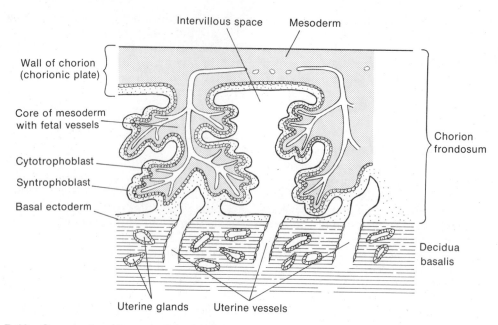

Figure 7–16. Cross section (diagram) of the human placenta. (After Arey: *Developmental Anatomy: A Textbook and Laboratory Manual of Embryology.* Revised 7th Edition. Philadelphia, W. B. Saunders Co., 1974.)

it may contain a single artery rather than two. The baby should then be inspected carefully, since there is a higher risk of anomalies in infants with a single umbilical artery.

The fetal circulation system is uniquely designed to meet fetal needs. Blood from the placenta, with oxygen and nutrients, enters the fetus through the umbilical vein. About half of the blood flows to the liver; the remainder bypasses the liver through the *ductus venosus* and enters the inferior vena cava, where it mixes with blood from the lower part of the fetus' body and then enters the right atrium. A second fetal structure, the foramen ovale, allows most of the blood to pass directly into the left atrium, then to the left ventricle via the ascending aorta to the head and neck, ensuring a supply of well-oxygenated blood to those areas. The blood that goes from the right atrium to the right ventricle then enters the pulmonary artery; most will pass through the *ductus arteriosus* into the descending aorta. Thus both the foramen ovale and the ductus arteriosis permit all but 10 to 15 per cent of the fetal circulation to bypass the lungs, which will not function as respiratory organs until after birth. From the descending aorta most blood passes into the umbilical arteries and returns to the placenta for the exchange of gases. Some blood circulates through the lower part of the body. Fetal circulation is diagrammed in Chapter 20 for comparison with neonatal circulation.

Production of human placental lactogen is evident by the sixth week and continues to rise throughout pregnancy.

As the placenta continues to develop, maternal blood supply to the pelvis increases. This results in two changes that may be observed about the sixth week.

Hegar's sign is considered the most reliable sign of pregnancy during the first trimester. The isthmus of the lower uterine segment becomes softened and can be compressed between two fingers inserted in the anterior fornix and a hand placed on the abdomen behind the uterus (Fig. 7–17). In multiparas Hegar's sign appears about the sixth week; it is noted approximately 8 weeks following con-

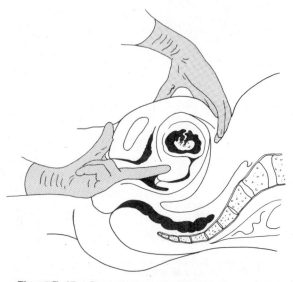

Figure 7–17. Detecting Hegar's sign. The softened isthmus of the uterus is easily compressed between the hand placed on the abdomen and the fingers inserted in the vagina anterior to the cervix.

ception in primigravidas and is most fully developed in all women about the tenth week.

Softening of the cervix, along with succulence of the vagina and an increase of leukorrheal discharge, is called *Goodell's sign*. Goodell stated that if the cervix felt like the mucous membrane of the lip, pregnancy was possible. Goodell's sign can be observed as early as 6 weeks in primiparas and even earlier in some multiparas. Thick mucus fills the cervical canal, becoming a *mucous plug,* which will remain in place until the time of labor.

Because other conditions can result in findings similar to those of Hegar and Goodell, they are considered probable signs of pregnancy but not positive signs.

Some women experience nausea, either in the morning or at some other time during the day, from about the fifth to the twelfth week of pregnancy, and occasionally longer. The reason for nausea is uncertain, but by no means every pregnant woman is nauseated. Some women will have nausea during one pregnancy and not at all during another. In some societies apparently no pregnant women have nausea. (See also Chapter 11.)

The *corpus luteum* may begin to regress as early as the sixth week, although well-developed corpora lutea have been found at term. During the first weeks of pregnancy progesterone produced by the corpus luteum is essential for the maintenance of pregnancy, but this function is assumed by the placenta soon after implantation.

Mother

Chadwick's sign.
  Cardiovascular changes.
  Basal metabolism falls.
  Blood sugar low.
  Increased salivation; mouth secretions acid.
  Ureters and renal pelves begin to dilate about tenth week.
  Enlarging anteflexed uterus rises above pelvic brim.
  Fetal heart tones heard by ultrasound by 10 to 12 weeks (page 194).
  Weight gain for first trimester: 2 pounds (1 kg.).

Eighth Through Twelfth Weeks

Beginning in the eighth week the embryo is considered a fetus. He is now a recognizable human being (Fig. 7–18). In contrast to the embryonic period in which new structures are continually developing, the fetal period is primarily a time of growth and maturation. Because of this the fetus is less at risk than the embryo to many teratogens (Chapter 8).

EIGHTH THROUGH TWELFTH WEEKS

Fetus

At twelve weeks weighs 14 grams (½ ounce) and is 7 cm. (2.75 inches crown to heel).
  Head ⅓ of total length.
  Fetal movements begin at about 8 weeks.
  Thin skin develops.
  Bones developing.
  External genitalia become distinctively male or female in third month.
  Eyelids develop and fuse.
  Fingers and toes begin nail growth.
  Liver becomes major producer of red blood cells.
  Intestine returns to abdomen.
  Supporting structures:
  Placenta continues to grow; high maternal blood pressure (40 to 60 mm. Hg) in central intervillous spaces.
  Amnion fills the chorionic cavity.
  Chorion almost fills the uterine cavity.
  Amnion and chorion remain in contact for the remainder of pregnancy.

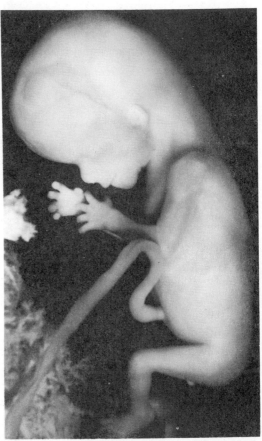

Figure 7–18. Eight-week-old embryo. (From Moore: *The Developing Human: Clinically Oriented Embryology.* 2nd Edition. Philadelphia, W. B. Saunders Co., 1977.)

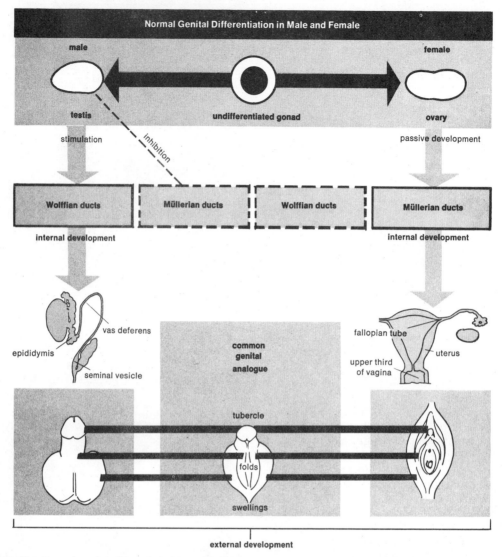

Figure 7–19. Normal genital differentiation in male and female. (From Hill: *AJN,* 9:811, 1977. Copyright May, 1977, The American Journal of Nursing Co. Reproduced with permission from the *American Journal of Nursing,* Vol. 77, No. 5.)

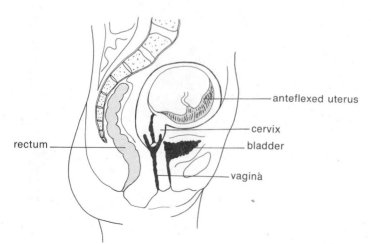

Figure 7–20. At the end of the third month, the corpus of the enlarged uterus rises out of the pelvis and becomes an abdominal organ. Note the sharp anteflexion of the uterus.

The crown-rump length more than doubles between the eighth and twelfth weeks, but head growth slows down, so that at twelve weeks the head represents only one-third of the total body length, rather than half.

The greatest noticeable change in the fetus is in the external genitalia. Until the end of the ninth week, the external reproductive organs of both males and females, which develop from analogous structures (Fig. 7–19), appear similar. Distinctive external genitalia are not present until the twelfth week.

In the mother enlarged blood vessels increase the blood supply of the vagina, which results in *Chadwick's sign,* a deep red-to-purple coloration ofthe vaginal mucosa. Other vaginal changes that are preparatory for vaginal distention at the time of delivery include muscle hypertrophy, mucosal thickening, and a loosening of connective tissue. Vaginal discharge becomes thicker and more profuse and is usually white to yellowish in color and crumbly in consistency. Because of an increased lactic acid content, this secretion is believed to help resist pathogens; douching will interfere with this protection. A douche should be used during pregnancy only when it is specifically prescribed.

During the third month the uterus rises out of the pelvis to become an abdominal organ. Note how the anteflexed uterus compresses the bladder (Fig. 7–20). The fundus is about midway between the symphysis pubis and the umbilicus at the end of the third month of gestation (Chapter 10).

Thirteenth Through Sixteenth Weeks

In relation to the individual's future potential, the period of the thirteenth to sixteenth week is highly significant, for it is the time when the number of neurons is increasing most rapidly. Insults during this period (rubella, for example) limit neuronal development and hence intellectual capacity.

Meconium begins to be present in the intestines, where it will remain, under ordinary circumstances, until birth when it forms the first stools (Chapter 21). Meconium in the amniotic fluid is a sign of fetal distress.

Lanugo, a fine, downy hair, covers the fetal body. It gradually decreases toward term. The amount of lanugo present at birth is one useful measure of gestational age.

SEVENTEENTH THROUGH TWENTIETH WEEKS

Fetus

At 20 weeks the fetus weighs approximately 460 grams (16 ounces) and is 25 cm. (10 inches) long.

Lower limbs reach final relative proportions.

Bone marrow becomes increasingly important in blood formation.

Iron deposits begin to be stored.

Vernix caseosa begins to form.

More frequent and stronger movements.

Enamel and dentine for teeth deposited.

Eyelashes and eyebrows forming.

Brown fat begins to be formed.

Myelinization of the spinal cord begins.

Mother

Fetal heart tones may be heard by an examiner.

Fetal movements may be felt by an examiner and by the mother (quickening).

Fundus reaches the level of the umbilicus at approximately the fifth month.

Lower uterine segment drawn into body; anteflexion disappears.

Skin changes (see following sections).

Ballottement (16 to 32 weeks).

Desirable weight gain at twentieth week: approximately 8 pounds (3.75 kg.).

THIRTEENTH THROUGH SIXTEENTH WEEKS

Fetus

A period of very rapid growth; at 16 weeks weighs 120 grams (4 ounces) and length is approximately 15 cm. (6 inches).

Period of rapid growth in the number of neurons in the brain.

Ossification widespread; evident on x-ray by 16 weeks.

Meconium present in intestines.

Lanugo growing on body; hair growing on head.

Fetus can suck thumb, swallow, make respiratory movements, protrude upper lip on stimulation, and has grasp reflex.

Mother

Desirable weight gain; ¾ to 1 pound per week (0.34 to 0.45 kg.).

Seventeenth Through Twentieth Weeks

In the fetus the storage of iron during pregnancy is important for the subsequent well-being of the baby. Since most iron storage occurs after the twentieth week, it is not difficult to understand that the baby of low gestational age will have limited iron stores and a high risk of developing iron deficiency anemia. Preterm babies usually receive supplemental iron at some time during the first year. Another factor limiting iron stores is maternal intake, which usually must be supplemented during the second half of pregnancy (Chapter 12).

Vernix caseosa is a material that looks a little like white cheese. It is formed from the fatty secretions of the fetal sebaceous glands and dead epidermal cells. Vernix caseosa covers much of the skin during the second half of pregnancy and is thought to have a protective function. It can be seen on the baby at the time of birth (Chapter 21).

Brown fat is fatty tissue found principally on the back of the neck, behind the sternum, and around the kidneys, the subclavian area, and the carotids. Brown fat plays a role in newborn heat production (Chapter 20).

For the mother this period, approximately the midpoint of pregnancy, is the time during which pregnancy may be positively confirmed by the fetal heart tones heard and fetal movements felt by the examiner. Mothers are also becoming aware of fetal movement, a phenomenon called *quickening,* a term dating from the time when the word "quick" meant living. Thus the pregnancy, nearly halfway complete, is now confirmed both by others and by the mother herself.

Fetal heart tones are heard by the nonamplified stethoscope between 16 and 20 weeks of pregnancy. With ultrasonic auscultation, sounds may be heard as early as 10 to 12 weeks. Fetal heart sounds have been described as resembling the rapid "tick-tock of a watch heard through a pillow." The "tick," representing systole of the fetal heart, is followed by a short pause and then by the "tock," which is the sound of the closure of the valves in the fetal heart. The normal range of the fetal heart rate is from 120 to 160 beats per minute. If the rate heard is considerably lower, it may be the maternal heart rate instead; this can be ascertained by simultaneously checking the maternal pulse. Although rates outside of this range may indicate fetal distress, increased rates may also be related to fetal movement, palpation of the fetus, maternal fever, or to no specific cause. Pressure on the fetal skull leads to a decreased rate, a fact that becomes important during labor.

The best site for hearing fetal heart tones in the sixteenth to twentieth weeks is at the midline on the edge of the pubic hair. As the fetus becomes larger and his outline is palpable, heart sounds are heard best through the fetal back. Many nurses prefer to use a fetoscope (Fig. 7–21) because the sound of fingers

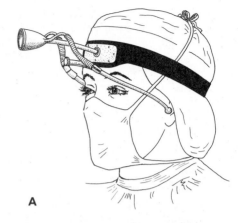

A

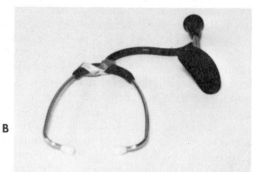

B

Figure 7–21. *A,* The fetoscope allows the examiner to hear fetal heart tones through air and bone conduction while eliminating the noise of the examiner's finger holding a stethoscope. *B,* A second type of fetoscope, one which does not strap onto the examiner's head.

holding the traditional stethoscope is eliminated.

Two sounds other than fetal heart rate and maternal heart rate may be heard: fetal (funic) souffle and uterine souffle. The fetal souffle is caused by the rush of blood through the umbilical arteries and is synchronous with *fetal* heart sounds. Uterine souffle is a soft, blowing sound, synchronous with the *maternal* pulse, caused by blood flowing through the large arteries at the sides of the uterus. If the uterine souffle is sufficiently loud, it may be difficult to hear fetal heart tones. Other obstacles to auscultation are excessive amniotic fluid, external noise, and the location of the placenta on the anterior wall of the uterus.

The shape of the uterus continues to change during the fifth month. By the twentieth week anteflexion disappears, relieving the pressure on the bladder and thereby relieving urinary frequency for the next months. (Frequency returns late in pregnancy, as the large uterus again encroaches on the bladder space.)

Ballottement is a sign elicited when the examiner places two fingers in the mother's vagina and gives the fetus a gentle push (Fig. 7–22). The fetus is felt leaving and returning to

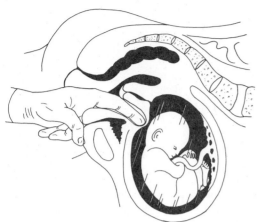

Figure 7–22. Eliciting ballottement. The fetal head or breech is pushed gently; it is felt moving away and quickly returning to the fingers. In short, the fetus "bounces."

the examiner's fingers; he bounces in the amniotic fluid like a beach ball in a swimming pool. Prior to 16 weeks the fetus is too small for ballottement; after 32 weeks he is too large in relation to the amount of amniotic fluid.

TWENTY-FIRST THROUGH TWENTY-FOURTH WEEKS

Fetus

At 24 weeks, weight is 720 to 960 grams (1½ to 2 pounds); length is 30 cm. (12 inches).

Alveolar cells beginning to make surfactant at about 24 weeks.

Skin pink to red because of visibility of blood in capillaries.

Primordia of permanent teeth begin to develop.

Nostrils reopen.

IgG levels rise, reaching maternal values at about 24 weeks.

Mother

Desirable weight gain: from ½ to ¾ pound per week (0.24 to 0.34 kg.).

Twenty-first Through Twenty-fourth Weeks

The fetus' lungs come closer to the point at which survival following birth will be a possibility with the beginning of surfactant production (see section below).

Levels of IgG, the only immunoglobulin produced by the fetus under normal conditions, will protect the fetus and newborn from those diseases for which his mother has immunity. Included are most blood-borne viruses, bacteria, parasites, and fungi. The IgM molecule is too large to cross the placenta; when IgM is found in the newborn, it is considered to be

the response of the fetus to intrauterine infection.

TWENTY-FIFTH THROUGH THIRTY-SECOND WEEKS

Fetus

Approximately 35 cm. (14 inches) and 1200 grams (2½ pounds) at 28 weeks; 40 cm. (16 inches) and 1900 grams (4 pounds) at 32 weeks.

Bone marrow becomes a major site of blood formation (28 weeks).

Subcutaneous fat minimal.

Moro's reflex at 30 weeks.

Alveoli appear in lungs; capillaries proliferate around alveoli; gas exchange possible at about 28 weeks.

If born, one in ten fetuses viable at 28 weeks gestational age; one in three viable at 32 weeks gestational age.

Glial cell formation and myelinization of brain.

Mother

Desirable weight gain: from ½ to ¾ pound per week (0.24 to 0.34 kg.).

Fundus halfway between umbilicus and ensiform process at 7 months gestational age; three-fourths of the way at 8 months gestational age.

Striae gravidarum may develop.

Increased pigmentation may develop.

Twenty-fifth Through Thirty-second Weeks

The exchange of gases (oxygen and carbon dioxide) is not possible until: (1) alveoli develop and (2) capillaries develop around the alveoli. This occurs at approximately 28 weeks, although it may be accelerated by stress, or delayed, as in the infant of a diabetic mother (Chapter 23).

A second stage of brain development, beginning about the twenty-eighth week and lasting into the year following birth, involves glial cell formation and myelinization. Poor nutrition, either prenatally or following delivery, during this period may result in learning disabilities, poor hand-eye coordination, and similar problems.

Mothers may note several skin changes in the third trimester. Red, slightly depressed streak marks on the abdomen and occasionally on the breasts, called *striae gravidarum,* occur in approximately half of all pregnant women. Within a few months following delivery, the marks will become silvery in color, but they will not entirely disappear.

Text continued on page 200

Table 7–11. SIGNS OF PREGNANCY

Sign	When Appears	Basis	Other Possible Causes
PRESUMPTIVE SIGNS			
Amenorrhea	Approximately 2 weeks after conception	Endometrium retained	Hormonal imbalance, emotional factors; physical disease
Breast changes	As early as fourth week	Development of duct system; hormonal	Hormonal; not as valuable in multiparas
Nausea	Second and third months, primarily	Uncertain. Related factors may be reverse peristalsis, decreased gastrointestinal motility, decreased carbohydrate levels, psychosocial influences	
Quickening	16 to 20 weeks	Movements of fetus	Intestinal activity may stimulate fetal movement, especially in nulliparous women very desirous of child
Chadwick's sign	8 to 12 weeks	Increased vascularity of pelvic organs	Any cause of pelvic congestion
Urinary frequency	6 to 12 weeks	Enlarging uterus	Urinary tract infection; emotional factors
Sleepiness, fatigue	First trimester		Many possible reasons
PROBABLE SIGNS			
Enlarged uterus		Growing fetus	Tumor; ascites
Hegar's sign		Hyperemia of pelvis	
Braxton Hicks contractions	From as early as 8 weeks throughout pregnancy	Normal uterine contractions	Hematomas; myomas
Ballottement	From 16 to 32 weeks	Fetus in amniotic fluid	
Palpation of fetal outline			Myomas, occasionally
Laboratory tests	7 to 14 days	Presence of human chorionic gonadotropin	
Goodell's sign	By the sixth week; may be earlier in multigravida	Pelvic congestion	Other causes of pelvic congestion
POSITIVE SIGNS			
Fetal movement felt by examiner	About 20 weeks		
Fetal heart heard by examiner	Doppler: 10 to 12 weeks; stethoscope: 16 to 20 weeks		
Fetal outline seen on X-ray or sonography			

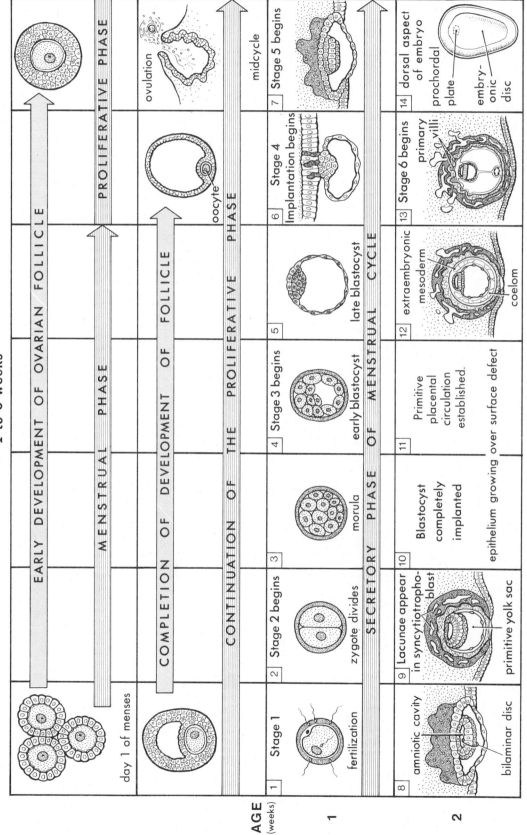

Figure 7–23. Development of a follicle containing an oocyte, ovulation, and phases of the menstrual cycle are illustrated. Development begins at fertilization, about 14 days after the onset of the last menstruation. Cleavage of the zygote in the uterine tube, implantation of the blastocyst, and early development of the embryo are also shown. The main features of the developmental stages in human embryos are illustrated. (From Moore: *The Developing Human: Clinically Oriented Embryology.* 2nd Edition. Philadelphia, W. B. Saunders Co., 1977.)

Illustration continued on following page

TIMETABLE OF HUMAN PRENATAL DEVELOPMENT
1 to 6 weeks

3

15 first missed menstrual period

primitive streak

16 Stage 7 begins

notochordal process

17 intra-embryonic mesoderm

trilaminar embryo

18 Stage 8 begins

neural plate

primitive streak

length: 1.5 mm

19 neural fold

notochord

embryonic coelom

20 Stage 9 begins

brain

neural groove

somite

Thyroid begins to develop.

21 neural groove

somite

Heart tubes begin to fuse.

4

22 Stage 10 begins

Heart begins to beat.

Neural folds fusing.

23 rostral neuropore

primordia of eye and ear present.

caudal neuropore

24 Stage 11 begins

heart bulge

rostral neuropore closes

2 pairs of branchial arches

25 otic pit

3 pairs of branchial arches

26 Stage 12 begins

arm bud

→ indicates actual size

27 4 pairs of branchial arches, arm & leg buds present.

C R = crown-rump length.

28 Stage 13 begins

C.R: 4.0 mm

5

29

C R: 5.0 mm

30 Lens pits, optic cups, nasal pits forming.

31 developing eye

nasal pit

primitive mouth

32 Stage 14

Hand plates (paddle-shaped)

Lens pits and optic cups formed.

33 Stage 15 begins

hand plate

C R: 7.0 mm

34 Head much larger relative to trunk.

cerebral vesicles distinct

leg buds (paddle-shaped)

35 C R: 8.0 mm

6

36 Oral & nasal cavities confluent.

37 Stage 16 begins

foot plate

C R: 9.0 mm

38 Upper lip formed.

39 C R: 10.0 mm

40 Arms bent at elbow.

Finger rays and auricular hillocks distinct

Palate developing.

41 Stage 17 begins

finger rays

ventral view

42 C.R: 13.0 mm

TIMETABLE OF HUMAN PRENATAL DEVELOPMENT
7 to 10 weeks

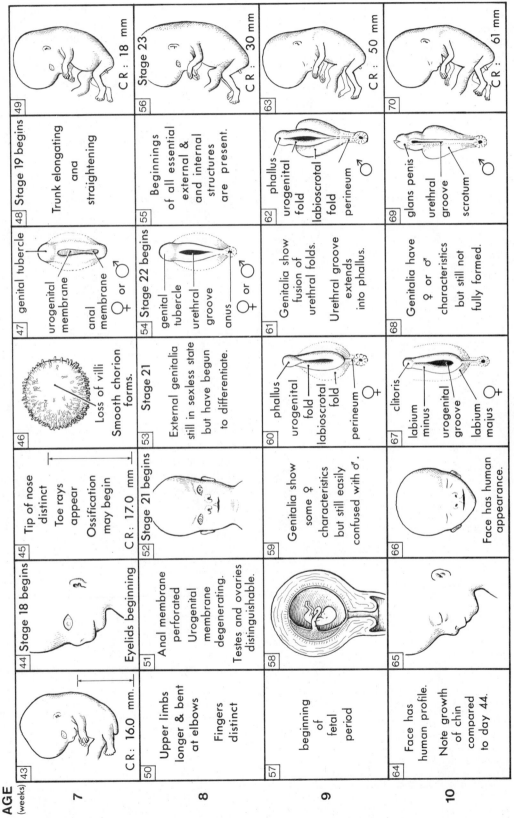

AGE (weeks)

7

43 — CR: 16.0 mm.
44 — Stage 18 begins
45 — Tip of nose distinct / Toe rays appear / Ossification may begin
46 — Loss of villi / Smooth chorion forms.
47 — genital tubercle / urogenital membrane / anal membrane / ♀ or ♂
48 — Stage 19 begins / Trunk elongating and straightening
49 — CR: 18 mm

8

50 — Upper limbs longer & bent at elbows / Fingers distinct
51 — Eyelids beginning / Anal membrane perforated / Urogenital membrane degenerating. / Testes and ovaries distinguishable.
52 — CR: 17.0 mm / Stage 21 begins
53 — Stage 21 / External genitalia still in sexless state but have begun to differentiate.
54 — Stage 22 begins / genital tubercle / urethral groove / anus / ♀ or ♂
55 — Beginnings of all essential external and internal structures are present.
56 — Stage 23 / CR: 30 mm

9

57 — beginning of fetal period
58 — (image)
59 — Genitalia show some ♀ characteristics but still easily confused with ♂.
60 — phallus / urogenital fold / labioscrotal fold / perineum / ♀
61 — Genitalia show fusion of urethral folds. / Urethral groove extends into phallus.
62 — phallus / urogenital fold / labioscrotal fold / perineum / ♂
63 — CR: 50 mm

10

64 — Face has human profile. / Note growth of chin compared to day 44.
65 — (image)
66 — Face has human appearance.
67 — clitoris / labium minus / urogenital groove / labium majus / ♀
68 — Genitalia have ♀ or ♂ characteristics but still not fully formed.
69 — glans penis / urethral groove / scrotum / ♂
70 — CR: 61 mm

Figure 7–23 *Continued.*

Increased pigmentation also occurs along the *linea alba,* which is then termed the *linea nigra;* the vulva; and the face (the latter termed *chloasma,* the mask of pregnancy). Chloasma, usually most pronounced in Caucasian brunettes, is often aggravated by exposure to the sun. Protecting the face from the sun may make it less noticeable. A change of cosmetics will also be helpful, as will the assurance that changes in facial pigmentation will not persist after delivery.

THIRTY-THIRD THROUGH THIRTY-EIGHTH WEEKS

Fetus

Approximately 45 cm. (18 inches) and 2900 grams (6 pounds) at 36 weeks; 50 cm. (20 inches) and 3350 grams (7 pounds) at 38 weeks.
  Viable.
  Flexed limbs; well-developed muscle tone.
  Testes descend at 36 weeks.
  Lanugo mostly disappearing.
  Pulmonary branching about two-thirds complete.
Placenta:
Cellular growth ceases at about 34 weeks.
Placenta at term weighs about 500 grams (approximately 1 pound); is ⅙ weight of fetus.

Mother

Fundus reaches level of ensiform process at about 32 weeks gestational age.
  Lightening may occur about 36 weeks after conception (38 weeks gestational age).
  Desirable weight gain: from ½ to ¾ pound per week (0.24 to 0.34 kg.)

Thirty-third Through Thirty-eighth Weeks

Babies born during these weeks are potentially viable, although development continues for many years. Newborn characteristics and the significance of these characteristics in assessing gestation age are described in Chapter 20.

Lightening describes the descent of the uterus when the baby's presenting part (i.e., the part that will deliver first, most frequently the head) becomes fixed in the pelvis. Because lightening is more frequent in women who have good abdominal muscle tone, it is more likely to occur in primiparas, usually 1 to 2 weeks before labor begins. Many multiparas and some primiparas never experience lightening until after labor begins. Following lightening, the fundus is approximately at the height it reached during the eighth month, about three-quarters of the distance between the umbilicus and the ensiform process. Abdominal contour changes, with the lower abdomen becoming more prominent. A mother finds that she breathes more easily, a welcome sign, but pressure can cause frequent voiding and leg cramps. Walking may be more difficult.

Figure 7–23 summarizes the development of the embryo-fetus and Table 7–11 summarizes the signs of pregnancy.

Summary

The months of gestation are a dynamic, constantly changing period for the mother and the embryo-fetus. An understanding of the physiologic changes described in this chapter and of the psychological and social changes described in the chapter that follows is essential to nursing assessment and intervention in the care of pregnant women and their families.

REFERENCES

1. Arey, L.: *Developmental Anatomy,* 7th Edition. Philadelphia, W. B. Saunders Co., 1965.
2. Bell, G., Davison, J., and Scarborough, H.: *Textbook of Physiology and Biochemistry,* 7th Edition. Edinburgh, E & S Livingstone, 1968.
3. Bruce, N.: Gestational Adaptation: Major Systems. In Iffy, L., and Kaminetzky, H. (eds.): *Principles and Practice of Obstetrics and Perinatology.* New York, John Wiley, 1981.
4. Davison, J., and Hytten, F.: The Effect of Pregnancy on the Renal Handling of Glucose. *Journal of Obstetrics and Gynaecology of the British Commonwealth 82:*374, 1975.
5. Ginsburg, J., and Duncan, S.: Peripheral Blood Flow in Normal Pregnancy. *Cardiovascular Research, 1:*132, 1967.
6. Marchant, D.: Alterations in Anatomy and Function of the Urinary Tract During Pregnancy. *Clinical Obstetrics and Gynecology, 21:*855, 1978.
7. Moore, K.: *The Developing Human: Clinically Oriented Embryology,* 2nd Edition. Philadelphia, W. B. Saunders Co., 1977.
8. Osathanondh, R., and Tulchinsky, D.: Placental Polypeptide Hormones. In Tulchinsky, D., and Ryan, K. (eds.): *Maternal-Fetal Endocrinology.* Philadelphia: W. B. Saunders Co., 1980.
9. Page, E., Villee, C., and Villee, D.: *Human Reproduction,* 3rd Edition. Philadelphia, W. B. Saunders Co., 1981.
10. Ryan, K.: Placental Synthesis of Steroid Hormones. In Tulchinsky, D., and Ryan, K. (eds.): *Maternal-Fetal Endocrinology.* Philadelphia, W. B. Saunders Co., 1980.
11. Thompson, A., Hylten, F., and Billewicz, W.: The Epidemiology of Oedema During Pregnancy. *Journal of Obstetrics and Gynaecology of the British Commonwealth 74:*1, 1967.

Hazards to the Developing Embryo-Fetus

OBJECTIVES

1. Define teratogen.
2. Identify the organisms of the TORCH group. Describe the potential effect of each on the embryo, fetus, or newborn.
3. Identify chemicals that are harmful to the embryo-fetus, including abused drugs.
4. Describe the potential effects of the following on the embryo-fetus or newborn.
   - a. Alcohol
   - b. Cigarette smoking
   - c. Caffeine
   - d. Nutrition
   - e. Radiation
5. Describe ways in which a knowledge of the hazards to the developing embryo-fetus can be used in nursing practice.

Developing within the mother's uterus, the embryo-fetus is not in safe and secure isolation, as was once supposed. He is, in fact, subject to a variety of hazards. Some are a result of conditions within his mother; maternal diabetes is an example. Some are a result of substances taken into his mother's body and subsequently transferred to his own, such as certain medications. Still others are a part of his mother's own external environment—a virus that she may have contracted or a chemical that may be present in the air she breathes or in her water supply.

Some of these hazards, such as radiation and the ingestion of certain drugs, can be controlled to a large degree. Others, such as some maternal infections, may pass unnoticed during pregnancy and be recognized only in retrospect, following the birth of a child who is not normal.

Teratogen is the term used to describe any environmental factor, chemical or physical, that affects the embryo-fetus adversely. Either too much or too little of almost any physical or chemical agent can have a teratogenic effect on mammals of some species. However, not every agent that affects one species or even one subspecies will necessarily affect a different species in the same way or even in a way that is harmful. This means that there are limits to what we can learn about the effects of teratogens on humans from animal research. A substance may prove teratogenic in some animal studies but be safe for humans. Perhaps even more important, a substance may appear safe in animal studies yet prove deleterious to human embryos. An example of the latter is the drug thalidomide, which did not harm embryos in animal studies but produced phocomelia (malformed limbs) in human infants (Fig. 8–1). On the other hand, dilantin has caused cleft palate in mice and cortisone has caused both cleft palate and cardiac defects in mice and rabbits, but no human association has been demonstrated.

Timing is important in the way in which a teratogen may affect the embryo. A teratogen that comes in contact with the embryo during the third to eight week of development, the period during which major organ system are being formed, will usually have a more devastating effect than the same substance introduced in the third trimester (Fig. 8–2). However, certain teratogens can affect the fetus even late in pregnancy; syphilis is an example of a disease that can cause late malformations in previously normally developed organs.

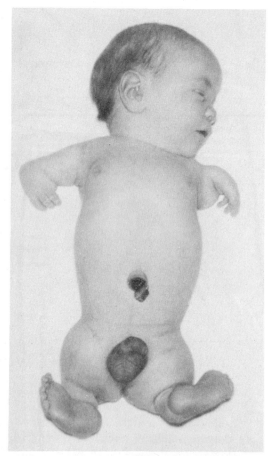

Figure 8–1. Newborn male infant showing typically malformed limbs (phocomelia) caused by thalidomide. (From Moore: *Manit. Med. Rev., 43*:306, 1963.)

Certain teratogens appear to have a predilection for specific organs or systems, while others are more general in their action. Thalidomide, already mentioned, affected the limbs. Other agents may affect a broad range of systems.

Fetal tissues may respond to teratogens in several ways. They may atrophy or hypertrophy. Structures may fuse, or they may split. There may be a general inhibition of normal growth and development because of failure of induction or failure of competence.

In order to provide care for the pregnant woman and her developing child, nurses must be specifically aware of teratogens, which include infectious organisms, certain medications and other ingested substances, and radiation. Maternal conditions that may also affect the fetus adversely are discussed in Chapter 13.

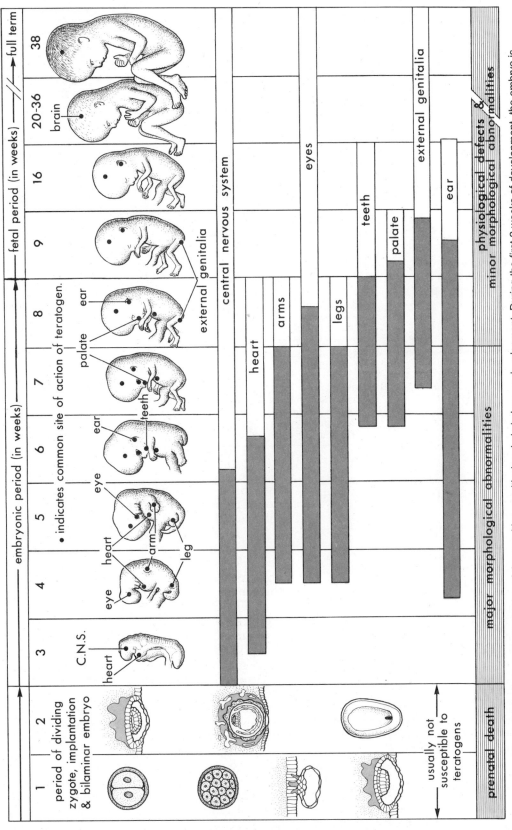

Figure 8–2. Schematic illustration of the sensitive or critical periods in human development. During the sensitive or critical periods in human development. During the first 2 weeks of development, the embryo is usually not susceptible to teratogens. During these predifferentiation stages, a substance either damages all or most of the cells of the embryo, resulting in its death, or it damages only a few cells, allowing the embryo to recover without developing defects. The left side of the bars denotes highly sensitive periods; the right sides indicate stages that are less sensitive to teratogens. (From Moore: *The Developing Human: Clinically Oriented Embryology.* 2nd Edition. Philadelphia, W. B. Saunders, 1977.)

Table 8–1. THE TORCH DISEASES

Infectious Disease	Principal Sources	Transmission	Symptoms and Related Signs
Toxoplasmosis	Eating undercooked meats; cat litter; warm, moist soil	Transplacental passage; mother's infection may be unnoticed	Small for gestational age (SGA); central nervous system (CNS) damage; triad: chorioretinitis, hydrocephaly, cerebral calcification
Syphilis	Sexual activity of mother	Transplacental passage; contact with active maternal genital lesions	Premature labor; purulent nasal discharge (snuffles); skin eruptions: symmetrical rash—oral, anogenital, palms of hands and soles of feet; osteochondritis on X-ray; no signs may be present
Rubella	Infection of mother	Transplacental passage particularly during first 8 weeks following conception	Many organ systems may be affected: microcephaly, congenital heart disease, cataracts, deafness, etc.
Cytomegalic inclusion disease (CID)	Person-to-person contact—respiratory and venereal routes: virus probably persists in host tissues indefinitely; virus is worldwide—most adults have CMV at some time in life	Transplacental	SGA; petechiae (blueberry muffin baby); microcephaly; deafness; blindness
Herpes simplex—Type I (oropharynx), Type II (genital) (HSV)	Genital herpes in mother; transmission in nursery from other infected infants or nursery personnel	At or immediately preceding birth from exposure to infected genital secretions	May be asymptomatic at first; fever; vomiting; lethargy; meningoencephalitis

Infectious Organisms as Teratogens

The most important organisms known to be teratogens are those of the TORCH group (Table 8–1):

T for toxoplasmosis
O for other (syphilis)
R for rubella
C for cytomegalovirus
H for herpes simplex

In many instances the fact that the mother has been exposed to the organism may not be evident until after the baby is born because the disease is nonsymptomatic in the mother.

Toxoplasmosis, a disease caused by a protozoan, is nearly always unrecognized in the mother until the baby is born. Yet it has been estimated that as many as 4 to 6 of every 1000 mothers in the United States may contract toxoplasmosis during pregnancy and that as many as 1 of every 1000 infants may have congenital toxoplasmosis. In a small proportion of these babies, the result is severe mental retardation.

The incidence of toxoplasmosis varies from one population to another. In Paris, the maternal infection rate is as high as 50 of 1000 pregnancies. Principal routes of infection are the consumption of raw or undercooked meat (frequent in Paris) and direct or indirect contact with cat feces. Thus, cooking methods, exposure to cats, and warm, moist soil conditions that favor the survival of the protozoan oocytes are factors in the incidence of the disease and also suggest preventive measures.

Congenital infection appears to be a result of a primary infection of the mother during pregnancy. Frequently the mother has no symptoms; when symptoms are present infection of the lymph nodes is most common. Spread of the infection of the fetus varies with the stage of pregnancy; fetal infection was found to occur in 20 per cent of first trimester infections, 30 per cent of second trimester infections, and 66 per cent of third trimester infections. Thus, early education of mothers

Table 8–1. THE TORCH DISEASES (*Continued*)

Treatment	Possible Outcome	Special Points
No satisfactory treatment	CNS damage (76 to 100% if infant has disease symptoms); visual impairment	Instruct pregnant women about sources of disease
Treat mother with penicillin if diagnosed prior to delivery; treat baby with penicillin if diagnosed after delivery	CNS damage; hearing loss; mortality 10 to 30% if untreated	Serology determination for all women early in pregnancy important in prevention
Treatment of sequelae when possible	Severity and systems involved depend on time of disease; most serious in first 8 weeks after conception; less serious after 20 weeks	Infant may shed virus for a year or more following birth; nurses should know their rubella titer
No effective treatment	75% of infants will have CNS damage	Pregnant nurses should not care for these babies; virus excreted in saliva and urine of baby
Isolate baby	CNS damage; untreated mortality: 75 to 80%	Delivery by cesarean section when genital herpes diagnosed; personnel with herpes infections should not work in nursery

concerning prevention should be of value in reducing the incidence.

Even when the fetus is infected, only 10 per cent of infected infants will have symptoms in the newborn period. Signs and symptoms may occur in the central nervous system (abnormal cerebrospinal fluid, convulsions, hydrocephalus, microcephalus) or the eyes (chorioretinitis), or they may be more general (anemia, jaundice). In infants with CNS or eye disease, there is a strong possibility that the infant will be severely mentally retarded. When toxoplasmosis is identified, infants are treated for 30 days with oral sulfadiazine and pyrimethamine. Since pyrimethamine is an antifolate agent that affects cell growth, folic acid is also given to the baby.

In the initial assessment of pregnant women, ascertaining exposure to cats, especially cats who spend much time out of doors, provides instruction.

Specific suggestions to all pregnant women should include the following:

1. Eat no raw or undercooked meat during pregnancy.

2. Wear gloves and/or wash hands thoroughly when handling raw meat to ensure against inoculation through breaks in the skin.

3. Feed house cats only dry, cooked, or canned meat; do not allow them to hunt.

4. Let someone else handle the cat litter; clean cat litter pans daily.

5. Avoid soil potentially contaminated with cat feces. Cover sand boxes to prevent their use by cats.

Serologic tests for *syphilis* should be a part of prenatal care for every woman, and in many states these are required by law. However, not all mothers receive prenatal care, and some may acquire syphilis following testing or may reacquire the disease after initial treatment. Moreover, because of the characteristics of the test, it will not become positive until 4 to 6 weeks after the initial infection. And because the mean length of time between treatment and a negative serologic reaction is 245 days, the test may remain positive following delivery, even though the mother has been treated and is no longer infected. Thus, important as serologic testing is, it must be supplemented by the education of mothers and their sexual partners about the significance of syphilis during pregnancy and by the development of trust between nurses and patients, so that patients will tell us if they suspect they might have become infected. If initial tests are negative, repeat testing during the third trimester is often recommended.

Regardless of when syphilis is discovered during pregnancy, it is treated. Effective treatment with penicillin prior to the eighteenth week of pregnancy prevents fetal infection because the organism apparently does not cross the placenta until after that time. Treatment after 18 weeks is also highly effective, however, as penicillin also crosses the placenta to reach the fetus quickly and in adequate amounts. Fortunately, penicillin has never been associated with teratogenicity in spite of frequent use during pregnancy for many years. For patients sensitive to penicillin, erythromycin or tetracycline is used. Failure to treat syphilis may lead to abortion, stillbirth, premature labor, and symptoms in the infant, as described in Table 8–1 and illustrated in Figure 8–3.

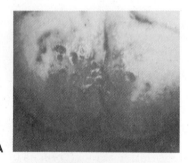

A

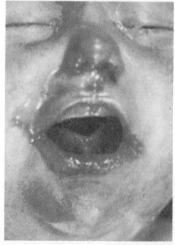

B

Figure 8–3. *A,* Syphilis. Eroded anogenital maculopapular skin lesions in the newborn. (Courtesy of the U.S. Department of Human Services.) *B,* Snuffles in a syphilitic infant. Note split infections papule on left. (Courtesy of the U.S. Department of Human Services.)

Rubella is certainly the best known of the teratogenic viral infections; it is the one that first alerted researchers to the concept that there could be an environmental source of congenital deformity. The discovery followed rubella epidemics in Australia in 1939 and 1940. Because there had been no major rubella outbreak in Australia in the previous 17 years, the vast majority of young, pregnant women had no immunity and contracted rubella in large numbers, with a high incidence of what are now recognized as the classic sequelae in their newborn infants: cardiac defects (particularly patent ductus arteriosus and pulmonary stenosis), cataracts, deafness, mental and motor retardation, dental and facial defects, retarded intrauterine growth, and several others. (Fig. 8–4).

Through what mechanism the rubella virus affects development remains a mystery. It is known that the virus enters the fetus through the placenta and that it may persist in the newborn for as long as 4 years. Thus a newborn with evidence of congenital rubella may himself be a source of infection to susceptible individuals.

Although rubella immunization for all children between 1 year of age and puberty has been recommended since the rubella vaccines were first licensed in 1969, only 60 to 70 per cent of infants and children in the United States receive rubella vaccines. This level of immunization has led to a continuous decline in the incidence of rubella, congenital rubella, and therapeutic abortion performed because of rubella during pregnancy. However, many unimmunized children now reach adolescence with no exposure to rubella, so that the disease occurs primarily in persons older than 15. Approximately 20 to 25 per cent of women of childbearing age are susceptible.[23]

To prevent congenital rubella syndrome, several solutions are worthy of consideration.

1. If rubella immunization were required for admission to school, as DPT (diphtheria-pertussis-tetanus), polio, and measles immunizations are now, the unimmunized segment of the future childbearing population would be decreased.

2. The Advisory Committe on Immunization Practices of the U.S. Public Health Service recommends that educational and training institutions, such as colleges and military bases, require proof of rubella immunity from all women of childbearing age and vaccinate those who lack proof. Proof consists of a positive serologic test or documentation previous rubella vaccination.[31]

3. Many health agencies and hospitals

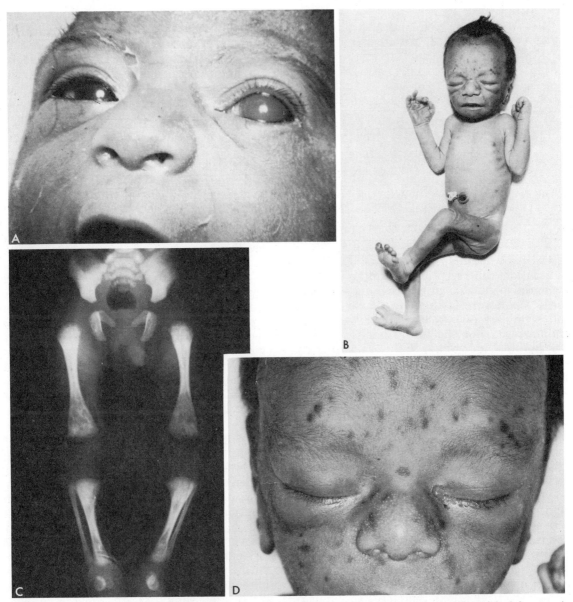

Figure 8–4. Newborn with congenital rubella. *A,* Note the prominence of the eyes and the clouding of the left eye typical of advanced congenital glaucoma. *B,* Term infant, underweight, with "blueberry muffin" rash over the face. *C,* Bone lesions in congenital rubella. The provisional zones of calcification are poorly defined. Multiple radiolucent defects are apparent. *D,* Closeup of rash shown in *B.* (From Schaffer and Avery: *Diseases of the Newborn,* 4th Edition. Philadelphia, W. B. Saunders Co., 1977. Figure courtesy of Dr. A. J. Rudolph.)

screen certain personnel for rubella immunity but not others (some states require that all female employees in hospitals be screened). For example, nurses who work on pediatric units may be routinely screened, a policy that protects the nurse herself but not nurses who work in other areas. Given the changing age range of rubella patients, such a policy may not protect the nurse most at risk. Pediatric patients may be the least in need of protection from a nurse who might have rubella.

4. Little consideration has been given to males who work in hospitals. In July 1978 a male house officer in New York contracted rubella; 170 staff members and 11 prenatal patients, 3 of whom were susceptible to rubella, were exposed to the disease. None of the prenatal patients contracted rubella, but the potential seriousness of even a single infection suggests that men as well as women who work in hospitals and clinics should be screened and immunized.[21]

Since the rubella vaccine may be teratogenic to the fetus, it is important that no one be

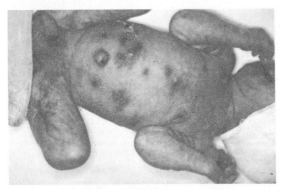

Figure 8–5. Disseminated herpes simplex. (From Solomon and Esterly: *Neonatal Dermatology.* Philadelphia, W. B. Saunders Co., 1973.)

vaccinated who might be pregnant. Following vaccination, contraception should be used for 3 months to guard against pregnancy. Nurses need to be aware of their own rubella titers and should receive vaccine if they are not immune, both for the future health of their own families and so they will not unwittingly transmit the virus to patients if they should acquire an asymptomatic infection.

Cytomegalovirus (CMV) rarely produces symptoms, yet it is apparently fairly common. The effects of CMV are summarized in Table 8–1.

Herpesvirus is classified as either Type I, causing disease above the waist, or Type II, causing disease below the waist. Herpes infection in newborns results in overwhelming systemic infection (Fig. 8–5) and often in death. It is believed that most newborn herpes infection is acquired from the mother's vaginal tract during delivery (and therefore is Type II). In recent years genital herpes has become the second most prevalent veneral disease among young Americans. It is therefore most important to identify the presence of this infection, especially late in pregnancy. When herpes is identified prior to delivery, this is an indication for cesarean section. Herpes is also the cause of common fever blisters (Type I), and therefore no one should be allowed in the nursery or in the mother's room who has such a blister.

Other Maternal Infections

Two additional maternal infections, gonorrhea and *Chlamydia* infection (due to *C. trachomatis),* while they are not teratogenic, can be transmitted from an infected mother to her baby at the time of delivery. Both gonorrhea and *Chlamydia* can cause ophthalmia neonatorum; *Chlamydia* infection can also result in pneumonia in infants (Chapter 21). Assess-

ment of sexually transmitted disease is discussed in Chapter 10; nursing intervention in Chapter 11.

Other infections (rubeola, mumps, chickenpox, and infectious hepatitis) do not appear to be teratogenic. They may cause an increase in fetal death and premature labor.

Drugs and Hormones as Teratogens

No individual should practice self-medication at any time, but it is essential that a pregnant woman take no medication unless specifically prescribed by a physician who knows she is pregnant. Even then, it is a good idea for the woman to double check with the physician or nurse who is responsible for her maternity care. Morever, women who might be pregnant must also be careful of the medicine they ingest because of the rapid embryologic development during the first weeks.

In spite of publicity about the harmful effects of some drugs in pregnant women, the use of medications appears widespread during pregnancy. Doering and Stewart (1978)[9] and Brocklebank and colleagues (1978)[4] reviewed the use of medications in over 3000 pregnant women. The number of drugs taken averaged from 4 to 11 per woman. In the Brocklebank study, 82 per cent of 2528 women received prescriptions; pregnant women received as many prescriptions for medications as nonpregnant women.

A variety of factors affect the way in which a specific drug will affect a particular mother and her fetus. Drug characteristics that will influence placental transfer include molecular weight, fat solubility, the degree to which inonization occurs, and the degree to which the drug binds to albumin in maternal blood. Compounds with a molecular weight greater than 1000 do not readily pass to the fetus. Increased fat solubility and decreased binding to albumin enhance the likelihood of transplacental passage. Maternal acid-base balance and placental blood flow also influence transfer. Acid-base balance may be particularly important during labor. If the mother hyperventilates and blood pH rises (alkalosis), the fetus becomes acidotic; drugs may cross the placenta and become trapped in the fetus. Certain genetic characteristics of the mother or fetus can also be important; for example, nitrofurantoin (Furadantin) may cause hemolytic anemia in mothers with glucose-6-phosphate dehydrogenase (G-6-PD) deficiency.

The effects of drugs taken during pregnancy will not necessarily be evident at the time of birth. The best known example of a long delayed effect are findings associated with diethylstilbestrol (DES). Of more than 200 case histories of young women with clear-cell adenocarcinoma of the genital tract, more than 80 per cent were daughters of mothers who had been given DES or a related synthetic hormone to reduce the incidence of spontaneous abortion. Although the number of women in whom adenocarcinoma has been detected and reported is small in relation to the total number of mothers receiving DES or related hormones, failure to detect or report the adenocarcinoma or its development later in the daughter's lifetime may decrease the reported incidence.

Most women who develop adenocarcinoma of the genital tract have symptoms of abnormal bleeding or discharge; approximately 10 per cent have no symptoms, however. Since a Pap smear may fail to identify the cancer cells, Schiller's test, in which the walls of the vagina are coated with an iodine stain, and colposcopy are essential for women at risk.[36]

Women exposed to DES should be closely followed during pregnancy. Genital tract abnormalities have also been detected in 41 of 163 *men* whose mothers received DES during pregnancy, compared with 11 of 168 male controls. Further studies have shown reduced sperm counts, lowered sperm mobility, and abnormal appearance of sperm.[26]

DES may also produce the more immediate effect of masculinization of the female fetus.

Although teratogenesis was originally thought of in terms of major physical malformation, drugs taken by the mother may also affect behavior in the infant or child. Phenytoin (Dilantin), heroin, and alcohol are examples discussed in this chapter. Because many behavioral difficulties are not recognized until several years after birth, it is difficult to establish a cause-and-effect relationship. Ongoing research with animal models, however, suggests that certain drugs may produce behavioral abnormalities without any physical changes.[44] As a general principle, this work, along with the findings related to DES, strongly suggests that immediately discernible effects are not the only ones with which responsible professionals must be concerned.

Effects of Specific Drugs

In Table 8–2 a number of drugs associated with problems before or after birth are summarized.

Anesthetic gases may present a hazard to nurses and other health care professionals. Epidemiologic studies in both the United States and the United Kingdom have shown an increase in spontaneous abortion and congenital abnormalities not only among women working in operating rooms but among the children of male anesthetists. Similar findings have been reported among dentists who use anesthetic gases in their practice compared with those who do not. A 16 per cent rate of spontaneous abortion in 887 pregnacies in wives of exposed dentists compares with a rate of 9 per cent in 1541 pregnancies in wives of unexposed dentists.[7]

It has been estimated that *acetylsalicylic acid* (aspirin) is taken at some time during pregnancy by approximately 80 per cent of women. The role of aspirin in congenital anomalies in humans has not been proved, although salicylates do cause anomalies in animals. However, salicylates taken within 10 days before delivery can cause platelet dysfunction and thereby interfere with clotting in the newborn. A U.S. Food and Drug Administration (FDA) advisory panel has suggested that no aspirin-containing compound be used during the third trimester of pregnancy.

Four antimicrobial drugs may cause problems. *Chloramphenicol* in the third trimester may cause "gray syndrome," an anemia due to bone marrow suppression in the newborn infant. *Tetracycline* inhibits bone growth and stains teeth. Brocklebank and his coworkers found, in their study of drug-prescribing during pregnancy, that tetracycline was prescribed for 6.2 per cent of pregnant women. *Streptomycin* may cause damage to the eighth cranial nerve and skeletal anomalies. It has already been noted that in mothers with G-6-PD deficiency, nitrofurantoin (Furadantin) may cause a hemolytic anemia in the fetus and the mother. Given at term, *sulfonamides* may decrease bilirubin binding and lead to hyperbilirubinemia in the newborn.

Benzodiazepines, of which diazepam (Valium) is the most widely used, have been associated with cleft lip and palate. Diazepam in the third trimester may lead to thrombocytopenia, hypothermia, and hypotonia in the infant. Lithium, also used as a tranquilizer, has been related to irritability and goiter in the newborn.

Glucocorticoids (e.g., methylprednisolone, dexamethasone) may inhibit cell growth or cause cell death in a variety of tissues. In a study by Reinisch and colleagues (1978), women receiving as little as 10 mg. of prednisone per day delivered infants weighing 200 to

Table 8–2.   DRUGS THAT MAY HARM THE HUMAN FETUS

Drug	Consequence	Comments
Abused drugs	Varies with drug	See text—Drugs That Are Abused
Alcohol	Fetal changes associated with chronic alcoholism	See text
Aminopterin Amethopterin	Gross deformity or death	8 of 41 infants affected in one study*
Anesthetic gases	Possibility of increased spontaneous abortion	See text
Benzodiazepines (e.g., diazepam, lithium)	Cleft lip, cleft palate, neonatal problems	See text
Busulfan	Spontaneous abortion and prematurity	10 of 30 infants affected in one study
Glucocorticoids (e.g., methylprednisolone, dexamethasone, prednisone)	Inhibition of cell growth	
Chloramphenicol	If used near term may result in gray-baby syndrome (i.e., sudden collapse and death)	
Diethylstilbestrol	Possible masculinization of female fetus; clear-cell adenocarcinoma of genetic tract in daughters of some women receiving DES	See text
Ethacrynic acid	Fetal and neonatal jaundice; thrombocytopenia	
Hydantoin anticonvulsants (e.g., phenytoin)	"Fetal hydantoin syndrome"	See text
Iodides (potassium iodide, radioactive iodine, propylthiouracil)	Congenital goiter, with possible respiratory distress from pressure of enlarged thyroid on trachea	Iodides may be found in over-the-counter cough medicines
Metronidazole (Flagyl)	Considered teratogenic, particularly in the first 16 weeks of gestation	
Mineral oil	Regular use may lead to reduced absorption of fat-soluble vitamins A, D, E, and K; reduced absorption of vitamin K may cause hypoprothrombinemia	
Nicotine	May affect fetal growth	See text—Maternal Smoking and the Fetus
Nitrofurantoin (Furadantin)	Hemolytic anemia in fetus or mother with G-6-PD deficiency	

*Shepard, T., and Fantel, A.: Teratology of Therapeutic Agents. In Iffy, L., and Kaminetzky, H. (eds.): *Principles and Practice of Obstetrics and Perinatology*. New York, John Wiley, 1981.

300 g. less than those of control mothers. Further research is necessary to evaluate the mechanism and long-term effects of prednisone and related compounds.

Hydantoin anticonvulsants (e.g., phenytoin, Dilantin) appear to produce a constellation of defects in some infants called the "fetal hydantoin syndrome." Signs include craniofacial, digital, and nail anomalies, intrauterine growth retardation, and mental deficiency. It has been suggested that folate deficiency may be related to the use of phenytoin as well as phenobarbital and alcohol, and thus mothers who receive anticonvulsants should begin folic acid supplementation prior to conception so that adequate folic acid will be available during implantation and organogenesis.

Oral contraceptives, discontinued in the cycle immediately prior to pregnancy, have been suspected as teratogens.[15] Ovulation is commonly delayed in the first cycle after oral

contraceptives are stopped, and it is suspected that fertilization of an aging ovum leads to malformation. This problem might be avoided if the couple used another form of contraception for one or two cycles after discontinuing oral contraceptives.

Propranolol (Inderal), which is considered a safe drug for nonpregnant women with thyrotoxicosis and cardiac arrhythmias, may be associated with intrauterine growth retardation, hypoglycemia, respiratory depression, and bradycardia in the newborn if the drug is present in the infant at the time of birth.

Thiazide diuretics, given in the third trimester, have been associated with thrombocytopenia and neonatal death. *Indomethacin* (Indocin), an anti-inflammatory drug, may also cause thrombocytopenia.

Sodium warfarin, a coumarin anticoagulant, may cause congenital anomalies if given in the first trimester. "Warfarin embryopathy" in-

Table 8–2. DRUGS THAT MAY HARM THE HUMAN FETUS

Drug	Consequence	Comments
Novobiocin	Near delivery associated with thrombocytopenia and hyperbilirubinemia	
Oral contraceptives	Both positive and negative findings	See text
Propranolol (Inderal)	Intrauterine growth retardation, neonatal hypoglycemia, respiratory depression, bradycardia if present at time of birth	
Reserpine	Nasal discharge, respiratory distress, lethargy, anorexia in newborn	
Rubella vaccine	Congenital rubella syndrome	No immunizations should be given during pregnancy
Salicylates	Neonatal bleeding; possible salicylate intoxication in high doses	
Sodium warfarin (coumadin)	Several types of deformities in individuals	
Streptomycin, dihydrostreptomycin, chloroquine	May affect inner ear of fetus	
Sulfonamides	Avoid during last trimester; possible hyperbilirubinemia, thrombocytopenia, kernicterus if given near term	
Testosterone, synthetic progestins (e.g., ethisterone, norethisterone)	Masculinization of the female fetus	At one time given to prevent spontaneous abortion
Tetracycline and derivatives	Inhibition of bone growth; discoloration of teeth	
Thalidomide	Phocomelia (seal-like limbs), amelia (absence of limbs), and other deformities	
Thiazides	Long-term use may lead to hyponatremia, diabetogenic effect on mother may have an effect on infant	
Trimethadione (Tridione) Paramethadione (Paradione)	A variety of defects may occur including facial defects, cardiac defects, cleft palate, and intrauterine growth retardation	

*Shepard, T., and Fantel, A.: Teratology of Therapeutic Agents. In Iffy, L., and Kaminetzky, H. (eds.): *Principles and Practice of Obstetrics and Perinatology.* New York, John Wiley, 1981.

cludes hypoplastic "saddle" nose, abnormalities of bones and hands, eye problems, and mental retardation. Warfarin administered during the third trimester has been associated with increased perinatal mortality.

Caffeine

Caffeine, in the form of beverages primarily, is one of the drugs most frequently consumed by pregnant women. The Food and Drug Administration has issued a warning about the use of caffeine during pregnancy, largely on the basis of multiple animal studies showing caffeine to be both mutagenic and teratogenic.[40] There are no large, well-controlled human studies. In a retrospective study, Weathersbee (1977)[45] found increased fetal loss in families in which caffeine intake in mothers was more than 600 mg. per day and in families in which the father's intake was more than 600 mg. per day while the mother's intake exceeded 400 mg. per day (Table 8–3).

When 220 mg. of caffeine are ingested, circulating catecholamines are released that can lead to vasoconstriction of uterine and placental blood vessels. Caffeine does cross the placenta and also enters breast milk; effects on the fetus/newborn are unknown.

The average intake of caffeine for pregnant women has been estimated at 144 mg./day,[11] the equivalent of one strong cup of coffee (Table 8–4). Parents should certainly be informed of the potential risks of caffeine, and when the drug is used in moderate to large quantities they should be encouraged to decrease their intake. Based on Weathersbee's data, four strong cups of coffee may be too much, even though the mother may not consider her intake excessive. It would also appear advisable to limit or even eliminate caffeine from the diet of mothers who are experiencing placental insufficiency; there is no research data to support this idea at this time.

Both coffee and tea products without caffeine are available. Since large amounts of caffeine

Table 8–3. FETAL LOSS AND CAFFEINE INTAKE*

Caffeine Intake	Maternal ≥600 mg./day	Paternal ≥600 mg./day (Maternal ≥400 mg./day)
Number	16	13
Spontaneous abortions	8	4
Stillbirths	5	2
Preterm deliveries	2	2
Uncomplicated term delivery	1	5

*Data from Weathersbee at al., 1977.

are usually not detectable to taste in soft drinks, soft drink manufacturers could be urged to limit caffeine. The FDA requires small amounts of caffeine in colas but not in diet colas.

Drugs That Are Abused

A wide variety of drugs, heroin and cocaine, LSD and cannabis (marijuana), prescribed barbiturates, tranquilizers and amphetamines, and nonprescription preparations (over-the-counter stimulants, sleep inducers, tranquilizers) are subject to abuse. Maternal use of these drugs is discussed in Chapter 13.

The effects of many of these drugs on the fetus have not been documented in humans but have been noted in animals. In other drugs such as heroin, specific changes in the fetus, either as a direct effect or as a corollary to drug use, have been noted.

Table 8–4. CAFFEINE CONTENT OF BEVERAGES AND SELECTED SUBSTANCES

Beverage/Substance	Caffeine Content (mg.)
Coffee (5 oz. cup)*	53–146
Tea (5 oz. cup)	20–46
Cocoa (water mix, 5 oz. cup)	10
Diet Mr. Pibb, Mountain Dew, Mellow Yellow†	51–52
Tab, Sunkist Orange, Shasta Cola	42–44
Dr. Pepper, Pepsi Cola, Coca Cola, Mr. Pibb	33–38
Seven-Up, Sprite, Diet 7-Up, RC-100, Diet Sunkist Orange, Patio Orange, Fanta Orange, Fresca, Hires Root Beer	0
Anacin‡	64
Midol	65
No Doz	200
Weight control aids (e.g., Dexatrim, Dietac)§	200

*Individuals vary greatly in the way they prepare coffee. Drip coffee generally contains more caffeine than instant coffee.
†Per 12 oz. can (based on tests by Consumer's Union).
‡Standard dose.
§Daily dose.

The fetus exposed to heroin typically has a decreased number of total cells and thus suffers intrauterine growth retardation. In addition, gestation is frequently shorter with a heroin-exposed fetus, leading to the birth of a preterm, small-for-gestational-age infant. Other potential risks include increased intrauterine infections due primarily to maternal life style and increased meconium staining of amniotic fluid. Should heroin withdrawal occur during the pregnancy, the fetus will also suffer withdrawal. Because withdrawal increases the mother's metabolic rate and oxygen needs, she may be unable to meet the oxygen needs of the fetus, which are also increased because of fetal withdrawal. The fetus demonstrates fetal distress, meconium is released into the amniotic fluid and hypoxia and intrauterine death may occur. Heroin does increase the maturation of both the glucuronyl transferase system and the pulmonary surfactant system in the fetus, so that hyperbilirubinemia and respiratory distress syndrome are less likely to occur (see Chapter 23 for description of these systems). The risk of congenital anomalies does not appear to be increased in mothers who use heroin. Heroin withdrawal in the newborn is discussed in Chapter 24.

Methadone may also affect fetal growth, but the effect is apparently somewhat less than in a fetus exposed to heroin. This may be because mothers on methadone maintenance are more involved in prenatal care and have better nutrition.

Cannabis (marijuana) has been shown to produce malformations in rats, hamsters, and rabbits, but there is no evidence at this time of increased defects in humans. It has been suggested that cannabis may adversely affect immunologic development in the fetus; there is concern about the effect on maturational processes in the fetal brain.

Lysergic acid diethylamide (LSD) has shown teratogenic properties in animal studies but not in human studies. The prenatal effects of *cocaine* are also unknown.

Barbiturates have produced deformities in several animal species. Retrospective studies of the infants of epileptic mothers taking phenobarbital with or without phenytoin (Dilantin) have suggested the possibility of an increased incidence of anomalies and growth retardation, but the extent to which phenobarbital is responsible is unclear. Phenobarbital may potentiate the action of phenytoin. Barbiturates in the mother can produce respiratory distress at the time of birth and withdrawal symptoms in the newborn (Chapter 00).

Benzodiazepines, a group of hypnosedatives that includes *diazepam* (Valium) and *chlordiazepoxide* (Librium), are considered by some to be the most abused drugs in American society. Diazepam has been associated with cleft lip and palate and if used in the third trimester, with thrombocytopenia, hypothermia, and hypotonia in the infant.

Lithium, also used as a tranquilizer, has been related to irritability and goiter in newborn infants.

Amphetamines, haloperidol, mescaline, methaqualone, and morphine are other drugs that have produced deformities in animal studies and have also been associated with neonatal withdrawal symptoms. Compounding the problem is the fact that many women who use one "hard" drug use others as well. In one survey, only 4 of 144 women (2.8 per cent) were found to use only one drug when carefully documented drug histories were taken.[29]

Alcohol and the Fetus

In 1973, Jones and colleagues first reported a "pattern of craniofacial, limb, and cardiovascular defects associated with prenatal onset growth deficiency and developmental delay" that has become known as the *fetal alcohol syndrome.*[16] In addition to this specific pattern of defects, maternal alcohol consumption appears to be related to more general conditions such as intrauterine and infant growth retardation and delays in behavioral development (Fig. 8–6).

In a study of 305 women in Boston, five of 15 babies born to women who drank heavily had congenital anomalies.[27] Forty-four per cent of the surviving children of 23 alcoholic women in a perinatal collaborative project showed mental deficiency.[12]

Other effects of alcohol use during childbearing include: (1) decreased birth weight among children of some women who average only 1 ounce of absolute alcohol (two standard drinks) per day during pregnancy[20]; (2) increased spontaneous abortion in women with alcohol consumption as low as 1 ounce of absolute alcohol twice a week[14]; (3) decreased lactation with heavy alcohol consumption; transmission of alcohol in breast milk.

In addition, alcohol compromises maternal nutrition by interfering with the absorption and utilization of a number of nutrients and with the synthesis of proteins. The alcoholic woman is frequently malnourished before she becomes pregnant and may continue to be malnourished during pregnancy. Because thiamine is metabolized at an accelerated rate, the need for that vitamin is increased. Alcoholic women often have iron deficiency or macrocytic anemia. A high-protein–high-iron diet, appropriate for the woman with iron deficiency anemia, also aids in preventing growth retardation. Folic acid is the therapy for macrocytic anemia. Increased intake of vitamin C enhances therapy in both anemias.

Questions about the type, frequency and amount of alcohol intake should be part of the initial prenatal assessment for every patient. Not only will these questions help in the early identification of mothers at risk, but they may also alert all mothers to the dangers of alcohol consumption during pregnancy. The presence of alcohol-related diseases, such as hepatitis and cirrhosis, suggests the possibility of alcoholism and the need for further assessment.

In July 1981 the Surgeon General advised women who were pregnant or considering pregnancy not to drink alcoholic beverages and to be aware of the alcohol content of food. This information should be shared with all women.

Maternal Smoking and the Fetus

Since Simpson[35a] first reported an association in 1957 between birth weight and smoking during pregnancy, a large body of subsequent research has confirmed his findings. Results have been consistent from a wide variety of nations, races, and cultures in both prospective and retrospective studies. The effects of smoking are independent of race, parity, maternal size, socioeconomic status, infant sex, and other variables.

Infants born to women who smoke are, on the average, 150 to 250 g. lighter than infants born to control women who do not smoke. Smokers have twice as many babies weighing less than 2500 g. than nonsmokers. Moreover, the more a mother smokes, the greater the reduction in fetal size, body length, and head and chest circumference as well as weight.

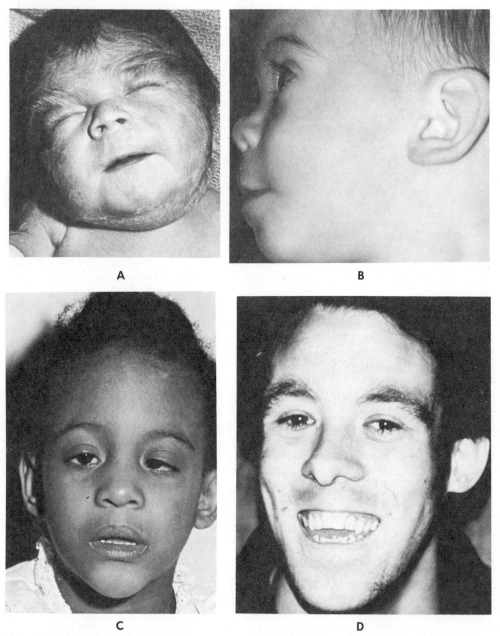

Figure 8–6. Affected children of chronic alcoholic women. *A,* Infant at birth. Note facial hirsutism and short palpebral fissures. *B,* Profile of an infant showing short upturned nose, thin upper lip, relatively small mandible, and prominent ridge across external ear. *C,* Affected child at 3¾ years. Note short palpebral fissures, also strabismus and ptosis of the eyelid. *D,* Twenty-two-year-old with fetal alcohol syndrome, still showing short palpebral fissures, smooth philtru, and smooth upper lip. He is a pleasant individual with an IQ of 65. (From Smith: *Recognizable Patterns of Human Malformation.* Major Problems in Clinical Pediatrics Series, Vo. VII. Philadelphia, W, B. Saunders Co., 1982.)

Since gestation is not shortened by smoking, these lower birth weights are due to intrauterine growth retardation rather than to decreased gestational age.

The mechanism by which smoking inhibits intrauterine growth has not been discovered. Wilson (1972),[46] Wingerd and colleagues (1976),[47] and others have noted a significantly higher ratio between placental weight and infant birth weight and have suggested that the increase may be a response by the placenta

to chronic hypoxia. Like birth weight, the placental weight was related to the level of maternal smoking. Other research has focused on the effects of smoking on placental metabolism, carbon monoxide or cyanide, maternal vitamin B_{12} and vitamin C levels, vascular damage, or indirect effects on maternal weight gain.

The effects of maternal smoking on long-term growth, development, and behavior are less clear. The largest long-term follow-up, of

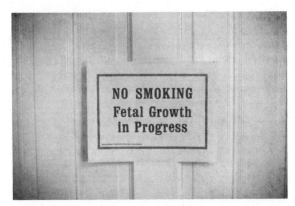

Figure 8–7. This no smoking sign on the door of a maternity center reminds expectant mothers of the effects of smoking on the unborn child. (Photograph by David Miller.)

17,000 births in the British Perinatal Mortality Study, did find differences in physical and mental growth at ages 7 and 11 ($p < 0.0001$) when social and biologic factors were controlled.

Additional studies suggest a relationship between maternal smoking and placenta previa,[42] abruptio placentae,[1, 22, 25] bleeding during pregnancy,[32] premature rupture of membranes,[42] and pre-eclampsia.[1]

In a study of 51,490 births, 701 fetal deaths, and 655 neonatal deaths, perinatal mortality rates per thousand births were 23.5 for nonsmokers, 28.2 for smokers of less than a pack per day (a 20 per cent increase), and 31.8 for smokers of more than a pack per day (a 35 per cent increase). Maternal smoking during pregnancy has also been associated with sudden infant death syndrome (SIDS).[2, 30, 38]

One troublesome question is whether fetal outcome is improved when the mother stops smoking during pregnancy; the answer is unclear at this time. With even a slim possibility that ceasing to smoke would benefit the baby, it seems important to encourage each mother to stop or reduce her smoking. Educating the public so that women who smoke stop prior to pregnancy would be even more valuable.

Nutrition and the Developing Embryo-Fetus

Animal experimentation has produced a variety of malformations related to nutritional deficiency of such elements as vitamin A, riboflavin, zinc, and manganese. The only proven congenital malformation related to a specific dietary deficiency in humans is cretinism, which is related to a lack of iodine in the diet. Cretinism and adult iodine deficiency are prevalent in several areas of the world where soil and water do not contain sufficient iodine.

Recently there have been reports that goiter is increasing in some parts of the United States because of a decrease in the use of iodized salt. Since mountainous and inland areas are most likely to be affected, pregnant women in these sections of the country should use iodized salt.

A general level of malnutrition has been correlated with low birth weight in babies; these babies are less likely to thrive after birth and have a higher incidence of infant mortality. Fetal malnutrition may be due to malnourishment in the mother or to failure of transport of necessary nutrients across the placenta. Maternal nutrition is discussed in detail in Chapter 12.

Radiation as a Teratogen

For many years it has been obvious that radiation is a direct cause of a number of congenital malformations. The specific organs affected depend upon the stage of fetal development at the time of exposure. The chance of defect is associated with the dose, but the range of safety is not known. Therefore, it is recommended that fertile women be exposed to X-rays only during the first 10 days following the onset of menstruation, except in an emergency.

Stewart and Kneale[39] suggest that X-rays during pregnancy may increase the risk of cancer in children under the age of 10. After an analysis of 15,000 children, they felt that "among one million children exposed shortly before birth to one rad of ionizing radiation, there would be an extra 300 to 800 deaths before the age of ten due to radiation induced cancer." A number of X-ray studies that might once have been felt necessary may now be avoided by the use of sonography, which has not been found harmful to the fetus. One example would be the confirmation of a twin pregnancy.

Lead as a Teratogen

Around the beginning of the century it was recognized that women employed in trade or industry involving lead often produced infants who were small, weak, and neurologically damaged. It was discovered that lead crossed the placental border, resulting in retarded intrauterine growth and postnatal failure to thrive. Industrial exposure is now controlled, but lead poisoning can result from other substances such as moonshine liquor, which is still commonly used in the southeastern United States.

Drinking from unglazed pottery or using pitchers made from unglazed pottery, (e.g., some cups and pitchers purchased from craftsmen) can be a source of lead. Acid foods (e.g., fruits, juices, tomatoes) left in opened cans may cause some lead to enter the food. Unused portions should be transferred to glass containers for storage.

The Role of the Father in Teratogenicity

Research has focused attention on the effects of the mother's practices on the fetus. In the late 1970's animal studies at the University of Vermont College of Medicine investigated and found some association between drug intakes in male rats and adverse effects on offspring such as low birth weight and increased mortality. Methadone, morphine, caffeine, and propoxyphene (Darvon) have been used in experiments. The process by which drug use in males affects the fetus is unknown; speculated causes include changes in sperm or seminal fluid or alterations in male mating behavior that may effect female hormonal levels.[16] Sperm mobility has been found to be lower in men who use heroin and methadone.[6]

In humans, the teratogenicity of anesthetic gases when the father alone has been exposed has already been noted. The birth of an infant with fetal alcohol syndrome, with the father rather than the mother as the alcohol consumer, has been reported.

Applying a Knowledge of Teratogens in Nursing Practice

Nursing assessment of pregnant women on both initial and subsequent contacts must be designed to consider the possible exposure to or use of teratogenic substances (Table 8–5). Assessment must be specific. For example, the word "drug" has a different meaning for each

Table 8–5. TERATOGENS AND NURSING ASSESSMENT

Teratogens or Factors Affecting Fetus-Newborn	Nursing Assessment
Toxoplasmosis	Cooking of meat, cats as pets
Syphilis	Serologic testing
Rubella	History, titer, if possible
Herpes simplex, gonorrhea, *Chlamydia* infection	Physical examination
Medications	Medication history
Alcohol, nicotine, caffeine, abused drugs	Use of substances
Anesthetic gases	Employment data, including father's employment

woman. Few would consider their cough medicine or aspirin a drug; for some persons only illegal "street" drugs are drugs. "Medicine" may mean a prescribed drug but not an over-the-counter preparation. Asking "What do you do when you have a headache?" or "What do you take for a cold?" may provide more accurate answers.

Questions about alcohol and illegal drugs require particular skill; they may be better deferred until some trust has developed between nurse and client. They may also not be answered truthfully by the client. Yet the mere asking of the question, along with prenatal teaching about the significance of these substances for the developing fetus, may lead to a modification of behavior.[3]

From the perspective of intervention the nurse's position is that of educator. We cannot mandate a change in a women's behavior; we can only inform, support, and encourage.

Continuing education is essential not only for prenatal patients but all individuals about the potential dangers of medications other than those for which there is a specific need as well as other substances. This is particularly important for women during the childbearing years because these substances may be used early in pregnancy before the existence of the embryo is even recognized.

REFERENCES

1. Andrews, J., and Mcgarry, J.: A Community Study of Smoking in Pregnancy. *Journal of Obstetrics and Gynaecology of the British Commonwealth,* 79:1057, 1972.
2. Bergman, A., and Weisner, L.: Relationship of Passive Cigarette-Smoking to Sudden Infant Death Syndrome. *Pediatrics,* 58:665, 1976.
3. Bishop, B.: *The Maternity Cycle: One Nurse's Reflections.* Philadelphia, F. A. Davis, 1980.
4. Brocklebank, J., Ray, W., Federspell, C., and Schaffner, W.: Drug Prescribing During Pregnancy.

American Journal of Obstetrics and Gynecology 132:235, 1978.
5. Chavez, C., Stryker, J., and Ostrea, E.: Sudden Infant Death Syndrome (SIDS) Among Infants of Drug-Dependent Mothers (IDDM) (abstract). *Pediatric Research,* 12:403, 1978.
6. Cicero, T., Bell, R., Wiest, W., et al.: Function of the Male Sex Organs in Heroin and Methadone Users. *New England Journal of Medicine,* 292:882, 1975.
7. Cohen, E., Brown, B., Bruce, D., et al.: A Survey of Anesthetic Health Hazards Among Dentists.

Journal of the American Dental Association, 90:1291, 1975.

8. Davie, R., Butler, N., and Goldstein, H.: *From Birth to Seven.* The Second Report of the National Child Development Study. London, Longman, 1972.

9. Doering, P., and Stewart, R.: The Extent and Character of Drug Consumption During Pregnancy. *Journal American Medical Association, 239:*843, 1978.

10. Evans, M., and Harbison, R.: Cocaine, Marihuana, LSD: Pharmacological Effects in the Fetus and Newborn. In Rementaria, J. (ed.): *Drug Abuse in Pregnancy and Neonatal Effects.* St. Louis, C.V. Mosby Co., 1977.

11. Graham, D.: Caffeine—Its Identity, Dietary Sources, Intake and Biological Effects. *Nutritional Review, 36:*97, 1978.

12. Hanson, G., Jones, K., and Smith, D.: Fetal Alcohol Syndrome. *Journal of the American Medical Association, 235:*1458, 1976.

13. Harbison, R., and Evans, M.: Teratogenic Aspects in Pregnancy. In Rementeria J. (ed.): *Drug Abuse in Pregnancy and Neonatal Effects.* St. Louis: Mosby, 1977.

14. Harlap, S., and Shiono, P.: Alcohol, Smoking and Incidence of Spontaneous Abortions in First and Second Trimester. *Lancet, 2:*183, 1980.

15. Janerich, D., Piper, J., and Glebatis, D.: Oral Contraceptives and Congenital Limb Reduction Defects. *New England Journal of Medicine, 291:*697, 1974.

16. Joffe, J.: Influence of Drug Exposure of the Father on Perinatal Outcome. *Clinics in Perinatology, 6:*21, 1979.

17. Jones, K., and Smith, D.: Recognition of the Fetal Alcohol Syndrome in Early Infancy. *Lancet 2:*999, 1973.

18. Jones, K., Smith, Ulleland, C., and Streissguth, A.: Pattern of Malformations in Offspring of Chronic Alcoholic Mothers. *Lancet, 1:*1297, 1973.

19. Langer, A., and Caghan, E.: Drug and Alcohol Abuse During Pregnancy. In Iffy, L., and Kaminetzky, H. (eds.): *Principles and Practice of Obstetrics and Perinatology.* New York, J. Wiley, 1981.

20. Little, R.: Moderate Alcohol Use During Pregnancy and Decreased Infant Birth Rate. *American Journal of Public Health, 67:*1154, 1977.

21. McLaughlin, M., and Gold, L.: The New York Rubella Incident: A Case for Changing Hospital Policy Regarding Rubella Testing and Immunization. *American Journal of Public Health, 69:*287, 1979.

22. Meyer, M., and Tonascia, J.: Maternal Smoking Pregnancy Complications, and Perinatal Mortality. *American Journal of Obstetrics and Gynecology, 128:*494, 1977.

23. Mennefor, A., and Oleske, J.: Rubella Infection During Pregnancy. In Iffy, L., and Kaminetzky, H. (eds.): *Principles and Practice of Obstetrics and Perinatology.* New York, Wiley, 1981.

24. Morris, M., and Weinstein, L.: Caffeine and the Fetus: Is Trouble Brewing? *American Journal of Obstetrics and Gynecology, 140:*607, 1981.

25. Naeye, R., Harkness, W., and Utts, J.: Abruptio Placentae and Perinatal Death: A Prospective Study. *American Journal of Obstetrics and Gynecology, 128:*740, 1977.

26. Offspring of Women Given DES Remain Under Study. *Journal of the American Medical Association, 238:*932, 1977.

27. Ouellette, E., and Rosett, H.: The Effect of Maternal Alcohol Ingestion During Pregnancy on Offspring. In: Moghissi, K., and Evans, T. (eds.): *Nutritional Impacts on Women.* Hagerstown, Md.: Harper & Row, 1977.

28. Reinisch, J., Simon, N., Karow, W., et al.: Prenatal Exposure to Prednisone in Humans and Animals Retards Intrauterine Growth. *Science, 202:*436, 1978.

29. Rementeria, J., and Marrero, G.: Drug-Addicted Family (Mother, Father, and Infant): Some Sociomedical Factors. In Rementeria, J. (ed.): *Drug abuse in pregnancy and neonatal effects.* St. Louis, C. V. Mosby Co., 1977.

30. Rhead, W.: Smoking and SIDS. *Pediatrics, 59:*791, 1977.

31. Rubella Vaccine: Recommendation of the U.S. Public Health Service Advisory Committee on Immunization Practices. Morbidity and Mortality Weekly Report, 27:451, Nov. 17, 1978.

32. Russell, C., Taylor, R., and Maddison, R.: Some Effects of Smoking in Pregnancy. *Journal of Obstetrics and Gynecology of the British Commonwealth, 73:*742, 1966.

33. Safra, M., and Oakley, G.: Association Between Cleft Lip With or Without Cleft Palate and Prenatal Exposure to Diazapam. *Lancet, 1:*478, 1975.

34. Shaul, W., and Hall, J.: Multiple Congenital Anomalies Associated With Oral Anticoagulants. *American Journal of Obstetrics and Gynecology, 127:*191, 1977.

35. Shepard, T., and Fantel, A.: Teratology of Therapeutic Agents. In Iffy, L., and Kaminetzky, H.(eds.): *Principles and Practice of Obstetrics and Perinatology.* New York, John Wiley, 1981.

35a. Simpson, W.: A Preliminary Report on Cigarette Smoking and the Incidence of Prematurity. *American Journal of Obstetrics and Gynecology, 73:*808, 1957.

36. Stafl, D., Dottingly, R., et al.: Clinical Diagnosis of Vaginal Adenosis. *Obstetrics and Gynecology, 43:*118, 1974.

37. Schachter, J., Grossman, M., Holt, B., et al.: Prospective Study of Chlamydial Infection in Neonates. *Lancet, 2:*(8139), 377, 1979.

38. Steele, R., and Langworth, J.: The Relationship of Antenatal and Postnatal Factors to Sudden Unexpected Death in Infancy. *Canadian Medical Association Journal, 94:*1165, 1966.

39. Stewart, A., and Kneale, G.: Radiation Dose Effects in Relation to Obstetric X-ray and Childhood Cancers. *Lancet, 1:*1185, 1970.

40. Thayer, P., and Palm, P.: A Current Assessment of the Mutagenic and Teratogenic Effects of Caffeine. *CRC Critical Review of Toxicology, 3:*345, 1975.

41. Underwood, P., Hester, L., Laffette, T., and Gregg, K.: The Relationship of Smoking to the Outcome of Pregnancy. *American Journal of Obstetrics and Gynecology, 91:*270, 1965.

42. Underwood, P., Kesler, K., O'Lane, J., and Callagan, D.: Parental Smoking Empirically Related to Pregnancy Outcome. *Obstetrics and Gynecology, 29:*1, 1967.

43. U.S. Department of Health, Education and Welfare, Office of Smoking and Health: *Pregnancy and Infant Health.* A reprint of Chapter 8 in *Smoking and Health: A Report of the Surgeon General.* Rockport, Md., Office of Smoking and Health, 1979.

44. Vorhies, C., Brunner, R., and Butcher, R.: Psychotropic Drugs as Behavioral Teratogens. *Science, 205:*1220, 1979.

45. Weathersbee, P., Olsen, L., and Lodge, J.: Caffeine and Pregnancy—A Retrospective Study. *Postgraduate Medicine, 62:*64, 1977.

46. Wilson, E.: The Effect of Smoking in Pregnancy on the Placental Coefficient. *New Zealand Medical Journal, 74:*384, 1972.

47. Wingerd, J., Christianson, R., Lovitt, W., and Schoen, E.: Placental Ratio in White and Black Women: Relation to Smoking and Anemia. *American Journal of Obstetrics and Gynecology, 124:*671, 1976.

Psychosocial Change Following Conception: The Beginnings of Transition to Parenting

Just as the mother's body undergoes physiologic change to meet the demands of the growing embryo-fetus, so too do the lives of parents change as they prepare for new responsibilities. This is true not only for a first pregnancy but for every pregnancy. Psychosocial change involves work; the work of becoming parents has been labeled a crisis by some investigators. The more knowledgeable we are about the social and emotional work of men and women during the months of pregnancy, the more helpful we can be in assisting them as they make their plans for parenting.

In this chapter we will explore psychosocial changes, including the beginnings of attachment and the changes that occur in roles and relationships, as well as some of the ways in which culture interfaces with and affects these changes.

Pregnancy as a Crisis

Many authors have described pregnancy as a crisis in the lives of the woman and man who are to become parents of a child. Crisis, in this sense, is defined as a turning point in the life of the individual.[4] Hill describes a crisis as "any sharp or decisive change for which previous patterns are inadequate."[18] Koos[20a] refers to "situations which block usual patterns of action and call for new ones." Loesch and Greenberg describe "acute disequilibria which under favorable conditions result in specific maturational steps toward new functions."[24] Each of these definitions can give us, as nurses, insight into the psychologic meaning of pregnancy for women and men about to become parents.

Pregnancy does represent a point from which there is no turning back. (Even if the decision is made to end the pregnancy in abortion, the fact of having become pregnant remains.) New patterns of action, i.e., behavior, will be necessary. Marital routines will change. The mother's employment outside the home will in some ways be affected, even if she continues to be employed. If this is a second or subsequent pregnancy for a couple, adjustments must be made for other family members.

At each of the crises of life (for example, going to school for the first time, going away to college, marriage), successfully dealing with the crisis leads to a more mature level of behavior. As the 6- or 7-year-old child successfully adapts to school, many "baby ways" are left behind. One need only compare first graders with second graders on the first day of school in September to observe such maturation.

The ability to cope with the crisis of pregnancy will also lead to maturation, which enables one to become a successful parent of either a first or a subsequent child. However, not every pregnancy leads to maturation. Factors that affect the developmental processes in pregnancy include:

1. The meaning of the pregnancy for the individual.
2. The individual's stage of development, i.e., readiness for pregnancy.
3. The acceptance or denial of the pregnancy.
4. The resources that the individual has to deal with the pregnancy.

Pregnancy as a Developmental Process

A number of professionals in the fields of nursing, medicine, and the behavioral sciences have considered pregnancy from a developmental perspective and have identified developmental *tasks*.

A developmental task is defined as "a task which arises at or about a certain period in the life of an individual, successful achievement of which leads to happiness and success with later tasks, while failure leads to unhappiness in the individual, disapproval by the society, and difficulty with later tasks."[16] Through the successful accomplishment of developmental tasks, women both prepare for parenthood and mature personally.

Rubin[37] identifies the following as maternal tasks during pregnancy: (1) "seeking safe passage for herself and her child through pregnancy, labor and delivery," (2) "ensuring acceptance of her child by significant persons in her family," (3) "bending-in to her unknown child," and (4) "learning to give of herself."

Klaus and Kennell have looked at tasks within the context of attachment.[20] They define attachment as "a unique emotional relationship between two individuals which is specific and endures through time." They have identified the tasks important to attachment as: (1) planning the pregnancy, (2) confirming the pregnancy, (3) accepting the pregnancy, (4) perceiving fetal movements, (5) accepting the fetus as an individual, (6) birth, (7) seeing the baby, (8) touching the baby, and (9) giving care to the baby.

Task number one, planning the pregnancy,

is completed prior to pregnancy. Tasks six through nine follow birth and are discussed in Chapters 20 and 26.

Caplan[6] identified two tasks: (1) acceptance of the pregnancy and (2) perception of the fetus as a separate individual.

Confirming and Accepting the Pregnancy

Confirmation of the fact of pregnancy begins the developmental process for those couples who did not plan the pregnancy beforehand.

Acceptance of the pregnancy, and ultimately of the baby, is multifaceted. First the "idea" of being pregnant must be accepted, and then the fetus must be seen and accepted as an individual, separate and apart from the mother. The perception and acceptance of the fetus as a separate individual usually does not occur until fetal movements are perceived (quickening) after the twentieth week of pregnancy.

Acceptance not only by the mother but by other people significant to her is necessary. These "significant others" include her husband, her baby's father if not married, and her own mother. This acceptance means that there will be a reorientation of basic roles and relationships—a major aspect of the psychologic work of pregnancy.

Accepting New Roles and Reorienting Basic Relationships

The role of father or mother is added to that of husband or wife during the couple's first pregnancy. Subsequent pregnancies also bring role change—from the parent of one child to the parent of two, and so on. Both single and married parents also have additional roles, son or daughter, occupational roles, roles in the community, and so on. Although more attention has been focused on the transition to wife-mother and husband-father, other role transitions are important as well. The couple's relationship with their own parents assumes new dimensions as those parents become grandparents of their child. The changing relationship of an unmarried mother to her own mother can affect the way in which the child grows.

The process of assuming a new role involves grief, fantasy, observation, and role playing.

Grief is felt for the role left behind. No matter how desirous a couple is for a child, there is still the knowledge of the irrevocability of the occasion, as mentioned previously. This is true not only during the first pregnancy but as each new baby is anticipated. Grief may be for loss of independence, financial loss, loss of the relationship with the previous child who

will no longer be the baby, or other factors important to a particular mother. Perception of this grief in herself may make an expectant mother feel guilty; this isn't the way she thinks she is supposed to feel. Knowing that these feelings are both common and "normal" can be reassuring.

Fantasy involves trying on the new role in one's mind. A mother imagines herself holding the baby, rocking him, and singing to him. Perhaps she pictures teaching a daughter to cook or sew. The father may fantasize playing ball with his son and taking him hunting or seeing his daughter in a school play. It is not unusual for the fantasy to involve not a newborn infant but a much older child. Both parents are trying to feel what it is like to be a mother or a father. During second and subsequent pregnancies both parents and siblings fantasize what life will be like with the expected baby.

In addition to fantasies of their own roles, parents also fantasize the roles of one another. The prospective father may imagine behavior by his wife that plays no part in her idea of her role, and vice versa. He may, for example, see her as breast-feeding their baby because that is traditional in his family, only to find that the idea has no appeal to her. She may have visions of his playing football with their son while she prepares dinner; she knows that he is highly unathletic now, but she imagines that having a son will change this. Both mother and father need to share their fantasies with each other.

The *observation* of other mothers and fathers is also a significant part of the development of parental role behavior. It is not unusual for couples, and particularly for mothers, to find that they are more interested in parents who are pregnant or who have recently had a baby. Old interests are changing; new values and ideas are being considered.

The opportunity to *play the role* of parents, with the infants of friends and relatives, is more difficult to arrange in nuclear families than in extended family living, in which infants are almost always present and many chances to care for them exist.

The period of preparation for childbearing is an ideal time for helping individuals and couples think about the way in which they view the roles of mother and father. Roles are a conglomeration of perceptions. We all have idealized, stereotyped ideas of what it means to be a mother or a father. Stereotypes have always existed, but television, viewed almost constantly since childhood by the current generation of parents, has probably affected our perception of what a father or a mother "ought to be" to an even greater extent. Role behavior is a result of reality impinging upon these stereotypes.

As roles change, basic relationships are altered. Consider the following example:

Prior to the birth of their first child, the end of the working day had been a time for Jan and Tom to share happenings—good and bad—with each other. A few weeks following the baby's delivery, Tom came home to find Jan too tired from the demands of mothering to give him the attention he had once received. He had hoped dinner would be ready so that he could make an evening business meeting. Not only had dinner not been started but Jan felt that (1) it was unfair of him to expect her to have dinner ready when the baby had been fussy all afternoon and (2) it was also unfair of him to leave her at home with the baby while he went out for an evening, even if it were business.

Jan wondered, "Doesn't my role as mother (caring for her fussy infant) come before my role as wife (having dinner ready)? After all, he's an adult; he should understand." She would also like him to assume the role of father (as she views that role) and help care for the baby now that he is home, but he may see his business meeting as even more significant to his father role, because for Tom a father's primary role is that of breadwinner.

Two basic problems are illustrated: differing perceptions of appropriate role behavior (e.g., how Tom and Jan perceive the priorities of the role of being a father) and conflict between the former role (wife) and the new role (wife-mother). If we can bring up these issues before they become problems, i.e., in the period before birth, and say, "This is a situation that all couples must deal with," some of these conflicts may be minimized.

Siblings and the Coming of a New Baby

The coming of each newborn affects the relationship of parents and every other child in the family. The changes that a new baby brings to the total family structure inevitably affect other children, as well as parents. There are changes in space, such as sharing a room or changing rooms. Possessions may change hands—the crib may be painted for the baby. A mother may be too tired during certain stages of pregnancy to participate in some formerly shared activities.

Siblings at every age, from the small baby to the adolescent, are affected. Very small children may not, however, perceive changes during the prenatal phase, unless their own activities change, as when a baby is weaned from the breast fairly rapidly.

Seeking Safe Passage

Rubin suggests that as a mother accepts the idea of her pregnancy, she also plans a safe passage for herself and her fetus.[37] As she becomes increasingly protective of the fetus, she becomes careful in her actions. She often tries hard to eat the foods suggested as being appropriate. She may avoid activities that she believes to be dangerous.

Seeking care that she believes to be competent and questioning even practices that formerly were taken for granted (riding in a car, hanging clothes) are further manifestations of her concern.

Learning to Give of Herself

The concept that during pregnancy the mother must learn to give of herself is also a contribution of Rubin's. Rubin sees giving in four contexts:

1. The fetus as a gift to the mother.
2. The mother's giving to the fetus in utero.
3. The mother's giving of the fetus in utero as a gift from herself to others.
4. The mother's exacting of gifts from the father and from friends as symbols of their concern.[37]

The theme of giving is evident in accounts of pregnancies in other cultures. Obeyesekere describes a craving, termed *dola-duka,* in Ceylon, which is a craving for specific types of food.[29] To deny the mother what she desires is considered a sin sufficiently grave to damage one's chances of rebirth. More immediately, it is believed that the ears of the fetus will rot if the woman's cravings are not satisfied.

Within the context of giving and receiving, perhaps the demands for gifts are preparatory to being able to give of oneself. We then need to question whether the mother who does not perceive of herself as being cared for, who is not "given gifts," may then have difficulty in meeting the many demands for giving that are placed upon a new mother.

Variables that Influence Achieving Developmental Tasks During Pregnancy

A number of factors may enhance or impede the achievement of the developmental tasks of pregnancy and ultimately of the tasks of parenting.

Success or Failure in Achieving Prior Developmental Tasks. A major block to the successful achievement of the developmental tasks of pregnancy is the failure to achieve prior tasks. For the individual or couple who has not yet resolved the tasks of adolescence and early adulthood, the intrusion of parenthood on uncompleted tasks may bring resentment of the pregnancy and rejection of the child.

Care by and Relationship to the Mother's and Father's Own Parents. From our own parents and our relationship with them, all of us develop, consciously and unconsciously, our understanding of what it means to be a parent and strategies for parental behavior. The fact that most parents who abuse their children were themselves abused as children points to this concept rather emphatically.

Expectations of Family and Society. The expectations of family and friends that developmental tasks will be achieved enhance their achievement. Conversely, the young mother or father who is told, or to whom it is implied, that for one reason or another she or he is not ready for pregnancy (too young, too immature, and so on) faces an added barrier.

When family and societal expectations become social pressures to become pregnant (the desire of the couple's own parents for grandchildren, pregnancy because one's peers are pregnant, and so forth) or when the pregnancy results in social disapproval (unwed pregnancy, pregnancies too closely spaced, too many children, for example) the achievement of tasks may be hindered.

The Relationship Between the Mother and Father. The relationship between the mother and father may also enhance or hinder the achievement of developmental tasks. If the father is supportive of the mother; if she, in turn, recognizes that he also has concerns and needs during the pregnancy (see below); and if their communication is effective most of the time, their relationship is likely to be a positive factor in achieving the developmental tasks of pregnancy. When serious problems exist in this relationship, however, not only is it more difficult to cope with the pregnancy, but the pregnancy is likely to put a further strain on the relationship. Parenthood is sometimes undertaken to strengthen a shaky relationship; however, the desired result is almost never achieved (see also motivation for pregnancy, Chapter 6).

Some couples do find themselves closer as a result of parenthood, but these are nearly always couples who have had a good relationship and good interpersonal communication prior to the pregnancy. Other couples begin to coexist, each in his or her separate world, as a result of pregnancy and parenthood—the mother becoming more absorbed in the world of her child or children while the father becomes absorbed in affairs outside the home.

Feelings about Femininity and Masculinity. The mother who is ambivalent about or unsure of her own femininity may have difficulty accepting motherhood. Equally, the man who is unsure of his masculinity may find the idea of fatherhood threatening.

High Risk Pregnancy. When the mother has some condition, such as diabetes mellitus or previous difficult pregnancies, that puts the outcome of the pregnancy at risk, there may be major problems in achieving developmental tasks. This issue is discussed in Chapter 13.

Emotional Reactions to Pregnancy

Culture and the Emotional Changes of Pregnancy

Before we examine the emotional changes that have been observed in both men and women in our society, we must recognize that we do not really know whether they apply to prospective mothers and fathers everywhere or whether they are part of Western society. We do not even know if they apply to everyone in our own society. They may indeed be applicable, but systematic studies have not been done to confirm this.

The recognition of this fact has very practical significance. We cannot assess the emotional reactions of individuals of one cultural group by using norms for another group, just as in many instances we cannot judge the physiologic status of one group by norms established for another.

For example, in some societies or subsocieties it is expected that the father will become involved in pregnancy far more than in others. The middle class American father may thus attend prenatal classes with his wife; because the Chinese-American father does not behave in the same way does not mean that he does not care for his wife or child-to-be. Many examples of the role of culture have been given in Chapter 2 and elsewhere, and will be encountered in your practice.

Changes Occur in Both Mothers and Fathers

When researchers and caretakers first became interested in the emotional changes that accompany pregnancy, attention was focused almost exclusively on the expectant mother. Several cultural factors are undoubtedly related to this bias, including the idea that pregnancy is "women's business" and a long-standing concept that men in our society are not supposed to react to events in an emotional way, but solely in an intellectual manner. Thus only recently have the reactions and needs of fathers received much attention.

If we examine the evidence that is now accumulating, it is interesting to observe that many characteristics exhibited by women during pregnancy are directly or inversely related to characteristics in their mates. The mother's attitude about pregnancy will influence the father's attitude and vice versa. It is in this context that we will examine some of the major emotional components of pregnancy.

The extent to which these reactions are experienced by an individual man or woman will depend upon many factors, including the individual's age and level of maturity (not necessarily equal), the relationship of each with his or her own parents and particularly with the parent of the same sex, the couple's relationship to one another, the meaning of the pregnancy for each of them, their desire for the baby, and the reason for that desire.

Ambivalence

The popular belief that each mother and father is overjoyed when she or he learns about the pregnancy is not supported by investigation. This is true for married couples as well as for couples who are not married. There is no one reaction typical of expectant parents. Yet a degree of ambivalence seems very prominent in our society, and perhaps in all societies as we come to know more about them.

Sears[38] reported that as high as 25 per cent of women were ambivalent or displeased when they first discovered they were pregnant; Caplan[6] found as many as 80 per cent of the women in his group were at first unhappy when they found themselves pregnant.

Ambivalent feelings may be present even when the child has been planned and is desired. The mother (and father) may feel, "Oh yes, we want this baby, but maybe not quite yet." The feeling is similar to that experienced at any major change of lifestyle—graduation from school, or marriage, for example. We count the days until the Big Day finally arrives, and then we feel, "No, not quite yet." This is because once the change occurs, nothing will be quite the same. It may be better; it may be worse, but it will never be the same

and that is frightening. We know how to cope with the known; will we be able to cope with the unknown? And so the couple feel as they face parenthood that nothing will ever be quite as it was before. Most couples expect their lives to be even better, but there are no guarantees.

Guilt about Ambivalence. Feelings of ambivalence are often unacceptable to men and women who are expectant parents, and because of this, such emotions may lead to feelings of guilt. Our myths tell us that, except in unusual circumstances, one should be delighted about the child who has been conceived. Because our ambivalent feelings are unacceptable to us, they are frequently not shared—even between the prospective mother and the prospective father. Each feels the other would think her (him) silly.

Helping Couples Cope with Ambivalence. For most couples all that is necessary is to communicate that (1) feelings of ambivalence are common and very normal reactions, for reasons described above, and (2) feelings of ambivalence usually disappear as pregnancy progresses. One has time to become accustomed to thoughts of a new lifestyle and to make specific plans in terms of finances, housing, and all the multiple logistical details that accompany parenthood—not just at the time of the first pregnancy but at each succeeding pregnancy.

Concern for Change in Body Image

The concern of the pregnant woman about her changing body image is often paralleled by the reaction in her mate to her change in form. The changing shape is very tangible evidence for both men and women of the occurrence of sexual intercourse, and therefore feelings about intercourse and sexuality can be related to feelings about body image during pregnancy. If intercourse is felt in some way to be shameful, then the announcement to the world that intercourse has occurred may pose some difficulties, even when the child is desired.

Some mothers appear to deny their changing body. Adolescents, particularly, may continue to wear their regular clothes long past the time when they fit properly, as if to continue their identification with their nonpregnant peers. (Before concluding that denial is always the reason for this behavior, however, we need to determine whether there is a financial problem in acquiring maternity clothes.)

For many mothers the changing body image

is confirmation that the pregnancy does indeed exist. Preparations for the coming baby, which may have seemed foolish and unnecessary when the pregnancy was first suspected, now become important. If the mother-to-be is employed outside of her home, the visible evidence of her pregnancy forces her to make plans with her employer for a leave of absence, perhaps, or for a "retirement," either temporary or permanent.

Men may react in varying ways to the changing shape of their mate. Some men find great satisfaction in this evidence of pregnancy, while others appear to be very uneasy around women who are pregnant, including their own wives. Husbands who are uncomfortable about their wives' changing anatomy may avoid prenatal classes in which anatomy is discussed and films of delivery and breast-feeding are shown. They may resist being, or be very uncomfortable as, participants in labor and delivery. Rarely is there an opportunity for them to discuss their concerns; most men will find it difficult to confide to either their mate or their buddies that they don't like the appearance of their pregnant mate.

Physical Symptoms as Emotional Reactions

Surprisingly similar physical symptoms can occur in both men and women during pregnancy, including nausea and vomiting, heartburn, indigestion, loss of appetite, and abdominal pain. We have been able to explain many of a mother's symptoms on a physiologic basis. Yet it appears that these symptoms have a social and emotional component as well, in that they vary markedly from one society to another, from one woman to another, and even from one pregnancy to another in an individual woman.

The "Sick Role." In 1951 sociologist Talcott Parsons[30] suggested that being sick involved not just physical symptoms but also circumstances in which certain behaviors were expected or permitted. If one were defined as "sick," one was then (1) exempt from normal social role responsibilities, relative to the nature and severity of the illness; (2) not expected to get well by an act of decision or will; (3) obliged to want to get well; and (4) obliged to seek technically competent help in relation to the severity of the illness.

These concepts are familiar to all of us. We say, "I can't go to work today because I'm sick" (exemption from normal responsibilities). "I wish I were well and could work" (obligation to want to get well and recognition that one

does not get well by just wishing it were so). Someone may then say to us, "If you're sick, why don't you see the nurse or doctor?" (obligation to seek competent help).

Rosengren, in 1962, suggested a "sick role in pregnancy."[34] He postulated that a woman who had no organic illness during pregnancy but who considered herself ill:

1. Expected to be exempt from her usual social obligations and responsibilities.

2. Regarded pregnancy as a condition of abnormality that one should get over and return to the "normal round of life."

3. Expressed worry and concern about body changes during pregnancy and possible organic complications.

4. Considered that pain and suffering were anticipated corollaries of "being ill" and of "getting better."

5. Expected to act in the subordinate role vis-a-vis her attending physician.[35]

In a study of 76 pregnant women (44 clinic patients and 32 private patients), none of whom had any pathologic disorder, Rosengren reports the following: "Women of comparatively low social status tended to regard themselves as more 'sick' during pregnancy than did women of higher social class standing."[34]

Rosengren had hypothesized that this would be so, in that he considered low social status an index of greater social disturbance than high social status. There was one exception to this:

Women who were or who had been employed in higher status occupations tended to regard themselves as more "sick" than those who held lower status jobs. . . . Those women with higher educational levels than their husbands had significantly higher sick role scores than those with similar or lower educational levels.[34]

One might speculate that in both of these instances pregnancy would be more disruptive of a specific way of life.

Rosengren also reported that there appeared to be an inverse relationship between social aspirations and sick role expectations. "Women who defined pregnancy as illness tended to express many negative social aspirations and many aspirations for material acquisition."

He further postulated that high sick role expectations would be found among the downwardly mobile while correspondingly lower sick role expectations would be found among the upwardly mobile. However, no significant difference was found between the upwardly and downwardly mobile. Nevertheless, when those women who were mobile in either direction were compared with those who were stable, those who were stable had a lower tendency to take the sick role. The disruption of life, rather than the direction of the mobility, seemed to be the significant factor.

Brown[5] found that there were a number of differences when he compared 148 consecutive primiparas who had a high number of bodily symptoms with those who had few or no physical symptoms during pregnancy. All of the women were from working and lower class backgrounds. In general, the mothers with a high number of symptoms:

1. Had had different experiences with their own mothers and fathers, with frequent inadequacy and social disorganization during their "growing-up" years.

2. Reported more problems in interpersonal relationships, particularly with their husbands and close relatives.

3. Appeared socially isolated.

4. Were more dependent upon and insecure about their husbands.

5. Were more anxious and less able to cope with their anxiety.

6. Had a less favorable reaction to their pregnancy.

7. Had a greater incidence of sexual malfunctioning and difficult menstrual periods.

Brown concluded that in the women with many physical symptoms during pregnancy, a difficult pregnancy appeared to be a further incident in a troubled life.

The studies reported above examine social/cultural correlates of physical symptoms during pregnancy. Individual emotional correlates are more difficult to document. For example, how important is the role of the mother's feelings about her pregnancy in causing nausea and vomiting during pregnancy, and particularly in producing the prolonged vomiting called *hyperemesis gravidarum*? Are these physical symptoms a coping mechanism?

Physical Symptoms in Fathers. Trethowan suggests that one in five expectant fathers has one or more physical symptoms during his wife's pregnancy.[42] Curtis found that 65 per cent (42 men) of his study group of fathers, all of whom were considered to be psychologically normal, demonstrated physical symptoms.[8]

Nausea and vomiting have been reported as beginning at about 6 to 8 weeks, even in men whose wives did not complain of nausea. Loss of appetite is fairly common for some men, while other expectant fathers increase their food intake and may gain from 10 to 20 pounds during pregnancy. Some men change their diet patterns, such as increasing their milk intake "for the baby." An interesting parallel is found in many traditional societies in which it is felt that the father, as well as the mother, is personally responsible for the growth of the fetus and that his actions during pregnancy will affect the unborn child's normal development. In some of these societies diet restrictions are applied to both the father and the mother.

Restlessness, anxiety, and sleeplessness, especially as the time of labor approaches, are not uncommon in expectant fathers. Films and television situation comedies that frequently picture the distraught father and the calm mother are a reflection of the recognition of this situation in our society. As nurses working with couples in the last weeks of pregnancy and in labor and delivery rooms, we need to be conscious of the potentially high level of paternal anxiety at a time when everyone is expecting the father to be supportive of the mother. (See the discussion of the father's supportive role below.)

Here again many traditional societies have provided for this anxiety by the practice of *couvade* (French, couver, to hatch, and Latin, cubare, to lie down). The couvade ritual takes various forms, all of which provide for male participation in childbirth. Among the Mohave Indians, transvestites mimic childbirth by being ceremonially delivered of stones. The Arapesh father shares his wife's childbirth bed. In other societies men may go to bed and enact the birth process in a ritualistic way. In our own society until relatively recently, twentieth century fathers have not been permitted a role in pregnancy and birth (other than conception).

Lacking a ritual or a role, many men responded to approaching delivery with physical symptoms. Trethowan found that it was not uncommon for either soldiers in the British army or civilians to experience abdominal cramps at the time of their wife's confinement.

Heightened Sense of Dependency

Both men and women commonly exhibit an increased need for dependency, a "desire to be mothered," during some phase of pregnancy.

Benedek[2] theorizes that the mother's heightened sense of dependency, her need to feel loved, enables her, in turn, to transfer love to the fetus and thus paves the way for the development of motherly feelings.

What happens, then, if the mother's dependency needs are not fulfilled? If she herself feels unloved, it may be very difficult for her to love her fetus or her child after birth. If her husband is unable to meet her needs for dependency, she is likely to be disappointed in him, and their relationship can become strained.

If there is no husband, if the husband is not supportive, or if there is no extended family or other group, nurses may find that women are very emotionally dependent upon them, as these mothers struggle to cope with their need for security.

As the woman turns to her husband or mate to fulfill her dependency needs, he may also be looking for "mothering," frequently from his wife but also from his own mother. Liebenberg[23] found that during pregnancy a number of husbands expressed a wish to be home on Mother's Day and wrote or called their own parents more frequently. This desire for mothering may make both husband and wife feel neglected. His need may coincide with a period during which his wife not only may be doing less for him because of her own decreased energy and self-absorption but may also be making increased demands upon him to meet her own dependency needs. In our society in which many young couples may live far from parents, relatives, and long-time friends, the husband may be the only source of support (other than professional) available to his wife. And although he may feel neglected and angry, he may also feel guilty because he feels (and society indicates to him) that he should be supportive of his wife since she is the one who is pregnant. If these feelings go unresolved during pregnancy, they may be heightened after the baby is born, as the demands of the baby further interfere with the attention that the father formerly received and still desires from his baby's mother.

"Turning Inward"

Closely related to dependency needs is a "turning inward," described by Benedek as a "vegetative calmness."[2] Even the busy extrovert usually finds herself "slowing down." One mother said, "I found myself quite content to sit and wash dishes, a job I've always hated. But now I'm not in a hurry to get on to other things. It gives me time to think about what it will be like when the baby comes."

For the mother who is busy completing her education or who has a career of her own, passivity may be distressing, particularly if she does not understand that her changing feelings are part of the normal process of pregnancy.

There does not appear to be a similar passivity in fathers. Often, in our society at least, he turns outward, becoming more concerned with his job or career as he feels increased financial responsibility, In Wapner's study of 128 first-time middle class fathers, the men's concern was not about income, per se, but about their ability to feel comfortable with the added responsibility.[45] We would suspect that for many fathers income itself might be a source of concern.

This apparent tendency for mothers and fathers to "go in different directions" can be stressful to a marriage. Maternal passivity, when not understood, may also be interpreted by the father as a rejection of him.

Anxiety

Few women experience pregnancy without some degree of anxiety at some stage. This appears to be true whether the pregnancy is planned or unplanned and whether the baby is wanted or unwanted.

Normal defense mechanisms seem to be relaxed, bringing old, unsettled conflicts closer to the surface. This is a useful function that enables the mother to resolve old conflicts in order to prepare for a new stage in her psychologic development.

Some fears will be old fears, fear of the dark, for example. Others will be related to the pregnancy itself. Will the baby be normal? Will delivery hurt? How will I behave if it hurts? Will I die? Fears about adequacy as a parent are a part of pregnancy for some mothers; for others this concern may not be important until after the birth of the baby.

Fears may appear during dreams. Mothers find it frightening to dream that their baby is born deformed or dead. They are usually relieved when they learn that many other prospective mothers have similar dreams.

If these anxieties are ridiculed rather than accepted, they are likely to be suppressed and to appear as physical or emotional symptoms.

Some mothers never mention fears or anxieties to nurses during the prenatal period. If they do not, the issue should be raised with a statement such as, "Most mothers find themselves worried at some time during their pregnancy about their health or the health of their baby," assuring them that such worries are quite common. This kind of permission to talk about concerns will often lead to a sharing of feelings.

The anxieties of fathers are less well documented but center primarily on their ability to provide financially, already discussed, and their ability to be a "father," i.e., to fulfill their image of the role of a father.

Sexual Needs During Pregnancy

Physiologic and psychologic factors interface in human sexual relationships; this is as true during pregnancy as it is at other times.

Physiologic Changes

The research of Masters and Johnson[26] has increased our understanding of the physiologic changes in sexual response that occur during pregnancy. Thorough anatomic and physiologic evaluation of six women and interviews with 111 women and 79 of their husbands during the second, sixth, and eighth months of their pregnancy and again 3 months after delivery were the basis of their findings.

As already noted in Chapter 6, during pregnancy there are physiologic changes in both breasts and genitalia. An increase in breast size, because of changes in the vascular and glandular bed, is one of the earliest signs of pregnancy, particularly in the primipara. Sexual tension in the nulliparous woman also results in vasocongestion, which can increase breast size by 20 to 25 per cent. When these changes in relation to sexual stimulation are superimposed on the changes of pregnancy, it is not surprising that many women, particularly primiparas, complain of tenderness and pain in their breasts during intercourse. The area of the areola and nipple is especially sensitive. It is helpful for the mother to know that this discomfort is greatest during the first trimester and that it will be reduced considerably during the remainder of her pregnancy.

Pregnancy affects the normal female genital response to sex in three major ways. First, as with the breasts, the vascular bed of the genitalia is increased. During the first and second trimesters, there is additional engorgement caused by sexual tension. In the third trimester the genitalia are so chronically engorged that sexual tension appears to bring little change.

Second, the increased production of vaginal lubrication and light mucoid discharge, beginning toward the end of the first trimester, appears to be greater in multiparas than in primiparas.

Third, using both intrauterine and abdominal electrode placement, Masters and Johnson have demonstrated that uterine muscle contractions occur during the orgasmic phase of the female sexual cycle.[26] During the third trimester, tonic spasm, lasting as long as 1 minute, may occur during orgasm rather than the regular contractions that normally occur. Fetal heart rate may slow at this time, but it quickly returns to normal levels. In some instances uterine contractions were observed to last as long as half an hour after orgasm during the last month of pregnancy.

Changes in Female Sexual Drive During Pregnancy

A second major consideration is the way in which pregnancy affects the emotional component of sexuality for women, recognizing that the emotional and physical components are very closely interrelated. Many factors certainly influence a woman's feelings about sexual intercourse when she is pregnant, including the beliefs of her cultural group, the attitudes of the significant people around her, and her own fears and misconceptions.

Table 9–1 summarizes the findings of three separate studies.

In the women interviewed by Masters and Johnson, decreased interest in sex was reported by three-quarters of the nulliparous women during the first trimester, but there was little change for most of the multiparas. Nausea and vomiting, sleepiness, and fatigue were present in many of those women who expressed a decreased interest. Others said they feared harming the baby.[26] In Falicov's group[12] 10 of 19 women expressed a fear of harming the fetus or of provoking miscarriage, a fear that is generally felt to be unrealistic for mothers who have no history of miscarriage. Couples may recognize this fear as groundless on an intellectual level but may still feel an emotional constraint. Some had pressing concerns about finances or other social problems that encroached on sexual interest.

Interest in sex markedly increased during the second trimester for virtually all of the women in the Masters and Johnson study. Sexual fantasies and dreams also increased. Falicov reported a slight increase in both coital frequency and sexual satisfaction although not to prepregnancy levels, while Solberg found a continuous decrease in interest. Falicov suggests that the difference in the results of Masters and Johnson may be related to the fact that women who enroll themselves in a study of sexuality may have a high level of sexual interest. There is an apparent association be-

Table 9–1. CHANGES IN SEXUAL PATTERNS DURING PREGNANCY

	Masters and Johnson[26]	Falicov[12]	Solberg, Butler, and Wagner[41]
Population studied	111 primiparas and multiparas; self-enrolled	19 primigravidas (16 college graduates)	260 women
When interviewed	4 interviews: 2nd, 6th, 8th month of pregnancy and 3 months postpartum	5 interviews: beginning in first trimester through 8 weeks postpartum	One interview 2nd or 3rd day postpartum
Sexual practices and feelings in first trimester	Decrease in sexual desire and coital frequency	Moderate to marked decrease in coital frequency	Decreased coital frequency
Sexual practices and feelings in second trimester	Marked increase in desire and coital frequency	Slightly increased coital frequency; below pregnancy levels	Continued decrease in coital frequency
Sexual practices and feelings in third trimester	Diminished interest	Fluctuation in desire in 7th and 8th months; 15 of 18 women* ceased intercourse by 8th month; 17 of 18 by 9th month (only 5 of 18 so advised by physician)	60 per cent abstained from intercourse during last month (only 29 per cent so advised by physician)

*One infant was delivered prior to 3rd trimester.

tween the level of sexual interest prior to pregnancy and the level of sexual interest during pregnancy; high prenatal interest correlates with a higher level of interest during pregnancy. Women with low prenatal interest have a correspondingly lower interest during pregnancy, although the removal of the fear of pregnancy sometimes makes intercourse more appealing. During the second trimester, the increasing size of a woman's abdomen means that changes in coital position and movements will become necessary.

By the end of the third trimester, the frequency of coital activity is markedly diminished and often has ceased. Even women who are not advised by nurses or physicians to limit intercourse often do so because they have heard from others that sexual abstinence is advisable to prevent infection or premature labor (Chapter 11).

Pregnancy and the Male Partner's Sexual Activities

It is inevitable that pregnancy will have some effect on the male partner's sexual activities. Fear of harming the fetus causes some men to lessen the frequency of coitus. A variety of personal reasons influences others. But by far the most frequent reason for limiting intercourse is the constraint of their mate's physician. Of 71 men studied by Masters and Johnson whose partners' physicians limited intercourse for varying periods during and after pregnancy:

1. Twenty-one understood the reason and agreed with and honored the prohibition.

2. Twenty-three did not understand the reason, were not sure the doctor had really said it, or wished the doctor had explained the reason to them as well as to their wives.

3. Eighteen found other sexual partners; twelve during the prenatal and postnatal periods and six during the postnatal period only. Three of these men stated that this was the first time they had sought extramarital sex.[26]

Nursing roles in helping couples meet their sexual needs during pregnancy are discussed in Chapter 11.

Summary

Psychologic and social change is as much a part of pregnancy as physiologic change. Understanding psychosocial changes is therefore essential to the care of all childbearing families.

REFERENCES

1. Bell, R. R.: *Marriage and Family Interaction.* Homewood, Ill., The Dorsey Press, 1971.
2. Benedek, T.: Psychological Aspects of Pregnancy and Parent-Child Relationships. *In* Leibman, S. (ed.): *Emotional Problems of Childhood.* Philadelphia, J. B. Lippincott Co., 1958.
3. Benedek, T.: The Psychology of Pregnancy. *In* Anthony, E., and Benedek, T. (eds.): *Parenthood: Its Psychology and Psychopathology.* Boston, Little, Brown and Co., 1970.
4. Bibring, G.: Some Considerations of the Psychological Processes in Pregnancy. *In* Eissler, R. (ed.): *The Psychoanalytic Study of the Child.* Vol. XIV. New York, International University Press, 1959.
5. Brown, L. B.: Social and Attitudinal Concomitants of Illness in Pregnancy. *British Journal of Medical Psychology, 35*:11, 1962.
5a. Caplan, G.: Patterns of Parental Response to the Crisis of Premature Birth. *Psychiatry, 23*:365, 1960.
6. Caplan, G.: Psychological Aspects of Maternity Care. *American Journal of Public Health, 47*:25, 1957.
7. Cohen, M., and Friedman, S.: Nonsexual Motivation of Adolescent Sexual Behavior. *Medical Aspects of Human Sexuality.* September, 1975, p. 9.
8. Curtis, J. L.: A Psychiatric Study of 55 Expectant Fathers. *United States Armed Forces Medical Journal, 6*:937, 1955.
9. Deutsch, H.: *The Psychology of Women.* New York, Grune and Stratton, 1945.
10. Duvall, E.: *Family Development.* 2nd Edition. Philadelphia, J. B. Lippincott Co., 1962.
11. Dyer, E. D.: Parenthood as Crisis: A Re-Study. *Marriage and Family Living,* May, 1963, p. 196.
12. Falicov, C. T.: Sexual Adjustment During First Pregnancy and Post Partum. *American Journal of Obstetrics and Gynecology, 117*:991, 1973.
13. Foltz, A., Klerman, L., and Jekel, J.: Pregnancy and Special Education: Who Stays in School. *American Journal of Public Health, 62*:1612, 1972.
14. Gordon, L.: National Survey of Legislation Relative to Schoolage Parents. National Alliance Concerned with Schoolage Parents. Unpublished, 1971.
15. Grinder, R. G.: *Adolescence.* New York, John Wiley and Sons, Inc., 1973.
16. Havighurst, R.: *Human Development and Education.* New York, Longmans, Green and Co., 1953.
17. Hendricks, C.: Delivery Patterns and Reproductive Efficiency among Groups of Differing Socioeconomic Status and Ethnic Origins. *American Journal of Obstetrics and Gynecology, 97*:608, 1967.
18. Hill, R.: *Families Under Stress.* New York, Harper Books, 1949.
19. Katchadourian, A., and Lunde, D. T.: *Fundamentals of Human Sexuality.* New York, Holt, Rinehart and Winston, Inc., 1972.
20. Klaus, M., and Kennell, J.: *Maternal Infant Bonding.* St. Louis, C. V. Mosby Co., 1976.
20a. Koos, E. L.: *Families in Trouble.* New York, Kings Crown Press, 1946.
21. LeMasters, E. E.: Parenthood as Crisis. *Marriage and Family Living.* November, 1957, p. 352.
22. Lenocker, J., and Daugherty, M.: Adolescent Mothers' Social and Health-Related Interests: Report of a Project for Rural, Black Mothers. *JOGV Nursing, 5*:9, 1976.
23. Liebenberg, B.: Expectant Fathers. *Child and Family, 8*:3, Summer, 1969.
24. Loesch, J., and Greenberg, V.: Some Specific Areas of Conflicts Observed during Pregnancy: A Comparative Study of Married and Unmarried Pregnant Women. *American Journal of Orthopsychiatry, 32*:624, 1962.
25. Marquart, R.: Expectant Fathers: What Are Their Needs? *Men, 1*:32, 1976.
26. Masters, W., and Johnson, V.: *Human Sexual Response.* Boston, Little, Brown and Co., 1966.
27. Mercer, R.: Becoming a Mother at Sixteen. *MCN 1*:44, 1976.
28. Newton, H.: *Maternal Emotions.* New York, Harper Books, 1955.
29. Obeyesekere, G.: Pregnancy Cravings (Dola Duka) in Relation to Social Structure and Personality in a Sinhalese Village. *American Anthropologist, 65*:323, 1963.
30. Parson, T.: *The Social System.* Glencoe, Ill., The Free Press, 1951.
31. Quirk, B., and Hassanein, R.: The Nurse's Role in Advising Patients on Coitus During Pregnancy. *Nursing Clinics of North America, 8*:501, 1973.
32. Rice, E. P.: Social Aspects of Maternity Care. *Obstetrics and Gynecology, 23*:307, 1964.
33. Richardson, L.: Unwed Mother. *American Journal of Nursing, 68*:2617, 1968.
34. Rosengren, W.: Social Sources of Pregnancy as Illness or Normality. *Social Forces, 39*:260, 1961.
35. Rosengren, W.: Social Status, Attitudes toward Pregnancy, and Child Rearing Attitude. *Social Forces, 41*:127, 1962.
36. Rubin, R.: Cognitive Style in Pregnancy. *American Journal of Nursing, 70*:502, 1970.
37. Rubin, R.: Maternal Tasks in Pregnancy. *Maternal-Child Nursing Journal, 4*(3):143, 1975.
38. Sears, R. R., Maccoby, E., and Levine, H.: *Patterns of Child Rearing.* New York, Harper and Row, 1957.
39. Silberg, D., Butler, J., and Wagner, N.: Sexual Behavior in Pregnancy. *New England Journal of Medicine, 288*:1098, 1973.
40. Siler, M.: The Ministry of a Southern Baptist Church to Families at the Event of the Birth of a Child. Unpublished doctoral dissertation. Louisville, Ky., Southern Baptist Theological Seminary, 1967.
41. Solberg, D., Butler, J., and Wagner, N.: Sexual Behavior in Pregnancy. *New England Journal of Medicine, 288*:1098, 1973.
42. Trethowan, W., and Conlon, M.: The Couvade Syndrome. *British Journal of Psychiatry, 111*:57, 1965.
43. Turner, E. K.: The Syndrome in the Infant Resulting from Maternal Emotional Tension During Pregnancy. *The Medical Journal of Australia,* 1956(a), p. 221.
44. Vincent, C.: *Sexual and Marital Health.* New York, McGraw-Hill Book Co., 1973.
45. Wapner, J.: The Attitudes, Feelings, and Behaviors of Expectant Fathers Attending Lamaze Classes. *Birth and the Family Journal, 3*(1):5, 1976.
46. Waters, J.: *The Atlanta Adolescent Pregnancy Program: Program Director's Report.* Atlanta, Emory University School of Medicine, 1971.
47. Ziegel, E., and Van Blarcom, C.: *Obstetric Nursing.* 6th Edition. New York, The Macmillan Co., 1972.

10

The Prenatal Family: Nursing Assessment of the Mother

OBJECTIVES

1. Define
   gravida
   abortion
   nulligravida
   nullipara
   primigravida
   primipara
   multigravida
   multipara
   mean arterial pressure
   Papanicolaou's test
   diagonal conjugate
   true conjugate
   pelvimeter
   intertuberous diameter
   pelvic inlet
   pelvic outlet
2. Identify the goals of the initial assessment.
3. Describe the varied tests used to confirm pregnancy as well as the advantages and disadvantages of each.
4. Identify potential risk factors that may be recognized during psychosocial assessment and the assessment of parent-infant interaction.
5. Explain the purpose of each of the following during pregnancy:
   a. general health history and physical assessment
   b. reproductive history and physical assessment
   c. laboratory studies
   d. nutritional assessment

Objectives continued on page 231

6. Describe the normal rise and fall of blood pressure during the course of pregnancy. Indicate all the signs of hypertension.
7. Identify the bones of the pelvis.
8. Explain the method of measurement, normal dimensions, and significance of the following pelvic measurements:
   a. diagonal conjugate
   b. conjugata vera
   c. intertuberous diameter
   c. posterior sagittal measurement
   e. shape of the suprapubic arch
9. Describe the common pattern of prenatal visits for mothers with no apparent major problems.
10. Identify physical signs in a pregnant woman that indicate a need for immediate further assessment and intervention.
11. Discuss desirable weight gain during pregnancy including the rationale for gaining adequate weight. Describe the distribution of the weight gained in pregnancy.

The nursing process—assessment, planning, intervention, and evaluation—is the framework for care of childbearing families. *Assessment*, beginning at our first contact with the mother and other members of her family, and continuing throughout pregnancy, is the theme of this chapter. Fetal assessment will be discussed in Chapter 14.

The First Contact

Mother and Nurse

Consider the woman coming for her initial maternity examination. She may have only recently missed a menstrual period for the first time, or she may have considered herself pregnant for many months. She may suspect that she is pregnant and that is why she has come, but her pregnancy has probably not been confirmed. Her feelings about the possibility of pregnancy may easily be ambivalent, as noted in Chapter 9. If she has never had an obstetric evaluation, or perhaps even a pelvic examination, she will almost always be anxious and fearful; many mothers show some anxiety at the time of initial examination during second and subsequent pregnancies as well. For many young women this visit may be their first contact with health care since they were children. Childhood fears of nurses and physicians may influence them unconsciously, if not consciously.

We will probably not be able to alleviate all of a woman's anxiety, but we can do a great deal to lessen it by the way in which we interact with her during this first visit. Although there is a great deal that we will be trying to accomplish at this visit, a first essential is allowing adequate time to make each woman feel comfortable in the clinical environment and to give us the opportunity to establish a relationship with her.

The physical environment must be planned so that we can talk with her in some place that assures privacy. An arrangement of furniture that allows nurse and patient to sit facing one another directly is far better than the barrier of a desk between them. Attempting to establish a relationship with a patient in a crowded waiting room or while she is lying on her back on an uncomfortable examining table is poor nursing care.

How can we make a mother more relaxed and comfortable during her first visit? Our approach, our manner, and our "therapeutic use of self" are difficult to codify into a set of rules. We can begin by introducing ourselves by name and by encouraging the woman to tell us something about herself before we begin to deal with specific questions. We want to

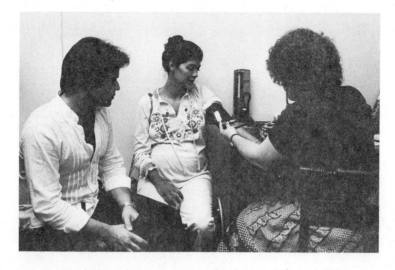

Figure 10–1. Measurement of blood pressure by nurse during prenatal assessment. Note that fathers may wish to be present also. (Courtesy of The Maternity Center Association, New York.)

convey the feeling that she is the focus of our concern at the moment and that we will take the time to answer any questions she may have.

The *goals* of the initial contact are eight:

1. To make the mother feel more comfortable by demonstrating our interest in her as a person and in her concerns, and by explaining to her what will happen during the rest of the initial visit (anticipatory guidance), along with the reason for each phase of the examination (these explanations will be reinforced as each step occurs).

2. To confirm the pregnancy by laboratory testing, if indicated.

3. To assess whether pregnancy is desired.

4. To assess factors in the social, medical, and reproductive history that are pertinent to the course and outcome of this pregnancy.

5. To assess general and reproductive health by physical and laboratory examination.

6. To assess nutritional needs.

7. To assess pertinent social needs.

8. To assess the mother's feelings about the pregnancy and also those of other significant people, usually the baby's father or other family members.

Father and Nurse

Note that we are discussing this first visit in relation to the mother, because many women come to clinics and offices without their husbands. We believe that the ideal situation is one in which both parents come together. Not only will both receive the same information, but we will have the opportunity to assess the needs and feelings of both man and woman. Often our only information about the father comes from the mother; what we hear, of course, is her perception of his feelings and attitudes. Her perception is important because it is a reality for her, but it should not be confused with the father's own perception of his feelings and concerns. In addition, observation of interaction between the couple, only possible if both are present, is important in understanding the couple's response to the pregnancy.

There is no reason why a father should automatically be banished to a waiting room even during the physical examination (Fig. 10–1). Just as many fathers sit at the head of the delivery table, talking with and supporting their wives, fathers can sit at the head of the table during the physical examination and support their wives during this initial assessment. Single mothers who desire to maintain a close relationship with their baby's father should have this same privilege.

Other Family Members

What about the mother of the unmarried daughter who comes with her for her initial visit? Vincent[29] suggests that we remember *who* the patient is, that it is the young woman who is pregnant and not her parents. If one or both of the young woman's parents are present during the initial interview, if indeed they are the major participants, their daughter may see us as an extension of her parents and her parents' attitudes. This may make it difficult for us to establish a relationship with her (see Chapter 9).

Confirmation of Pregnancy

Jokes about pregnancy detection, particularly in old movies, often center on the rabbit test, in which urine from the woman is injected into a rabbit. Human chorionic gonadotropin (HCG), a hormone produced by the syncytiotrophoblast, is found only in the presence of trophoblastic tissue. If a woman is pregnant, the HCG in her urine causes formation of corpora lutea in the ovaries of the test animal.

Biologic tests for pregnancy include the Aschheim-Zondek test, first developed in 1928, which uses mature mice, the Friedman rabbit test, and others using young mice, frogs, and toads. Biologic tests are almost never used today.

HCG, discussed in Chapter 6, is the basis for contemporary pregnancy testing. Three types of testing, the urine agglutination-inhibition test, a radioreceptor assay, and a radioimmunoassay, are used.

The agglutination-inhibition test utilizes (1) antiserum against HCG, prepared by producing an antibody response in animals; (2) antigen, which consists of latex particles coated with HCG; and (3) urine from the mother.

There are two steps in pregnancy testing. In the first step, if urine from a woman containing HCG is exposed to anti-HCG serum, the HCG in the urine will combine with the antiserum and form a bond. In the second step, sheep cells coated with HCG (the antigen) are then added to this solution. If HCG has already bonded with the antiserum, the antigen will have no cells with which to bond and thus will not agglutinate (clump). The test is positive. In a negative test, the woman's urine will not contain HCG, and therefore when the antigen is added, the antigen cells will bond with the antiserum and agglutinate.

In order to reduce false positive results to less than 5 per cent, the lower limit of detection is set so that HCG of less than 1000 to 2000 ml U/ml will not be detected. This means that pregnancy will not be detected until the sixth week after the last menstrual period (the fourth week after conception). Some clinics ask that women miss two menstrual periods before testing to reduce the likelihood of a false negative test.

Urine for testing should be collected in a clean urine specimen container; any substance in the container (such as a jar of urine brought from home) could cause an inaccurate, falsely positive test.

Radioreceptor assay and β-subunit radioimmunoassay tests utilize serum rather than urine. The radioreceptor assay measures the ability of the blood sample to inhibit the binding of radiolabeled HCG to receptors.[21] Only 100 to 200 ml U/ml of HCG are required, and thus the test is far more sensitive and may be performed as soon as a menstrual period is missed (the second week after conception). The radioreceptor assay does not distinguish HCG from luteinizing hormone, which may be disadvantageous. One hour is required for the test.

Still more sensitive is the measurement of the β-subunit of HCG through radioimmunoassay. Because only 5 to 10 ml U/ml of HCG are required, the test may be diagnostic as early as 8 to 9 days after ovulation, before a menstrual period has been missed. Maternal serum HCG (unlabeled) and HCG that has been radioactively bound to antibody (labeled) compete for binding sites. The higher the concentration of HCG in the mother's serum, the greater the number of binding sites that will be occupied by the unlabeled HCG. The one disadvantage of radioimmunoassay is the time required (12 to 24 hours) for results to be obtained.

If pregnancy is suspected but the urine agglutination-inhibition test is negative, a positive β-subunit radioimmunoassay test may mean that (1) it is too early in the pregnancy to detect HCG, or (2) there has been a prior pregnancy in the recent past. In serum, HCG may be detected up to 4 weeks following an abortion.

A persistently low level of HCG may indicate an ectopic pregnancy or an intrauterine pregnancy in which the placenta is abnormal.

Home Pregnancy Testing

Beginning in 1976 and accelerating markedly in 1978, home pregnancy testing kits have become a multimillion dollar industry in the United States. Home pregnancy testing kits are urine agglutination-inhibition tests. On the basis of limited clinical data, the Food and

Table 10–1. PREGNANCY TESTING

Method	Specimen	Period of Gestation (Time Since Last Menstrual Period)	Time Required for Test
Agglutination-inhibition	Urine	6 weeks	2 minutes
Radioreceptorassay	Serum	4 weeks	1 hour
Radioimmunoassay	Serum	3 + weeks	12–24 hours

Drug Administration has determined that the manufacturers' claims that home pregnancy testing kits are 95 to 98 per cent reliable are valid.[15]

Women who use home pregnancy testing kits should be aware of the following information:

1. Product accuracy claims are based on tests done approximately 15 days after the last menstrual period, although the kits advertise diagnosis of pregnancy as early as 7 to 9 days following the last menstrual period.

2. Urine should be clear, "strawlike" in color, and without particles. If urine is cloudy and appears to contain blood or other material, the woman should have a health evaluation for possible causes. In addition, pregnancy testing will not be accurate.

3. Because the HCG level is usually very low in the early weeks of ectopic pregnancy (pregnancy outside the uterus—Chapter 10), home pregnancy testing frequently will not detect ectopic pregnancy.

4. Factors that can alter results include
   a. detergent or dirt in the urine container;
   b. movement, including vibration from a refrigerator or air conditioner or children running through the room;
   c. placing the container in direct sunlight;
   d. improper timing; evaluating the test too early or too late.

Women should be encouraged to seek health care immediately when a home pregnancy test is positive. A second test will be done in the health care facility to confirm pregnancy.

Assessment: Is Pregnancy Desired? The confirmation of pregnancy is a joyous moment for some women, a time of mixed emtions for others, and a source of distress to still others. Failure to confirm pregnancy also has varying meanings for individual women. The meaning of pregnancy is assessed for each woman so that appropriate counseling can be provided. A model incorporating various alternatives is found in Figure 10–8 at the end of this chapter.

Psychosocial Assessment

Psychosocial assessment, like physical assessment, begins by gathering a data base at the first prenatal visit. Table 10–2 lists some basic questions that may be included in the initial data, along with some of the risk factors that may be associated with those questions.

Once the basic assessment is completed, potential problems can be identified and re-

corded, along with physical data, so that intervention can occur or referral can be made.

Horsley[13] has developed a system by which points are assigned to various risk factors. Two points are given for the following: unmarried mother, attempted abortion or miscarriage, bereavement during this pregnancy, no emotional support, no financial support, and isolation. One point is accorded for: old for childbearing, shotgun wedding, relative infertility, serious illness or abnormality, maternal or sibling obstetric complications, broken home in childhood, economic insecurity, or concealed fears.

Horsley considers mothers with 0 or 1 point as being at low risk of severe emotional stress in pregnancy; two points indicate a high risk mother, and three or more points a very high risk mother. Such an evaluation does not indicate that attention to the emotional needs of the *low* risk or *no* risk mothers is not important but that special attention is necessary for mothers recognized as being at high risk.

A potential risk factor must be evaluated within the total context of each woman's life. For example, a woman who has no communication with her parents, or whose parents are dead, may lack other support systems or may have many other sources of support. The potential problem is a red flag that says, "Explore this further!" (See also Assessment of Potential Parent-Infant Interaction, below.)

Health History Assessment

A mother with a lifelong history of good physical and mental health is far more likely to have a healthy pregnancy with a successful outcome than is the mother with a chronic disease or frequent acute illnesses. Just as healthy mothers produce healthy babies, healthy babies, with proper care, are likely to grow to become healthy parents. Unfortunately, the opposite is also true. Mothers who are not healthy produce babies who are less likely to be healthy and who will grow to be parents who are not healthy. Generation after generation of poor or marginal health is hard to correct during the months of pregnancy. Good health (and good health care) prior to conception and in the period between pregnancies could probably improve pregnancy outcome for many mothers. Those of us who are concerned about the outcome of pregnancy need to focus attention on both research and designs for care during these periods, as well as during pregnancy itself.

Table 10–2. PSYCHOSOCIAL ASSESSMENT

Data	Potential Risk Factors

MARITAL STATUS
1. Married, single, separated, divorced, widowed
2. Date of marriage
3. Husband's age, health, occupation, employed or unemployed
4. Husband's attitude about pregnancy
5. Separation due to:
  a. Frequent need to travel (husband)
  b. Absent in military service
  c. Desertion
	1. Single parent, bereavement, potential lack of emotional support
	2. Shotgun wedding
	3. Disparity in age, stress of illness in family, economic problems
	4. Source of conflict
	5. Potential lack of emotional support

FAMILY HISTORY 1. Parents' ages, health; siblings' ages, health 2. Death, divorce, remarriage of parents 3. Relationship with mother, father 4. Obstetric problems of female relatives 5. Communication with parents	1. Familial illness, stress of current family illness, fear of hereditary problem 2. Broken home, bereavement 3. Effect on perceptions of parent role 4. Fear of complications 5. Isolation
CURRENT PREGNANCY 1. Planned/unplanned 2. How long attempting to conceive	1. Either may be associated with psychosocial risks but of different type (see text) 2. Relative infertility
STATUS OF MOTHER 1. Employed: plans for continuation of employment 2. Feelings about bodily changes* 3. Physical symptoms* 4. Relationship to fetus (see Table 10–6)	1. Economic problems, baby as interference in career plans 2. Denial of bodily changes 3. Possible relationship between marked physical symptoms and attitudes and feelings

*Depending on the stage of pregnancy during which initial assessment takes place, may not be evident until later.

General Health History

Some disease states are known to have specific effects on pregnancy; they include diabetes mellitus, chronic hypertension, severe anemias and other blood dyscrasias, obesity, heart disease (including a past history of rheumatic fever), and venereal disease. A family history of certain of these conditions, diabetes mellitus for example, will alert us to the possibility that the disease itself may appear during pregnancy, even though it has not been previously detected. Pregnancy may have a deleterious effect on some of the mother's health problems. The mother with valvular damage from rheumatic fever may have difficulty because of the increased cardiac workload of pregnancy.

Other factors in the general health history that should be noted include urinary tract disease; chronic lung problems such as asthma, emphysema, and tuberculosis; ulcers; phlebitis; varicosities; thyroid disease; hepatitis; gallbladder problems; seizure disorders; allergies and drug sensitivities; and major surgery or accidents.

Note should be made of what immunizations the woman has had, particularly for rubella (Chapter 8). In women who are not sure whether they have had either rubella or rubella immunization the rubella titer should be evaluated. Rubella vaccine is not given to women who are pregnant. Any medications taken by the mother, either self-prescribed or prescribed by a physician, must be noted and evaluated, as should the use of alcohol, caffeine, cigarettes, and illegal drugs (Chapter 8).

Reproductive History

In addition to general health, reproductive health is assessed during the initial visit. Menstrual history includes the date of menarche (i.e., the onset of menstruation), a description

Nursing Care Plan 10–1. Initial Prenatal Visit*

NURSING GOALS:
To assist the woman who is pregnant in entry into the health care system

OBJECTIVES: At the completion of the first prenatal visit the woman who is pregnant will:
1. Begin to develop a trust relationship with her care providers
2. Begin to understand her responsibilities in regard to pregnancy and self-care
3. Be informed of her health and psychosocial status as it relates to her pregnancy
4. Receive guidance regarding physical and emotional aspects of the childbearing experience
5. Begin to understand the role of the care provider
6. Be informed of resources available to her during the childbearing experience

ASSESSMENT	POTENTIAL NURSING DIAGNOSIS	NURSING INTERVENTION	COMMENTS/RATIONALE
A. Initial contact (usually by phone)	Need for information about entry into the health care system for prenatal care	Determine reason for contact	
		Schedule appointment time that is convenient for client and care provider	
		Determine approximate estimated date of conception (EDC)	
		Ask that urine specimen (1st A.M. voided) be brought for pregnancy test, if needed	Urine specimen should be refrigerated after it is collected
		Answer immediate questions, if asked	
		Discuss financial arrangements, if desired	Cost discussion promotes informed consent
		Restate appointment date and time	
		Encourage client to bring support person, if desired	
B. Initial visit	Need for information about health care activities during pregnancy	See at appointed time. Introduce self and other staff, care provider	Begins trust relationship. Informed consent promotes trust
	Need for information about own rights and responsibilities and those of care provider	Describe activities for this visit (i.e., pregnancy test, intake interview, history, physical exam, laboratory procedures)	
		Explain clinic (office) visits: Up to 28 wks—every 4 weeks. 28–36 wks.—every 2 wks. 36 wks. to delivery— every wk.	
		Determine EDC based on subjective data (i.e., last menstrual period, last normal menstrual period)	
		Explain "weeks of gestation"	
		Determine need for information regarding alternatives to pregnancy if indicated	Provide abortion counseling or referral, if indicated
1. Subjective data	Need for information about relationship of assessment factors and pregnancy course and outcome	May be collected by interview or by form provided to client	Determine client's reliability. May need to include support person in data collection
a. Family history—parents, siblings, "blood" relatives (1) health status			

Nursing Care Plan 10–1. Initial Prenatal Visit* (*Continued*)

ASSESSMENT	POTENTIAL NURSING DIAGNOSIS	NURSING INTERVENTION	COMMENTS/RATIONALE
(2) history of TB, cancer, diabetes, vascular disease, neuromuscular disease, allergies, multiple gestations, deformities, congenital diseases		If form used, clarify any questionable areas and record as needed	
b. Client's past medical history (1) age (2) racial origin (3) ethnic background (4) Childhood diseases and other illnesses and diseases (5) surgical procedures (6) Gynecologic history—infections; age of menarche; regularity, flow, and duration of menses; history of dysmenorrhea; contraceptive history			Black race—screen for sickle cell trait or disease. Jewish race—screen for Tay-Sachs syndrome.
c. Past obstetric history (1) number of pregnancies and outcome (2) history of previous pregnancies including any complications—antepartum, intrapartum, postpartum			
d. Current pregnancy (1) date of last menstrual period (and last normal menstrual period) (2) presence of cramping, spotting, bleeding (3) attitude toward pregnancy. Partner's attitude (4) Weight—usual and prepregnant (5) Medications taken since pregnant (6) Alcohol, drug, tobacco use (7) allergies (drug, food, etc.) (8) exposure to teratogens (viral infections, x-ray, pollutants) (9) presence of any abnormal symptoms (10) other concerns client may have about own history and condition			
e. Father's history (1) presence of genetic conditions or diseases (2) age (3) significant health problems (4) previous or present alcohol intake (5) blood type and Rh (if known)			
f. Personal information (1) educational level (2) cultural patterns (3) religious beliefs (if they have implications for health care)			

	Nursing Care Plan 10–1.	Initial Prenatal Visit* (*Continued*)	
ASSESSMENT	**POTENTIAL NURSING DIAGNOSIS**	**NURSING INTERVENTION**	**COMMENTS/RATIONALE**

(4) economic status
(5) support systems
(6) coping mechanisms
2. Objective data
  a. Physical examination
    (1) temperature, pulse, respirations, BP, weight, and height
    (2) general appearance, skin
    (3) head, eyes, ears, nose, throat
    (4) chest, lungs, heart, breasts
    (5) abdomen
    (6) extremities
    (7) neuromuscular reflexes
    (8) pelvic examination
      (a) vulva, perineum, vaginal discharge, vaginal muscle tone
      (b) uterus, cervix, adnexa, height of fundus
      (c) rectovaginal exam
      (d) clinical pelvimetry measurements
	Need for information about relationship of assessment data to pregnancy status
	
	Need for information about examination procedures and their purpose
	
	Discomfort, pain, or anxiety related to diagnostic procedures
		Instruct client in preparing for exam. Promote relaxation and participation
		
		Assist care provider as needed
		
		Provide privacy
			Physical exam and laboratory tests may be delayed until another day. Intake process may be exhausting and informational overload can easily occur

b. Laboratory tests
    (1) chest x-ray or tine test
    (2) cervical smears—Pap and GC
    (3) blood—VDRL, Hg6, hematocrit, type, Rh, sickle cell (if indicated)
    (4) urinalysis—glucose, albumin, microscopic, culture, and sensitivity if indicated
    (5) rubella titer
    (6) antibody screen
    (7) sickle cell screen (if indicated)
		Collect specimens as needed
		
		Provide information to client as needed
			If Pap smear done within past 3 months it may be omitted. Obtain results for record

of usual periods (interval, duration, amount of flow), and the date of the last menstrual period. Any gynecologic problems or surgery should be noted.

Certain specific terms are used to describe reproductive history. *Gravida* refers to the number of times a woman has been pregnant, regardless of the outcome of the pregnancy.

Para refers to the number of pregnancies that last beyond 20 weeks; it does not refer to the number of infants born. A woman who is para III has had three pregnancies that lasted at least 20 weeks. She may have more than three children; multiple births, such as twins, are counted as a single pregnancy. She may have no living children if, for example, she delivered three stillborn infants after 20 weeks of pregnancy.

The following terms are used:

Abortion: a pregnancy that terminated prior to the twentieth week (miscarriage).

Nulligravida: a woman who has never been pregnant.

Nullipara: a woman who has never delivered a viable infant (legally an infant of 20 weeks' gestation or more).

Primigravida: a women during her first pregnancy (gravida I, para 0).

Primipara: a woman who has delivered one viable infant (gravida I, para I).

Multigravida: a woman pregnant for the second or subsequent time (gravida II, para I).

		Nursing Care Plan 10–1. Initial Prenatal Visit* (Continued)	
ASSESSMENT	**POTENTIAL NURSING DIAGNOSIS**	**NURSING INTERVENTION**	**COMMENTS/RATIONALE**

3. Informational needs assessment
  a. personal hygiene
  b. diet
  c. rest and exercise
  d. dental care
  e. use of medications
	Need for information about course of pregnancy and effects
	
	Anxiety related to changes occurring during pregnancy
		Provide information as needed
		
		May need to anticipate some needs and provide guidance as indicated
		
		Encourage client to take vitamin and iron preparations if prescribed.
		
		Discourage use of non-prescribed and over-the-counter medications
			Written instructions are very helpful and can be reviewed at home when anxiety level has decreased

f. minor discomforts of pregnancy (see Nursing Care Plan 11–1)
  g. emotional responses to pregnancy
  h. danger signs of pregnancy
    (1) vaginal bleeding
    (2) persistent vomiting
    (3) chills and fever
    (4) sudden loss of fluid from vagina
    (5) abdominal pain
  i. fetal growth and development
  j. resources available to the pregnant family
		Encourage support person's participation in discussions
		
		Provide information about community resources as needed or requested.	

C. Subsequent prenatal visits (see Nursing Care Plan 10–2)		Review routine visits, schedule next appointment Provide phone number and information about after hours calls Encourage open communications	

*Contributed by Elizabeth K. Dickson.

Multipara: a woman who has delivered two or more viable infants (gravida II, para, II, etc.).

In practice, one may hear the terms primigravida and primipara interchanged, as well as the terms multigravida and multipara. For example, a woman pregnant for the second time (gravida II, para I) is often referred to as a multipara.

Each pregnant woman, thus, is described briefly as gr____, p____, a____. A woman pregnant for the fifth time who has had two miscarriages and two pregnancies that lasted beyond 20 weeks, one of which resulted in a stillborn infant and one of which resulted in a live infant, would be described as gr V, p II, a II.

An alternate system has been suggested, using four digits—first digit: full term deliveries; second digit: premature deliveries; third digit: abortions; and fourth digit: living children. Thus 2102 would mean two full-term deliveries, one premature birth, no abortions, and two living children. This system gives more information than the system in common use.

It is equally important to know if the mother had complications during a previous pregnancy and if she had any pregnancy terminated by induced abortion.

Factors in a mother's reproductive history that suggest the possibility of a problem during pregnancy or the birth of a high risk infant include:

1. Two or more consecutive spontaneous abortions.
2. A previous perinatal death.
3. Previous premature labor.
4. Five or more pregnancies.
5. Previous cesarean section.
6. Multiple pregnancy (twins, triplets, and so on).
7. A previous baby with a major congenital anomaly.
8. Rh_D incompatibility in a previous pregnancy.
9. A previous baby weighing 4000 grams or more.
10. A previous baby with intrauterine growth retardation.
11. Two or more years of infertility.

In addition to the mother's own reproductive health, some aspects of reproductive health in other members of her family—mother, aunts, sisters—may also be significant. For example, if there have been frequent miscarriages in her family, there may be some genetic basis. If several women relatives have had cesarean delivery because of a small pelvis, she may share this characteristic. She may not know why they have had a cesarean birth but may report that all women in her family have had cesarean deliveries.

Physical Assessment

General Health

Key factors in the general physical examination include assessment of height and weight, temperature, pulse, blood pressure, heart, lungs, and abdomen. Although this examination is ideally performed early in pregnancy, in reality it may occur at almost any time, so it is important to try to establish the prepregnancy weight as well as the weight at the time of the examination. In general, mothers who weigh less than 100 pounds or more than 250 pounds prior to pregnancy are at higher risk for problems (Chapter 12). Each woman's weight must be evaluated in relation to her height.

Evidence of heart disease or thyroid disease may be noted on physical examination, even though no previous history has been reported.

An examination of the teeth and gums should be included in the general physical examination, not as a substitute for an evaluation by a dentist but to emphasize the importance of dental care during pregnancy. Because many women believe that dental care is con-

traindicated during pregnancy, this brief check-up gives us the opportunity to assure them that this is not true. For patients unable to afford private dental care, appropriate referral should be made.

Assessment of Blood Pressure

Blood pressure evaluation will be important throughout pregnancy. Early identification and correction of hypertension are essential if serious problems are to be averted.

Although the assessment of blood pressure has been a part of the care of women in all phases of childbearing for many years, failure to recognize such factors as the effect of maternal position on blood pressure results in inaccurate assessment. Brachial artery pressure is highest when the woman is in a sitting position; it is considerably lower when she is in the lateral recumbent position. In the supine position, blood pressure is lower for some women than in the lateral recumbent position (supine hypotensive syndrome, Chapter 6) but higher for other women. It is recommended that blood pressure be assessed in either the lateral recumbent or the sitting position; thus the position should always be noted on the chart along with the blood pressure.

In addition to position, maternal anxiety is another factor that affects blood pressure. Blood pressure is frequently assessed upon arrival at the clinic, office, or hospital when anxiety is highest. Allowing the mother time to rest and to become more comfortable may result in more accurate measurement. If blood pressure is elevated, it should be rechecked after a period of time in which the mother is helped to relax.

Utilizing a cuff of the proper size (approximately 20 per cent wider than the diameter of the arm) and wrapping the cuff snugly around the arm are basic principles of blood pressure measurement that apply to childbearing women as well as to all other persons.

In addition to routine assessment two screening tests, the evaluation of mean arterial pressure and the roll-over test, are noninvasive and simple to perform.

Recent studies have shown that *mean arterial pressure* has value in predicting which mothers are likely to have hypertension. Normally, mean arterial pressure reaches its lowest point about 22 weeks after the last menstrual period and then rises slowly until term (Chapter 7).

In a prospective study of 710 women carried out in several different clinics, the *roll-over test* was found to be a good predictor of pregnancy-induced hypertension (Chapter 13).[8] The roll-over test is performed at 28 to 32 weeks' gestation. A gravida first lies in the left lateral position, and her blood pressure is measured until it is stable. She then turns to her back, and blood pressure is again measured. If there is an increase of 20 to 30 mm Hg in systolic pressure or 15 to 20 mm Hg in diastolic pressure, the test is considered positive, and the likelihood of later hypertension is significantly increased.

Interpretation of Blood Pressure. As noted in Chapter 7, changes in blood pressure are a part of maternal adaptation to pregnancy. Interpretation of blood pressure measurement is related to (1) absolute value, (2) length of gestation, and (3) relation to pattern throughout pregnancy.

1. Absolute Values. A systolic blood pressure of greater than 140 mm Hg or a diastolic blood pressure of greater than 90 mm Hg indicates hypertension.

2. Length of Gestation. A mean arterial pressure greater than 90 mm Hg in the second trimester or greater than 105 mm Hg in the third trimester is associated with an increased risk of hypertension in the third trimester.

3. Relation to Pattern Throughout Pregnancy. An increase in systolic blood pressure of 30 mm Hg or more over the base line as assessed in early pregnancy, or an increase in diastolic blood pressure of 15 mm Hg or more is considered significant even if the evaluation

is lower than the criteria given above. Therefore, individual assessments must always be compared with previous assessments.

Breast Examination

Careful examination of the breasts provides an opportunity for evaluation and for some beginning instruction in self-examination. Because breast changes begin early in pregnancy, we can assure the mother that the increased size and tenderness, the darkening of the areola, and so forth, are normal. We will want to observe the protrusion of the nipples (are they protruding, flat, or inverted?), the general contour of the breasts, and the presence of any lumps or painful areas.

Laboratory Studies

Significant laboratory studies include urinalysis, a complete blood count, blood typing and Rh determination, a serologic test for syphilis, and both a smear for gonorrhea and a Papanicolaou smear.

Urinalysis for the detection of asymptomatic bacteriuria, glucose, and protein is an important part of prenatal assessment. Urine is generally collected by the clean-catch technique (Table 10–3). While urethral catheterization produces fewer false positive (contami-

Table 10–3. COLLECTING A CLEAN-CATCH URINE SPECIMEN

Equipment needed	Comments
Sponges with green soap	
Sponges with sterile distilled water	
Sterile container for urine	
Technique (as explained to woman)	
1. Wash your hands thoroughly and dry them.	
2. Prepare soap and sterile water sponges as directed and place where easily accessible.	Do not use soap containing pHisoHex or Benzalkonium; antibacterial action will influence culture results.
3. Sit on toilet. Separate labia (lips) with one hand and keep open until specimen is obtained.	
4. Wash from front to back with soap sponge. Rinse with water sponge.	Failure to rinse soap will affect results of test.
5. Pass a small amount of urine into toilet.	Clears urethral canal of any contaminated urine.
6. Hold specimen container without touching rim. Pass a small amount of urine into container.	
7. Finish urinating and wash hands. Give container to nurse, handling with care.	
Technique (nurse handling specimen)	
1. Culture immediately or refrigerate.	Specimens not refrigerated are of no value after 2 hours.

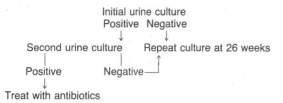

Figure 10–2. Screening for asymptomatic bacteriuria. As noted in Chapter 6, glycosuria is increased during pregnancy; glycosuria fluctuates markedly and appears to bear little relation to levels of serum glucose. Protein in the urine may be a sign of pre-eclampsia (Chapter 13).

nated) specimens, the risk of introducing infection is considered to be 2 to 6 per cent at a single catheterization[17] and thus is rarely done. Suprapubic aspiration of the urinary bladder is occasionally utilized when repeated bacterial counts are equivocal or when anaerobic organisms are suspected.[18] Obtaining the urine specimen affords an excellent opportunity to review personal hygiene with each woman, emphasizing the importance of always wiping the vulva from "front to back" to prevent infection.

Asymptomatic bacteriuria is the presence of a single species of bacteria with a concentration equal to or greater than 100,000 organisms per milliliter (or 10^5/ml) of urine on two consecutive cultures. The dip-slide method (Bacturcult) is simple, accurate, and inexpensive. A variety of other methods are reviewed by Mocarski (1980).

In 90 per cent of positive cultures, *Escherichia coli* is the causative organism; other organisms include *Klebsiella-Enterobacter, Proteus*, and *Enterococcus*. If the initial culture is negative, reculture at the beginning of the third trimester is suggested. If the the first test is positive, a second urinalysis is performed. If the second culture is positive, antibiotic treatment is started. If the second culture is negative, a repeat culture at the beginning of the third trimester is advised (Fig. 10–2).

Blood Tests.   Iron deficiency anemia is the most common nutritional complication of pregnancy. All mothers should have a complete blood count, including hemoglobin and hematocrit, during their initial prenatal visit. Norms for these indices are summarized in Table 10–4. The slight decrease in the norms for hemo-

globin and hematocrit during pregnancy reflects expanded blood volume; the number of red cells is actually increased. When values fall below these levels, further studies are important to discover the reason for anemia. In addition to iron deficiency anemia, the mother may have megaloblastic anemia due to folate deficiency (fairly common in combination with iron deficiency anemia) or she may have anemia due to blood loss or infection, hemolytic anemia, or anemia due to other causes.

Black women should be tested for sickle cell disease or sickle cell trait.

The mother's blood type and Rh status are determined to identify those mothers who are potentially at risk for problems of Rh and ABO incompatibility. Should the mother be Rh negative and the father Rh positive, antibody titers will be followed throughout pregnancy (Chapter 13).

A laboratory test for tuberculosis is frequently performed, and cases may be discovered in this way, probably because pregnancy is the first contact the mother has with the health care system in a number of years.

Venereal Disease Testing.   Since both syphilis and gonorrhea affect the fetus and the newborn infant, a serologic test for syphilis and a vaginal smear for gonorrhea should be part of the initial examination of all pregnant women. The laws of many states require testing for syphilis, both during pregnancy and prior to marriage. (See Sexually Transmitted Diseases, below.)

Papanicolaou Test.   The Papanicolaou test (Pap smear) for cervical cancer, introduced by Papanicolaou and Traut in 1943, is an important part of the prenatal examination because for many women pregnancy may be their only contact with health care during this period of their lives. Ideally, Pap smears should be performed each year for women over 18 years old and for young women who are sexually active. After 35 years of age a semiannual test is often recommended. Moreover, it is not enough to perform the test; we need to explain its purpose and the importance of annual tests to each woman. Because of the strong emotions of most women during this initial examination, which may interfere with learning, our teaching needs to be reinforced at a later date.

The test consists of "scraping" the ectocervix,

Table 10–4.   NORMAL RED BLOOD CELL VALUES

	Nonpregnant	Pregnant
Hemoglobin	>12 grams/100 ml	>11 grams/100 ml.
Hematocrit	>36%	>33%

the endocervix, and the vaginal pool in the posterior fornix with a wooden spatula and spreading the material obtained on slides that are then sprayed with a fixative. Analysis of the cervical scrapings is about 98 per cent accurate in detecting cervical dysplasia, carcinoma in situ, and invasive cancer. Analysis of the vaginal pool scrapings is about 75 per cent accurate in detecting adenocarcinoma of the endometrium and will detect cancer of the ovary 25 per cent of the time. Certain vaginal infections can also be recognized.

Pap specimens were originally grouped into five classes: today they may be described rather than classified, but many institutions still report in terms of these classifications:

Class I: Absence of atypical or abnormal cells.

Class II: Atypical cytology but no evidence of malignancy.

Class III: Cytology suggestive of, but not conclusive for, malignancy.

Class IV: Cytology strongly suggestive of malignancy.

Class V: Cytology conclusive for malignancy.

Evaluation of the External and Internal Genitalia

Many women dread examination of their genitalia, in part because of lifelong conditioning that tells them (and us) that genitalia should not be exposed, and in part because of the fear of discomfort or the experience of discomfort during a previous examination. In some parts of the world pelvic examinations are not performed during pregnancy or are performed only by women. Because of these feelings, many women fear and even postpone an initial pregnancy examination.

How can we support and reassure women in preparation for a vaginal examination? As already noted, we can explain what will happen and why. We can give them an opportunity to express their fears and bring them into the open by a statement such as, "Many women have told me that they do not look forward to a vaginal exam. How are you feeling about it right now?" We can assure them of our presence during the examination. We can drape them to provide minimum exposure. Examining-room furniture can be placed so that the woman does not lie facing in the direction of a door that could possibly be opened during the examination. The number of people in the room can be minimized, a somewhat difficult task in a teaching clinic of a large medical center but not impossible with good planning. Techniques of relaxation, breathing, and fo-

cusing that are helpful to mothers during labor are also valuable in making mothers more comfortable during examinations (Chapter 12).

An empty bladder is essential before the examination begins. Examination of the external genitalia includes inspection for the presence of a cystocele or rectocele (Chapter 4) and palpation of Bartholin's glands and the urethra. The character of any vaginal discharge is noted. Although there is normally an increase in vaginal discharge late in pregnancy (Chapter 11), certain types of discharge are characteristic of sexually transmitted diseases (see below).

The vaginal speculum, used for the internal examination, is always warmed before insertion. The cervix is examined through the speculum (Chapter 4). After the speculum is removed, two gloved, lubricated fingers are inserted into the vagina for palpation of size, shape, and consistency of the uterus. With the middle finger in the rectum and the index

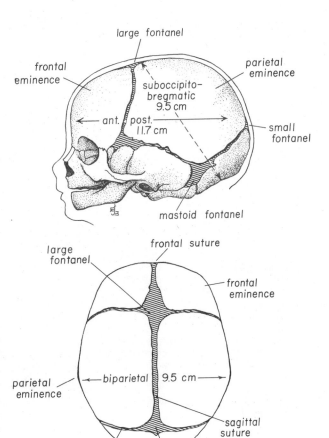

Figure 10–3. Average measurements of the full-term fetal head. (From Page, Villee, and Villee: *Human Reproduction: Essentials of Reproductive and Perinatal Medicine.* 3rd Edition. Philadelphia, W. B. Saunders Co., 1981.)

Table 10–5.   MAJOR PELVIC MEASUREMENTS

Measure	Area Measured	Method	Normal Measure	Comment
True conjugate (conjugata vera)	Upper margin of symphysis pubis to sacral promontory (Fig. 10–4)	Subtract 1.5 to 2.0 cm. from diagonal conjugate measurement (below).	11 cm.	Can not be measured directly.
Diagonal conjugate	Inferior margin of symphysis pubis to sacral promontory	First two fingers in vagina until tip of 2nd finger touches sacral promontory (Fig. 10–5). Point at which lower margin of symphysis pubis rests on finger is marked with fingernail and measured.	12.5 cm.	Examiner must know own reach. Not all examiners will be able to reach sacral promontory; record "diagonal conjugate reached at 12.0 cm." or "diagonal conjugate not reached at 11.5 cm." May be uncomfortable for patient; reassure.
Intertuberous diameter	Plane of the outlet. Distance between ischial tuberosities	Measured with pelvimeter (Fig. 10–6) or with four knuckles of hand.	Should be 9 cm. or greater; average is 11 cm.	Measurement of outlet is best indication of midplane diameters, through which passage may be most difficult.
Posterior sagittal	Distance between midpoint of intertuberous diameter and tip of sacrum	Measured with pelvimeter	7.5 cm.	—
Shape of the suprapubic arch	—	Palpation	Arch should be wide (Fig. 10–7)	A narrow arch, as found in male pelvis, may indicate other characteristics of narrow male pelvis.

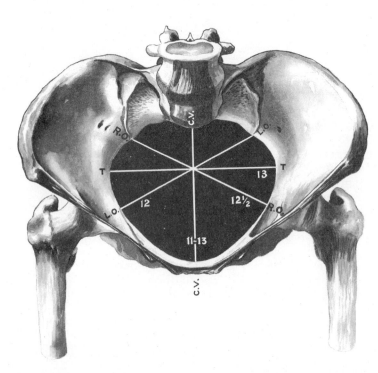

Figure 10–4.   The pelvic inlet. *C. V.,* conjugata vera; *T,* widest transverse; *L.O.,* left oblique; and *R.O.,* right oblique. (From Greenhill and Friedman: *Biological Principles and Modern Practice of Obstetrics.* Philadelphia, W. B. Saunders Co., 1974.)

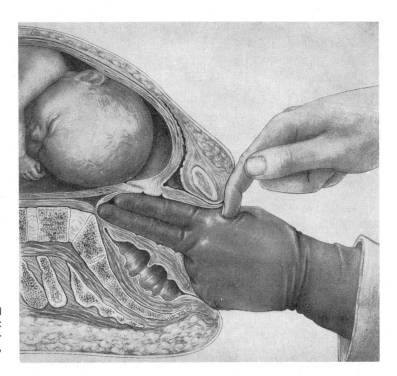

Figure 10–5. Measuring the diagonal conjugate. (From Eastman and Hellman: *Williams Textbook of Obstetrics*. 13th Edition. New York, Appleton-Century-Crofts, 1966.)

finger in the vagina, the examiner palpates the lateral pelvic walls and the parametrial areas.

Evaluation of the Bony Pelvis

For vaginal delivery to be possible, the bony pelvis must be large enough to accommodate the passage of the baby. The pelvis is often evaluated early in pregnancy as an aid for planning delivery. Sometimes measurement of the diagonal conjugate is deferred until the vagina and perineum become more elastic at midpregnancy. Evaluation of pelvic capacity can be repeated near term when fetal size can also be estimated.

Three areas, the inlet, the midpelvis, and the outlet, must be adequate for the descent of the fetal head. The two largest diameters of the head in the flexed position, in which it usually passes through the pelvis, are the biparietal and the suboccipitobregmatic (Fig. 10–3). Both of these diameters measure approximately 9.5 cm. in a fetus weighing approximately 3400 grams (7.5 pounds).

The major measure of the pelvic inlet is the *diagonal conjugate*. From this measure the true conjugate is estimated (Table 10–5 and Figures 10–4 to 10–7). The average measure of the true conjugate, 11 cm., is adequate for the 9.5 cm. fetal head.

Direct measurement of the midpelvis is possible only by x-ray; because of the danger of radiation to the fetus, x-ray is usually deferred until the time of labor. Such x-ray is necessary only when there is a question about the adequacy of the pelvis for delivery. During vaginal examination, however, the examiner can feel the prominence of the ischial spines, the way in which the walls of the pelvis slope, the curve of the sacrum, and the width of the sacrosciatic notch.

The outlet is measured by the distance between the ischial tuberosities, which averages 11 cm. If the distance is 8 cm. or less, the posterior sagittal measurement is particularly important. The sum of the intertuberous and the posterior sagittal measurements should be at least 15 cm. if the pelvis is adequate for vaginal delivery. The mobility of the coccyx, which is pressed back during delivery, and the shape of the suprapubic arch are also noted in the evaluation of the outlet.

Nutritional Assessment

Nutritional assessment begins at the first prenatal visit with evaluation continuing throughout pregnancy. Factors in general and reproductive health that are associated with nutritional status are discussed in Chapter 12 (Table 12–1). Nutritional assessment also includes data about the mother's eating patterns and food preferences, a comparison of her food intake with recommended practices (Chapter 12), evaluation of weight gain, and laboratory evaluation including hemoglobin levels and hematocrit.

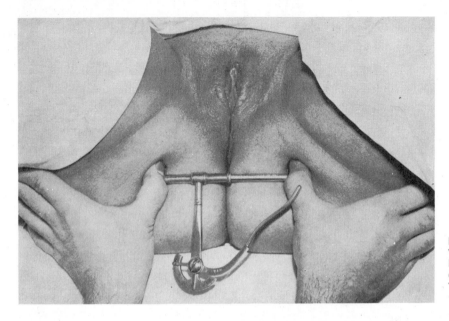

Figure 10–6. Measuring the pelvic outlet with the Thoms pelvimeter. (From Eastman and Hellman: *Williams Textbook of Obstetrics.* 13th Edition. New York, Appleton-Century-Crofts, 1966.)

Assessment of Feelings

Chapter 7 has described many feelings of pregnant women and their partners. The myths of our culture suggest that women should be happy that they are pregnant, although studies indicate that both women and men may be at least initially ambivalent and that some may continue to have mixed feelings or be unhappy through much of their pregnancy. Certainly many other women and couples accept the idea of pregnancy and the birth of their child with joy.

Since few of us are going to share deep feelings with strangers, the verbal expression of feelings about pregnancy during an initial visit may be infrequent. Nonverbal cues, such as facial expression and posture, may be helpful but are not as easy to interpret as they will be when we know the woman better.

As noted previously, it is customary to ask if the pregnancy was planned, and the answer may give us some clue about the woman's feelings. However, unplanned pregnancies are not always unwelcome, nor is a planned pregnancy necessarily a happy one (as, for example, a pregnancy planned by a woman to hold a

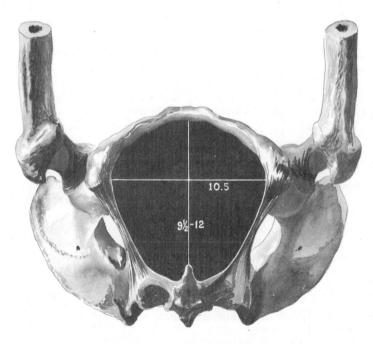

Figure 10–7. The pelvic outlet viewed from below. It passes through the arch of the pubic rami, the ischial tuberosities, and the tip of the coccyx, forming two triangles bent at their mutually shared base, the intertuberous diameter. (From Greenhill and Friedman: *Biological Principles and Modern Practice of Obstetrics.* Philadelphia, W. B. Saunders Co., 1974.)

shaky marriage together). One way to elicit this information in a manner nonthreatening to the patient is to ask if she was using contraceptives at the time that she conceived. Questions about desired family size may also lead to some indication from the mother about her feelings regarding the pregnancy.

Assessment of Potential Parent–Infant Interaction

Even prior to the conception of an infant, factors in the history of the parents may indicate a potential for excellent parenting or for disturbances in parenting. These factors include their beliefs about appropriate methods of child rearing, treatment received when they were themselves children, and individual characteristics of parents.

Because the most familiar model of parenting to most of us is the model set by our own parents, it is important to know something about the expectant parents' perception of the way their parents cared for them. Steele[27a] quotes a mother as saying "babies' butts are built to be busted," a somewhat emphatic version of the widely believed dictum "spare the rod and spoil the child." These parents may not perceive harsh treatment as being extraordinary. Moreover, the harsh treatment they received as children may lead them to believe that they deserved to be so treated, resulting in an image of themselves as unworthy. Gil[9] also found that widespread acceptance of physical discipline was a characteristic of families who abused their children.

Although the maternal or paternal history may not indicate harsh punishment or overt abuse or neglect, the lack of "sympathetic mothering" is felt by Steele[27a] to be more important than any other *single* factor (italics mine). Benedek[1] has repeatedly cited the relationship between mother and infant in the future development of the child; she believes that memories of one's own experience of being a child surge up when the baby is born and influence one's parental behavior.

Because many parents may initially feel ambivalent about pregnancy (Chapter 9), it may be best to defer assessment of attitudes and behavior until after quickening or the beginning of the third trimester. This is a time when many parents have started to make realistic plans for their coming infant: buying items, considering names, and the like.

Gray and her associates[11] suggest the following as "high risk signals" (Table 10–6). No

Table 10–6. HIGH RISK SIGNALS IN THE PRENATAL CLINIC*

A. Overconcern with the unborn baby's sex
B. Expressed high expectations for the baby
C. "Too many" children or children too closely spaced
D. Evidence of the mother's desire to deny the pregnancy
E. Depression over pregnancy
F. Serious consideration of abortion by either parent
G. Consideration of relinquishment by either parent
H. Support systems lacking
I. Evidence that the mother is very frightened
J. Avoidance of eye contact

*After Gray et al., 1976.

single item is considered conclusive, but a combination of these signs, together with observations of affect and an understanding of the sociocultural milieu of the parents, can be of value.

When there is undue concern about the baby's sex, the infant may be expected to fulfill strong needs of the mother, or the mother may feel that she must please the father by giving him a child of the sex he prefers. The expectation that the child must fulfill expectations or needs of the parents may result in abuse or neglect when the infant fails to do so, as he inevitably must, if not in terms of gender then in some other way. This phenomenon, called *role reversal,* is not unusual in reports of parents who abuse or neglect their children.[19]

Indications that the mother may be denying her pregnancy include refusal to gain weight, failure to dress appropriately, and lack of "nesting behavior" such as planning for baby clothes or equipment. Conversation with the mother may also indicate denial of pregnancy.

Signs of depression during pregnancy include sleep disturbances other than those that may be related to the physical discomforts of pregnancy, dropping of many former activities, and lack of affect or attempted suicide. Relating the time of onset of depressive symptoms to the time of pregnancy may be the clue that pregnancy rather than some other factor is the cause of the depression.

If either abortion of relinquishment of the child has been considered, it is important to know why there was a change of mind. Was abortion not performed because the decision was delayed until a therapeutic abortion was no longer possible?

A further characteristic of many families with dysfunction in parent–infant interaction is family isolation. The nuclear family or single mother has few family members and friends upon whom they can rely for help or emotional support. Kennell, Voos, and Klaus[14] suggest that the following questions should be a routine part of the prenatal assessment:

1. How long have you lived in this immediate area?

2. Where does most of your family live?

3. How often do you see your mother or other close relatives? (Noting who accompanies the mother to prenatal visits, if anyone, and whether she is receiving supportive help from any community agencies.)

Parental fears may be a result of lack of understanding of pregnancy; if so, education may help to dispel them. It is deep-seated fear, unrelieved by information, that is considered a high-risk indicator. Signs of such fears may include overdependence on health care professionals, and frequent visits to the emergency room or calls to the clinic or office with complaints for which no organic basis can be found. Such frequent visits may indicate a level of stress felt by the mother. In Elmer's study[5] contrasting mothers of 17 infants who had accidents with 17 infants who were abused (from a sample of 101 infants), five abusive mothers but only one accident mother saw the pregnancy with the index baby as stressful. Objective data from their medical records

showed no difference in complications, indicating that the stress was in the mother's perception.

Sexually Transmitted Diseases: Assessment and Treatment

The significance of certain sexually transmitted diseases (syphilis and herpes simplex type II) in relation to the health of the mother or her infant has been discussed in Chapter 6 and is summarized in Table 10–7. All pregnancy women should be screened for syphilis using blood tests that measure antibody reaction, either the VDRL (Venereal Disease Research Laboratory) test or the newer, more sensitive RPR (rapid plasma reagin) test. Testing is usually performed during the initial prenatal visit and again in the eighth month of pregnancy. If the VDRL or RPR test is positive, the diagnosis is confirmed by the FTA–ABS (fluorescent treponemal antibody absorption) test. This confirmation is important because occasional false positive results occur (1 in 2000) with both the VDRL and RPR tests, particularly following acute infection, mononucleosis, systemic lupus erythematosus, immunization, and exposure to some drugs.

Table 10–7.   SEXUALLY TRANSMITTED DISEASES IMPORTANT IN THE CHILDBEARING CYCLE

Disease	Effect on Pregnancy or Infant	Screening	Treatment During Pregnancy	Mode of Transmission to Infant
Syphilis	Abortion, stillbirth, premature labor; Neonatal syphilis, CNS damage, hearing loss, possible death	Serologic tests	Penicillin	Transplacental contact with active maternal genital lesions
Gonorrhea	Ophthalmia neonatorum	Culture of endocervix	Penicillin–erythromycin base	Mother to infant postnatally
Chlamydia trachomatis infection	Ophthalmia neonatorum, pneumonia in newborn	Gram stain of endocervical smear if symptoms present	Penicillin–erythromycin base	Vaginal tract at time of delivery
Trichomonas vaginitis	Metronidazole (Flagyl), commonly used for treatment, considered potentially teratogenic	Microscopic examination of vaginal discharge (saline wet smear)	During pregnancy only topical agents to relieve symptoms	Uncommon
Candida albicans vaginitis	Thrush in infant if *Candida* present at time of vaginal delivery	KOH slide; Nickerson culture	Monistat, sporostacin, mycostatin	Vaginal tract at time of delivery
Herpes simplex	Abortion, premature labor CNS damage and possible death (75–80 percent if untreated)		No known effective treatment	Vaginal tract at time of delivery (majority); transplacental

If a woman acquires syphilis shortly before, during, or soon after conception and is not treated, fetal infection is nearly certain. The result may be fetal death, premature labor and birth, or congenital syphilis. The spirochetes cross the placenta between the eighteenth week of pregnancy and the time of delivery.

Not every instance of maternal syphilis is detected, and congenital syphilis continues to occur. Reasons include absence of prenatal care, failure to perform the screening test, failure to treat the mother after a positive test, and infection or reinfection after the initial testing.

Penicillin (2.4 million units of benzathine penicillin G divided in two equal doses) is the treatment for primary and secondary syphilis in the first 16 weeks of pregnancy. After 16 weeks aqueous procaine penicillin, 2.4 million units, is given on alternate days for a total of six doses.[20] If the mother is allergic to penicillin, erythromycin is used. Although tetracycline is given in place of penicillin for treatment of syphilis in nonpregnancy women, it is not recommended during pregnancy because it is widely deposited in the fetal skeleton and teeth and may cause inhibition of bone growth and discoloration of fetal teeth. Since the efficacy of drugs other than penicillin in the treatment of syphilis has not been established, careful documentation of penicillin allergy is important.

After the pregnant woman has been treated for syphilis, she should have monthly serologic tests for the remainder of pregnancy. Many months may elapse before a negative serology is obtained (245 days is the average), but some drop in titer should be evident. (This is why a mother may come to delivery with a positive test for syphilis, yet her baby will not be syphilitic.) Treatment early in pregnancy will prevent fetal infection; penicillin given late in pregnancy will cross the placenta and treat the fetus as well as the mother. A fourfold rise in titer for syphilis indicates reinfection and the need for retreatment.

Herpes simplex type II (HSV–2) infections occur three times more frequently in pregnant women and are frequently more severe during pregnancy. This condition is recognized by vesicular lesions that rupture, leaving shallow, painful ulcers on the labia, perineum, vulva, vagina, or bladder. Painful urination, pain and tenderness at the site of ulceration, systemic symptoms of uremia (fever, headache, chills, and so on), and secondary bacterial infection may occur. Herpes can recur throughout the individual's lifetime; the virus is believed to be dormant in sensory nerve ganglia. Recurrence may be triggered by emotional stress, another infectious disease, or some other factor that destroys the body's equilibrium, but it may also occur spontaneously. There is no known cure, nor is there any known way to protect the fetus in utero. Women with herpes infections have an increased incidence of cervical cancer.

Neisseria gonorrhoeae, the causative organism of gonorrhea, is a gram-negative bacteria that invades mucosal surfaces; in women the urethra, endocervix, and Bartholin's and Skene's glands are primary sites. Both men and women may be affected; the disease is spread through direct physical contact, most often sexual contact.

In women gonorrhea is frequently asymptomatic. This is one important reason for screening all women in prenatal and family planning care, which is a time when screening is both economically and logistically feasible. When symptoms occur, they may include a yellow vaginal discharge, urinary frequency or burning on urination, involuntary loss of urine, redness and itching of the vulva (from contact with the vaginal discharge), or pain (if there is obstruction of Bartholin's or Skene's glands).

Intramuscular penicillin is the preferred treatment (4.8 million units of aqueous procaine penicillin G, one-half of the dose in each buttock). Approximately 30 minutes prior to the administration of penicillin, 1 gram of probenecid may be given orally; probenecid decreases the excretion time of penicillin in the urine, thus allowing increased blood levels.[6]

Smears and cultures for gonorrheal organisms are repeated monthly when gonorrhea has been detected, and the woman is re-treated if gonococci reappear. When a woman with known, untreated, or resistant gonorrhea is in labor, vaginal exploration is kept as minimal as possible.

The baby is most likely to be affected by gonorrhea during the passage through the birth canal at the time of delivery. Ophthalmia neonatorum, a gonococcal infection of the infant's eyes, was formerly a major cause of neonatal blindness. Prophylactic treatment for ophthalmia neonatorum is mandatory in most states at the time of birth (Chapter 20). The infant of an untreated mother is treated with penicillin and additional silver nitrate.

Chlamydia trachomatis is isolated more frequently in clinics for sexually transmitted disease than either *N. gonorrhoeae* or *Treponema pallidum* (the causative organism of syphilis).

Formerly called by a variety of names (e.g., *Trachoma* inclusion conjunctiva agent), a form of *C. trachomatis* causes the eye disease trachoma, the most common form of preventable blindness in the world; it is rarely seen in the United States. *Chlamydia trachomatis* is a gram-negative intracellular organism that is able to replicate only within the host cell; it differs from a virus in that a virus contains either DNA or RNA but not both, whereas *C. trachomatis* contains both.

It has been estimated that the incidence of *Chlamydia* infections in infants is 28 per 1000 live births. This rate far exceeds the infection rate of many of the other diseases discussed here (e.g., 1 per 6000 births for herpes simplex, 1 to 6 per 1000 for toxoplasmosis). Others estimate that 5 to 12 per cent of all pregnant women may harbor the virus. Prenatal screening and treatment of infected pregnant women has been suggested.[25a] These authors believe that such screening could prevent 42,000 instances of inclusion conjunctivitis and 24,000 cases of chlamydial pneumonia each year. Currently, however, screening is not a part of prenatal care.

Symptoms in women include cervicitis, pelvic inflammatory disease, and postpartum endometritis; the disease may be asymptomatic in both men and women. In looking at the cervix, it is hard to distinguish chlamydial infection from gonorrhea; both present a beefy red surface with purulent discharge.

In both men and women a Gram stain of a smear (urethral or cervical) showing polymorphonuclear leukocytes (polys) is the basis of diagnosis. The smear is 60 to 70 per cent accurate in women, and approximately 90 per cent accurate in men. Accuracy in the cervical smear is improved by wiping any discharge from the cervix and then obtaining the culture from material deep in the endocervix. The specimen should then be gently rolled on the slide; rubbing the applicator on the slide will destroy the polys.

If a pregnant woman is found to have a chlamydial infection, her sexual partner should have an examination of a urethral smear. Males and nonpregnant women may be treated with tetracycline or erythromycin. A common regimen is 500 mg. of either drug four times a day for 7 days. If patients find this course difficult to tolerate because of gastrointestinal distress, enteric-coated tablets or doxycyline may be helpful. As noted in the discussion of syphilis, tetracycline and erythromycin are contraindicated during pregnancy. Erythromycin *base* may be used.

A thin, greenish-gray, foul-smelling discharge that is very irritating is a symptom of a *Trichomonas vaginalis* infection (trichomoniasis vaginitis). Microscopic examination of the discharge (saline wet smear) will show motile trichomonads. Metronidazole (Flagyl), used to treat *Trichomonas* infection in nonpregnant women, is contraindicated in pregnancy because it is a potential teratogen. Topical agents will relieve symptoms, but recurrence and the necessity for retreatment are not uncommon. As in other sexually transmitted diseases, sexual partners must also be treated; he can, of course, take metronidazole.

Because of the high glycogen content of the vaginal mucosa during pregnancy, *candidal* vaginitis, caused by *Candida albicans,* may occur. There is intense burning and itching but not necessarily a discharge. When a discharge is present, it tends to be thick and tenacious, resembling cottage cheese. White patches are seen on the vaginal walls about 50 per cent of the time.

Treatment is topical, with Monistat (miconazole) or Sporostacin (chlordantoin) applied twice a day for 2 weeks. Mycostatin (nystatin), the traditional treatment, is considered less effective but is still used. Gentian violet is still used occasionally; if it is prescribed, the mother must be alerted to protect clothing and linens. Candidiasis is difficult to relieve during pregnancy. Should a mother have candidiasis at the time of vaginal delivery, her baby may develop thrush, an oral candidal infection (Chapter 21).

Counseling Women with Sexually Transmitted Disease

When physical examination or screening indicates that a pregnant woman has a sexually transmitted disease, time and attention must be given to providing both education and support as well as physical treatment. Although the specific information given will vary with the individual pathogen, there are general topics that should be discussed with all women (Table 10–8). Privacy is important with all clients but especially with these women. Some women are particularly sensitive about reporting their sexual partners. They may be fearful of their partner's reaction to being "reported." Other women are very angry at their partner for having "given them the disease," or they are angry at themselves. It should be obvious that nurses must be nonjudgmental as they talk with and care for these women.

Table 10–8. COUNSELING WOMEN WITH SEXUALLY TRANSMITTED DISEASE

Topic	Subjects of Discussion
Treatment	Mode of transmission
	Possibility of reinfection or recurrence
	Relation to other conditions (e.g., HSV-2 and cervical cancer)
	Drugs (action, effectiveness, and side effects)
	Efficacy of treatment
	Need to follow up
Sexual partners	Investigation of contacts
	Treatment of contacts
Sexual intercourse	Abstinence during treatment to avoid reinfection
	Use of condom if abstinence impossible
Local relief	Sitz bath
	Topical steroid creams
	Wet compresses (e.g., boric acid)
Facilitating treatment	Avoidance of tampons (may absorb medication)
Prevention of recurrence	Treatment of sexual partners
	Good personal hygiene
	Proper wiping after bowel movements
	Avoidance of douching (changes in vaginal mucosa)
	Avoidance of chemicals that irritate vaginal mucosa

Continuing Maternal Assessment

At the conclusion of her first visit, the course of a mother's pregnancy may be considered "normal" or "high risk." The plan of care during pregnancy will vary according to each mother's special needs. Continuing evaluation will designate some mothers as high risk later in pregnancy or may remove other mothers from the high risk category. Continuing assessment for the high risk mother is discussed in Chapter 13.

For mothers with no apparent major problems during pregnancy, a common pattern of return visits is: monthly until the twenty-eighth week, biweekly from 28 to 36 weeks, and weekly from 36 weeks until delivery.

A return visit within a week of the initial visit is ideal to begin implementation of a nursing care plan early in pregnancy. This visit need not include a physician examination but gives nurses a chance to begin a teaching program after the mother and father have had a few days to become accustomed to the idea of pregnancy.

Assessment during these visits follows a plan similar to the initial assessment, in that nurses will be concerned with general health, course of pregnancy, nutritional status, and social and emotional status.

The Mother's Assessment of Her Pregnancy

As important as the physical examination or laboratory testing is what the mother tells us about her reactions to the pregnancy since the time of her last visit.

Has she been "feeling well" since her last visit, or has she been tired and listless? Has nausea limited her diet? Has she been constipated? Has she been having marital problems or problems with her children? Or is she finding this pregnancy to be one of the most satisfying times of her life?

We want particularly to note any danger signs that she may report (summarized in Table 10–9) and to refer these to her physician for immediate care. The significance of these symptoms is discussed in Chapter 13.

Other aspects of the mother's evaluation are mentioned in the sections below.

Certain specific assessment procedures will be a part of each return visit.

Continuing Physical and Laboratory Assessment

A great deal of attention has been focused on *weight gain* during pregnancy in the last three decades. It is believed now that the limitations placed on weight gain in the 1950's and 1960's, and still to a large extent in the 1970's, are harmful to the developing fetus. Because there is a close relationship between the total weight gain of the mother and the birth weight of the baby, a weight gain of 22

Table 10–9. SUMMARY OF SIGNS INDICATING NEED FOR IMMEDIATE FURTHER ASSESSMENT

Genital bleeding
Puffiness in face and hands, or feet and legs in morning
Sudden increase in abdominal size
Sudden weight gain
Decrease in urinary output
Persistent or severe headache
Blurred vision, spots or flashes of light, abdominal pain, back pain, epigastric pain
Chills and fever
Muscle twitching or torpor

Nursing Care Plan 10–2.   Subsequent Prenatal Visits

NURSING GOALS:
OBJECTIVES:

To provide continuing asessment of the woman who is pregnant and her adaptations to pregnancy.
At the completion of assessment and guidance visits the woman who is pregnant will:
1. Have developed a trust relationship with her care providers.
2. Understand her responsibilities regarding pregnancy and self-care.
3. Understand the care provider's role in providing continuing assessment and guidance.
4. Continue to be informed of her health and psychosocial status as it relates to her progressing pregnancy.
5. Have received guidance regarding physical and emotional aspects of the childbearing experience.
6. Have explored resources available to her during the childbearing experience.
7. Be prepared to begin assumption of role transition to incorporate a new member into the expanding family.

ASSESSMENT	POTENTIAL NURSING DIAGNOSIS	NURSING INTERVENTION	COMMENTS/RATIONALE
Subsequent physical assessment 1. Vital signs:	Alteration in physiologic status that could compromise client or fetus	Evaluate for signs of infection. Refer to care provider. Note irregularities; evaluate stress or anxiety.	Elevated pulse rate may indicate cardiac disorders. Marked elevation may indicate respiratory disease. Blood presure decreases in second trimester. Blood pressure increase of more than 30 mm Hg systolic and more than 15 mm Hg diastolic may indicate developing pre-eclampsia.
a. Temperature (98–99.6°F.)		Check blood pressure carefully. Observe for edema and proteinuria.	
b. Pulse (60–90 per minute)			
c. Respirations (16–24 per minute)			
d. Blood pressure 90–140 systole; 60–90 diastole; blood pressure decreased in second trimester			
e. Weight gain 1st trimester: 2–4 pounds 2nd trimester: 11 pounds 3rd trimester: 11 pounds		Discuss appropriate weight gain. Provide nutritional counseling as needed and desired. Observe and elicit information from mother and significant other.	Too little as well as too much weight gain may have implications for outcome.
f. Edema (small amount of dependent normal edema normal, especially in last weeks of pregnancy).			If edema accompanies raised blood pressure and proteinuria, it may indicate pre-eclampsia.
g. Uterine size consistent with length of gestation		Measurements are done by same examiner if possible to provide consistency.	Unusually rapid uterine growth may indicate multiple gestation, hydatidiform mole, miscalculation of estimated date of conception.
h. Fetal heartbeat (120–160 beats per minute)		Evaluate carefully. May elect to use doptone to allow client and other family members to hear fetal heart tones.	Use of doptone or ultasound for normal pregnancy is controversial owing to unknown effect on fetus. Client may prefer not to use unless clearly indicated.

Nursing Care Plan 10–2.   Subsequent Prenatal Visits (*Continued*)

ASSESSMENT	POTENTIAL NURSING DIAGNOSIS	NURSING INTERVENTION	COMMENTS/RATIONALE
Subsequent laboratory evaluation			
1. Hemoglobin/hematocrit (11–16 g./100 ml., 30–40 per cent)	Alteration in physiologic status that could compromise client or fetus	Provide nutritional counseling. Notify practitioner if less than 11 g. or less than 30 per cent. Encourge consistent use of prenatal vitamins or iron preparations if prescribed. Explain reason for continuing follow-up.	Anemia may be due to iron deficiency or other hemoglobinopathy. May need further laboratory assessment—i.e., morphology, electrophoresis.
2. Antibody screen (negative)			Antibody screen usually done at 4-week intervals after 28th week of pregnancy. If positive, further testing is indicated (Nursing Care Plan 13–6).
3. Urinalysis—glucose and protein		Instruct client in how to obtain clean specimen. Obtain information if symptoms of urinary tract infection (UTI).	If glucose is more than 1 + refer to practitioner; may indicate diabetes. If protein is more than 1 + refer to practitioner; may indicate vaginal discharge, UTI, orthostatic proteinuria, pre-eclampsia.
Subsequent psychosocial assessment			
1. Emotional status of client a. First trimester: Mother incorporates idea of pregnancy, ambivalence, looks for signs to validate pregnancy. Anxiety related to impending labor and parenting role and responsibilities.	Need for information about normal psychosocial adaptations to pregnancy Alteration in normal adaptation to pregnancy		
b. Second trimester: Baby becomes reality with increase in abdominal size and fetal movement; mother becomes introspective.			
c. Third trimester: Begins to think of baby as separate being, eager for labor to begin, self-centered, makes preparation for baby's arrival.			
2. Emotional status of expectant father a. First trimester: Excitement and assurance of virility, concerned with financial responsibilities, may identify with some discomforts of pregnancy.		Encourage expectant father to come to prenatal visits, encourage communications, establish trust relationship. Counsel regarding normality of behavior and feelings. Assure confidentiality. Include expectant father in pregnancy activities as he desires. Provide education, information, and support. Encourage participation in preparatory classes.	Remain alert for increasing and abnormal stress and anxiety, such as: inability to communicate, inability to accept pregnancy, lack of support or abandonment

Nursing Care Plan 10–2. Subsequent Prenatal Visits *(Continued)*			
ASSESSMENT	**POTENTIAL NURSING DIAGNOSIS**	**NURSING INTERVENTION**	**COMMENTS/RATIONALE**
b. Second trimester: May have increasing confidence, concern over partner's physical and behavioral changes.			
c. Third trimester: May feel competitive toward fetus, concern about sexual activity, may take more interest in himself, fantasizes about child, fears about safe passage for woman and child.			
Subsequent informational needs assessment			

1. Self-care measures and knowledge
  a. Breast care
  b. Hygiene
  c. Rest
  d. Exercise
  e. Nutrition
  f. Minor discomforts and relief measures
	Need for information about self-care and alternations in pregnancy	Teach or suggest appropriate relief measures. Provide atmosphere conducive to expression of concerns.	

2. Sexual activity		Provide information and counseling.	Ideal to include both partners if possible.
3. Preparation for parenting	Anxiety related to role transition	Counsel as needed, provide information regarding community resources.	
4. Sibling preparation		Encourage inclusion of other children in prenatal visits and home preparations. Suggest anticipatory techniques and role play if appropriate.	
5. Infant feeding 1. Breast preparation	Anxiety related to parenting capabilities	Provide information as needed.	Bottle-feeding mothers need information and support just as do breast-feeding mothers.

to 27 pounds is considered advisable for *all* patients, even those who are obese. The highest incidence of low birth weight babies occurs in mothers who gain less than 11 pounds.

The distribution of the weight gain in pregnancy is summarized in Table 10–10.

Weight gain should follow a pattern: a graph as illustrated in Figure 10–8 should be on each patient's chart to aid in evaluating weight gain. Approximate rates of gain at various stages of pregnancy have also been noted in Chapter 7.

When weight gain varies from the standard pattern, the cause should be assessed and an attempt made to correct it. It is particularly important to differentiate between acute weight gain, which is caused by fluid retention and may be related to pre-eclampsia (Chapter 13), and long-term weight gain, which is normal. A gradual, long-term weight gain of as much as 30 pounds may be perfectly healthy, while a total gain of 22 pounds, if 10 of those pounds are gained in a 2- to 3-week period, is potentially dangerous. Weight gain is discussed further in Chapter 12.

Urine is checked at each visit for sugar and acetone, which may indicate gestational diabetes, and for protein, an indication of pre-eclampsia. These high risk conditions are discussed in Chapter 13.

Nursing Care Plan 10–2. Subsequent Prenatal Visits (*Continued*)

ASSESSMENT	POTENTIAL NURSING DIAGNOSIS	NURSING INTERVENTION	COMMENTS/RATIONALE
2. Breast-feeding techniques 3. Bottle feeding		Suggest community resources, books. Provide information about formula and preparation.	
6. Danger signs of pregnancy 　a. Sudden gush of fluid from vagina 　b. Vaginal bleeding 　c. Abdominal pain 　d. Temperature above 101°F. and chills 　e. Dizziness, blurred vision, double vision, spots before eyes 　f. Persistent vomiting 　g. Severe headaches 　h. Edema of hands, face, legs, and feet		Provide appropriate information; written information helpful. Encourage client to report danger signs.	e.–h. are signs of potential eclampsia (Nursing Care Plan 13–10)
7. Preparation for childbirth 　a. Prepared childbirth techniques 　b. Normal processes and changes during childbirth 　c. Pain relief measures and their effects	Anxiety related to ability to succeed during childbirth.	Provide information about community resources. Individual counseling if needed. Provide reading list.	Stress that no one fails in childbirth. Different techniques are appropriate for different people.
8. Impending labor 　a. Uterine contractions increasing in frequency, duration, and intensity 　b. Bloody show 　c. Expulsion of mucus plug 　d. Rupture of membranes 　e. Alternate care providers	Need for information about signs of labor	Provide appropriate information. Encourage reporting of signs to practitioner. Explain call schedule if primary provider not available. Introduce alternate practitioners.	
Subsequent situational stress evaluation 1. Family 2. Lifestyle 3. Financial	Anxiety related to situational stress	Encourage open communication. Provide support and referral as needed.	

Contributed by Elizabeth K. Dickson.

Table 10–10. DISTRIBUTION OF WEIGHT GAINED IN PREGNANCY

	Pounds (Approximate)	Grams (Approximate)
Fetus	7–8	3200–3600
Placenta	1.5	700
Amniotic fluid	2.0	900
Uterine mass	2.0	900
Blood volume	3–4	1400–1800
Breasts	1–3	450–1400
Maternal stores	7.5–8.5	3400–3800
	24	11,000

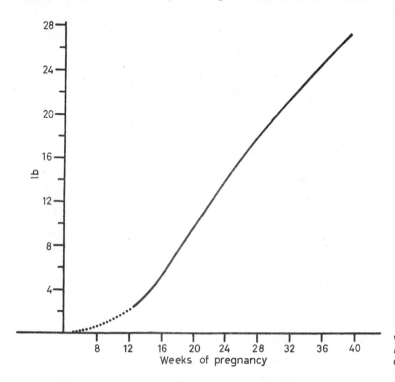

Figure 10–8. Graph charting prenatal weight gain. (From Greenhill and Friedman: *Biological Principles of Obstetrics*. Philadelphia, W. B. Saunders Co., 1974.)

Blood pressure elevation, as noted earlier, is also a warning sign; therefore blood pressure is carefully monitored at each visit.

Continuing Social Assessment

The primary nurse caring for each mother needs to keep herself informed about social problems that may have been referred to other professionals. For example, has a plan been made for a teenager's continuing education, and is it being followed? Is the eligible mother receiving food stamps? Have financial arrangements been made for hospital delivery? It is not unusual for the best of ideas to get lost in bureaucratic red tape if someone—the primary nurse—does not continue to monitor them.

New social problems, unanticipated at the initial interview, also arise during the months of pregnancy. The illness of another family member, the unexpected loss of a job, or a sudden need to move one's residence are examples. Anxiety related to such changes may affect feelings about pregnancy and may make the period of pregnancy a most difficult time.

Continuing Emotional Assessment

As noted in Chapter 9, a woman's feelings about pregnancy, and those of her husband, may change appreciably during the course of 9 months. Finding time at each visit to talk at least briefly about feelings not only is essential to evaluation but indicates to the woman (or couple) that changes in feelings are normal. When a woman's comments, or her husband's, indicate particular stress, more time from us or perhaps referral to another professional may be indicated. We might say, "You seem particularly concerned about _____. Would you like to make an appointment to discuss this on Wednesday afternoon?" or "_____ has talked with many women (couples) with similar concerns. Would you like an appointment to talk with her?"

Expanding Mother-Father Role in Prenatal Assessment: A New Scenario

Traditionally, the majority of prenatal assessments have been provided by nurses and other health care providers. An innovative program developed at the Maternity Center Association in New York has involved parents actively in many activities in which they are generally passive recipients of care. Consider the usual scenario of a prenatal visit. A woman steps on the scale to be weighed; a nurse records the weight. She holds out her arm to have her blood pressure assessed; she may not even be told the result. She presents a urine specimen. She lies on the examining table for assessment of fetal position and heart rate and a measurement of fundal height. The father may not be present in the room even if he has accompanied her on the prenatal visit.

Table 10–11. PASSIVE VS. ACTIVE PARENT PARTICIPATION

Assessment	Passive	Active
Weight	Mother is weighed; nurse records height	Mother weights herself and records weight
Blood pressure	Nurse assesses blood pressure and records	Father assesses blood pressure; mother or father records
Urinalysis	Mother gives urine specimen to nurse	Mother or father tests urine for sugar and protein, and records
Fundal height, fetal position, fetal heart rate	Assessed by nurse	Father assesses and records

If the nurse sees her role as an educator and facilitator of a person's participation in her own care, that person can be a far more active partner with her health care provider. At the Maternity Center Association a course called Self-Help Education Initiated in Childbirth teaches expectant parents assessment skills early in pregnancy so they can actively assume increased responsibility for their own health and, after birth, for the health of their baby. In addition to the skills described in Table 10–11, expectant parents learn other physical examination skills, such as ear and throat assessment and assessment of the newborn. The program believes that active participation is a unifying force between mother, father, and their unborn child.

Summary of Nursing Process in the Prenatal Phase

The model shown in Figure 10–9 summarizes the course of the nursing process when a woman believes she is pregnant and interacts with nurses. Some elements of this model were discussed in this chapter. Other elements are discussed in chapters throughout this book.

Summary

Nursing assessment is the basis of care of the prenatal family. This assessment is multifaceted, involving physical, reproductive, nutritional, social, and emotional aspects on an initial and a continuing basis.

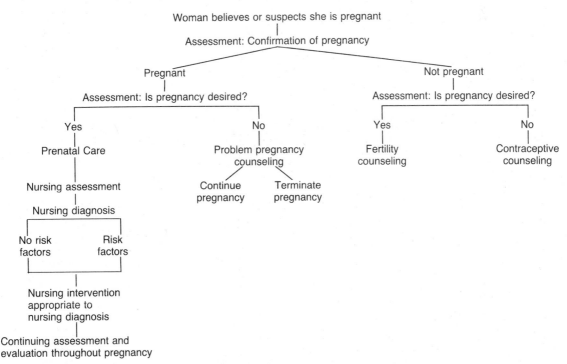

Figure 10–9. Nursing process for pregnancy.

REFERENCES

1. Benedek, T.: Parenthood as a Developmental Phase: A Contribution to the Libido Theory. *Journal of the American Psychoanalytic Association: 7,* 389, 1959.
2. Benson, R. C., Berendes, H., and Weiss, W.: Fetal Compromise During Elective Cesarean Section. *American Journal of Obstetrics and Gynecology, 105*:579, 1969.
3. Brock, D. J. H., and Sutcliffe, R G.: Alpha-fetoprotein in the Antenatal Diagnosis of Anencephaly and Spina Bifida. Lancet, *II*:197, 1972.
4. Chard, T.: Monitoring of High-Risk Pregnancies by Alpha-Fetoprotein. *In* Spellacy, W. N. (ed.): *Management of the High-Risk Pregnancy.* Baltimore, University Park Press, 1976.
5. Elmer, E.: *Fragile Families, Troubled Children.* Pittsburgh, University of Pittsburgh Press, 1977.
6. Fogel, C.: The Gynecologic Triad: Discharge, Pain and Bleeding. *In* Fogel, C., and Woods, N. (eds.): *Health Care of Women: A Nursing Perspective.* St. Louis, C. V. Mosby, 1981.
7. Gant, N. F., Chand, S., Warley, R. J., et al: Clinical Test Useful for Predicting the Development of Acute Hypertension in Pregnancy. *American Journal of Obstetrics and Gynecology, 120*:1, 1974.
8. Gant, N., Worley, R., Cunningham, F., et al.: Clinical management of Pregnancy-Induced Hypertension. Clinical Obstetrics and Gynecology, *21*:397, 1978.
9. Gil, D.: *Violence Against Children.* Cambridge, Harvard University Press, 1970.
10. Gluck, L.: Fetal Maturity and Amniotic Fluid Surfactant Determinations. *In* Spellacy, W. N. (ed.): *Management of the High-Risk Pregnancy.* Baltimore, University Park Press, 1976.
11. Gray, J., Cutler, C., Dean, J., et al.: Perinatal Assessment of Mother-Baby Interaction. *In* Helfer, R., and Kempe, C. (eds.): *Child Abuse and Neglect.* Bollinger, Cambridge, 1976.
12. Greenhill, J., and Freedman, E.: *Biological Principles and Modern Practice of Obstetrics.* Philadelphia, W. B. Saunders Co., 1974.
13. Horsley, S.: Psychological Management of the Pre-Natal Period. *In* Howells, J. (ed.): *Modern Perspectives in Psycho-Obstetrics.* New York, Brunner/Mazel, 1972.
14. Kennell, J., Voos, D., and Klaus, M.: Parent-Infant Bonding. *In* Helfer, R., and Kempe, C., (eds.): *Child Abuse and Neglect,* Cambridge, Bollinger, 1976.
15. Maio, J.: Pregnancy Test Kits. FDA Consumer. Washington, D.C., U.S. Department of Health, Education and Welfare, 1979.
16. Mandelbaum, B., LaCroix, G., and Robinson, A. R.: Determination of Fetal Maturity by Spectrophotometric Analysis of Amniotic Fluid. *Obstetrics and Gynecology, 29*:471, 1967.

17. Mead, P., and Gump, D.: Asymptomatic Bacteriuria in Pregnancy. *In* de Alvarez, R. (ed.): *The Kidney in Pregnancy.* New York, John Wiley, 1976.
18. Mocarski, V.: Asymptomatic Bacteriuria—A "Silent" Problem of pregnant women. *MCN, 5*(4): 238, 1980.
19. Morris, M., and Gould, R.: Role Reversal: A Concept in Dealing With the Neglected/Battered Child Syndrome. In The Neglected-Battered Child Syndrome. New York, Child Welfare League of America, 1963.
20. Noller, K.: Sexually Transmitted Diseases in Pregnancy. *In* Iffy, L., and Kaminetzky, H. (eds.): *Principles and Practice of Obstetrics and Gynecology.* New York, John Wiley, 1981.
21. Osathanondh, R. and Tulchinsky, D.: Placental polypeptide hormones. *In* D. Tulchinsky and K. Ryan (eds.): *Maternal-Fetal Endocrinology.* Philadelphia: W. B. Saunders, 1980.
22. Page, G., Villee, C., and Villee, D.: *Human Reproduction: The Core Content of Obstetrics, Gynecology and Perinatal Medicine.* 3rd Edition. Philadelphia, W. B. Saunders Co., 1981.
23. Pitkin, R. M.: Fetal Maturity: Nonlipid Amniotic Fluid Assessment. *In* Spellacy, W. N. (ed.): *Management of the High-Risk Pregnancy.* Baltimore, University Park Press, 1976.
24. Pitkin, R. M., and Zwirek, S. J.: Amniotic Fluid Creatinine. *American Journal of Obstetrics and Gynecology, 98*:1135, 1967.
25. Sabbagha, R. E.: Ultrasound in Managing the High-Risk Pregnancy. *In* Spellacy, W. N. (ed.): *Management of the High-Risk Pregnancy.* Baltimore, University Park Press, 1976.
25a. Schachter, J., Grossman, M., Holt, B., et al.: Prospective study of chlamydial infection in neonates. *Lancet,* 2:377, 1979.
26. Seller, M.: Alpha fetoprotein and the Prenatal Diagnosis of Neural Tube Defects. *Developmental Medicine Child Neurology, 16*:369, 1974.
27. Spellacy, W. N.: *Management of the High-Risk Pregnancy.* Baltimore, University Park Press, 1976.
27a. Steele, B.: Psychodynamic Factors in Child Abuse. *In* Kempe, H. B., and Helfer, R. (eds.): *The Battered Child.* 3rd Edition. Chicago, University of Chicago Press, 1980.
28. Tulchinsky, D.: The Value of Estrogens in High Risk Pregnancy. *In* Spellacy, W. N. (ed.): *Management of the High-Risk Pregnancy.* Baltimore, University Park Press, 1976.
29. Vincent, C.: *Sexual and Marital Health.* New York, McGraw-Hill Book Co., 1973.
30. Wager, G.: Sexually Transmitted Disease. Presentation at Workshop *Ob-Gyn Emergencies,* Cook County Graduate School of Medicine, October, 1981.

The Prenatal Family: Teaching and Counseling

When the mother is physically and emotionally healthy throughout pregnancy, nursing care is focused on teaching and counseling. Antenatal teaching and counseling involve three basic areas:

1. Coping with the physical, social, and emotional changes and needs related to the pregnancy itself.

2. Preparing for the process of labor and delivery.

3. Preparing for parenting.

How Nurses Can Help Parents Learn to Be Parents

Classes taught in high school and colleges, and many of the textbooks that accompany these courses, seem to stress preparation for and adjustment to marriage much more thoroughly than they explore pregnancy and parenthood. Popular media often romanticize the lives of young mothers and fathers. And with relatively few large and/or extended families in our society, most of us come to pregnancy with neither a realistic idea of what will be demanded of us nor the knowledge that will help us cope.

Mothers (and fathers, as well) are seeking different kinds of information at various stages of pregnancy. During the first weeks and months, principal concerns are for the woman herself—the changes that are occurring within her body, the changes in her feelings, and the fluctuations in the couple's relationship. Later, particularly after quickening, interest in the baby will heighten, and she will be more interested in learning about infant needs and care. Some mothers, especially adolescents, may not show any interest in baby care until after the time of delivery; their own needs seem to outweigh those of an infant who hardly seems real. At this later stage of pregnancy, a mother will also be concerned about the process of labor and delivery—about what is going to happen to her. In the days following delivery, interest in baby care and in her own recovery is intensified. Table 11–1 summarizes learning interests by trimester.

We teach best when we take these general interests into account, always individualizing them for each mother or couple. Although that seems to be only common sense, how often we hear of a mother with whom contraception is discussed during the initial visit at which the pregnancy is confirmed, as if to say, "Why didn't you know better?"

How do parents learn best? Obviously there is no single answer. At times a one-to-one relationship is very important. Groups, either of mothers alone or of couples, are ideal at other times; the sharing of feelings as well as of information makes the classes themselves assets to learning. Nurses leading groups need to watch for the shy mother who never asks a question or volunteers a comment; she may need some individual attention at another time.

The length of a group session will vary with the setting and the needs and interests of the group. Classes for couples that are held in the evening are frequently 2 hours long. On the other hand, classes for a group of mothers waiting their turn for examination will often be as short as 15 minutes and rarely longer than 30 minutes.

Many childbirth education classes have focused on the middle class couple. Attendance is dependent on knowledge that the classes exist, the value to be gained from them, transportation, and often a fee, which is small ($20 to $30, for example) but nevertheless prohibitive for many poorer people. One of the challenges of the next years in maternity nursing will be to extend classes to a broader group—mothers from lower income groups, teenaged

Table 11–1.   LEARNING INTERESTS DURING PREGNANCY

First Trimester	Second Trimester	Third Trimester
Learning Needs Centered on Mother	*Interest in Fetus Grows*	*Preparation for Labor and Parenting*
The expected date of delivery	Fetal growth	Fetal growth
Fetal growth	Physiologic changes of second trimester	Physiologic changes of third trimester
Physiologic changes of first trimester	Alleviation of maternal discomfort related to growing fetus	Alleviation of maternal discomfort
Emotional changes of men and women during first trimester	Emotional changes of second trimester	Emotional changes as time of labor approaches
Changes in family relationships	Maternal nutrition	Labor: signs, progress, the experience of labor
Nutritional needs	Infant feeding plans and other preparation for baby	Preparation for labor: relaxation and breathing techniques
Exercises for comfort and conditioning	Danger signs	Analgesia and anesthesia
Danger signs		Hospital tour; hospital policies
Available resources		Provision for others in family (e.g., other children) during hospitalization
		Preparation for homecoming
		Care of new baby

mothers, unwed mothers, and mothers in rural areas, for example.

Nurses may not always be the best persons to teach classes when the socioeconomic background of the parents is vastly different from their own. For example, if a mother in a Mexican-American community can be trained to teach parents in ways that are both in harmony with their cultural beliefs and consistent with our best knowledge, she may be far more effective than the nurse who is an "outsider."

Another type of prenatal learning experience described by Flapan and Schoenfeld,[15] is a "maternal role practicum" in which pregnant women visit homes of women with infants "to observe, ask questions, practice child care tasks, and experience the realities of ministering to an infant." Each woman visits a number of different homes in order to observe many different styles of mothering and thus to feel more free to develop a pattern that suits her best. Regular group meetings with other mothers give them a chance to discuss their reactions.

By visiting and volunteering to babysit for friends with small children, prospective parents accomplish much the same objective. We can encourage this trying on of the role of mother and father and can use it as a basis for both individual and group teaching.

Basic Principles for Prenatal Classes

1. Because women in prenatal classes are usually pregnant and often in their third trimester, sitting for long periods of time is uncomfortable. There should be a break after 45 or 50 minutes of class. Moreover, mothers should be encouraged to get up and walk around or go to the bathroom whenever they need to do so.

2. One of the greatest values of prenatal classes is the chance to share feelings with other mothers and couples. A mother-to-be said, "None of my friends have been pregnant yet, and it's hard to talk with them about the way I feel sometimes. It's been great to be with other couples who are pregnant." Ten to 12 couples, or 15 mothers, is an ideal group size for discussion. The physical arrangement of the room, with group members facing one another rather than sitting in rows facing an instructor, is also important.

Most childbirth instructors have couples wear name tags; first names are used in class to promote an atmosphere of informality and cohesiveness. The use of first names avoids embarrassment for unmarried couples.

3. Most childbirth education series last six to eight sessions, sometimes meeting once a week, sometimes twice a week. Couples' classes meet in the evening; classes for women only meet in the daytime as a rule. This type of scheduling tends to overlook the woman who will be coming to classes alone for any of a variety of reasons (single, husband travels in his work, husband chooses not to come) but who works during the daytime as well as the couple who works evenings.

It has been our practice to include both couples and mothers whose husbands cannot be present in our classes. A woman will often ask, "Is it all right to come even if my husband can't (won't)?" Once they are assured that every class has both couples and individual women, they seem quite comfortable in being present. In our own practice women of all ages (including teens), married and single, are welcome. Partners include husbands, boyfriends, girlfriends, sisters, mothers—any person important to the expectant mother (Fig. 11–1).

Sometimes a pregnant woman may have no one who would be willing or able to attend childbirth education classes with her or be with her during labor. In some communities women volunteer to serve as labor companions to other women who are alone. Nurses interested in developing a program for labor companions can obtain further information from the Community Outreach Committee, ICEA (see address in Appendix I). If a woman is comfortable attending classes alone, she is, of course, welcome.

The Nurse's Role in Prenatal Classes

The most effective role for nurses in parent education classes is not that of an authoritative teacher but of a group facilitator. This does not mean that the nurse has no plan for the series of classes, but rather that her plan is flexible and can be adapted to the needs and interests of the class. For example, she will plan at some point to talk about signs of labor, but she would not interrupt a very active discussion about how relationships in marriage change when the couple become parents because her preplanned schedule says she must discuss signs of labor that particular evening.

Nurse leaders need to be accepting of opinions and lifestyles different from their own and at times may need to help the group accept the right of an individual to express a point of view that is different from that of the majority.

Nurse leaders need to be comfortable in discussing sexuality (see below). If the nurse is obviously uncomfortable, the entire class will have difficulty in discussing their feelings.

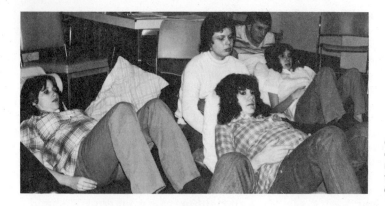

Figure 11–1. Classes in preparation for childbirth involve active participation on the part of both the women and their coaches and the nurse. Coaches may be husbands or boyfriends, women friends, or anyone the mother chooses to be with her during labor.

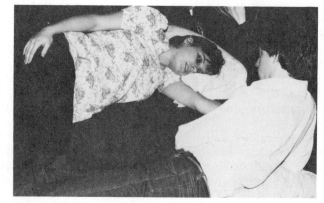

Figure 11–2. Mothers and coaches practice focusing, relaxation, and breathing techniques in a variety of positions. The woman in this photograph is focusing, with her eyes open and her body relaxed, as we can see from the way her hand is resting loosely on her hip.

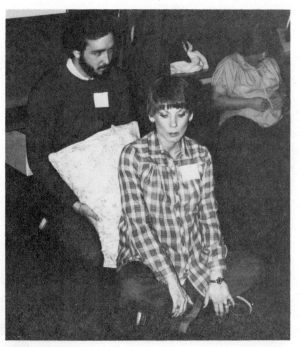

Figure 11–3. The coach in this couple is providing support to the woman by propping a pillow behind her back. She is tailor sitting and focusing. Note that the woman in the background is using effleurage. Name tags help everyone to get to know one another.

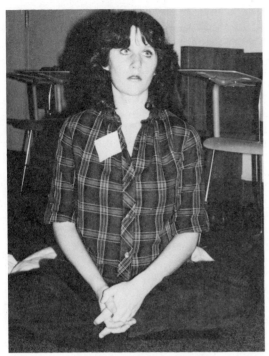

Figure 11–4. This woman is using relaxation with focusing and much concentration while tailor sitting.

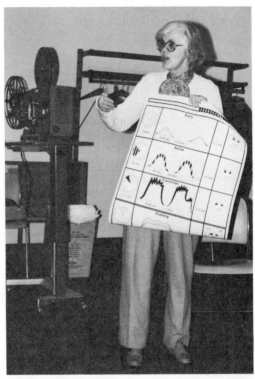

Figure 11–5. An instructor using a chart to illustrate stages of labor. Childbirth education films can be useful way to help prepare mothers and coaches for the birth experience. Note movie projector in the background of this photograph. (See Appendix H for a list of films and audiovisual aids.)

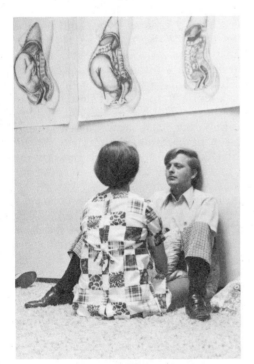

Figure 11–6. A couple practicing breathing. Notice the father's intense concentration. Anatomic drawings on the wall in the background illustrating pregnancy are used by the instructor as a visual aid (available from the Maternity Center Association, New York).

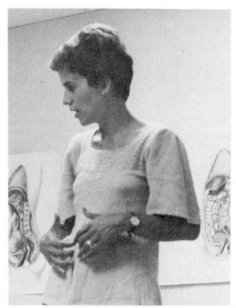

Figure 11–7. Nurses use their bodies and visual aids to facilitate learning. Brenda McBride, R.N., demonstrates effleurage to a class of mothers and fathers.

Helping the Mother Cope with Physiologic Changes

In Chapter 7 the physiologic changes produced by pregnancy in the mother's body were discussed. As a result of these changes, many mothers have symptoms that are often described as "minor" discomforts of pregnancy (Nursing Care Plan 11–1). Although these symptoms are minor in that they are not life-threatening to either mother or fetus, they can be a *major source of discomfort* to an individual woman.

Gastrointestinal Problems

Gastrointestinal problems are often major sources of discomfort to women during pregnancy. In addition, they can interfere with a woman's ability to meet her nutritional needs. Nursing Care Plan 11–1 summarizes the relationship between the gastrointestinal problems discussed below, nutrition, and the relief of symptoms.

Nausea and Vomiting

Nausea, with or without vomiting, is closely associated with pregnancy in the minds of most people in our society, so much so that "morning sickness" constitutes a confirmation of pregnancy for many women. It is important, however, to recognize that nausea of pregnancy seems totally absent in some societies. Burrows and Spiro[5] report that they were unable to find any evidence of nausea among Ifaluk women of the South Pacific, either by listening to their conversation or by direct questioning. Holmberg,[19] who lived among the Siriono of eastern Bolivia for many months, was unable to observe any cases of "morning sickness" or to find any recognition of it among pregnant women he interviewed. In our society, some women never experience nausea, while others may have nausea and vomiting during one pregnancy but none at all in another.

No one knows why nausea occurs in pregnancy. Two persistent theories suggest that nausea:

1. Is caused by hormonal imbalance, involving human chorionic gonadotropin and/or estrogens and/or progesterone.
2. Is related to emotional factors and perhaps to a rejection of pregnancy. (Remember that a high percentage of women are initially ambivalent about being pregnant.)

Slight to moderate nausea during the first trimester has been widely regarded as "normal" in Western society and is thought to be primarily of endocrine origin. The occurrence of nausea with use of oral contraceptives as well as in pregnancy is further support for an endocrinologic origin.

Studies of emotional factors and nausea in pregnancy are conflicting. Although Uddenberg et al.[36] found a significant association between severe nausea and marital status and attitudes toward pregnancy, others have found no association. Women with moderate nausea, however, were found to have the fewest adjustment difficulties.

Although nausea and/or vomiting may begin as early as the second week of pregnancy, they are most common during the fifth to twelfth weeks.

Nausea may occur in the morning ("morning sickness"), at which time it may be aggravated by an empty stomach, or at any time during the day. Frequently it is associated with excess salivation.

A dry carbohydrate snack before getting out of bed may help the mother with early morning nausea. Fatty foods and fluids exacerbate nausea and vomiting for many women; fluids can be taken between meals rather than with meals. Cooking odors are often enough to stimulate feelings of nausea.

Bendectin, a combination of doxylamine succinate and pyridoxine hydrochloride, has been approved by the Federal Drug Administration (FDA) since 1956 for the relief of nausea of pregnancy. (Bendectin is marketed as Debendox outside the United States.) Doxylamine, an antihistamine, provides the antinauseant and antiemetic activity. Pyridoxine (vitamin B_6) also has antinauseant activity. Because doxylamine may cause drowsiness and vertigo, it is taken at bedtime; the enteric coating of the tablet delays absorption so that the medication is active in the early morning when nausea is most common. When nausea is severe, an additional tablet in the morning and midafternoon may be prescribed. Women should be aware of the potential for drowsiness; many women already experience drowsiness during the first trimester because of increased levels of endogenous progesterone.

As is appropriate with any medication used during pregnancy, questions have been raised about the safety of Bendectin. At least one court case involving Bendectin as a teratogen is in litigation at the time of writing.

Those who argue for Bendectin's safety believe that Bendectin has been given to more than 30 million women with no conclusive evidence of a causal relationship to birth de-

Text continued on page 280

Nursing Care Plan 11–1. Minor Discomforts of Pregnancy

NURSING GOALS: To assist the woman who is pregnant in understanding and coping with minor discomforts. To screen possible pathologic conditions related to minor discomforts experienced by the woman who is pregnant.

MINOR DISCOMFORT	BASIS FOR DISCOMFORT	TIME PERIOD	PREVENTIVE AND RELIEF MEASURES (MEDICAL AND NURSING MANAGEMENT AND RATIONALE)	INDICATION OF PATHOLOGY
		Skin		
1. Pigmentation changes a. Striae	1. Mechanical stretching of skin over abdomen and breasts 2. Increased levels of estrogen and progesterone	Late second through third trimester and into postpartum period. Usually remain permanently with some change in color	1. Gradual weight gain; increased stretching 2. Provide moisture to skin, i.e., lanolin, cocoa butter creams, and massage; increase elasticity by increasing surface tension and health of skin. May or may not be effective 3. Support to abdomen decreases sag and stretch. 4. Recognize that striae may occur regardless of counter measures. Body image changes during pregnancy may create alterations in emotional adjustment for women or partners	
b. Vascular spider nevi; palmar erythema c. Chloasma Linea nigra Areola and nipple darkening	High levels of estrogen and progesterone produced by placenta have a melanocyte-stimulating effect. Melanocyte-stimulating hormone, a polypeptide similar to ACTH, is remarkably elevated from the end of second month of pregnancy until term.	Second month through postpartum period; may continue permanently. Most begin at 5 to 6 months' gestation.	1. Explain, recognize that changes may happen, discuss feelings and self-image. 2. Stay out of direct sun, use screening agents.	

Continued on following page

Nursing Care Plan 11-1.   Minor Discomforts of Pregnancy (Continued)

MINOR DISCOMFORT	BASIS FOR DISCOMFORT	TIME PERIOD	PREVENTIVE AND RELIEF MEASURES (MEDICAL AND NURSING MANAGEMENT AND RATIONALE)	INDICATION OF PATHOLOGY
		Skin (Continued)		
2. Pruritus a. Vulva	1. Increased blood supply and metabolic rate cause perspiration, which may lead to itching. 2. Leukorrhea—increase in pH favors proliferation of organisms and thus itching (e.g., Döderlein's bacilli)	Throughout pregnancy, increasing in third trimester	1. Cotton underwear 2. Bathe daily to decrease bacteria and remove leukorrhea. 3. Avoid douching—may alter pH 4. Loose clothing to decrease perspiration. 5. Avoid prolonged sitting—this prevents drying of perspiration. 6. Cornstarch or bath powder may prevent intertrigo and increase drying. 7. Avoid scratching and excoriation.	Rule out: 1. Monilia (may be associated with diabetes mellitus) 2. *Corynebacterium vaginalis* 3. Trichomonas 4. Gonorrhea 5. Herpes II 6. Hair follicle cyst (folliculitis) 7. Urinary tract infection
b. Skin	1. Possibly due to retention of bile salts induced by estrogens 2. Increased perspiration and sebaceous gland activity. 3. Possibly related to slightly elevated bilirubin level or other liver function alterations in pregnancy		Cleaniness; avoid drying soaps, perfumed lotions. Lotions are of little value, but some get temporary relief from calamine lotion. Nonperfumed bath oil may help.	1. Scratching may lead to infected excoriations. 2. Intertrigo—red, scaly, irritated rash 3. Gestational herpes manifest by erythematous spots, urticaria, papules, vesicles (on side of extremities, scapular and sacral regions) Jaundice—indication of gallbladder disease, liver pathology, or hyperbilirubinemia.
		Head and Neck		
1. Dental Caries a. Pain	1. Alteration in food choices and variations in salivary pH lead to dental caries. 2. Pain due to increased hyperemia from increased blood volume	Throughout pregnancy	1. Reassurance regarding normality of condition. Dental check-up and removal of plaque when necessary. 2. Dental repair under local anesthesia when necessary.	If abscessed, follow up with antibiotics prior to delivered increased incidence of endometritis and postpartum infection.

	Cause	Timing	Nursing Actions/Teaching	Complications
b. Gums—sore, bleeding, hyperplasia	Hyperemia from increased blood volume during pregnancy	Midpregnancy	3. Dental x-ray and extensive dental work should wait until after pregnancy unless absolutely necessary. 4. Regular flossing and tooth brushing. 5. Use soft brush; brush gums also. 1. Dental check-up to remove plaque early in pregnancy. 2. Soft-bristle toothbrush; brush gums gently. 3. Rinse mouth with warm saline several times per day. 4. Explain normalcy of this happening.	1. Gingivitis 2. Epulis (gingival lesion) 3. Oral cancers
2. Headaches	1. In most cases, no cause can usually be found. Possibly hormonal, ocular strain, sinusitis, emotional factors 2. Vasoconstriction with low CO_2 levels 3. Cerebral edema from increased fluid levels	Beginning to middle of pregnancy (headaches usually frontal and mild)	1. Tylenol, if severe 2. If wearing contact lens, may need eye exam.	1. Eye problems. 2. Pre-eclampsia (after 20 weeks) 3. Neurologic complications
3. Nasal stuffiness, nose bleeds	1. Vasomotor response to local disturbance of the autonomic nervous system; increased engorgement 2. Nosebleeds due to increased blood flow to the nasal mucous membranes		1. Increase fluids; use saline nose drops 2. Vaporizer to produce moist air 3. Avoid blowing nose vigorously 4. Elevate position of trunk and compress soft outer portion of nose against midline septum for 5–10 minutes.	1. Hypertension can result in severe nosebleeds 2. Trauma 3. Acute sinusitis 4. DIC 5. Drug addiction
4. Ptyalism	Theories vary. 1. May be related to increased dietary starch, which itself may be related to nausea and vomiting 2. Hysterical inability to swallow the normal amount of saliva produced daily (2–3 pints). Nausea may play a part in inability to swallow.	First trimester or until about time of quickening	1. Relieve nausea and anxieties and therefore causes of condition. 2. Mouthwash may help foul taste that may accompany symptoms. 3. Decreases dietary starch. 4. Carry Kleenex and container for expectoration. 5. Tincture of belladonna may aid by blocking secretion of saliva.	1. Observe for parotitis. 2. Excess nausea and vomiting can lead to electrolyte imbalance and weight loss. 3. Pica for starch can be related to anemia.

Continued on following page

Nursing Care Plan 11–1.   Minor Discomforts of Pregnancy (Continued)

MINOR DISCOMFORT	BASIS FOR DISCOMFORT	TIME PERIOD	PREVENTIVE AND RELIEF MEASURES (MEDICAL AND NURSING MANAGEMENT AND RATIONALE)	INDICATION OF PATHOLOGY
Head and Neck *(Continued)*				
6. Taste or olfactory distractions	1. Ptyalism caused by increased acidity may affect taste and smell. 2. Pyrosis and regurgitation may affect sensory system. 3. Nasal stuffiness may be due to increased estrogen. 4. More acute sense of smell in pregnancy	Throughout pregnancy	1. Reassure regarding normality; tell partner. 2. Correct pyrosis. 3. Correct nasal stuffiness.	Tumors
Respiratory System				
1. Dyspnea	1. Increased progesterone affects the respiratory center, lowering levels of CO_2 and raising O_2, often causing a feeling of hyperventilation. 2. Pressure of growing uterus on diaphragm 3. Increased engorgement of nasal mucosa 4. Elevation of diaphragm approximately 4 cm.	First to second trimesters	Good posture	Possibility of bronchitis, pneumonia, embolus
		Third trimester	1. Reassure regarding normality of occurrence. 2. Do "reaching" exercise to expand the thoracic cavity to its maximum and allow fullest expansion of lungs. 3. Sleep in semisitting position, propped with pillows or blocks under bed, if necessary. 4. Eat small, frequent meals to avoid crowding lungs with full (too full) stomach. 5. Good posture 6. Inform woman that neither her nor baby's life is threatened; relief will occur when baby "drops." 7. Saline drops if necessary	
Cardiovascular, Peripheral Vascular, and Cerebrovascular Systems				
1. Dizziness	1. Vasomotor instability associated with	Early in pregnancy primarily	1. Avoid sudden changes in motion.	Be alert for: 1. Anemia

	hypotension results in transient cerebral oligemia with pooling of blood in legs and in visceral and pelvic areas, especially after prolonged sitting or standing in warm room. 2. Hypoglycemia before or between meals can cause light-headedness.		2. Employ slow, deep breathing, vigorous leg motions, elastic stockings. 3. Eat frequently, carry food in purse for periods of hunger between meals. 4. Stimulants such as coffee or tea, as well as spirits of ammonia, may be helpful. 5. Avoid constricting garments.	2. Blood pressure problems 3. Hypoglycemia 4. Pre-eclampsia
2. Edema	1. Increased blood volume and decreased circulation due to pressure on vessels from growing uterus 2. Sodium and water retention due to ovarian, placental, and adrenal steroid hormones.	Second to third trimesters	1. Elevate feet and legs several times a day. Sleep in slight Trendelenburg position. 2. Get proper rest. 3. Avoid binding clothing—garters, tight slacks, knee socks. 4. Position self on left side when lying down. 5. Increase protein intake and encourge fluids, especially water. 6. Assess blood pressure; assess urine for protein.	1. Swelling of face and fingers may be a sign of pre-eclampsia. 2. Kidney, cardiac problems

3. Hemorrhoids	1. Pressure from enlarging uterus, specifically in the hemorrhoidal veins
	2. Tendency toward constipation in pregnancy
		Third trimester	1. Avoid constipation:
			  a. Adequate fluid intake
			  b. Warm liquids on rising
			  c. Foods containing roughage
			  d. Establishment of good bowel habits
			2. Sitz baths—heat of the water gives comfort and increases circulation
			3. Witch hazel compresses for reduction
			4. Ice packs for pain and reduction
			5. Epsom salt compresses for reduction
			6. Reinsertion of hemorrhoids into rectum in conjunction with Kegel exercises.
			7. Bed rest with hips and lower extremities elevated
			8. Analgesic ointments or topical anesthetics
			9. Topical hemorrhoid preparation
				Thrombosed vein leads to severe pain, considerable bleeding.

Continued on following page

Nursing Care Plan 11–1.   Minor Discomforts of Pregnancy (Continued)

MINOR DISCOMFORT	BASIS FOR DISCOMFORT	TIME PERIOD	PREVENTIVE AND RELIEF MEASURES (MEDICAL AND NURSING MANAGEMENT AND RATIONALE)	INDICATION OF PATHOLOGY
Cardiovascular, Peripheral Vascular, and Cerebrovascular Systems (Continued)				
			10. Stool softeners (e.g., Colace)	
			11. When trying to have bowel movement place feet on stool (10–12 inches high), take two deep cleansing breaths, and exhale as if pushing.	
4. Leg cramps (shooting pain in thighs, buttocks)	1. Enlarged uterus exerts pressure on pelvic blood vessels, impairing circulation, or on nerves supplying lower extremities.	Late months of pregnancy	1. Have the woman straighten affected leg and dorsiflex foot.	
	2. Imbalance of calcium/ phosphorus/magnesium ratio in the body		2. General exercise and good body mechanics	
			3. Legs should be elevated periodically throughout the day.	
			4. Avoid lying in prone position and pointing the toes.	
			5. Increasing the amount of calcium in the diet while decreasing phosphorus may help.	
			a. Decrease milk and take calcium lactate to elevate ionized calcium level of plasma.	
			b. Continue to drink 1 quart of milk daily and take aluminum hydroxide, which will trap the dietary phosphorus in the intestinal tract.	
5. Perspiration, hot flashes, increased feelings of warmth	Increased levels of progesterone and vasodilatation lead to increased warmth and increased metabolic rate.	Throughout pregnancy and postpartum period	1. Wear appropriate clothing—layers that can be removed	1. If accompanied by fever—infection may be present.
			2. Frequent baths or showers	2. If accompanied by fainting—safety of women should be discussed.
			3. Adjust temperature of home.	
			4. Inform of normality; explain to pregnant woman and significant others.	
6. Supine hypotensive syndrome	1. Compression of the vena cava by large uterus when woman is in supine position	Second and third trimesters	1. Turn on to left side from supine position.	
			2. If in supine position, maintain 45-degree angle.	

7. Varicosities—leg and vulvar	2. Increased progesterone levels 3. Vasodilatation 1. Increased vascularity of the pelvic organs leads to turgescence of tributary veins of pelvis. Vessels in pelvis and legs relax and dilate in response to progesterone. 2. Later in pregnancy, the enlarging uterus may occlude some venous return in inferior vena cava. 3. Gravity causes some stasis when standing. 4. Familial tendency may predispose to development of varicosities.	As early as fourth week and throughout pregnancy Last trimester	1. Full length support stockings should be put on before arising, keeping leg elevated. 2. Lie flat on bed or floor and prop legs on wall vertically for 15 minutes. 3. Avoid restrictive clothing, stockings, or garters. 4. Avoid prolonged standing or sitting. 5. Do not cross legs. When sitting, elevate legs. 6. Avoid constipation (see constipation and hemorrhoids) 7. A supportive foam pad may be worn to support vulvar varicosities. 8. Elevate hips on a pillow or use knee-chest position. Varicosed vessels may need to be drained. 9. Thrombosed vessels may or may not require surgical intervention. 10. Do not rub legs because this may dislodge a thrombus.	1. Severe calf, vulvar, or femoral pain indicates thrombosis (positive Homan's sign, localized warmth, redness). 2. Dyspnea, pallor, sweating, rales, rhonchi, anxiety, cardiac arrest may indicate pulmonary embolus.

Breasts

Breast enlargement: tingling and tenderness	1. Occurs as a result of increased sex hormones: progesterone, estrogen, and human chorionic somatomammotropin 2. Venous stasis	First and third trimesters	1. Well-fitted bra should be worn 24 hours a day. 2. Ice packs and cold compresses may help. 3. In late pregnancy, express colostrum to relieve engorgement, (if planning to breast-feed). Do not express colostrum if there is a history of premature labor.	1. Check for palpable mass. 2. Check for fever or other signs of infection.

Continued on following page

Nursing Care Plan 11–1.　Minor Discomforts of Pregnancy *(Continued)*

MINOR DISCOMFORT	BASIS FOR DISCOMFORT	TIME PERIOD	PREVENTIVE AND RELIEF MEASURES (MEDICAL AND NURSING MANAGEMENT AND RATIONALE)	INDICATION OF PATHOLOGY
		Gastrointestinal System		
1. Constipation	1. Suppression of smooth muscle motility by increased progesterone and by pressure upon and displacement of intestines by enlarging uterus. 2. Nausea and vomiting may cause diet changes (such as eating bland foods).	Throughout pregnancy; increases as uterine size and pressure increase	1. Stress good bowel habits; attempt bowel movement at same time each day. 2. Diet: bulk foods, roughage, fruits, liberal fluid intake 3. Encourage exercise. 4. Stool softeners or bulk laxatives that are not irritating to bowel may be used. *Avoid* mineral oil—interferes with absorption of fat-soluble vitamins. 5. Avoid strong purgatives that might initiate labor. 6. Drink warm liquids in morning.	Possibility of intestinal obstruction or impaction
2. Flatulence	1. GI motility is decreased owing to increased progesterone. 2. Uterus displaces and compresses bowel mechanically.	Throughout pregnancy but increased in third trimester	1. Dietary modifications: avoid large meals, fats, gas-forming foods, and chilled beverages. Exercise and frequent change of position may help. 2. Regular bowel function important.	1. Milk intolerance 2. Gallbladder problem
3. Heartburn (pyrosis)	Regurgitation of acidic gastric contents into lower esophagus by reverse peristalsis is caused in pregnancy by: 1. Relaxation of the cardiac sphincter of the stomach due to effects of increased amounts of progesterone. 2. Decreased gastrointestinal motility leading to delayed gastric emptying results from smooth muscle relaxation—which is caused by increased amounts of progesterone. 3. There is lack of room for stomach because of its	Begins toward end of second trimester and extends through third trimester.	1. Small, frequent meals are helpful to avoid overloading the stomach. 2. Avoid fats with meals since fat depresses both motility of stomach and secretion of gastric juices. 3. Decrease amount of beverages with meals since they tend to inhibit gastric juices. 4. Avoid very cold foods with meals because they inhibit gastric juices. 5. Drink cultured milk (e.g., buttermilk) rather than sweet milk, drink milk between meals.	1. If heartburn persists and becomes severe with pain radiating into neck and is increased in supine position, hiatal hernia may be present. 2. Differentiate from epigastric pain, which precedes eclampsia. 3. Ulcers

	Etiology	Occurrence	Interventions	Signs
	upward displacement and compression by enlarging uterus.		6. Good posture gives stomach more room to function. 7. Avoid specific foods that are identified as causing heartburn. 8. Remain upright for 3–4 hours following a meal; avoid bending over immediately after mealtime. 9. Low sodium antacids may be taken as ordered. 10. No preparations containing sodium bicarbonate should be taken.	

4. Nausea and vomiting	Not known; several theories have been proposed.
	1. Hormonal changes of pregnancy:
	  a. High levels of circulating steroids such as estrogen
	  b. High level of HCG present during first trimester
		5–13 weeks' gestation	1. Small, frequent meals instead of three large meals
			2. Dry crackers before getting up in the morning, since emptying stomach seems to precipitate the condition.
			3. Eat or drink something sweet (e.g., fruit, fruit juices) before getting up in the morning.
			4. Avoid foods with strong or offensive odors.
			5. Restrict fats in diet; fat slows peristalsis.
			6. Separate liquid and solid intake by ½ hour.
			7. Medication: controversy exists because of unknown possible teratogenetic effects of drug on fetus.
			8. Reassure mother that it will usually end during the 4th month.
				Persistent nausea and vomiting beyond first trimester may indicate:
				a. Severe emotional problem.
				b. Hyperemesis gravidarum.
				c. Hydatidiform mole.

5. Pica and food cravings	1. Increased appetite may be stimulated by estrogen and progesterone.
	2. Etiology unknown; may be related to
	  a. Psychologic factors
	  b. Social factors
	  c. Iron deficiency
		Throughout pregnancy	1. Maintain adequate diet to ensure appropriate nutrition.
			2. Check for anemia and decreased intake as needed.
			3. Reassure that occurrence is not uncommon.
			4. Indulge reasonable cravings.
			5. Increase psychological well-being.
			6. Validate intake.
				1. Anemia
				2. Intrauterine growth retardation

Continued on following page

Nursing Care Plan 11–1.   Minor Discomforts of Pregnancy (Continued)

MINOR DISCOMFORT	BASIS FOR DISCOMFORT	TIME PERIOD	PREVENTIVE AND RELIEF MEASURES (MEDICAL AND NURSING MANAGEMENT AND RATIONALE)	INDICATION OF PATHOLOGY
Urinary System				
1. Urinary frequency	1. Pressure of the growing uterus on bladder compresses it against pubic bone. 2. Presenting part presses bladder after engagement.	First trimester Third trimester, especially after engorgement occurs	1. Avoid drinking large amounts of liquid within 2–3 hours of bedtime. 2. Ingest required intake of liquid earlier in the day. 3. Instruct woman about signs and symptoms of UTI and tell her to report these to care providers. 4. Reassure her about normality and causative factors.	Burning, hematuria, fever, pyuria, CVA tenderness, lower abdominal pain may indicate UTI.
2. Nocturia	1. Supine position at night causes better renal perfusion. 2. Mobilization of dependent edema 3. Increased renal filtration	Throughout pregnancy	As above	As above
Reproductive System				
1. Braxton Hicks contractions	Rhythmic tightenings of uterus; occur as part of preparatory changes for labor.	Occur approximately every 5–20 minutes throughout pregnancy; most noticeable in last 6 weeks for primipara, last 3–4 months for multipara	1. Reassure woman about normality—the uterus is "getting ready" for labor and birth. 2. Advise mother to try slow deep breathing to enhance relaxation; if active, stop and rest; massage the abdomen lightly. 3. Differentiate between true and "false" labor (page 287).	Possibly associated with: 1. Leg cramps due to low calcium levels 2. Abruptio placentae 3. Appendicitis 4. UTI 5. Gallbladder problem 6. Other abdominal problems
2. Dyspareunia	1. Physiologic: a. Pelvic/vaginal congestion due to pressure and impaired circulation b. Related to enlarging uterus and pressure of presenting part	First and third trimesters depending on cause Postpartum, especially if breast-feeding	1. Positional changes for sexual expression 2. Alternate sexual expressions; avoid cunnilingus. 3. Accessible congestion may be reduced with ice but imposes own restrictions. 4. Provide explanation and	Excessive pain

	Physiology	Time	Interventions	Signs to report

	2. Physical alterations:
	  a. Enlarged abdomen in way
	  b. Engagement
	3. Psychologic alterations:
	  a. Misconceptions and fears (hurting baby)
	  b. Alterations in libido
	4. Postpartum: decreased vaginal secretions due to decreased estrogens.
			discussion of misconceptions and fears, substituting facts and knowledge; this can be helpful and reassuring.
			5. Education of both partners needed; encourage communication.
			6. Lubrication if necessary.
			7. Anticipatory guidance with breast-feeding.	

3. Leukorrhea	1. Increased vascularity of the cervix and increased mucus formation by the cervical glands due to increased levels of estrogen.
	2. Increased desquamation from the cervix and increased transudation through the vaginal walls
	3. Secretions are acidic because of the conversion of an increased amount of glycogen in the vaginal epithelial cells by Döderlein's bacilli into lactic acid.
		Begins first trimester and occurs again in third trimester	1. Good hygiene necessary
			2. Frequent change of soft cotton-crotch panties
			3. Use bath powder sparingly.
			4. In extreme cases use vinegar douche (2 quarts warm water to 3 T. vinegar)
			  a. Never use hand bulb syringes.
			  b. Never allow bag to hang higher than about 2 feet above level of hips.
			  c. Nozzle is inserted no further than 2 inches into vagina.
				Acidic secretions foster growth of organisms responsible for vaginitis.
				1. *Trichomonas*
				2. *Candida*
				3. *Gonorrhea*
				4. *Hemophilus*

4. Perineal pressure pain	1. Pressure of fetal presenting part 2. Vascular engorgement of tissues due to estrogen and stasis of blood 3. Constipation 4. Bulging membranes if woman is in labor 5. Imminent delivery	Third trimester	1. Side-lying position to relieve stasis 2. Some practitioners disagree about knee-chest position. 3. Elevate hips on pillows.	1. Constipation 2. Late stages of labor
5. Pubic pain	1. Progesterone and relaxin cause softening of cartilage of pubic symphysis. 2. Increased joint motility can lead to muscle and ligament strain, and thus pain.	32–40 weeks	1. Girdle or maternity corset decreases mobility and lends support. 2. Correct posture relieves excess strain. 3. Avoid activities that require balance and coordination.	1. Rule out lower abdominal pain, urinary tract infection, contractions. 2. Severe pain 3. Inability to walk 4. Complete separation of symphysis on x-ray

Continued on following page

Nursing Care Plan 11–1. Minor Discomforts of Pregnancy (Continued)

MINOR DISCOMFORT	BASIS FOR DISCOMFORT	TIME PERIOD	PREVENTIVE AND RELIEF MEASURES (MEDICAL AND NURSING MANAGEMENT AND RATIONALE)	INDICATION OF PATHOLOGY
Reproductive System (*Continued*)				
6. Round ligament pain	Round ligaments stretching as uterus enlarges.	Sometimes occurs in latter part of first trimester but most commonly at 16–32 weeks.	1. Pelvic rock and pelvic tilt relieve stretch. 2. Avoid prolonged sitting; pain can occur on standing after sitting. 3. Use heat—hot pad, warm moist soak. 4. Use rest, side-lying position to relieve stretch.	Rule out 1. Urinary tract infection 2. Labor 3. Appendicitis 4. Other abdominal infections 5. Constipation
Musculoskeletal, Neurologic Symptoms				
1. Backache (high)	Increase in size and discomfort of breasts	All trimesters	1. Reassure woman about normality during pregnancy. 2. Wear well-fitting and supportive bra. 3. Maintain good posture; attempt to hold shoulders back instead of giving in to weight of breasts. 4. Stretch arms over head to exercise muscles of upper back.	1. CVA tenderness 2. Cervical disk problems 3. Gallbladder problem 4. Predisposition to flu 5. Pleurisy
2. Backache (low)	1. Muscular fatigue and strain due to changes in body balance is caused by growing uterus. 2. Pressure on nerve roots causes muscle spasm. 3. Pelvic joints are relaxed owing to sex hormones.	Increases as pregnancy progresses, especially in third trimester	1. Reassure woman about normality during pregnancy. 2. Improve posture; stress "tall" posture with pelvis tilted forward, buttocks "tucked under." 3. Instruct about good body mechanics—squatting (to avoid bending and stress on lower back); rolling to side before sitting up from prone or supine position; tailor-sitting. 4. Perform moderate daily exercise to "tone" and maintain muscle strength—	1. Bladder or kidney infection 2. Nerve compression or intervertebral disk syndrome 3. Possible sign of premature labor

Discomfort	Etiology/Rationale	Timing	Interventions
			pelvic rock or alternative positions.
			5. Heels of shoes should be medium, not high, to avoid increasing the spinal curvature.
			6. A firm mattress or bed board under mattress can be used to aid support.
			7. Maternity girdle or alteration in regular girdle may be indicated for patient with extreme lordosis or kyphoscoliosis, obesity, or multiple pregnancy.
			8. Local heat or light massage helps.
			9. Assume side-lying position with upper leg supported on pillow(s) for sleep and rest.
			10. Proper arrangement of household appliances at good working level avoids undue stooping or stretching.
			11. Analgesics such as Tylenol can be used for pain relief.
			12. Pelvic tilt stretches and tones side and back muscles.
			13. Rest with legs bent and elevated in chair or on bed.
3. Gait alterations	1. Increased endocrine hormone relaxin affects sacroiliac joints and pubis. 2. Increased motility of joints is characterized by "waddle" gait.	Late in third trimester	1. Maintain good body mechanics and good posture. 2. Wear low-heeled shoes. 3. Watch safety factors. 4. Use girdle for stabilization.
4. Paresthesias (numbness and tingling of fingers and toes)	Various theories are suggested: 1. Fingers and upper extremities are affected if lordotic posture is extreme; the head and neck are flexed, putting strain on the brachial nerves and causing tingling of hands and arms. 1. Edema in hands may indicate onset of pre-eclampsia. 2. If lower extremity numbness, and weakness are present, rule out herniated disk. (This can also occur higher, producing upper extremity symptoms.)	Third trimester / Anytime	1. Prevent or relieve edema (see Edema, above). 2. Remove rings and constricting jewelry. 3. Exercise hands to relieve edema. 4. Correct lordotic posture (see Backache, above). 5. Correct vitamin deficiency with diet and prenatal vitamins.

Continued on following page

Nursing Care Plan 11–1. Minor Discomforts of Pregnancy (Continued)

MINOR DISCOMFORT	BASIS FOR DISCOMFORT	TIME PERIOD	PREVENTIVE AND RELIEF MEASURES (MEDICAL AND NURSING MANAGEMENT AND RATIONALE)	INDICATION OF PATHOLOGY
Musculoskeletal, Neurologic Symptoms *(Continued)*				
	2. Toes and lower extremities are affected if gravid uterus presses on femoral veins and nerves supplying lower extremities, thus interfering with circulation and causing paresthesias.		6. Inform patient that she may have to tolerate a certain amount of numbness or tingling.	3. Generalized tingling and hypertonus of muscles may indicate severe calcium-phosphorus imbalance.
	3. Edema may cause pressure and tingling of hands or feet, especially in hands when rising in morning.		7. Discuss safety measures to prevent dropping objects or skin injury. 8. Avoid hyperventilation. 9. Maintain adequate but not excessive calcium intake (milk and dairy products).	
	4. Carpal tunnel syndrome (edema causes pressure on nerves and ligaments within the carpal tunnel).		10. Maintain good bra support. 11. Try vitamin B_6 (pyridoxine) supplement with orange juice or banana.	
	5. Vitamin B deficiency. 6. Hypocalcemia (see Leg cramps, above).	Anytime	12. Wrist splint while sleeping may reduce pain.	
	7. Hyperventilation leads to decreased CO_2 normally in pregnancy. This can cause systemic vasoconstriction, which causes tingling.			
Emotional Status				
1. Anxiety	Normal concerns during pregnancy about health of baby, ability to be a parent.	Throughout pregnancy	Encourage open communications with parents about fears and anxiety; openly accept whatever they say.	
2. Fatigue	1. Initial fall in basal metabolic rate is of unknown etiology.	First trimester	1. Reassure them of normality and improvement as pregnancy progresses.	May be anemic. Check 1. Hemoglobin and hematocrit. 2. Mucous membranes. 3. Nailbeds. 4. Pulse rate.
	2. Altered posture and extra weight may contribute to fatigue.	Second and third trimesters	2. Frequent rest periods needed. 3. Encourage adequate nutrition. 4. Prenatal vitamins, iron needed 5. If mother is still working outside the home, she may need assistance or restructuring of chores at home.	

3. Insomnia	1. Concerns, anxieties or excited anticipation of an event the next day as in non-pregnant state. 2. Physical discomforts from the enlarged uterus. 3. Fetal movement especially when extremely active.	Anytime, but particularly during latter part of pregnancy	1. Warm bath 2. Warm drink (milk, tea with milk) 3. Nonstimulating activity before going to bed 4. Use of relaxation positions; extra pillows to support body parts. 5. Use techniques of progressive relaxation. 6. Short rest periods and naps during the day, since extreme exhaustion can make sleep difficult. 7. No exercise 2 hours before going to sleep.	Severe emotional problem.
4. Mood swings	1. Major hormonal and general metabolic changes due to influence of progesterone. 2. Hypo/Hyperglycemia 3. Shifting of the id-ego relationship	Throughout pregnancy Second and third trimesters	Explain normalcy of such feelings	

5. Libido alterations	1. First trimester is heavily influenced by fatigue, nausea, depression, sore and enlarged breasts, worries, anxieties, ambivalence toward pregnancy.
	 2. Second trimester is relatively free of physical discomfort:
	   a. Size of abdomen not yet a problem
	   b. Vaginal lubrication increased.
	   c. Ambivalence toward pregnancy usually resolved.
	 3. In third trimester:
	   a. Physical discomforts have returned.
	   b. There is abdominal enlargement.
	   c. There is fear of harming the baby.
		Generally, in first trimester there is decreased interest in sexual expression.
		
		 Second trimester—increased interest in sexual expression
		
		 Third trimester—decreased interest in sexual expression
			1. Explain normalcy of varying sexual desires during pregnancy.
			
			 2. Discuss alternate position for intercourse and alternate methods of achieving sexual satisfaction.	

Contributed by Elizabeth K. Dickson.

fects. In opposition, some of the epidemiologic studies, formerly used to support Bendectin's safety, have been recently questioned on a variety of methodological issues.[4, 27, 31]

In a series of investigations involving rat and rabbit experiments,[16] the malformation ratio was 4:70 in treated rabbits. However, the reporting of all observed deformities has been questioned. In the rat studies, no defects were reported, although rat mothers were treated for 80 days prior to conception as well as during pregnancy. The question is whether there is decreased teratogenicity in rats if a drug is given for a sufficient period prior to conception and the rat metabolism "adjusts."[8] Limb development has been a main concern with Bendectin, which may produce a teratogenic effect like that of thalidomide. The critical period for limb formation is from the twentieth to the thirty-fifth day of gestation; studies have not examined the timing of Bendectin doses in relation to the incidence of possible defects.

The FDA position on Bendectin, restated in February, 1980, affirmed its belief in the safety of Bendectin. In 1981, Merell Dow, the manufacturer of Bendectin, decided voluntarily to include a package insert that would include information about nausea and vomiting of pregnancy, nondrug measures to relieve symptoms, and the effects of Bendectin.

How do we as nurses utilize this information? It would seem that nondrug measures should be suggested to and tried by mothers with nausea and vomiting prior to the prescription of medication. For many women, these measures will suffice, and medication can be avoided entirely. For women with severe nausea and vomiting that are unrelieved by other measures, Bendectin *may* be appropriate if it is recognized that severe vomiting may present problems of nutritional and electrolyte depletion and that even severe nausea may interfere with adequate nutrition. Certainly all mothers should be given information about the possible disadvantages as well as the advantages of Bendectin.

When nausea is so prolonged and severe that no food is retained, the condition is known as *hyperemesis gravidarum*. Complete anorexia may also be present. Women with hyperemesis will lose weight, become dehydrated, and eventually become severely ill if their vomiting is not stopped. Years ago hyperemesis could lead to death, but this would be highly unusual today. As with nausea and vomiting, the basis is unknown, although many feel that there is a major emotional component to hyperemesis.

Initial treatment is similar to that for nausea and vomiting—small, frequent meals and fluids taken between meals. Rest after meals may be helpful. Tranquilizers are sometimes prescribed. If these measures are inadequate, the mother may be hospitalized, with oral intake stopped and intravenous fluids given. Feeding by mouth is gradually resumed 48 hours after vomiting has ceased.

Nausea and vomiting that *begin* after the first trimester probably have some basis other than the pregnancy; pyelonephritis is one possibility. This should never be ignored as "just nausea of pregnancy."

Heartburn

The combination of decreased gastric motility, increased intra-abdominal pressure caused by the enlarging uterus, and relaxation of the cardiac sphincter may allow gastric contents to reflux into the esophagus (gastroesophageal reflux). The mother experiences "heartburn" and indigestion, which may be relieved, at least partially, by eating smaller meals containing fewer fatty or highly sweetened foods.

Remaining upright for 3 to 4 hours following a meal or resting propped with pillows may alleviate some discomfort. Bending over shortly after mealtime should be avoided. Some women will find sleeping with additional pillows (a semi-Fowler's position) helpful.

If antacids are taken, those that contain sodium, including baking soda, should be avoided. Aluminum antacids are considered safe (Maalox, Amphojel, milk of magnesia, or Gelusil, for example). Often the other methods described can eliminate the need for antacids.

Constipation

Decreased muscle motility together with the pressure of the enlarging uterus on the descending colon and rectum are factors in constipation. The oral iron preparation commonly (and appropriately) taken by pregnant women also contributes to this common problem.

Mineral oil (which depletes the body of fat-soluble vitamins) and enemas and harsh laxatives (which may stimulate premature labor) are contraindicated in pregnant women.

Effective remedies for constipation during pregnancy include daily exercise such as walking, an adequate fluid intake (6 to 8 glasses each day), and menus that include foods with fiber and laxative properties (Nursing Care Plan 11–1). A bulk-producing agent or "wetting agent," for example, dioctyl sodium sulfosuccinate (Colace), is safe to use if proper diet and exercise do not resolve the problem.

Flatulence, also common, is again related to

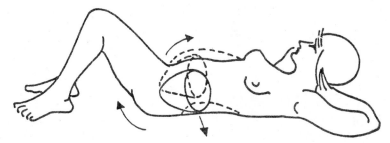

Figure 11–8. Pelvic rocking with the small of the back against the floor. (From Noble, E.: *Essential Exercises for the Childbearing Year.* Boston, Houghton Mifflin Co., 1976.)

decreased motility, which retards peristalsis and allows gas to accumulate (just as it may after surgery). Avoiding gas-producing foods (fried foods, members of the cabbage and bean families, and highly sweetened foods are the major offenders) and having daily bowel movements should be helpful.

Musculoskeletal Problems

Backache

The center of gravity progressively shifts during pregnancy. In addition, an increased level of hormones leads to a softening of ligaments and pelvic joints, which is important in preparation for labor and delivery. These changes lead to a characteristic walk during the later months of pregnancy (the waddle) and often to backache, as pelvic ligaments are stretched.

Women who have maintained good posture since they were girls are likely to have fewer problems with backache. Good posture during pregnancy will also be helpful. Because high-heeled shoes increase the pressure on the already strained pelvic ligaments, wearing shoes with moderate heels will also help to prevent backache.

Tailor sitting and pelvic rocking are two exercises that we can teach mothers that can be helpful in minimizing backache. Tailor sitting (Fig. 11–3) involves sitting on the floor with the feet crossed at the ankles. A woman can sit "tailor style" during some of her everyday activities, such as sewing, preparing fruits or vegetables for a meal, or watching television. In the tailor position, knees can be pushed toward the floor to stretch the thigh muscles in preparation for delivery. Stretching three times, twice a day, is adequate.

Pelvic rock may be performed in several positions. In the most common, the woman lies on her back with her legs bent and her feet flat on the floor (Fig. 11–8). The buttocks are

contracted, the back is pushed against the floor, and the abdominal muscles are contracted to tip the pelvis forward. The woman then relaxes. Practicing pelvic rock three times, twice a day, can relieve a good proportion of back strain.

Rocking is also possible in a standing position or with the hands and knees on the floor (Fig. 11–9).

Leg Cramps

Painful spasm of the gastrocnemius muscle in the back of the calf may occur during the late months of pregnancy. Such spasms are likely to occur when the woman has been lying down and pointing with her toes. As a preventive, each woman should be taught to always stretch her leg by pointing with her heel rather than with her toe.

The level of ionizable calcium in the woman's plasma has been implicated in leg cramps. If calcium intake is too low, calcium levels will obviously be low. However, an excessive intake of milk, with its high levels of phosphorus as well as of calcium, may also lead to low levels of ionizable calcium. If leg cramps become a major problem, calcium lactate may be given at bedtime.

When a cramp occurs, straightening the muscle will alleviate it. Standing on the affected leg is the easiest way to relieve the cramp. Any way in which the toe can be forced upward while the knee is kept straight will be helpful.

Respiratory Symptoms

Dyspnea

As the fetus grows larger and the uterus begins to encroach on the thoracic cavity, a feeling of shortness of breath occurs. As noted in Chapter 7, this feeling may be due to a decrease in functional residual capacity or to a perception of increased respiratory rate, even

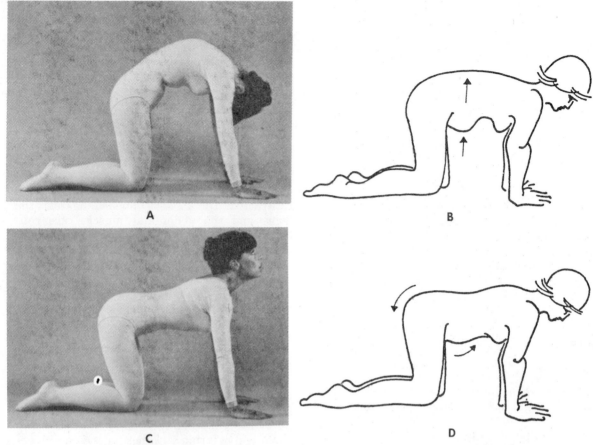

Figure 11-9. Pelvic tilt (pelvic rock) may also be practiced on "all fours." The woman pulls the pelvis up to make a "cat-back" (*A* and *B*) and then relaxes to a neutral position (*C* and *D*). The back must never be allowed to sag. (*A* and *C* from Prudden, S. and Sussman J.: *Suzy Prudden's Pregnancy and Back-to-Shape Exercise Program.* New York, Workman Publishers, 1980. *B* and *D* from Noble, E.: *Essential Exercises for the Childbearing Year.* Boston, Houghton Mifflin Co., 1976.)

though the respiratory rate does not normally increase. For some mothers dyspnea becomes sufficiently marked to make lying flat in bed difficult and to limit certain activities. The mother may need to sleep in a semi-Fowler's position with her head elevated.

Lying on her back with her arms stretched out above her head will maximize the area of the mother's thorax and allow the fullest possible lung expansion. This position will frequently relieve dyspnea.

Genitourinary Symptoms

Urinary Frequency

It was noted in Chapter 7 that urinary frequency occurs early in pregnancy as the growing uterus presses on the bladder, is relieved during the third month as the uterus rises into the abdomen, and reappears late in pregnancy as the greatly enlarged uterus again compresses the bladder.

Frequency cannot be avoided; limiting fluids

is not healthy. We can, however, explain the reason for frequency to the mother and, during the early period of pregnancy, assure her that the condition will improve.

Vaginal Discharge

A normal increase of white or yellowish vaginal discharge is to be expected during the last months of pregnancy, caused by an increase in mucus produced by the cervical glands, increased cervical vascularity, and increased cervical desquamation. These secretions are less acid than the vaginal secretions of nonpregnant women.

Douching is not recommended for removing these normal secretions. Daily bathing and wearing cotton underpants, rather than nylon, will help keep the mother-to-be comfortable.

Vaginal secretions caused by infection are summarized in Chapter 10. Herpes, one of the TORCH organisms that can lead to fetal damage, is discussed in Chapter 8.

Because of the tremendous discomfort

caused by trichomoniasis, a douche prepared with 3 tablespoons of vinegar to 2 quarts of warm water may be recommended. A douche bag should be used to hold the solution; bulb syringes may cause an air embolus and death. The bag should not be more than 2 feet above hip level, nor should the nozzle be inserted more than 3 inches into the vagina. These instructions should be given to the mother in a clearly understood form. It is never adequate to tell her "to take a vinegar douche" and send her home.

General Symptoms

Edema of the Feet and Legs

Edema of the feet and legs toward the end of the day can be frightening to the mother who has been told that "swelling" is a danger sign during pregnancy. This dependent edema is not unusual during late pregnancy and is often prevented or relieved by resting, with the feet elevated, several times during the day.

Edema that causes concern is present in the early morning as well as the late afternoon, is found in the face, hands, and pretibial area, and may be accompanied by sudden weight gain (Chapter 13).

Pruritus (Itching) of the Skin

Pruritus is not uncommon; it may be due to overactive sebaceous glands. Daily bathing, adequate fluid intake, and the use of bland soaps usually will relieve pruritus. A starch bath or some baking soda in the bath water may also be helpful.

Varicosities of the Legs and of the Anus (Hemorrhoids)

Increased pressure from the enlarging uterus that may obstruct venous return from the legs and perineal area, combined with decreased tone in the smooth muscles of vein walls, predisposes about 20 per cent of all pregnant women to varicosities in the legs or around the anus (hemorrhoids). The vulva and perineum may also be affected.

Varicosities may be prevented or their severity decreased by some simple measures that should be suggested to all mothers:

1. Garters or stockings with elastic bands around the calf should not be worn during pregnancy (or at all). Maternity garter belts are available. Support hose should be worn if previous varicosities have occurred or if the woman must stand for long periods. Support hose should be put on before arising and worn throughout the day.

2. Do not wear clothes that are too constricting.

3. Standing for long periods of time causes blood to pool in the lower veins. Sit when possible, with feet elevated.

4. Avoid crossing legs in such a way as to restrict blood flow. Crossing legs at the ankles with the barest of touching is all right.

5. Try to find some time each day to lie on the floor or on a bed next to a wall with your legs at right angles to your body resting against the wall. Elevating hips on a pillow may help avoid hemorrhoids and varicosities of the vulva.

Surgery for either hemorrhoids or leg varicosities is not performed during pregnancy. Occasionally, a clot in an external hemorrhoid may be evacuated as an office procedure. Hemorrhoids usually improve so markedly following delivery that no further treatment is necessary. Varicose veins should be evaluated and, if necessary, treated after the baby is delivered, or they may continue to be a source of problems for the mother, particularly during subsequent pregnancies.

Variations in Sleep Patterns: Excessive Sleep and Insomnia

During the early weeks of pregnancy, some mothers find themselves constantly tired and sleepy. The desire is strong to spend most of the day and night sleeping. A mother may report feeling very disgusted with herself. Our assurance that many other mothers experience the same fatigue and that this excess fatigue will usually disappear near the end of the first trimester is important.

By contrast, other mothers, and even the same mother at a different stage of pregnancy, may have periods of insomnia. The cause may be a combination of physical discomfort, especially during the last trimester, and a measure of anxiety, which may be present at any stage. Dreams are not unusual. Many babies become very active just as the mother lies down and begins to be comfortable.

The most comfortable position for sleeping for many mothers is a side-lying position (Fig. 11–2). Old remedies such as warm milk or cocoa at bedtime and limited tea, coffee, or "cola" after dinner may help. If anxiety is the problem, an alert nurse may be able to note this and help the mother express her concerns.

Short rest periods and naps during the day can help, because extreme exhaustion can make sleep difficult. Sleeping medications should be avoided.

Activities of Daily Living During Pregnancy

Many of the changes in a mother's activities of daily living during pregnancy have been noted in the section immediately preceding. These needs are summarized in Table 11–2.

Rest

Many women who consider themselves to be in excellent health during pregnancy nevertheless find that they tire more easily. During the first trimester, a desire to sleep more than usual is not uncommon. Extra rest may also be required during the third trimester.

Exercise

As noted in Table 11–2, daily exercise in some form is desirable during pregnancy, just as it is during all of life. The amount and kind of exercise will vary with a woman's lifestyle. Women who have been active in sports such as swimming and golf, for example, may continue to enjoy these activities throughout most of their pregnancy. It would be a mistake, however, for a woman who has led an extremely sedentary life to begin strenuous exercise. Walking is one example of an exercise more appropriate for her. For some women, the exercise involved in caring for a home may be adequate.

How much exercise? Exercise that leads to fatigue exhaustion is *too much*. Moderate exercise, on the other hand, often results in a feeling of both physical and mental well-being.

As the woman's center of gravity shifts during the last months of pregnancy, she should avoid exercise in which she might lose her balance; active tennis is an example. A woman with a previous history of spontaneous abortion or premature labor is usually advised to limit her activity for part or all of her pregnancy.

Employment

Employment during pregnancy is common today; many women work away from their home until very close to their expected delivery date with no apparent adverse effects. For some women the income from the job is vital; for others the satisfaction of the job itself is equally important. We do, however, want to discuss certain precautions for each mother.

1. Becoming overly tired should not be allowed.

2. Heavy lifting and straining must be avoided.

3. Good body mechanics are as important on the job as at home. If the mother is asked to describe the activities involved in her job, we may be able to suggest ways in which she can utilize good body mechanics.

4. Both prolonged sitting and prolonged standing in one spot should be avoided.

5. Pregnant women should not work around radiation or chemicals. Women with jobs that expose them to these potential teratogens should discuss the possibility of hazard with their employers.

6. Some arrangement for rest periods during the working day should be planned. Is it possible for her to lie down or sit with her feet elevated during coffee break?

Table 11–2.   CHANGES IN ACTIVITIES OF DAILY LIVING

Need	Meeting the Need
Proper clothing	Nonrestrictive clothing Moderately low-heeled shoes Maternity garter belt Support hose, if varicosities present
Adequate rest	Frequent rest periods, with feet elevated, during day A minimum of 8 hours sleep at night
Daily exercise	Exercise should not be carried to the point of fatigue* Formal exercises, such as pelvic rock, may alleviate backache
Bathing	Tub bathing allowed throughout pregnancy; care must be taken to avoid slipping Daily bathing aids comfort

*See section on exercise.

Nurses might begin to become aware of employers' attitudes toward and provisions for pregnant employees by examining practices in hospitals and health agencies. An awareness of policies of other community employers, particularly those that employ large numbers of women, is also important for nurses who care for childbearing couples.

Travel

The basic principle governing travel is the same as that for exercise and employment: fatigue should be avoided.

For women with a history of spontaneous abortion, travel is usually contraindicated in the early months of pregnancy. As the date of delivery approaches, travel may mean delivery in another community if labor begins earlier than expected.

Sexual Relationships During Pregnancy

Basic physiologic and psychologic factors influencing sexual relationships during pregnancy are discussed in Chapter 9.

The Nurse's Feelings About Discussing Sexuality

"I'm not sure I can discuss sex with a group of expectant mothers and fathers," a very excellent nurse told me as we were planning a series of prenatal classes. Many nurses, as well as others in and out of the health field, share these feelings, although not everyone is as open about confessing their discomfort.

The ability to discuss sexual concerns with patients is related to: (1) feeling comfortable about our own sexuality and (2) experience in talking about sexual feelings and practices.

Providing an opportunity for students and registered nurses to discuss their own feelings about sex is an important facet of basic and continuing education, not only for nurses who care for couples during childbearing but for all nurses. Fortunately, this need is becoming more widely recognized in both the nursing literature and in conferences, workshops, and other continuing education programs.

Role playing, on a one-to-one or a group basis, can help nurses gain experience and feel more comfortable. The following example of the beginning of a discussion with a group of expectant parents could be used as a role play.

Nurse: "Many couples find their sex life changes during pregnancy. I wonder if any of you have noticed changes?" (No one responds verbally, but couples exchange glances with one another, indicating that the nurse's comments are appropriate to their concerns.)

Nurse (continuing): "While every couple's experience is unique in some ways, many couples find they have intercourse less frequently during pregnancy. This does not mean that they care less about each other, although they may be afraid that it does."

The nurse can go on to talk about specific fears, such as fear of harming the baby or fear of beginning premature labor (see below). Her manner can convey, or she may verbally indicate, that anyone in the group may interrupt at any time. In our own experience, we find many glances and even whispered comments shared by couples, but some reluctance to share comments with the group as a whole. How often the group has met together, how much they feel they have in common, and other variables will influence their participation.

Similar comments can be used to introduce sexual counseling with individual mothers or, ideally, with couples.

Specific Concerns

Some specific concerns are so common that they are worthy of close scrutiny to separate fear from fact.

The Fear of Harming the Baby. There is no indication that intercourse is harmful to the fetus. However, when the presenting part has become engaged, intercourse is not recommended.

The Fear of Infection. The possibility of infection as a result of coitus was largely discounted in the decade of the seventies. A recent review of data from the U.S. Collaborative Perinatal Project, a prospective study in which data were gathered during antenatal visits and through placental and autopsy examinations, shows an increase in mothers who have intercourse one or more times per week in the month before delivery. Table 11–3 summarizes that information in relation to maternal age. Note that increases in infection occur in both groups as age increases.

These data do not indicate whether pregnant women from all socioeconomic groups are equally at risk. It does seem important for nurses to share this information with expecting couples to aid their decision-making. Once the membranes have ruptured, no pregnant woman should have intercourse.

The Fear of Premature Labor. As already mentioned, sexual intercourse does indeed cause uterine contractions. Some women who are *near term* have reported that labor

Table 11–3. EFFECTS OF MATERNAL AGE AND COITUS ON PERINATAL MORTALITY DUE TO AMNIOTIC FLUID INFECTIONS*

	Amniotic Fluid Infections	
Mother's age	*No Coitus*	*Coitus*[a]
14–34 years		
Cases/1000 births	114 (2508)	174 (578)
Deaths/100 cases	9.3 (234)	30.8 (178)
Perinatal mortality rate	10.7	53.7
35–39 years		
Cases/1000 births	159[e] (206)	209 (32)
Deaths/100 cases	12.6 (26)	37.5 (12)
Perinatal mortality rate	20.1[d]	78.4
Over 39 years		
Cases/1000 births	135 (47)	233 (7)
Deaths/100 cases	21.3[c] (10)	71.4 (5)
Perinatal mortality rate	28.8[d]	166.7[b]

*From *Perinatal Infections* (Ciba Foundation Symposium 77, new series). New York, Elsevier North Holland, Inc., 1980.

Perinatal mortality rates increased with maternal age, mainly due to increases in case fatality rates from the amniotic fluid infections. Perinatal mortality rates were also several times higher with than without coitus up to the time of delivery. Figures in parentheses denote no. of cases.

[a]Coitus once or more per week in the month before delivery.

[b]$P < 0.05$ compared with figure in same coitus category, 14–34 years of age.

[c]$P < 0.03$.

[d]$P < 0.005$.

[e]$P < 0.001$.

began following intercourse. In the study of Solberg et al.[32] of 260 women, not one woman reported the onset of labor following intercourse.

However, there are currently no good data concerning sexual practices and the onset of premature labor, a very significant question that needs to be investigated. When intercourse is limited, many women substitute masturbation and/or other sexual manipulation. However, these activities produce more intense contractions than does intercourse. In oral sex there is a danger of air embolism.

Currently, it is suggested that women who have a history of miscarriage or premature labor should limit intercourse during pregnancy. Intercourse may be permissible for these women at certain stages of pregnancy; the decision is based on individual physician evaluation.

A woman who is bleeding should refrain from intercourse.

Preparation for Labor and Delivery

Preparation for labor and delivery has many components. Mothers and fathers need to know:

1. The signs of labor and delivery.

2. What happens during each stage of labor and delivery.

3. Preparation for coping with labor and delivery.

4. Practices in local hospitals.

Some parents have questions about alternatives to labor and delivery in the hospital that should be discussed.

The Signs of Labor and Delivery

Signs indicating that the time of labor is approaching but is not necessarily immediately imminent include lightening, intensifying of Braxton Hicks contractions, cervical changes, and the presence of *show*. Occasionally rupture of the membranes may occur several days before true labor begins, although spontaneous rupture may not occur until well after labor has begun.

Bloody show and rupture of the membranes, together with regularly spaced contractions that increase in frequency and duration, are usually signs of true labor.

Lightening. Lightening, the process that indicates that the presenting part has descended into the pelvis, has been described in Chapter 9. Since lightening may not occur in multiparas and does not always occur in primiparas, the absence of lightening has little significance. The presence of lightening indicates that the time of labor is approaching, but

DIFFERENTIATION OF TRUE AND FALSE LABOR		
	True Labor	**False Labor**
Contractions	Regular Increase in intensity Increase in frequency May intensify with activity	Irregular Fail to increase in intensity Fail to increase in frequency Often lessen with activity
Discomfort	Most of discomfort in back	Most of discomfort in abdomen
Cervix	Cervix becomes thinner and dilates	Cervix does not change in thickness or dilate

it may yet be a week or more in the future. Urinary frequency, due to the pressure of the uterus on the bladder, usually occurs after lightening.

Intensifying of Braxton Hicks Contractions. Contractions of the uterine muscles occur throughout pregnancy, but in the early months they are so slight that they are usually not noticed by the mother. During the last trimester, and chiefly during the last 6 weeks of a first pregnancy, Braxton Hicks contractions become more frequent and more intense. As the time of labor approaches, mothers may find it difficult to distinguish Braxton Hicks contractions, termed false labor, from the contractions of true labor. These differences are summarized herewith.

Many mothers enter the hospital with false labor. Prenatally, we can reassure mothers that no one will be angry with them if they come to the hospital in false labor and that it is, in fact, quite a common occurrence. Labor room nurses must be supportive of the often highly embarrassed mother with false labor.

Cervical Changes. As the time of labor approaches, the cervix becomes shorter and softer; it may begin to dilate 1 to 2 cm. prior to the actual beginning of labor.

Show. Vaginal secretions increase as the time of labor approaches. As the cervix softens and shortens, the mucous plug that has occupied the cervical canal is discharged; this discharge is called *show*. Show may be blood-streaked or blood-tinged. The appearance of show usually indicates that labor will begin within 1 to 2 days; however, show may not appear until after labor has begun.

The bloody tinge of show, which is from the rupture of superficial blood vessels, must be differentiated from true bleeding, which may be due to a placenta previa or abruptio placentae, very serious complications (Chapter 13).

Rupture of the Membranes. In about 15 per cent of patients, membranes rupture an hour or more before the onset of the first stage of labor. In another 15 per cent, rupture occurs about the time that painful contractions begin. For the remaining 70 per cent, spontaneous or artificial rupture will occur late in the first stage of labor or early in the second stage. (Stages of labor are discussed in Chapter 15.)

The rupture of the membranes may be accompanied by a sudden gush of amniotic fluid, or occasionally, fluid may only "dribble" out slowly. Since amniotic fluid continues to be produced until delivery, the myth of a "dry labor" if the amniotic sac ruptures early is unfounded.

Once membranes have ruptured, the mother should come to the hospital. If labor has not started, it is frequently initiated, because the incidence of infection in the newborn infant increases when membranes have been ruptured more than 24 hours.

Coming to the Hospital

Mothers are told to be prepared to come to the hospital or birthing center (1) when membranes rupture or (2) when they believe they are having contractions of true labor. A common question is, "How close together should the contractions be before I come to the hospital?" Although a frequent recommendation is "every 5 minutes," the time will vary widely with parity, the distance to be travelled, and other individual factors. Some women may be so anxious at home that hospitalization early in labor facilitates relaxation. Other mothers will feel more comfortable at home during the first hours of labor.

Hospitals differ in determining what the mother should bring with her. Some prefer that her personal suitcase be brought after the time of delivery because they have no place to keep it while she is in the labor room. In other hospitals the mother brings her own clothes with her but is advised to wait until the time of discharge to bring her baby's clothes. In either event, she does need to have everything ready prior to the time she herself goes to the hospital. Basic needs for mother and baby are listed below.

BASIC NEEDS FOR MOTHER AND BABY IN HOSPITAL

Mother

Gowns
Robe
Firm slippers or shoes
Toilet articles
Nursing brassieres

Baby

Two diapers
Safety pins
Shirt
Gown
Blankets
(Fancy dresses, shoes are not necessary)

Useful articles to bring include: hard candy, such as lollipops; Chapstick, because lips get dry during long hours of labor; talcum powder, for effleurage; warm socks, because feet often feel cold during labor; and a rolling pin for back massage. Depending on hospital facilities and policies, food for the father may be brought along. Many hospitals will not permit food to be brought into the labor area. Couples should know about this and similar policies in advance (see hospital tour, below).

The Stages of Labor

The stages of labor are discussed in detail in Chapter 15, along with suggestions about information that is helpful to prenatal families.

Films of Labor and Birth

Because couples experiencing pregnancy for the first time will rarely have witnessed the process of labor and delivery, many nurses who teach prenatal classes use films to help parents anticipate what their experience may be like. Individuals and couples have varying reactions to films of birth. Some parents find birth films very helpful; others seem to feel more anxious about labor and delivery than they did before seeing the film. Sometimes it is hard for a nurse who has seen both films and births many times to appreciate the impact of these films on some prospective parents. Student nurses who may be witnessing birth and/or birth films for the first time can evaluate their own feelings and, in sharing them with their classmates and with faculty, gain an appreciation of how a first-time parent may feel.

In general, it has been found that films (whatever their subject) that reinforce previous knowledge and attitudes are influential in attitude change, while films that are antagonistic to attitudes held by the viewer are less influential.[25] This would indicate several important considerations:

1. Films of labor and delivery must be preceded by a discussion of labor and delivery and by a very clear explanation of what will be seen in the film. (All films should be presented in this way.)

2. The film itself should be chosen carefully. Films helpful to medical personnel (student nurses, for example) are not necessarily the best for parents. Films emphasizing husband participation would not be a good choice for a group of single mothers. In general, we have found films with a minimal number of views of the perineum most acceptable to parents.

3. The instructor should know her class and have a "feeling" for their attitudes about labor and birth.

4. Class participants should feel comfortable in choosing not to see a particular film. Usually we have to give them "permission" to refrain from witnessing a showing. For example, labor and delivery may be discussed during one class meeting. During this period the film can be discussed and announced (a) for a special time other than class time or (b) for a specific hour of the next class. Mothers and fathers can be told that sometimes couples choose not to see birth films and that this is quite all right or that some couples prefer to wait until closer to the time of delivery. By scheduling the film at a particular time, couples are free to come or not to come without feeling the need for explaining their reasons to other class members or to the instructor.

5. Films should be followed by a discussion that involves both questions about the material portrayed and a sharing of feelings about what was seen. Sometimes scenes viewed are misconstrued and need to be clarified. After seeing a film, couples may have questions that they had not previously considered. Both women and men need a chance to express what the film meant to them in terms of their own experience.

Following these guidelines, our own experience in using birth films in prenatal classes has been very good. But we are aware of other situations in which the showing of similar films has been distressing, so we continue to urge thoughtfulness in planning this teaching.

Specific Preparation for Labor

In the decade of the seventies, more and more women have sought to be awake, aware, and in control of themselves during labor and at the time of delivery. In response to these desires, several methods and systems of preparation for childbirth, although not new, have become far more popular and widespread.

The basis of each of these methods is a combination of physical and psychologic techniques that help each pregnant woman, with the help of her mate or another person, cope with labor and delivery in a manner acceptable to her. The normality of childbirth is emphasized as the mother is helped to prepare herself to participate consciously and effectively in birth. The term *psychoprophylaxis,* which literally means prevention (prophylaxis) by the mind (psyche), is used to described Lamaze training, probably the most popular method in the United States. The Bradley method and the Read method are other examples of psychophysical preparation for birth.

Historical Background

Methods practiced today are an outgrowth of a search that began over 50 years ago (or many centuries ago, if the varied proscriptions of tribal and folk medicine are considered). Although contemporary psychoprophylaxis as practiced in the United States neither guarantees painless childbirth nor rules out the use of medication, the techniques did evolve from a search for a method of painless childbirth that began in the Soviet Union in the 1920's.

Hypnosis was first investigated as a possible answer. The researchers were strongly influenced by Pavlov's principles of conditioned response, and when hypnosis as a general method proved disappointing, the basic principles of psychoprophylaxis were developed in 1930, although the applications were not introduced into practice until 1947 to 1949. The sociocultural climate of the Soviet Union in these years following World War II was ideal for the acceptance of these new ideas. Both money and physicians were limited, emphasizing the necessity of making childbirth easier for the mother. Initially, the Russians taught the mother during labor itself, but this made demands upon hospital staff time that were difficult to meet. The current method of training before labor was then developed.

The Work of Grantly Dick-Read

It was in the 1930's that an English physician, Grantly Dick-Read, suggested that childbirth was a beautiful emotional experience, divinely intended, and as such was never meant to be painful. Read observed childbirth in both traditional and contemporary societies. He suggested that at some point in history, anxiety and fear became a part of childbirth. Because of this, muscle tension resulted, which made dilatation more difficult and caused pain by tension-stimulation of nerve endings in the uterus—a syndrome of fear leading to tension leading to pain.

Read believed that by replacing fear and tension with a calm attitude and the ability to relax, childbirth would become the wonderful experience it was meant to be. This childbirth would be "natural," i.e., as nature intended.

To eliminate fear, Read began to educate mothers about birth and brought them to the hospital to visit before the time of labor. To eliminate tension, he developed a series of exercises in mental and physical relaxation and breathing.

The Read method has been helpful to many women since its introduction. The concepts of education, relaxation, and breathing were a tremendous advance.

One difficulty with the Read method is the tendency to deny the possibility of pain altogether rather than assisting women to cope with discomfort. Both women and labors vary widely; the woman who has a difficult labor or the woman who does not find labor to be the joyous, spiritual experience described in a Read class may feel disappointed and cheated.

Bradley Method

The Bradley method of childbirth, developed by Dr. Robert Bradley, emphasizes "true natural childbirth." This method stresses relaxation, a quiet environment, and a slow breathing technique throughout labor. Bradley has observed that this is the way all mammals with sweat glands give birth. An unmedicated birth is a goal. The American Academy of Husband Coached Childbirth provides certification for teacher preparation.

Table 11–4. PSYCHOPROPHYLACTIC PREPARATION: INSTRUCTOR'S GOALS

1. Make each couple feel comfortable about being in the class.
2. Explain what prepared childbirth means.
3. Dispel myths about prepared childbirth.
4. Review reproductive anatomy and physiology.
5. Describe embryo-fetal development.
6. Discuss pain during labor.
7. Introduce the topic of relaxation and teach three types of relaxation—progressive relaxation, touch relaxation, and controlled relaxation.
8. Review basic concepts of prenatal care including diet, rest, exercise, emotional changes, sexuality, keeping appointments, and symptoms to be reported to health-care providers.
9. Encourage attendance at hospital tour.
10. Encourage exercise and teach specific body-building exercises.
11. Describe the stages and phases of labor. Discuss roles of mother and coach at each phase.
12. Teach appropriate breathing in combination with relaxation, focal point, and effleurage for each stage and phase of labor.
13. Describe hyperventilation, its cause and remedy.
14. Discuss the signs of labor, distinguishing between true and false labor. Discuss the actions of parents when they believe the mother is in labor.
15. Discuss fetal monitoring, so that the monitor will not be a source of anxiety to parents.
16. Discuss obstetric intervention—episiotomy, forceps, and types of anesthesia.
17. Describe back labor and ways of coping with back labor.
18. Describe and discuss breech and Cesarean birth.
19. Discuss pushing—when and how not to push, when and how to push.
20. Discuss the immediate postpartum period in the hospital.
21. Discuss the needs of newborn infants (physical, emotional, social) and ways to meet them.
22. Discuss the needs of parents of newborn infants and ways to meet them.
23. Discuss the needs of siblings of newborn infants and ways to meet them.
24. Help couples integrate all they have learned through a rehearsal of the labor experience.
25. Discuss the postpartum experience with particular attention to sexuality, contraception, fatigue, and infant feeding.
26. Invite a recently delivered couple to share the experience of childbirth with the class.
27. Allow those couples who so desire to listen to the baby's heartbeat with a Doppler ultrasound device.

Table 11–5. EXERCISES IN PSYCHOPROPHYLACTIC PREPARATION

Type of Exercise	Specific Exercise	Purpose	Frequency
Body building	Good posture		At all times
	Kegel	Firms muscles in front of and behind vagina	
	Pelvic floor muscles	Firms muscles of pelvic floor	3 times, twice a day
	Pelvic rock	Relieves backache	3 times, twice a day
	Blowing out the candle	Strengthens abdominal muscles	3 times, twice a day
Stretching	Tailor position		
Controlled relaxation	Contraction of specific muscle groups along with relaxation of other groups	Learning to consciously relax specific muscle groups	Twice a day
Controlled breathing	Effacement breathing (slow, deep)	Learning to respond to contractions with controlled breathing	Daily
	Dilation breathing (shallow accelerated-decelerated)		
	Transition breathing (shallow with forced blowing out)		
	Expulsion breathing		
Massage	Effleurage (light massage)	Aid in relaxation	Daily
	Deep massage		

Hypnosis

Hypnosis has been used as a method of inducing relaxation and reducing the discomfort of labor and birth. Successful use of hypnosis also involves prenatal preparation, but in a one-to-one relationship of therapist (usually an obstetrician or anesthesiologist) and mother. The father or other supportive persons are not included, which is frequently seen as a disadvantage. Initially, prenatal preparation involves an extended period of hypnotic induction; during labor, cues (posthypnotic suggestions) enable the mother to relax quickly and to feel diminished or no pain. Hypnotized women are never unconscious. Not every woman is a potential candidate for hypnotism, and the technique is not in common use. (See Chapter 17 for the care of the hypnotized woman in labor.)

Psychoprophylaxis: The Lamaze Method

The goal of contemporary Lamaze training is the preparation of parents to participate actively and knowledgeably in their baby's birth. Based on the principle of the conditioned response, preparation substitutes controlled breathing, focusing, massage, and relaxation for tension as an automatic response to uterine contractions. By working with a contraction, mothers are better able to control their bodies during labor.

Lamaze training does not guarantee childbirth without pain; many factors influence the amount of discomfort an individual mother may experience (Chapter 17). However, the trained mother is better able to cope with the discomfort of contractions.

Some "Lamaze mothers" may need no medication for pain or no anesthesia; other mothers may choose to have medication. A mother does not "fail" Lamaze by asking for medication; this concept needs to be emphasized in prenatal training and affirmed during labor.

Appendix K contains a course outline for Lamaze classes. Table 11–4 lists typical instructor objectives. Every class will vary according to the needs of the individual participants as well as the instructor.

Exercises in Psychoprophylactic Preparation

Exercises are an important part of psychoprophylactic preparation for childbirth. There are different types of exercises that serve different purposes; they are summarized in Table 11–5. The role of posture, pelvic rock, and tailor position have been described previously.

Because understanding the role of breathing during labor is so closely related to understanding labor itself, breathing exercises are described in Chapter 17 and are shown in Figure 11–5.

Kegel Exercise. The Kegel exercise for strengthening of the vaginal muscles is not just for pregnancy and the postpartum period but for all women during their lifetime. Fortunately, it can be practiced while washing dishes, watching television, talking on the phone, riding in a car—almost any time and any place. One only has to remember to do it. The result should be improved muscle tone that may add to sexual enjoyment and prevent gynecologic difficulties later in life.

The Kegel exercise is valuable as a preparation for vaginal examinations and for labor because a woman learns to consciously relax her vaginal opening.

One of the easiest ways to learn the Kegel exercise is to practice stopping the flow of urine during voiding. The actual exercise involves simply relaxing, as if voiding, and then contracting, as if to stop the flow. Often it is taught so that the woman gradually tightens the muscle and them gradually releases it. The analogy of an elevator is used: Tighten (elevator on the first floor); still tighter elevator on the second floor); still tighter (elevator on the third floor); then gradual relaxation—"second floor," "first floor," "basement" (very relaxed), and a slight tightening (first floor) to finish.

Exercising the Muscles of the Pelvic Floor. This exercise is done lying on the back with arms at the side and legs crossed at the ankles. Contract the buttocks and hold. Squeeze the legs together, contracting the thigh muscles, and hold. Contract the muscles of the urethra, vagina, and rectum. Hold all muscle groups contracted and then relax.

Exercising the Abdominal Muscles. An exercise called "blowing out the candle" is helpful in strengthening the abdominal muscles. The mother lies on the floor with her legs bent, her feet flat against the floor, and a pillow beneath her head. She holds her finger, as if it were a lighted candle, about 12 inches from her lips, takes a deep breath, and exhales. Then, without taking another breath, she continues to "blow out the candle," blowing and blowing as she feels her abdominal muscles contract.

Exercising to Achieve Relaxation Through Neuromuscular Control

Relaxation is a skill that, once learned, is useful in many situations and can become a daily part of one's lifestyle. Many childbirth educators emphasize this long-term value of relaxation techniques as well as the benefits of being able to relax during labor. A variety of relaxation techniques have been developed. Couples preparing for childbirth usually learn several, one each week, enabling them to choose the one or the combination that is most helpful to them. Whatever technique is used, complete support of the individual's body with pillows is essential (Fig. 11–3).

Imagery encourages a woman to concentrate her thoughts on a favorite quiet location, perhaps in the mountains or at the beach, or to imagine such a place. As she sees that place in her mind, hears sounds associated with it, smells it, she excludes other thoughts and begins to relax mentally as well as physically.

Progressive relaxation is the conscious relaxation of the body's muscles. After the women are in a comfortable position with joints supported (the pregnant woman should be on her side rather than her back), the leader quietly gives instructions similar to those below. (At home, individuals can think the instructions for themselves.)

> Relax your forehead . . . let the tension go . . . feel your eyes relax . . . feel your jaws go loose . . . relax your neck . . . relax your shoulders . . . feel the tension from your arms leave through your fingers . . . relax your elbows . . . relax your wrist . . . your fingers . . . your arms feel heavy . . . let your back sink . . . relax your chest . . . your abdomen . . . feel the tension leave your legs through your feet . . . relax your ankles . . . let your feet flop . . . your legs feel very heavy . . . do you feel any tension anywhere? . . . let it go.

At the end of a relaxation period, a person is encouraged to experience the feeling of being relaxed first and then slowly to sit up and become active. Pregnant women, particularly, should sit or stand slowly after practicing relaxation.

In *touch relaxation,* touch rather than a verbal cue is the stimulus for relaxing the area touched. In practice, the mother contracts a set of muscles (an arm, for example) and then releases to the warmth of her partner's touch as he or she strokes the muscles, always drawing tension out and away from the body. During actual labor, as the partner sees or feels tension in a set of muscles, stroking will help the mother to relax toward her partner's touch.

Controlled relaxation (neuromuscular control) involves the alternate tensing and relaxing of muscle groups, and subsequently the tensing of some groups. It enables persons to recognize the feeling of tension in muscles. The pattern used for progressive relaxation can be used, but the instructions are changed so that a muscle is first tensed and then released. For example:

> Tense your forehead . . . make lots of wrinkles . . . hold the tension . . . now relax . . . tense your jaw . . . really grit your teeth . . . now relax . . . and so on . . . tense your entire body . . . now relax . . . experience the feeling of relaxation.

After women or couples have practiced controlled relaxation, they practice tensing specific muscles while relaxing the rest of the body. This simulates the situation during a labor contraction when the uterus is contracting but all the other muscles of the body should be relaxed. This is practiced with one's partner. The sequence of instructions is similar to that in the following example:

> Contract your left arm; relax the rest of your body (partner checks relaxation in remainder of the body); relax left arm. Contract right arm, then left leg, right leg, both arms, right arm and left leg, and so on. A variety of combinations can be used in different practice sessions.

As Braxton Hicks contractions become more noticeable, mothers can use them as a stimulus to practice relaxing other areas of the body. By the time labor has started, the mother will be able consciously to relax the other muscles of her body instead of tensing them (the "natural" response to a painful stimulus). The smooth, involuntary muscles of the uterus cannot be controlled by relaxation techniques. But concentrating on relaxation, along with concentrating on breathing, effectively helps women to control their bodies during contractions.

Further reading on relaxation is included in Brown, 1977; Gregg and Frazier, 1972; Jacobson, 1965, 1978; Tanner et al., 1977.

Massage

Both light massage (effleurage) and deep massage are helpful to many women in coping with labor. Husbands and others who stay with the mother during labor often help by using both massage techniques.

Effleurage is a light massage that can be felt by the mother but is not so heavy as to irritate the uterus. The movement of the hands is from the pubic area upward and outward toward the hip bones (Fig. 11–7). During a contraction that lasts about a minute, from 10 to 20 effleurage movements are average. The massage should begin as the contraction begins and should continue until it is completed.

Deep massage of the back from the coccyx to the lower back is very comforting during labor. Both of these techniques will be more effective if practiced antenatally.

Focusing and Breathing. Focusing and breathing patterns, taught in prenatal classes, are discussed in Chapter 17 in relation to the care of the intrapartum family.

A Hospital Tour in Preparation for Labor and Delivery

Rarely have first-time parents ever seen a labor and delivery suite. Many have never seen a newborn nursery. In our mobile society many parents may have a second baby delivered in a city far removed from the area of their first delivery. Thus a valuable part of preparation for childbirth can be a visit to the maternity unit of the hospital at which the couple will deliver. This tour can be particularly helpful if many of the following points are observed:

1. Give mothers or couples an overview of what they will see before they go. If the hospital is a large medical center with many parking areas and entrances, arrange for them to enter at the same entrance they will use when they come for delivery. Very specific directions and/or a map may be necessary. Be sure to note if entrances used at night are different from those used during the day.

2. Point out the place and procedure for registration and admission.

3. Show them the labor and delivery rooms. Explain how various pieces of equipment may make them more comfortable and protect the mother and baby. Receiving a warm greeting from nurses in various areas, and especially in the labor and delivery suites, helps to lessen the anxiety some parents feel about the approaching delivery.

4. Seeing babies in the nursery helps to prepare parents for the appearance of newborn infants—an appearance that surprises many of them. (Even in hospitals with rooming-in, there are still usually some babies in the nursery at most times.) Many questions about newborns and newborn care arise from even a brief view of the nursery.

5. On the postpartal unit, policies about visiting, rooming-in, and learning opportunities can be reviewed.

Following the tour, there are often many questions. The ideal time to answer them is immediately, but this is not always possible. The nurse who is teaching childbirth preparation classes many not be able to participate in the tour if the mothers in her classes are to be delivered at many different hospitals. The nursing staff in the hospital may be having a busy day and may be unable to spend as much time with touring couples as they would like. Couples can be encouraged to have a note pad and pencil with them so that they can write down questions that occur to them at the time or after they return home. These questions can then be a basis for discussion at a subsequent class.

Because all parents will forget some of the information they have heard discussed on a hospital tour, written information about the policies of the hospital is also essential. A booklet, which reviews policies from admission to discharge, is helpful. The more specific this information is, the more helpful it will be. Here is an example of introductory paragraphs from one such booklet.

It is our pleasure to welcome you to our maternity unit. Our aim is to provide physical and emotional support during your hospitalization. We value your cooperation and suggestions as we work together.

Before your expectant admission date, you will receive pre-admission forms that should be completed and returned to the hospital. This preparation will hasten and simplify the admission process.

When labor starts you do not have to call the hospital. Come to the hospital using the emergency entrance. There a nurse will direct you or have someone take you to the labor and delivery suite.

All jewelry, valuables and other personal items should be left at home. Neither is it necessary for you to bring your luggage with you when you are admitted since you will not need any personal items until after your baby is born. The hospital cannot assume the responsibility for valuables brought with you to the hospital.

Upon arrival at the labor and delivery suite on the second floor, notify the nursing staff that you are ready to be admitted by using the buzzer at the door. A nurse will talk with you through the intercom system and will ask you if she can help you. Please respond by telling her your name and that you need to be admitted.[26]

This 18 page booklet, developed by nurses working in the maternity unit, describes all phases of the hospital experience. Photographs complement the text.

Preparing the Expected Baby's Siblings for Childbirth

The words *sibling* and *rivalry* commonly go together in many societies. It is hard for an older child, particularly a child who is not very much older, to hold on to the "specialness" he

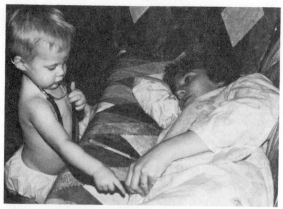

Figure 11–10. The toddler is using a stethoscope to "listen to the baby inside Mommy." Pregnant mothers may want to encourage their children to feel the baby move inside or put their ears on mother's abdomen to "hear" the baby. In this way, siblings can be prepared for the eventual arrival of their new brother or sister.

feels when a new baby with needs of his own becomes a part of the family. Jealousy can begin even before the birth of the baby. "If I were only good enough, Mommy wouldn't have to go to the hospital to have a new baby," the child may feel but rarely articulates.

Nurses can suggest to parents a number of ways to prepare a child for a new member of the family. Obviously, the age of the child (or children) is important. Children under the age of 6, and particularly children 3 years old and under, seem most vulnerable to the birth of a new baby because their own world is centered around their parents.

1. Children should be told about the new baby early in the pregnancy, by 4 months at the latest. Many mothers feel comfortable allowing their children to pat their abdomen or pretend to listen to the baby (Fig. 11–10) or to help them practice for labor (Fig. 11–11). Telling the child well in advance of the baby's

birth gives the child time to become accustomed to the idea. A mother in my postpartum unit asked, "How can I 'sneak' this new baby into the house?" She had never told her son, then 16 months old, about the baby. During prenatal visits, nurses need to ask parents if they have discussed the new baby with their other children. This question provides an opportunity for us to answer questions they may have.

2. Telling children early in pregnancy also allows for changes in the child's environment (different room, different bed) well in advance of the new baby's birth; the older child will then be less likely to feel displaced.

3. In talking about the new baby, parents need to present the baby from the child's point of view—the difficulties (babies cry, sometimes smile, smell bad, take a lot of Mommy's and Daddy's time) as well as the joys. All too frequently, when the idea of a new baby is introduced, it is suggested that the baby will be a "playmate" or "someone you can help take care of." Realistically, a new baby is not much of a playmate, and there are certainly limits to the extent to which the older child (toddler or preschool child) will be able to participate in the baby's care.

Somewhat more realistic is the comparison of the new baby with the baby experience of the older child. Pictures are very helpful. "This is what you looked like when you were in the hospital (or when you first came home)." Tell the child how he was fed and held and cared for as a baby, emphasizing that he is still cared for, but in his special, more "grown-up" way: Visiting in a home with a young baby will also help the child be more realistic about a newborn sibling.

4. Children can help prepare for the new baby in ways commensurate with their age. If children participate in shopping trips for the baby, purchases for them should be included too. These purchases need not be toys; if mom or dad is buying shirts or diapers for the baby, shirts and underwear for the sibling are appropriate corollaries.

5. Books about new babies, either purchased or borrowed from a public library, are helpful (Table 11–6).

6. In talking about the new baby, children need to expect either a sister or a brother, unless the sex is known (because of amniocentesis—see Chapter 14).

7. Planning for the period of hospitalization requires special attention. Because young children have no accurate sense of time, telling them that their mother will be away in the hospital for 4 days means little. Christensen[7]

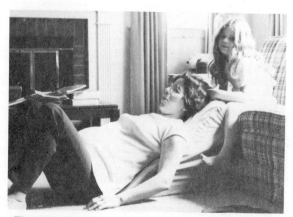

Figure 11–11. Practicing for labor can be a family affair.

Table 11-6. BOOKS TO PREPARE CHILDREN FOR CHILDBIRTH

A Baby Sister for Frances, by Russell Hoban (New York, Harper & Row, 1964).
Berenstein Bear's New Baby, by Stanley and Janice Berenstein (New York, Random House, 1974).
Billy and Our New New Baby, by Helene Arnstein (New York, Human Sciences Press, 1973).
Go and Hush the Baby, by Betsy Byars (New York, Viking Press, 1971).
Hi, New Baby, by Andrew Andry and Suzanne Kratka (New York, Simon and Schuster, 1970).
Hush, Jon!, by Joan Gill (Garden City, N.Y., Doubleday, 1968).
A New Baby, by Terry Berger (Milwaukee, Raintree Publications, 1974).
A New Baby is Coming to My House, by Chihiro Iwasaki (New York, McGraw-Hill Book Co., 1970).
Nicky's Sister, by Barbara Brenner (New York, Knopf, 1966).
Nobody Asked Me If I Wanted a Baby Sister, by Martha Alexander (New York, Dial Press, 1971).
On Mother's Lap, by Ann Herbert Scott (New York, McGraw-Hill Book Co., 1972).
Peggy's New Brother, by Eleanor Schick (New York, Macmillan, 1970).
Peter's Chair, by Ezra Jack Keats (New York, Harper & Row, 1967).
She Came Bringing Me That Little Baby Girl, by Eloise Greenfield (Philadelphia, J. B. Lippincott Co., 1974).
Sometimes I'm Jealous, by Jane Werner Watson, Robert E. Switzer, and J. Cotter Hirschberg (Racine, Wis., Golden Press, 1972).
Someone Small, by Barbara Borack (New York, Harper & Row, 1969).
That New Baby, by Peggy Mann (New York, Coward, McCann and Geoghegan, 1967).
We Are Having a Baby, by Vicki Holland (New York, Scribner's, 1972).
Where Do Babies Come From?, by M. Sheffield (New York, Knopf, 1974).
The Wonderful Story of How You Were Born, by S. Greenberg (New York, Doubleday, 1970).

suggests wrapping four dinners for the freezer (or four small packages) in advance. The child opens one package each day; when all are gone it is time for Mom to come home.

If possible, children should stay in the familiar environment of their home while their mother is in the hospital. They need to know who will be caring for them. The hospital telephone number can be posted in big numbers on the refrigerator door. Prior to hospitalization, the mother should talk on the phone to the children. Voices sound different on the phone; the mother's voice may not be recognized if the child has never heard it on the telephone before. Because the mother may go to the hospital at an unexpected time—in the middle of the night or while the child is in school, for example—a child needs to know this ahead of time.

Many hospitals allow siblings to visit during the postpartum period. For young siblings, the need to see mother is usually far more important than the desire to see the baby; baby may receive only a passing glance from preschoolers. For years the problems associated with separation of young children from parents when the child is hospitalized have been recognized; we need to recognize that hospitalization of a parent can also be upsetting to a young child.

In some units siblings may visit at the mother's bedside; in others, visiting may occur only in a waiting room. One concern has been the potential effect of young children on the incidence of bacterial colonization in the newborn. Umphenour[37] reports on a study in which nasal and umbilical cord swab specimens were obtained in each newborn (N = 214) at birth and at discharge prior to the institution of sibling visiting policy. In addition, infant records were examined for evidence of infection at 2 to 3 weeks of age. In this institution (Dwight David Eisenhower Army Medical Center, Fort Gordon, Georgia), siblings visit at the mother's bedside with the baby present for 2 hours every evening and are allowed unrestricted contact with the mother and new baby after hand washing with an iodine scrub preparation. No significant difference was found in bacterial colonization, infection, or illness. Only three instances of illness were discovered in 89 mothers on follow-up examination: two cases of monilial diaper rash and one case of conjunctivitis that cultured *Staphylococcus epidermidis.*

In some communities a prehospital sibling orientation program is provided. In one program (Hampton General Hospital, Hampton, Virginia) the Prepared Siblings Program for children of all ages includes a hospital tour to see the birthing room, postpartum floor and newborn nursery, slide presentation showing activities surrounding childbirth (e.g., checking into the hospital, baby being weighed, Mother talking on the phone to the child at home, children visiting Mother in the hospital, family going home together), stories and pictures to color for young children, dolls for the child to practice holding, diapering, and other care giving. Children wear pediatric gowns on the tour; they are given a mask and disposable scrub cap to wear and take home with them afterward. Each child has a chance to talk about his feelings about having a new baby in his family. While the children are touring, their parents see a film on prepared childbirth. Afterward, the whole family comes together for punch and cookies. Children receive certificates, postpartum gift packs, and buttons that say "I am a Prepared Sister (Brother).*

8. Parents need to know that not everything will go smoothly with siblings in the first weeks at home with a new baby. Parents often feel torn between the needs of older children and those of the baby. Siblings often regress in behavior, especially if a behavior is recently learned (e.g., toilet training). The older brother or sister may wonder why everyone is mad at him or her for "messing in my pants" when no one is mad at the baby for doing the same thing.

Siblings can be reassured that parents are in control and that their angry feelings will destroy neither parents nor baby. Parents can say, "I see you don't like babies very much today," thereby giving the children an opportunity to verbalize or play out their feelings.

Siblings need to feel "special" just as the baby is special. Pointing out that they have their special foods (babies don't get hamburgers) and activities (babies don't have wagons or whatever is the child's favorite toy) shows that each age has its rewards. The opportunity to spend some time away from home for parents and older siblings while someone babysits with the new baby is important.

9. Discussing realistically how much a child can "help" with the new baby is useful. Even young children can hold out a finger for the baby to grasp or can hold up a shiny foil pie pan for the baby to look at; thus they may feel they are helping with infant care (consider the importance of touch in parent attachment to infants). Young children can bring mom or dad a diaper and perform many similar activities. When siblings are school-aged or teen-agers, they may be asked to assume too much responsibility for the new baby; it is helpful to discuss this issue in the prenatal period.

---

*At Hampton General, the program is sponsored by the hospital and the Peninsula Chapter of ASPO (American Society for Psychoprophylaxis in Obstetrics). For further information, write Peninsula ASPO, Box 5689, Parkview Station, Newport News, Va. 23605.

Preparation for the Labor/Birth Experience

If a child is to be present at birth (usually at home, in an alternative birthing site, or a birthing room), additional preparation is necessary. Someone must be available to care for and support the child other than mother or dad. As labor progresses, mother will become more centered in the sensations of her body, and dad, if he is serving as labor coach, will be involved in supporting mother. They will be limited in the attention they can give to a child.

During much of the labor, the child will probably be in another room, "checking" on the progress of the labor from time to time. Preparation for birth should include a basic knowledge of what the child will see, appropriate to his age level; the child should see the mother's perineum prior to the time of birth. He should also know that mother may make "noises" during pushing that may sound frightening but are just part of having a baby.

Preparation for Cesarean Birth

The cesarean birth rate has tripled in the United States in the decade between 1970 and 1980 (Chapter 19). Approximately one mother in six will have a cesarean birth; the incidence is higher in some populations. Prenatal education, to be complete, must include preparation for cesarean birth. Such education must be developed for two groups of women: the woman who is expecting to have a vaginal delivery and the mother who is expecting to have a cesarean birth.

Cesarean Birth Preparation for the Mother Expecting Vaginal Delivery

Prospective parents who attend childbirth preparation classes are anticipating a vaginal delivery, often with a minimum of obstetrical "interference" with a process they view as "natural". Because of this, they may disregard what is said about cesarean birth, feeling that it may apply to others but not to them. Nurses who work with prenatal families, particularly families considered "low risk," may also believe that preparation for cesarean birth is not particularly important. Nurses sometimes feel that giving too much emphasis to cesarean birth legitimizes an increasing cesarean birth rate about which they have serious concerns. As a result, mothers and families may come to delivery with high expectations for a particular style of delivery and, if that delivery is not possible, may feel anger, disappointment, and guilt if they have a cesarean birth.

In the author's childbirth education classes, cesarean birth is mentioned at nearly every session. For example, early in the first class, couples talk about their expectations of childbirth. Rarely does anyone mention the possibility that they might have a cesarean birth. So I ask if they have considered that possibility, pointing out that (1) of 12 couples, the statistical probability is that 2 will have a cesarean birth and (2) that I have never had a class in which at least one mother did not have a cesarean birth. At the same time I tell them of excellent cesarean birth experiences and explain that most of the techniques they learn in class will be useful to them. The words that are used are important, I believe. Sometimes cesarean birth is contrasted with a "normal" birth; it is important to use the terms vaginal birth and cesarean birth. Many other terms nurses frequently use, such as cut you open, section, take the baby, malpresentation, and failure to progress can be replaced by terms such as make an incision, cesarean birth, deliver the baby, unusual position, and slow progress.

As we look at models of presentations, we talk about the possibility of a cesarean birth. When we talk about the length of labor, about medications used in labor, about the postpartum period, about breast-feeding, cesarean delivery as well as vaginal delivery is discussed. In the class following the one in which a birth film is shown, a cesarean birth film is shown, and cesarean birth is discussed in more detail. Because cesarean birth has been mentioned throughout the series of classes, class participants are much more open to the information presented at this time.

Many pregnant women never attend a childbirth education class. Cesarean birth should be one of the topics discussed with them through whatever means is used to meet their other educational needs: one-to-one conferences, waiting-room group discussions, posters and written materials, for example. Nurses who care for mothers during labor should assess the couples' knowledge of cesarean birth so that teaching during labor can build on prior knowledge.

Cesarean Birth Preparation for the Mother Expecting Cesarean Birth

Women who have had previous cesarean births or surgery that has resulted in a uterine scar have, until recently, rarely attended child-

birth education classes because they felt that the information shared in these classes was not applicable to them. Because of this, they frequently missed information important for all childbearing families, from a better understanding of the anatomy and physiology of childbearing and prenatal and postpartum exercises, to discussions of parenting. Special classes for parents expecting cesarean births are not available in many communities. In addition, there are now classes for parents who are planning vaginal birth after prior cesarean births. Appendix K outlines possible class content for these groups of parents.

A Postural Exercise for a Breech Presentation

One reason for cesarean birth is a breech presentation (Chapter 15). The following exercise is recommended to gravidas by a number of practitioners, including the author, when the breech is ascertained to be the presenting part. There is currently no scientific evidence to prove that this technique is successful. A number of practitioners report clinical success, but since some infants spontaneously turn from a breech to a cephalic presentation, it is difficult to gauge the effect of positioning. However, the exercise appears to cause no ill effects.

The mother is instructed to lie on her side on a firm surface, with her hips elevated about 9 to 12 inches by pillows, for 10 minutes twice a day. Her stomach should be empty to avoid gastric reflux. If the mother believes that the baby has turned, she should discontinue the exercise and check with her care-provider to confirm the change in presentation.

Prenatal Preparation for Parenting

As parents become more comfortable with the process of labor and birth, they are able to give some attention to the tasks of parenting and the needs of their expected infant. Information about preparation for infant feeding is given in Chapter 12; the characteristics and needs of newborn infants are described in Chapter 17; preparation for the role changes in parenting is discussed in Chapter 9. This information is presented first as a part of prenatal education and reinforced in the postpartal period when it can be applied to the needs of a particular infant and family. A record of prenatal teaching is very helpful to nurses who care for mothers in the postpartum period.

Preparation for Home Birth

The current and controversial area of home delivery is discussed in Chapter 30. In areas where planned home deliveries occur, there may be classes that prepare parents. A series of classes in the Washington, D.C. area, sponsored by H.O.M.E. (Home Oriented Maternity Experience) include five meetings:

1. Positive aspects of home birth.
2. Practical aspects of home birth.
3. Psychologic aspects of home birth.
4. Medical aspects of home birth, including contraindications and emergencies.
5. Postpartum care and breastfeeding.

Home Oriented Maternity Experiences: A Comprehensive Guide to Home Birth[14] is recommended to nurses who would like additional information about preparation for home delivery.

Summary

For the woman whose pregnancy is progressing without major complications, a primary nursing function is teaching and counseling. As teachers and counselors, nurses first assess what women and their families already know and their particular learning needs and then adapt the information they provide to these specific requirements. Throughout the pregnancy—at prenatal visits, home visits, and in prenatal classes—learning is continually evaluated, and plans for further teaching are made jointly by nurses and families. Information about the prenatal education that has been provided should be a part of a woman's prenatal record and should be available to those who will care for her and her family in the intrapartum and postpartum periods.

REFERENCES

1. Bing, E.: *Six Practical Lessons for an Easier Childbirth.* New York, Bantam Books, 1969.
2. Bradley, R.: *Husband-Coached Childbirth.* New York, Harper & Row, 1965.
3. Brown, B.: *Stress and the Art of Biofeedback.* New York, Harper & Row, 1977.
4. Bunde, C., and Bowles, D.: A Technique for Controlled Survey of Case Records. *Current Therapeutic Research, 5:*245, 1963.
5. Burrows, E., and Spiro, M.: *An Atoll Culture. Ethnography of the Ifaluk in the Central Carolines.* New Haven, Human Relations Area Files, 1957.
6. Chabon, I.: *Awake and Aware.* New York, Dell Publishing Co., 1966.
7. Christensen, V.: *Sibling Adjustment to the Newborn.* Paper presented at a conference. Childbirth: A Family Experience. February 23, 1980. Charlotte, North Carolina, Charlotte ASPO, 1980.
8. Congress Investigating Bendectine. *Federal Monitor, 3*(5):1, July 1, 1980.
9. Dick-Read, G.: *Childbirth Without Fear.* 2nd Revised Edition. New York, Harper & Row, 1959.
10. Doering, S. C., and Entwisle, D. R.: Preparation During Pregnancy and Ability to Cope with Labor and Delivery. *American Journal of Orthopsychiatry, 45:*825, 1975.
11. Emerson, K., Saxena, B., and Poindexter, E.: Caloric Cost of Normal Pregnancy. *Obstetrics and Gynecology, 40:*768, 1972.
12. Enkin, M.: An Adequately Controlled Study of the Effectiveness of P.P.M. Training. *In* Morris, N. (ed.): *Psychosomatic Medicine in Obstetrics and Gynecology.* Basel, S. Karger, 1972.
13. Ewy, D., and Ewy, R.: *Preparation for Childbirth.* New York, New American Library, 1972.
14. Fitzgerald, D., Herman, E., Ventre, F., et al.: *Home Oriented Maternity Experience. A Comprehensive Guide to Home Birth.* Washington, D.C., H.O.M.E., Inc., 1976.
15. Flapan, M., and Schoenfeld, H.: Procedures for Exploring Women's Childbearing Motivations, Alleviating Childbearing Conflicts and Enhancing Maternal Role Development. *American Journal of Orthopsychiatry, 42:*389, 1972.
16. Gibson, J., Staples, R., Larson, E., et al.: Teratology and Reproduction Studies with an Antinauseant. *Toxicology and Applied Pharmacology, 13:*439, 1968.
17. Gregg, R., and Frazier, L.: Relaxation Training Effects on Childbirth. *In* Schwartz, G. and Beatty J. (eds.): *Biofeedback: Theory and Research,* New York, Academic Press, 1972.
18. Hawkins, M.: Fitting a Prenatal Education Program into the Crowded Inner City Clinics. *MCN, 1:*226, 1976.
19. Homberg, A.: *Nomads of the Long Bow.* New York, Natural History Press, 1969.
20. Jacobson, E.: *How to Relax and Have Your Baby.* New York, McGraw-Hill Book Co., 1965.
21. Jacobson, E.: *You Must Relax.* 5th Edition. New York, McGraw-Hill Book Co., 1978.
22. Karmel, M.: *Thank You, Dr. Lamaze.* Philadelphia, J. B. Lippincott Co., 1959.
23. Laird, M., and Hogan, M.: An Elective Program on Preparation for Childbirth at the Sloane Hospital for Women. *American Journal of Obstetrics and Gynecology, 72:*641, 1956.
24. Lamaze, F.: *Painless Childbirth: The Lamaze Method.* New York, Pocket Books, 1972.
25. Leppert, P., and Williams, B.: Birth Films May Miscarry. *American Journal of Nursing, 68:*2181, 1968.
26. *Maternity Care Book.* Winston-Salem, Forsyth Memorial Hospital OB-GYN Ongoing Education Committee (Ollie S. Taylor, R. N., Chairperson), 1976.
27. Milkovich, L., and van den Berg, B.: Evaluation of teratogenicity of certain antinauseant drugs. *American Journal of Obstetrics and Gynecology, 125:*244, 1976.

28. Naeye, R.: Factors in the mother/infant dyad that influence the development of infections before and after birth. In *Perinatal Infections* (Ciba Foundation Symposium 27). New York, Excerpta Medica, 1980.
29. Recommended Treatment Schedules for Syphilis. *Resident and Staff Physician.* p. 60, September, 1976.
30. Roberts, J.: Priorities in Prenatal Education. *JOGN,* 5(3):17, 1975.
31. Smithells, R., and Sheppard, S.: Teratogenicity Testing in Humans: A Method Demonstrating Safety of Bendectine. *Teratology, 17*:31, 1978.
32. Solberg, D., Butler, J., and Wagner, N.: Sexual Behavior in Pregnancy. *New England Journal of Medicine, 288*:1098, 1973.
33. Sumner, G.: Giving Expectant Parents the Help They Need: The ABCs of Prenatal Education. *MCN* 1:220, 1976.
34. Tanner, J., Roper, J., Fredrick, A., et al.: *Are You Ready? A Guide For Prepared Childbirth.* Columbia, S.C., Columbia Association for Prepared Childbirth, 1977.
35. Thomas, J., and Wyatt, R.: One Thousand Consecutive Deliveries Under a Training for Childbirth Program. *American Journal of Obstetrics and Gynecology, 61*:205, 1951.
36. Uddenberg, N., Nilsson, A., and Almgren, P.: Nausea in Pregnancy: Psychological and Psychosomatic Aspects. *Journal of Psychosomatic Research, 15*:269, 1971.
37. Umphenour, J.: Bacterial Colonization in Neonates with Sibling Visitation, JOGN 9(2):73, 1980.

12

Nutrition During Pregnancy

OBJECTIVES

1. Define:
   a. pica
   b. lactose intolerance
2. Explain why meeting the nutritional needs of pregnant women is a complex problem.
3. Identify nutritional factors that may affect the outcome of pregnancy.
4. Describe the specific nutrient needs of pregnant women and the foods that will enable women to meet those needs. Identify needs that cannot generally be met by diet alone.
5. Explain how the needs of pregnancy can be met in the diets of various cultural and ethnic groups, of women with special physiologic needs, and of women with limited incomes.
6. Describe changing trends in breast-feeding over the past decade.
7. Cite advantages of breast-feeding.
8. Describe specific prenatal preparation for breast- and bottle-feeding.

Nutrition is a keystone of health at any period in life, but particularly so during pregnancy. Both maternal health and fetal development, including brain development, may be affected by malnutrition.

Currently, nutritional guidance during pregnancy is delegated mainly to nurses. Few physicians take the time or have the practical knowledge of foods and their preparation that can be helpful to a mother. Nutritionists are not currently available in adequate numbers to see each pregnant woman even once during 9 months, much less on a continuing basis. Patients of private physicians may have no access at all to a nutritionist.

Nutritional guidance for pregnant women begins with general and nutritional assessments (Nursing Care Plan 12–1). A number of factors in general and reproductive health that may be related to nutritional status are summarized in Table 12–1.

Nutritional guidance during pregnancy serves not only to help both mother and fetus during the months of pregnancy but ideally will help to establish patterns that will carry over into the period of lactation, if the mother is breast-feeding, and into the care of her children as they grow.

The problems of helping mothers with nutritional needs are complex for several reasons:

1. Her diet during her entire life, as well as during the 38 weeks of gestation, has a bearing on the outcome of pregnancy.

2. There is no clear indication of just what the nutritional needs of pregnancy are for a number of important food constituents.

3. Eating patterns are cultural practices that are often deeply ingrained and difficult to change.

4. Economic factors, physiologic status, cooking facilities, and other related factors limit the diets of many women.

In order to help mothers meet their nutritional needs during pregnancy, nurses need to know:

1. The relationship between nutrition and the outcome of pregnancy.

2. The specific nutritional needs of mothers and what foods will meet these needs within the framework of the mother's cultural, physiologic, and economic enviroment.

3. How to assess the nutritional needs of women during pregnancy (Chapter 10).

Nutrition and the Outcome of Pregnancy

Several specific concepts describe the relationship between nutrition and the outcome of pregnancy.

1. There is a strong positive association between the total weight gain of the mother and the birth weight of the baby. This concept has been discussed in Chapter 10 in relation to assessment of maternal weight gain.

2. There is a strong positive association between the prepregnancy weight of the mother and the birth weight of the baby. The highest incidence of low birth weight babies occurs when infants are born to mothers with a nonpregnancy weight of less than 100 pounds or more than 10 per cent below the standard weight for height.

Low prepregnancy weight may indicate long-term malnutrition and depleted stores. The mother who has severely restricted her diet during her teen-aged and early adult years in order to be fashionably slim may have inadequate nutritional stores, as may the mother who is underweight from chronic malnourishment.

It has been postulated that adults with severe nutritional depletion require 16 weeks of good diet to return to their level of function prior to nutritional deprivation. This emphasizes the importance of adequate nutrition not only from the beginning of pregnancy but at every stage of life, a point we can emphasize in all of our nutritional teaching.

Mothers with a prepregnancy weight of greater than 200 pounds or more than 20 per cent above the standard weight for their height are also at higher risk of developing complications. However, no attempt at reduction should be undertaken during pregnancy; these mothers should gain between 22 and 27 pounds during their pregnancy. Although obese women consume large quantities of food, the quality of their diet is often poor. If good nutritional practices can be developed during pregnancy, they may form the basis of a sound postpregnancy reduction diet. Breast-feeding can also contribute to postpartum weight reduction. No other postpartum weight reduction should be undertaken until the baby is off the breast.

Nursing Care Plan 12–1.   Nutritional Assessment and Counseling

NURSING GOAL: To provide every pregnant woman with information that will enable her to meet her own nutritional needs and those of her growing fetus.

OBJECTIVES:
1. Individual nutritional needs will be determined on the basis of physical and sociocultural assessment.
2. Specific counseling to meet nutritional needs will be provided within the context of each woman's individual and cultural preferences and economic resources.
3. Women who qualify will receive supplementary food assistance (women infants and children—WIC) where available.
4. Maternal weight gain will be 25 to 30 pounds.
5. Hemoglobin will be maintained at a level of ≥12 g./dl.; hematocrit will be maintained at a level ≥33 per cent.
6. Infant weight will be appropriate for gestational age.

ASSESSMENT	POTENTIAL NURSING DIAGNOSIS	NURSING INTERVENTION	COMMENTS/RATIONALE

1. Physical baseline
  a. Age; age of menarche
  b. Height
  c. Nonpregnant weight
  d. Small, medium, or large frame
  e. Weeks gestation at time of assessment
  f. Weight at time of assessment.
  g. Activity level (very active, moderately active, sedentary)
  h. Physical evidence of good nutrition (alert, good posture, pink mucous membranes, vitality).
	Nutritional risk during pregnancy related to various factors (e.g., age, [adolescence], weight [underweight, overweight], inadequate weight gain, etc.).	Counsel to meet any identified deficits—e.g., to provide additional nutrition for adolescent mother who is underweight, in addition to meeting basic pregnancy needs as described in text.	Adolescents less than 3 years postmenarche are considered at particular risk because of their own growth needs. Prepregnant weight of less than 100 pounds, height less than 60 inches, or weight greater than 120 per cent of standard weight for height are nutritional risk factors.

2. Laboratory assessment
  a. Iron deficiency anemia
    1. Hemoglobin
    2. Hematocrit
    3. Additional tests as indicated
  b. Folate deficiency
    1. Serum folate
    2. Mean corpuscular volume
    3. RBC folate
    4. Serum protein
	Nutritional risk during pregnancy related to (specific condition)	In addition to including foods rich in iron and folic acid (see text), supplementation is recommended for all pregnant women, and especially for women with nutritional deficiencies.
		Elemental iron 30–60 mg./day
		Folacin 400–800 µg./day
			Even though supplementation supplies needs during pregnancy, including iron and folic acid, rich foods in diet may lead to improved eating habits for mother and other family members.

Health History 1. Diabetes mellitus 2. Chronic hypertensive disease 3. Heart disease	Nutritional risk during pregnancy related to (specific condition).	Diabetes mellitus (see Nursing Care Plan 13–3) Chronic hypertensive disease (see page 349) Heart disease (see Nursing Care Plan 13–4)	

4. Lactose intolerance		Supplement calcium and vitamin D. Increase intake of other protein foods.
a. Reported by woman		
b. Bloated feeling, flatulence, cramps, diarrhea following milk ingestion.		
5. Drug abuse		Frequently associated with poor nutrition. Nutritional counseling a part of total care (Nursing Care Plan 13–13)
6. Obstetrical factors	Nutritional risk related to (specific condition).	Hospitalization usually necessary.
a. Hyperemesis with weight loss, fluid–electrolyte imbalance.	Risk of dehydration, ketosis, hypokalemia, or hypochloremia is related to hyperemesis.	Intravenous therapy to correct fluid–electrolyte problems. Oral feedings initiated after vomiting ceases. Provide emotional support. Provide opportunity to talk about feelings concerning pregnancy.
b. Frequently closely spaced pregnancies (less than 1 yr. apart or three in 2 yrs.)		Explain important of adequate weight gain. Help plan meals with adequate calories and protein.
c. Limited weight gain in prior or current pregnancy (use of weight chart)		
d. Multiple pregnancy		No published studies document increased needs. Larger blood volume, increased fetal and placental mass suggests need for increased nutrients.
e. History of pregnancy loss, pregnancy complications, low birth weight infants		
7. Social-cultural-economic factors	Risk during pregnancy related to (specific factors derived from assessment).	See texts for examples of variations of specific ethnic group. Nutritional intervention must be within context of ethnic group preference and individual preference. Refer to appropriate resource for economic assistance in food purchases.
a. Ethnic group: Assess individual variations from traditional group practice.		
b. Economic factors: Assess funds available for food purchase, possible eligibility for assistance (WIC, food stamps).		

Continued on following page

Nursing Care Plan 12–1. Nutritional Assessment and Counseling (Continued)

ASSESSMENT	POTENTIAL NURSING DIAGNOSIS	NURSING INTERVENTION	COMMENTS/RATIONALE
7. Social-cultural-economic factors (Continued)			
c. Vegetarianism 1. Strict 2. Lactovegetarian 3. Lacto-ovo-vegetarian		Vegetarians will need specific nutritional counseling, usually from nutritionists experienced in working with vegetarians.	Some practicing vegetarians are very knowledgeable about combining proteins for complete protein intake; others have limited nutritional understanding. Seventh-Day Adventist Church has specific materials about nutrition for pregnant and lactating vegetarians.
d. Pica (starch, flour, cracked ice, clay, and other nonfood substances)		Provide information about potential dangers. Encourage substitution of other foods for pica.	
e. Smoking (number of packs per day)		Encourage cessation of smoking; explain relationship of smoking and fetal growth (Chapter 8).	
f. Regularity of meals (meals on a regular basis or snacking throughout day)		Some pregnant women have little control over some or all of the food they eat (e.g., adolescent living at home with parents).	
g. Person who buys and prepares food for household			
8. Nutrition in current pregnancy a. Food intake in a "typical" day. Identify areas of need, if any. (If 24 hr. recall is the basis of assessment, determine if the day recalled was typical of usual diet.)		If changes are to be made, address one change at a time— e.g., the addition of citrus fruit or juice. Counsel within framework of other assessed factors.	
b. Alcohol consumption		Explain rationale for deletion of alcohol during pregnancy.	
	Continuing Assessment		
1. Weight gain a. Inadequate: gain of 1 kg.) (2.2 pounds) per month during second and third trimesters		Continue to review importance of weight gain. Review dietary intake; help to modify.	Inadequate weight gain increases risk of low birth weight newborn.
b. Excessive: gain of 3 kg. (6.6 pounds) or more per month		Review dietary intake, methods of preparing foods. Identify "empty" calories.	Excessive weight gain may be due to edema. Excessive fat deposits may contribute to later obesity.
2. Improvement in problems identified in earlier assessment			

Table 12–1. FACTORS IN GENERAL AND REPRODUCTIVE HEALTH THAT MAY BE RELATED TO NUTRITIONAL STATUS

Factors	Relation to Nutritional Status
Age	Young adolescents have increased nutrient needs for growth; often have poor food habits.
Age at menarche	Average age at menarche: 12.5 years. Delayed onset may be associated with poor childhood nutrition.
Prepregnancy weight	Weight less than 100 pounds or greater than 200 pounds correlates with poor pregnancy outcome. Recent substantial weight loss from dieting may deplete nutritional reserves.
Addiction to drugs, alcohol, cigarette smoking	Women addicted to drugs and alcohol often have nutritional deficiencies; cigarette smoking correlates with low birth weight.
Chronic disease	Effects of metabolic diseases are intensified during pregnancy; nutrient requirements of some disease states may affect pregnancy.
Weight gain in previous pregnancies	Previous patterns of low or excessive weight gain may indicate special nutritional learning needs.
Outcome in previous pregnancies	Low birth weight may suggest previous nutritional problem that is still present; large-for-gestational-age infant (Chapter 20), stillbirths, congenital malformations may suggest pregestational or gestational diabetes.
Length of interconceptual period	Interval between end of lactation and subsequent pregnancy of less than a year may deplete nutritional stores in undernourished mothers.
Steroid contraception	May inhibit folic acid absorption.
EDC (estimated date of confinement)	Nutritional planning is keyed to stage of pregnancy.
Anemia: iron deficiency or megaloblastic	Inadequate nutrition.

In addition to compromising essential intake, attempts at weight reduction during pregnancy can lead to acidosis, which may place the fetus at risk.

3. Improved nutrition during pregnancy is associated with decreased perinatal mortality.

4. Improved nutrition or supplementation of the maternal diet has been associated with improved mental and motor development and behavior in infancy.[2, 5, 13, 18]

5. The concept that the fetus will be able to supply its needs from maternal stores, regardless of the nutritional status of the mother, is invalid. As noted above, the mother may not have adequate stores.

6. Pregnancies involving more than one fetus (twins, for example) increase nutritional needs, particularly for iron and folic acid.

7. When pregnancies are closely spaced, particularly if there is reason to believe that nutritional needs have been unmet or marginally met in prior pregnancies, the mother is nutritionally at risk.

Meeting Nutritional Needs

During pregnancy, women have specific needs for calories, protein, fats, iron, calcium and phosphorus, sodium, iodine, trace elements, vitamins, and folic acid. The need for many of these essentials is increased during adolescence, when growth needs for the adolescent mother as well as for the fetus must be considered, as indicated in the tables that follow. For convenience, the needs of the lactating mother are also included.

Table 12–2. DAILY CALORIC NEEDS*

Age	Normal	Pregnancy	Lactation
11–14	2200	2500	2700
15–18	2100	2400	2600
19–50	2000	2300	2500

*Food and Nutrition Board, National Research Council, 1980.

The Need for Calories

The need for adequate calories to provide optimal weight gain has already been discussed. Calories are needed for the growth of the fetus, placenta, and associated maternal tissues. An increased maternal basal metabolism also requires additional calories. If the mother's daily activities become more limited, this will partially offset her caloric needs. Calories are also important to protect protein. When calorie intake is not adequate, the body will utilize protein for energy; protein then becomes unavailable for necessary growth. In addition, the breakdown of protein leads to acidosis. Caloric needs are summarized in Table 12–2. Higgins[6] suggests that a number of specialized conditions increase caloric needs (Table 12–3).

Table 12–3. CALORIC AND PROTEIN SUPPLEMENTATION*

Criteria	Additional Calories per Day	Additional Protein per Day (g)
20 weeks gestation or more	500	25
Protein deficit[a]	10/g of deficit	equal to deficit
Underweight by 5% or more[b]	500[c]	20
Nutritional stress (per condition)		
Pernicious vomiting	200	20
Less than 1 year between pregnancies	200	20
Poor previous obstetrical history	200	20
Failure to gain 10 lbs by week 20	200	20
Serious emotional problems	200	20

*From Moore: *Newborn, Family, and Nurse.* 2nd ed. Philadelphia, W. B. Saunders Co., 1981.
[a]Difference between actual dietary intake and requirement.
[b]Metropolitan Life Insurance weight tables.
[c]Permits gain of 1 lb per week; mother is to gain the difference in her weight and the norm for her height.

The Need for Protein

It should not be surprising that the need for protein, so essential for all growth, is increased during pregnancy (Table 12–4). Proteins are the only food substances that contain nitrogen, phosphorus, and sulfur; fats and carbohydrates do not. Protein is essential for the synthesis of hemoglobin; iron alone will not alleviate anemia.

Proteins consist of 22 known amino acids, the amount of a single amino acid and the combination of amino acids varying from one protein to another. Nine of these amino acids are called "essential" because they cannot be synthesized within the adult human body. Of the nine essential amino acids, the need for histidine for adults has not yet been established. It is necessary for infants. Not only must the essential amino acids be ingested, they must be ingested *simultaneously* and in *proper balance*

Proteins that contain all eight essential adult amino acids in a balance usable by the body are called *complete* proteins. In general, animal proteins are complete proteins. When one or more amino acids are limited in amount, the usefulness of all the other amino acids is limited in the same proportion. Proteins lacking or having a limited amount of an essential amino acid are called *incomplete*; most plant protein is incomplete. However, all eight essential adult amino acids are contained in one plant or another, so that it is possible to eat meals containing the necessary amino acids using plant sources rather than animal sources by a proper combination of foods. When the amino acids in one protein complete the amino acids in another, these are called *complementary* protein combinations. Basic complementary combinations are grains and legumes, grains and milk, and seeds and legumes. Table 12–5 illustrates some complementary combinations using commonly available foods. It is interesting that the traditional dishes of many cultures combine plant foods that complement one another to make a complete protein. For example, Latin American black beans and rice, Creole red beans and rice, the hopping John of the Carolina low country (cow peas and rice),

Table 12–4. PROTEIN*

Recommended Daily Dietary Allowance (Grams)

	11–14 Years	*15–18 Years*	*19–50 Years*
Nonpregnant	48	52	44
Pregnant	78	82	74
Lactating	68	72	64

Foods	Size of Serving	Approximate Grams of Protein
Turkey (combination dark and light)	3 ounces (3 pieces)	26.8
Chicken	Thigh or half breast	25.7
Tuna fish[a]	3½ ounces (small can)	27.7
Great northern dried beans (raw)	½ cup dried (raw)	20
Canned salmon (various kinds)	1 cup	47
Cottage cheese (large or small curd)	½ cup	16.6
Beef (e.g., chuck roast)	3 ounces (1 slice)	19–26
Fish (e.g., perch, haddock; not seafood)	3½ ounces (1 piece)	17–19
Hamburger (cooked)	3 ounces	19–23
Milk[a]	8 ounces (1 cup)	8.5
Eggs	1 medium	5.7
	1 large	6.5
	1 extra-large	7.4
Peanut butter	1 tablespoon	4.0
Bread	1 slice	2.2–2.4

*From Adams: *Nutritive Value of American Foods in Common Units*. Agriculture Handbook #456, Washington, D.C., United States Department of Agriculture, November 1975.

[a]Most economical in terms of amount and quality of protein in relation to cost.

Table 12–5. COMPLEMENTARY VEGETABLE PROTEIN

Serve	At the Same Meal with One of These Foods
Rice	Beans Soy products Sesame seeds Milk Wheat and soy combinations
Whole wheat	Milk Beans Soy products Peanuts and milk Peanuts and soy products Soy and sesame products
Cornmeal	Beans Soy products and milk
Peanuts	Milk Sunflower seeds Soy and sesame products
Beans	Rice Cornmeal Milk Whole wheat bread
Potatoes	Milk

New England baked beans and brown bread, and the corn bread and pinto beans of the South.

Although knowledge of complementary proteins is essential in counseling women who choose to be vegetarians (see below), it is also useful in helping any mother supplement the protein in her diet. Many plant proteins are less expensive than animal proteins and can be used to stretch animal proteins for maximum effectiveness. Just adding milk, for example, to a meal that contains rice, whole wheat, peanuts (peanut butter), beans or potatoes complements the incomplete protein in these foods and boosts the mother's intake of usable protein.

The Need for Fats

Large amounts of fats are not tolerated well by many women during pregnancy (see section on gastrointestinal disturbances above), nor are large amounts necessary. Some fat is necessary to supply essential fatty acids and fat-soluble vitamins; margarine on a piece of toast will supply this need. Many popular foods, such as peanut butter, contain fat as well as protein.

The Need for Iron

Iron is essential during pregnancy for both mother and fetus. Few mothers have iron stores sufficient to meet their own needs and those of the fetus. Beginning in the fifth month, the fetus begins to store iron that will serve him during the first 4 to 6 months of his life. If the mother's iron intake is inadequate or if the baby is born prior to term, the newborn's iron stores will be inadequate, and he will be at risk of developing iron deficiency anemia during his first year of life. Inadequate iron intake during pregnancy will also leave the mother with iron deficiency anemia in the weeks following delivery; she may find herself weak and chronically tired and find mothering a difficult task.

The increased need for iron during pregnancy is caused by:

1. Increased maternal red cell volume—300 mg.
2. Fetal iron stores—300 mg.
3. Iron stored in the placenta—70 mg.
4. Iron in blood lost at the time of delivery—50 mg.

A small amount of iron (about 150 mg.) is conserved by the body during pregnancy because of the cessation of menstruation.

Iron is available in small quantities in a large variety of foods (Table 12–6). When the diet habits of many Americans are considered, these foods are not eaten in quantities sufficient to meet iron needs. Since these needs are greater during pregnancy, mothers should be encouraged to eat foods high in iron. An iron supplement (30 to 60 mg. per day) is also recommended during pregnancy to help the mother meet these increased needs. However, supplements should not be relied upon to correct improper food habits. Good eating patterns formed during pregnancy can be the basis for good eating patterns that will last after pregnancy and that can influence the food habits of other family members.

The Need for Calcium and Phosphorus

Calcium needs during pregnancy are increased by 50 per cent because of the needs of the fetus for calcium in skeletal development and because of the role of calcium in muscle function and blood coagulation.

Four glasses of milk will meet the need for calcium; a piece of cheddar cheese weighing 1¼ ounces substitutes for 8 ounces of milk. Green leafy vegetables are also good sources of calcium (Table 12–7). Outside of these foods, calcium amounts in single servings are more limited. For the woman who does not drink milk or utilize sufficient quantities of milk in her cooking, calcium supplementation, usually calcium gluconate (1000 mg. in the first and second trimesters; 1500 mg. in the third trimester), is necessary. The mother with lactose intolerance has a dual problem because of low calcium intake and decreased calcium absorption.

Maternal stores of calcium are more difficult to monitor than iron stores unless the deficiency is severe because the body maintains equilibrium of calcium and other minerals in the plasma.

Needs for phosphorus are met when calcium needs are adequately served.

The Need for Sodium

Sodium needs are adequately met through normal eating patterns. The problem with sodium intake is *iatrogenic* (i.e., caused by faulty health care), in this instance the result of faulty health teaching. For several decades we have urged women to restrict their salt intake as a precaution against edema and pre-eclampsia. It is now recognized that:

1. Some edema of the ankles and feet is normal during pregnancy and is not a sign of impending pre-eclampsia.
2. Sodium is essential to maintain normal

Table 12–6.   IRON

Recommended Dietary Allowance		
Adolescent and Adult (Ages 11–50)		
Nonpregnant	18 mg. per day	
Pregnant	18 plus mg. per day plus supplement[a]	
Lactating	18 mg. per day plus supplement[a]	
Foods	**Size of Serving**	**Mg.**
Liver, pork	3 ounces	24.7
Liver, beef	3 ounces	7.5
Variety meats:		
Kidney	4 ounces	14.8
Heart	4 ounces	6.8
Turkey (combination light and dark)	3 ounces	1.5
Beef (chuck)	3 ounces	2–3
Soybean flour (low fat)	½ cup	4
Grits[b]	½ cup	0.4 (based on minimum level of enrichment)
Dark green vegetables:		
Mustard greens	½ cup cooked	1.2
Turnip greens	½ cup cooked	0.8
Spinach	½ cup cooked	2.0
Bread (enriched)	1 slice	0.3–0.7
Eggs[a]	1 extra-large	1.3
	1 large	1.2
	1 medium	1.0
Cereals—may be fortified (see individual packages)		

[a]The Committee on Maternal Nutrition, National Research Council, recommends supplementation with 30 to 60 mg. of elemental iron per day. Adequate iron intake cannot be met by traditional diet.

[b]Can be blended with other flours in making breads and used as ground meat extender.

sodium levels in plasma, bone, brain, and muscle, as both tissue and fluid expand during the prenatal period.

Sodium restriction is now considered potentially hazardous. Therefore, sodium *should not be restricted*. Diuretics, which can lead to sodium loss, should not be used.

The Need for Iodine

The need for iodine, an essential nutrient, can be met be encouraging the use of iodized salt. Women who buy most of their foods at "natural food" stores should know that sea salt is not iodized. However, seafoods such as

Table 12–7.   CALCIUM

Recommended Daily Dietary Allowance		
Adolescent and Adult	*11–18 Years*	*19–50 Years*
Nonpregnant	1200 mg.	800 mg.
Pregnant	1600 mg.	1200 mg.
Lactating	1600 mg.	1200 mg.
Foods	**Size of Serving**	**Mg.**
Milk	1 cup	288
Cheese, cheddar	1 ounce	213
Dark green vegetables		
Mustard greens	½ cup cooked	97
Turnip greens	½ cup cooked	134
Broccoli	½ cup cooked	68
Spinach	½ cup cooked	84
Soybean flour	½ cup	116
Grits (cooked) enriched[a]	½ cup	1

[a]Can be blended with other flours in making breads and used as ground meat extender.

Table 12–8.   VITAMIN A

Recommended Daily Allowance	
Adolescent and Adult (Ages 11–50)	
Nonpregnant	800 mg RE[a]
Pregnant	1000 mg RE
Lactating	1200 mg RE

Foods	Size of Serving	Vitamin A Content RE
Spinach (cooked)	½ cup	1100–2300[b]
Other leafy green vegetables	½ cup	Up to 1200
Broccoli	½ cup	190–240
Liver (beef)	3 ounces	500–1000
Sweet potatoes	1 medium	900–1100
Squash, yellow	½ cup	79–106
Carrots	½ cup	760–1200
Apricots (dried or fresh)	2	157–220
Peaches, fresh yellow	1 medium	100–200
Nonfat dry milk:		
Vitamin A added	1 cup reconstituted	200
No added vitamin A	1 cup reconstituted	3
Whole milk (not fortified with vitamin A)	1 cup	35

[a]Content varies; in general, the deeper the color, the more vitamin A.
[b]RE = Retinal Equivalent. This is the recommended unit of measure. 1 RE = 10 IU.

shrimp, scallops, and clams are good sources of iodine.

The Need for Trace Elements

There is a great deal yet to be learned about trace elements, those nutrients that appear in foods in small "traces" but that are nevertheless essential. One of the fallacies of relying on vitamin preparations rather than foods to supply essential nutrients is that we may not even be aware of all of our needs. For example, when breads and cereals are enriched, intake of B vitamins and iron may be sufficiently increased, but the content of magnesium and zinc will be less than that in whole grain products.

The Need for Vitamin A

Vitamin A is abundant in a number of foods (Table 12–8). Many of these foods are not included in American diets, which tend to skimp on liver and dark green and yellow vegetables. Whole milk contains limited amounts of vitamin A, but nonfat dry milk to

which vitamin A has been added can be a good source.

The fetus stores about 7000 I.U. of vitamin A in his liver during the last half of pregnancy, a need met adequately if the required intake is achieved. The increased need for vitamin A during lactation provides for the vitamin A excreted in breast milk.

The Need for B Vitamins

Thiamine, riboflavin, niacin, B_6 and B_{12} are components of the B complex vitamins. During pregnancy, the need for these vitamins is increased slightly as caloric intake is increased because of their essential role in metabolism. When foods are cooked properly and eaten in the recommended amounts for pregnancy, the needs for B complex vitamins will be met (Table 12–9).

Good food sources of thiamine are pork, dried beans and peas, liver, and nuts. Up to 50 per cent of thiamine may be destroyed by heat. From 12 to 24 per cent of the thiamine in meat may be in the gravy by the time the meat is served.

Table 12–9.   B VITAMINS

	Thiamine (mg.)			Riboflavin (mg.)			Niacin (mg.)		
Ages	*11–14*	*15–18*	*19–50*	*11–14*	*15–18*	*19–50*	*11–14*	*15–18*	*19–50*
Nonpregnant	1.2	1.1	1.0	1.3	1.4	1.2	16.0	14.0	13.0
Pregnant	1.5	1.5	1.4	1.6	1.6	1.5	17.0	16.0	15.0
Lactating	1.6	1.6	1.5	1.8	1.8	1.7	20.0	20.0	20.0

Riboflavin, like thiamine, is affected by heat, with 10 to 30 per cent being lost in the cooking liquid of vegetables. The old custom of dunking cornbread in the liquid in which greens were cooked ("pot-licker") saved vitamins for our grandfathers' generation, but is rare today. Riboflavin is also lost when foods are left in the light. Foods that are high in riboflavin are liver, milk, meat, and cottage cheese.

Although niacin is not affected by heat, it is still lost in the water in which vegetables are cooked. Liver, fish, poultry, meat, and peanut butter are all good sources of niacin, The body is also able to convert a small amount of the amino acid tryptophan into niacin.

Vitamin B_6 (pyridoxine) plays an essential role in metabolism; it is required by all animals. The need is increased as protein needs are increased, because it is a coenzyme in many phases of amino acid metabolism. Meat, cereals, nuts, lentils, and some fruits and vegetables are good sources of vitamin B_6.

Vitamin B_{12} plays an important role in normal growth and in the maintenance of epithelial cells and the myelin sheath of the nervous system. It helps to maintain erythropoiesis (in combination with folic acid) and leukopoiesis. Like several other vitamins, it is heat labile and some is lost in cooking. Vitamin B_{12} is found primarily in animal products. Therefore, a strict vegetarian must receive supplementary B_{12}. A serum B_{12} determination is advisable for women who are vegetarians.

The Need for Vitamin C

Because water-soluble vitamin C is not stored in the body, daily intake is essential (Table 12–10). Meeting the requirement for vitamin C is not as difficult as for some other vitamins, at least for middle class mothers, who choose daily citrus fruits and juices. Fortunately, in the summer when citrus fruit is more expensive, tomatoes, cabbage, and green peppers are fairly abundant. Heat affects vitamin C.

The Need for Vitamin D

Vitamin D is necessary to ensure calcium absorption and utilization. The normal need for vitamin D, 400 I.U., is apparently not increased during pregnancy or lactation. Ever since margarine, butter, and milk have been fortified with vitamin D, and because even a few minutes of sunshine each day will lead to the manufacture of vitamin D in the body, deficiencies of this vitamin are not a major problem in the United States unless the diet is very severely limited.

The Need for Vitamin E

Vitamin E plays a role in both growth and metabolism. Vitamin E is found chiefly in vegetable and seed oils. When food needs have been properly met, vitamin E needs will be met as well.

The Need for Folic Acid (Folacin)

Folic acid is involved in a number of metabolic processes. A deficiency of folic acid leads to several types of anemia, including megaloblastic anemia, which is relatively common in pregnancy. Folic acid deficiency also affects the normal response of female reproductive organs to estrogens. Folic acid is provided by intestinal synthesis in man. Of the folic acid ingested, 75 per cent is excreted in the urine.

Serum folacin levels are measured in some pregnant patients. The desired level is 6 nan-

Table 12–10. VITAMIN C

Recommended Daily Allowance		
	Age 11–14	*Age 15–50*
Nonpregnant	50 mg.	60 mg.
Pregnant	70 mg.	80 mg.
Lactating	90 mg.	100 mg.
Foods	**Size of Serving**	**Mg.**
Orange juice	4 ounces (½ cup)	50–60
Grapefruit	½	30–67
Green vegetables:		
Broccoli	½ cup	50–70
Green, leafy vegetables	½ cup	20–50
Green peppers	½ cup	20–50
Tomatoes	1	20–40
Cabbage, raw	½ cup	15–35

Table 12–11. FOLIC ACID (AGES 11–50)

Nonpregnant	400 mg.
Pregnant	800 mg.
Lactating	500 mg.

ograms per ml. Folic acid is available in a wide variety of foods, especially liver, leafy vegetables, fruit, and yeast. Folic acid requirements during pregnancy are greatly increased (Table 12–11). Many nutritionists and the American College of Obstetrics and Gynecology (ACOG) advise supplementation of the diet with folic acid (200–400 mg. per day).

A Diet Plan

Nurses must understand basic food needs before they can counsel patients. But basic needs must be translated into the kind of meals that patients eat. The following pattern (Table 12–12) is suggested because it can be adapted by women from every cultural background (Table 12–13).

Applying Principles to an Individual Patient

Doris C. is 20 years old, a black woman pregnant for the first time. She finished eleventh grade before dropping out of school. Ms. C. is 5′3″ tall and weighs 133 pounds in her fifth month of pregnancy. She says that her prepregnancy weight was "about" 125 pounds, which is slightly overweight for her height. A weight gain of 8 pounds at 20 weeks is "right on target."

Breakfast:	1	slice toast
	1	soda (soft drink)
Lunch:	2	beef sandwiches
Dinner:	2	pork chops
	½	cup snap beans
	2	slices light bread
Snacks:	2	sodas
	3	donuts
	4	cups cracked ice
	¼	cup starch
		(laundry starch)

She reports that she has approximately $22 to spend each week on groceries for herself and her husband. She is eligible for and uses food stamps.

An analysis of Doris C.'s diet indicates an adequate intake of protein and an excessive intake of grains. She had one nonleafy green vegetable. Milk, a vitamin C fruit or vegetable, and leafy green vegetables are lacking.

This mother indicated, however, that she likes milk and often drinks as much as 6 glasses a day; that she eats oranges and apples

Table 12–12. BASIC MEAL PLAN

Vitamin C fruit or vegetable	1 serving
Vitamin A fruit or vegetable	1 serving
Other fruits or vegetables	2 servings
Meat	3 servings
Milk	3–4 cups
Grain	3–4 servings

two to three times a week, and that she likes both broccoli and spinach. Using foods she likes, it should not be too difficult to modify her diet to meet her basic needs. The amount of money she has to spend for food would be a real constraint without food stamps; however, with stamps and careful spending, she can manage adequately.

One of the biggest problems for Doris C. is the large number of "empty" calories she consumes from laundry starch (see pica, below), sodas (soft drinks), and donuts. These habits will be difficult to change, but if they are not changed, her baby will probably also be eating these foods before his first birthday.

A follow-up interview 2 weeks later showed the addition of orange juice, milk, and "greens" to the day's menus, but continued to show intake of both starch and "junk food."

Mothers with Special Needs

Many mothers will need special help in planning meals during pregnancy. The reason may be cultural, economic, or physiologic (lactose intolerance, gastrointestinal problems during pregnancy, or a medical complication such as diabetes or toxemia). Nutritional problems related to high risk conditions such as diabetes are discussed in Chapter 13.

Cultural Variations in Food Preferences

There is no standard diet in the United States. Many groups of peoples have special foods and special ways of preparing food that add welcome variety to our dining.

During pregnancy, some ethnic variations in diet may present problems in achieving optimum nutrition. Several large ethnic groups are discussed here by way of example. In our practice, we must become familiar with both customs in our communities and also with the ways in which each individual woman conforms to or varies from the cultural practice of her group.

The Spanish-American Mother. The Spanish-speaking mother may be a Mexican-American in California or Texas, a Cuban-

Table 12–13. ADAPTATION OF BASIC NEEDS IN SELECTED CULTURES

	Basic	Southern	Mexican-American	Oriental
Breakfast				
Fruit or vegetable containing vitamin C[a]	Orange	Orange	Orange	Orange
Grain product (bread, cereal)	Cereal or toast	Grits or biscuits	Tortilla	Rice
Milk product	Milk	Buttermilk	Milk in coffee	(Limited milk taken as beverage)
Protein food	Egg	Egg	Egg	Egg
Lunch				
Grain product (2 servings, e.g., 2 slices bread)	Grilled cheese sandwich	Cornbread	Tortillas[b]	Rice
Protein food	Apple	Pinto beans	Pinto beans	Fish
Fruit or vegetable	Milk	Greens	Apple or tomatoes	Bean sprouts
Milk product		Milk	Custard	Tofu[c]
Dinner				
Protein food (2 servings)	Hamburger	Chicken	Chicken	Chicken
Leafy green vegetables (2 servings)[a]	Spinach (2)	Collards	(Few green and yellow vegetables eaten; suggest carrots)	Chinese broccoli
Grain product	Roll	Broccoli		Mustard greens
Milk product	Milk	Biscuits		Rice
		Milk	Rice pudding	Cheese
Between Meals and at Bedtime				
Milk product	Cottage cheese or milk	Cottage cheese or milk	Cheese	Tofu

[a]Could be eaten at another meal.
[b]Suggest nonfat dry milk in preparing tortillas.
[c]Tofu is soybean curd; it contains protein and also calcium, the latter often deficient in Oriental diets because of low milk intake.

American in Miami, or an American of Puerto Rican descent in New York City (Chapter 5). Although food preferences vary, there are some similar areas. Special considerations concerning Spanish-American diets are:

1. Milk is not commonly used as a beverage, and only fairly small amounts are used in cooking. Cheese, however, is popular, but the amount is often not adequate for calcium needs. Some milk is used in puddings.

2. Consumption of carbonated beverages and other foods with high calories but low nutritive value is common.

3. Tomatoes and chili peppers are popular vegetables. Few yellow and green leafy vegetables are used. Vegetables may be cooked for long periods of time.

The Mother of Asian Heritage. Mothers of Asian heritage—Japanese, Chinese, Filipino, and Indian, for example—like Spanish-speaking mothers, represent a diverse heritage but may share some characteristics.

Oriental cuisine varies from one nationality to another; the longer a family has been in the United States, the less strict is adherence to traditional diet patterns. There are some common practices that are important to note when planning a diet during pregnancy and lactation.

1. Milk is used in limited quantities; it is rarely used as a beverage. Thus calcium and vitamin D intake may need to be supplemented. Six ounces of tofu (soybean curd), a popular dish, contains the same amount of calcium as a cup of milk.

2. Since rice is such a basic staple, it is important that enriched rice be used and that it not be washed before cooking.

3. A large assortment of fruits and vegetables are used.

4. Stir frying, a popular method of preparing vegetables, meats and fish, results in minimal vitamin loss.

5. Meats and fish may be eaten in such small quantities that protein and calorie intake is often inadequate.

American Indian Mother. Every American Indian tribe has had its own traditional diet modifications in years gone by. Today Indian diets tend to be "Americanized" and vary with location. Coastal Indians will eat more seafood, for example, but so do non-Indian peoples living in coastal areas.

Poverty (Chapter 5) rather than Indian traditions may limit the diets of many American Indian mothers. Protein, fruits, vegetables, and milk may be limited, and carbohydrate intake may be high.

Traditional Southern Cooking. All of the necessities of excellent basic nutrition are present in the traditional Southern diet. Proteins are available not only in meats but in popular pinto beans, black-eyed peas, and the like. Probably few people eat as many leafy green vegetables (collards, mustard greens, and turnip greens, for example) as do Southerners. Unfortunately, these vegetables are cooked for a long period of time, and if the cooking water (pot-licker) is discarded, much food value is lost. The old custom of dipping bread in the pot-licker was commendable from a vitamin standpoint. Both buttermilk and "sweet milk" are popular. Peaches, strawberries, and apples are grown and eaten.

Disadvantages include a high consumption of carbonated beverages and a somewhat limited intake of citrus fruits. The popularity of pica among many Southern black women is discussed below.

The Mother Who Is a Vegetarian. Vegetarianism is popular with many young couples. Unknowledgeable vegetarianism, with limited intake of complete proteins, can present hazards to the growing fetus and to the mother herself. Ideally, women who are vegetarians should be counseled by nutritionists during pregnancy and lactation. The aim of counseling is not to convince the mother to give up vegetarianism but to be sure that she is eating combinations of plant products that will assure adequate nutrition.

There are three basic types of vegetarian diets:

1. The strict or pure vegetarian diet, which excludes all foods of animal origin.

2. The lactovegetarian diet, which includes milk, cheese, and other diary products, but not eggs, meats, poultry, and fish.

3. The lacto-ovo-vegetarian diet, which includes eggs and sometimes fish, as well as dairy products, but excludes meat and poultry.

Obviously the more limited the diet, the greater the potential hazard. The macrobiotic diet eaten by some families, which contains no fresh fruits or vegetables as well as no animal protein, is extremely limited and dangerous. Vegetarian diets lack vitamin B_{12} unless four glasses of cow's milk are consumed daily; otherwise vitamin B_{12} (4 micrograms) must be given as a supplement, An iron supplement is recommended, as it is for all pregnant women. Vegetarians who do not drink milk must have supplemental calcium (see calcium, above) and vitamin D (400 I.U. per day). Iodized salt should be used during pregnancy.

Special Physiologic Needs

The Mother Who Is Lactose Intolerant. In talking with patients about diet, it is not unusual for a woman to tell us, "I can't drink milk; it makes me sick." For many years this was translated as either (1) the individual just didn't like milk or (2) she was allergic to milk. A third possibility is the presence of lactose intolerance.

Lactose is the sugar in milk; lactase is the enzyme that breaks down lactose into simple sugars (glucose and galactose) that are then utilized by the body. Adult mammals other than man lack lactase; kittens and puppies drink milk, for example, but cats and dogs do not. Many humans after the age of 2 to 4 years are also lactase deficient and therefore lactose intolerant. The reason that this has not been recognized widely until very recently is that approximately 90 per cent of individuals of nothern European ancestry are exceptions, and much of scientific research has dealt with northern Europeans. Another exception is the members of certain pastoral tribes in Africa, tribes that use fresh milk as a major contribution to their diet; about 8 per cent of the people in these tribes are lactose intolerant.

Why this difference in lactose tolerance? There are two theories, each of which may be a partial explanation. In terms of evolution, those individuals who were able to digest milk in societies in which milk was available has a survival advantage over those individuals who were not able to do so. It may also be that the drinking of milk by men and women in those societies stimulated lactase activity. Experiments in rats suggest that this may be so.

In the United States one might expect to find more lactose intolerance among blacks than among whites. Most of the black people brought to the United States were West Africans, people originally intolerant to lactose. Kretchmer[8] suggests that in the 10 to 15 generations that black men and women have been in this country a certain amount of northern European genes have entered the black population; he estimates that approximately 70 per cent of American blacks may be lactose intolerant. So, too, may white persons from many areas of the world, and Indian and Asian peoples as well.

Symptoms of lactose intolerance include a bloated feeling, flatulence, cramps and watery diarrhea after the ingestion of milk. (These symptoms are also seen in some newborns who are lactose intolerant either because of a congenital deficiency or as a secondary reaction to a variety of conditions, including surgery, drugs, or even nonspecific diarrhea).

Some lactose intolerant people can drink small amounts of milk or eat milk products, which can be helpful in planning their diets. In Nigeria, for example, pastoral Fulani drink fresh milk and prepare a partially fermented yogurt-like milk drink, with reduced lactose content, for sale in the marketplace to villagers who cannot digest milk. Mothers who tell us they cannot drink milk may be able to include cheeses in their diet in order to receive the nutrients contained in milk.

An awareness and appreciation of lactose intolerance is important not only in helping people in the United States but in nutrition assistance to peoples in other parts of the world. Large scale dissemination of standard powdered milk to a lactose intolerant people is of no value; lactose-free powder would be far more useful.

Mothers who are lactose intolerant should receive supplemental calcium (1200 mg.) and vitamin D (400 I.U.) each day during pregnancy. They will also need to increase their intake of other protein foods, since milk is such a major source of dietary protein.

The Mother with Food Allergies. Mothers who have specific food allergies must have meals planned or supplements provided to supply the nutrients in the foods they must avoid. Orange juice is a fairly common allergen, as are yeast, wheat, eggs, and milk. Although it is important to help women recognize the difference between their dislikes and true allergies, the practical results of both are the same—the food will not be eaten, and the nutrient will therefore be missed.

The Mother Who Ingests Pica. Nonfood substances that are eaten are called *pica*. Varieties of pica common in the United States include laundry starch, white flour (considered a nonfood in the raw form), and clay. The excessive consumption of cracked ice is a similar practice.

The ingestion of pica is increased during pregnancy but occurs at other times as well. It is also practiced by men, although apparently less frequently in the United States than in other countries. The ingestion of pica is high among poor black women in both the South and in northern cities. Li and White[10] found that 45 of 49 pregnant teenagers, all black, admitted having eaten starch at one time or another. Twelve had also eaten clay or expressed a preference for clay over starch.

In a smaller sample of 13 women in another community, Hochstein[7] found that one-fourth ate clay, half favored starch, and the remaining women preferred raw flour.

Various reasons have been offered to explain the phenomenon of pica. They include the relief of spasms due to hunger, the relief of menstrual cramps or uterine sensations that occur during pregnancy, and the belief that the clay may contain substances essential to the well-being of mother or child. Hochstein points out that just as the physician may recommend soda crackers to the middle class mother who is nauseated during early pregnancy, neighbors and relatives of the poorer mother may guide her to clay or starch for the same purpose.

Regardless of the historically reported reasons for pica, Li[10] found that the girls in her study ate clay because it was "good," "gummy," "crunchy," or "bitter." Their descriptions of starch included "good, "smooth," "sweet," "bitter," and "thick." In short, they enjoyed eating the clay or the starch, just as the woman who smokes or chews gum enjoys that particular habit. In no way did the girls in the study attribute any special food value to either starch or clay. The habit seemed so natural to them that there was no reluctance to discuss it; it was no different from expressing a preference for a candy bar. The findings of other researchers support this matter-of-fact attitude.

Is the ingestion of pica harmful? One potential harm is the substitution of "empty calories" for food that contains essential nutrients. Anemia is not unusual among mothers who ingest pica, probably due in part to socioeconomic status as well as to the pica itself. Eating clay is thought to interfere with the absorption of iron in the gastrointestinal tract; anemia in a mother who continues to eat clay is treated with parenteral rather than oral iron. Fecal impaction is a potential hazard to clay eaters; the attempt to relieve the impaction with enemas may lead to premature labor.

It is not easy to persuade a woman to give up the ingestion of pica, just as it is not easy to persuade many people to give up cigarettes.

The Mother with a Limited Income

The foods that pregnant women need most— foods high in animal protein and rich in vitamins and minerals—often appear to be the most expensive in the grocery store. Certainly though, when one looks at food value in relation to cost, they are not; a quarter spent for a soft drink is wasted in terms of nutrition. However, many people on limited incomes, with little knowledge of nutritional needs, eat foods that fill their stomachs and keep them from feeling hungry—usually foods high in carbohydrate and often little else.

It is more difficult for the mother with a limited income to buy the foods she needs, not only because of the number of dollars she has to spend but because of several other related factors. She may be forced to shop in a neighborhood "Mom and Pop" store, in which prices are higher as a result of small volume, because she has no transportation to a less expensive supermarket. In addition, she may be charging food at the small neighborhood grocery and, as a result, spending part of her food dollars paying interest on the bills she owes for last month's food. She may not have proper storage facilities for what she buys, which not only limits her purchase of "specials" at reduced prices but may also mean spoilage and waste. The low income mother may also not have cooking facilities to prepare a variety of foods.

Changing any of these factors involves a change in lifestyle that may not be possible for many women. The time required to bring about such change may not be available to the nurse working with a large number of women, all of whom need help. Resource people are essential. In addition to a nutritionist who may be attached to the same facility where the nurse is working, homeworkers from extension services or the county agricultural services are available in many urban as well as rural communities. These home economists welcome referrals from obstetric clinics and have more time than we usually do to help families improve their practices of buying, storing, and preparing food.

Concurrently, as we assess nutritional needs (see below), we may be able to begin to make one or two changes within the framework of the mother's budget. Information, of the kind described below, that is related to the specific community can be incorporated into information given to patients during pregnancy.

Milk. In reviewing the nutritional components of food, it is obvious that milk plays a major role in meeting the nutritional needs of pregnancy. Some low income mothers receive milk free through federally sponsored programs such as WIC (Women, Infants and Chil-

dren Supplemental Food Program). Nonfat dry milk, now fortified with fat-soluble vitamins A and D, is very useful for the mother who does not like to drink milk, because it can be so easily incorporated into cooking. For example, if a recipe for pudding or macaroni and cheese calls for a cup of milk, ½ cup of powder can be used instead of the ⅓ cup of powder that is ordinarily used to reconstitute a cup of milk. Hence, milk intake is increased by using the most inexpensive variety of milk. For women who drink milk but who do not enjoy the taste of reconstituted powdered milk, the powder can be combined with fresh whole milk (1:1 ratio) for good taste at a reduced price.

Cheeses. Many processed cheese foods have the nutritional value of more expensive varieties. Cheese is a good value because there is no waste; even the smallest scrap can be used in salads or sauces, for example.

Meats. Comparing meat prices should be on a cost per *serving* basis, not cost per pound. There are approximately four servings per pound in boneless meat and fish (hamburger, canned tuna, or canned chicken), two servings per pound in meat and fish with moderate bones (chicken, turkey, pot roast of beef) and one serving per pound in meats with a large amount of bone (spare ribs, short ribs).

Eggs. Eggs can be the protein food at lunch or dinner, as well as at breakfast.

Fish. Fish often gives more protein per ounce and per unit cost than meat and can be a big help in stretching budgets. (See Meats, above for serving information.)

Fruits and Vegetables. Farmer's markets, seasonal specials, and home gardens can help provide these foods, sometimes more difficult to include in the diet than the high protein foods in some parts of the country. Fruits and vegetables may be particularly difficult for the inner city mother to find at a good price at certain times of the year.

Cereals. Cooked cereals, many of which require only the briefest of cooking or merely the addition of hot water, are not only less expensive but are usually better sources of nutrition than cold cereals. They are excellent and economical foods for a growing baby, another important reason for making the mother more aware of them during pregnancy.

Preparation for Infant Feeding

As parents prepare for birth, one significant decision that they must make is the manner in which they will feed their infant—a decision that should be made in advance of the day of delivery.

What influences the choice of breast- or bottle-feeding? The choice is almost always a cultural decision rather than a medical one. In societies that are just beginning to develop technologically, there is no real choice but breast-feeding, either by the infant's own mother or by another lactating female. But even in traditional societies, breast-feeding is on the decline as mothers become aware of Western practices. This is hardly surprising; cultural change in some aspects of life does not take place in isolation from the rest of life. But it is unfortunate that the switch from breast- to bottle-feeding has taken place in many instances before water has become safe and before adequate sanitary conditions and practices are established. Thus gastrointestinal disease remains the major cause of infant mortality in many developing nations.

There was also little choice in the manner of feeding infants in our own country until late in the nineteenth century when technology made bottle-feeding a reasonably safe alternative to breast-feeding. As recently as 1946 approximately 65 per cent of American infants were breast-fed during the newborn period. By 1965 the figure had dropped to 26 per cent.

However, since 1971 breast-feeding has become increasingly common, with 33 per cent of infants of 1 week of age reported to be breast-fed in 1975 and 45 per cent reported to be breast-fed at 1 week in 1978.[12] Although the actual percentages are based on responses to mailed questionnaires and thus may not reflect the exact incidence in the population, the fact of an increased incidence of breast-feeding does seem evident.

Not only are more mothers initially breast-feeding, but many mothers seem to be breast-feeding for longer periods of time (Table 12–14). In 1971 only 5.5 per cent of infants were breast-fed at 5 to 6 months of age. By 1978 over 20 per cent of mothers continued to breast-feed at 5 to 6 months. These data suggest that support for breast-feeding mothers must not be limited to a brief period in the hospital (when one mother in three continues to breast-feed for 2 months and one in four continues for 3 to 4 months).

Although the incidence of breast-feeding remains higher in women with at least some college education, between 1971 and 1978 the most rapid increase in breast-feeding, both initially and at 2 months, was in mothers with less education and mothers living in rural areas. The percentage of mothers with incomes of less than $7,000 and those with incomes of between $7,000 and $14,999 who were breast-feeding at 2 months postdelivery doubled between 1971 and 1978. Primiparous mothers breast-feed more frequently than multiparous mothers. The reasons for this finding need to be explored.

A variety of studies indicate that several factors influence the decision to breast- or bottle-feed. These factors include being breast-fed as an infant, having friends who breast-feed, a successful previous breast-feeding experience, and support from husband and health-care providers.[16]

Schmitt[17] emphasizes that the cultural values of nurses, as articulated by the nursing literature, are strongly in favor of breast-feeding. She feels that such strong predispositions can interfere with good nursing care, and in this we feel she is correct. If a mother who prefers to bottle-feed feels that nurses expect her to breast-feed, she may do so while she is in the hospital, but will switch very quickly to bottle-feeding when she returns to her own home.

There are several disadvantages to this. Having changed her baby to the bottle, the mother may subsequently feel uncomfortable in the presence of nurses who favor breast-feeding. She may equate the attitudes of hospital nurses with those nurses in the clinic or doctor's office or with the public health nurse who comes to her home. It is not too difficult to imagine that the mother will fear the nurse's disapproval in other aspects of child care. Thus a barrier arises between mother

Table 12–14. PERCENTAGE OF INFANTS BREAST-FED AT VARYING AGES IN 1971 AND 1978*

Age of Infant	1971	1978	Percentage of Change (1971–1978)	Seven-Year ARG[a]
1 week	24.7	46.6	21.9	9.5
2 months	13.9	34.9	21.0	14.1
3 to 4 months	8.2	26.8	18.6	18.4
5 to 6 months	5.5	20.5	15.0	20.7

*From Moore: *Newborn, Family, and Nurse*, 2nd ed. Philadelphia, W. B. Saunders Co., 1981; developed from data in Martinez and Nalezienski: *Pediatrics*, 64:686, 1979.
[a]ARG = average annual rate of gain.

and nurse, and the infant receives less than the best of medical care.

Moreover, too strong an insistence on breast-feeding may create some nagging measure of guilt or feeling of inadequacy in mothers who really prefer bottle-feeding, particularly in the mother whose feelings are ambivalent to begin with. Since the mother who has really decided to bottle-feed will probably do so shortly after she returns home, regardless of what she has done in hospital, it would be much wiser to spend the time that is available in the prenatal clinic, office, or hospital instructing her about bottle-feeding rather than teaching her a technique that she plans to discard.

Recognizing the validity of these arguments, it is also important to face some other realities. It is easy to say that breast-feeding from the standpoint of infant health is important today only in developing nations in which environmental standards in terms of water and sanitation are low. This argument fails to recognize that for a significant proportion of our own population, both sanitary and economic resources are limited. There are homes, both rural and urban, in which mothers feed their babies from "coke" or whiskey bottles topped with nipples because these are the only kinds of bottles available; in which a hungry, runny-nosed toddler drinks from the baby's bottle that has dropped from the crib to the floor and then puts the bottle back in the baby's mouth; and in which refrigeration is inadequate and a pan for sterilization of equipment just doesn't exist, even if the mother had the time, energy, and knowledge to carry out daily formula preparation. The fact that presterilized, individually packaged formula is available to some middle and upper class mothers is virtually as remote for these mothers as it is for a Southeast Asian tribeswoman or an Australian aborigine mother. The babies of these mothers suffer a high rate of neonatal and postneonatal mortality and could certainly benefit from breast-feeding during their early months, but as we have already pointed out, they are the least likely to be breast-fed.

It would be tremendously worthwhile if we could find some effective way to encourage more poor mothers to breast-feed their babies, not only because poor techniques of bottle-feeding increase the likelihood of introducing infection into milk but also because the lactobacillus flora in the gastrointestinal tract of breast-fed babies produces an environment unfavorable to *Escherichia coli*, the organism most commonly associated with infection in infants. Low pH produced by the lactobacillus is thought to be the primary inhibiting factor. Cow's milk, on the other hand, produces an environment favorable to the growth of enteric bacteria.

Perhaps the kind of techniques used by cultural-change agents (public health nurses, agriculturalists, sanitary engineers, anthropologists, and others), who work in developing nations, can offer some ideas. One or two key members of a neighborhood group are won to the new idea, and it is they, rather than the change agent, who bring about change on a larger scale. Nurses who work with programs that aim to bring about significant change need to know the neighborhoods in which they work; they need to be able to recognize who the leaders in the neighborhood are, and they need to have a large measure of rapport with the people for whom they care.

Prenatal Education About Infant Feeding

All parents deserve to have information about the relative advantages and disadvantages of different methods of infant feeding during the prenatal period (Nursing Care Plan 12–2).

Advantages of Breast-Feeding

No formula can duplicate exactly the composition of human milk. Not only do the nutritional components vary, but there are nonnutritional components, such as macrophages and immunoglobulins that can never be incorporated in formulas. (See Chapter 22 for comparison of human milk and cow's milk.)

For the baby with a family history of allergy, there is the possibility of allergy to formula but not to breast milk. Occasionally a baby may develop an allergic reaction to some food his nursing mother has eaten that is transmitted in the milk, but the symptoms subside when the mother discontinues the food.

Breast-feeding is less expensive. The small additions to the mother's diet are not as expensive as are infant formula and equipment. In some areas, supplemental feeding programs for mothers and infants will provide food to nursing mothers for a longer time than to mothers who are bottle-feeding.

Not only is it virtually impossible for breast milk to become contaminated, there is also a marked difference in the intestinal flora of the breast-fed baby. The *Lactobacillus bifidus* nonpathogenic organism is the major bacteria in the gastrointestinal tract of the breast-fed baby; a variety of bacteria may be found in the stools of bottle-fed infants.

The different growth rate of the breast-fed infant, once considered a possible disadvantage, seems now to be still another advantage, as we examine the relationship between infant feeding and adult obesity (Chapter 22).

Sucking at the breast varies from sucking at the bottle in a manner that appears to be significant for tooth and jaw development. The energy required to suck at the breast is as much as 60 times greater than that required to suck from a bottle. This muscle exercise encourages the development of the jaws and teeth. Not only does sucking a nipple fail to require as strong exercise as nursing at the breast, but the easy flow of milk from the bottle's nipple may cause the baby to use his tongue to protect himself from a too rapid flow of milk. Dentists have suggested that this forward thrust of the tongue may lead to a variety of problems, including mouth breathing, disease of the gums, and problems in tooth alignment. An "orthodontic nipple" has been designed to help correct the problem of "tongue thrust."

The physiologic benefits of breast-feeding to the mother are described in Chapter 25. I emphasize these benefits along with the benefits to the baby.

For both mother and baby, the experience of breast-feeding is often immensely satisfying. The emotional benefits are difficult to quantify but are reflected in the statements of many mothers and in the apparent contentment of their infants.

The Environmental Contamination of Milk

In recent years there has been growing concern for potential environmental contamination of everything that humans eat and drink. The level of contaminants present in human milk is included in that concern. From time to time articles in newspapers and magazines and programs on television have suggested that human milk may be a potential cause of cancer, genetic defects, liver damage, and central nervous system disorders in breast-fed infants. There have been hearings by a subcommittee of the United States Senate about the possible dangers of human milk. Many parents are puzzled and confused by conflicting information.

Some pollutants do appear to exist in greater concentration in human milk than in cow's milk. This is because animals, including poultry and fish, store certain chemicals in their tissues and pass them on to humans. Some chemicals are also secreted in higher concentration in human milk. Even after a specific pollutant has been banned, it may continue in the food chain for many years.

However, no one at this time is suggesting that women abandon breast-feeding. Other foods contain many of the same pollutants that have been found in human milk. Some of these pollutants (DDT, for example) also cross the placenta, so that even prior to birth they may be stored in the baby's tissues.

Moreover, the content of milk varies from one woman to another, and even from the beginning of a particular feeding until the end, the last part of the feeding having the highest fat content and therefore the highest level of contaminants.

Infant formulas are also subject to most of the pollutants suspect in human milk.

As nurses, we need to be aware of the continuing research in this field and of efforts to reduce environmental pollution for all individuals. Without more concrete data than are presently available, we believe we can continue to recommend breast-feeding to mothers who are interested.

Breast-feeding and the Working Mother

In our society, in which many mothers return to work, often within 4 to 6 weeks after the birth of their infants, a very frequent question is, "Can a mother who works away from home breast-feed her baby?"

Certainly she can for a few weeks, and this is worthwhile for both mother and baby. Breast-feeding is usually well established by the time the mother returns to work at 4 to 6 weeks. She may then nurse while she is at home and express her milk during the hours that she is at work (see Expression, Chapter 26). If refrigeration is available, the expressed milk can be given to the baby in her absence the next day. If necessary, the expressed milk can be discarded and formula given when the mother is at work. She should continue to express her milk about midway through her work period, however, to maintain her supply.

A mother who prefers to wean her baby as she returns to work should do so gradually, one feeding at a time. For example, she may first switch the baby to formula at feedings when she will be away, then an early morning feeding, and then evening and night feedings. Not only will the gradual change be easier for the baby but it will be much more comfortable for her.

Breast Care During Pregnancy

Whether or not a mother plans to breast-feed her baby, her breasts will enlarge during pregnancy. By the fifth month, and sometimes earlier, she will need a larger bra. If she is planning to breast-feed, it is more economical to buy nursing bras and wear them for the rest

Nursing Care Plan 12–2.   Prenatal Preparation for Breast-Feeding

NURSING GOALS: To provide the mother with knowledge that will prepare her to breast-feed her infant

OBJECTIVES: The mother planning to breast-feed:
1. Will be identified in the prenatal period.
2. Will gain basic information about breast-feeding.
3. Will prepare her breasts for breast-feeding.
4. Will identify sources of support.

ASSESSMENT	POTENTIAL NURSING DIAGNOSIS	NURSING INTERVENTION	COMMENTS/RATIONALE
1. Identify mother as planning to breast-feed.	Need for information about breast-feeding	Provide information (below).	
2. Identify reasons for breast-feeding; is breast-feeding planned to please others or because mother desires to breast-feed?		Provide opportunity to discuss reasons for breast-feeding, express concerns, fears, expectations.	
3. Identify sources of support. a. Husband, male partner b. Mother, husband's mother c. Friends d. Organized support groups (e.g., La Leche League) e. Hospital and community health nurse, nurse midwife, nurse practitioner	Lack of support for breast-feeding	Encourage mother to discuss desire to breast-feed with husband and other family members; provide information about support available in community.	Lack of support from husband and other family members can be a significant barrier to successful breast-feeding.

4. Assess knowledge of breast-feeding.
 a. Breast-fed previous child successfully.
 b. Attempted to breast-feed another child but unsuccessfully
 c. Self or siblings were breast-fed as infants.
 d. Peers have successfully breast-fed.
	Need for information about breast-feeding	1. Provide basic information:
		 a. Breast development during pregnancy
		 b. Maternal nutrition to facilitate breast-feeding
		 c. Breast preparation
		   1. Handwashing before the breasts are touched
		   2. Avoidance of any drying substance, including soap, hair spray, and spray deodorant on breast
		   3. After washing breasts with plain water, gently rub dry with a towel or dry washcloth.
			If breasts are uncovered when sprays are used, some may get on breast.

4. Allow clothes to rub against nipples during a part of the day by leaving bra off, flaps down, or cutting a nipple hole in old bra.

5. Nipple rolling with nipple held between thumb and forefinger and gently pulled out and rolled.

These exercises help the woman become comfortable in handling her breasts.

6. Breast massage: fingers and thumbs of both hands encircle breast, massage toward nipple.

Breast massage in the prenatal period will enable mother to learn technique and become comfortable in handling her breasts.

7. If nursing bra is worn, plastic liners should be removed to prevent accumulation of moisture; cup of bra should support entire breast; straps should not leave pressure marks.

8. Old handkerchiefs or old diapers make excellent and inexpensive liners for bra if colostrum leaks (and during the nursing period following birth).

9. Lanolin may be used on breast, but many feel it is unnecessary.

10. Anticipatory guidance for early breast-feeding should be given as soon possible after delivery. For content, see Nursing Care Plan 26–5.

5. Identify potential physical problem: nipples inverted. Assess inverted nipples by asking mother to place thumb and forefinger on areola and compress. If nipple retracts rather than protrudes, nipple is inverted.

Inverted nipples

a. Instruct in the use of Woolwich breast shields to increase protractility of nipples. Shields are worn 1 to 2 hr. per day at first; later can be left in place throughout day.

b. Hoffman's exercise (Fig. 12–1) will make nipple more protractable.

of pregnancy, rather than purchase a larger size of a regular bra now and nursing bras later. The cup of the bra should support the entire breast in a comfortable natural position. If there are pressure marks on the shoulders or under the arms or breasts, the bra is too tight. Wide straps are more comfortable and offer better support than narrow straps.

Nursing bras have plastic liners that trap moisture and will often cause sore nipples even before the baby is born, as well as afterward. It is a good idea to remove these liners.

Striae appear on the breasts, just as they do on the abdomen; there is no way to prevent them.

Prenatal Preparation for Breast-Feeding

Throughout most of the world, women do nothing to prepare their nipples for breast-feeding and have no problems after the baby is born. But because of our lifestyle, some special preparation may be helpful.

During the last trimester (and as long as the baby is nursing) washing the breasts with plain water, rather than with soap, is preferable. Soap is drying; if the mother insists on using soap, it must be thoroughly rinsed away.

After washing, the nipples can be rubbed with a rough washcloth or towel. In contrast to many societies, our custom of wearing brassieres prevents nipples from receiving any friction. Rubbing with a towel and allowing clothing to rub against the nipple by not wearing a bra during part of the day or cutting a nipple hole in a bra will help "toughen" the nipple in preparation.

If nipples are inverted, a Woolwich breast shield (not a nipple shield) can be placed inside the bra; the nipple will eventually be drawn into the shield. The Woolwich shield should be worn for 1 or 2 hours at first; later it can be left in place all day. If not available locally, Woolwich shields may be ordered from La-Leche League (address in Appendix I).

Nipple rolling is also helpful in preparing breasts for nursing. The nipple is held between opposing thumbs and gently pulled out and rolled for 1 to 2 minutes (Fig. 12–1).

Opinions differ on the value of breast massage in prenatal preparation. Massage is done for the purpose of bringing colostrum from alveoli into the lactiferous sinuses (see Figure 4–14 in Chapter 4). The mother encircles the breast with the fingers and thumbs of both hands and closes them together gently.

Massage may be followed by hand expression of colostrum with the hands held at the edge of the areola. Again, the value of regular

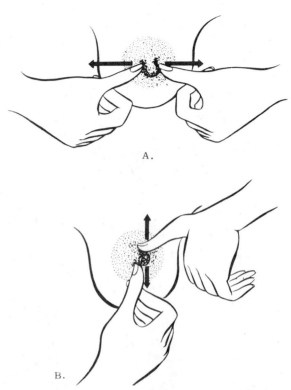

Figure 12–1. Hoffman's exercise to make the nipple more protractile. *A,* The nipple is stimulated by opposing thumbs in a horizontal plane. *B,* The procedure is repeated with thumbs in a vertical plane. (From Applebaum: *Pediatric Clinics of North America, 17*:207, 1970.)

manual expression prenatally is debated, but the prenatal period is an excellent time to learn the technique that will be useful to many mothers at some time after the baby is born.

Prenatal Preparation for Bottle-Feeding

Just as women planning to breast-feed their babies need prenatal instruction, women who plan to bottle-feed also need help in prenatal planning (Nursing Care Plan 12–3). The formula they will use will generally be recommended by a nurse midwife, nurse practitioner, or physician. However, most formulas come in a variety of forms (premixed, powdered, already bottled, and so on). There is a considerable cost difference in these various preparations, and nurses can help parents select the way of preparation that is most cost-effective for them. Saving time may be a prime requisite for a mother returning to work, whereas a mother who plans to remain at home may find that a less expensive method that takes somewhat more time is more suitable. Allowing parents to experiment in prenatal classes with various preparations and to ex-

Nursing Care Plan 12–3. Prenatal Preparation for Bottle Feeding

NURSING GOALS: To provide the mother (and family) with knowledge that will prepare her to bottle-feed her infant.

OBJECTIVES: The mother planning to bottle-feed:
1. Will be identified in the prenatal period.
2. Will gain basic information about bottle-feeding.
3. Will identify hazards related to inappropriate bottle-feeding practices.

ASSESSMENT	POTENTIAL NURSING DIAGNOSIS	NURSING INTERVENTION	COMMENTS/RATIONALE
1. Identify mother as planning to feed by bottle.	Need for information about bottle-feeding.	Provide information about various forms of formula (e.g., powdered, liquid, ready to feed).	
		Explain advantages and disadvantages (cost, time, etc.) of each.	
2. Assess knowledge of bottle-feeding. 1. Bottle-fed previous child successfully. 2. Complications in previous child (e.g., failure to thrive, bottle caries, frequent otitis media).		Provide information about other equipment (e.g., bottles, sterilizers) that will be needed. Help parents choose form of prescribed formula and equipment that best meets their needs.	
		Provide information about relative costs.	Many parents choose a form of preparation more expensive than necessary or buy excess amounts of equipment.
3. Assess facilities for preparation of formula, e.g., source of water, lack of running water.	Need to modify formula preparation information.	Provide instructions that are realistic in relation to family resources. Families without hot or running water cannot wash bottles in hot, running water. Community health nurse may provide instruction on formula preparation in home using available equipment and resources.	
4. Assess mother's knowledge of potential complications. a. Decreased parent–infant interaction b. Bottle caries c. Otitis media	Risk for complications of bottle-feeding is related to inadequate knowledge.	Encourage mother to hold infant during bottle-feeding and provide skin contact.	
		Never allow infant to take bottle to bed with anything but water in it. Hold infant for bedtime bottle; then rinse mouth with gauze sponge dipped in water.	

amine various types of bottles is helpful. Up-to-date local cost figures are also welcomed by expectant parents. The amount of equipment each family needs will vary with the method they select.

The prenatal period is not too early for parents to become aware of the dangers of allowing a baby to take a bottle to bed, teaching that will be reinforced after the baby's birth. Bottle mouth (bottle caries, nursing bottle syndrome) and increased incidence of ear infections are potentially serious problems (Chapter 22).

Because some mothers wish to breast-feed for several weeks and then gradually wean the baby to a bottle as they prepare to return to work, the following suggestions are offered:

1. You can pump your breast milk or manually express it to be given to your baby while you are at work. This method is the most satisfactory in terms of maintaining milk supply.

2. If you are going to substitute formula for the feedings you will miss while you are away, begin by substituting formula at just one feeding for several days. This will be less uncomfortable for you and enables the baby to adapt gradually. After several days you can substitute at a second feeding. Some mothers will be able to continue breast-feeding at other feedings after this change. The increased activity demands and diminished rest times, as well as the stress associated with some jobs, may diminish milk supply. However, many mothers successfully return to work and continue breast-feeding. If further weaning is desired, continue in the same gradual manner.

Summary

The importance of nutrition in pregnancy cannot be overemphasized. Because nurses have more interaction with many women during pregnancy than any other health-care provider, they must work actively to achieve the goal of optimum nutrition for every pregnant woman.

REFERENCES

1. Adams, C.: *Nutritive Value of American Foods in Common Units* (Agricultural Handbook #456). Washington, D.C., U.S. Department of Agriculture, 1975.
2. Delgado, H., Lechtig, A., Yarbrough, C., et al.: Maternal Nutrition: Its Effects on Infant Growth and Development and Birthspacing. In Moghissi, K., and Evans, T. (eds.): *Nutritional Impacts on Women*. Hagerstown, Harper & Row, 1977.
3. Eiger, M., and Olds, S.: *The Complete Book of Breastfeeding*. New York, Bantam Books, 1973.
4. Food and Nutrition Board, National Research Council: *Recommended Dietary Allowances*. 9th ed. Washington, D.C., National Academy of Sciences, 1980.
5. Herrera, M.: Malnutrition and Psychologic Development. The Section on Nutrition and Growth of the Clinical Nutrition and Early Development Branch. *In A Report to the National Advisory Child Health and Human Development Council*. Washington D.C., 1979.
6. Higgins, A.: Nutritional Status and the Outcome of Pregnancy. *Journal of the Canadian Dietary Association, 37*:17, 1976.
7. Hochstein, G.: Pica: A Study in Medical and Anthropological Explanation. *In* Weaver, T. (ed.): *Essays in Medical Anthropology*. Athens, University of Georgia Press, 1968.
8. Kretchmer, N.: Lactose and Lactase. *Scientific American, 227*:71, October, 1972.
9. Lappe, F.: *Diet for a Small Planet*. New York, Ballantine Books, 1971.
10. Li, S., and White, R.: The Presence of Geophagy in North Carolina. (Unpublished manuscript), 1970.
11. Luke, B.: Lactose Intolerance During Pregnancy: Significance and Solutions. *MCN, 2*:92, 1977.
12. Martinez, G., and Nalezienski, J.: The Recent Trend in Breast-Feeding. *Pediatrics, 64*:686, 1979.
13. Moghissi, K., Churchill, J., and Kurrie, D.: Relationship of Maternal Amino Acids and Proteins to Fetal Growth and Mental Development. *American Journal of Obstetrics and Gynecology, 123*:398, 1975.
14. *Nutrition During Pregnancy and Lactation*. Sacramento, California Department of Health, 1975.
15. *Nutrition Services in Perinatal Care*. Washington, D.C., National Academy Press, 1981.
16. Saul, H.: Potential Effect of Demographic and Other Variables in Studies Comparing Morbidity of Breast-Fed and Bottle-Fed Infants. *Pediatrics, 64*:523, 1979.
17. Schmitt, M. H.: Superiority of Breast-Feeding: Fact or Fancy. *American Journal of Nursing, 70*:1488, 1970.
18. Vuori, L., Mora, J., Christiansen, N., et al.: Nutritional Supplementation and the Outcome of Pregnancy. II. Visual Habituation at 15 Days. *American Journal of Clinical Nutrition, 32*:463, 1979.

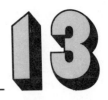

The High Risk Mother

1. Define:
   a. maternal mortality rate
   b. fetal mortality rate
   c. neonatal mortality rate
   d. perinatal mortality rate
   e. infant mortality rate
   f. spontaneous abortion
   g. threatened abortion
   h. inevitable abortion
   i. incomplete abortion
   j. missed abortion
   k. habitual abortion
   l. induced abortion
   m. abruptio placentae
   n. placenta previa
   o. amniocentesis
   p. alpha-fetoprotein
   q. estriol
   r. surfactant
   s. creatinine

2. Discuss the way in which the developmental tasks of pregnancy and the meaning of pregnancy may be altered for high risk mothers.

3. Describe specific effects of each of the following on the pregnant woman or fetus. Identify assessment factors and appropriate nursing intervention.
   a. maternal age greater than 35
   b. diabetes mellitus
   c. heart disease
   d. urinary tract disease
   e. essential hypertension
   f. Rh$_d$ isoimmunization and ABO incompatibility
   g. hypertensive states of pregnancy
   h. bleeding
   i. hydatidiform mole
   j. infection
   k. trauma
   l. abuse
   m. alcoholism
   n. addiction to drugs

4. Identify the special problems of multiple pregnancy.

Who is the high risk mother? In the broadest sense, any mother who has a problem or condition—physiologic, emotional, or social—that may adversely affect the delivery of a healthy, full term infant may be considered high risk.

Physiologic conditions that designate a mother or newborn as high risk may exist before the mother becomes pregnant (diabetes mellitus, heart disease, and hypertension are three examples) or may be directly related to the pregnancy (eclampsia, for example). Certain conditions, such as ectopic pregnancy or a spontaneous abortion, prevent the completion of pregnancy. Others, such as the TORCH diseases described in Chapter 8, go unnoticed by the mother until a baby is born with characteristic problems. Mothers who have a multiple gestation (twins, for example), mothers who have previously delivered a child with a congenital abnormality, and mothers who have been trying to conceive for a number of years prior to becoming pregnant are examples of women who are classified as high risk because *statistics* indicate that their chances of having difficulty in their current pregnancy are greater than the chances of the mother who has had no previous reproductive problems.

Psychosocial factors are equally as important as physiologic factors as criteria for identifying potentially high risk mothers. Psychosocial factors are usually interrelated with physiologic factors, as, for example, in the adolescent mother who may have poor nutritional stores, poor dietary habits, and at the same time a psychologic denial of the fact of her pregnancy.

The purpose of this chapter is to examine:

1. The major factors that designate a pregnancy as high risk.

2. The ways in which the special needs of high risk mothers can be met.

3. The concept of regionalization as a strategy for improving the care of high risk mothers.

Identifying High Risk Mothers

A variety of studies, each approaching the issue in a somewhat different perspective, have attempted to identify the percentage of all mothers who can be considered high risk. Table 13–1 summarizes findings of several studies. Note that in the Harbor Hospital study,[20] a total of 55 per cent of mothers were considered at risk at some time during the prenatal or intrapartum period. Moreover, these studies indicate only risk associated with physiologic morbidity or mortality. They do not include emotional and social risks that are far more difficult to measure but are highly important in caring for whole families during childbearing.

The number of women at risk will vary from one population to another. Socioeconomic factors, for example, appear to be an important influence. There are likely to be more high

Table 13–1.   HIGH RISK MOTHERS AND INFANTS

Study	Date Published	No. of Pregnancies	Time Included	Criteria	Per Cent at Risk	
					Mother	*Infant*
Prechtl[40a]	1967	1378	Prenatal, intrapartum, neonatal	7 or more non-optimum conditions	12	
Nesbitt and Aubry[34]	1969	1001	Prenatal	Weighed 29 adverse prenatal factors	29	
Stembera, Zezvlakova, and Dittrichova[48]	1975	3500	Prenatal, intrapartum, neonatal		23	20
Harbor Hospital[20]	1976	1417	Prenatal, intrapartum, neonatal		Prenatal risk only—16 Intrapartum risk only—23 Prenatal and intrapartum risk—16	12.5 to prenatal only 23.2 to intrapartum only 39.9 to both

risk mothers, even in a strictly physiologic sense, in an inner city clinic than in a suburban private office.

Mortality and Morbidity

Mortality indicates death; morbidity indicates illness. Measurements of mortality and morbidity are one parameter of care given to mothers and infants.

In order to communicate with others who care for childbearing families, we must understand certain commonly used terms and use these terms in the same way.

Maternal mortality is expressed as the number of maternal deaths per 100,000 live births. (Prior to 1960, maternal mortality was expressed in deaths per 10,000 live births. The rates are now so low that the higher base is used. In comparing maternal mortality rates, it is important to note the way in which the rate is expressed.)

Several terms are used to describe fetal and neonatal deaths. Unfortunately, these terms are not defined identically by all professionals, which makes comparisons very difficult.

Fetal death (stillbirth) refers to the death of a fetus or an infant weighing at least 500 grams or of at least 20 weeks gestation. Weight is felt to be a preferable criterion because estimates of gestational age vary. A fetus weighing less than 500 grams is considered an abortus. The *fetal death rate* is the number of fetal deaths per 1000 births.*

Neonatal death is death of a newborn who has shown any sign of life (such as heartbeat or respiratory effort) within 28 days following birth. The *neonatal death rate* is the number of neonatal deaths per 1000 births.*

The term *perinatal death* is frequently used today, reflecting the concept that both fetal and neonatal deaths are often related to similar problems. The *perinatal death rate* is the sum of the fetal death rate plus the neonatal death rate.

On a worldwide basis, perinatal and neonatal statistics are not always available for comparison. *Infant mortality* rates are more readily available. The infant mortality rate is the number of deaths in the first year of life per 1000 live births. A comparison of infant mortality in the United States with that in other nations is discussed in Chapter 30.

*These rates are sometimes expressed per 100 *live* births, rather than births. Before rates can be compared, it is essential to ascertain that one is comparing identical rates.

What Does Being a High Risk Mother Mean?

Considering the emotional and social tasks of pregnancy when the pregnancy is viewed as "normal" (Chapter 9), one might easily suspect that the mother designated as "high risk" must face even more complex feelings. In the terms of adaptation theory, adaptation may be more difficult physiologically. Self-esteem, role perceptions, and important relationships can all be affected (see Nursing Care Plan 13–1).

As these feelings are explored, remember that our designation of a mother as being at risk does not necessarily mean that she feels herself at risk. The teenager who is pregnant and considered at risk from a health point of view may feel herself quite normal, particularly if she has friends who are also pregnant. Moreover, if *her* mother was also a teen-aged mother, the mother may not feel that her daughter's pregnancy is particularly unusual or hazardous.

Some mothers enter pregnancy knowing they are at risk—the mother with diabetes who has had a previous pregnancy, for example. (The diabetic mother who has not previously been pregnant may not be aware of all the implications that her diabetic condition may have for her pregnancy.) For other mothers, events during the course of pregnancy may classify her as high risk, sometimes quite suddenly.

Thus, pregnancy for the high risk mother, as for all mothers, will have varied meanings. Nevertheless, it is possible to identify feelings that many of these mothers and fathers may share.

Grief Reactions

Like the person who learns that he has a serious or terminal illness or like parents who deliver a malformed or sick infant, high risk parents exhibit many of the same manifestations of grief: anger, guilt, questions of "why me," and, in time, acceptance.

"Why me," for the mother with a chronic condition, may revive old feelings present when the diagnosis of the condition (diabetes, for example) was originally made. Self-esteem, threatened then, is now again attacked. "Other women are able to have normal pregnancies; it is unfair for me to have these problems," will not often be spoken but will underlie behavior.

The mother or father may express guilt feel-

Nursing Care Plan 13–1.   High Risk Pregnancy: General Model

(This Nursing Care Plan is incorporated into the plan for all high risk mothers, along with plans for high risk indicators)

NURSING GOALS:
To provide optimum care for the mother and her fetus when alterations in health status exist that place the pregnancy at risk of complications.
To assist the woman who has a high risk pregnancy and her family to understand and cope with variations in pregnancy and health care associated with her health needs.
To assist the woman who has a high risk pregnancy and her family to cope with feelings about her high risk status.

OBJECTIVES:
The woman with high risk pregnancy will:
1. Participate in health care appropriate to her physiologic needs.
2. Become knowledgeable about her health status and the reasons for variations in her health care.
3. Verbalize her feelings about her high risk status and feel that health-care providers accept her feelings.
4. Be aware of the need for continuing health supervision.

ASSESSMENT	POTENTIAL NURSING DIAGNOSIS	NURSING INTERVENTION	COMMENTS/RATIONALE
1. Assessment as in all pregnancies (Nursing Care Plans 10–1, 10–2)	Risk of complications for mother and/or fetus related to (specific indicator[s])	Basic care as for all pregnant women	Outcome in previous pregnancy (positive or negative) will affect physical, emotional, social aspects of this pregnancy.
2. Previous high risk pregnancies and outcome	Alterations in self-care ability	Provide time for thorough discussion of any previous pregnancy, maternal perception, family perception, health history.	
3. Assessment related to high risk indicators (See Nursing Care Plans in this chapter related to specific high risk indicators)	Knowledge deficit related to effect of high risk status on pregnancy	Obtain health records.	
	Disruptions in fetal placental unit	See Nursing Care Plans in this chapter for intervention related to specific high risk indicators.	
	Risk for abnormal fetal development related to (specific conditions)		
4. Gravida's feelings about high risk status	Negative self image related to complications of pregnancy	Allow adequate time to provide continuing opportunities to verbalize fears, anger, and other emotions.	Cultural factors, (e.g., religious beliefs, beliefs about health care) are the context within which emotional and social issues develop and must be addressed.
a. Anger	Anxiety related to high risk pregnancy		
b. Denial			

c. Guilt d. Diminished self esteem e. Anxiety or fear f. Acceptance g. Other	Guilt related to high risk pregnancy Fear related to high risk pregnancy Anger related to high risk pregnancy Denial of high risk of pregnancy Ineffective coping with high risk pregnancy	Accept feelings as presented. Help woman explore reasons for her feelings. Group discussions (e.g., gravidas with diabetes) may be helpful to some women. Refer for additional counseling when appropriate (e.g., abused mother, woman addicted to narcotics, prolonged inability to cope with high risk pregnancy).
5. Effect of high risk status on family relationship a. Mother's perception of effects b. Perception of other family members c. Nursing observations	Ineffective family coping patterns	Include family in prenatal visits, teaching, counseling. Arrange home visits when other family members are present, if possible. Assessment and intervention of community health nurse who makes home visits is particularly valuable.
6. Family support for mother's special needs (e.g., bed rest, diet modification)	Lack of support system	Include family in teaching; explain importance of modifications. Provide opportunity for family to question, express concerns.
7. Effect of high risk status on developmental tasks of pregnancy (see Table 13–2)	Threat to developmental tasks of pregnancy associated with high risk pregnancy Lag in prenatal attachment behavior related to fear of fetal or infant death	As in 3 (above), provide continuing opportunities for mother to express concerns. Accept basis of lag in attachment behavior—"I know it's hard to prepare for your baby when you're afraid something might happen."

Continued on following page

Nursing Care Plan 13–1.   High Risk Pregnancy: General Model (Continued)

8. Gravida's knowledge of care related to high risk status	Knowledge deficit	Provide information about specific condition related to: a. Nutrition b. Rest c. Exercise d. Medication e. Special tests f. Symptoms to be reported See Nuring Care Plans in this chapter for each high risk condition for specific information.
9. Skills necessary for gravida's participation in own care	Knowledge or skills deficit	Teach appropriate skills (e.g., urine testing, use of Dextrostix for mother with diabetes, count-to-ten chart).
10. Social and economic problems a. Transportation to clinic, office, hospital for frequent visits b. Inability to work because of need for additional rest c. Additional costs of high risk pregnancy	Need for supportive services	Refer to appropriate supportive services when available (e.g., transportation service, social services, supplementary nutritional services [food stamps, WIC]).
11. Preparation for childbirth and parenting for mother (couple) unable to attend childbirth/parenting classes because of hospitalization or bed rest at home	Need for information about childbirth and parenting	Explore alternatives for mother unable to attend classes; preparation in home or in hospital on an individual basis.
12. Prenatal record		Ensure that fully documented health record is available to hospital at any admission. Record should include information from community health nurse(s) and referral agencies as well as information about physiologic, emotional, and social aspects of health status.

ings through questions ("What did I do to cause this?") or statements ("I suppose this is my punishment—for not wanting a baby—for having sex when I wasn't married," and so on). "I am going to eat properly during *this* pregnancy" or "we are not going to have intercourse this time" are statements indicating guilt for an unhappy outcome in a prior pregnancy.

Anger may be directed at nurses or physicians, or at one another. It may be expressed directly in relation to the care during pregnancy ("If my care had been better, *this* might not have happened") or less directly ("The nurses don't care about me" or "I have to wait too long"). Anger may lead to blaming the partner ("I didn't want another baby but *he* insisted" or "If *she* would rest when she should, she wouldn't be sick").

Before there can be any degree of acceptance of high risk pregnancy, these feelings must be recognized—a major nursing goal. Because they may not be verbalized directly, a primary nurse who can come to know a couple is very important. She may be the nurse in the high risk clinic, the public health nurse, or the school nurse, who may be the one most likely to see adolescents on a continuing basis.

Good records that describe feelings as well as physiology are also essential to helping families recognize and cope with these feelings.

Communication between the mother and father and the nurse is important; communication between the mother and the father themselves is even more significant and is behavior that we can encourage. It would be ideal, perhaps, to have the father present at each prenatal visit, but this is rarely possible. But we can encourage the mother to share her feelings with her partner, a suggestion that may seem obvious but that, in actuality, may be unusual for some couples. Galloway suggests role playing between the mother and the nurse as preparation for a discussion with her husband, if the mother feels this will be difficult for her.[12]

Developmental Tasks in High Risk Pregnancy

In Chapter 9 maternal developmental tasks were identified as accepting the pregnancy, assuring safe passage, acceptance of the child by significant others, attachment, and giving of oneself. Each of these tasks has special meaning for the high risk mother, although every mother and couple will not necessarily achieve each task with the same degree of difficulty (Table 13–2).

Accepting the Pregnancy. Accepting a pregnancy that involves risks means accepting the idea of being a less than perfect bearer of children; this can be a blow to feelings about oneself as a woman. For a woman who defines her femininity in terms of childbearing, the possibility that she will not be successful is difficult to accept. For some mothers there will have been previous unsuccessful pregnancies—pregnancies that ended in spontaneous abortion or stillbirth or a malformed infant. The anxiety that this pregnancy may also come to a less than perfect conclusion is ever present.

Denial is one way that a mother or father may fail to accept the fact of high risk pregnancy. In denying the reality of the pregnancy with risk, the mother or father may behave as

Table 13–2. COMPARISON OF DEVELOPMENTAL TASKS FOR ALL MOTHERS AND FOR HIGH RISK MOTHERS

Tasks for All Mothers	Special Tasks for High Risk Mothers
Accepting the pregnancy	Pregnancy may not be successfully completed
Assuring safe passage	Long term hospitalization
	More frequent outpatient visits
	Special proscriptions
	Added expense
	Fear of potential problems
Acceptance of the child by significant others	Fear that the baby may die or may be abnormal and thus unacceptable
Attachment	Fear of attachment because child may die or be abnormal.
	Postponement of nesting behavior
Giving of oneself	Extensive sacrifice to protect fetus
	Need for recognition of her sacrifice

if there were no problem. Specific needs in terms of rest or diet or keeping appointments may be ignored.

Once the pregnancy has been accepted, the mother is ready to deal with additional tasks.

Assuring Safe Passage. For the high risk mother, assuring safe passage for her baby is a major task. It may involve inconvenience and a considerable expenditure of time and money. The mother living in a small community may need to travel to a medical center for specialized care. Hospitalization may be required for 1 or more weeks, or even months, during the course of the pregnancy. The mother, and the father as well, may have to make major adjustments in their lives.

The willingness of mothers to do this—to spend sometimes days in the hospital awaiting the appropriate time for delivery, to submit to multiple amniocenteses and other tests, and to comply with all the other proscriptions we place upon them—testifies to the strong drive of most mothers to assure safe passage for their baby.

We can reinforce this need by recognizing the mother's efforts and praising her for them. This can also be helpful later, if the pregnancy does not result in the birth of a healthy infant, by assuring the mother that she did everything she possibly could.

Acceptance of the Child by Significant Others. It is important to all mothers to feel that the father of their child, the grandparents, or whoever else is important to them accepts their unborn child. People important to the high risk mother may be reluctant to talk with the mother about her coming child or to become too attached to the idea of the child's birth lest something happen to the baby.

Added to the mother's anxiety about rejection of her baby is the concern that she too may be rejected if she is unable to produce a healthy child.

Although these thoughts may be almost continually on the mother's mind, the father may not even suspect her concern. Our opportunity to talk with both parents together may help her share her concern; lacking this, we can encourage her communication.

Attachment. Just as the mother fears that others may not accept her baby if he is less than perfect, she may also be afraid to become attached to him during the prenatal period. The assessment of prenatal attachment behavior (described in Chapter 9) is an important tool in recognizing this fear. Once recognized, it is appropriate to help the mother cope with her feelings. We believe that attachment to the baby after birth, even if the baby is going to die, is necessary to healthy grieving (Chap-

ter 28); we wonder if prenatal attachment may also be important to a healthy grief process—grief for the baby who was not born, should the baby have some type of abnormality, as well as grief for the baby who dies, either in utero or following delivery.

Not every baby born to a high risk mother will die or will even be ill following delivery. What effect might failure to form a prenatal attachment have on the mother's relationship with her subsequently healthy infant?

Giving of Oneself. Pregnancy makes certain demands on all women, but the demands placed upon the high risk mother to give may be overwhelming. She may have to give up time for favorite or necessary activities for hospitalization or for periods in bed at home. She may have excessive costs for care. The experience of the fetus as her gift to others may be tempered by concerns about the status of the fetus.

Her need for evidence of concern from those around her—husband, friends, relatives—is frequently heightened. Yet at the same time, she may reject some of the traditional signs of concern and affection (a baby shower, for example) because of her fear of attachment.

Thus, just as the high risk mother has specific and special physiologic needs, she also has particular social and emotional needs. Helping her to cope with these needs is as important as the care we give to support the physiologic demands of her pregnancy.

Home vs. Hospital for the High Risk Mother

Before considering specific problems that identify the mother as high risk, the environment in which care is provided (i.e., home or hospital) deserves exploration. It is obvious that acute high risk conditions, such as moderate to severe pre-eclampsia or abruptio placentae, require immediate hospitalization. Women with other conditions, however, can care for themselves at home; their success is related in part to our ability to teach each woman what she needs to know about her condition and to enable her to find resources to provide the necessary support.

A nurse as educator must assess (1) what the woman already knows about the required self-care, (2) what she needs to know, and (3) how she feels about what is required of her.

Consider the gravida with diabetes mellitus, for example. If she has had diabetes prior to pregnancy, she is probably already familiar with at least the basics of the disease process, of urine testing, and perhaps of insulin use. However, we cannot assume her level of knowledge but must determine the extent of her understanding of both the mechanics of care and the importance of that care. If the woman has not previously been diabetic, information about diabetes per se and the teaching of basic skills will be required. No matter how excellent our teaching skills, if a woman is denying or having difficulty accepting the idea that she both has diabetes and is pregnant, she may not participate in the needed self-care.

Family members may also be able to learn skills, for example, blood pressure assessment. Skills taught in a clinic, office, or hospital to either a woman or a member of her family should be evaluated at home by a visiting or public health nurse. It is easy to forget a newly learned skill when one attempts it in a different environment. A visiting nurse can also aid in the assessment of the home and family support and help to evaluate the success of the plan of care. Obviously, any success requires close cooperation between all care-givers—nurses in a variety of settings, physicians, and frequently nutritionists and social workers.

As facilitators, nurses must assess the mother's ability to comply with the plan of care and help assure the needed resources whenever possible. Assessing family support and understanding is equally important. For example, a mother with hypertension may require several hours of bed rest a day (see section on Chronic Hypertensive Disease below). Will this be possible at home? Are there small children for whom she is the only caretaker for much of the day? Who can do the shopping? Who is able to prepare the meals? It is irresponsible to tell a woman she must rest in bed without addressing these questions. In some communities resources like a Homemaker Service may be available at a cost that varies with family income. In smaller communities there may be no organized support services, but informal support networks may be available through neighbors or church or civic groups. Some women may find support within their nuclear or extended family.

Special plans need to be made for childbirth education for a couple when the mother is confined to her home (or when she spends much of her last trimester in the hospital). The information normally provided in classes (Chapter 11 and Appendix I), including preparation for Cesarean birth, is just as important for the high risk mother as for other mothers. Because of the anxiety associated with her high risk status, it could be considered even more essential. Close cooperation between childbirth educators, visiting nurses, and

nurses who care for high risk antepartum women in hospital is essential. Arrangements may be made for childbirth educators to visit the home or the hospital unit or to provide films and film equipment, relaxation practice on casette tapes, and other material appropriate to the needs of individual patients.

One common concern for mothers who require bed rest is a need to leave employment earlier in pregnancy than originally planned. Either directly or working through social services we may be able to communicate with her employer so that she is not penalized for her prolonged absence. Some mothers may qualify for disability insurance payments.

Age As A Risk Factor

From a biologic perspective, and in many ways from social and psychologic perspectives, the ideal age range for reproduction is the twenties to early thirties. Although many women, both younger and older, may successfully bear and care for children, there is good evidence that at either end of the reproductive years both mortality and morbidity are increased. For this reason, the particular needs of adolescents and women over 35 require special attention. The needs of adolescent mothers are described in Chapter 29.

The Mother Over 35

Approximately 4 per cent of all births in the United States are to women 35 years of age and older; most of these women are between the ages of 35 and 42. It is estimated that 3 per cent of all primagravidas are over 35. The United States Bureau of the Census has projected that the number of births to women over 35 will increase by more than 40 per cent in the decade 1978–1988. This projection is based on societal changes such as later marriage and postponement of childbearing until after careers have been established. Infertility is an additional factor in late childbearing.

Although it is certainly possible for a mother older than 35, and even older than 40, to deliver a healthy infant, the mathematical possibility that there may be a problem is increased.

As the hormonal regulation of the menstrual cycle becomes less regular, the internal environment becomes less optimal for the development of both egg and endometrium. The incidence of multiple pregnancy increases because more than one egg is released. The egg itself may be defective, with chromosomal abnormalities.

Table 13–3. RISK OF DOWN'S SYNDROME

Age of Mother	In Any Pregnancy	After Birth of Baby with Down's Syndrome
–29	1 in 3000	1 in 1000
30–34	1 in 600	1 in 200
35–39	1 in 280	1 in 100
40–44	1 in 70	1 in 25
45–49	1 in 40	1 in 15
All mothers	1 in 665	1 in 200

Down's syndrome, described in Chapter 3, is due to a chromosomal abnormality. The risk increases dramatically with age (Table 13–3). Because of this, some physicians suggest that all mothers over 35 have an amniocentesis to screen for Down's syndrome. There does not appear to be an increased risk of other congenital malformations.

Trophoblastic disease (hydatidiform mole, below) is more common in older women (and in women younger than usual). Multiparas with previous children born prior to 1968 who are Rh_d negative will not have received Rh immune globulin and must be assessed for the possibility of erythroblastosis in the baby.

Because the incidence of diabetes mellitus and hypertension is increased in women over 35, these conditions are potential complications to pregnancy but are not necessarily a problem for an individual woman.

In Kessler's[24] review of 298 women (98 primaparas over 35 and two control groups), premature rupture of the membranes (PROM) was the most common complication, with toxemia of pregnancy in second place. Statistically significant differences were found between older primiparas and younger primiparas. The incidence in older multigravidas fell between that of the other two groups (Table 13–4).

Increased risks of abortion, anemia, and cardiac disease have been attributed to older gravidas in the past, but there does not seem to be empirical support for these concerns.

Just as individual women of all ages may have varying feelings about pregnancy, women over 35 will display a variety of emotions. A woman who has been intensely involved in a career may desire pregnancy because she feels her "biological time clock" is running out and it is "now or never," yet she may be ambivalent about the effect of a baby on her career. A woman who has been infertile and desirous of pregnancy for many years may feel differently about the parenthood from the mother of three teen-aged children.

Many older mothers are aware of the increased risks, and this is a source of concern during their pregnancy. Although most mothers worry about whether their baby will be normal, older mothers feel they have added reason for concern. Even though amniocentesis assures them that their baby is not likely to have Down's syndrome, they are concerned about other possible problems.

Some older mothers are very self-conscious about their pregnancy. They sit in the office or clinic waiting room with women much much younger. They joke half-heartedly about being the grandmother at the Parent-Teachers' Association or about reaching retirement age when the child is still in college. Careful listening to small comments will help us to assess

Table 13–4. PROBLEMS DURING PREGNANCY*

Problem	Older Primipara (> 35)	Older Multipara (> 35)	Younger Primipara (< 35)
PROM	13	9	4
Toxemia of pregnancy	11	4	2
Hemorrhage in months 2 to 8 of pregnancy	4	9	5
Other complications	11	9	2
Total complications	39	31	13
Total in group	98	100	100
Per cent complications	40%	31%	13%

*From Kessler, Lancet, Borenstein, et al.: The Problem of the Older Multipara. Obstetrics and Gynecology, *56*:165, 1980.

this mother's needs realistically and thereby to help her cope with her pregnancy.

Nursing Assessment and Intervention Based on Special Needs: Prenatal Phase. The special characteristics of mothers over 35 are the basis of nursing interaction beyond that provided to all other mothers (see Nursing Care Plan 13–2). Because ovulation becomes more irregular as women become older, documentation of gestational age may be more difficult. Fundal measurements are less accurate if twins are present. Documenting the time at which fetal heart tones are first heard by Doppler ultrasound (10 to 12 weeks) and by stethoscope (18 weeks) is particularly important. The presence of fetal heart tones also rules out the possibility of trophoblastic disease.

Other important ways in which nurses can provide special care to mothers over 35 during the prenatal phase are summarized in Nursing Care Plan 13–2. Meeting these special needs may require more frequent prenatal visits, although Kessler[24] argues that these mothers are not necessarily a high risk group.

High Risk Pregnancy Due To Pre-existing Maternal Conditions

Diabetes Mellitus

The number of mothers with diabetes mellitus is increasing steadily. It has been estimated that there are 18,000 women with diabetes pregnant each year, and 30,000 women with gestational diabetes.[23] Prior to the discovery of insulin in 1923, most women with diabetes were sterile. Young girls who acquired diabetes early in childhood often did not live to their reproductive years. For those who did become pregnant, there was a 25 per cent maternal mortality and a 50 per cent fetal mortality.

Now mothers with diabetes rarely die when they are pregnant; maternal mortality is less than 1 per cent. But mortality for the fetus and infant remains far higher than for the general population (see below). Moreover, as the number of mothers with diabetes increases, the number of potential diabetic mothers in succeeding generations increases. For these reasons, an understanding of the relationship between diabetes and pregnancy is extremely important.

Table 13–5 describes the classifications that are commonly used to group mothers with diabetes. The term *gestational* diabetes is used for mothers who have chemical diabetes during pregnancy (i.e., an abnormal glucose tolerance test). Mothers who have babies that resemble infants of diabetic mothers (IDM) or who have a history of stillborn infants and who subsequently develop diabetes at some later time in their life are, in retrospect, considered *prediabetic,* although the diagnosis is not made at the time. Recognizing the possibility of future diabetes in these mothers is important in health counseling.

The goal in the care of a mother with diabetes is good health for both mother and baby (Nursing Care Plan 13–3). The mother may have problems because of the effect of her diabetes on the pregnancy or because of the effect of the pregnancy on her diabetes. The fetus faces multiple risks (see below).

The frequency of complications for both mother and baby is reduced when excellent care is given by nurse-physician-nutritionist teams. The large, fat baby still considered typical of Group A, B, and C diabetic mothers is less frequent with proper prenatal care and is now considered an unnecessary outcome by many.

Gestational Diabetes

Gestational diabetes is not always apparent; it may be recognized only after the birth of an infant who resembles the infant of a diabetic mother (Chapter 23). A careful health history during the initial nursing assessment combined with physical and laboratory assessment is important in identifying women at risk for gestational diabetes (Nursing Care Plan 13–3). These women can then be further screened with a glucose tolerance test, usually at 26 to 28 weeks gestation because glucose tolerance is most evident at that time. Other women who should be carefully evaluated are those with polyhydramnios (excess amniotic fluid), pregnancy-induced hypertension, and excessive pregnancy weight gain. These conditions can be related to a variety of factors discussed in this chapter, but the possibility of gestational diabetes should not be overlooked.

A glucose tolerance test (GTT) may be oral (oral glucose, 50 or 100 grams) or intravenous (25 grams of glucose given intravenously over 2 minutes). Several studies have indicated that many women with an abnormal oral GTT will have normal intravenous tests.[25] Standard results for a 3-hour 100-gram oral test compared with results in nonpregnant women are shown in Table 13–6. Note that the initial peak values are higher during pregnancy and remain

Nursing Care Plan 13–2.   Gravidas Over 35 Years of Age

NURSING GOALS:
1. To provide care for the gravida over 35 that protects the mother and the fetus.
2. To recognize the special needs of gravidas over 35 years of age.
OBJECTIVES:
1. The gravida will meet the basic objectives of prenatal care (see Nursing Care Plans 10–1, 10–2)
2. Problems associated with age will be prevented or identified quickly.
3. Appropriate intervention will correct identified problems.

ASSESSMENT	POTENTIAL NURSING DIAGNOSIS	NURSING INTERVENTION	COMMENTS/RATIONALE
Establish gestational age.	Uncertain gestational age related to irregular ovulation	Document first fetal heart tones by Doppler ultrasound device (10 to 12 weeks) and stethoscope (18 weeks).	
		Gravida should have frequent appointments during the time of assessment for first fetal heart tones.	
		Document fetal movement perceived by mother (18 to 20 weeks).	
		Possible referral for ultrasound to document gestational age.	
Evaluates for Down's syndrome in fetus (12 to 14 weeks' gestation).	Risk for Down's syndrome in fetus related to maternal age.	Refer for amniocentesis to test for Down's syndrome. If negative, parental anxiety is diminished.	
		If positive, refer for genetic counseling to provide information base for decision about possible pregnancy termination.	
Assess for multiple gestation.	Risk for multiple gestation related to irregular ovulation.	Careful assessment of fetal heart tones, fundal height	Hearing fetal heart tones rules out hydatidiform mole, for which older mothers are at increased risk.
		Possible ultrasound	
Antibody titer	At risk of sensitization prior to development of Rh immune globulin.	If antibody present, follow plan as in Nursing Care Plan 13–6.	

Assessment	Nursing Diagnosis	Nursing Intervention	Rationale
Screen for diabetes mellitus.	Risk for diabetes related to age.	Glucose tolerance test (see Nursing Care Plan 13–3).	
Evaluate blood pressure on continuing basis; assess history of hypertension.	Risk for hypertension related to age.	If chronic hypertension exists, medications currently evaluated. Hydralazine (Apresoline) causes vasodilation and increased blood flow.	Pre-eclampsia and eclampsia occurs in 15 to 30 per cent of women with chronic hypertension.
Edema, proteinuria	At risk for pre-eclampsia	See Nursing Care Plan 13–7.	
Identify signs of premature rupture of membranes. Test fluid with nitrazine paper.	At risk for premature rupture of membranes	Explain the importance of contacting health-care provider if she suspects membranes have been ruptured. Explain symptoms: gush of fluid (rupture below presenting part), or trickle (rupture above presenting part).	The risk of neonatal infection increases when membranes are ruptured more than 24 hours prior to delivery. Nitrazine paper (Phenophthazine) tests pH; alkaline amniotic fluid turns paper dark blue; acidic urine or pus turns paper yellow.
Assess for signs of infection: maternal fever, malodorous vaginal drainage.	At risk of infection secondary to premature rupture of membranes	Decision for possible induction of labor based on gestational age of fetus. Explain course of treatment to mother and family. Betamethazone may be given to mother to enhance fetal lung maturity. Dispel myth of "dry labor"; explain that amniotic fluid is constantly forming. Prepare (personnel and equipment) for resuscitation of preterm infant if gestational age less than 38 weeks.	If fetus very immature labor may be delayed. Occasionally membranes become intact.
Attitude of woman, family about pregnancy	Anxiety about risk to baby and self; ambivalence about pregnancy	Provide opportunities to verbalize concerns; encourage verbalization. Provide primary nurse to develop relationship and trust over time.	

Table 13–5. WHITE'S CLASSIFICATION OF DIABETES IN PREGNANCY*

Group A:	Abnormal glucose tolerance test only.
Group B:	Onset of clinical diabetes after age 20, duration less than 10 years, no demonstrable vacular disease.
Group C:	Onset between ages 10 and 20, duration 10 to 19 years, no x-ray evidence of vascular disease.
Group D:	Onset before age 10 or duration over 20 years, x-ray diagnosis of vascular disease in legs, retinal changes.
Group E:	Same as Group D with addition of calcifications of pelvic arteries by x-ray examination.
Group F:	Diabetic nephropathy.
Group G:	Many pregnancy failures.
Group H:	Cardiopathy.
Group R:	Active retinitis proliferans.

*Adapted from White: *Medical Clinics of North America,* 49:1015, 1965; and White: *American Journal of Obstetrics and Gynecology,* 130:228, 1978.

elevated longer. A 3-hour test in pregnancy is important because of prolonged gastric emptying time (120 minutes compared with 75 minutes in nonpregnant women). The test is considered abnormal if two of four values are exceeded. Consider the following two examples:

Mrs. A. is given an oral glucose tolerance test because her two previous babies weighed 3900 grams (8.6 pounds) and 4100 grams (9 pounds). Her blood glucose values (mg./dl.) are fasting, 8.4; 1 hour, 174; 2 hours, 140; 3 hours, 121. The test is considered normal because only one value exceeds the standard.

Ms. B., who is being tested because of a strong family history of diabetes, has the following blood glucose values: fasting, 94; 1 hour, 170; 2 hours, 145; 3 hours, 127. Three values exceed the standard, and the diagnosis of gestational diabetes is made.

A diagnosis of gestational diabetes can be a major stress to a pregnant woman. Many women are visibly distressed at the time they are told and need a great deal of support. They are encouraged to cry if they want to (many do), and time is provided to answer their questions. Many fear having to take "shots" and are relieved to hear that insulin will probably not be necessary. The initial plan of care includes dietary control and urine testing (see below) and prenatal visits at least every 2 weeks. Women with gestational diabetes, as well as women with Class B-R diabetes, are at increased risk of infection and pregnancy-induced hypertension. Should dietary management fail to control blood glucose, insulin will be required.

The Effect of Pregnancy on Diabetes

We have noted in earlier chapters that pregnancy affects the hormonal system of the body. One of the effects of the mother's accelerated endocrine activity is increased insulin production by the islet cells of the pancreas. If this increased insulin output were to go unchecked, progressively increased hypoglycemia would result. The mother's body, however, is also producing estrogen, progesterone, cortisol, and human chorionic somatomammotropin (HCS, or placental lactogen), all of which are antagonistic to insulin. Moreover, glucocorticoids from the adrenal cortex and human growth hormone from the anterior pituitary are produced in increased amounts; these hormones increase the mother's tendency to hyperglycemia.

The net result of all of these changes is an increased insulin requirement in most mothers who have diabetes; some diabetic mothers have

Table 13–6. ORAL GLUCOSE TOLERANCE TEST (WHOLE BLOOD)

	Pregnant[a] Glucose (md./dl.)	Non-Pregnant[b] Glucose (mg./dl.)
Fasting	90	80
One hour	165	125
Two hours	145	60
Three Hours	125	80

Criteria for abnormal test: Two of four values exceeded.

[a]O'Sullivan and Mahan[36]
[b]Wallach[51]

Nursing Care Plan 13–3. The Pregnant Woman with Diabetes Mellitus

NURSING GOALS:
To ensure optimum care to meet the needs of the pregnant woman with diabetes mellitus and her fetus, through early identification and appropriate management.
To assist the woman and her family in understanding and coping with the modification her condition requires and her feelings about her high risk status and those modifications.

OBJECTIVES:
As a result of nursing care:
1. Women with diabetes mellitus (Class B-R) will be identified on the first prenatal visit.
2. Women with gestational diabetes will be identified.
3. Woman and her family will become knowledgeable about the effects of diabetes mellitus on pregnancy and the effects of pregnancy on diabetes mellitus.
4. Woman will become knowledgeable about the need for and practices involved in self-assessment, insulin administration, and diet modification.
5. Woman will keep a record of diet, insulin administration, urinalysis, blood glucose levels, and exercise.
6. Fetal and maternal well-being will be assessed on a continuing basis.
7. The birth of an infant who is large or small for gestational age will be avoided.
8. Complications of diabetes (e.g., ketoacidosis, retinopathy, nephropathy) will be avoided, and pre-existing complications will not increase in severity.
9. Woman and her family will verbalize their feelings about diabetes, and the woman will feel that her feelings are accepted.
10. Social and economic needs will be met as far as possible.

ASSESSMENT	POTENTIAL NURSING DIAGNOSIS	NURSING INTERVENTION	COMMENTS/RATIONALE
1. Determine classification if diabetes mellitus present prior to pregnancy (Table 13–5).			
2. Identify mother with gestational diabetes.	At risk for gestational diabetes		Suggest Medic-Alert bracelet or tag to ensure identification.
a. Risk factors			
1. Family history of diabetes mellitus			
2. Unexplained stillbirth			
3. Unexplained habitual abortion			
4. Previous birth of infant weighing > 4000 g. (8.8 pounds)			
5. Previous birth of infant with congenital anomaly			
6. Diabetes or glycosuria in previous pregnancy			
7. Maternal weight > 180 pounds			
b. Glucose tolerance test			
1. Screening for pregnant women at 28 weeks: oral 1-hour test. If glucose in whole blood exceeds 165 mg./dl. at 1 hour, test is abnormal. May be followed by 3-hour test.			

Continued on following page

Nursing Care Plan 13–3.   The Pregnant Woman with Diabetes Mellitus (Continued)

ASSESSMENT	POTENTIAL NURSING DIAGNOSIS	NURSING INTERVENTION	COMMENTS/RATIONALE
2. Screening for women at risk of gestational diabetes: 3-hour oral glucose tolerance test (normal values, Table 13–6).			
3. Knowledge of modification in prenatal care a. Diet 1. Reasons for modification during pregnancy 2. Effect of ketosis on fetus	Knowledge deficit Need for information about (specific area identified in assessment)	Refer for nutrition counseling. Diet: 30–50 calories/kg. body weight; 2 g. protein/kg. body weight; 3.5 g. carbohydrates/kg. body weight; sufficient fat to meet caloric needs. Even distribution of calories, including snacks. Encourage use of "diet diary."	Gravida may be hospitalized for a brief period early in pregnancy to adjust diet and insulin needs; provide teaching opportunity.
b. Self assessment 1. Urinalysis 2. Glucose (e.g., Dextrostix)	Need for practice	Provide opportunity to discuss importance of urinalysis, glucose assessment, and insulin therapy. Review or teach skills; observe mother in performance of skills. Refer to community health nurse for assessment of performance at home and further teaching.	
c. Regular exercise		Teach mother to keep a record of results of self-assessment (urinalysis, blood glucose, insulin, diet, exercise) to bring at each prenatal visit and for community health nurse assessment between visits. Explain that insulin requirements will change as pregnancy progresses and following birth (see text).	
d. Administration of insulin (if required)		If insulin is required by mother who has not previously taken insulin, total teaching program is necessary. In some settings, refer to diabetic teaching nurse. Community health nurse reinforces teaching in home.	
4. Complications of diabetes a. Hypoglycemia: weakness, hunger, nervousness, pallor, per-	At risk for complications of diabetes mellitus	Provide sugar (e.g., glucagon, orange juice).	

Assessment	Nursing Diagnosis	Intervention	Rationale
spiration, headache; blood glucose levels ≤ 60 mg./dl.; urine negative (sugar and acetone)		Obtain specimens (urine and blood) for laboratory analysis if not previously available. Notify physician. Provide supportive care.	
b. Ketoacidosis: abdominal pain, nausea and/or vomiting, dry skin, acetone odor to breath, flushed, thirsty, constipation, drowsiness, blood glucose level ≥ 250 mg./dl., urine positive (sugar and acetone)		Anticipate the need for intravenous therapy. Obtain specimens (urine and blood) for laboratory analysis if not previously available. Record intake/output. Notify physician.	
5. Signs of infection a. Urinalysis at each vist to assess urinary tract infection b. Mother's recognition of signs of infection (e.g., fever)	Increased risk of prenatal infection related to diabetes	Explain rationale for immediate notification of health-care provider at first sign of infection; insulin.	
6. Pregnancy-induced hypertension (PIH) (see Nursing Care Plan 13–9)	Increased risk of pregnancy-induced hypertension related to diabetes		
7. Fetal growth a. Ultrasound measurement: fetal biparietal diameter at 16–24 weeks	Need for information about fetal surveillance	Explain reason for ultrasound at this time. Describe examination to mother.	Ultrasound will aid in verifying gestational age; women with diabetes may have irregular menses.
8. Fetal well-being (Chapter 14) a. Nonstress test (NST) b. Contraction stress test (CST) c. Estriol levels		Explain rationale for tests and procedures (see Nursing Care Plan 14–1).	
9. Fetal lung maturity (Chapter 14) a. Lecithin/sphingomyelin ratio b. PG			
10. Assess social and economic needs (see Nursing Care Plan 13–1).		See Nursing Care Plan 13–1.	
11. Preparation for labor and birth	Need for information about labor and birth	Mother may be hospitalized prior to onset of labor; may want to attend childbirth preparation classes in sixth or seventh month. If no prior preparation, preparation should be provided in hospital.	
If hospitalized, assess prior preparation, inclusion of cesarean birth preparation.			

a decreased requirement, however, so that all mothers must be individually evaluated throughout pregnancy (see below).

The increase in glomerular filtration rate, which occurs in all pregnant women, along with a decrease in glucose reabsorption (i.e., a decreased renal threshold), makes glycosuria rather common in all pregnant women and makes the evaluation of the meaning of urine sugar more difficult.

The Effect of Diabetes on Pregnancy

Diabetes mellitus may affect pregnancy in several specific ways. Even with good care, perinatal mortality for the fetus-infant is as much as eight to ten times higher than in normal pregnancy. More than 10 per cent of fetuses may die in utero, and neonatal mortality is greater than 8 per cent. In addition, the likelihood of the infant's having one or more congenital anomalies is three times greater than that in the general population, and brain damage from hypoglycemia following birth does occur, although this is largely preventable with proper care (Chapter 23). Respiratory distress syndrome is far more common in infants of diabetic mothers (Chapter 23). Vaginal delivery is complicated when the infant is oversized. Perinatal mortality is increased when maternal diabetes is uncontrolled, when the mother also has a urinary tract infection or pregnancy-induced hypertension, and when the mother does not follow a plan of care devised for her.

The likelihood of pregnancy-induced hypertension (below) is five times greater in mothers with diabetes than in the general population; approximately one diabetic mother in every four will have pre-eclampsia, eclampsia, or hypertensive disease.

Maternal hydramnios (amniotic fluid in excess of 2000 ml.) occurs about 20 per cent of the time. Hydramnios may cause maternal distress because of the pressure of an enlarged uterus on the diaphragm, the gastrointestinal tract, or the venous system returning blood from the lower extremities.

The Basic Plan of Care

The prevention of hyperglycemia is the basic principle underlying the plan of care for pregnant women with diabetes. Women with Group A through Group C diabetes who maintain blood sugar levels between 80 and 110 mg. per 100 ml. usually have babies with normal weight and low morbidity. About 10 per cent of women with Class D-R diabetes have infants

small for gestational age, probably due to decreased placental perfusion.

When a woman with diabetes becomes pregnant she is usually hospitalized for several days. During this period her diet and insulin needs will be adjusted. A large part of her day will be devoted to assessing her knowledge of her condition and providing additional information she will need to care for herself.

The more a woman is able to participate in the development of her plan of care, the more likely she will be to participate in that plan. Nursing Care Plan 13–3 lists the components of a care plan for women who are pregnant and diabetic.

During this hospitalization other body systems affected by diabetes (optic fundi, kidney, heart) are evaluated. Between 16 and 24 weeks ultrasonic measurement of fetal biparietal diameter (Chapter 14) is performed because menstrual irregularity in many women with diabetes makes gestational age uncertain, and third trimester evaluation of gestational age is complicated by the increased size (macrosomia) of some infants of diabetic mothers. In addition, the lecithin/sphingomyelin (L/S) ratio (below) is less reliable as an index of fetal lung maturity. The mother, especially if this is her first pregnancy and she is feeling well, may have difficulty understanding the reason for and the importance of this hospitalization. Both before her admission and while she is in the hospital, we can help her by encouraging her to express her feelings about this hospitalization and by using her time and ours to teach her as much as possible about the special requirements of her pregnancy. She should not remain in bed during the time she is in the hospital but should be as normally active as possible while diet and insulin requirements are being regulated. Diabetic mothers who have experienced difficulties during a previous pregnancy may better recognize the reason for early hospitalization.

Diet.   Diet is important for anyone who has diabetes and for any woman who is pregnant; it should therefore not be surprising that good diet control is essential for the pregnant diabetic woman.

For the diabetic mother with normal weight and activity, a diet of approximately 38 to 50 calories/kg. of body weight is usually recommended; about 400 additional calories per day are needed for mothers under 18 years of age. Calories are never restricted, whatever the mother's weight; the resulting ketonemia can cause irreversible central nervous system damage to the fetus. Protein is calculated at 1.5 grams per kg. of body weight per day (roughly

90 grams for a 130 pound woman), carbohydrate at 3.0 grams per kg. per day, and fat in quantities sufficient to make up the total caloric needs. (Note that the protein intake is considerably higher than that of the average pregnant woman, for whom approximately 65 grams of protein are recommended.)

The diet plan includes meals, between-meal snacks, and a bedtime snack. Even distribution of the calories is important so that blood glucose will remain as constant as possible, and fetal equilibrium will be maintained with no marked episodes of either hypoglycemia or hyperglycemia.

A "diet diary" will help the mother become aware of what and when she is eating; it will help us in assessing her diet and in counseling her about subsequent planning. Again, this may seem like a lot of extra trouble to the mother unless she understands the reason and the importance. She is not likely to keep records accurately just because we ask her to do so.

Insulin. Insulin is regulated so that the fasting blood sugar level is maintained between 80 and 110 mg. per 100 ml. or the 2-hour postprandial blood sugar level between 110 and 145 mg. per 100 ml. Values considered acceptable will vary somewhat from one institution to another. Testing is usually done once every 2 weeks, although a specific plan will be made for each patient.

A common insulin regimen combines intermediate or long-acting insulin plus regular insulin taken in the morning, with only regular insulin taken again in the evening. Insulin requirements may be lower for some women in the first trimester; by the third trimester insulin will usually be increased by as much as 50 to 75 per cent, although again there are individual variations.

Oral hypoglycemic agents are not used during pregnancy, even if the mother has taken them previously. These agents stimulate the beta cells, not only in the maternal pancreas but in the fetal pancreas as well.

Because insulin is inactivated by the placenta, failure to require an increased amount of insulin after the first trimester or a sudden drop in insulin requirement may mean some problem in placental function.

Urine Checks. Diabetic mothers are asked to check urine sugar levels four times a day and to keep a record of urine tests, insulin taken, exercise, and blood glucose levels (below). These records can be used to help the mother recognize variations that affect her, such as the interaction between a favorite activity and her urine sugar level, and thus

can help her become better able to plan for herself. Sugar levels of 4+ should be reported to her nurse or physician immediately.

Blood Glucose. Diabetic gravidas are frequently taught to use a Dextrostix to assess blood glucose levels at home as an adjunct to urine testing, and to record these results. Some women are asked to monitor glucose daily while others may be asked to use Dextrostix bi-weekly as long as urine tests are stable.

Monitoring the Fetus

In the third trimester, beginning at 32 to 34 weeks, urinary estriol levels and oxytocin challenge testing to determine fetal well-being and evaluation of the lecithin/sphingomyelin (L/S) ratio and creatinine levels to assess fetal maturity become a part of care. These procedures, important to high risk mothers with many kinds of problems, are discussed below.

Note in the discussion of the L/S ratio in Chapter 14 that a ratio of 2.0 or greater is usually considered an indication of lung maturity. Experience indicates that in certain laboratories, at least, the infant of a diabetic mother may need a higher ratio (at least 2.5 to 3.0) to indicate lung maturity.

Heart Disease

The cardiac-related changes that occur in all pregnant women have been discussed in Chapter 7. To review these briefly, there is an increase in both blood volume and heart rate, with a resultant increase in cardiac output of from 40 to 50 per cent. For the mother who has a diseased heart, this increased workload may compromise her health.

About 1.5 to 3 per cent of all pregnant women have some form of heart disease. As a cause of maternal mortality, heart disease ranks fourth or fifth, depending on the study. The most common cardiac problem of women who become pregnant is rheumatic heart disease, with mitral stenosis the most common lesion. Over 80 per cent of pregnant women with heart disease will have rheumatic heart disease. Ten to 15 per cent (figures vary from study to study) will have some form of congenital heart defect. All other forms of heart disease account for only 2 per cent of cardiac maternity patients.

For some mothers with heart disease, there may have been no prior symptoms; the diagnosis of cardiac disease is made during the pregnancy. This is not always an easy diagnosis because:

1. The apex of the heart rotates laterally

during pregnancy, and therefore, it is normal for the heart to *appear* larger in an x-ray film.

2. A systolic murmur is common in pregnant women (as frequent as 96 per cent of the time in some studies) and a diastolic murmur may be present as often as 18 per cent of the time.

3. Tachycardia is not unusual.

It is not difficult to imagine the anxiety of a woman who must adjust not only to pregnancy but also to the possibility of heart disease as well. Difficulty in diagnosis will add to her anxiety; it is essential that we understand and explain why the diagnosis is not always easy. Symptoms that clearly indicate heart disease include:

1. A continuous diastolic or presystolic murmur.

2. A loud, harsh systolic murmur, especially with a thrill.

3. Definite heart enlargement.

4. Severe arrhythmia, such as bigeminy.

The Effect of Heart Disease on Pregnant Women

In assessing the status and needs of the mother with heart disease, the classification of the New York Heart Association is commonly used (Table 13–7). This classification is one indication of the extent to which pregnancy will affect the mother.

Also important is the mother's age. The incidence of congestive heart failure increases with age; mothers over 30 often do not tolerate pregnancy as well as younger mothers. Ther-

apeutic abortion may be suggested for some older mothers.

The longer the mother has had heart disease, the greater her likelihood of problems. Previous atrial fibrillation, previous heart failure, and cardiomegaly are also serious signs.

Although we cannot change the mother's age or cardiac status, there are a number of other factors that can be controlled in helping her to experience a safe pregnancy. If the mother is obese, weight reduction prior to pregnancy will improve her chances for a good outcome. Anemia must be prevented; anemia alone can lead to congestive heart failure.

Toxemia (below) can also cause congestive failure, even if the mother has mild heart disease (and can, in fact, cause congestive failure in the mother with no heart disease). Many physicians will digitalize a woman with heart disease who shows signs of toxemia. Infection may also contribute to heart failure. Congestive heart failure is a cause of death in pregnant women with heart disease.

Cardiac Workload in Pregnancy

Cardiac output increases slightly during the first 8 weeks of pregnancy and then increases more sharply until the period of maximum output, about 28 to 32 weeks. It then levels off from 32 weeks until the time of delivery.

During labor, cardiac output increases slightly with each uterine contraction. Following delivery, cardiac output increases markedly within the first day or two, as fluid in the mother's tissues returns to the circulatory sys-

Table 13–7. CLASSIFICATION OF HEART DISEASE IN PREGNANCY*

Class	Criteria	Possible Course of Pregnancy
I	No discomfort during normal activity.	Generally few problems during pregnancy.
II	May have transient angina during normal activity.	Generally few problems during pregnancy.
III	Activity brings discomfort (fatigue, angina, dyspnea). Comfortable only at rest.	Often advised against pregnancy, but may choose to become pregnant. Should be hospitalized if signs of cardiac decompensation develop.
IV	Barely comfortable even at rest; may have symptoms of angina or congestive heart failure at rest. Unable to perform any activity without discomfort.	High maternal mortality. Postpartum period particularly hazardous. Usually advised against pregnancy.

*Adapted from New York Heart Association: *Nomenclature and Criteria for Diagnosis of Diseases of the Heart and Blood Vessels.* 5th Edition. New York, Peter F. Mallon, Inc., 1953.

tem (Chapter 25). The first days postpartum are critical, and the mother must be watched closely for the signs of congestive heart failure described below. By the third to fourth postpartal day, marked diuresis has occurred, and the risk of heart failure decreases.

The Plan of Care during the Prenatal Period

The goal of care for the pregnant woman with heart disease is reduction of the workload on the heart (Nursing Care Plan 13–4).

Activity is limited in relation to the extent of the heart disease. If the mother is short of breath and dyspneic or tachypneic, she is doing too much. For mothers in Classes I and II, limitation may mean a midmorning and midafternoon rest period. Ten hours of sleep are recommended at night, as well as a rest period after each meal. Mothers in Class IV may require complete bed rest throughout pregnancy.

Reduced physical activity is so important, particularly for Class III and IV mothers, that time spent in helping the mother plan her daily schedule is a significant part of her care. If appropriate, perhaps some type of household help can be arranged; many communities have "homemaker" services as part of the Department of Social Services or of another community agency. Another resource is a home economist (a county extension agent, for example), who will visit the home and help the mother plan her work with a minimum amount of effort.

The frustration of inactivity, particularly for the mother who must have complete bed rest, must also be faced. She will need frequent opportunities to share her feelings about this pregnancy and the changes it is making in her family life. For many mothers hospitalization for rest may be required at some time during pregnancy.

Sodium intake is usually limited to 2 grams. If a mother is restricting her sodium intake and still gaining excessive weight, a diuretic such as hydrochlorothiazide may be prescribed.

Any *infection* is promptly treated with antibiotics. Upper respiratory infections, if complicated by bronchitis and pneumonia, are important as contributory causes of heart failure. Infection may also lead to bacterial endocarditis in a patient with diseased heart valves. Because of this, prophylactic antibiotics may be given during labor and following delivery.

The avoidance of *anxiety* is important. A certain amount of anxiety is present during every pregnancy. That anxiety is easily compounded when the mother knows she has "complications." Frequent visits to the clinic or office, careful explanations of what is happening and the reasons for care, and, again, the opportunity to talk with a concerned and interested listener are essentials. Frequent visits are particularly important as the period of maximum cardiac output is reached. Output increases rapidly beginning about 20 weeks and peaks from 28 to 32 weeks.

Assessment of the Gravida with Heart Disease

Weight gain—A gain in weight in excess of the normally expected gain may indicate accumulating fluid and the potential for congestive heart failure.

Heart rate—A heart rate of 110 or more when the woman is resting may be a sign of early heart failure or of infection.

Respiratory rate—Respirations greater than 20 to 24 per minute may be a preliminary to heart failure. Ask about dyspnea, orthopnea, and coughing.

Unexplained cough—An unexplained cough may be a first sign of congestive failure.

Hemoptysis, distention of neck veins, rales and *wheezes,* and *pulmonary edema*—These are signs of congestive heart failure.

The treatment for congestive heart failure is medical; it is almost never the termination of the pregnancy. As in the nonpregnant patient, treatment includes rest, digitalis, diuretics, oxygen, sedatives, and restricted sodium and fluids.

The Woman with a Cardiac Valve Prosthesis

Since a cardiac valve prosthesis is only inserted in patients with significant cardiac impairment, these patients are not particularly good candidates for successful pregnancy. In addition, such a woman has special problems during pregnancy. She normally uses an anticoagulant because thrombosis and thromboembolism are problems with all prostheses currently available. The coumarin derivatives, often prescribed for these patients, cross the placenta and (1) may be teratogenic (Chapter 8) and (2) may cause bleeding in the newborn infant (especially cerebral bleeding) if given to the mother late in pregnancy. Heparin is the anticoagulant of choice during pregnancy because it does not cross the placenta. (Oral anticoagulants are sometimes used after the first trimester until the thirty-seventh week.)

Mothers with a cardiac prosthesis are at increased risk of endocarditis; they may be

Nursing Care Plan 13–4.   The Pregnant Woman with Heart Disease

NURSING GOALS:
To ensure optimum care for the pregnant woman with heart disease through early identification and management appropriate to the severity of her cardiac status.
To assist the woman and her family in understanding and coping with necessary modifications in activity.

OBJECTIVES:
1. Women with heart disease will be identified early in pregnancy.
2. The gravida and her family will understand and comply with necessary modification in care.
3. Congestive heart failure will be prevented.

ASSESSMENT	POTENTIAL NURSING DIAGNOSIS	NURSING INTERVENTION	RATIONALE/COMMENTS
1. Identify signs of heart disease (physical) a. Continuous diastolic or presystolic murmur b. Loud, harsh systolic murmur, especially with a thrill c. Definite heart enlargement on x-ray d. Severe arrhythmia, such as bigeminy			
2. Identify signs of heart disease (subjective) a. Transient angina during activity b. Fatigue, dyspnea, angina during activity c. Dyspnea, angina at rest	Activity intolerance related to heart disease and pregnancy	Intervention based on classification of heart disease (Table 13–4). Activity is limited as necessary to prevent dyspnea, tachypnea. Help mother plan daily schedule to allow adequate rest; enlist family cooperation. Gravida should rest 8–10 hours at night and after each meal. Additional rest is related to symptoms.	Activity limits will vary from morning and afternoon rest periods to complete bed rest.
3. Identify other relevant factors a. Maternal age b. Duration of heart disease, previous heart failure, cardiomegaly, atrial fibrillation c. Obesity	Risk of cardiac decompensation related to (maternal age, etc.).	More frequent ambulatory and home visits for close supervision. In obese women, help with weight reduction *prior* to pregnancy.	Frequent visits are of particular importance as maximum cardiac output is reached (28 to 32 weeks)

d. Hemoglobin/hematocrit to detect anemia
e. Infectious disease
f. Signs of pre-eclampsia
  (1) Edema
  (2) Proteinuria
  (3) Hypertension
	Correction of anemia through diet and supplemental iron.
	
	Discuss prevention of infection (avoiding crowds, persons with infections; good nutrition).
	
	Instruct woman to notify clinic or physician at first sign of infection.
	
	Instruct mother in signs of pre-eclampsia.
		Edema may be related to pre-eclampsia or to cardiac decompensation.

4. Medications woman is currently using
  1. Digoxin, digitoxin
  2. Anticoagulants (coumarin, heparin)
  3. Diuretics (e.g., chlorothiazide, hydrochlorothiazide, furosemide, ethacrynic acid)
  4. Prophylactic antibiotics
  5. Propranolol (Inderal)
  6. Quinidine
	Need for information about medications and pregnancy
	Anxiety about use of medications during pregnancy
	
	Explain reason for each medication and for medication changes.
	Reassure about effects on fetus on basis of available information.
	
	1. Digoxin, digitoxin: cross placenta; no known harm to fetus. Expansion of body water may lower circulating level, may require increased dosage. Blood levels must be determined. Explain reason for increased dosage to gravida and family.
	2. Anticoagulants: coumarin changed to heparin. Heparin does not cross placenta (large molecule).
	Teach heparin administration. Foods high in vitamin K (e.g., raw green leafy vegetables) are avoided because vitamin K inactivates heparin.
	3. Diuretics: Used occasionally when congestive heart failure is uncontrolled by rest and decreased sodium intake. Fluid and electrolyte balance must be carefully monitored.
		Many women and families are aware of information about taking medications during pregnancy; this may be a source of anxiety.
		
		Coumarin may cause congenital malformation (early pregnancy) and fetal hemorrhage (late pregnancy). Coumarin is also contraindicated in women planning pregnancy because congenital anomalies most likely in very early pregnancy.

Continued on following page

Nursing Care Plan 13–4.   The Pregnant Woman with Heart Disease (Continued)

ASSESSMENT	POTENTIAL NURSING DIAGNOSIS	NURSING INTERVENTION	RATIONALE/COMMENTS
		4. Prophylactic antibiotics. Women with rheumatic heart disease continue antibiotic prophylaxis during pregnancy.	
		5. Propranolol: potential for initiating premature labor; causes sustained increase in uterine tone that may compromise uterine circulation.	
		6. Quinidine: no harmful effects known.	Beta-sympathomimetic drugs (e.g., ritodrine, terbutaline) are contraindicated in women with heart disease.
5. Signs of cardiac decompensation a. Weight gain in excess of norms for trimester (Chapter 10) b. Heart rate greater than 110 b.p.m. when woman is at rest c. Respiratory rate greater than 20–24 r.p.m.; dyspnea, orthopnea d. Unexplained cough e. Hemoptysis, rales, wheezes, pulmonary edema	Alterations in cardiac output secondary to cardiac decompensation Anxiety of woman and family related to heart failure	Bed rest; digoxin or digitoxin; sodium restriction. Reassure woman, family about care.	Congestive heart failure is the normal cause of maternal mortality in gravidas with heart disease.
6. Knowledge of labor and birth; attitudes about labor and birth	Need for information about labor and birth Anxiety related to labor and birth	Prenatal education to reduce anxiety (if mother at bed rest, education must be provided in home). Reassure that necessary analgesia and anesthesia will be provided; "pushing" in second stage of labor may be contraindicated; only gentle pushing with woman exhaling during pushing may be allowed.	Anxiety and pain may, in themselves, lead to cardiac decompensation and possible heart failure (anxiety → tachycardia → pulmonary edema → heart failure). Scopolamine never used (restlessness, tachycardia). Atropine rarely used.

given prophylactic antibiotics during labor for this reason.

Prostheses may limit the blood flow and make it difficult to meet the higher tissue needs for oxygen during pregnancy.

Valve prostheses also cause some trauma to red blood cells, which may be sufficiently extensive to cause anemia.

Urinary Tract and/or Renal Disease

Urinary tract infections are a fairly common complication of pregnancy (see Infection and the Pregnant Woman, below).

Renal disease, in which there is impairment of kidney function, is associated with both eclampsia and premature labor. Some studies indicate that asymptomatic bacterial infections also may be associated with premature labor, while others find no similar relationship.

The effect of chronic renal disease on pregnancy is related to the presence of hypertension. When there is no hypertension, a successful pregnancy and good fetal outcome are possible even if there is impaired renal function. However, if the mother is hypertensive, intrauterine growth retardation is common, and the incidence of pre-eclampsia and perinatal mortality is very high.

Chronic Hypertensive Disease

Chronic hypertensive disease is not always easy to recognize during pregnancy unless the woman is aware of her hypertension. If the woman is first seen for prenatal care in the second trimester when blood pressure is at its lowest, hypertension may not be recognized. A diastolic pressure greater than 80 mm. Hg at midtrimester is suggestive of chronic disease.

What happens when the woman with essential hypertension becomes pregnant? Approximately 15 to 30 per cent of gravidas with essential hypertension will develop preeclampsia. The higher the blood pressure, the greater the risk of both pre-eclampsia and a poor fetal outcome.

For some women, pregnancy is a stimulus to the development of latent essential hypertension, just as pregnancy may stimulate latent diabetes (gestational diabetes). The hypertension may disappear following delivery only to reappear during subsequent pregnancies, eventually becoming chronic hypertension.

Bed rest with the mother lying on her side is most important. Two hours in the morning and 2 hours in the afternoon are recommended (see Home vs. Hospital for the High Risk Mother, above).

Unlike the mother with pregnancy-induced hypertension (below), table salt is eliminated for mothers with chronic hypertension. Diuretics are not used, however, because a decreased intravascular volume is undesirable. Antihypertensive drugs (hydralazine) are used only for blood pressure levels above 160 mm. Hg (systolic) or 110 mm. Hg (diastolic). The goal is not to return blood pressure to normotensive levels, because this would decrease blood flow to the uterus and placenta, but to maintain the diastolic pressure at 100 mm. Hg.

The fetus, like the fetus of a woman with PIH, is at risk of growth retardation; fetal assessment is essential (Chapter 14).

Sickle Cell Disease

No condition complicating pregnancy carries as great a risk as sickle cell disease. Maternal mortality is as high as 10 to 20 per cent, and perinatal mortality is in the range of 50 per cent in the severe forms of the disease. (There are several forms of sickle cell disease, such as sickle cell disease (SS), hemoglobin SC disease, homozygous hemoglobin C disease, and so on, the description of which is beyond the scope of this book.)

Approximately 8 per cent of black gravidas have sickle cell trait (SA) (Chapter 3). Although they do not have the severe problems of the mother with sickle cell disease, their fetuses may be at risk of hypoxic stress.

The mother with sickle cell trait or sickle cell disease should ideally be identified prior to pregnancy by community screening programs. (The mother with sickle cell disease may have been identified because of recurrent illness throughout her life.) If a woman has never been tested, this should be a part of her prenatal assessment, along with testing of the baby's father for purposes of genetic counseling (Nursing Care Plan 13–5).

Care of the mother with sickle cell disease who wishes to complete a pregnancy includes careful observation of hemoglobin levels. A hemoglobin level in the range of 6 to 8 grams per 100 ml. is normal for these mothers; no attempt is made to raise the hemoglobin level beyond the mother's normal range during the course of pregnancy. A rapidly falling hemoglobin value is a sign of sickle cell crisis. At term or during labor, transfusions of whole blood or packed red blood cells are usually given as a measure of protection for mother and infant.

Iron is not given to mothers with sickle cell disease. Folic acid needs are increased during and following crises.

Nursing Care Plan 13–5.   The Mother with Sickle Cell Trait, Sickle Cell Disease, or Related Hematologic Disorders

NURSING GOALS:
To identify the gravida with sickle cell trait, sickle cell disease or related hematologic disease.
To provide care that protects both mother and fetus.

OBJECTIVES:
1. The gravida with sickle cell trait will be identified.
2. Appropriate genetic counseling will be provided; fetal testing will be provided as available.
3. The gravida with sickle cell disease will receive such care that complications will be prevented or, if they occur, will be recognized and treated promptly.
4. The gravida with another hematologic disorder will be identified and appropriate care provided to protect mother and fetus.

ASSESSMENT	POTENTIAL NURSING DIAGNOSIS	NURSING INTERVENTION	COMMENTS/RATIONALE
1. Identify gravidas at risk of sickle cell trait (AS). a. Hemoglobin electrophoresis b. History (1) Gravida (2) Family	Risk of pregnancy complications related to sickle cell trait.	If trait (AS) is present, screening of partner is necessary. If both woman and partner have AS, genetic counseling concerning risk of fetal sickle cell disease (SS) is needed. Amniotic fluid analysis for fetal SS first available in 1982.	Approximately 8 per cent of American black women have sickle cell trait. Sickle cell disease may also occur in women of Mediterranean ancestry. Screening should be done prior to pregnancy and involve the woman and her partner so that appropriate genetic counseling can be provided.
2. Potential complications of AS. a. Bacteriuria b. Hematuria c. Fetal hypoxia	Risk of urinary tract infection related to AS. Risk of possible fetal hypoxia.	Prompt treatment of urinary tract infections (Nursing Care Plan 13–4) Fetal assessment: Nonstress test (NST) (Nursing Care Plan 14–1)	
3. Identify mothers with sickle cell disease (SS). a. History (1) Gravida (2) Family b. Hemoglobin electrophoresis	Risk of pregnancy complications related to SS.		

4. Identify complications. a. Hemoglobin/hematocrit (hct <25–30 per cent)	At risk of anemia	Prepare gravida for transfusion or exchange transfusion when hematocrit less than 25 per cent. Diuretic may be given with transfusion to avoid congestive heart failure. Folic acid supplementation to avoid megaloblastic anemia.	Hemodilution of pregnancy increases anemia. Severe anemia associated with fetal hypoxia; folic acid requirements increased in women with chronic disorders.
b. Pulmonary infarction (chest pain; symptoms similar to lung infection)	At risk of pulmonary complications	Early identification of pulmonary infarction	Pulmonary disease in 15 per cent of women with SS
c. Signs of infection, including bacteriuria	At risk of infection (including pyelonephritis)	Early identification and prompt treatment of infections (Nursing Care Plan 13–4)	Infection may precipitate SS crisis.
d. Signs of congestive heart failure (edema, dyspnea, tachycardia)	At risk of congestive heart failure	Early identification and prompt treatment of congestive heart failure (Nursing Care Plan 13–3)	
e. Signs of pre-eclampsia (1) Proteinuria (2) Edema (3) Hypertension	At risk of pre-eclampsia	Frequent monitoring of urine, blood pressure, signs of edema (Nursing Care Plan 13–7)	Risk of pre-eclampsia 3 to 4 times greater than normal
f. Signs of spontaneous abortion	At risk of spontaneous abortion	Instruct mother to contact health-care provider at first sign of bleeding, cramping.	Abortion markedly increased; rates as high as 25 per cent
g. Signs of premature labor	At risk of premature labor	Teach signs of premature labor. Instruct mother to contact health-care provider at first sign of labor (contractions, ruptured membranes, show)	Rates of spontaneous premature labor are higher.
h. Sickle cell crisis	At risk of SS crisis	Ensure adequate hydration. Provide analgesia.	Exchange transfusions may be part of the treatment for crisis.
5. Preparation for labor	Need for information about relationship of labor and SS disease	Encourage childbirth preparation to reduce need for medication and risk of hypoxia.	General anesthesia avoided in labor because of danger of hypoxia; conduction anesthesia is used for Cesarean birth or labor.

Continued on following page

Nursing Care Plan 13–5.   The Mother with Sickle Cell Trait, Sickle Cell Disease, or Related Hematologic Disorders (*Continued*)

ASSESSMENT	POTENTIAL NURSING DIAGNOSIS	NURSING INTERVENTION	COMMENTS/RATIONALE
6. Following delivery a. Signs of infection (fever, foul-smelling lochia)	At risk for post-partum infection.	Careful preventive techniques needed. Teach mother self-care to prevent infection. Frequent assessment for early signs of infection and prompt treatment if recognized.	
Other Hematologic Disorders			
1. Hemoglobin SC disease a. Identify	Risk of complications related to SC		Risk of mortality, morbidity as great or greater than in SS disease
b. Potential complications (1) Infection (prenatal and postpartum) (2) Pulmonary infarction (3) Pre-eclampsia (4) Crises (5) Decreasing hemoglobin, hematocrit (6) Postpartum hemorrhage		As in SS disease	
2. Sickle cell beta-thalassemia a. Identify: distinguish from women with iron deficiency anemia	At slight risk of complications		
b. Potential complications (1) Bone pain (2) Anemia (3) Infection		As in SS disease	Fetal loss, maternal complications less than with conditions above

Sterilization is frequently recommended for a mother with severe sickle cell disease because of the risk pregnancy carries to her own life.

Rh Isoimmunization

When a mother lacks the D factor in her blood, she is said to be Rh negative. If her fetus has the D factor and is thus Rh positive, Rh isoimmunization is possible.

The genetic basis of Rh disease has been discussed in Chapter 3.

In about 10 per cent of all pregnancies, an Rh negative mother is carrying an Rh positive fetus. Theoretically, each Rh positive fetus of an Rh negative mother is a candidate for *erythroblastosis fetalis,* in which the red blood cells of the fetus and newborn are destroyed by a process described below. However, in only 5 per cent of pregnancies in which there is a potential problem does the mother develop antibodies to the fetal red blood cells.

Erythroblastosis occurs in from 4 to 10 pregnancies per every 1000. The problem could be eliminated in the large majority of these babies by applying our current knowledge (Nursing Care Plan 13–6).

The physiologic basis of erythroblastosis is an antigen-antibody reaction. The Rh_D negative mother (genotype dd) has no Rh_D antigen in her body. When her fetus is Rh_D positive, any fetal blood (containing D antigen) that enters her system is treated as a "foreign substance," i.e., she develops antibodies to protect her system against the "intruder." Her antibodies attach themselves to the fetal red blood cells and destroy them.

Since fetal blood and maternal blood do not mix, normally fetal red blood cells do not enter the maternal system during the prenatal period. Thus the first D-positive infant of a D-negative mother does not usually have problems, *unless* at some prior time the mother was transfused with D-positive blood (rare) or has had a spontaneous or an induced abortion of a D-positive fetus without the use of passive-antibody (RhoGAM), as described below.

At the time of delivery (or abortion), fetal red blood cells do enter the maternal circulation. The mother's immune system develops anti-Rh_D antibodies. Once the immune response begins, antibody production may continue for many years without additional stimulus.

When the Rh_D negative mother next becomes pregnant with an Rh_D positive fetus, those antibodies cross the placenta, coat the red blood cells of the fetus, and cause their destruction.

In the most severe form of erythroblastosis, red blood cell destruction in the fetus results first in marked anemia and subsequently in an attempt to raise red cell production and in heart failure, as the heart tries harder and harder to oxygenate the body with a limited number of red blood cells. The fetus develops edema with pleural effusion and ascites. Intrauterine hypoxia, hypoproteinemia, and lowered oncotic pressure probably are factors in causing edema, in addition to the anemia. This condition is termed *hydrops fetalis.* The fetus may die in utero or, if born alive, frequently dies in the first days after birth. Once a mother has delivered a stillborn infant whose death was caused by Rh sensitization, the chances are less than 30 per cent that she will ever be able to deliver a living child.

Fortunately, not every infant of a sensitized mother is so seriously affected. With a more moderate course, the infant may be delivered and then develop erythroblastosis fetalis postnatally, with characteristic jaundice and anemia caused by the breakdown of red blood cells. The needs and care of the infant with erythroblastosis are discussed in Chapter 24.

Caring for the Sensitized Mother

Determination of the level of anti-D antibody in the serum of an Rh_D negative mother (when the father is Rh_D positive) is basic to her continued assessment. This test, known as the antibody-titer or anti-Rh titer, is repeated every 4 weeks, even if there is no indication of antibody. As long as there is no antibody present, the mother's prenatal care and delivery will be the same as that of any woman with no special problems.

If antibodies are detected but titers remain below or at low levels throughout pregnancy (the critical levels will vary according to the laboratory technique used), again pregnancy care is essentially "normal." The mother will, however, need information and reassurance about the meaning of antibody testing. She needs to understand why testing is important and why she should return for testing at prescribed intervals, without being unduly alarmed.

If titers rise above a level determined as critical in a particular laboratory (commonly 1:32 or 1:64), amniocentesis is performed to determine the level of bilirubin in amniotic fluid by a technique called spectrophotometric analysis. The amount of bilirubin in amniotic

Nursing Care Plan 13–6.   The Gravida with Rh Isoimmunization

NURSING GOALS:
To protect the fetus at risk of erythroblastosis fetalis from illness and possible death.
To provide information that will enable the mother and her family to understand Rh isoimmunization.

OBJECTIVES:
1. Mothers at risk of isoimmunization will be identified early in pregnancy.
2. Care of mothers at risk will include antibody titers and, when indicated, amniocentesis.
3. The mother and her family will understand the condition and the reason for the care she receives.
4. A healthy infant will be delivered.

ASSESSMENT	POTENTIAL NURSING DIAGNOSIS	NURSING INTERVENTION	COMMENTS/RATIONALE
1. Identify mothers at risk. 　a. Mothers who are Rh$_D$ negative 　b. Mothers who lack other Rh antigens (Kell, C^w,C, E)	Fetus at risk of erythroblastosis fetalis; need for information about erythroblastosis.	Explain Rh isoimmunization to gravida and family; explain purpose of Rh immune globulin, time of administration, and when it should be given if mother has not been previously sensitized.	Even in first pregnancy or when mother has previously received Rh immune globulin (RhoGram) mother is considered at risk because (1) dosage of Rh immune globulin may have been insufficient; (2) mother may have unknowingly become sensitized e.g., prior to delivery, at her own birth, etc.
2. Antibody titer		Explain reason for frequent blood tests.	
3. If antibody titer exceeds 1:8 or 1:16, amniocentesis is done to measure amount of bilirubin present.		Explain purpose of amniocentesis. Support during procedure (see Nursing Care Plan 14–1).	

4. Assessment of gestational age through L/S ratio, PG (Chapter 14)

If OD_{450} indicates fetal illness, early delivery or intrauterine transfusion may be indicated; explain purpose of testing to parents.

5. Feelings of gravida and family

Anxiety, fear, etc. related to Rh isoimmunization

Encourage verbalization of fears. Give appropriate support.

If mother not previously sensitized, prognosis is good. If there was previous sensitization and/or death of previous infant, prognosis is more guarded.

Following Delivery

Rh immune globulin is given within 72 hours of delivery to all mothers not previously sensitized. (Also given following spontaneous or elective abortion.)

No prophylaxis available for Kell, C^w,C, E antigens.

Inform mother of results; counsel about future pregnancies.

Test for the presence of antibody in maternal blood at 4 to 6 months postdelivery or postabortion.

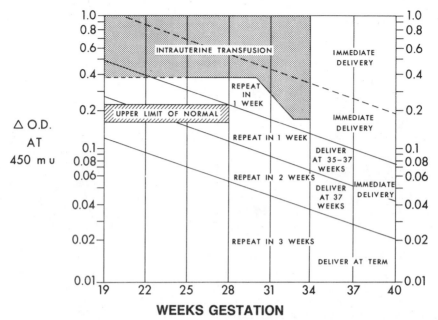

Figure 13–1. A modified Liley graph which correlates the 450 nm. peak at each week of gestation with the recommended method of management. The phrase "repeat in 1 week" refers to a repeat spectrophotometric analysis of the amniotic fluid. (From Jennings: *Family Health Bulletin.* Suppl. 4, Winter 1970–71, State of California Department of Public Health.)

fluid more accurately reflects fetal involvement than does the mother's antibody titer. The optical density (expressed as ΔOD_{450} and read delta OD_{450}) of the amniotic fluid indicates the amount of bilirubin and thus the severity of fetal disease (Fig. 13–1).

If the ΔOD_{450} is low, the fetus will probably be only mildly affected. If the ΔOD_{450} is moderate at the time of the first amniocentesis, amniotic fluid analysis will be repeated every 2 to 3 weeks thereafter. It may subsequently:

1. Fall to a low zone, with a mildly affected infant delivered at or near term.

2. Fall slowly, but remain in a middle zone, with a moderately affected infant delivered at approximately 37 weeks.

3. Increase to a high level.

When the ΔOD_{450} is at a level deemed critical on initial or subsequent examination, one of two courses is chosen. If the parameters of gestational age indicate that the baby could survive, he is delivered, and preparations are made to care for a very sick infant. When it is at all possible, the mother should be transferred to a major medical center for delivery rather than attempting to transfer a very sick newborn after delivery.

If the baby is too immature for extrauterine survival, he may receive an intrauterine transfusion. Intrauterine transfusion does not always save the baby's life. If the fetus already has hydrops fetalis, the infused blood is not absorbed. Fetal organs such as the liver or

bladder may be perforated. However, since transfusion is used only for a fetus already severely sick and in danger of death, any success is welcomed.

Radiopaque material is injected into the amniotic fluid approximately 5 hours prior to the transfusion. Because the fetus is continually swallowing amniotic fluid, the radiopaque material will concentrate sufficiently in the fetal bowel to outline the bowel. A needle is then inserted into the fetal peritoneal cavity, further dye is injected, and the position of the needle is verified by roentgenography. From 80 to 150 ml. of fresh O-negative packed red blood cells that have been cross-matched with the mother's serum is injected, the amount being approximately 15 per cent of the estimated fetal weight.

It is believed that the injected red blood cells enter the fetal circulation by way of the lymphatics below the diaphragm. Fetal hemoglobin levels rise. The procedure can be repeated every 1 to 2 weeks, if necessary, until the fetus has reached a gestational age at which extrauterine existence is possible.

Nursing Support for the Sensitized Mother

The sensitized Rh_D negative mother has realistic fears that her unborn or newborn infant may die or may be neurologically damaged (see Chapter 10). She may have lost one or more infants in previous pregnancies.

She may feel guilty or angry about her baby's condition. For example, if she became sensitized as a result of an induced abortion after which she was not given RhoGAM, she may feel that sensitization was her fault for having had the abortion, or she may be angry at the caretakers who failed to give her RhoGAM.

Like the mother of any sick fetus or newborn, she needs the opportunity to talk out her feelings and feel our concern. She needs to be informed about what is happening to the fetus, and hope for survival should be offered as long as it is appropriate.

The Prevention of Sensitization

Techniques for treating the affected fetus and newborn of sensitized mothers have certainly improved during the past decade. Far more significant in terms of eliminating the problem is the successful prevention of antibody formation.

The product RhoGAM, already mentioned, is gamma globulin containing anti-D antibody. Remember that when the fetal Rh_D positive cells enter the mother's circulation, she produces antibodies to destroy the positive cells. If she is given antibodies to destroy these cells, her system will not produce antibodies. The antibodies given in this way are not permanent; the positive red blood cells are destroyed, and the antibodies, as in all passive immunization, are short-lived. With certain exceptions described below, sensitization can be prevented, and each pregnancy for an Rh_D negative mother can be as safe as a first pregnancy.

Treatment with RhoGAM is required within 72 hours of delivery. We do not know the exact time at which the mother's body begins to produce anti-D antibodies; it is apparently longer than 72 hours. Some researchers believe that if the mother has not been given RhoGAM in the first days following delivery, it may be given up to 3 to 4 weeks postpartum. Mothers should be tested for the presence of antibodies 4 to 6 months postpartum (or postabortion). Once a mother has been sensitized, RhoGAM is of no value. RhoGAM can only prevent sensitization; it cannot eliminate actively acquired anti-D antibodies.

Two types of problems prevent the elimination of Rh sensitization as a cause of infant mortality and morbidity. The first is physiologic; the second is a problem of utilization of RhoGAM.

Physiologic Problems. About 10 per cent of women given RhoGAM are sensitized nevertheless. This may be caused by bleeding from the mother to the fetus prior to delivery—during a threatened abortion, for example, or during amniocentesis in which the placenta is entered by mistake. A massive hemorrhage at the time of delivery, so large that the amount of RhoGAM given is inadequate to destroy the large numbers of cells that have entered the circulation, may also result in sensitization.

The Rh_D negative daughter of an Rh_D positive mother may become sensitized at the time of her own birth if some maternal cells enter her bloodstream; there may be no indication that she has been sensitized until Rh titers are performed, perhaps 20 years later when she herself becomes pregnant.

Some women may become sensitized without even knowing they have been pregnant. For example, a woman may have a spontaneous abortion during the early weeks of pregnancy and believe she has had a delayed, heavy menstrual period.

Problems in Utilization of RhoGAM. It is estimated that 15 to 20 per cent of the women who should receive RhoGAM each year do not. The rate of utilization is poorer in women following abortion than in women following delivery. Nurses play a vital role in making certain that every woman who should get RhoGAM is treated.

ABO Incompatibility

If the husband is blood type A or B and the wife is type O, ABO incompatibility is possible. Severe anemia, hydrops, and stillbirth are rare in ABO incompatibility. No special antenatal care is necessary. Care of the baby is discussed in Chapter 24.

If both Rh_D and ABO incompatibility exist in a mother-infant pair, the ABO incompatibility may act as a protection for Rh sensitization. The mechanism may be the destruction of the fetal red cells in the mother before they can stimulate Rh antibody formation.

Other Pre-existing Conditions

In addition to the pre-existing conditions described above, any mother with a health problem, physical or emotional, needs special attention. It would be impossible to catalog all possible problems. Table 13–8 lists some of the more common conditions other than those already described. When any condition is identified, nurses have the obligation to be knowledgeable about the relationship between the condition and pregnancy. This may mean library research and conferences with colleagues when a less common problem is noted.

Table 13–8. SELECTED HEALTH PROBLEMS RELATED TO PREGNANCY OR CHILDBEARING

Condition	Incidence in Pregnant Women	Effect of Health Problem on Pregnancy	Effect of Pregnancy/ Childbearing on Health Problem	Effects on Fetus/ Newborn	Comments
Hyperthyroidism	1:500	Anovulation	Incidence of thyrotoxicosis similar to nonpregnant women (1:2500)	Radioactive iodine (diagnosis and treatment) can harm fetal thyroid; increased incidence of premature labor.	Goal of therapy: in hyperthyroidism and hypothyroidism, maintain maternal T_4 index in normal range: 0.75–2.5 units.
Hypothyroidism	Rare	Anovulation	Need for thyroid hormone may be increased.	Spontaneous abortion, fetal anomalies, fetal goiter	
Seizure disorders (epilepsy)	1:1000	Unpredictable		Dilantin, diazepam may affect fetus/ newborn (Chapter 8).	Must differentiate seizures from eclampsia; history, absence of proteinuria and edema, normal plasma uric acid suggest seizure disorder.
Asthma	1:100 to 1:200	Unclear	Summary of studies:[16] 36 per cent improve; 41 per cent unchanged; 23 per cent worsen.	Use of epinephrine, isoproterenol, terbutaline, aminophylline considered safe. Long-term steroid therapy	Desensitization considered safe during pregnancy. Steroids not continuously given to women with pre-eclampsia/eclampsia.
Tuberculosis	From 6:1000 to 5:100 (in indigent populations); 10–20 per cent of above active	Increased spontaneous abortions, pre-eclampsia, hyperemesis[2]	Relapse rate less than 1 per cent of patients on drug therapy.	No teratogenic effects known for isoniazid, ethambutol, rifampin; vestibular and auditory defects in some mothers treated with streptomycin.	If tuberculosis is *active*, isolation precautions are taken in hospital (isolation of infant from mother). Breast-feeding contraindicated if disease is *active* but not if converted. Infant followed with tuberculin testing.

Complications of Pregnancy That Contribute to Risk

Hypertensive States of Pregnancy

One of the terms most commonly used by nurses, physicians, and others who care for childbearing families is *toxemia*. The use of this term is discouraged today because it has long been used, and misused, to mean many different things to different people. Old habits are hard to change, however, and student nurses may hear the word frequently.

More appropriate is the phrase *hypertensive states of pregnancy*. Pregnancy-induced hypertension (PIH) is a term used to describe hypertensive conditions occurring in pregnancy (Nursing Care Plan 13–7). Some pregnant women were hypertensive before they became pregnant; these women have chronic hypertensive disease and may have pregnancy-induced hypertension superimposed upon chronic hypertensive diseases (Table 13–9). Hypertension is the leading cause of perinatal death in the United States; an estimated 25,000 fetal and neonatal deaths each year result.

Table 13–8. SELECTED HEALTH PROBLEMS RELATED TO PREGNANCY
OR CHILDBEARING (*Continued*)

Condition	Incidence in Pregnant Women	Effect of Health Problem on Pregnancy	Effect of Pregnancy/ Childbearing on Health Problem	Effects on Fetus/ Newborn	Comments
Viral hepatitis (acute viral hepatitis A)	Most common cause of jaundice in pregnancy	If nutritional support adequate, no effect. Severe disease may lead to preterm labor.	No effects noted.	Adequate fetal growth with good nutrition; offspring generally do not have liver disease.	Disease treated with nutritional support, vitamins, rest; complete remission usual in hepatitis A.
(acute viral hepatitis B)		Good nutritional support essential.	No effects noted.	Neonate may contract disease or become chronic carrier if infected after 28 weeks' gestation; samples of cord blood tested for hepatitis B antigen	Chronic liver disease and chronic hepatitis more common than with hepatitis A.
Cholestasis of pregnancy		Pruritus may be severe; baths and creams of little value.	A disease of pregnancy; clears following delivery.	Perinatal mortality 10 per cent, preterm birth 30 per cent. Fetal death in utero from anoxia; close fetal observation required after 35 weeks. More serious for fetus than mother.	Second most frequent cause of jaundice in pregnancy. Mild to severe pruritus and jaundice. No chronic liver disease following pregnancy. May recur in subsequent pregnancies.
Systemic lupus erythematosus (SLE)		Increased spontaneous abortion; more serious for mother than fetus	Adverse outcome possible in severe disease; less likely in mild disease.	Increased incidence of stillbirth, prematurity, IUGR. Transient lupus for 3 months after birth (rare).	Acute postpartum exacerbation frequent and often severe. SLE may be clinically evident for the first time during or following pregnancy.

Pre-eclampsia and Eclampsia

Approximately 90 per cent of hypertension in pregnancy is related to pre-eclampsia.

Etiology and Predisposing Factors

The etiology of pre-eclampsia and eclampsia is unknown, although many theories exist. Pre-eclampsia:

1. Requires the presence of trophoblastic tissue but not necessarily of a fetus (pre-eclampsia often occurs when there is a hydatidiform mole).

2. Occurs after the twentieth week of pregnancy, characteristically in the third trimester.

3. Is most common in young nulliparas and women over 35.

4. Most frequently occurs in the southern states.

5. More frequently occurs in multiple gestation pregnancies.

6. Disappears after delivery or fetal death.

7. Seldom recurs in subsequent pregnancies.

Other pregnant women who are at increased risk of hypertension are those with diabetes,

Text continued on page 364

Nursing Care Plan 13–7. The Woman with Pregnancy-Induced Hypertension (PIH)

NURSING GOALS:
To assure optimum care for the woman at risk of PIH and her fetus through identification of women at risk, early identification of PIH, and early treatment.
To assist the woman and her family in understanding and coping with the modifications her condition requires and her feelings about her high risk status and those modifications.

OBJECTIVES:
As a result of nursing care
1. Women at risk of PIH will be identified early in pregnancy.
2. Early signs of PIH will be recognized and bed rest initiated.
3. Woman and family will learn appropriate self-assessment measures.
4. Signs of increasing severity will be recognized and appropriate intervention, which may include hospitalization, instituted.
5. Fetal and maternal well-being will be assessed on a continuing basis.

ASSESSMENT	POTENTIAL NURSING DIAGNOSIS	NURSING INTERVENTION	COMMENTS/RATIONALE
1. Identify women at increased risk: a. Young nulliparas b. Women over 35 c. Multiple gestation d. Diabetes mellitus e. RH incompatibility f. Chronic hypertensive disease g. Chronic renal disease h. Significant malnutrition	At increased risk of pregnancy-induced hypertension	Careful assessment of blood pressure at each prenatal visit; note woman's position (e.g., seated, lying on left side) and assess in same position Roll-over test at 28–32 weeks (Chapter 10, page 240) Assess proteinuria, edema, weight gain. Provide nutritional counseling and referral. More frequent prenatal visits may be necessary.	

2. Identify signs of pregnancy-induced hypertension:
 a. Physical assessment of edema
  (1) Does not disappear after 12 hours bed rest
  (2) Pitting edema
  (3) Weekly gain of 3 pounds or more
	Edema related to possible PIH	Bed rest in side-lying position
		
		Help gravida identify ways of meeting family needs when bed rest required.
		
		Help gravida plan ways of relieving the boredom of bed rest.
			It is possible to have significant edema without PIH, or PIH without edema.
			
			Unless issues such as boredom and family needs are discussed, mother may have difficulty in maintaining bed rest.

b. Hypertension (1) Roll-over test between 28 and 32 weeks to identify women at risk (page 240)	Hypertension related to pregnancy at risk of eclampsia		

(2) Blood pressure > 125 mm. Hg systolic or 75 mm. Hg diastolic prior to 32 weeks
(3) Blood pressure > 140 mm. Hg systolic or 90 mm. Hg diastolic
(4) Elevation in blood pressure > 30 mm. Hg systolic or 15 mm. Hg diastolic
(5) Mean arterial pressure > 90 mm. Hg diastolic
(6) Hypertension increased during sleep

c. Laboratory assessment
(1) Proteinuria
  (a) two specimens at 6-hour intervals 1+ or greater
  (b) > 300 mg./liter in 24-hour specimen
  (c) specimen: clean, midstream, voided specimen

Proteinuria related to possible PIH

Monitor administration of hydralazine (see text).

If mother is receiving care at home, teach mother and a family member to monitor blood pressure, proteinuria, weight.

Community health nurse should be closely involved in care of all women with PIH; frequent home visits important for assessment and family teaching.

Provide teaching to mother and family concerning signs of increasing illness:
1. Decreased urine output
2. Increased edema
3. Headache
4. Blurring of vision
5. Clouding of consciousness
6. Epigastric pain
7. Nausea and/or vomiting
8. Jaundice
9. Seizures

Mother and her family must know how to contact health-care provider quickly on a 24-hour basis if any of these symptoms occur.

(2) Hematocrit
  (a) Baseline hematocrit after 20 weeks
  (b) Comparison of hemoglobin and hematocrit (when hematocrit is less than 3 times hemoglobin, hemoconcentration exists).

3. Assess fetal status (Chapter 12)
a. Ultrasound
b. Nonstress test; contraction stress test if nonreactive
c. Estriol determination
d. L/S ratio, PG for fetal lung maturity

Disruptions in fetal-placental unit

If mother's or fetus's condition progressively worsens, early delivery may be necessary.

Bed rest on side enhances placental perfusion.

Avoid lying on back; vena caval compression decreases uterine blood flow.

Uterine blood flow and thus blood flow to fetal-placental unit is further compromised if mother's condition deteriorates.

Continued on following page

Nursing Care Plan 13–7. The Woman with Pregnancy-Induced Hypertension (PIH) (Continued)

ASSESSMENT	POTENTIAL NURSING DIAGNOSIS	NURSING INTERVENTION	COMMENTS/RATIONALE
4. If PIH requires hospitalization, assessment includes: a. Blood pressure on 24-hour basis (arterial blood pressure, central venous pressure and/or pulmonary artery pressure) b. Vital signs c. Intake/output d. Edema e. Daily weight f. Hematocrit g. Urine creatinine, protein levels h. Reflexes i. Symptoms included in prenatal teaching (headache, blurring vision, etc.) j. Fetal assessment (Chapter 14) 5. If mother receives magnesium sulfate a. Blood pressure, pulse, respiration (marked decrease in blood pressure and pulse, respirations <12–14/minute) indicate toxicity. b. Reflexes: 0 to 4+ clonus (number of beats) c. Urine output: retention catheter is inserted. d. Monitor serum magnesium levels (Table 13–16)		Nursing care is carefully planned to provide extended periods of rest with mother in side-lying position. Sedatives (e.g., phenobarbital) may be given. As symptoms improve, activity is gradually increased. Magnesium sulfate: 1. Warn mother of discomfort of IM injection. 2. Use Z-tract technique. 3. Local anesthetic may be used prior to injection (requires prescription or standing order). 4. Calcium gluconate (20 ml. of a 10 per cent solution) must be immediately available as antidote for magnesium toxicity. 5. Women receiving magnesium sulfate are never left unattended. 6. Withhold dose and notify physician unless: a. Respirations > 12/minute b. Deep tendon reflexes are present c. Urinary output is 30 ml./hour or greater.	

6. Assess for signs of labor (Chapter 11, page 286)
   a. Contractions
   b. Rupture of membranes
   c. Show

7. If mother becomes eclamptic (one or more seizures) assess:
   a. Urine output (Foley catheter)
   b. Urine protein level
   c. Vital signs
   d. Intravenous fluid intake
   e. Pulmonary artery or central venous pressure
   f. Chest for moist respiration
   g. Optic fundi
   h. Reflexes and clonus above
   i. Describe seizure:
      (1) Length
      (2) Prodromal signs (e.g., twitching of facial muscles)
      (3) Convulsion stage: parts of body involved, tonic, clonic, respiration
      (4) State of consciousness following seizure

Early labor

7. Contraindications to use of magnesium sulfate (in addition to above):
   a. Heart block
   b. Myocardial damage
   c. Impaired renal function

Notify physician.

Monitor contractions.

Provide care as in labor (Nursing Care Plans 17-1 through 17-4)

1. Immediate care:
   a. Ensure adequate ventilation; oxygen may be necessary; place plastic airway if possible.
   b. Give magnesium sulfate to control seizure activity.
   c. Position mother on side to prevent aspiration and improve cardiac output.
   d. Pad side rails of bed.
   e. Have suction equipment immediately accessible; suction as necessary.
   f. Elevate foot of bed to facilitate drainage of mucus.
2. Following stabilization:
   a. NPO, IV fluids to maintain fluid intake
   b. Provide dark quiet environment.
   c. Keep family members informed; visitors are not allowed in room.
   d. Anticipate delivery within 6 to 12 hours following stabilization of mother's condition.

Mother receiving medications such as phenobarbital may not be aware of labor contractions.

Table 13–9. CLASSIFICATION OF HYPERTENSIVE STATES OF PREGNANCY

Condition	Definition	Time of Occurrence	Incidence	Comments
Pregnancy-Induced Hypertension				
Pre-eclampsia	Hypertension with protein-uria, edema, or both	After the 20th week	6 to 7 per cent of pregnant women in U.S., primarily in primigravidas	May occur earlier than 20 weeks in presence of trophoblastic disease
Eclampsia	Occurrence of one or more convulsions, not attributable to other cerebral conditions (e.g., epilepsy) in woman with pre-eclampsia	After 20 weeks	1:2000 women	
Chronic hypertensive vascular disease	Persistent hypertension from whatever cause	Before pregnancy; before the 20th week of gestation; beyond the 42nd postpartum day		Incidence is three times higher among black gravidas than white gravidas
Superimposed pre-eclampsia or eclampsia	Proteinuria and/or edema; a rise in blood pressure of 30 mm. Hg systolic or 15 mm. Hg diastolic in a woman with chronic hypertensive vascular disease	After 20 weeks		

Rh incompatibility, chronic hypertensive and chronic renal disease, and significant malnutrition.

Theories of the cause of pre-eclampsia include speculations that the condition may be related to such factors as inadequate nutrition, metabolic disease, or an immunologic process. None of these theories adequately explains the characteristics of the condition. For example, if poor diet is the basis, why is pre-eclampsia primarily a disease of a first pregnancy?

Some societies are apparently free of pre-eclampsia. Soichet[46] reports little or no evidence of toxemia in certain African societies, Eskimo tribes in Greenland, and some tribes in the South Pacific. He suggests that in these societies:

1. Fertility is cherished by everyone in the society.
2. No stigma is attached to children born out of wedlock.

3. Babies of both sexes are welcomed.
4. Pregnant women are treated with tenderness and love.

We believe that the role of psychosocial factors is worthy of further exploration. In the interrelationship of psychosocial and physiologic antecedents, clues to cause and thus to prevention may be discovered.

Pathophysiology

An understanding of the pathophysiology of pre-eclampsia and eclampsia is essential to understanding both the medical plan of care and the nursing intervention.

Blood vessel spasm is postulated as the underlying mechanism. When vessels are in spasm, less blood perfuses all body tissues. This basic problem leads to a number of other physiologic changes that account for the classic symptoms of edema, hypertension, and proteinuria as well as symptoms of progressive disease if the process is not interrupted (Table 13–10, Fig. 13–2).

1. Vasospasm leads to an increase in resistance in the peripheral circulatory system.

2. Resistance leads to an increase in peripheral blood pressure and a decreased volume of blood in the decreased vascular bed. Decreased blood volume also affects the renin-angiotensin system, increasing blood pressure (Fig. 13–3).

3. Fluid shifts from the vascular compartment (i.e., from within the blood vessels) to the intracellular space. Protein and electrolytes also shift into the intracellular space. Particularly significant is the leakage of sodium.

4. Because of the fluid shift, the blood becomes "thicker," with a tendency to sludge and

coagulate. Intravascular coagulation leads to diminished blood flow to all organs, including, of course, the uterus, placenta, and fetus. In addition, peripheral resistance is increased when blood is thicker; the heart must work harder and the blood pressure becomes high. The increased workload of the heart in the presence of a decreased blood supply may lead to heart failure.

5. Decreased blood supply to the kidneys leads to a loss of integrity in the glomeruli and a consequent spillage of protein into the urine, and to oliguria.

6. Decreased uterine and therefore placental blood flow can lead to intrauterine growth retardation and an infant small for gestational age (SGA, see Chapter 23), fetal hypoxia, and possible fetal death.

7. Cerebral vasoconstriction may lead to

Table 13–10. RELATIONSHIP BETWEEN SYMPTOMS AND PATHOPHYSIOLOGY OF PRE-ECLAMPSIA AND ECLAMPSIA

Symptom	Pathophysiologic Basis	Criteria for Assessment[a]
Edema	Fluid moves from intravascular to intracellular space.	Pitting edema after 12 hours rest in bed; weight gain of 3 pounds or more in 1 week.
Hypertension	Increased peripheral vascular resistance, increased blood viscosity leads to increased cardiac load.	Elevation of blood pressure of 30 mm. Hg systolic and 15 mm. Hg diastolic or levels above 140/90. Levels of 125/85 at 32 weeks or at term. Blood pressure must be abnormal on at least two occasions 6 hours apart.
Proteinuria	Loss of integrity in the glomeruli from decreased blood supply allows spillage of protein.	Urine protein 1+ or greater (Ketostix) on two occasions 6 hours apart; protein in excess of 300 mg. in 24-hour urine specimen.
Signs of progressive disease Central nervous system signs (headache, vertigo, apprehension, nausea, vomiting) Visual disturbances Hemoconcentration	Vasoconstriction→cerebral edema→hypoxia→cerebral cortical hyperirritability. Vasoconstriction→retinal edema, spasm. Shift of fluid from intravascular to extravascular space.	Careful attention to mothers' complaints. Assessment of fundi; ophthalmologic consultation. Hematocrit rises.
Signs of impending eclampsia Oliguria (urine output less than 30 ml./hr.) or anuria Epigastric pain Hyperactive reflexes, decreased pulse and respirations (less than 14 per minute) Increased restlessness Convulsions (presence indicates eclampsia) Semicoma, coma	Decreased renal circulation→impaired renal function. Stretching of liver capsule or subcapsular hemorrhage. Decreased cerebral blood flow→CNS irritability. Decreased cerebral blood flow.	Urine output 30 ml. less than RBC; casts in urine. Evaluation of liver function. Assess reflexes. Assess level of consciousness.

[a]See text also.

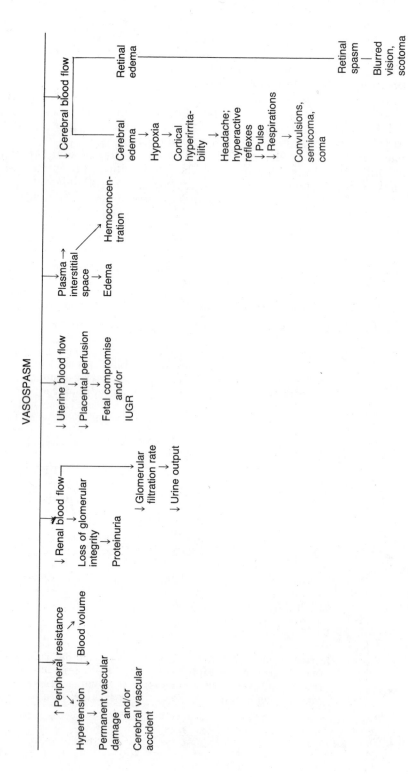

Figure 13–2. Pathophysiology of pregnancy-induced hypertension.

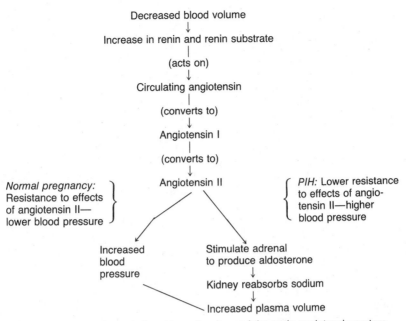

Decreased blood volume

↓

Increase in renin and renin substrate

|

(acts on)

↓

Circulating angiotensin

(converts to)

↓

Angiotensin I

|

(converts to)

↓

Angiotensin II

Normal pregnancy: Resistance to effects of angiotensin II— lower blood pressure ⎫

PIH: Lower resistance to effects of angiotensin II—higher blood pressure ⎫

Increased blood pressure

Stimulate adrenal to produce aldosterone

↓

Kidney reabsorbs sodium

↓

Increased plasma volume

Figure 13–3. Pregnancy-induced hypertension and the renin-angiotensin system.

cerebral and retinal edema, hypoxia, and irritability of the cerebral cortex. Headache, blurring of vision and scotomas (areas of depressed or absent vision) are signs of progressive disease. Untreated, convulsions or coma may result.

Major Signs: Assessment and Intervention

The principal signs of pre-eclampsia, already noted, are edema, proteinuria, and hypertension. Any one or a combination of signs may be present.

Edema. In Chapter 11 the normal dependent edema of pregnancy was described. This normal edema usually disappears with elevation of the feet or after a night in bed. Physiologic edema may also be present in the hands and face. Edema that does not disappear after 12 hours of rest in bed, or *pitting* edema of the face, hands, sacral area, abdominal wall, or legs (Fig. 13–4), a weekly gain of more than 3 pounds or a daily weight gain of 0.5 to 1.0 pound suggests a need for careful evaluation of a woman's condition. However, it is possible to have even extensive edema without pre-

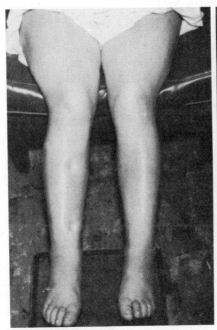
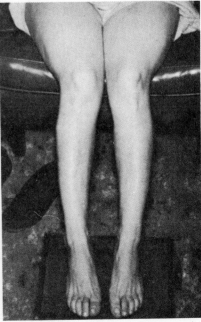

Figure 13–4. Acute peripheral pitting edema of the lower extremities in a patient with severe pre-eclampsia at term *(left)* and seven days post partum *(right)*. (From Greenhill and Friedman: *Biological Principles and Modern Practice of Obstetrics.* Philadelphia, W. B. Saunders Co., 1974.

eclampsia, just as it is possible to have pre-eclampsia without edema. About 10 per cent of women who have eclampsia (i.e., convulsions) do not have pitting edema.

The classic treatment of edema (i.e., diuretics) is *not* of value in pre-eclampsia or eclampsia, and may even be harmful.

Because excess body fluids and electrolytes are in the tissues rather than within the blood vessels (intravascular compartment), giving diuretics without expanding blood volume and supplying electrolytes will further complicate electrolyte imbalance and lead to possible neonatal hyponatremia and other complications. Diuretics may also mask the appearance of early warning signs of pre-eclampsia by preventing fluid retention and edema, thus postponing detection until the condition is further advanced. In addition, the use of diuretics may result in decreased perfusion of the placenta, thus further compromising the fetus.

Salt, like fluid, is in the tissues, not the vascular tree. Low serum sodium levels lead to increased sodium reabsorption in the kidney tubules.

The progress of edema is evaluated by daily recording of weight taken at the same time each day because of diurnal variation, by determinations of hematocrit, and by careful intake/output records, which will indicate decreased intravascular fluid. Changes in hematocrit are best evaluated by comparison with a hematocrit value determined after 20 weeks gestation but prior to the onset of disease, because hematocrit varies individually. For example, a woman with pronounced anemia and a hemoglobin of 9 may have a hematocrit of 27, while another woman, with a hemoglobin of 12, may have a hematocrit of 36. In the second woman a hematocrit of 27 would indicate marked hemoconcentration.

Bed rest, in a side-lying position, will allow an increase in cardiac output and a subsequent increase in glomerular filtration rate. Output is improved most when the woman lies on her left side, but it is difficult for anyone to maintain one position hour after hour. As fluid is excreted in the urine, fluid from the interstitial tissues enters the circulation and the process continues. Bed rest alone may lead to a weight loss of as much as 4 pounds in 24 hours.[53]

Proteinuria. Small quantities of protein (less than 1+ by Ketostix) are found in the urine of many pregnant women. Strenuous exercise or work, exposure to cold, and other factors tend to increase proteinuria. Two specimens at 6-hour intervals that are 1+ or greater or more than 300 mg./liter of protein in a 24-hour specimen is considered beyond the range of normal (Table 13–10).

Urine that is to be tested for protein must be either a clean, midstream voided specimen or obtained by catheterization, because contamination with either blood or vaginal discharge will give falsely high protein determinations. Women should not drink quantities of fluid to obtain a urine specimen that is to be tested for protein. The reagent strip measures the quantity of protein in a given quantity of urine; increase of fluid intake will dilute the urine and cause a falsely low reading. If the specimen is voided in a routine manner (as a specimen taken at home may be), a protein level of 1+ is acceptable, and the woman is asked to notify her health-care provider when the specimen is 2+ or greater after checking a second clean-catch specimen. (Directions for obtaining a clean-catch specimen are given in Chapter 10.)

Hypertension. Several criteria are helpful in identifying hypertension during pregnancy:

> 1. An elevation of 30 mm. Hg or more systolic or 15 mm. Hg diastolic blood pressure.
> 2. A blood pressure level above 140 mm. Hg systolic or 90 mm. Hg diastolic.
> 3. A blood pressure level above 125 mm. Hg systolic or 75 mm. Hg diastolic prior to 32 weeks, or at term.
> 4. A mean arterial pressure greater than 90 (Chapter 10).
> 5. A positive response to the rollover test (Chapter 10).

There is a tendency in pregnant women toward a reversal of the usual pattern of higher blood pressure during waking hours and lower blood pressure during sleep. Particularly in women with severe pre-eclampsia, hypertension is more common during the nocturnal hours of sleep.[4]

Hydralazine (Apresoline) may be given for blood pressure control. Hydralazine causes arteriolar vasodilation, thus specifically addressing the problem of vasoconstriction. Cardiac output, cerebral blood flow, uterine blood flow, and renal blood flow are increased. Diastolic blood pressure is usually decreased more than systolic pressure.

Hydralazine is completely absorbed after oral administration (100 mg./day in two to four divided doses) with peak serum levels occurring within 1 to 2 hours. If a rapid decrease in blood pressure is required, intravenous injection of a bolus with repeated doses every 15 to 20 minutes may be given. Slow intravenous infusions, using an infusion pump, are also used. When intravenous hydralazine is given, blood pressure is checked every minute for the first 5 minutes, and then every 5 minutes for the next 30 minutes.[53] The diastolic pressure is maintained between 90 and 110 mm. Hg because of the danger of sudden hypotension for both the mother and fetus, the latter from suddenly reduced placental blood flow. This level of diastolic pressure allows adequate urinary output.[4] Fetal heart rate is continuously monitored during administration; fetal hypoxia from decreased placental blood flow will result in a pattern of late decelerations (Chapter 18).

Tachycardia is the most common side effect of hydralazine; if tachycardia progresses to cardiac arrhythmia, propanolol (Inderal) is given. The intravenous dose is 1 to 3 mg., diluted to a volume of 50 ml. and given at a rate of no more than 1 mg./minute. If there is no response within 2 minutes, a second dose may be given; 0.15 mg./kg. of body weight is the maximum 6-hour dose.[9]

Other side effects include tachycardia, headache, and nausea and vomiting. Chronic administration of hydralazine in doses exceeding 200 mg./day may result in rheumatoid-like symptoms, but this would be highly unusual during pregnancy.

Progression of Pre-eclampsia

Pre-eclampsia may progress from mild to severe symptoms over a period of weeks or within a period of hours. Signs of a more severe pre-eclampsia are described in Nursing Care Plan 13–7.

Once seizures have occurred, the condition is eclampsia. With optimum care, many instances of eclampsia are probably preventable by early recognition of symptoms of pre-eclampsia, when pre-eclampsia is mild and more easily treatable.

Caring for the Mother with Pre-eclampsia

When pre-eclampsia is recognized in a woman, she is usually hospitalized. Bed rest is the principal treatment for mild pre-eclampsia.

Mild pre-eclampsia is sometimes treated at home when adequate care appears possible (see Home vs. Hospital for the High Risk Mother, above). With guidance, families can learn to monitor the woman's blood pressure, weight, and proteinuria and provide the opportunity for adequate rest. In hospital, careful assessment of blood pressure, urinary output, weight, and hematocrit is essential. Deep tendon reflexes and ocular fundi are evaluated.

Sedation may be prescribed to ensure quiet rest. Whether medication for sedation is prescribed or not, nursing care must be carefully planned so that vitally important assessment does not conflict with the need for rest. Examinations, for example, should be performed shortly before the time that medication is given for sedation, not afterward. Not only must nurses plan their own care to provide maximum periods of rest, but they must coordinate the actions of physicians, laboratory technicians seeking blood specimens, and others who might enter the woman's room.

As diuresis occurs and symptoms return to more normal levels, the woman is allowed out of bed. If the fetus is assessed to be mature (Chapter 14), the mother will be delivered (vaginally unless there are obstetric indications for Cesarean delivery). If the fetus is not sufficiently mature, both mother and fetus must continue to be followed closely (fetal assessment is described in Chapter 14). Labor is induced when the fetus has matured on the premise that pre-eclampsia has not been "cured."

If more severe symptoms of pre-eclampsia appear, magnesium sulfate is given intramuscularly or, more frequently, intravenously. Magnesium sulfate decreases neuromuscular irritability by depressing action at the myoneural junction (i.e., the junction of muscle and nerve) and at nerve-nerve junctions within the central nervous system. In addition, magnesium sulfate frequently has a transient hypotensive effect, but this is not the primary reason for its use. The dosage of magnesium sulfate is summarized in Table 13–11.

Table 13–11. DOSAGE SCHEDULES FOR MAGNESIUM SULFATE

	Intravenous	Intramuscular
Initial dose	2–4 gm $MgSO_4$ (USP) as 10% solution injected slowly over 2- to 4-min period	10 gm $MgSO_4$ (USP) as 50% solution in H_2O: divided doses. 10 ml in each buttock: 1% procaine may be added to reduce pain of injection
Maintenance dose	20 gm $MgSO_4$ in 1,000 ml 5% dextrose in H_2O; usual maintenance dosage, 1 gm/hr, depending on reflexes, respirations, urinary output, etc.	5 gm $MgSO_4$ as 50% solution every 4 hr (administered same as initial dose), depending on reflexes, etc.

From Cavanagh, Woods, O'Connor: *Obstetric Emergencies.* New York, Harper & Row, 1978.

Intravenous administration utilizes an infusion pump to maintain constant dosage. Intramuscular injection, deep in the upper outer quadrant of the buttock by two-track technique, is painful. A local anesthetic such as lidocaine may be given prior to the magnesium sulfate. The woman should be forewarned of the discomfort. The risk of overdosage is considered more likely with intravenous administration because of the constant infusion.

Assessment of the mother receiving magnesium sulfate includes the following:

1. Blood pressure, pulse, and respiration are measured and recorded before and after the initial dose and every 15 minutes thereafter. A marked decrease in blood pressure and pulse and a decrease in respirations below 12 to 14 per minute indicates toxicity and the need to discontinue the drug.

2. Patellar reflexes (kneejerk) are assessed; absence of reflexes is in indication of potential toxicity. To elicit the patellar reflex the mother should be sitting (if her condition allows) or lying with the knee supported in a slightly flexed position. The patellar tendon is tapped just below the patella. Reflexes are usually graded on a scale of 0 to 4+:

0   no response
1+ somewhat diminished; low normal
2+ average
3+ brisker than average
4+ very brisk; hyperactive

Clonus, the rhythmic oscillation of the extremity between flexion and extension, is associated with 4+ reflexes. Clonus is recorded as number of beats—i.e., the number of times the muscle contracts. Urine output should be at least 30 ml./hour. Because magnesium sulfate is excreted almost entirely through the urine, diminished output may alter the action of the drug significantly.

3. Serum magnesium levels can be helpful. Table 13–12 relates serum magnesium levels to clinical observations. Note that there is a greater difference between therapeutic levels

Table 13–12. SERUM MAGNESIUM LEVELS AND RELATED CLINICAL OBSERVATIONS

Serum Levels (mEq/liter)	Clinical Observation
1.5–3.0	Normal serum magnesium
4.0–7.5	Anticonvulsant therapeutic blood levels
4.0	Deep tendon reflexes decreased
5.0	Cardiac conduction prolonged (prolonged P-R interval and QRS restoration)
10.0–12.0	Loss of patellar (knee-jerk) reflex
12.0–15.0	Respiratory paralysis; possible complete heart block

and the loss of the patellar reflex than between the loss of the patellar reflex and respiratory paralysis and the possibility of complete heart block.

Respiratory and cardiac failure occur because magnesium decreases the amount of acetylcholine released in response to a nerve action potential; impulses are not conducted. Calcium gluconate (20 ml. of a 10 per cent solution) is the antidote for magnesium toxicity and must always be available for slow intravenous administration. The initial dose may be repeated hourly until symptoms are relieved up to a maximum of eight doses in 24 hours.

Women who have heart block, myocardial damage, or impaired renal function should not receive magnesium.

Traditionally, once women with severe preeclampsia were stabilized for a period of 24 hours, the fetus was delivered by Cesarean section; this practice is still common.

However, in institutions with staff and facilities for perinatal intensive care, more vigorous treatment of the mother, along with the assessment of fetal maturity and well-being, is possible if the baby is less than 34 to 35 weeks gestational age.

Caring for the Mother with Eclampsia

Should one or more convulsions occur, the condition is eclampsia. The treatment of a woman with eclampsia requires constant and excellent nursing care closely correlated with medical management. The goals are:

1. Prevention of further convulsions.
2. Insurance of adequate ventilation.
3. Control of blood pressure.
4. Prevention of cardiac failure.
5. Continuing assessment of the fetus.

A woman with eclampsia is cared for in a quiet room. She lies on her side to prevent possible aspiration of vomitus and other secretions as well as to improve cardiac output. Side rails on the bed are padded; the use of a padded tongue blade has become controversial because of potential oral trauma during insertion. If a tongue blade is used, it must be inserted very carefully.

The foot of the bed is elevated to prevent drainage of mucus. Suction equipment must be immediately available as an additional precaution against aspiration. Oxygen may be necessary. Magnesium sulfate (see section above) is used to control seizures. Urine output, urine protein, intravenous fluid intake, vital signs, reflexes, and frequently central venous or pulmonary artery pressure are continuously assessed.

Once a woman is stable for 2 to 4 hours, delivery by cesarean section or induction is initiated. Further continuation of the pregnancy places both mother and fetus at risk. (See Chapter 19 for intrapartum care of the mother with pregnancy-induced hypertension.)

Long-Term Prognosis

Is a woman who has pregnancy-induced hypertension at increased risk of hypertension in subsequent pregnancies or later in her life? Chesley,[6] in long-term studies, found that:

1. Women with pre-eclampsia did not have subsequent hypertension.

2. Women with eclampsia in more than one pregnancy did ultimately become hypertensive.

3. Most women with pre-eclampsia or eclampsia in a first pregnancy were normotensive in subsequent pregnancies; a few had hypertension in all subsequent pregnancies.

Infection and the Pregnant Woman

Infection in women who are pregnant is of concern because it may affect the fetus, the newborn, and the course of the pregnancy as well as the woman herself. Infections that are potentially harmful to the fetus and newborn have been discussed in Chapter 8. Major infections that are of concern include urinary tract infections, chorioamnionitis, and sexually transmitted diseases (Nursing Care Plan 13–8).

The fetus in utero is at far greater risk from bacterial and viral organisms than was once suspected. Whether exposure results in a deleterious infection seems to be related to both maternal factors and fetal factors (Table 13–13), including maternal and fetal resistance, the stage of development of the fetus, and the nature, number, and route of the infecting organism.[33]

Preventing infection is a major goal of nursing care in the prenatal period. A part of prevention is recognizing those factors that appear to predispose women to infection at any stage of the childbearing year.

Nutritional deficiency may come from inadequate maternal nutrition during pregnancy or from inadequate placental blood flow (uteroplacental insufficiency). Chandra[5a, b] and Ferguson[10a, b] found that the infants of mothers with malnutrition during pregnancy not only suffered a decreased immunologic response as newborns but that some features of that decreased response persisted into childhood.

Maternal undernutrition may also lead to metabolic acidosis as maternal fat stores are utilized to meet energy needs, resulting in acetone production and possibly in the reduction of glucose to the fetus, which may be the mechanism leading to increased mortality. Naeye[33] reported that the excessive number of fetal and neonatal deaths from urinary tract infections are often accompanied by maternal acetonuria. He has suggested that the temporary decrease in the mother's food intake combined with the increase in metabolic rate that is concurrent with fever lead to metabolic acidosis.

The relation between maternal age, coitus, and increased amniotic fluid infection is discussed in Chapter 11; drug addiction and multiple gestation are described in this chapter.

In some pregnant women, amniotic fluid is deficient in antimicrobial activity, perhaps related to a dietary deficiency in zinc.[42] This is an area requiring additional research before recommendations for practice are made.

Urinary Tract Infections

Urinary tract infections are the most common infections complicating pregnancy. The anatomic and physiologic changes that occur in the renal system during pregnancy are probably one etiologic factor (Chapter 7). Unrecognized and untreated asymptomatic disease may become more serious in the mother and may increase the potential for increased congenital malformation and premature labor in the fetus. Particularly at risk are women with sickle cell trait, with multiple sexual partners, with previous urinary tract infections, and with frequent pregnancies. These women can be identified by nursing history.

Screening for asymptomatic bacteriuria is discussed in Chapter 10. Asymptomatic bacteriuria, by definition, requires the presence of 100,000 (10^5/ml.) organisms on two consecutive cultures. The incidence of asymptomatic bacteriuria is estimated at 3 to 8 per cent of all pregnant women. Untreated, from 20 to 30 per cent of pregnant women with asymptomatic disease will develop symptomatic infections of either the lower or upper urinary tract (cystitis or pyelonephritis).

Signs of lower urinary tract infection include dysuria, frequency, urgency, lower abdominal pain and tenderness, and a low grade fever or chills. Upper tract infection may be characterized by any of the signs associated with lower tract infection and, in addition, a more significant fever, lumbar pain, tenderness, nausea, vomiting, or diarrhea. Pyuria may be present, and urine activity may increase. Women who have asymptomatic bacteriuria should be

Nursing Care Plan 13–8. The Woman with Prenatal Infection

NURSING GOALS:
To prevent infection in pregnant women.
To identify early symptoms and provide prompt treatment if infection occurs.

OBJECTIVES:

As a result of prenatal care
1. Women at increased risk of infection will be identified early in pregnancy.
2. Urine will be kept sterile throughout pregnancy; when infection (asymptomatic or symptomatic) occurs it will recognized and treated promptly.
3. Premature rupture of the membranes will be recognized immediately and appropriate treatment instituted.
4. Sexually transmitted infection will be recognized when possible and treated early.
5. The effects of sexually transmitted infection in the newborn will be prevented.

ASSESSMENT	POTENTIAL NURSING DIAGNOSIS	NURSING INTERVENTION	COMMENTS/RATIONALE
1. Identify women at increased risk of developing infections during pregnancy. a. Inadequate maternal nutrition b. Maternal diabetes mellitus c. Multiple partners d. Sickle cell trait	Risk of infection during pregnancy related to (specific indication).	Correct factors amenable to intervention—e.g., continuing nutritional counseling, referral to WIC, food stamps if eligible.	
e. Frequent pregnancies f. Previous urinary tract infection g. Addiction to alcohol, drugs h. Maternal age 39 or over i. Multiple gestation	Need for treatment due to two positive urine cultures	Antibiotic therapy (Table 13–18) Be sure woman understands need for full course of therapy as prescribed and the importance of therapy. Because she is asymptomatic, cost of medication and remembering to take medication may not have high priority.	3 to 8 per cent of all pregnant women develop asymptomatic bacteriuria; 20 to 30 per cent of these women will develop symptomatic urinary tract infection.
Urinary Tract Infection (UTI)			
1. Screen all gravidas for asymptomatic bacteriuria Two positive consecutive cultures ≥ (10^5 organisms/ml.) require treatment (clean-catch specimen).		Provide information about symptoms of UTI, importance of seeking prompt treatment.	
2. Signs of lower urinary tract infection a. Dysuria b. Frequency c. Urgency		Antibiotic therapy Continue urine cultures throughout pregnancy and after delivery for 1 year.	Approximately 20 per cent of women with complicated UTI may develop premature labor.

   d. Pain or tenderness in lower abdomen
   e. Low-grade fever of chills.

3. Signs of upper urinary tract infection
   a. Any signs of lower tract infection
   b. Increased fever
   c. Lumbar pain, tenderness
   d. Nausea, vomiting, diarrhea
   e. Pyuria

Explain need for continuing care to prevent future urinary tract impairment.

Antibiotic therapy

Continue urine cultures throughout pregnancy and after delivery for 1 year.

Explain need for continuing care to prevent future urinary tract impairment.

Chorioamnionitis

1. Identify woman at risk:
   a. Premature rupture of membranes (confirm by mitrizine test)

Risk for development of chorioamnionitis related to premature rupture of membranes

Provide information to all pregnant women about:
1. Signs of ruptured membranes (from trickle to gush of amniotic fluid)
2. Need to notify health-care provider immediately when mother suspects membranes ruptured

2. If membranes ruptured:

Anticipate culture of maternal blood and amniotic fluid.

Assess signs of infection—increasing maternal fever, foul-smelling vaginal discharge.

Antibiotic therapy

Induction of labor (Nursing Care Plan 19–1) or cesarean delivery (Nursing Care Plan 19–3)

Infant will be at risk of sepsis; communicate maternal history to nurses caring for infant.

Sexually Transmitted Infections (STD)

1. Screen all pregnant women for:
   a. Blood for VDRL, RPR, STS (syphilis) tests at initial prenatal visit; repeat in third trimester of exposure.
   b. Vaginal smear for gonorrhea; repeat in third trimester of exposure.
   (Some clinics routinely repeat vaginal smear in third trimester.)

Risk of complications (mother and fetus or newborn) related to sexually transmitted disease

Penicillin, 4.8 million units, for syphilis or gonorrhea

Encourage treatment of sexual partner to prevent reinfection.

Explain potential effects of fetus and newborn.

Untreated maternal syphilis may cause congenital neonatal syphilis.

Gonorrhea untreated may cause ophthalmia neonatorum in infant (Chapter 20).

Continued on following page

Nursing Care Plan 13–8.   The Woman with Prenatal Infection (Continued)

ASSESSMENT	POTENTIAL NURSING DIAGNOSIS	NURSING INTERVENTION	COMMENTS/RATIONALE
	Sexually Transmitted Infections (STD) (Continued)		
2. Assess for other STD on basis of physical assessment. a. Trichomonas (gray-green discharge)		*Trichomonas:* 1. Symptomatic treatment for mother in first 20 weeks of pregnancy; metronidazole (Flagyl) may be used in second 20 weeks. 2. Male partner treated. Intercourse avoided until infection cured (1 to 2 weeks).	
b. Herpes (culture of lesion; cervical smear)		*Herpes:* 1. No cure 2. Cesarean delivery needed if active lesion at time of birth or in month preceding; explain to mother. 3. Weekly viral cultures and Pap smears following initial diagnosis 4. Acyclovir *not* recommended for use during pregnancy. 5. Topical anesthetic, sitz baths may relieve discomfort.	Neonatal herpes, a life-threatening illness, is transmitted to infant during passage through vagina.
c. *Candida albicans* (burning; thick white discharge)		*Candida albicans:* 1. Nystatin (Mycostatin) suppositories or vaginal tablets, or 2. Gentian swabs. 3. Sodium bicarbonate solution aids in relieving discomfort of vulva. 4. Avoid intercourse until cured.	Common in mothers with diabetes mellitus if diabetes is not well controlled. If *Candida* is present at time of delivery, inspect infant carefully for thrush.

Table 13–13. FACTORS INFLUENCING THE DEVELOPMENT OF INFECTION IN THE CHILDBEARING YEARS*

Factor	Possible Effect on Mother	Possible Effect on Fetus/Newborn
Inadequate nutrition	Acetonuria; metabolic acidosis Decreased antimicrobial activity of amniotic fluid	Increased incidence of infections Immunoincompetence
Fever and decreased food intake	Acetonuria; metabolic acidosis	
Maternal age greater than 39 Coitus Drug addiction	Increased amniotic fluid infection	
Population differences	Decreased antimicrobial activity in amniotic fluid	
Multiple gestation	(?) Increased demands on maternal nutrition	Increased mortality from amniotic fluid infection

*Based on data from Naeye, and from Ross et al.: *In Perinatal Infections.* Ciba Foundation Symposium 77. New York, Excerpta Medica, 1980.

taught to recognize the signs of urinary tract infection as well as the importance of seeking prompt treatment. Sometimes it is difficult for women to differentiate the symptoms of cystitis from feelings of urgency and pelvic pressure due to pregnancy, or from the symptoms of vaginitis and urethritis.

Approximately 20 per cent of those with a complicated urinary tract infection may develop premature labor, probably owing to high fever or increased metabolic rate.[45] Other fetal effects include increased congenital malformation,[10] amniotic fluid infection, and placental growth retardation.[33] Mothers may develop urinary tract abnormalities and abnormal intravenous pyelograms.[28]

Because of these potential complications, a goal of prenatal care is to keep urine sterile throughout pregnancy. Antibiotic treatment is the means of achieving this goal (Table 13–

14). Some antibiotics that might be used to treat urinary tract infections in women who are not pregnant, such as tetracycline and aminoglycosides (e.g., kanamycin, gentamicin) are not used because of their potential teratogenicity (Chapter 8).

Any woman who has a urinary tract infection during pregnancy should have follow-up care throughout pregnancy (monthly cultures until delivery) and after delivery (cultures and a pyelogram) for a year.

Chorioamnionitis

By precise definition, chorioamnionitis is an inflammation of the fetal membranes, the chorion, and the amnion. Clinically, the term frequently includes infection in the uterus, the fetus, or the amniotic fluid, or a combination

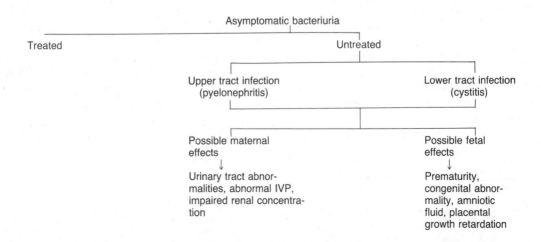

Table 13–14. ANTIBIOTIC TREATMENT OF URINARY TRACT INFECTION

Drug	Initial Dose	Maintenance Dose	Comments
Initial Course			
Sulfonamide (Sulfisoxazole)	1 g.	0.5 g. q 6 hr. × 8 days	Sulfa drugs not given during final weeks of pregnancy; risk of hyperbilirubinemia and kernicterus in newborn (sulfa displaces bilirubin from albumin binding sites) (Chapter 23).
and			
Nitrofurantoin	100 mg.	100 mg. q 12 hr. × 8–10 days	
			Nitrofurantoin not used in persons with glucose-6-phosphate dehydrogenase deficiency (10 per cent of American black population and some Mediterranean ethnic groups). Discontinued in final weeks; causes hemolytic anemia in newborn.
Second Course (failure to respond to first course)			
Ampicillin	250 mg.	250 mg. q 6 hr. × 10 days	See comments above.
or			
Nitrofurantoin	100 mg.	100 mg. q 8 hr. × 10 days	Antibiotics not used: streptomycin, tetracycline, gentamicin, kanamycin, chloramphenicol.
or			
According to sensitivities			

of these. Infection may be histologic only (e.g., seen only upon examination of tissue) or may cause symptoms in the mother and fetus. Maternal fever is the most frequent sign, usually accompanied by fetal tachycardia (a fetal heart rate of 180 beats per minute or more).

The most common cause of chorioamnionitis is premature rupture of the membranes with a subsequent ascending infection if membranes are ruptured for more than 24 hours. In one study, when membranes were ruptured less than 24 hours prior to delivery, the incidence of infection was found to be 19.7 per cent; after 24 hours the incidence increased to 54.5 per cent.[11a] Common causative organisms are those already in the lower genital tract— *Escherichia coli*, anaerobic and aerobic streptococci, *Lactobacillus, Staphylococcus epidermidis*, and others.

Based on this knowledge, an essential nursing action is the explanation to all pregnant women of both the signs of membrane rupture and the necessity for prompt notification of the health-care provider. Subsequent medical management will include culturing of the maternal blood and amniotic fluid and antibiotic therapy (for mild infection, ampicillin or cephalothin intravenously until afebrile, then orally for a total of 7 days; for severe infection, a combination of two or three antibiotics for 7 days).

Labor is induced medically if infection is mild and is allowed to continue if delivery seems possible in 6 to 8 hours. When infection is severe, when the fetus is distressed, or when delivery does not seem likely within 8 hours, cesarean delivery is chosen.

Trauma and the Pregnant Woman

The major cause of death and illness in women of childbearing years is not disease (such as diabetes and heart disease) but traumatic injuries, primarily motor vehicle accidents, with gunshot and stabbing wounds the second most frequent source. When a mother with major trauma arrives at the emergency room, the concern is for both mother and fetus. Fetal death is most commonly the result of maternal death, and therefore, efforts are directed toward stabilizing the mother in a manner that will best meet the needs of the fetus as well (Nursing Care Plan 13–9). The unique characteristics of women who are pregnant are important in the assessment and treatment of trauma during pregnancy. Because trauma may occur at any stage of pregnancy, continual changes in the mother's cardiovascular and respiratory systems must be considered in assessment.

In motor vehicle accidents, the most common injury above the waist is head injury. Below the waist, hemorrhage, bladder trauma, ruptured spleen, and fracture of the anterior rami of the pelvis are frequent problems. Hemorrhage is the major problem in knife and gunshot wounds. Infection is always a potential problem, not only for the mother but also because it may lead to premature labor.

Maternal blood volume is increased markedly in pregnancy (Chapter 7); by 24 weeks' gestation a pregnant woman can lose 30 to 35 per cent of her blood volume before blood pressure changes are evident. Moreover, the gravida's blood pressure must be maintained at a level higher than is necessary for many trauma patients in order to maintain a blood supply to the uterus; blood is shunted away from the uterus in shock. Vasoconstricting drugs, frequently used to elevate blood pressure in trauma patients, will also shunt blood away from the uterus. A maternal blood pressure of 130/80 is recommended. A pulse rate greater than 140 or a diastolic blood pressure of less than 80 indicates shock. The phenomenon of supine hypotensive syndrome (Chapter 7) must also be considered; the mother should be tilted toward her left side, if possible, with a pillow. She should not be allowed to lie flat on her back. Aggressive replacement of blood with whole blood and packed red blood cells through a large bore intravenous needle (not a butterfly) is important to provide fetal oxygenation as well as maternal stabilization.

If cardiac massage is necessary, it should be remembered that the heart is rotated "up and out" during pregnancy (Chapter 7).

The respiratory changes of pregnancy, with increased respiratory rate and increased functional residual capacity (Chapter 7), will be particularly important if assisted ventilation is required.

In evaluating maternal pH, remember that fetal pH is lower than maternal pH. If maternal pH is 7.1, fetal pH may be as low as 6.9. Treatment should be directed toward keeping maternal pH greater than 7.2.

Unnecessary x-ray exposure to the fetus is avoided by using ultrasound when possible and by directing x-rays, when necessary, to specific areas based on clinical assessment.

The fetus is also assessed through continuous fetal monitoring. In many hospitals a nurse familiar with fetal monitoring may need to assist those who are caring for the mother. If there is a possibility of fetal maturity, confirmation by amniocentesis (Chapter 14) and subsequent delivery can spare the fetus the trauma resulting from maternal treatment. Signs of impending labor, such as rupture of the membranes, should also be assessed. Fetal monitoring should continue for at least 48 hours after the mother is no longer seriously ill.

In a critically ill mother who may die, the possibility of *postmortem cesarean delivery* must be considered if the fetus is of 26 weeks' gestation or more. Even discussion of the possibility is uncomfortable both for the family and for professionals caring for the mother because it requires both groups to face the issue of the mother's death before it occurs. Reedy[41] has suggested that considering the issue from the mother's point of view may be helpful—i.e., she would want someone to be concerned for her baby. Should the mother die, there is a 25-minute period during which the fetus can be delivered safely. A plan on the chart and family permission in advance will allow that time to be utilized to best advantage in behalf of the fetus. A classic cesarean incision while maintaining maternal cardiopulmonary resuscitation, combined with prompt neonatal resuscitation, is essential to allow the best possible neonatal outcome.

Prenatal Bleeding

One of the most feared symptoms during pregnancy is bleeding. Bleeding has meant "something is wrong" to most of us throughout our lives. Vaginal bleeding during pregnancy, other than the slightest spotting, is a serious or potentially serious complication that deserves immediate attention.

From a physiologic standpoint, hemorrhage may be sufficiently serious to be life-threatening to the mother, requiring rapid intervention. From an emotional standpoint, bleeding often indicates the potential or actual loss of the fetus and demands skilled care to deal with the associated anxiety and grief.

In this segment we will examine some major causes of bleeding during pregnancy and the appropriate interventions to meet physiologic and psychosocial needs (see Nursing Care Plan 13–10).

Ectopic Pregnancy

First trimester bleeding is usually related to *ectopic* pregnancy or to the potential or actual loss of the fetus by spontaneous abortion. Ectopic or extrauterine pregnancy refers to gestation outside of the uterine cavity, most commonly in the uterine tube and in the distal portion of the tube.

Initially, the ovum burrows into the muscular wall of the tube. As the ovum grows, the wall at the placental site becomes weakened and eventually bursts from overdistention. This occurs in the second or third month after conception if the ovum is in the isthmus of the tube, and somewhat later if the ovum is in the ampulla or in the interstitial portion of the tube because those areas are more easily distended.

Signs of Ectopic Pregnancy. The woman may complain of cramping pains on *one side* of her lower abdomen. Pregnancy may have been diagnosed, or she may only have noticed

Text continued on page 388

Nursing Care Plan 13–9. Traumatic Injury in the Pregnant Woman

NURSING GOALS:
To provide care to the pregnant woman with a traumatic injury that protects mother and fetus.
To recognize the relationship between the unique physiologic status of the pregnant woman and care given subsequent to traumatic injury.

OBJECTIVES:
1. Care appropriate to the mother's injury will be provided.
2. Both mother and fetus will be protected from additional injury.
3. The fetus will be delivered in the event of the mother's death if gestational age is 26 weeks or more.
4. The family will be supported through the maternal or infant illness.
5. The family will be supported during grieving for the mother or infant.
6. Attachment to the infant following birth will be facilitated.

ASSESSMENT	POTENTIAL NURSING DIAGNOSIS	NURSING INTERVENTION	COMMENTS/RATIONALE
	Maternal	**Maternal**	
1. Blood pressure: diastolic < 80 = shock		Maintain blood pressure:	
2. Pulse rate > 140 = shock		1. Position mother on side to avoid supine hypotensive syndrome.	
3. Respiration (rate, characteristics)		2. Replace blood loss immediately.	
4. Temperature		3. Provide oxygen, ventilation to maintain fetal as well as maternal oxygenation, pH.	
5. Blood gases < 7.2 may compromise fetal pH		4. Keep family informed of maternal status.	
6. Signs of labor (contractions, rupture of membranes, show)			
	Fetal	**Fetal**	
1. Continuous electronic fetal monitoring done until 48 hours past serious maternal illness.	At risk for fetal distress	Note indications of fetal distress: variable or late decelerations, tachycardia, bradycardia (Chapter 18).	
2. Ultrasound rather than radiation in maternal/fetal assessment to protect fetus when possible			
3. Assess fetal gestational age.			
4. Assess fetal maturity (L/S ratio, etc. [Chapter 14]).			
5. Assess fetal well-being (estriol, etc. [Chapter 14]).			If fetus is mature, early delivery may protect fetus from further trauma.

Labor and Birth

Assessment	Nursing Diagnosis	Intervention	Rationale
Continuous maternal and fetal assessment	Mother or fetus may be at extreme risk during labor and birth.	Nursing care related to severity of mother's condition, mode of delivery (vaginal or cesarean) Support family throughout labor and birth.	The choice of vaginal delivery or cesarean birth will be made with consideration of both maternal and fetal status.
Assess attachment behaviors	Lag in attachment	If mother's condition does not allow her to touch and hold infant immediately, encourage attachment as soon as possible (see, hold, care for infant). Provide opportunity for father or other support persons to bond to infant.	Concern for mother's condition may interfere with bonding.
Need for post mortem cesarean delivery	Mother at risk of dying	1. Written plan on chart for delivery if mother should die 2. Permission for delivery obtained from family in advance 3. Personnel and equipment immediately available to maintain maternal cardiopulmonary resuscitation and provide neonatal resuscitation	If fetus is at 26 weeks' gestation or more and there is a possibility that the mother may die, the need for post mortem cesarean delivery should be considered. Delivery must occur within 25 minutes after maternal death.
Expressions of grieving (denial, anger, etc. [page 393])	Family grief: inadequate coping	Support family throughout; do not leave alone if at all possible. Encourage to cry, verbalize feelings, bond with infant.	If infant also dies, grief is magnified. If infant survives, grief for mother may inhibit bonding to infant.
Attachment behavior (verbal and nonverbal)	Lag in attachment	Gently encourage touching, holding, caretaking attachment. Continue to follow after hospitalization (community health nurse and others).	Father, other family members may need to grieve for mother before they become attached to infant.

Nursing Care Plan 13–10.　The Mother with Prenatal Bleeding

NURSING GOALS:
1. To identify the cause of prenatal bleeding.
2. To protect the mother's well-being during and following prenatal bleeding.
3. To protect the fetus when possible.
4. To support the woman and other family members during grieving when pregnancy loss occurs.

OBJECTIVES:
1. All pregnant women will report prenatal bleeding immediately.
2. The cause of bleeding is determined.
3. Hemorrhage is prevented or quickly controlled and blood is replaced.
4. Care appropriate to the source of bleeding is provided
5. Rh immune globulin is provided to Rh_D negative woman.
6. The woman and her family receive counseling about future reproductive capability.

ASSESSMENT	POTENTIAL NURSING DIAGNOSIS	NURSING INTERVENTION	COMMENTS/RATIONALE
All gravidas should have knowledge of action to be taken if bleeding should occur.	Need for information about prenatal bleeding	Provide information to all gravidas about action to be taken if prenatal bleeding occurs.	
Determine the cause of bleeding. 1. Early pregnancy: ectopic pregnancy; spontaneous abortion; hydatidiform mole 2. Late pregnancy: placenta previa, with premature separation; abruptio placentae; disseminated intravenous coagulation	Bleeding related to (specific cause)	Based on specific etiology (see below)	
Ectopic Pregnancy			
Identify woman at risk. 1. History of pelvic inflammatory disease 2. Prior treatment for gonorrhea 3. Previous ectopic pregnancy 4. Previous abdominal surgery 5. Prior spontaneous or elective abortion	Risk for ectopic pregnancy related to (specific condition)	Instruct gravida to report bleeding, unilateral pain, other symptoms to health-care provider immediately.	
Identify signs of ectopic pregnancy. 1. Missed menstrual period 2. Tenderness, fullness, or mass in adnexa 3. Pain on *one side* of lower abdomen; pain may be excruciating following rupture.		Immediate hospitalization required. Explain reasons for hospitalization and course of treatment to woman and family.	
5. Shoulder pain (referred pain if pain reaches level bleeding of diaphragm)		Prepare woman for surgery: intravenous fluids; type and cross-matching for blood, oxygen, and emergency medications available Keep family informed.	Note Rh factor in blood type: Rh immune globulin given to Rh negative mother (Nursing Care Plan 13–6)

Assessment	Nursing Diagnosis	Intervention	Rationale
Following surgery 1. Postsurgical physiologic support: vital signs, bleeding, etc. 2. Hemoglobin, hematocrit	At risk of anemia secondary to blood loss	Woman may continue to receive blood in postoperative period. Counsel to increase iron and folic acid in diet.	
3. Woman's and family's reaction to pregnancy loss	Grief related to pregnancy loss Diminished self-esteem related to pregnancy loss	Provide opportunities to verbalize grief, cry. Provide opportunity for baptism of conceptus, if desired.	
4. Understanding of future reproductive capacity: determine woman's and family's perception of information already provided.	Need for information concerning future reproductive capacity Fear related to future reproductive ability	Future reproduction is related to status of remaining tube.	Approximately 50 per cent of women have at least one normal gestation following ectopic pregnancy.

Spontaneous Abortion

Assessment	Nursing Diagnosis	Intervention	Rationale
Identify mother at risk. 1. History of abortions	Risk of spontaneous abortion related to (specific reason)	Couples with history of repeated abortions may be referred for genetic counseling (Chapter 3).	Risk of spontaneous abortion increases in relation to the number of previous spontaneous abortions.
2. Maternal disease (e.g., sickle cell anemia, lupus erythematosus) 3. Cervical incompetence 4. Previous fetus or newborn with abnormal karyotype (Chapter 3) 5. Congenital anomalies of the reproductive tract		Provide information to couples related to specific condition, e.g., possibility of surgical intervention for certain congenital anomalies, cervical incompetence. Provide referral if appropriate.	
Identify signs of abortion: 1. Vaginal bleeding (passage of clots or tissue fragments, number of pads used) 2. Abdominal cramping Pregnancy test may be negative, depending upon length of gestation; usually negative or inconclusive.		Value of bed rest and sedation inconclusive If abortion becomes inevitable, prepare woman and family for evacuation of the uterus in hospital. 1. Medical (oxytocin) 2. Surgical (dilatation and curettage) Following evacuation, ergonovine is administered to ensure uterine contractions.	
Hemorrhage Maternal hemoglobin, hematocrit at risk of anemia related to blood loss		Blood replacement may be necessary.	

Continued on following page

Nursing Care Plan 13–10.   The Mother with Prenatal Bleeding (Continued)

ASSESSMENT	POTENTIAL NURSING DIAGNOSIS	NURSING INTERVENTION	COMMENTS/RATIONALE
Spontaneous Abortion (Continued)			
Following abortion and evacuation of uterus: 1. Vital signs 2. Bleeding 3. Signs of infection Reactions to pregnancy loss (Nursing Care Plan 13–1 and ectopic pregnancy above)	Nursing Care Plan 13–1	Nursing Care Plan 13–1	
Understanding of future reproductive capacity	Need for information related to reason for abortion and possible outcome in future pregnancy Fear related to future reproductive ability	Provide or reinforce information provided about suspected reason. May include referral for genetic counseling, surgery, etc., as noted above.	
Hydatidiform Mole			
Identify signs of hydatidiform mole. 1. Bloody discharge (often brownish) beginning at tenth to twelfth week of pregnancy; continuous or intermittent 2. Enlargement of uterus out of proportion to estimated gestational age of fetus 3. Absence of fetal heart tone 4. High level of HCG 100 days or more after last menstrual period 5. Signs of pre-eclampsia 6. Hyperemesis	Need for information about hydatidiform mole	Explain possibility of hydatidiform mole and necessary treatment. Refer to physician for evacuation of uterus or possible hysterectomy. Following evacuation: care related to procedure employed (medical induction, dilation and curettage, hysterectomy)	
Reaction of woman and family (e.g., view mole as pregnancy loss?)	Grief related to pregnancy loss Diminished self-esteem	Provide opportunity for expressions of grief. Provide opportunity to see and hold fetus if desired; encourage but do not force this action. Provide memento of fetus—picture, lock of hair, footprint. If parents do not desire memento, let them know it will be available to them when they wish.	Frequently parents do not wish reminder of infant immediately but cherish it later.

Assessment	Nursing Diagnosis	Intervention
Woman's and family's understanding of necessity for continuing care	Need for continuing care	Explain reason for continuing assessment and care: early detection of possible choriocarcinoma.
1. HCG levels:	Need for information about continuing care	Continuing high or rising HCG levels suggest choriocarcinoma; treatment by chemotherapy.
a. Weekly until three negative weekly tests, then		Oral contraceptives to prevent pregnancy until HCG negative for 1 year
b. Monthly for 6 months, then		Choriocarcinoma metastasizes rapidly if treatment is inadequate or unsuccessful.
c. Bimonthly for 6 months, then		Lungs are a common site for metastasis.
d. Every 6 months		
2. Chest x-ray		
a. Monthly until negative HCG, then		
b. Bimonthly for 1 year		

Placenta Previa

Assessment	Nursing Diagnosis	Intervention
Identify mothers with placenta previa:	Risk of hemorrhage related to placenta previa	Hospitalize mother for evaluation. Intervention depends on extent of bleeding.
1. May be discovered incidentally during ultrasound examination for another purpose prior to symptoms	Anxiety related to hemorrhage	Expectant management when fetus is immature (less than 36 weeks) and bleeding is minimal.
2. Bright red bleeding: assess woman's estimate of amount, number of pads used.		a. Bed rest
Following hospitalization, nursing assessment of amount of bleeding		b. Observation for bleeding
3. Ultrasound examination to identify placental location		c. Blood replacement as indicated (hemoglobin, hematocrit)
		d. Emotional support: opportunity to verbalize fears; reassurance about care

Additional Assessment Following Diagnosis of Placenta Previa

Assessment	Nursing Diagnosis	Intervention
1. Pain or abdominal tenderness	When bleeding is severe there is risk of shock; maternal mortality or morbidity; fetal or neonatal mortality or morbidity	Management in severe bleeding
2. Uterus: contractions, irritability, size, contour, fetal life		a. Explain each action to woman and family—encourage questions and verbalization of fears
3. Estimated gestational age of fetus		b. NPO
4. Fetal heart tones: use external fetal monitor		c. Bed rest with head elevated
5. Urinary output		d. IV fluids; blood as indicated by laboratory values and extent of bleeding
6. Maternal vital signs: CVP line may be indicated. Note character as well as rate of pulse		e. *Do not* give enema.
7. Laboratory assessment: hemoglobin, hematocrit, blood type and cross match, urinalysis		f. Prepare for "double set-up" (see text)
8. *Do not* attempt rectal or vaginal examination		Pain is not common in placenta previa. Pain may indicate labor or abruption of placenta.
		Fetal presenting part may exert pressure to control bleeding.
		Blood must be available in delivery room before any examination is attempted. Rectal or vaginal examination may precipitate massive hemorrhage.

Continued on following page

Nursing Care Plan 13–10.   The Mother with Prenatal Bleeding (Continued)

ASSESSMENT	POTENTIAL NURSING DIAGNOSIS	NURSING INTERVENTION	COMMENTS/RATIONALE
Additional Assessment Following Diagnosis of Placenta Previa (Continued)			
		g. Be prepared (personnel and equipment) for infant resuscitation. In severe hemorrhage neonatal mortality and morbidity high. Infant may also be preterm.	
		h. In total previa, delivery will be Cesarean; vaginal delivery may be attempted if previa is small (less than 30 per cent) and bleeding is minimal.	
Post Delivery			
1. Maternal bleeding	At risk for postpartum bleeding secondary to myometrial trauma and atony		
2. Hemoglobin and hematocrit following delivery and prior to discharge	At risk of anemia secondary to hemorrhage	Additional transfusions may be necessary.	
3. Signs of infection	At risk of infection secondary to hemorrhage and delayed healing of abdominal placental site		
4. Neonatal hemoglobin hematocrit	At risk of anemia secondary to maternal hemorrhage		
5. Woman's and family's understanding of experience	Need for information about placenta previa	Review information provided earlier. Answer questions. Encourage verbalization.	
6. Grieving response if infant is seriously ill or dies	Grief related to neonatal illness, death (anger, denial, guilt, etc.). See Nursing Care Plan 13–1.	Provide opportunity for expression of grief. Accept feelings of anger, etc.	
Abruption of the Placenta			
Identify conditions placing women at risk.	At risk for placental abruption		Clinical classification:
1. Pre-eclampsia or eclampsia			*Grade 0:* No symptoms (diagnosis following delivery); 35 per cent of abruptions
2. Hypertension			
3. Multiple gestation			*Grade 1:* External bleeding; no signs of shock or fetal distress; 55 per cent of abruptions
4. Multiparity (five or more gestations)			
5. Advanced maternal age			
6. Diabetes mellitus			
7. Short umbilical cord			

8. Prolonged gestation (particularly in multiparas)
9. Deprived socioeconomic status
10. Previous reproductive loss

Identify signs.

Signs	Nursing Diagnosis	Intervention	Comments
			Grade 2: External bleeding, uterine tetany, fetal distress; 10 per cent of abruptions *Grade 3:* External or internal bleeding, uterine tetany, maternal shock, fetal death, DIC; 5 per cent of abruptions
1. Sudden, severe abdominal pain: knifelike, dull, colicky 2. Nausea or vomiting 3. Hypotension (may not occur in mother with hypertension with tachycardia, pallor, dyspnea	Abdominal pain secondary to possible abruption of placenta	Rapid hospitalization (ambulance) if not in hospital Notify attending physician. Explain actions to woman and family. CVP line ensures accurate assessment of pressure. Replace fluid, blood loss.	Pain may not be present if vaginal bleeding occurs and area of abruption is small.
4. Bleeding may be concealed (internal) or vaginal. Vaginal bleeding frequently dark red. *Do not attempt rectal or vaginal examination.*	Vaginal bleeding related to possible abruption of placenta		Note that bleeding is usually dark, compared with bright red bleeding of placenta previa.
5. Uterus may be rigid, "boardlike" (uterine tetany); inability to feel fetal parts; uterus does not relax between contractions.			If vaginal bleeding occurs and blood does not accumulate in uterus, abdominal rigidity is unlikely. Couvelaire uterus: bleeding into myometrium → rigidity, pain
6. Laboratory assessment: hemoglobin/hematocrit—initial hemoconcentration (elevated hematocrit); subsequent anemia (decreased hemoglobin). Clotting time, prothrombin time (see DIC, below). Type and cross-match fibrinogen levels.	Hemoconcentration secondary to decreased intravascular fluid Anemia secondary to blood loss	Replace fluid, blood loss. Prepare for possibility of DIC (below).	
7. Urinary output and fluid intake (IV)	Oliguria related to poor kidney perfusion secondary to depleted intravascular fluid.	Replace fluid, blood loss.	
8. Backache	Backache related to retroplacental hemorrhage.		
9. Signs of amniotic fluid embolism (Chapter 19)		See Nursing Care Plan 19–7.	
10. Signs of fetal distress (variable, late decelerations; see Chapter 18)	Fetus at risk of oxygen deprivation secondary to placental detachment	Use electronic fetal monitor for continuous fetal monitoring. If decelerations noted, provide O$_2$ (face-mask); increase IV rate. Prepare for immediate delivery. Be prepared (personnel and equipment) for infant resuscitation (Nursing Care Plan 23–1).	

Continued on following page

Nursing Care Plan 13–10.   The Mother with Prenatal Bleeding (Continued)

ASSESSMENT	POTENTIAL NURSING DIAGNOSIS	NURSING INTERVENTION	COMMENTS/RATIONALE
	Abruption of the Placenta (Continued)		
11. Reactions, emotional status of woman, family	Anxiety related to symptoms (pain, bleeding, etc.)	Provide opportunity to verbalize fears for self, infant.	Guilt about actions causing abruption may be implicit in some questions.
		Answer questions.	
		Reassure woman that she will not be alone.	
Following delivery			
1. Assessment as in vaginal delivery (Nursing Care Plan 17–4) or Cesarean delivery (Nursing Care Plan 19–3).		See Nursing Care Plan 17–4 or 19–3, as appropriate.	
2. Additional assessment related to extent of bleeding and secondary problem (DIC, below) acute renal tubular necrosis (assess oliguria, hematuria).	At risk for DIC At risk for acute renal tubular necrosis	Heparin and cryoprecipitate should be immediately available (see DIC, below).	
3. Signs of infection	At risk for infection		
4. Note if hysterectomy performed			
5. Status of newborn	Infant at risk related to intrauterine asphyxia	Infant may be transported to regional center; ascertain that parents are in contact with infant's care-givers.	
		If infant remains in same hospital, provide for maternal-paternal-infant contact as soon as possible.	
6. Family response a. Infant mortality or morbidity b. Hysterectomy	Grief related to (specific reason)	Continue to provide opportunity for grieving, verbalization, questions.	
	Disseminated Intravascular Coagulopathy		
Identify conditions that place woman at risk: 1. Abruptio placentae 2. Retention of fetus following intrauterine fetal death 3. Retention of placenta 4. Amniotic fluid embolism 5. Septicemia 6. Eclampsia	At risk of DIC secondary to (specific reason)	Careful evaluation of women at risk for early signs of DIC.	

7. Massive hemorrhage for any reason
8. Oxytocin induction
9. Tumultuous labor
10. Difficult delivery

Identify signs of DIC.
1. Bleeding from gums, nose
2. Bleeding from injection sites, other areas of slight trauma
3. Tachycardia
4. Restlessness, anxiety
5. Diaphoresis

Laboratory assessment:
1. Clot observation: no clot
2. Coagulation time: no clot
3. Plasma fibrinogen less than 100 mg./100 ml.
4. Platelets: decreased
5. Fibrinogen-fibrin degradation products (FDP-fdp) increased
6. Thrombin time, prothrombin time, partial thromboplastin time increased

During treatment and for a minimum of 24 hours thereafter assess:
1. Vital signs: elevated pulse and respirations, low blood pressure indicate increased risk of shock
2. CVP: maintain between 6 and 12 mm. H_2O
3. Urinary output: maintain between 30 and 60 ml./hour.
4. Cyanosis, pallor
5. Cool, clammy skin indicates shock.
6. Level of consciousness: restlessness, confusion indicate cerebral hypoxia.
7. Fetal status prior to delivery if fetus is viable; continuous electronic fetal monitoring

During and following treatment assess woman's and family's understanding and response.

Suspect DIC
Blood drawn for studies
Heparin or fibrinogen (or both) available
Prompt intervention to remove cause:
1. Prepare for immediate delivery if there is placental abruption, retention of dead fetus.
2. Action to remove retained placenta
3. Treatment for amniotic fluid embolism, eclampsia, sepsis
4. Control of hemorrhage

Provide physiologic support:
1. Oxygen; mechanical ventilation may be necessary.
2. IV fluids
3. CVP monitoring
4. Lateral position or elevation of right hip
5. Whole blood or blood components
   a. Platelets
   b. Cryoprecipitate
   c. Fresh frozen plasma
6. Heparin (IV administration)

Need for information about DIC
Anxiety related to maternal condition

Provide information. Encourage questions.

Expect anxiety, grief reaction. Encourage verbalization.

Normal plasma fibrinogen in pregnancy is greater than 300 mg./100 ml.

Cryoprecipitate is the most effective source of fibrinogen currently available.

The use of heparin is controversial; used primarily prior to resolution of obstetrical problem.

Heparin is not given if woman is not bleeding.

menstrual irregularity. If the ectopic pregnancy ruptures, more definite symptoms are sudden, excruciating pelvic pain, dizziness, and/or shock. The woman often appears pale and slightly cyanotic; her pulse is rapid and thready. Bleeding occurs at the placental site; when blood reaches the level of the diaphragm, shoulder pain may occur.

Rupture may be more gradual, with symptoms including abdominal pain and tenderness, nausea, vomiting, and diarrhea.

Intervention. Surgical intervention is the treatment for an ectopic pregnancy. Ideally, the condition is recognized before rupture, and the affected tube is removed. If the woman has only one functioning tube, occasionally the surgeon may try to remove the ovum and leave the tube, but this is uncommon because the risk of a subsequent ectopic pregnancy is high.

If the tube has ruptured, a salpingectomy is performed immediately. When the abdomen is opened, the intestines may be found floating in blood. Blood loss is replaced during and following surgery.

Spontaneous Abortion

The term *abortion* refers to the process by which a nonviable fetus is expelled from the uterus. By convention, a fetus of less than 20 weeks' gestation or less than 500 grams in weight is considered an *abortus*.

Probably one in every five to seven conceptions ends in abortion. In many instances the abortion occurs in the first weeks at a time when the mother may not even know she is pregnant. The bleeding may appear to be a somewhat delayed and perhaps heavier than normal menstrual period.

A variety of terms are used by laymen and professionals to describe events related to abortion.

Miscarriage is the word most commonly used by laymen to describe a spontaneous abortion. The word abortion, for many, implies an event that is sinful or criminal. A mother or couple may be terribly upset to hear their problem referred to as an abortion. If we ask a mother if she has ever had an abortion, she will assure us that she has not.

Spontaneous abortion occurs with no apparent interference.

Threatened abortion refers to transcervical bleeding. Uterine contractions may or may not be present, but the cervix is not dilated, and the conceptus has not been expelled.

In *inevitable abortion,* bleeding, uterine contractions, and progressive cervical dilatation are present.

Abortion is *incomplete* when only part of the products of the conception are expelled. For example, the fetus may be expelled, but portions of the fetal membrane may remain.

In *complete abortion,* all of the uterine contents are expelled.

Missed abortion refers to the situation in which the fetus dies but is retained in the uterus for 8 weeks or longer following death.

When a woman has three or more consecutive spontaneous abortions, she is said to have *habitual abortions*.

Deliberate interruption of pregnancy is termed *induced abortion*.

Why Spontaneous Abortion? A major concern of mothers who have had a spontaneous abortion is "Why did this happen to me?" In most spontaneous abortions the cause is unknown. Trauma is rarely a cause. Abnormalities of the fetus and of the umbilical cord, fetal chromosomal abnormalities, inadequate levels of progesterone to support implantation and development, acute maternal infection, diseases of the decidua, and an incompetent cervix (see below) are some factors that have been shown to cause abortion.

An incompetent cervix begins to dilate for no apparent reason, often during the second trimester. Once an incompetent cervix has been diagnosed as the cause of abortion, a cerclage surgical procedure is performed, either between pregnancies or when the cervix begins to dilate.

Intervention. The traditional advice to a woman in whom abortion is suspected is to go to bed and to avoid coitus. Although these prohibitions may be harmless, there is no evidence that they are effective. Nor is there good evidence that bleeding or abortion is more likely at the time that menstruation would normally occur, which is another popular belief.

If bleeding continues in spite of bed rest, the woman may be allowed to be out of bed on the premise that the gestation may best be terminated. If and when the abortion occurs, it is important that the uterus be completely emptied; remaining fragments of fetal or placental tissue can cause infection and/or continued bleeding. The method used varies with such factors as the length of gestation.

Aftercare. Following spontaneous abortion, observation for bleeding and signs of sepsis is important. Equally critical is emotional support, described at the conclusion of this section on bleeding problems.

Hydatidiform Mole

In one of 2000 pregnancies, hydatidiform mole will be the cause of bleeding. Hydatidi-

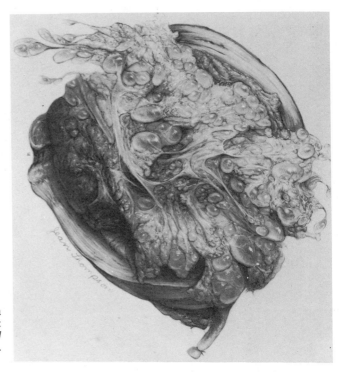

Figure 13–5. Drawing of a uterus containing a hydatidiform mole. (From Page, Villee, and Villee: *Human Reproduction: Essentials of Reproductive and Perinatal Medicine.* 3rd Edition. Philadelphia, W. B. Saunders Co., 1981.)

form mole is a developmental anomaly of the placenta. Some or all of the chorionic villi degenerate into transparent vesicles (Fig. 13–5) that may fill the uterus. This anomaly is classified as a trophoblastic disease.

Signs that a possible mole may be present include:

> 1. Bloody discharge beginning at the tenth to twelfth week of pregnancy.
> 2. Enlargement of the uterus out of proportion to the estimated gestational age of the fetus.
> 3. Absence of fetal heart tone.
> 4. A high level of serum human chorionic gonadotropin (HCG) 100 days or more after the last menstrual period.
> 5. An ultrasound evaluation unique and characteristic of a mole.
> 6. The edema, proteinuria, and hypertension of pre-eclampsia.

The bleeding of a molar pregnancy may be bright red, but is frequently brownish and often not profuse. It may be continuous or intermittent.

Human chorionic gonadotropin is produced in the second week of pregnancy (Chapter 7). In normal pregnancy, HCG declines after 100 days. However, when trophoblastic tissue proliferates, levels of HCG continue to be high or to rise further.

The treatment for hydatidiform mole is evacuation of the uterus. If the woman is already undergoing spontaneous abortion, it will be completed. Otherwise a procedure appropriate to the size of the uterus, such as dilatation and curettage, suction curettage, or intra-amniotic saline (Chapter 30), is used.

Evacuation does not end the mother's need for care, however. Trophoblastic tissue may remain and may metastasize to other areas of the body. The continued presence of trophoblastic tissue is indicated by the presence of HCG in the urine. Metastases are most frequent to the lung and may be apparent on chest x-ray; the vagina, liver, kidneys, and brain are other possible sites. Treatment of metastasis is most commonly performed by chemotherapy today.

The finding of a negative HCG level is recommended strongly for 1 year before another pregnancy is planned.

Placenta Previa

Placenta previa is the development of the placenta in part of, or entirely in, the lower uterine segment. A placenta previa occurs in approximately 8 of 1000 pregnancies; about 75 per cent occur in multiparas, although the age of the mother, rather than parity, appears to be more significant.

Figure 13–6 illustrates the difference between (A) low implantation of the placenta, in which the edge of the placenta can be palpated through the cervix but the placenta itself

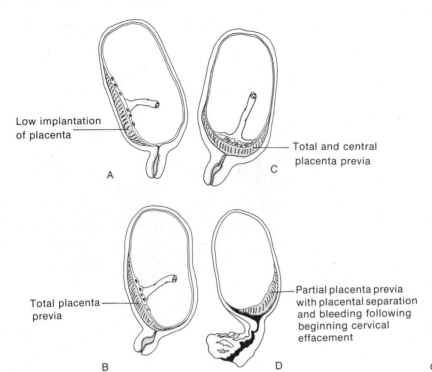

Low implantation
of placenta

A

Total and central
placenta previa

C

Total placenta
previa

B

Partial placenta previa
with placental separation
and bleeding following
beginning cervical
effacement

D

Figure 13–6. Some variations of placenta previa.

barely extends to the margin of the internal os; (B) partial placenta previa, in which the placenta partially covers the internal os; and (C) total placenta previa, in which the placenta entirely covers the internal os.

Why does placenta previa occur? It is probable that the ovum is implanted low in the uterus. Because the nutritional support of the lower urine segment is not as great as that of the body of the uterus, the placenta will spread further in its search for nourishment. A placenta previa is usually both larger and thinner than the usual placenta.

Symptoms of Placenta Previa. The first and only symptom of a placenta previa may occur when the woman awakens one morning and finds herself lying in a pool of blood. Or she may first notice blood in the toilet bowl. The bleeding is painless. Although bleeding caused by placenta previa is most commonly in the third trimester, particularly in the eighth month, bleeding may begin before this time. The earlier bleeding occurs, the more likely it is that the placenta previa is total. Partial placentia previa may not cause bleeding until the cervix dilates during labor.

Dangers of Placenta Previa. Placenta previa presents major dangers to the mother both before and after delivery and to the fetus. For the mother, the loss of large amounts of blood can lead to hemorrhagic shock, fibrinogenopenia (see below), thrombocytopenia, and marked anemia.

Other complications that may be related to placenta previa are:
1. Premature rupture of the membranes.
2. Premature labor.
3. Malposition and/or malpresentation of the fetus.
4. Air embolism (because the uterine sinuses are exposed to external air).
5. Rupture of the uterus (because the uterine musculature is weakened by placental ingrowth).
6. Postpartum hemorrhage (because the thin, weakened uterine wall does not contract firmly and quickly to prevent hemorrhage from the large venous sinuses at the placental site).
7. Postpartum infection (because pieces of placenta may adhere to the uterine wall and become infected as a result of the close proximity of the placental site to the cervix and vagina).

The fetus is also at risk. Anoxia resulting from the premature separation of the placenta is the most common cause of fetal death. There may also be fetal blood loss, largely preventable if proper care is given (see below). Because a bleeding placenta previa may force early delivery, prematurity is an additional problem.

The Recognition and Immediate Care of a Mother with Suspected Placenta Previa. As noted in Chapter 10, mothers should be told early during their pregnancy to call the physician or nurse if bleeding occurs. The mother should be hospitalized immediately.

She should not be examined in a clinic or office first. Rectal or vaginal examination can lead to uncontrollable hemorrhage. An ambulance is preferred for transportation to the hospital.

When the mother arrives at hospital, blood is immediately typed, and a minimum of 1000 ml. of blood is matched. If the mother is anemic, she is immediately transfused. Even though the mother may not be bleeding profusely at the time she is admitted, she should be treated as if she might begin to hemorrhage.

A rapid physical assessment is necessary, both to establish the woman's status at admission and to evaluate any future changes. This assessment includes:

> 1. Vital signs, with particular attention to the character as well as the rate of the pulse. A central venous pressure line may be inserted for continuous assessment.
> 2. The condition of the abdomen. Is pain present? Is the abdomen tender?
> 3. The condition of the uterus: size, contour, irritability, relaxation, fetal presentation.
> 4. Engagement of the presenting part.
> 5. Presence of a placental souffle just above the symphysis pubis.
> 6. Urinary output, a measure of both fluid and kidney perfusion.

The placenta is localized by an ultrasound technique. Placental localization is necessary before the course of action can be determined.

No vaginal examination is done until:

1. Blood for transfusion is available.
2. The delivery room is totally prepared for both abdominal and pelvic delivery (called a "double set-up"). Not only must all equipment and personnel be available, including a physician or nurse competent to manage anesthesia, but equipment must be ready for use (i.e., trays and tables "opened" so that their contents are instantly available).

At this point a speculum may be inserted into the vagina; sometimes a reason for bleeding other than placenta previa (a cervical polyp or a laceration, for example) is detected.

Intervention Following the Definite Diagnosis of Placenta Previa. Medical intervention will vary with the severity of the bleeding. If bleeding is profuse and the mother has signs of shock (decreasing blood pressure and increasing pulse rate), emergency measures are undertaken. Blood must be replaced, and blood pressure, cardiac output, and tissue perfusion must be maintained. Oxygen is administered. Simultaneously, Cesarean section is performed. Obviously, these mothers must

be carefully observed following delivery for signs of shock, hemorrhage, and infection for reasons already noted.

Fortunately, the majority of mothers with placenta previa do not arrive with such life-threatening symptoms. For these other mothers, *expectant management* has improved fetal survival, mainly by allowing the fetus to become more mature. Expectant management involves putting the mother to bed, close observation for signs of bleeding, and both physiologic (e.g., blood replacement) and emotional support.

Should the mother begin to hemorrhage at any time, surgical intervention will be necessary.

The Newborn Infant of a Mother with Placenta Previa. Anemia is possible in the infant of a mother who has had placenta previa. Hemoglobin and hematocrit levels should be checked during the first days and weeks of life.

Abruptio Placentae

Abruptio placentae is defined as premature separation of a normally implanted placenta. Studies indicate that major abruption occurs in from 1 in 85 deliveries to 1 in 139 deliveries.

What Causes Abruptio Placentae? The mechanism of abruptio placentae is apparently degeneration of the spiral arterioles that nourish the endometrium and supply blood to the placenta (Chapter 4). This degeneration leads to necrosis of the decidua beneath the placenta; hemorrhage follows, and the placenta becomes detached.

The area of detachment may be a small one at first; the resulting hemorrhage may then further separate the placenta from the decidua.

The more basic question of why changes occur in the spiral arterioles has not been answered definitely. Similar changes have been experimentally produced by elevating venous pressure; this would explain why mothers with pre-eclampsia and eclampsia have a higher rate of abruption.

Abruption may occur during labor because of a sudden loss of a large amount of amniotic fluid, a shearing effect that may follow the birth of a first twin, or traction on the placenta.

Types of Abruptio Placentae. Table 13–15 summarizes types of abruptio placentae. Note that in the first three instances, vaginal bleeding is unlikely, at least initially (Fig. 13–7). The flow of blood may be blocked by the fetal head or by a clot. In most patients, external hemorrhage eventually follows internal bleeding (Fig. 13–8).

Table 13–15. TYPES OF ABRUPTIO PLACENTAE

Type	Description	Hemorrhage
I	Placenta edges attached to uterus (most rare)	Concealed (internal)
II	All membranes around placenta severed from uterine wall	Concealed (internal)
III	Hemorrhage into the amniotic sac	Concealed (internal)
IV	Hemorrhage outward under the edge of the placenta	Apparent (external)

Assessing the Symptoms of Abruptio Placentae. Abruption of the placenta may be so mild that there are no recognizable symptoms in the antepartum period; the sole evidence may be a scar on the maternal surface of the placenta, indicating a separation that may have occurred weeks or months before. The woman may or may not have reported symptoms such as uterine tenderness or pain and vaginal bleeding at the time. The fetus apparently had not been jeopardized.

In more serious instances of abruption, sudden and severe abdominal pain is usually the first sign. The pain is often at the site of the placenta and is often described by mothers as "knifelike" at first and later as varying between "dull" and "colicky." The mother may be nauseated or may vomit.

Blood pressure readings may indicate shock, but if the mother has pre-eclampsia or eclampsia, blood pressure may remain high.

Abdominal examination will usually reveal an enlarged uterus; repeated examinations will indicate that the uterus is enlarging each hour as blood collects behind the placenta. The uterus is often boardlike; fetal parts cannot be palpated. The mother reports uterine tenderness when palpation is attempted.

In severe abruption, fetal movement may no longer be felt by the mother, nor can fetal heart tones be heard by the examiner.

Laboratory examination reveals increasing anemia.

Intervention. Unlike placenta previa, in which expectant management is often appropriate, moderate to severe abruptions of the placenta require rapid intervention. Time is important. Delay may result in severe hemorrhage with anemia and fibrinogenopenia, leading to shock and fetal and maternal death.

The mother who is admitted with potential abruptio placentae is often in pain and always anxious. She may not understand exactly what has happened, but she feels that it is "something terrible." In our haste to perform the many tasks that her physiologic condition requires, we must not forget her or her husband's emotional concerns.

Blood is drawn for examination (hemoglobin, hematocrit, clotting time, prothrombin time, type and cross match) and from 4 to 6 units of blood are prepared for transfusion.

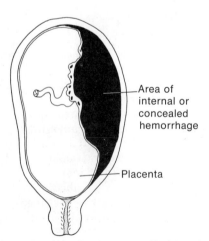

Figure 13–7. Abruptio placentae with internal or concealed hemorrhage.

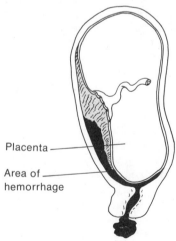

Figure 13–8. Abruptio placentae with external (revealed) hemorrhage.

A central venous pressure line is inserted to monitor blood pressure. A careful record of intake and output is essential; oliguria indicates poor kidney perfusion and depleted intravascular fluid.

Subsequent intervention varies with the condition of both mother and fetus.

If the fetus is alive but in apparent distress, if the bleeding appears to be increasing, if the mother has tachycardia and hypotension, or if fibrinogen levels are falling (see below), immediate Cesarean section is almost always performed.

However, if the condition of the mother and fetus appears good, if no coagulation problem is present, and if coagulation can be monitored closely, labor may be induced. No more than 6 to 8 hours should be allowed for the progress of labor, during which both mother and baby are intensively monitored. Any deterioration in the condition of either mother or fetus would indicate immediate Cesarean intervention.

If the fetus is known to be dead, the decision is made on the basis of the mother's condition, often allowing labor if the mother's physiologic status appears stable, or intervening with Cesarean section if the mother's life is in jeopardy.

Fibrinogenopenia. As fibrin forms in the retroplacental clot following an abruption of the placenta, the level of fibrinogen in the blood decreases and thus interferes with normal clotting mechanisms. Disseminated intravascular coagulation (DIC) may result, with widespread bleeding. Any woman in whom abruptio placentae is suspected should have levels of fibrinogen checked.

Rapid information is obtained from observing carefully drawn blood placed in a clean test tube. The blood should clot quickly; the clot should be firm and retract well. In many hospitals plasma fibrinogen levels are obtained. If the level is below 100 mg. per 100 ml., clotting mechanisms are abnormal. (Normal levels during pregnancy exceed 300 mg. per 100 ml.).

Intervention includes (1) prompt treatment of the cause, (2) replacement of lost blood, (3) use of heparin to block the consumption of fibrinogen, or (4) replacement of lost fibrinogen with 4 grams or more of fibrinogen.

It is obviously essential that fibrinogen be available in the delivery room.

Other obstetric conditions that may cause fibrinogenopenia include retention of a dead fetus, as in a missed abortion; amniotic fluid embolism; bacteremia; and any instance of massive hemorrhage.

Emotional Support of the Mother with Bleeding

The physiologic support of the pregnant woman with bleeding can be, in some instances, truly a matter of life and death. In every instance, considerable attention must be paid to blood loss and replacement, monitoring of vital signs, and the other care that has been described. In the necessary haste, it is easy to forget the monumental fear and sadness that the mother and her husband are experiencing. Mary Ross Osborn, a nurse and mother, describes her own feelings, "Frantic over my extreme discomfort and terrified of the bleeding, I called the nurse again."[26]

How can we help women and their families cope with this experience?

1. The mother should not be left alone if she is having contractions or active bleeding. Even if the father or another family member is with her, she needs close nursing attention. If no one else is present, a nurse should stay with her. Ideally, no mother should labor alone, but if staffing needs make it impossible for every mother to have constant attention, this mother has priority. She should be made as comfortable as possible; clean bedding, back rubs, and cool cloths can convey emotional support as well as physical support.

A woman may cry, quietly or loudly; she may moan softly or call out. This is appropriate behavior. She may talk about her feelings, but often she will be receiving medication for pain and will not be able to communicate effectively until the next day.

2. Should the mother see her dead baby? Only she should make that decision. Neither physicians nor nurses should make it, nor should the father decide for her. The decision need not be made immediately; it can be deferred until the next day. Consider the following conversation in the paper by Kowalski and Osborn:

> "Would you like to see the baby?" I asked.
> "I don't know, Karen," she replied hesitantly . . . "No, I don't think I want to."
> "Think about it, Mary. I'll do whatever you want. But please remember how angry you were that you did not see John" (a previous child who had died almost immediately after birth).
> There was a pause. Mary looked intently at me.
> "Would you like me to find her?" I asked.
> Mary nodded. I squeezed her hand and went in search of the baby.[26]

Are there advantages to a mother and father in seeing their dead fetus or baby? In Chapter

28 the importance of parents' becoming "attached" to their high risk newborns, even when it is highly likely that the baby is going to die, is discussed. Attachment under these circumstances is felt to lead to a more normal resolution of grief.

Can seeing and touching a formed but nonviable fetus, a fetus of 16 to 20 weeks' gestation, for example, serve a similar function? Kowalski and Osborn commented about "feelings of peace and calm after having seen the baby."[26]

The baby was wrapped in blankets to be taken to the mother. Before the nurse showed the baby to the mother, she prepared her for what she would see. The mother should be told that the baby will feel cold; he will probably be blue. If there is an abnormality or bruising, she should know this. But normality can be stressed. "Your baby is small but seems perfectly formed . . . or has perfect hands and feet . . . or a perfect face." Many parents fantasize a deformed fetus. Particularly in relation to abortion, they may have been told that a spontaneous abortion is nature's way of "getting rid of an imperfect fetus" or, more bluntingly, "getting rid of a mistake."

The mother and nurse then talked about similarities between the baby and other members of the family as the mother touched first the baby's hands and then her trunk and her back. They spent about 20 to 25 minutes examining the baby and then another 30 to 45 minutes talking about feelings after the baby was taken away.

The value of similar nursing intervention for other mothers who deliver a nonviable or dead fetus seems worth exploring.

3. A further pregnancy may or may not be possible for an individual mother. Even if a subsequent pregnancy is highly likely (as for example, a first spontaneous abortion), it is inappropriate at this point to say, "You can always have another baby." Parents need to resolve their grief for this baby before they can contemplate another.

Should the parents ask or appear to be anxious about the possibility of a similar occurrence in a future pregnancy, their questions should be answered. For many parents, followup counseling may be the best time to explore this issue.

For some parents, future pregnancy obviously may be impossible. A single functioning uterine tube may have been removed because of an ectopic pregnancy. Hysterectomy may have been performed following the rupture of the uterus. Self-image and lifetime goals may have been shattered in a few hours.

Not only must these parents grieve for their lost baby, but perhaps also for their hopes and dreams of a future family.

4. The resolution of grief may begin in the hospital, as we take the time to encourage and allow both the mother and father to talk about their feelings, to cry, to be angry. But further opportunities for expressing feelings must be available following discharge, and a plan for utilizing resources in each family's community should be a part of discharge planning. So acutely do some families feel this need that they travel many miles to have the opportunity to talk about their feelings.

Multiple Pregnancy

Approximately 1 in 90 births in the United States is a twin birth. The frequency of triplets is roughly 1 in 90 births and of quadruplets 1 in 90 births. The use of "fertility drugs" (Chapter 6) has somewhat increased the frequency of multiple births in recent years.

Twins, the most common multiple births, are more commonly born to black women (1 of 39 births) than to white women (1 of 54 births). Multiple births are more frequent as maternal age increases.

Monozygotic and Dizygotic Twins

Monozygotic twins, often called identical twins, occur when a single fertilized ovum divides to form two embryos at an early stage of development. Monozygotic twins will thus have the same genetic make-up, the same sex, and the same blood type and will be very similar in physical appearance. About one-third of twins are born monozygotic; the ratio of monozygotic twins to all births is similar throughout the world.

Dizygotic twins, often called fraternal twins, result when two eggs are fertilized. These twins have no more in common than siblings born at different times. They may or may not be of the same sex.

The frequency of dizygotic twins varies with ethnic group and maternal age. The tendency for multiple ovulation is governed by genotype, and thus dizygotic twins tend to recur in families.

It is not always possible to tell at the time of birth if twins are monozygotic or dizygotic. If there is a single placenta, amnion, and chorion, the twins are definitely monozygotic. But monozygotic twins may have two placentas and membranes. If the twins are of different sexes, they must be dizygotic, but dizygotic twins may also be of the same sex.

Prenatal Diagnosis of Multiple Birth

Not every multiple pregnancy is diagnosed prenatally. There are some indications during the prenatal period (see Nursing Care Plan 13–11). The uterus may be larger than expected for the gestational age or the rate of growth more rapid. Palpation may be difficult, but it may be possible to feel two heads or an excessive number of small parts. Two fetal heart rates may be heard.

When multiple pregnancy is suspected, ultrasound techniques may reveal two or more gestational sacs as early as the tenth week.

Intrauterine Development

The intrauterine environment is not necessarily identical for twin fetuses. Placental exchange may vary, with one twin receiving less than the other. Recently we saw a twin weighing approximately 700 grams while his brother weighed over 2500 grams. In all cases of disparate size the smaller twin is particularly at risk of hypoglycemia (Chapter 23) following birth.

In monozygotic twins with a circulatory connection between the two placentas, twin-to-twin transfusion occurs about 15 per cent of the time. The donor twin will be pale at birth and may be stillborn. Twin-to-twin transfusion is suspected in identical twins with a difference in hemoglobin levels of more than 5 grams per 100 ml.

Hydramnios is ten times as frequent in twin pregnancies as in single pregnancy, but often only one sac is involved.

When the combined weight of the fetuses reaches 7 to 8 pounds (about 32 weeks' gestation in twin pregnancies and even earlier when there are three or more fetuses), fetal growth is usually slowed because the placenta cannot nourish the babies adequately.

Antenatal Problems

Classically, the problems of multiple pregnancies have been described in terms of six *P's*: prematurity, pre-eclampsia, pressure, primary anemia, placenta previa, and postpartum hemorrhage. A seventh *P,* psychosocial concerns, is also significant.

Many of the psychosocial problems of the high risk mother described earlier in this chapter are applicable. She often recognizes that twins are premature and may be ill. One mother who knew she was to deliver twins wanted to see the intensive care nursery rather than the newborn nursery when she toured the hospital, because she expected her babies

to be there (they were). She also planned to attend Lamaze classes during the second trimester, in anticipation of restricted activity and early delivery during the third trimester.

Although each pregnant woman ponders her adequacy as a future mother, the mother expecting more than one infant often has appropriately heightened concerns about how she will be able to care for more than one baby.

The opportunity to talk with another mother who has twins (some communities have formed groups of mothers with twins) may be helpful. Increased costs, beginning with a potentially longer period of hospitalization and extending ad infinitum, will be a worry for many families and will make financial counseling desirable.

Pregnant Women Who Are Abused

The abuse of a woman by her male partner (legal husband, common-law husband, or cohabitee) was rarely discussed in the professional literature until the past decade. Research now indicates that woman-abuse is a health and social problem of great dimension. Conservative estimates are that over a million wives are battered each year. Strauss[49] applied the incidence rate from a national survey to the 47 million couples living in the United States and estimated the incidence at 1.8 million women each year. Women from all social and economic classes are abused.

Although empirical data are limited, pregnancy and the early postpartum months appear to be a period in a woman's life when abuse may escalate. Other women report less abuse during pregnancy; in one study a woman reported that she deliberately stayed pregnant to avoid violence.[19] Pregnancy is also a period when many battered women are in closer contact with health-care providers than during other periods of their lives.[50]

Pregnant women who are battered are high risk maternity patients both physiologically and psychologically (Nursing Care Plan 13–12). Physiologically, the abdomen becomes a frequent target; resulting abdominal trauma may lead to antepartum hemorrhage and premature labor. Gelles[15] quotes one woman: "Oh yea, he hit me when I was pregnant. It was weird. Usually he just hit me in the face with his fist, but when I was pregnant he used to hit me in the belly. It was weird."

Psychologically, women who are battered are likely to suffer loss of self-esteem, insecurity, loss of trust, and anger, among other feelings. Combined with feelings of vulnerability

Text continued on page 400

Nursing Care Plan 13–11.   Multiple Pregnancy

NURSING GOALS:
To ensure optimum care for the mother with more than one fetus through early identification and care designed to meet special needs.
To assist the woman and her family in understanding and coping with the modifications her condition requires and her feelings about multiple pregnancy.

OBJECTIVES:
1. Multiple pregnancy will be identified in the prenatal period.
2. Risk factors associated with multiple pregnancy will be identified and appropriate intervention will occur.
3. Attachment to two or more infants will develop.

ASSESSMENT	POTENTIAL NURSING DIAGNOSIS	NURSING INTERVENTION	COMMENTS/RATIONALE
Carefully assess length of gestation through dating, ultrasound.	High risk pregnancy related to multiple gestation Risk of prematurity related to multiple gestation	Explain need for careful dating of pregnancy; traditional methods (e.g., fundal height) are less accurate. Activity may be restricted, particularly in third trimester.	Ultrasound as early as 10 weeks may reveal multiple gestation. Mean duration of pregnancy: single: 280 days twins: 260 days triplets: 246 days quadruplets: 238 days
Assess hemoglobin, hematocrit.	Risk of anemia related to increased fetal demand for iron and folic acid	Dietary counseling: increase protein, supplemental iron, vitamins, folic acid.	
Carefully assess signs of pre-eclampsia: 1. Edema 2. Excessive weight gain	Risk of pre-eclampsia related to multiple gestation	See Nursing Care Plan 13–7 for care of mother with pre-eclampsia.	Pre-eclampsia occurs in 20 per cent of all twin pregnancies (4 times the incidence of singleton pregnancies)

3. Hypertension 4. Proteinuria			
Maternal sensations of pressure, particularly in last trimester	Discomfort to increased pressure	Suggest frequent changes of position, small frequent feedings rather than large meals, positioning of pillows to support uterus during rest. Instruct woman to report spotting or bleeding promptly.	Increased uterine size and increased incidence (10 times) of hydramnios lead to pressure.
Vaginal bleeding	Risk of bleeding related to placenta previa; at risk of placenta previa because of large area of placental attachment		
Feelings about multiple gestation pregnancy	Anxiety related to increased risk of complications in pregnancy, labor, and birth, and risk of prematurity. Anxiety related to ability to care for more than one infant (economic, emotional, physical aspects of care)	Encourage verbalization of concerns. Provide information about support groups in community (e.g., Mothers of Twins). Provide information or refer to appropriate source for financial counseling.	Financial needs may be increased by prenatal hospitalization for infants as well as costs of two infants.
Effect of multiple gestation pregnancy on family relationships		Include family in discussions of prenatal needs, anticipatory guidance.	
Desired method of feeding	Need for information about breast-feeding twins, if breast-feeding desired	Provide information about breast-feeding twins. Explain that milk supply equals demand. Provide contact with mother who has breast-fed twins successfully.	

Nursing Care Plan 13–12.   The Pregnant Woman Who May Be Abused

NURSING GOALS:
To provide an environment in which an abused pregnant woman will seek and receive help for problem related to abuse as well as pregnancy-related care.

OBJECTIVES:
In addition to the care given all pregnant women, a woman who is abused will:
1. Be identified.
2. Discuss abuse with her prenatal nurse.
3. Seek specialized help from individuals or agencies that specialize in helping women with problems of abuse.
4. Form an attachment with her infant.
5. Have a realistic plan for care of herself and her infant.

ASSESSMENT	POTENTIAL NURSING DIAGNOSIS	NURSING INTERVENTION	COMMENTS/RATIONALE
1. Physical signs of abuse: a. Hemorrhage b. Bruises c. Broken bones d. Abdominal trauma e. Burns (cigarette, liquid)	Abused woman Loss of self-esteem related to abuse Fear related to abuse	Provide privacy to explore suspected abuse with nurse woman trusts. Be patient; do not expect "instant" sharing. Provide continuity of care from primary nurse to build trust.	Woman may not initially discuss abuse because of shame, fear.
2. Psychosomatic signs of abuse: a. Chest pains b. Gastrointestinal symptoms c. Headache	Physical symptoms secondary to tension related to abuse	Provide information about community resources for abused women. Provide for specialized assistance as necessary (e.g., financial, nutritional).	

Assessment	Nursing Diagnosis	Intervention	Rationale
3. Prenatal attachment 　a. Acceptance of pregnancy 　b. "Nesting" behavior	Lag in attachment secondary to abuse	Follow-up failure to keep prenatal appointments. Provide opportunities for woman to verbalize feelings about self and infant. Document and communicate assessment of abuse and attachment to nurses providing intrapartum, postpartum care.	When self-concern is intense, it may be difficult to focus on fetus.
4. Willingness of abusing partner to consider counseling		Explore possibility of counseling for abusing partner. Provide information about resources available in community.	
5. Intrapartum, postpartum assessment 　a. Maternal attachment 　b. Family interaction 　c. Interaction of partner and infant	Lag in attachment	Facilitate attachment by opportunities for holding and care-giving. Provide referral to appropriate community resources for abused women. Ensure follow-up by community health nurse and Department of Social Services to provide assessment and support into early childhood.	Men who abuse their partners may also abuse their infants.

that may be heightened by pregnancy, battered pregnant women are very much in need of support.

The causes of family violence in general and wife abuse in particular appear to be multifaceted. No single factor accounts for violence in all situations. During pregnancy, possible causes of escalation in violence include sexual tension and frustration and the strain of pregnancy or impending parenthood, particularly when the pregnancy is unwanted. An abused mother stated: "Our problem was getting married and having a baby so fast . . . that produced a great strain. . . . I wasn't ready and he wasn't ready. I had the baby 6 months after we were married."[15]

Some wife abuse may be considered a form of prenatal child abuse. For wives who choose to remain with their abusing mate, there is also a potential for child abuse as well. The tensions caused by a baby with 24-hour needs may precipitate violence toward the wife, baby, or siblings by the husband, and also child abuse by the mother.

During any phase of childbearing, nurses may identify an abused woman by physical signs or by somatic symptoms related to tension (which may be due to factors other than abuse, of course). When abuse is suspected, an opportunity for privacy may enable the mother to talk with a nurse about the problem. Many abused mothers are reluctant to talk about abuse because of shame or fear; these mothers must first develop trust in a professional, which takes time.

The long-term counseling needed by abused wives requires referral to resources with specialized experience. In many communities crisis shelters as well as counseling services are available. Since the decision to seek counseling is an important step for the abused woman, many resources require the woman to make the contact herself. We can, however, make her aware of the resources and the process through which she can make contact.

Not every abused woman will affirm abuse, nor will every woman who affirms abuse seek counseling, at least initially. A woman may feel that occasional abuse is less threatening than being without her partner during pregnancy and childbirth. Unfortunately, there are fewer resources for abusing men.

A nurse who sees the mother prenatally and can develop a trusting relationship may, over time, be able to encourage her and perhaps the abusing spouse to seek counseling. Close follow-up of the infant after birth as well as the mother is important in the prevention or early detection of possible child abuse.

Maternal Alcoholism

The effects of alcohol on the fetus and newborn have been described in Chapter 8. Frequently, alcoholism is not recognized in pregnant women for a variety of reasons. Denial is probably important. The woman does not recognize the possibility that she may be, or is becoming, an alcoholic. Health professionals are also reluctant to recognize drinking in young women as well as in teenagers, in whom alcohol consumption is increasing.

Drinking may actually increase during pregnancy. For some women the stress of pregnancy or fears about approaching parenthood may justify increased drinking. For other women the need to "keep up" with boyfriend or husband, business associates, and other peers "in spite of" pregnancy may lead to intensified drinking.

Alcohol compromises maternal nutrition by interfering with the absorption and utilization of a number of nutrients and with the synthesis of proteins. The alcoholic woman is frequently malnourished before she becomes pregnant and may continue to be malnourished during pregnancy. Because thiamine is metabolized at an accelerated rate, the need for that vitamin is increased. Alcoholic women often have iron deficiency or macrocytic anemia. A high protein–high iron diet, appropriate for the woman with iron deficiency anemia, also aids in preventing growth retardation. Folic acid is the therapy for macrocytic anemia. Increased intake of vitamin C enhances therapy in both anemias.

A careful history of alcohol intake over the course of pregnancy is obviously important. Particularly when a woman indicates that she uses alcohol, changes in patterns of use should be assessed periodically throughout pregnancy. Providing information on fetal alcohol syndrome may be helpful, but it is unlikely that most women who are alcoholic will be able to stop drinking on the basis of such information alone. Referral to professionals skilled in the counseling of alcoholic persons will probably be necessary for the alcoholic gravida.

The Mother Addicted to Drugs (Street Drugs or Hard Drugs)

It is difficult to document the exact number of pregnant women who are addicted to street or hard drugs. At one New York City hospital (Metropolitan Hospital Center in East Harlem), Salerno[43] reported that 1 birth in 29 was to an addicted mother in 1973. There are other hospitals in the United States where an addicted mother is seldom if ever admitted. Chambers and Hunt[5] propose the following generalizations:

1. Drug use of all types seems to be increasing in all parts of the country and among all segments of the population.

2. The rate of increase is higher among women than men, and among young people.

Thus, women of childbearing age are among those most at risk for drug abuse, and, indeed, the use of drugs by pregnant women appears to be increasing significantly throughout the country.

Much of the research on addiction during pregnancy has been directed toward the woman addicted to heroin or on methadone maintenance. As noted in Chapter 8, most drug users take more than one drug.

Heroin-addicted women frequently do not seek prenatal care (Nursing Care Plan 13–13). Salerno[43] estimated that less than 15 per cent of these women receive adequate prenatal care (defined as six or more visits), and 75 per cent have none at all. There are probably several reasons for this. Intense drug dependency, in which a need for a "fix" every 3 to 4 hours is followed by a period of lethargy, does not allow these women to cope with clinic or office schedules. Attention is focused not on the pregnancy but on the drug need. Second, because irregular periods are common in heroin-addicted women, the gravida may not even realize that she is pregnant until several periods have been missed. Moreover, there is a common misconception that heroin use protects one from pregnancy. (Methadone appears to influence the ovulatory cycle less frequently.)

Passivity has been described as a characteristic of addicted women. Passivity in relation to birth control leads to pregnancy. Once pregnant, passivity frequently prohibits the evaluation of options such as adoption or termination of pregnancy as well as positive steps toward self-care. In addition, many addicted mothers are unrealistic about their pregnancy and the demands of parenting. Some hope that pregnancy or the new infant will solve their problems just as they hoped that drugs would solve their problems.

Addicted women have multiple health problems, including a high incidence of infectious disease (e.g., hepatitis, vaginal and urinary tract infections, abscesses at injection sites), nutritional deficits, and venereal disease. They are more likely than the general obstetrical population to deliver premature or growth-retarded infants (Chapter 8) and experience toxemia. Many addicted women are anemic; however, because some addicted women have increased erythrocytes, possibly due to stress, hematocrit is frequently not a good indication of nutritional status. Rates of spontaneous miscarriage and stillbirth are high. The infant is not only physically at risk from many of these factors but is also at risk of impaired bonding and neglect. (Further discussion of the newborn is found in Chapter 24.)

Mothers on methadone maintenance generally participate more actively in prenatal care than do heroin-addicted mothers and have a decreased incidence of toxemia. Nevertheless, they share many of the physical and emotional problems of heroin-addicted women.

How do addicted women react to pregnancy? Moriarity[30] found that some were pleased because their ability to "make" a baby contrasted with more common feelings of helplessness. Assurance of femininity, alleviation of loneliness and isolation, the feeling of being needed, and increased respect from consorts were other positive gratifications. On the negative side, other mothers feared that their baby would be addicted and worried about providing both material and emotional support for the infant.

The provision of care for addicted mothers requires cooperation not only within the team concerned for her pregnancy but also with those who can help her addiction problem. Few specialists in maternity care are also specialists in problems of addiction.

If the mother is willing to seek treatment for her addiction, several options are available. The mother using heroin may agree to participate in a methadone maintenance program; pregnancy outcome is usually improved, and for some women this is an incentive to change. She may do it for her baby when she wouldn't do it for herself. Detoxification (i.e., total withdrawal from drugs) is difficult during pregnancy because it is dangerous to the fetus (abortion in the first trimester and meconium aspiration and possible fetal death in the third trimester; see Chapter 8). If detoxification is requested, it is recommended that it be accomplished between the fourteenth and twenty-eighth weeks of gestation at a very slow rate.[11]

Because the addicted woman in labor is a high risk mother, a hospital is the appropriate place for her delivery. Addicted women may delay hospitalization because they fear the lack of access to drugs and the attitudes of staff toward addicted women. If the mother is using methadone, maintenance in the hospital should not be difficult. Providing narcotic therapy to the heroin user is more difficult; methadone is used for these mothers as well, in combination with analgesics to keep the

Nursing Care Plan 13–13.   Caring for the Pregnant Woman Addicted to Drugs

NURSING GOALS:
1. To provide an environment that encourages the woman addicted to drugs to participate in prenatal care and hospital delivery.
2. To encourage decision-making by the mother about keeping or relinquishing her baby and about realistic plans for infant care.
3. To facilitate attachment and care-giving behavior in drug-dependent mothers who plan to keep their babies.
4. To encourage the drug-dependent mother to seek help for her drug habit.

OBJECTIVES:
The drug-dependent gravida will be identified and will receive consistent prenatal care, beginning in the first trimester.
1. Utilize support services, including drug counseling.
2. Have concurrent health problems corrected (e.g., venereal disease, anemia).
3. Deliver in hospital.
4. Form an attachment with her infant and participate in infant care.
5. Have a realistic plan for care of herself and her infant following discharge.

ASSESSMENT	POTENTIAL NURSING DIAGNOSIS*	NURSING INTERVENTION	COMMENTS/RATIONALE

1. Prenatal assessment as for all pregnant women; particular attention paid to nutritional status, anemia, venereal disease, other infectious disease, EDC
2. Assess drug use
  a. History of drug use
  b. Current use
  c. Urine testing for drug at intervals during pregnancy
	Risk of complications (premature labor, intrauterine growth retardation, pregnancy-induced hypertension, miscarriage, stillbirths) is related to drug use.	Provide basic care as for all pregnant women; consider flexibility in scheduling.
		Provide specialized intervention as indicated from assessment:
		  a. Intensive dietary counseling
		  b. Food supplements (WIC) if eligible
		  c. Iron therapy for anemia
		  d. Treatment of venereal disease
		
		Refer for counseling and treatment of drug habit.
			EDC may be difficult to assess in heroin-addicted women because of irregular menses.
			Flexible scheduling may increase visits in women who cannot cope with rigid schedules.
			Some mothers may participate in treatment for the baby's sake.

3. Assess knowledge of pregnancy and effects of drug use.
4. Assess social/emotional status:
  a. Feelings about this pregnancy (planned, desired, fear for infant)
  b. Relationship with infant's father
  c. Plans for infant care
  d. Economic needs
  e. Support system
	Need for information about drug use and pregnancy	Provide information about relation of drug use and pregnancy.
		Provide opportunities to describe feelings about pregnancy.
		Refer to social worker for help with specific economic and social needs.	

5. Assess fetal growth and well-being (see Nursing Care Plan 14–1).
6. Assess knowledge of labor.

Fetus at risk for prematurity, intrauterine growth retardation

Need for information about labor; specific information about care of women using drugs during labor and postpartum

Explain reason for testing (see Chapter 14).

Provide information about hospital care of drug-dependent woman in labor (e.g., methadone maintenance)

Provide labor/delivery and postpartum nurses with health history, prenatal teaching record, woman's expectations about medication.

Drug-dependent women may avoid hospital for fear of withdrawal or staff attitudes.

In some communities maintenance therapy may not be immediately available without advance notice.

Intrapartum Period

1. Identify drug-dependent woman in labor.
   a. From prenatal history
   b. Possible signs
      (1) Limited or no prenatal care
      (2) Evidence of drug injection
2. Assess extent of prenatal care.
3. Assess current drug use:
   1. Type of drug
   2. Time of last use
   3. Dosage
4. Assess emotional status: may fear withdrawal more than labor.
5. Assess for complications that may affect fetus or mother during labor
   1. Anemia
   2. Infectious diseases, including venereal disease
   3. Preterm labor
   4. Intrauterine growth retardation
   5. Drugs currently in maternal system
   6. Pregnancy-induced hypertension
   7. Fetal malpresentation
   8. Abruptio placentae or placenta previa

Drug-dependent woman in labor

Reassure mother of support of staff; prevent withdrawal symptoms during labor through administration of methadone or other drugs. Provide pain relief.

Risk for fetal complications related to (specific factors).

Provide continuous fetal assessment; provide careful maternal assessment.

Continued on following page

Nursing Care Plan 13–13.   Caring for the Pregnant Woman Addicted to Drugs (Continued)

ASSESSMENT	POTENTIAL NURSING DIAGNOSIS*	NURSING INTERVENTION	COMMENTS/RATIONALE
	Puerperium		
1. Assess physical status of mother and infant. (See Nursing Care Plan 24–15 for care of infant of mother addicted to drugs; Chapter 25 for physical assessment of mother.) In addition, assess drug-related symptoms in mother and infant.	Behavior (specific) related to drug dependence	Encourage hospital stay of at least 3 to 5 days to provide opportunities for attachment, assessment of attachment, development of plans.	Drug-dependent woman may try to leave shortly after delivery. The supportive attitude of nurses is essential to prolong stay.
		Encourage good nutrition.	
		Prevent withdrawal symptoms through administration of methadone or other medication.	
		Provide ice packs and other comfort measures to relieve engorgement if not breast-feeding.	
		Encourage mother to participate in infant's care. Demonstrate infant's unique characteristics.	Mother must be able to focus on infant's needs to become competent caregiver.
2. Assess attachment and caretaking behavior (see also Nursing Care Plan 22–1). a. Feeding and other caretaking behaviors b. Naming infant c. Positive and negative comments about infant d. Hugs, kisses, smiles e. Response to infant crying	Infant at risk for neglect or abuse related to mother's drug dependence Lag in attachment	Provide information about infant development; provide opportunity to discuss feelings about self and body.	Unrealistic expectations are one factor in infant abuse.
3. Assess plans for self and infant. a. Relationship with infant's father b. Support system c. Economic needs d. Contraceptive counseling	Lack of realistic plans for care of self and infant Need for contraception	Refer to drug counseling if not currently in counseling and agreeable to woman. Ensure continuing health supervision by public health nurse. Refer to social worker for help with specific economic and social needs. Provide contraceptive counseling realistic for woman's lifestyle before discharge from hospital. Refer to family planning agency for follow-up.	

mother comfortable. Nurses may be uncomfortable with providing narcotics to an addicted mother; we must remember that withdrawal at this time can cause serious distress and possible death to the fetus.

Problems that are increased in addicted mothers include maternal and fetal infection, premature rupture of membranes, toxemia, placenta previa and abruptio placentae, and malpresentation.

Following delivery, many addicted mothers sign out of the hospital as soon as possible. Assurance that withdrawal symptoms will be prevented by medication and a supportive attitude from staff may convince the mother to remain for several days. This will provide the opportunity to assess withdrawal symptoms in the baby, facilitate initial bonding, and plan for follow-up after discharge. (Withdrawal symptoms of methadone do not appear until 4 to 12 days after birth; see Chapter 24.)

Most addicted women do not choose to breast-feed; since both heroin and methadone cross into breast milk, breast-feeding is not recommended. Nursing measures to relieve the discomfort of engorgement (Chapter 25) plus medication are appropriate.

Contraceptive counseling must be highly individual. Sufficient motivation for effective use of contraceptives is frequently lacking. Oral contraceptives may be contraindicated because of liver disease, phlebitis, or other concurrent health problem. The frequency of venereal disease makes an intrauterine device a problem for many women.

Maternal-infant attachment and the need for long-term intervention are discussed in Chapter 24.

Perinatal Regionalization

In this chapter's discussion of the needs of high risk mothers and their infants, hopefully it is obvious that optimum care for these mothers involves intensive professional nursing coordinated with medical care; a laboratory that is immediately available 24 hours a day, 7 days a week; and other supportive services.

This level of care is not available at every hospital in the United States, nor should it be. Even if it were possible to provide highly sophisticated care at every community hospital and outpatient clinic in order to serve one or two high risk mothers each month, the cost would be prohibitive and unwarranted.

The concept of regionalization is a strategy to provide each family with the level of maternity care they need in the most effective way.

The goal of regionalization is reduction in maternal and perinatal mortality and morbidity. Originally, regionalization developed as a neonatal program, transferring small or sick newborns from community hospitals to medical centers for specialized care. It is on this basis that regionalization exists in several states today.

It is increasingly apparent, however, that transfer of a high risk mother to a regional center in advance of delivery may prevent complications and reduce perinatal mortality and morbidity. Thus the concept of *perinatal regionalization,* rather than neonatal regionalization, is the goal of many states during the next decade.

Plans for regionalization vary somewhat from state to state, but the basic features are similar. A number of regions are designated within the state, taking population, geography, traditional patterns of care, and other factors into consideration. Within each region one center offers highly specialized inpatient and outpatient care for the most critically ill mothers and infants. This center (sometimes called a regional center or a Level III center) is also active in perinatal education for the entire region and in perinatal research. Level II or district centers offer an intermediate level of care for many complications of both the period of pregnancy and the neonatal period. Level I centers, usually located in smaller communities, care for mothers and infants without complications.

Implementing this concept is no easy task. Nurses, social workers, nutritionists, administrators, obstetricians, pediatricians, and consumers must work together to plan and coordinate regionalization on both state and regional levels.

Many issues must be faced:

Financial Support. Upgrading the quality of care costs money—money for equipment, money for additional professional personnel, money to help alleviate the very high cost of maternal and neonatal intensive care, and money for transportation for high risk mothers and infants from the communities in which they live to the regional or district center best able to serve them.

What are the sources for these large amounts of money?

(1) *Health and medical insurance:* Some types of health insurance do not provide coverage for newborn or high risk maternal care. State laws can be revised to require the inclusion of such benefits.

(2) *Public funds:* Federal, state, and local governments can have a direct influence on

the availability and quality of care through the budgeting of tax dollars. Although this expense is costly if one looks only at immediate expenditures, over a period of years there may be a saving, not only in human terms but even in terms of actual dollars. The cost of prenatal and newborn care, even the cost of high risk neonatal care, which may be as high as $50,000 to $100,000 for a baby, is still far lower than the cost of lifelong institutionalization for a severely mentally retarded individual. Actual cost figures will vary from one state to another but can be compiled as a part of the effort to convince legislators at all levels of government of the value of perinatal care.

(3) *Private funds:* Both national and local foundations, philanthropic organizations, and service clubs have in the past been, and continue to be, valuable resources for equipment purchases, for the sponsorship of educational seminars, and for a variety of other types of support. Often a single specific purchase, such as an infant warmer for a delivery room or nursery or a modern transport incubator for use in transferring a sick infant to a medical center, can significantly improve the quality of care. Nurses can effectively explain such needs to community lay groups.

The members of community organizations who understand perinatal needs are also very helpful in supporting perinatal requests to governing bodies, such as state legislatures.

Availability of Nurses with Special Education in the Care of Mothers and Infants. Without an adequate number of nurses who have had, and continue to have, special education in the care of mothers and infants, quality of care cannot improve. The most sophisticated transport incubator is of little value if there is no nurse to accompany the baby or if the nurse is not adequately prepared to care for a very sick infant.

This is a nursing problem that can only be solved by nurses themselves. The basic problem of numbers of nurses is beyond the scope of this book. Continuing education needs can be met in a variety of ways. Because many community hospitals do not have staff adequate to provide continuing education, regional planning is essential. The opportunity for clinical experience as well as for lectures and discussions in the field of continuing education is valuable. In one type of plan, nurses from community hospitals may spend 1 day each week for a specific number of weeks at a regional center, the day being divided between clinical practice and classroom discussion.

A second type of program allows nurses from community hospitals to spend a specific number of weeks at a regional center, again with both clinical and classroom experience.

Nursing internship programs offer opportunities for beginning practitioners to acquire specialized knowledge and skills. More extensive programs to prepare nurse clinicians, clinical nurse specialists, and certified nurse midwives must be evaluated. Nurses with this type of advanced training play an essential role in high quality care (see Chapter 30).

Both nurses in regional centers and nurses in community hospitals and health agencies must work together to plan and implement educational programs that meet their educational needs.

Continuing Education for Other Health Professionals. Although we have emphasized nursing education, continuing education for physicians, nutritionists, and all those who care for childbearing families is essential. Interdisciplinary programs meet a part of this need.

Establishment of Mechanisms for Coordinating Regionalization. Each state and region will coordinate regional activities in a somewhat different manner.

Summary

A team approach is essential to the care of high risk mothers and their families. Nurses join with nutritionists, social workers, and physicians to meet the physical, social, and emotional needs of this group of parents.

REFERENCES

1. Biggs, J.: Pregnancy at 40 Years and Over. *Medical Journal of Australia,* 1:542, 1973.
2. Bjerkedal, T., Bahna, S., and Lehmann, E.: Course and Outcome of Pregnancy in Women with Pulmonary Tuberculosis. *Scandinavian Journal of Respiratory Disease,* 56:245, 1975.
3. Butnarescu, G., Tillotson, D., and Villarreal, P.: *Perinatal Nursing: Reproductive Risk.* Volume 2. New York, John Wiley, 1980.
4. Cavanaugh, D., and Knuppel, R.: Preeclampsia and Eclampsia. *In* Iffy, L., and Kaminetsky, H. (eds.): *Principles and Practice of Obstetrics and Perinatology.* New York, John Wiley, 1981.
5. Chambers, C., and Hunt, L.: Drug Use Patterns in Pregnant Women. *In* Rementeria, J. (ed.): *Drug Abuse in Pregnancy and Neonatal Effects.* St. Louis, C. V. Mosby, 1977.
5a. Chandra, R.: Fetal Malnutrition and Postnatal Im-

munocompetence. *American Journal of Disease of Children, 129*:450, 1975.

5b. Chandra, R., Ali, S., and Kutty, K.: Thymus-Dependent Lymphocytes and Delayed Hypersensitivity in Low Birth Weight Infants. *Biology Neonate, 31*:15, 1977.

6. Chesley, L.: *Hypertensive Disorders in Pregnancy.* New York, Appleton-Century-Crofts, 1978.

7. Cohen, W., Newman, L., and Friedman, E.: Risk of Labor Abnormalities with Advancing Age. *Obstetrics and Gynecology, 55*:414, 1980.

8. Committee on Perinatal Health: *Toward Improving the Outcome of Pregnancy.* White Plains, N.Y., The National Foundation–March of Dimes, 1976.

9. Costrini, N., and Thompson, W.: *Manual of Medical Therapeutics.* 22nd Edition. Boston, Little, Brown & Co., 1977.

10. Elder, H. A., et al.: The Natural History of Asymptomatic Bacteriuria During Pregnancy: The Effect of Tetracycline on Clinical Course and Outcome of Pregnancy. *American Journal of Obstetrics and Gynecology, 111*:441, 1971.

10a. Ferguson, A., Lawlor, G., Neumann, C., et al.: Decreased Rosette-Forming Lymphocytes in Malnutrition and Intrauterine Growth Retardation. *Journal of Pediatrics, 85*:717, 1974.

10b. Ferguson, A.: Impairment of Cellular Immunity with Intrauterine Growth Retardation. *Journal of Pediatrics, 93*:52, 1978.

11. Finnegan, L., Schut, J., Flor, J., et al.: Methadone Maintenance and Detoxification Programs for the Opiate-Dependent Woman During Pregnancy: A Comparison. *In* Rementeria, J. (ed.): *Drug Abuse in Pregnancy and Neonatal Effects.* St. Louis, C. V. Mosby, 1977.

11a. Fox, 1977

12. Galloway, K.: The Uncertainty and Stress of High Risk Pregnancy. *MCN, 1*:294, 1976.

13. Gant, N., Worley, R., Cunningham, F., et al.: Clinical Management of Pregnancy-Induced Hypertension. *Clinical Obstetrics and Gynecology, 21(2)*:397, 1978.

14. Gant, N., Chand, S., Worley, R., et al.: A Clinical Test Useful for Predicting the Development of Acute Hypertension in Pregnancy. *American Journal of Obstetrics and Gynecology, 120*:1, 1974.

15. Gelles, R.: *The Violent Home.* Beverly Hills, Sage Publications, 1974.

16. Gluck, J., and Gluck, P.: The Effects of Pregnancy on Asthma: A Prospective Study. *Annals of Allergy, 37*:164, 1976.

17. Greenhill, J., and Friedman, E.: *Biological Principles and Modern Practice of Obstetrics.* Philadelphia, W. B. Saunders Co., 1974.

18. Gusdon, J., Anderson, S., and May, W.: A Clinical Evaluation of the "Roll-over" Test for Pregnancy-Induced Hypertension. *American Journal of Obstetrics and Gynecology, 127*:1, 1977.

19. Hilberman, E., and Munson, K.: Sixty Battered Women. *Victimology, 2*:460, 1977–1978.

20. Hobel, C. J.: Recognition of the High Risk Woman. *In* Spellacy, W. N. (ed.): *Management of the High Risk Pregnancy.* Baltimore, University Park Press, 1976.

21. Harger, G., and Smythe, A.: Pregnancy in Women Over Forty. *Obstetrics and Gynecology, 49*:257, 1977.

22. Jasper, M.: Pregnancy Complicated by Diabetes—A Case Study. *MCN, 1*:307, 1976.

23. Josimovich, J.: Endocrine Disorders and Pregnancy. *In* Iffy, L., and Kaminetsky, H. (eds.): *Principles and Practice of Obstetrics and Perinatology.* New York, John Wiley, 1981.

24. Kessler, I., Lancet, M., Borenstein, R., et al.: The Problem of the Older Primipara. *Obstetrics and Gynecology, 56*:165, 1980.

25. Kitzmiller, J.: The Endocrine Pancreas and Maternal Metabolism. *In* Tulchinsky, D., and Ryan, K. (eds.): *Maternal-Fetal Endocrinology.* Philadelphia, W. B. Saunders Co., 1980.

26. Kowalski, K., and Osborn, M.: Helping Mothers of Stillborn Infants to Grieve. *MCN, 2*:29, 1977.

27. Malkaslan, G.: Respiratory Diseases and Pregnancy. *In* Iffy, L., and Kaminetsky, H. (eds.): *Principles and Practice of Obstetrics and Perinatology.* New York, John Wiley, 1981.

28. Mocarski, V.: Asymptomatic Bacteriuria—A "Silent" Problem of Pregnant Women. *MCN, 5(4)*:238, 1980.

29. Moore, D., Bingham, P., and Keesling, O.: Nursing Care of the Pregnant Woman with Diabetes Mellitus. *JOGN Nursing, 10(3)*: 188, 1981.

30. Moriarity, J.: *The Psychological Understanding and Treatment of the Pregnant Drug Addict.* Proceedings of the Third National Drug Abuse Conference, New York, 1976.

31. Morrison, T.: The Elderly Primigravida. *American Journal of Obstetrics and Gynecology 121*:465, 1975.

32. Naeye, R.: Causes of the Excessive Rates of Perinatal Mortality and Prematurity in Pregnancies Complicated by Maternal Urinary Tract Infections. *New England Journal of Medicine, 300*:819, 1979.

33. Naeye, R.: Factors in the Mother/Infant Dyad that Influence the Development of Infections Before and After Birth. *In Perinatal Infections.* Ciba Foundation Symposium 77. New York, Excerpta Medica, 1980.

34. Nesbitt, R., and Aubry, R.: High Risk Obstetrics. Value of a Semiobjective Grading System in Identifying the Vulnerable Group. *American Journal of Obstetrics and Gynecology, 103*:972, 1969.

35. *Nomenclature and Criteria for Diagnosis of Diseases of the Heart and Blood Vessels.* 5th Edition. New York, The New York Heart Association, 1955.

36. O'Sullivan, J. B., and Mahan, C.: Criteria for the Oral Glucose Tolerance Test in Pregnancy. *Diabetes, 13*:278, 1964.

37. Page, E., Villee, C., and Villee, D.: *Human Reproduction: The Core Content of Obstetrics, Gynecology and Perinatal Medicine.* 3rd Edition. Philadelphia, W. B. Saunders Co., 1981.

38. Pardue, S.: Hydatidiform Mole: A Pathological Pregnancy. *American Journal of Nursing, 77*:836, 1977.

39. Perimutter, J.: The Pregnant Drug Addict in Labor. *In* Rementeria, J. (ed.): *Drug Abuse in Pregnancy and Neonatal Effects.* St. Louis, C. V. Mosby, 1977.

40. Petit, M.: Battered Women: A (Nearly) Hidden Social Problem. *In* Getty, C., and Humphreys, W. (eds.): *Understanding the Family: Stress and Change in American Family Life.* New York, Appleton-Century-Crofts, 1981.

40a. Prechtl, H.: Neurological Sequelae of Prenatal and Perinatal Complications. *British Medical Journal, 4*:763, 1967.

41. Reedy, N.: *Trauma During Pregnancy.* Presentation at Workshop on Obstetrical-Gynecological Emergencies, Cook County Graduate School of Medicine, October 5, 1981.

42. Ross, S., Naeye, R., Du Plessis, J., et al.: The Genesis of Amniotic Fluid Infections. *In Perinatal Infec-*

tions. Ciba Foundation Symposium 77. New York, Excerpta Medica, 1980.

43. Salerno, L.: Prenatal Care. *In* Rementeria, J. (ed.): *Drug Abuse in Pregnancy and Neonatal Effects.* St. Louis, C. V. Mosby, 1977.

44. Sammons, L.: Battered and Pregnant. *MCN, 6:*246, 1981.

45. Seebode, J., Kamat, M., and Apuzzio, J.: Urinary Tract Infections in Pregnancy. *In* Iffy, L., and Kaminetsky, H. (eds.): *Principles and Practice of Obstetrics and Perinatology.* New York, John Wiley, 1981.

46. Soichet, S.: Emotional Factors in Toxemia of Pregnancy. *American Journal of Obstetrics and Gynecology, 77:*1065, 1959.

47. Spellacy, W. N. (ed.): *Management of the High Risk Pregnancy.* Baltimore, University Park Press, 1976.

48. Stembera, Z., Zezvlakova, J., and Ditrichova, J.: Srovnani Vlivu Nekterych Faktorv Rizikoveho Teho-

tenstvi na Perinatalni Mortalitv a Morbiditv. *Cesk Gynekol, 40(6):*401, 1975.

49. Straus, M.: Wife Beating: How Common and Why? *Victimology, 2:*443, 1977–1978.

50. Walker, L.: *The Battered Woman.* New York, Harper & Row, 1979.

51. Wallach, J.: *Interpretation of Diagnostic Tests.* 3rd Edition. Boston, Little, Brown & Co., 1978.

52. Webster, H. D., Barclay, C., and Fischer, C.: Ectopic Pregnancy: A 17-Year Review. *American Journal of Obstetrics and Gynecology, 92:*23, 1965.

53. Wheeler, L., and Jones, M.: Pregnancy-Induced Hypertension. *JOGN Nursing, 10(3):*212, 1981.

54. White, P.: Pregnancy and Diabetes, Medical Aspects. *Medical Clinics of North America, 49:*1015, 1965.

55. White, P.: Classification of Obstetric Diabetes. *American Journal of Obstetrics and Gynecology, 130:*228, 1978.

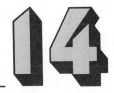

The Prenatal Family: Assessment of the Fetus

During the prenatal period, in addition to maternal and parental assessments described in Chapters 10 to 13, the condition, growth, well-being, and maturity of the fetus must be evaluated. Traditionally, the height of the uterine fundus has been used as an estimate of fetal growth, and the position of the fetus and the fetal heart rate have been evaluated in all pregnant women. These assessments continue to be an essential part of prenatal care. For certain women, additional evaluation is of great benefit. Although not all of these additional techniques involve nursing assessment, it is often from nurses that mothers seek information and reassurance. Additional techniques of fetal assessment are used primarily when mothers are identified as being at risk because of factors either in their reproductive history or in their present pregnancy. Table 14–1 lists the techniques and Nursing Care Plan 14–1 lists the goals and objectives of fetal assessment.

Basic Fetal Assessment

Abdominal Palpation

Because the assessment of both fundal height and fetal position requires abdominal palpation, basic principles of palpation are described first. The woman's bladder should be empty; this is more comfortable for her and aids in palpation of fetal structures, which are beneath the bladder. Relaxation of the abdominal muscles is aided by the use of relaxation

Table 14–1.   FETAL ASSESSMENT

Basic Assessment
  Fundal height
  Fetal outline (last trimester)
  Fetal heart rate
Additional Assessment as Indicated
  Before 20 weeks gestation
    Amniotic fluid for chromosomal or genetic
      abnormalities
    Amniotic fluid or serum for alpha-fetoprotein
    Fetoscopy
    Ultrasound
  After 20 weeks gestation
    Amniocentesis (bilirubin, L/S, creatinine,
      PG)
    Hormones in blood and urine
    Assessment of daily fetal movement
    Antepartum fetal heart rate (NST, CST)

techniques (Chapter 11), the calm manner and warm hands of the examiner, and explanations of each step of the examination. It is helpful to put a pillow under the woman's head or to keep her head elevated and her knees slightly bent to avoid stretching the abdominal muscles, thereby making them more tense (Fig. 14–1).

Fundal Height

After the thirteenth week pregnancy, abdominal palpation will ascertain the *height of the fundus*. To palpate the fundus, stand facing the woman's head with hands on both sides of the uterus. Using gentle pressure, with the

Text continued on page 416

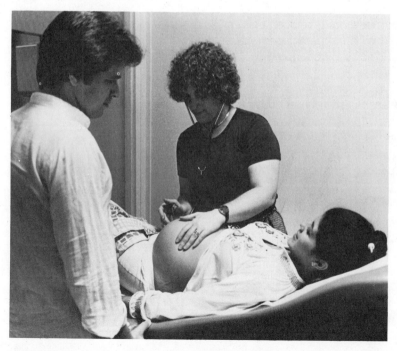

Figure 14–1. A nurse is using abdominal palpation to assess fundal height and fetal position. Note that the woman's head is elevated so that some of the strain is taken off her abdominal muscles, making palpation easier. (Courtesy of the Maternity Center Association, New York. Photography © by Raimondo Borea.)

Nursing Care Plan 14–1.   Nursing Care During Prenatal Assessment of the Fetus

NURSING GOALS: 1. To assess fetal growth and fetal heart rate in every gestation.
2. To further assess fetal well-being and fetal maturity in mothers at risk.

Objectives:
1. Fundal height will be assessed at every prenatal visit after the thirteenth week.
2. Fetal heart rate will be assessed at every prenatal visit following initial assessment at approximately 20 weeks.
3. Fetal position (lie) will be assessed in the third trimester.
4. Gravidas who may benefit from additional fetal testing will be identified.
5. Gravidas and families will understand the purpose of additional fetal testing, and will have any possible risks explained.
6. Gravidas and families will understand the results of fetal testing.

ASSESSMENT	POTENTIAL NURSING DIAGNOSIS	NURSING INTERVENTION	COMMENTS/RATIONALE
		Basic Assessment for All Gravidas	
Fundal height after 13 weeks: measure from symphysis pubis to top of fundus with tape measure.	Fundal height not consistent with gestational age. When fundal height is less than expected, at risk for intrauterine growth retardation. When fundal height is greater than expected, at risk for multiple gestation, hydramnios, hydatidiform mole, etc. Incorrect calculation of length of gestation by dates.	Explain reason for measurement of fundal height. Have measurements done by same person (if possible) throughout course of pregnancy to provide consistency. When measurements are inconsistent with gestational age. 1. Reevaluate gestational age; review history, last menstrual period, first fetal heart tones, first fetal movement. 2. Possible referral for ultrasound evaluation of gestational age. 3. Evaluate possible intrauterine growth retardation, multiple gestation, other causes for variation in fundal height.	
Fetal heart rate (FHR) (normal range, 120–160 beats per minute)		Note carefully *first* time fetal heart tones heard by Doppler (approximately 10 weeks) and stethoscope (or fetoscope), approximately 20 weeks). Provide opportunity for gravida, family to hear fetal heart tones.	Hearing heart tones confirms the reality of the fetus and may facilitate prenatal attachment.

Continued on following page

Nursing Care Plan 14–1.   Nursing Care During Prenatal Assessment of the Fetus (*Continued*)

ASSESSMENT	POTENTIAL NURSING DIAGNOSIS	NURSING INTERVENTION	COMMENTS/RATIONALE
	Basic Assessment for All Gravidas (*Continued*)		
Fetal lie and presentation (after 30 weeks gestation). Use Leopold's maneuvers (see text). Note engagement of presenting part.	Need for information about significance of fetal lie and presentation.	If lie continues to be transverse throughout third trimester, prepare parents for possible Cesarean delivery.	Although the benefits of this exercise are unproven in a controlled study, the experience of clinicians suggests it may be helpful and is not harmful.
		If presentation is breech, suggest the following exercise: gravida lies on her side with hips elevated on two pillows for 20 minutes, two times a day (never immediately following meals).	
Utilize serum alpha-fetoprotein (AFP) to screen for neural tube defects (NTD) at 16–18 weeks' gestation (not available in all areas).	Need for information about NTD screening.	Explain purpose of NTD screening; offer screening to gravida if available.	
		Requires sample of maternal blood; no risk to mother.	
	Anxiety related to elevated serum AFP.	If serum AFP is elevated, refer for further testing (repeat serum AFP, ultrasound evaluation, amniotic fluid AFP). Anticipate parental anxiety; provide opportunities for verbalization of fears; support during time they are waiting for results of tests.	Elevated serum AFP may indicate: 1. Neural tube defect 2. Abortion 3. Intrauterine fetal death 4. Multiple gestation 5. Miscalculation of length of gestation
	Additional Fetal Assessment for Mothers Identified at Risk		
Amniocentesis 1. Determine gravida's and family's understanding of: a. Reason *this* woman is having amniocentesis b. The procedure c. The information that will be derived d. When the information will be available e. Risks f. Discomfort g. Possible sequelae	Need for information about amniocentesis as it relates to individual fetal health.	Provide information as indicated under assessment. Remain with gravida to provide support throughout process. Assist in relaxation, focusing, and slow breathing. Explain that she may have lower abdominal cramping following amniocentesis.	Reasons for amniocentesis: 1. Prior to 20 weeks gestation: testing for chromosomal or genetic disorders. 2. After 20 weeks gestation: testing for bilirubin (in mother with Rh antibodies), evaluation of fetal maturity. Probability of risk: 1 per cent

2. Identify gravida who is Rh negative and is not sensitized.		Provide Rh-immune globulin to Rh negative mother not previously sensitized.	
Fetoscopy (not widely available) Determine gravida's and family's understanding (see above, under amniocentesis).	Need for information about fetoscope as it relates to individual fetal health.	As in amniocentesis	Reasons for fetoscopy: diagnosis of specific disorders.
Ultrasound examination Determine gravida's and family's understanding.	Need for information about ultrasound as it relates to individual fetal health.	Explain process: Mother should have a full bladder; ask her to drink 8 oz. water every 15 minutes beginning 1½ hours prior to test. During ultrasound evaluation, point out fetal structures (e.g., head, heart beating, etc.).	Reasons for ultrasound: 1. Evaluation of gestational age 2. Identification of specific disorders of fetus or placenta 3. Localization of placenta Seeing fetus during ultrasound evaluation may promote prenatal attachment.
Estriol studies 1. 24-hour urine specimen	Fetal maturity and well-being reflected in estriol levels.	1. Explain reason for urine collection and instruct regarding importance of collecting *all* urine voided during the 24 hours. 2. Provide container for specimen collection. 3. If gravida is not hospitalized, be sure she knows where to bring specimen and has transportation available at the appropriate time.	
2. Serum studies	Need for information about studies.	Explain reason for serum studies to determine estriol levels.	
Assessment of daily fetal movement	Need for information about self-assessment of daily fetal movement.	Provide information about reason for assessment. Explain how to do the assessment. Use written information to supplement oral discussion. Provide chart for her use. Provide phone number for her to call if she becomes confused after returning home.	Because this assessment is carried out entirely by the gravida herself, it is essential that she clearly understand the process.

Continued on following page

Nursing Care Plan 14-1.   Nursing Care During Prenatal Assessment of the Fetus (Continued)

Additional Fetal Assessment for Mothers Identified at Risk (Continued)

ASSESSMENT	POTENTIAL NURSING DIAGNOSIS	NURSING INTERVENTION	COMMENTS/RATIONALE
Antepartum fetal heart rate monitoring 1. Nonstress test (NST) Evaluate FHR in relation to fetal movement: a. Reactive: FHR more than 15 beats per minute for 15 sec two times in a 10-minute period b. Nonreactive: Above criteria unmet	Need for information about purpose, process of NST.	1. The purpose of this test and the procedure are explained to the mother. The mother is told she will be given a button to push each time she feels her baby move, and that the fetal heart rate will be recorded by the monitor. 2. The mother signs a consent form. 3. The mother lies in a semi-Fowler's position or in lateral tilt with her right hip elevated 3 to 4 inches to avoid supine hypotensive syndrome. 4. A fetal heart monitor is applied. 5. Maternal blood pressure should be assessed intitially and at frequent intervals throughout the procedure. 6. The mother is observed for 20 minutes or until two to five fetal movements have occurred. 7. If no fetal movements are observed in 20 minutes, the mother is observed for a second 20-minute period. Fetal movements may be induced by giving the mother a snack with readily available glucose. 8. If test is still nonreactive, mother may be referred for contraction stress test (CST). 9. The results of testing are explained.	If spontaneous uterine contractions occur during NST, note response of FHR. NST requires from 10 to 40 minutes. Glucose in the maternal blood-stream crosses the placenta and the fetus becomes active in response.

2. Contraction Stress Test (CST)
   Evaluate fetal heart rate in
   response to contractions:
   a. Negative: no late
      decelerations
   b. Positive: repetitive late
      decelerations
   c. Equivocal: occasional but not
      repetitive decelerations
   d. "10-minute window"—a
      period of 10 minutes that
      satisfies requirements of
      either negative or positive
      test; reduces the number of
      equivocal tests.
   e. Unsatisfactory: failure to
      stimulate sufficient uterine
      contractions or inadequate
      FHR data

Need for information about
purpose, process of CST.

1. The purpose of this test and the
   procedure are explained to the
   mother.
2. The mother signs a consent
   form.
3. The mother lies in a semi-
   Fowler's position or in lateral tilt
   with her right hip elevated 3 to 4
   inches to avoid supine
   hypotensive syndrome.
4. The fetal heart monitor is applied.
5. Maternal blood pressure is
   assessed initially and at frequent
   intervals throughout the
   procedure.
6. Intravenous infusion is started;
   low-dose oxytocin by infusion
   pump is "piggy-backed" into IV.
   The initial rate is 0.5 to 1.0
   milliunit per minute.
7. Oxytocin dose is increased,
   usually every 10 minutes, until
   there are three 40-second
   contractions in a 10-minute
   period.
8. Oxytocin is discontinued when
   the criterion of three contractions
   in 10 minutes has been met, and
   the mother is observed until
   contractions are at least 10
   minutes apart.
9. The results of the test are
   explained.

If mother finds contractions
uncomfortable, encourage
relaxation, focusing, breathing to
cope with contractions.
CST requires approximately 90
minutes.

Oxytocin is discontinued if any
contraction lasts longer than 90
seconds.

FHR recording:
   Negative: no late
      decelerations—indicative of
      fetal well-being
   Positive: repetitive late
      decelerations—indicative of
      fetal or placental problems
   Equivocal: occasional but not
      repetitive late decelerations;
      repeat test may need to be
      done after 24 hours.
   "10-minute window" (see text)
   Occasionally the oxytocin
      stimulus triggers onset of
      labor.

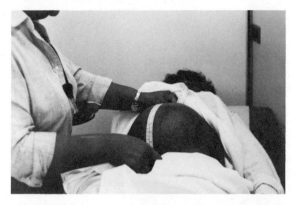

Figure 14–2. Nurse practitioner uses a tape measure to measure the distance from the top of the symphisis pubis to the top of the fundus (fundal height).

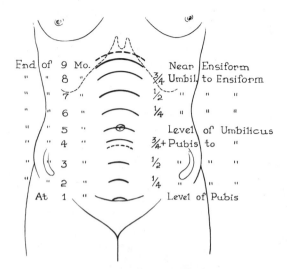

Figure 14–3. The relative level of the fundus of the gravid uterus during each successive month of pregnancy according to Bartholomew's "rule of fourths." Beginning with the uterus at the level of the pubis at the end of the first month of pregnancy, it is expected to grow one quarter of the way to the umbilicus each month until the fifth month (with slight positive variation from the dotted line at the end of the fourth month) and one quarter of the remaining distance to the ensiform process (with slight negative variation in the last month) during each succeeding month. (From Greenhill and Friedman: *Biological Principles and Modern Practice of Obstetrics*. Philadelphia, W. B. Saunders Co., 1974.)

palms of the hand and the fingers close together, palpate the abdomen upward until the hands meet at the fundus. The distance from the top of the symphysis pubis to the top of the fundus is usually measured by a tape measure stretched across the contour of the abdomen (Fig. 14–2). After 22 to 24 weeks' gestation, the number of centimeters should approximate the number of weeks of gestation. Calipers may be used to measure this distance; they are probably more accurate but also more cumbersome. It is important to use the same method consistently with each woman. Because the measurement varies even when different examiners use the same method, the most accurate assessment is achieved when the same professional assesses fundal height at each prenatal visit. This is particularly important when the fundal height varies from the norm (see below). An approximation of the correlation of fundal height with the duration of pregnancy is known as Bartholomew's "rule of fourths," which describes the uterus as being at the symphysis pubis at the end of the first month, one-quarter of the way to the umbilicus each successive month, at the level of the

umbilicus at the end of the fifth month (20 weeks), and then one-quarter of the distance of the ensiform process at the end of each of the following months (Fig. 14–3). There may be a slight drop in the height of the fundus in the ninth month as the time of delivery approaches. This method of evaluation is considered less accurate than measurement with a tape measure because the distances between symphysis, umbilicus, and xyphoid vary widely in different women.

When the height of the fundus does not

Table 14–2. A COMPARISON OF GESTATIONAL AGE, FUNDAL HEIGHT, AND FETAL WEIGHT

Gestational Age (Weeks Since First Day, Last Menstrual Period)	Approximate Fundal Height (Position)	Approximate Fundal Height (cm.)	Approximate Weight (g.)
12	Level of symphysis pubis	—	10
16	Halfway between symphysis and umbilicus	10	80
20[a]	Slightly below umbilicus	20	360
24	1 to 2 fingers above umbilicus	24	630
28	Halfway between umbilicus and xyphoid	28	1050
32	3 to 4 fingers below xyphoid	32	1700
36	1 finger below xyphoid	36	2500
40	2 to 3 fingers below xyphoid[b]	34	3400

[a]Fetal heart tones often first audible by stethoscope.
[b]Fundus is lower if lightening has occurred.

correlate with the mother's menstrual dates, the duration of pregnancy may need to be reevaluated. Ultrasound measurements (see below) may give additional information.

A more rapid increase in fundal height than would ordinarily be expected may indicate multiple pregnancy (e.g., twins); excess amniotic fluid (hydramnios), which in turn may be caused by one of several factors (Chapter 13); the presence of tumors or a hydatidiform mole (Chapter 13); or internal hemorrhage, as in abruptio placentae (Chapter 13).

When the fundal height is lower than expected, possibilities such as intrauterine growth retardation, a transverse lie (Chapter 15) death of the fetus, fetal abnormality, or decreased amniotic fluid (oligohydramnios) must be considered. Table 14–2 compares gestational age, fundal height, and approximate fetal weight.

Fetal Position (Leopold's Maneuvers)

By 30 weeks the fetal outline is also palpable. Note in Figures 14–4 through 14–8 that palpation is done with the fingers and palms and not with the fingertips.

In palpating for fetal position, first palpate the fundus as described above (Fig. 14–4). If you feel a hard, smooth, round body, this is likely to be the fetal head. If you feel an irregularly shaped structure, this is very likely the breech, i.e., the fetal buttocks and legs.

Verify your assessment by ascertaining what structure is over the inlet (Fig. 14–5). In either instance the fetus is said to have a *longitudinal lie* (Chapter 15). If neither the head nor the breech can be palpated, the lie is said to be *transverse;* one must palpate the head and breech at the sides of the uterus (Fig. 14–6).

After 32 weeks, most commonly the breech will be felt in the fundus, and the lie will be longitudinal.

When the lie is ascertained, the position of the fetal spine and "small parts" (hands and feet) may be felt (Fig. 14–7).

Next check for *engagement* of the *presenting part*. Engagement means that the largest section of the presenting part of the fetus has passed the pelvic inlet and entered the true pelvis. This usually occurs as time for delivery approaches. The extent of engagement can be determined by placing both hands on the presenting part (Fig. 14–8) and trying to move the part from side to side. If it is movable, or if the fingers can meet below the presenting part, the part is not engaged.

Fetal Heart Rate

At approximately 20 weeks, fetal heart rate (FHR) or fetal heart tones (FHT) can be heard by fetoscope (Fig. 14–9). (As noted in Chapter 7, FHR may be heard as early as 10 weeks by Doppler effect.) After the fetal outline is determined, FHR is best heard at the position of

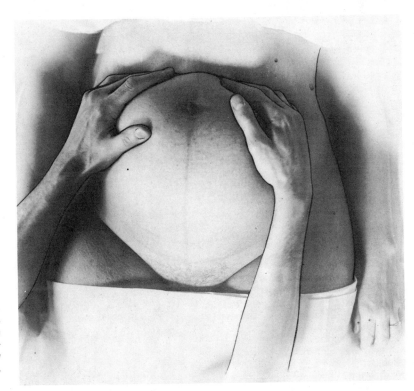

Figure 14–4. What is in the fundus? Palpation of the uterine fundus will disclose the presence of the breech or the head. (From Greenhill and Friedman: *Biological Principles and Modern Practice of Obstetrics.* Philadelphia, W. B. Saunders Co., 1974.)

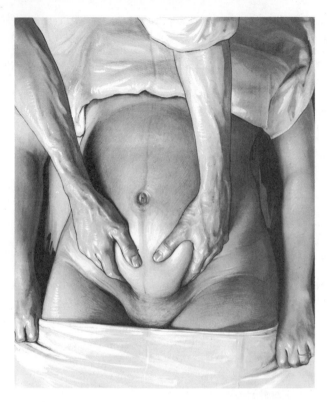

Figure 14–5. What is over the inlet? By pressing deeply into the pelvis on either side, one learns whether the hard fetal head or soft breech is presenting. (From Greenhill and Friedman: *Biological Principles and Modern Practice of Obstetrics*. Philadelphia, W. B. Saunders Co., 1974.)

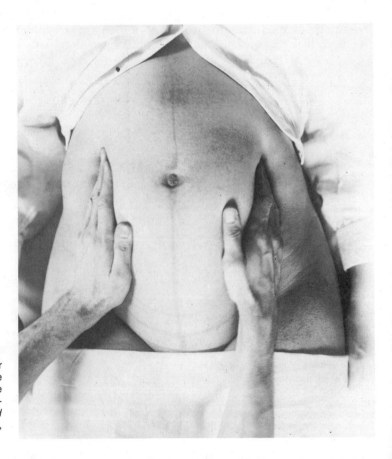

Figure 14–6. Is the ovoid longitudinal or transverse? Facing the patient's head, the nurse applies her hands to the sides of the uterus to determine the fetal lie. (From Greenhill and Friedman: *Biological Principles and Modern Practice of Obstetrics*. Philadelphia, W. B. Saunders Co., 1974.)

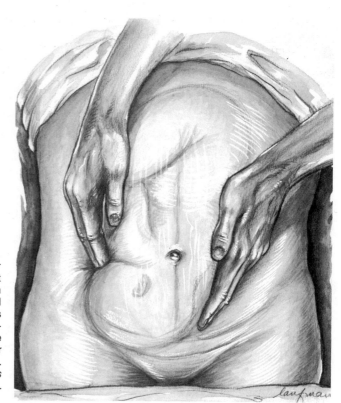

Figure 14–7. Method of determining the greater cephalic prominence, here shown on the mother's right side. As both hands are passed along the abdomen toward the pelvis, one is impeded by the fetal forehead and the other one descends until the occiput is reached. The forehead is the greater cephalic prominence in well-flexed vertex presentations, but in face and brow presentations, the occiput is the greater cephalic prominence because the head is deflexed. (From Greenhill and Friedman: *Biological Principles and Modern Practice of Obstetrics.* Philadelphia, W. B. Saunders Co., 1974.)

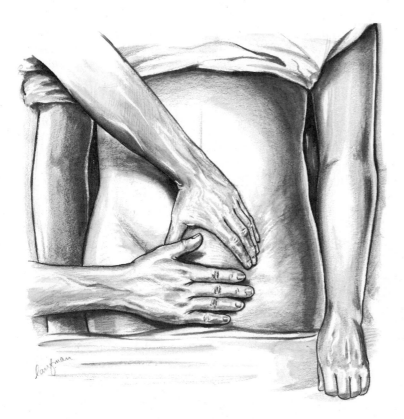

Figure 14–8. A method of determining overriding of the head. The head is grasped with one hand and pushed down toward the pelvic cavity, while with the other hand over the symphysis pubis, it is determined whether the head sinks into the pelvic cavity or overrides the symphysis. (From Greenhill and Friedman: *Biological Principles and Modern Practice of Obstetrics.* Philadelphia, W. B. Saunders Co., 1974.)

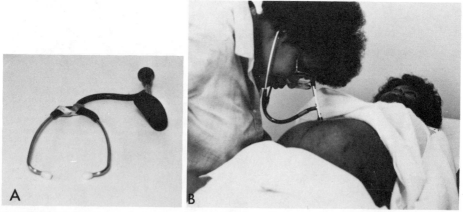

Figure 14–9. *A*, Fetoscope. *B*, A nurse practitioner using the fetoscope to determine the fetal heart rate.

the anterior shoulder. FHR is approximately 140 beats per minute with a normal range of 120 to 160 beats per minute. The FHR can be differentiated from the maternal heart rate by checking the mother's pulse simultaneously. The quadrant on the mother's abdomen where FHR is heard, as well as the rate, may be recorded as shown here.

$$\overline{145}\,\Big|$$

This indicates that a FHR of 145 is heard in the right lower quadrant.

The assessment of fetal heart rate offers a good opportunity to encourage bonding between parents and fetus by allowing the mother, and the baby's father if he is present, to listen to the baby's heart beat. Parents will say, "It makes the baby seem so much more alive and real." With the Doppler (Fig. 14–10) fetal heart tones can be heard many weeks before the mother feels the baby move (at 18 to 20 weeks). A Doppler can be available in childbirth education classes for the purpose of allowing couples to hear the fetal heart tones.

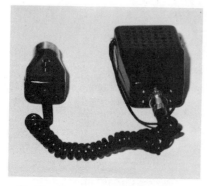

Figure 14–10. Portable Doppler, used to hear the fetal heart tones and determine the fetal heart rate.

Often the father has had no other opportunity for this experience if he has not accompanied the mother for her prenatal check-ups.

The assessment of fetal heart rate is helpful in confirming the gestational age of the fetus. The *first* time the fetal heart is heard by Doppler or by fetoscope should be recorded on the mother's chart. Later in pregnancy, if there is concern about the gestational age of the fetus, this information can be most helpful.

Further Assessment of the Fetus

In many pregnancies, the assessment techniques just described will be adequate to ensure both health-care providers and parents that the fetus is growing normally and is healthy. Prior to the twentieth week of pregnancy, additional fetal assessment is done principally for the purpose of detecting abnormalities in the fetus so that the parents may choose to terminate the pregnancy if a fetal defect is discovered. Methods of assessment are amniocentesis, maternal blood sampling, fetoscopy, and ultrasonography. After 20 weeks additional fetal assessment is done to determine fetal well-being and assess fetal maturity.

Assessment Prior to 20 Weeks' Gestation

Amniocentesis

The term amniocentesis is derived from the Greek words *amnion* (sac), the inner lining of the fetal membranes, and *kentesis* (puncture). Amniocentesis may be done in the clinic or the office; hospitalization is not required.

Common reasons for amniocentesis prior to 20 weeks include detection of chromosomal defects (e.g., Down's syndrome) or genetic de-

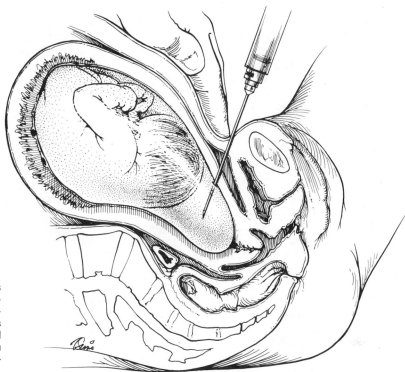

Figure 14–11. Amniocentesis late in pregnancy, performed suprapubically. During amniocentesis approximately 10 ml. of amniotic fluid is withdrawn. (From Pritchard and MacDonald: *Williams Obstetrics*, 16th Edition. New York, Appleton-Century-Crofts, 1980.)

fects (e.g., inborn errors in metabolism) or neural tube defects.

Amniocentesis involves the withdrawal of amniotic fluid from the intrauterine sac surrounding the baby. Before the procedure is carried out, the placenta is located by means of ultrasonography so that it can be avoided when the needle is inserted. In addition, ultrasonography aids in the identification of any uterine abnormality, such as a bicornuate uterus, that might complicate amniocentesis.

After the site is chosen, the abdominal skin is prepared with an iodine solution, and a local anesthetic is injected into the skin surrounding the site. Approximately 10 to 15 ml. of amniotic fluid is withdrawn through an 18- or 20-gauge spinal needle (Fig. 14–11). This volume of fluid is replaced within 3 to 4 hours following amniocentesis by newly formed amniotic fluid. Maternal blood pressure and fetal heart rate are checked before and after the procedure.

When considering the possibility of amniocentesis, parents most frequently ask: will it be uncomfortable for the mother, and will it hurt the baby, perhaps even causing a miscarriage?

The major maternal discomfort occurs during the injection of local anesthetic. Maternal anxiety can be relieved by helping the mother use relaxation techniques such as focusing and slow breathing (see Chapter 11). Some women experience cramps in the lower abdomen in the hours immediately following amniocen-

tesis. Women should be told in advance that this discomfort may occur.

The *potential* risks of amniocentesis for the fetus include miscarriage, fetal injury, infection, subsequent leakage of amniotic fluid, and Rh sensitization of the mother, which can jeopardize the fetus. In a prospective study evaluated by the National Institute of Child Health and Human Development,[15a] no significant difference was found in the rate of fetal loss between 1040 women who had amniocentesis and 922 matched controls who did not. There was no case of fetal injury. The probability of risk is considered to be less than 1 per cent.

Although amniocentesis is not advocated for mass screening, it is considered a safe diagnostic procedure when family history or maternal age suggests that there may be a potential problem.

When amniocentesis is performed on a mother who is Rh_D negative, the administration of anti-D immunoglobulin (RhoGAM) following the procedure is currently recommended to prevent possible sensitization.

The Detection of Chromosomal Abnormalities. Amniotic fluid cells grown in culture can be karyotyped (Chapter 3) to detect chromosomal abnormalities (such as Down's syndrome) approximately 3 weeks after the amniocentesis is performed. In a competent laboratory, accurate prediction rates are very high. Because the risk of Down's syndrome increases significantly with maternal age, many physicians and clinics now routinely screen mothers over 35 years old in the fourteenth to fifteenth week of pregnancy.

Timing is important in relation to the successful growth of the amniotic fluid cells in culture. Because of the 3-week time period necessary for cell growth and because the mother may choose abortion should the test show the fetus to have Down's syndrome, the test is not usually performed much later in pregnancy than the fourteenth to fifteenth week.

Chromosomal Studies to Detect Sex. Although many parents may wonder about the sex of their coming child, for those mothers known to be carriers of X-linked recessive traits, the baby's sex is especially important. Daughters will not inherit the condition (certain types of muscular dystrophy or hemophilia, for example) but sons have a 50:50 chance of inheritance (Chapter 3). Amniotic fluid studies to identify the fetal sex may be important to these parents.

The Detection of Genetic Defects. Cultured cells from amniotic fluid are used to detect the presence or absence of certain enzymes and thereby to predict such inborn errors of metabolism as galactosemia. Early detection combined with early treatment can prevent deleterious side effects.

Blood Sampling and Amniocentesis for Detection of Alpha-Fetoprotein. In 1972 Brock and Sutcliffe[3] first recognized that the level of alpha-fetoprotein (AFP), a protein produced by the yolk sac and the fetal liver, is as much as eight times higher when the fetus has an *open* neural tube defect (NTD) as when there is a closed NTD. The most common open defects are spina bifida (a congenital defect in which the vertebral canal does not close properly) and anencephaly (a congenital absence of the cerebrum and cerebellum). AFP moves from the fetal serum to the fetal cerebrospinal fluid and then through the open lesion into the amniotic fluid. When there is a closed defect of the neural tube, such as hydrocephalus (a condition in which there simply is an increased volume of cerebrospinal fluid), AFP does not enter the amniotic fluid. With an open NTD the level of AFP in amniotic fluid increases until 15 weeks' gestation and then decreases until term; hence, studies are done at 14 to 16 weeks' gestation.

Alpha-fetoprotein may be detected in blood or in amniotic fluid. In a large collaborative study done in the United Kingdom (1977),[14] serum studies were 79 per cent accurate in predicting myelomeningocele and 88 per cent accurate in predicting anencephaly. Screening for AFP is not widespread at this time in the United States, where many practitioners still consider the procedure experimental. Large studies are currently in progress. In the future mass serum screening for AFP may become a routine aspect of prenatal care.

Screening for neural tube defects by amniocentesis is a highly reliable procedure. Milunsky[15] reports experience with more than 14,000 pregnancies in which 110 neural tube defects were detected and none were missed. The false positive rate (i.e., diagnosing a neural tube defect when none is present) was below 0.1 per cent.

Amniocentesis for the detection of NTD is reserved for women who have previously delivered an infant with this anomaly or who have a positive serum AFP. Because the probability of risk from amniocentesis, even though less than 1 per cent, is greater than the risk of having a child with a NTD (approximately 0.2 per cent for women in general), the procedure is inappropriate for mass screening. In normal adults, serum AFP levels are very low; AFP from fetal sources, however, can be detected in maternal blood after the tenth week of pregnancy, with maximum levels between 16 and 18 weeks. Maternal blood for AFP testing is drawn at this peak time.

Elevated AFP levels may be related to factors other than an open NTD. Abortion, intrauterine fetal demise, and multiple gestation are recognized causes. False positive results are relatively common. When serum AFP is elevated, further evaluation is necessary before an open NTD can be confirmed; included in this evaluation are a repeat of the serum AFP analysis, ultrasound evaluation, and amniocentesis.

Fetoscopy for Confirmation of Suspected Fetal Problems

Fetoscopy is an experimental procedure in which a fetoscope is introduced into the amniotic cavity through the abdominal wall. Depending on the preference of the examiner, ultrasound examination to locate the fetus and placenta is done before or during the procedure. Fetoscopy is used at present for fetal blood sampling, fetal skin sampling, and direct visualization of the fetus.

The seventeenth week of pregnancy is the preferred time for fetoscopy, since the procedure is difficult to perform before this time. Examination during the seventeenth week allows 3 weeks for cell growth before re-examination (with therapeutic abortion, if indicated) in the twentieth week.

Prior to fetoscopy, the mother may be given Demerol, which will cross the placenta and quiet the fetus, because excessive fetal activity makes the procedure more difficult.

Fetal blood sampling permits the diagnosis of sickle cell anemia, beta-thalassemia (a type of hemolytic anemia), and hemophilia in the fetus as well as certain immunologic disorders, including Rh incompatibility. Fetal skin biopsies may indicate the presence of certain primary skin disorders such as ichthyosis, a condition in which the skin is harsh and dry with adherent scales. Through direct visualization, the diagnosis or confirmation of certain severe malformations such as NTD is possible.

Fetoscopy is available almost exclusively in large medical centers. It is a technically difficult procedure and is not without risk. As in amniocentesis, spontaneous abortion is possible following the procedure; stillbirth is a less common occurrence. Amnionitis has also occurred as a complication; prophylactic antibiotics may be used for 10 days following examination to prevent it.

Ultrasonography

Ultrasound is based on the piezo electric effect; sound too high to be heard causes the movement of crystals, generating electrical impulses. These impulses are directed toward the surface tissue and reflect back onto a screen, where a photograph of the tissue (a visualization of the reflection of the ultrasonic impulses) may be taken (Fig. 14–12B).

Different body tissues reflect sound waves in different ways, and thus as the sound waves "bounce off" or echo from different tissues, they cn be captured and displayed on an oscilloscope and, if desired, preserved permanently in Polaroid photographs.

Through ultrasonography, the fetus can be observed within the uterus approximately 5 weeks after the last menstrual period; with certain techniques, the beating of the fetal heart can be observed as early as 6 to 7 weeks.

Two types of ultrasound are used in fetal

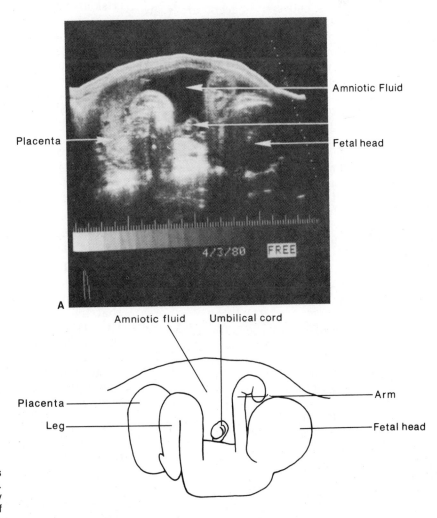

Figure 14–12. *A*, Fetus as seen on ultrasound at 32 weeks. (Ultrasound and photography by Dr. Lewis Nelson.) *B*, Outline of fetus seen in ultrasound photograph in *A*.

Table 14–3.   USES OF REAL TIME ULTRASOUND

Biparietal diameter
Crown-rump length
Placental localization
Fetal presentation
General screening for congenital anomalies
Prior to amniocentesis
Multiple gestation
Early signs of fetal life (after 9 weeks)
Early absence of fetal life
Bleeding (e.g., possible placenta previa)
Pelvic masses

assessment—real time and gray scale (B-scan) (Tables 14–3, 14–4). Real time is used most frequently; it is rapid, portable, and inexpensive in both initial cost and maintenance and is therefore less expensive to the patient. It is possible with real-time scanning to observe movement during the later stages of pregnancy, including cardiac and respiratory movements as well as fetal thumb-sucking. The chief disadvantage of real-time sonography is that distinctions between adjacent areas are difficult to make.

Many mothers say that seeing their baby move on the screen, perhaps sucking a thumb, makes the baby seem very real to them. Mothers are frequently given pictures of their fetuses made by ultrasound impressions after the examination. In one study using real-time scanning, many mothers reported a heightened sense of attachment; some mothers who feared fetal loss worried about this increased attachment to the fetus they might lose.[12]

A number of fetal anomalies have been diagnosed by ultrasound in the second or third trimester including anencephaly, meningomyelocele, hydrocephaly, renal agenesis and dysplasia, diaphragmatic hernia, gastroschisis, and omphalocele.[10] Current research projects are investigating the results of diagnosis prior to 20 weeks for a variety of conditions including cardiac defects and kidney abnormalities.

Ultrasound may also be used after 12 weeks' gestation to "date" the pregnancy when gestational age is in doubt; dating by measuring the fetal biparietal diameter (Chapter 10) is considered accurate between 12 and 34 weeks'

Table 14–4.   USES OF GRAY SCALE (B-SCAN) ULTRASOUND

Genetic screening
Some instances of placenta previa
Posterior placenta
When real time ultrasound is not available
Observation of gestational sac by 6 weeks
Early localization of the placenta (9 weeks)

gestation.[9] Because of the variability in ultrasound measurement of biparietal diameter, two or more examinations on separate occasions may be obtained. Ultrasound examination is also used to localize the placenta prior to amniocentesis; to diagnose placenta previa; to detect multiple pregnancy, polyhydramnios, and fetal anomalies; and to determine fetal death.

The ultrasound scan is not uncomfortable for the mother. A transducer is moved back and forth across the abdomen; the image is produced on the oscilloscope. Many parents request an explanation of what they are seeing on the oscilloscope.

Unlike many procedures that require a women to empty her bladder before examination, ultrasonography requires a full bladder, which then functions as an amplifier to transmit sounds. Beginning approximately 1½ hours before the test, the woman is asked to drink an 8 ounce glass of water every 15 minutes.

There is apparently minimal chance of any risk associated with ultrasonography. Any procedure must be evaluated in relation to potential fetal risks. The large majority of experiments on animals and human observations do not indicate any harmful or permanent effects from ultrasound used at diagnostic levels. In one study of the outcome of 1952 pregnancies, 303 of which included exposure to ultrasound, no physical or developmental differences were found in exposed or control groups of infants at 1 year of age. It is always possible, of course, that differences might appear at some future time.[22] No research has so far reported any harm from diagnostic ultrasonography.

Pregnancy Termination and Prenatal Assessment

Some diagnostic centers screen for fetal abnormalities, especially when screening involves amniocentesis, only if the parents agree that the pregnancy will be terminated if the fetus is abnormal. Others believe that screening should be offered even if the parents do not agree in advance that the pregnancy will be terminated if an abnormality is found. These workers suggest that (1) finding evidence of normality in the fetus can be reassuring to the parents; (2) if there is evidence of abnormality, parents who choose not to terminate the pregnancy can begin to plan for their infant's special needs; and (3) it is easier to make a decision when all the information is available.

Consider mothers over 40 (over 35 in some centers) who are screened for Down's syndrome. Even with the high probability (1 in

40) of having an infant with Down's syndrome at this age, 39 mothers out of 40 will not be carrying a fetus thus afflicted. Knowing this at 20 weeks' gestation can relieve a great deal of anxiety for parents in this situation. Parents must understand that amniocentesis is specific for the condition under consideration and is not a general test of fetal normality. Ultrasonography is more general but still does not guarantee absolute normality.

Fetal Assessment After 20 Weeks' Gestation

After 20 weeks' gestation fetal assessment is done primarily to evaluate fetal well-being or to determine gestational age prior to interruption of pregnancy because of maternal complications (e.g., PIH, diabetes; see Chapter 13) or prior to an elective cesarean delivery in which gestational age is uncertain. Amniocentesis is one of the most reliable methods of assessment, along with tests that measure the level of certain hormones in maternal urine and blood, maternal evaluation of fetal movement, and antepartum fetal heart rate monitoring.

Amniotic Fluid Studies of Fetal Well-Being

Bilirubin in Amniotic Fluid. Mothers with Rh isoimmunization (Chapter 13) will have a series of amniocenteses during the second half of pregnancy to follow the level of bilirubin pigment in the amniotic fluid. In this way the severity of their disease may be assessed, and the fetus can be identified as having (1) very mild disease or no problem, (2) moderate disease that may necessitate early delivery, or (3) severe disease.

Meconium Staining of Amniotic Fluid. Meconium is not normally present in amniotic fluid. If meconium is present, it is considered a sign of current or previous fetal anoxia that causes the anal sphincter to relax, thus indicating fetal distress.

Blood and Urine Studies of Fetal Well-Being

Estriol Determination. The measurement of estrogens in the urine and maternal blood is one method of determining fetal well-being. During the first 6 to 8 weeks of pregnancy, estrone (E_1) and estradiol (E_2) are produced by the corpus luteum. After the sixth week the corpus luteum begins to regress (Chapter 7), but the levels of estrogens continue to rise as the placenta becomes the producer. Estrogen precursors are produced in the mother's adrenal gland in the first trimester. These precursors are the basic substances from

which estrogen is produced; the principal precursor is dehydroepiandrosterone (DHEA).

In the third trimester, the fetal adrenal glands become a significant source of estrogen precursors; at term the fetal adrenals provide more than 60 per cent of E_1 and E_2 precursors. The placenta secretes E_1 and E_2 into the maternal and fetal circulation. In the maternal bloodstream, E_2 is further metabolized to estriol (E_3) and other estrogens that are excreted in the urine. Estradiol may also undergo further change in the fetal liver to form estetrol (E_4), which is transported to maternal circulation and excreted in maternal urine as estetrol glucuronide.

Because of this physiologic pathway (Fig. 14–13), measurement of estriol (E_3) is thought to be a measure of the activity of the fetal adrenals and thus of fetal well-being.

Estriol in urine is most commonly measured in a 24-hour specimen. When a 24-hour urine specimen is being collected, *all* the urine excreted in 24 hours must be included, or the reported estriol level will be inaccurate. The difficulty in accurately collecting urine for 24 hours and the delay in obtaining information when there is reason to suspect that the fetus is in jeopardy have led to increasing use of serum estriols. A single estriol level is of limited value, but serial estriol levels on consecutive days are helpful. Because E_3 levels normally continue to rise until delivery, a fall in these levels is one indication of fetal distress, especially if that fall is marked.

Estriol levels are not universally useful; they are evaluated along with other criteria described below. Table 14–5 lists some of the factors that may influence estriol levels.

Human Placental Lactogen. Human placental lactogen (HPL), also called human chorionic somatomammotropin (HCS; see page 178) is a hormone produced by the placenta. HPL can be detected in serum as early as the twenty-eighth to thirty-fourth day of pregnancy. Levels rise gradually until the thirty-sixth week of pregnancy. During the remaining weeks, levels tend to remain stable.

In normal pregnancy, values of less than 4 micrograms per 100 ml. are rarely found in the last 10 weeks of pregnancy. When HPL values are low, fetal distress is possible. This possibility is even more likely when other tests, such as estriol levels, also suggest fetal distress. There is evidence that using HPL values to recognize a fetus in distress can lower perinatal mortality.

HPL values can also aid in detecting other problems of both mother and fetus. Values are low in threatened abortion, toxemia, intrauterine growth retardation, and postmaturity.

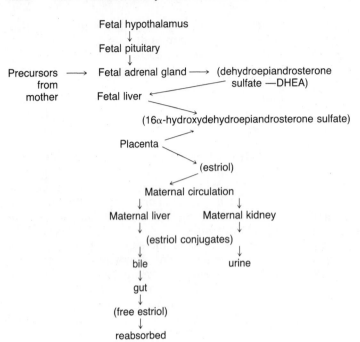

Figure 14–13. The pathway of estriol synthesis. (From Moore: *Newborn, Family, and Nurse,* 2nd Edition. Philadelphia, W. B. Saunders Co., 1981.)

Table 14–5.   FACTORS THAT MAY INFLUENCE ESTRIOL LEVELS IN MATERNAL SERUM AND URINE

Condition	Result	Estriol Level
Fetal anencephaly	Stimulatory portions of the brain absent	↓
Maternal corticosteroid therapy Hypoplasia or aplasia of fetal adrenal gland	Fetal adrenal gland suppressed	↓
Reduced function of placenta (e.g., infarction, growth retardation)	Limitation of conversion ability	↓
Maternal hepatic disease	Impaired estriol conjugation in liver	↓
Ampicillin administration	Decreased gut flora Decreased hydrolyzation and limited reabsorption	↓
Maternal obstructive gallbladder disease	Disturbed enterohepatic circulation; estriol lost in feces	↓
Impaired maternal renal function	Decreased excretion of estriol and decreased estriol levels in urine	↓
Increased fetoplacental size	Increased production of estriol	↑
Rh disease	Hypertrophy of placenta; increased efficiency in conversion of precursor	↑

They may be high in a multiple gestation, maternal diabetes mellitus, Rh sensitization, maternal liver disease, and maternal sickle cell disease.

Assessment of Daily Fetal Movement: The Count-to-10 Chart

Daily fetal movement begins at approximately the eighteenth week of pregnancy, reaches a peak between 29 and 38 weeks, and then decreases slightly until term. When there is marked placental insufficiency, there is a significant decrease in fetal movement that precedes intrauterine fetal death. However, there is a period of time during which fetal movement is decreased but fetal heart rate remains normal. These observations form the basis of the "count-to-10" chart.

The count-to-10 chart (Fig. 14–14) gives the mother an opportunity to help assess the well-being of her fetus. Beginning at 30 to 32 weeks' gestation she is asked to count the number of fetal movements beginning at 9:00 A.M.. When she has counted 10 discrete instances of fetal movement, she marks the time on her chart. If she has not felt 10 fetal movements by 9:00 P.M., she records the number of movements actually felt. If, for 2 days in a row, less than 10 movements are felt for each day, she is to notify her health-care provider, thus assessing her fetal well-being at no expense to either family or health-care system.

Antepartum Fetal Heart Rate Monitoring

In assessing fetal well-being, it is important to know how the fetus will respond to stress, particularly the stress of labor. The development of antepartum fetal heart rate (FHR) monitoring arose from the observation that the fetal heart rate dropped in the fetuses of some women after they had climbed one or more flights of stairs. Observers wondered if the stress involved in climbing stairs diverted blood from the placenta. In Europe, antepartum monitoring focused on spontaneous fetal heart rates, utilizing the nonstress test (NST); in the United States the contraction stress test (CST) was initially employed. The CST is frequently called an oxytocin challenge test (OCT), but this term is not quite accurate because, although oxytocin is usually given to the mother to stimulate uterine contractions, it does not challenge either mother or fetus. At present, NSTs are widely used in the United States as well as in Europe. Antepartum fetal heart rate monitoring is a regular part of the

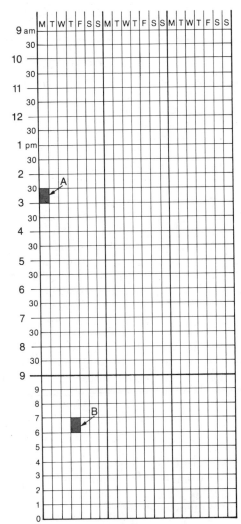

Figure 14–14. A count-to-ten chart. The date and number of weeks gestation are recorded at the top. Each day, starting at 9 A.M., the gravida counts the number of times she feels the fetus move. When she has counted 10 movements, she fills in the appropriate time square (A). If the number of movements felt is less than 10, she fills in the square opposite the exact number in the area below the heavy line (B). If no movements are felt on any day, or if less than 10 movements are felt on two successive days, she is instructed to contact her health-care provider immediately.

care of the many women with the high risk conditions described in Chapter 13.

Nonstress Tests

The NST evaluates a complex response of the fetal central nervous system. Babies born within 7 days of a reactive nonstress test are almost invariably in good health.

An NST is classified as either reactive or nonreactive (Table 14–6). Originally, an NST was considered reactive if, five times within a 20-minute period, the fetal heart rate increased 15 beats per minute or more, and the increased rate (acceleration) lasted for 15 seconds or longer. Now two accelerations of 15 beats for 15 seconds within any 10-minute

Table 14–6. NONSTRESS TESTING (NST) RESULTS*

| | Pattern | |
	Reactive	*Nonreactive*
Accelerations		
Number in 10 minutes	≥2	<2
Duration in seconds	≥15	≤15
Beats per minute	≥15	<15

*From Moore: *Newborn, Family, and Nurse*, 2nd Edition. Philadelphia, W. B. Saunders Co., 1981.

period constitute a reactive test. Failure to meet any of these criteria constitutes a non-reactive test. If no reactive pattern is recorded within 40 minutes, the test is also considered nonreactive. A 40-minute period is used because this is the average duration of the sleep-wake cycle of the fetus, although the cycle can vary considerably. When the fetus appears to be sleeping, stimulation by glucose or sound may induce activity. The result. The result in about two thirds of NSTs is reactive, which is interpreted as indicating fetal well-being.[15b] A false normal test occurs in only 1 per cent of cases, so the nonstress test is considered highly reliable when it is reactive. However, a non-reactive test does not necessarily indicate that the fetus is in jeopardy. When the NST is nonreactive, it is usually followed by a contraction stress test (Fig. 14–15). In one study of 2422 patients, 91 per cent of fetuses with a nonreactive NST also had a negative CST, indicating fetal well-being.[13a]

Directions for Nonstress Test

1. The purpose of this test and the procedure are explained to the mother. The mother is told she will be given a "button" to push each time she feels her baby move, and that the fetal heart rate (FHR) will be recorded by the monitor.

2. The mother signs a consent form.
3. The mother lies in a semi-Fowler's position or in lateral tilt with her right hip elevated 3 to 4 inches to avoid supine hypotensive syndrome (see page 171).
4. A fetal heart monitor is applied.
5. Maternal blood pressure should be assessed initially and at frequent intervals throughout the procedure.
6. The mother is observed for 20 minutes or until two to five fetal movements have occurred.
7. If no fetal movements are observed in 20 minutes, the mother is observed for a second 20-minute period. If they do not occur spontaneously, fetal movements may be encouraged by giving the mother a snack containing readily available glucose. Glucose in the maternal bloodstream crosses the placenta, causing the fetus to become active in response.

Contraction Stress Test

In the contraction stress test (CST) uterine contractions are stimulated, usually by the intravenous administration of oxytocin. The reaction of the fetus to the contractions is assessed by external fetal heart rate monitoring. Results are categorized as negative, positive, equivocal, or unsatisfactory (Table 14–7). If fetal oxygen reserve and placental function are satisfactory, there should be no late decelerations (see Chapter 18 for description of late decelerations) in the fetal heart rate, and the test result is *negative*. In a *positive* CST, repetitive late decelerations occur. If there are occasional but not repetitive late decelerations, the test is considered *equivocal* and is repeated, usually 24 hours later.

Recently, the concept of a "10-minute window"—a period of 10 minutes in which the criteria for either a positive or a negative test should be satisfied—has reduced the incidence of equivocal tests. If an occasional deceleration is followed by 10 minutes in which there are

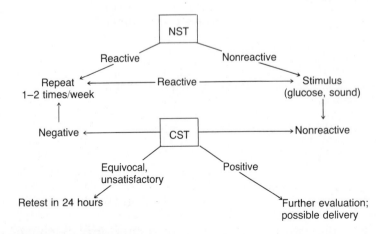

Figure 14–15. Nonstress test and contraction stress test. (From Moore: *Newborn, Family, and Nurse,* 2nd Edition. Philadelphia, W. B. Saunders Co., 1981.)

Table 14–7. CONTRACTION STRESS TESTING (CST) RESULTS*

Pattern	Criteria	Frequency of Occurrence (%)
Negative	Absence of late decelerations in three contractions within 10 minutes	85 to 90
Positive	Repetitive late decelerations	3 to 10
Equivocal	Occasional but not repetitive late decelerations; absence of a positive or negative "window"	5 to 10
Unsatisfactory	Inability to provoke sufficient uterine contractions; lack of adequate FHR data	5 to 10

*From Moore: *Newborn, Family, and Nurse*, 2nd Edition. Philadelphia, W. B. Saunders Co., 1981.

no decelerations during three contractions, this is a "negative window," and the test is considered negative. Conversely, a "positive window" is one in which there is a 10-minute period that satisfies the criteria of a positive test. Failure to stimulate sufficient uterine contractions or to collect adequate FHR data results in an unsatisfactory test.

As with a reactive NST, a negative CST is reassuring. The chances of the infant dying in utero are considered to be less than 1 per cent. Although antepartum deaths ranging from 5 to 10 in 1000 tests have been reported, analysis shows that these deaths are usually the result of factors that could not have been predicted, such as abruptio placentae.

A positive CST simply identifies a group of mothers and fetuses who are at risk. Evaluation and care of each mother and fetus is developed on an individual basis, and using the results of various other fetal assessments.

Directions for Contraction Stress Test

1. The purpose of this test and the procedure are explained to the mother.
2. The mother signs a consent form.
3. The mother lies in a semi-Fowler's position or in lateral tilt with her right hip elevated 3 to 4 inches to avoid supine hypotensive syndrome.
4. The monitor is applied.
5. Maternal blood pressure is assessed initially and at frequent intervals throughout the procedure.
6. An intravenous infusion is started, and a low-dose of oxytocin is administered "piggyback" by infusion pump. The initial rate is 0.5 to 1.0 milliunit per minute.
7. The oxytocin dose is increased, usually every 10 minutes, until there are three 40-second contractions in a 10-minute period. Oxytocin is discontinued if any contraction lasts longer than 90 seconds.
8. Oxytocin is discontinued when the criterion of three contractions in 10 minutes has been met. The mother is observed until any

residual contractions are at least 10 minutes apart.

Advantages and Disadvantages of NST and CST and Their Use in the Care of a Mother and Fetus

The NST offers obvious advantages for initial screening. It is easily administered wherever a fetal monitor is available, usually an outpatient clinic or office. As a result, it is less expensive than the CST. The time involved may be as little as 10 to 15 minutes and, following protocol, no longer than 40 minutes. If the test is reactive, a CST is unnecessary.

The CST requires at least 90 to 100 minutes and is usually performed in a hospital setting because of the administration of intravenous oxytocin. This increase in expense and time suggests that the CST is not as valuable in overall screening as it is useful in evaluation of the approximately 10 per cent of women who have a nonreactive NST. The use of a combined NST and CST has been shown to aid in reducing perinatal mortality (Fig. 14–14).[8]

Assessment of Fetal Maturity

We have already noted that fetal or maternal well-being must sometimes be balanced against fetal maturity. Estimates of fetal maturity are also important in selecting the date for an elective cesarean delivery. In a study published in 1969,[1] before the studies of fetal maturity described below were in use, it was found that 8.4 per cent of all infants delivered by *elective* cesarean delivery weighed less than 2500 grams. Thus a large number of newborns each year were unnecessarily exposed to the hazards of prematurity or low birth weight, and therefore were potentially exposed to problems in the immediate neonatal period and to longterm problems such as learning disability, which may not even become evident until the child is of school age.

It is probable that tests of fetal maturity

will be required before every elective cesarean delivery. This is already the practice in some centers.

Amniotic Fluid Studies

Amniotic Fluid Surfactant. When an infant is born prematurely he is able to synthesize a surface active material, *surfactant,* which lowers surface tension in the alveoli. If there is insufficient surfactant, alveoli collapse during exhalation, resulting in atelectasis and respiratory distress syndrome (RDS). RDS is a major cause of death in immature babies and is discussed in detail in Chapter 23.

Surfactant is synthesized by Type II cells lining each alveolus, beginning at 24 to 26 weeks' gestation. Phospholipids are the active components of surfactant; the most abundant of the phospholipid compounds is *lecithin.* After 32 weeks, concentrations of lecithin begin to rise rapidly, The concentration of a second phospholipid, *sphingomyelin,* changes very little.

In 1971 Gluck demonstrated that the relationship between lecithin and sphingomyelin in amniotic fluid could serve as an index of fetal lung maturity.[7] This discovery is the basis of a now widely used test of fetal maturity, the L/S ratio. When the ratio of lecithin to sphingomyelin is 2.0 or greater, the lung is considered mature. One exception, in some laboratories, has been testing the diabetic mother; her fetus may still have immature lungs until the ratio is higher than 2.0

The shake test is also an assessment of surfactant in amniotic fluid, the results of which have been correlated with the L/S ratio and the incidence of RDS. It requires no expensive laboratory equipment, and the results are available in less than 30 minutes. Although the technique is simple, errors can be easily made if care is not taken.

The shake test is based on the principle that the presence of surface active materials (e.g., surfactant) prolongs the stability of an emulsion. When amniotic fluid is diluted with saline, and alcohol is added to nullify the action of other surface active materials, the persistence of fine bubbles indicates the presence of surfactant. A positive test result, in which fine bubbles (foam) are present at dilutions greater than 1:2 (amniotic fluid:saline), indicates pulmonary maturity; the accuracy is considered high. If there is no foam in undiluted amniotic fluid, the risk for RDS is high and the test is judged negative. Results between 0 and 1:2 are considered intermediate, and a determination of the L/S ratio is indicated to predict more accurately the possibility of RDS.

An even more sensitive indicator of lung maturity is phosphotidyl glycerol (pg), a phospholipid that appears at 36 weeks and increases until term. When pg is present in amniotic fluid, RDS does not occur.[12a]

Creatinine Levels. Levels of creatinine in amniotic fluid rise gradually until the thirty-second to thirty-fourth week of pregnancy and then rise more rapidly until term, when levels are two to four times greater than at midpregnancy. This rise is generally believed to be related to the increasing muscle mass of the fetus; it may also be due to maturing renal function. Creatinine levels of 2 mg. per 100 ml. or greater are considered to indicate a fetal age of 37 weeks or more.

Cytologic Changes. Epithelial cells, probably from the skin of the fetus, are normally present in amniotic fluid during the second and third trimesters of pregnancy. As the fetus becomes more mature, the percentage of cells containing lipid increases. By staining amniotic fluid cells with Nile blue stain, lipid cells can be identified. At 34 weeks less than 1 per cent of the cells are lipid cells; by 38 to 40 weeks from 10 to 50 per cent are lipid cells. After 40 weeks' gestation, more than 50 per cent are lipid. One advantage of this test is that it can be done without sophisticated laboratory equipment.

Maturity is also assessed by identifying types of cells present. Basal cells are the major type of cell present until approximately 32 weeks; precornified cells predominate between 32 and 36 weeks. After 36 weeks cornified cells begin to appear; they predominate after 38 weeks.

Bilirubin Levels. In studying the amniotic fluid of mothers who were Rh-sensitized, it was recognized that in normal pregnancy bilirubin levels in amniotic fluid reach a peak between 20 and 24 weeks and then decline. When levels reach zero, the fetus is assumed to be mature.[13] This test is of no value if the mother is Rh-isoimmunized.

Utilizing a Knowledge of Fetal Assessment in Nursing Practice

Nurses caring for pregnant women in ambulatory or hospital settings are frequently the primary educators and supports of women during fetal assessment. A number of initial assessments are made by the nurse: fundal height, fetal outline, fetal heart rate (NST), and sometimes ultrasonography. Nurses explain to mothers the use of a "count-to-ten" chart and care for mothers during CST.

Explanations by nurses of the reason for testing and the benefits to mother and fetus are essential. Many of the tests described here are repeated once or twice a week during much of the last trimester of pregnancy; they require families to travel to the clinic, office, or hospital frequently at a cost of time, money, and the mother's energy. A mother and her family must feel that this extra "cost" is worthwhile in achieving the desired outcome—a newborn who is as healthy as he can possibly be.

In prenatal classes, mothers who are not having additional tests are often curious about the reasons for various types of assessments.

We explain that these decisions are based on the course of the pregnancy in each mother. We emphasize that for most mothers, additional testing as indicated provides reassurance of the continuing health of the fetus.

The use of fetal assessment techniques to enhance "bonding" has been noted. Allowing the mother to hear the fetal heart rate by means of a Doppler or during an NST or CST (because the woman is "attached" to the fetal monitor), to see the fetus during ultrasound evaluations, and to receive a picture of the fetus after ultrasound examination are all techniques that can be used by nurses to strengthen the mother's and father's attachment to their infant.

REFERENCES

1. Benson, R., Berendes, H., and Weiss, W.: Fetal Compromise During Elective Cesarean Section. *American Journal of Obstetrics and Gynecology,* 105:579, 1969.
2. Bonica, J. (ed.): *Principles and Practice of Obstetric Analgesia and Anesthesia.* Philadelphia, F. A. Davis Co., 1972.
3. Brock, D. J. H., and Sutcliffe, R. G.: Alpha-fetoprotein in the Antenatal Diagnosis of Anencephaly and Spina Bifida. *Lancet,* 2:197, 1972.
4. Chard, T.: Monitoring of High-Risk Pregnancies by Alpha-Fetoprotein. *In* Spellacy, W. N. (ed.): *Management of the High Risk Pregnancy.* Baltimore, University Park Press, 1976.
5. Douglas, C.: Tubal Ectopic Pregnancy. *British Medical Journal,* 2:838, 1963.
6. Calloway, K.: Placental Evaluation Studies: Their Procedures, Their Purposes and the Nursing Care Involved. *MCN,* 1:300, 1976.
7. Gluck, L.: Fetal Maturity and Amniotic Fluid Surfactant Determinations. *In* Spellacy, W. (ed.): *Management of the High Risk Pregnancy.* Baltimore, University Park Press, 1976.
8. Gordon, E., and Schifrin, B.: Antepartum Heart Rate Monitoring. *In* Kaminetzky, H., and Iffy, L. (eds.): *New Techniques and Concepts in Maternal and Fetal Medicine.* New York, Van Nostrand Reinhold, 1979.
9. Hissong, S.: Obstetric Ultrasound. *In* Iffy, L., and Kaminetzky, H. (eds.): *Principles and Practice of Obstetrics and Perinatology.* New York, John Wiley, 1981.
10. Hobbins, J., Grannum, P., Berkowitz, R., et al.: Ultrasound in the Diagnosis of Congenital Anomalies. *American Journal Obstetrics and Gynecology* 134:331, 1979.
11. Hogan, K., and Tcheng, D.: The Role of the Nurse During Amniocentesis. *JOGN Nursing,* 7(5):24, 1978.
12. Kohn, C., Nelson, A., and Weiner, S.: Gravidas' Responses to Realtime Fetal Image. *JOGN Nursing,* 9(2):77, 1980.
12a. Kulovich, M., Hollman, M., and Gluck, L.: The lung profile. I. Normal pregnancy. *American Journal of Obstetrics and Gynecology,* 135:57, 1979.
13. Mandelbaum, D., LaCroix, G., and Robinson, A.: Determination of Fetal Maturity by Spectrophotometric Analysis of Amniotic Fluid. *Obstetrics and Gynecology,* 29:471, 1967.
13a. Martin, C., Schifrin, B.: Prenatal fetal monitoring.

In Aladjem, S., and Brown, A. (eds.): Perinatal Intensive Care, St. Louis. C. V. Mosby, 1977.
14. Maternal Serum Alpha-fetoprotein Measurement in Antenatal Screening for Anencephaly and Spina Bifida. Report of a U.K. Collaborative Study on Alpha-fetoprotein in Relation to Neural-Tube Defects. *Lancet,* 2:1323, 1977.
15. Milunsky, A.: Alpha-fetoprotein and the Prenatal Tube Defects. *American Journal of Public Health,* 69:552, 1979.
15a. National Institute of Child Health and Human Development: Amniocentesis Registry Symposium. *JAMA* 236:171, 1976.
15b. Paul, R., and Miller, F.: Antepartum fetal heart rate monitoring. *Clinical Obstetric Gynecology,* 21(2):375, 1978.
16. Pilon, R.: Anesthesia for Uncomplicated Obstetric Delivery. *American Family Physician,* 9:113, 1974.
17. Pitkin, R. M.: Fetal Maturity: Nonlipid Amniotic Fluid Assessment. *In* Spellacy, W. N. (ed.): *Management of the High Risk Pregnancy.* Baltimore, University Park Press, 1976.
18. Pitkin, R. M., and Zwirek, S. J.: Amniotic Fluid Creatinine. *American Journal of Obstetrics and Gynecology,* 98:1135, 1967.
19. Prechtl, H. H.: Neurological Sequelae of Prenatal and Perinatal Complication. *British Medical Journal,* 4:763, 1967.
20. Sabbagha, R. W.: Ultrasound in Managing the High-Risk Pregnancy. *In* Spellacy, W. N. (ed.): *Management of the High Risk Pregnancy.* Baltimore, University Park Press, 1976.
21. Sadovsky, E., and Yaffe, H.: Daily Fetal Movement Recording and Fetal Prognosis. *Obstetrics and Gynecology,* 41:485, 1973.
22. Scheidt, P., and Lundin, F.: Investigations for Effects of Intrauterine Ultrasound in Humans. *In* Hazzard D., and Litz, M. (eds.): *Symposium on Biological Effects and Characteristics of Ultrasound Sources.* DHEW (FDA) Publication No. 78–8048. Washington, D.C., U.S. Government Printing Office, 1977.
23. Seller, M.: Alpha-fetoprotein and the Prenatal Diagnosis of Neural Tube Defects. *Developmental Medicine Child Neurology,* 16:369, 1974.
24. Tulchensky, D.: The Value of Estrogens in High Risk Pregnancy. In Spellacy, W. N. (ed.): *Management of the High Risk Pregnancy.* Baltimore, University Park Press, 1976.
25. Varney, H.: *Nurse-Midwifery.* Boston, Blackwell Scientific Publications, 1980.

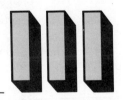

Labor and Birth

15

The Physiologic Basis of the Process of Labor

OBJECTIVES

1. Define the following in relation to the process of labor:

   a. increment
   b. acme
   c. decrement
   d. frequency
   e. duration
   f. intensity
   g. lie

   h. presentation
   i. molding
   j. breech
   k. position
   l. station
   m. engaged (presenting part)
   n. fixed (presenting part)

   o. dilatation
   p. effacement
   q. latent phase
   r. active phase
   s. transitional phase

2. Discuss current theories to explain the onset of labor.
3. Describe the physiology of a uterine contraction.
4. Explain the relationship between the shape of the mother's pelvis and the process of labor.
5. Identify the types of presentation.
6. Explain potential problems of presentations other than vertex.
7. Explain the way in which fetal position is described.
8. Describe the physiologic regulation of fetal heart rate; identify the effects of the sympathetic, parasympathetic, and central nervous systems, baroreceptors, chemoreceptors, and hormones.
9. Describe the major purpose and average length of each stage of labor and the changes that mark the beginning and end of each stage.
10. Identify the mechanism of labor when the baby is in cephalic presentation and in breech presentation.
11. Identify factors in maternal status and in fetal status that may affect the course of labor.
12. Describe ways in which maternal position may affect the course of labor and the fetus.
13. Describe the basic physiologic stimuli that may cause pain during labor.
14. Identify the neural pathway for the transmission of sensory stimuli from the uterus, cervix, and perineum.
15. Describe the physiologic effect of labor on the mother other than effects on her reproductive system.

A number of concepts are used to explain that complex set of processes that result in the birth of each human infant. Understanding these concepts is basic to the understanding of our nursing role in supporting parents and their infants in the hours surrounding birth. In this chapter we will consider the:

1. Possible causes of the onset of labor.
2. Interrelationship between uterine contractions, the maternal pelvis, and the fetus.
3. Physiologic basis of pain during labor.

What Causes Labor to Begin?

Roughly 40 weeks from the date of the last menstrual period (38 weeks after conception), human labor begins. The length of time varies for each mammalian species but is characteristic for that species. Why?

There is no satisfactory answer to this question, although there are a number of theories. The answer is important, however, not merely as a matter of academic curiosity but as a possible clue to better management for women who labor prematurely, women who do not labor spontaneously, and others. We will examine several theories briefly, keeping in mind that they are *theories*. It is probable that no one factor, but rather a combination of factors, is responsible for the onset of labor.

Uterine Distention. It is a fact that as the uterus expands, the muscles of the uterus become more irritable, and their contractility is enhanced. (This is also true of other muscle tissue.) When the uterus is more distended than usual at a given gestational age, as in the case of a twin pregnancy or *hydramnios* (excess amniotic fluid), early labor is frequent but not universal. As the uterus becomes increasingly distended, intrauterine pressure and intramural tension increase, which *may*, in turn, contribute to a decreased oxygen supply and subsequent "aging" of the placenta. The possible changes in the placenta may influence the length of gestation (below).

Placental Aging. It has been suggested that progesterone, or an analog of progesterone, may inhibit uterine activity. As term approaches, the placental production of progesterone falls, uterine inhibition is gradually decreased, and uterine contractions begin to increase. This parallels the menstrual cycle: when the corpus luteum begins to regress, blood levels of estrogen and progesterone fall, and menstruation occurs within a few days (Chapter 4). There is no evidence, however, that local tissue levels of progesterone fall prior to the onset of labor.

Endocrine Activity. Four hormones or classes of hormones are related to initiation of labor. *Oxytocin* and *prostaglandins*, termed effector hormones, act directly on the myometrial cells of the uterus to produce contractions, and *estrogens* and *progesterone* appear to modulate the action of oxytocin and prostaglandins (Table 15–1).

Estrogens increase both spontaneous and drug-induced myometrial activity and also stimulate the synthesis, release, and action of both oxytocins and prostaglandins. Progesterone, as noted in Chapter 7, often has the opposite effect from estrogens and does appear to inhibit the effects of estrogens. In explaining the onset of labor it would be convenient if levels of progesterone dropped before labor began, but this does not appear to happen. Estrogen levels do continue to rise, however; and a relative increase in estrogen in relation to progesterone *may* be a factor in the onset of labor.

Oxytocin and prostaglandins are believed to block both the rise of cyclic AMP and calcium sequestration, thus leading to the contraction of myometrial cells. One possible pattern is illustrated on the following page.

Other factors that may play a role in this process are a possible decrease in the destruction of oxytocin by oxytocinase or a change in the myometrial receptors to oxytocin.

Under certain circumstances the cycle described may be short-circuited. Trauma, tissue

Table 15–1. ENDOCRINE ACTIVITY IN RELATION TO THE ONSET OF LABOR (PROPOSED)

Hormone	Action
Modulating hormones	
Estrogens	Increase myometrial activity; stimulate synthesis, release, and action of oxytocin and prostaglandins
Progesterone	Decreases myometrial activity; inhibits synthesis, release, and action of oxytocin
Effector hormones	
Oxytocin	Stimulates myometrium to contract; stimulates release of prostaglandins from contracting muscle
Prostaglandins	Stimulate myometrial contractility; sensitize myometrial cells to oxytocin

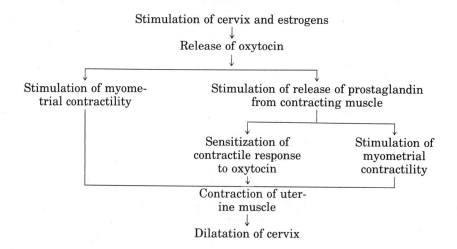

acidosis, excessive muscle stretching, or hemorrhage may lead to a release of lysosomal enzymes that stimulate oxytocin release without prior changes in estrogens and progesterone.

Sympathomimetic Amines. In animals epinephrine influences relaxation of the myometrium whereas norepinephrine influences activation. It is unclear what role these substances play in the onset of labor, but beta-sympathomimetric drugs are used to inhibit premature labor (Chapter 19).

Fetal Adrenal Production. Hippocrates thought that the fetus, when mature, initiated labor. The production of cortisone by the fetal adrenals may be a significant factor. Liggins[12] was able to manipulate the timing of the onset of labor in sheep by manipulating adrenal function. Anencephalic fetuses, who have retarded adrenal development secondary to hypofunction of their pituitary gland, have a delayed onset of labor about 40 per cent of the time.[18]

Physiologic Changes Prior to the Onset of Labor. Physiologic changes prior to the onset of labor (lightening, Braxton Hicks contractions, cervical changes, show, and/or rupture of the membranes) and the differentiation of true and false labor have been discussed in Chapter 11.

The Four P's

Traditionally, descriptions of labor have described 3 *p*'s: powers, passage, and passenger. To these three we believe a fourth should be added: psyche. The first three are discussed below: the role of the psyche is discussed in Chapter 16.

Powers

The power of labor comes from the force of contractions of the uterine muscles and the voluntary contractions of the abdominal muscles.

Uterine Contractions

The Physiology of a Uterine Contraction. A contraction begins as a result of "pacemaker" action in the myometrial cells near the right or left uterotubal junction. The contraction itself normally begins in one uterine cornu and spreads downward over a period of 15 seconds (Fig. 15–1). Although the contraction begins later in the lower uterus, it reaches its peak at the same time in all areas. The intensity of the contraction is directly proportional to the number of myometrial cells in that area of the uterus and is greatest at the fundus, less lower in the uterine body, and least at the cervix, where there are few muscle fibers. When contractions do not follow this normal pattern, various types of abnormalities are possible. *Rhythmicity* of uterine contractions is essential to effective labor. No matter how frequent, how intense, or how long contractions are, if they are irregular they will be ineffective and labor will not progress.

If the contraction begins in a lower segment and spreads upward, a *reverse gradient*, the cervix does not dilate and will contract during the contraction. This may be suspected if a woman complains of low back or low abdominal pain 5 to 10 seconds before the contraction is palpated at the fundus.

A *mild incoordination* occurs when there is more than one pacemaker and the pacemakers are asynchronous. Weak contractions may alternate with stronger ones. Mild incoordination is fairly common during early labor; often

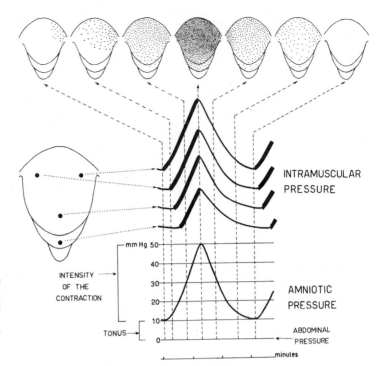

Figure 15–1. Schematic representation of the normal contractile wave of labor. Diagram of the uterus on the left shows the four points at which the intramyometrial pressure is recorded with microballoons. (From Caldeyro-Barcia: *Clinical Obstetrics and Gynecology,* 3:394, 1960.)

contractions become more coordinated as labor progresses.

If there are several pacemakers in various parts of the uterus, *severe incoordination* results. Labor does not progress; the mother is very uncomfortable and may become overly tired. Continued hypertonus can lead to fetal distress because of the interference with uteroplacental circulation. If sedation, analgesia, and regional anesthesia (Chapter 17) do not relieve the incoordination, cesarean delivery may be necessary.

Properties of Uterine Contractions. Uterine contractions have a number of specific properties.

Phases. There are three phases in a contraction, the *increment*, during which intensity increases; the *acme*, or height of the contraction; and the *decrement*, or period of decreasing intensity (Fig. 15–2).

Frequency, Duration, Intensity. In describing contractions, the terms frequency, duration, and intensity are used.

Frequency is measured from the beginning of one contraction to the beginning of the next (Fig. 15–2). The interval progessively decreases, and contractions become more frequent as labor progresses.

Duration is the length of the contraction. It is measured by abdominal palpation or by monitor from the time that the contraction is first perceived by the examiner (not the beginning of pain perceived by the laboring mother) until complete relaxation (Fig. 15–2).

Intensity, or strength, can be estimated by abdominal palpation or observed by monitor. When a contraction is strong, the uterus cannot be indented by examining fingers.

Early in labor, contractions are comparatively weak; the uterus is firm but not hard, and the duration may be about 30 seconds. As labor progresses, the duration increases to about 45 seconds, and firmness also increases. Strong contractions, of about 50 to 90 seconds' duration, occur as the time of birth approaches. (See also Stages of Labor, below.)

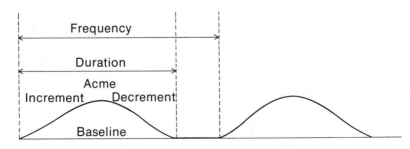

Figure 15–2. Terms used to describe uterine contractions.

Abdominal Muscle Contractions

During the second stage of labor (see below), the voluntary contractions of abdominal muscles, when coordinated with uterine contractions, are important in the expulsion of the baby. This coordination is facilitated by skilled coaching from the nurse caring for the woman, who tells her when to "bear down," i.e., when to contract her abdominal muscles (Chapter 17). As labor progresses and the fetus descends to the floor of the perineum, the mother feels such a great urge "to push" that abdominal muscle contractions become difficult for the mother to control.

The Passage: The Pelvis

The four types of female pelves were briefly described and illustrated in Chapter 4. Here we will consider the effect of each type of pelvis on labor more specifically.

1. *Gynecoid pelvis:* Considered the most satisfactory for normal labor, the gynecoid pelvis allows effective uterine contractions and spontaneous delivery. Because the pubic arch is wide, the frequency of perineal tears is reduced.

2. *Anthropoid pelvis:* The head often engages in an occiput posterior position and may deliver in that position. Labor and delivery are usually without difficulty, and the fetus has a good prognosis.

3. *Android pelvis:* The head engages in a posterior or transverse diameter and may not rotate; forceps are often needed for both rotation and extraction. This is a difficult vaginal delivery, and the prognosis for the baby is often poor. Because the pubic arch is narrow, perineal tears are common.

4. *Platypelloid pelvis:* Because of the short anteroposterior, posterior sagittal, and anterior sagittal diameters, the baby may never be able to enter the pelvic inlet. The outlook for the fetus is poor unless the condition is recognized and cesarean delivery performed.

The Passenger

The passenger is, of course, the fetus, who must travel from the uterus through the vagina to the world outside his mother's body.

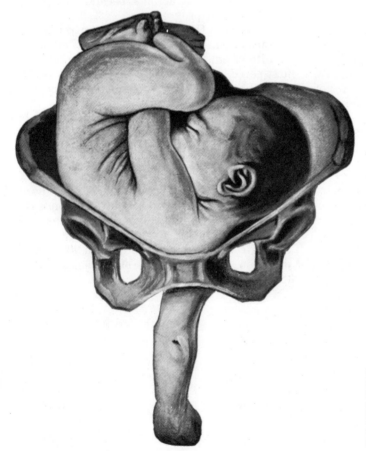

Figure 15–3. Schematic drawing of shoulder presentation, left acromion anterior position, in advanced labor with prolapsed right arm, head in the left iliac ala, and back down and anteriorly located. Lie is transverse. (From Greenhill and Friedman: *Biological Principles and Modern Practice of Obstetrics.* Philadelphia, W. B. Saunders Co., 1974.)

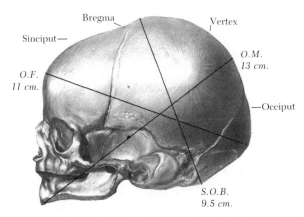

Figure 15–4. Lateral view of fetal skull showing cranial relationships, regional designations (reference points), and main diameters, including *O.F.,* occipitofrontal; *O.M.,* occipitomental: and *S.O.B.,* suboccipitobregmatic. (From Greenhill and Friedman: *Biological Principles and Modern Practice of Obstetrics.* Philadelphia, W. B. Saunders Co., 1974.)

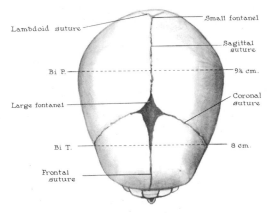

Figure 15–5. Top view of fetal skull, showing cranial bones, anterior (large lozenge shaped) and posterior (small triangular) fontanels and sutures. The important diameters, *Bi P.,* biparietal and *Bi T.,* bitemporal, are also designated. (From Greenhill and Friedman: *Biological Principles and Modern Practice of Obstetrics.* Philadelphia, W. B. Saunders Co., 1974.)

The fetus is described in terms of lie, presentation, position, and station.

Lie

Consider first the fetus within the uterus in the days immediately prior to delivery. The relationship between the long axis of the fetus and the long axis of the mother is the lie. Lie may be longitudinal or transverse (Fig. 15–3). Labor cannot progress to vaginal delivery when the lie is transverse (see discussion under Shoulder Presentation, below).

Presentation

The part of the fetus that first enters the vagina is the *presenting part.*

Cephalic Presentation. At term, 95 per cent of presentations are *cephalic.* In a cephalic presentation the presenting part may be the vertex (most commonly), the sinciput, the brow, or the face (Fig. 15–6). It is necessary to understand the structure of the fetal head in order to appreciate the process of labor.

The landmarks of the cranium are illustrated in Figures 15–4 and 15–5. At the time of birth the bones of the cranium are joined only by a membrane; they are thin and easily compressed. These characteristics make it possible for them to overlap, changing the shape of the head to fit the pelvis, a process known as *molding.*

The *sutures,* the membranous spaces between the bones, serve a useful function in addition to permitting molding. The sutures

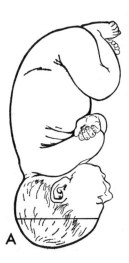
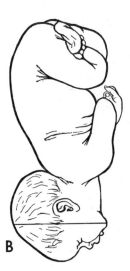
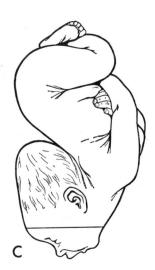

Figure 15–6. Gamut of deflexion attitudes from *A,* sincipital and *B,* brow presentation to *C,* face presentation, showing altered presenting fetal diameters from occipitobregmatic to mentobregmatic to trachelobregmatic. (From Greenhill and Friedman: *Biological Principles and Modern Practice of Obstetrics.* Philadelphia, W. B. Saunders Co., 1974.)

Table 15–2.   DIAMETERS OF THE FETAL SKULL

	Diameter	Location	Average Size at Term (in cm.)
Transverse diameters	Biparietal	Between parietal bosses	9.5
	Bitemporal	Between temporal bones	8.0
Anteroposterior diameters	Occipito-frontal	External occipital protuberance to glabella	11.0
	Suboccipito-bregmatic	Undersurface occipital bone to center of bregma	9.5
	Verticomental	Vertex to chin	13.5
	Submentobreg-matic	Junction neck and lower jaw to bregma	9.5

can be identified on vaginal examination, and in this way an examiner can determine the position of the baby's head. At the intersection of the sutures are the fontanels, which also aid in identifying the position of the fetal head.

The anterior fontanel (bregma), at the junction of the frontal, sagittal, and coronal sutures, is diamond-shaped. Measuring about 2 to 3 cm., it is much larger than the posterior fontanel.

The sagittal and lambdoidal sutures meet to form the triangular posterior fontanel.

Several diameters of the fetal skull are important. These diameters were illustrated in Figure 15–5 and are summarized in Table 15–2. The diameter presenting to the pelvic inlet varies with the baby's position.

Cephalic Presentations Other Than Vertex.   In the vertex presentation the head is flexed with chin on chest. A variety of maternal or fetal factors can cause deflexion (lack of flexion) or extension, although the reason is not always apparent. Among the maternal factors are uterine anomalies, a contracted pelvis, placenta previa, and a pendulous abdominal wall. Fetal factors include macrosomia, congenital anomalies, polyhydramnios, and malposition of the umbilical cord.

In a *sincipital* presentation (Fig. 15–6) the vertex is neither flexed nor extended; when the sinciput reaches the pelvic floor, flexion usually occurs. When the presenting part is the *brow* (1 in 2000 deliveries), the progress of labor is slow; cesarean delivery may be necessary. A *face* presentation (1 in 250 deliveries) also prolongs labor. The face becomes swollen and bruised, and the newborn may have laryngeal edema. Cesarean delivery is frequent in such cases unless the face presentation is diagnosed early; if the vertex has not entered the pelvis, external manipulation to a flexed position is possible.

Synclitism and *asynclitism* refer to the relationship of the fetal sagittal suture (the suture that runs between the anterior and posterior fontanels, Fig. 15–5) to the maternal sacrum and symphysis pubis. In synclitism the sagittal suture is midway between the symphysis pubis and the sacral promontory. Asynclitism is anterior when the sagittal suture is closer to the sacrum and posterior when the sagittal suture is closer to the symphysis. It is common for the head to enter the pelvic inlet with posterior asynclitism and then change to anterior asynclitism during descent, allowing the fetus the maximum space during the journey through the pelvis.

Breech Presentation.   In 3 to 4 per cent of deliveries, the presenting part is the breech. Figures 15–7 and 15–8 illustrate the types of breech presentation.

In a breech presentation, lightening is rare; the presenting part is not engaged until after labor begins. Early rupture of the membranes is more common than in vertex presentations because the breech fits unevenly into the pelvis.

A number of circumstances make labor and delivery in the breech presentation more complex than in the vertex presentation.

1. Because the breech is not as effective as the head as a dilating wedge, labor is usually longer.

2. The breech, born first, is smaller than the head; the head must then pass through the pelvis quickly, with no time to mold.

3. Assisted delivery, a *breech extraction*, is often necessary.

4. *Prolapse* of the umbilical cord is more frequent than in vertex presentation (Chapter 19).

Because of the complexity of breech delivery, fetal and neonatal mortality and morbidity are higher than in vertex presentation. Potential

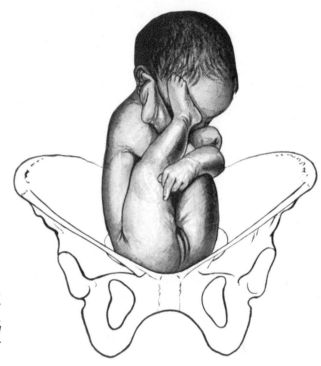

Figure 15–7. Fetus in frank or single breech presentation, right sacrum posterior position, with lower extremities extended fully across the abdomen, chest, and face. (From Greenhill and Friedman: *Biological Principles and Modern Practice of Obstetrics.* Philadelphia, W. B. Saunders Co., 1974.)

complications include intracranial hemorrhage, injury to the brachial plexus, and fracture of the humerus and clavicle.

In some centers, cesarean delivery may be recommended in many instances of breech presentation.

Shoulder Presentation. A shoulder presentation occurs when the lie is transverse,

about once in every 300 to 400 deliveries. Predisposing causes include the pendulous abdomen of a grand multipara, placenta previa (Chapter 13), a very narrow pelvis, or a uterine anomaly.

Spontaneous version (change of direction) occurs only occasionally, with the *lie* changing to a longitudinal one (cephalic or breech pre-

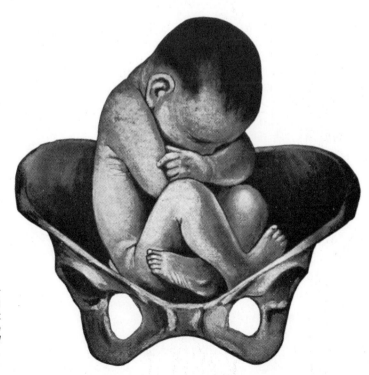

Figure 15–8. Fetus shown in complete or double breech presentation with buttocks and both feet presenting in the pelvic inlet, right sacrum posterior position. Compare with Figure 15–7. (From Greenhill and Friedman: *Biological Principles and Modern Practice of Obstetrics.* Philadelphia, W. B. Saunders Co., 1974.)

sentation) shortly before or after labor begins. The obstetrician may try to "turn" the baby to a longitudinal lie by *external version* early in labor or by *internal podalic version* under general anesthesia if the longitudinal lie is not recognized until the second stage. Cesarean delivery is more common than version today.

If for some reason a transverse lie is not recognized, the following sequence is likely:

1. Uterine contractions are of poor quality, and the cervix dilates slowly.

2. Membranes rupture early.

3a. The fetal shoulder enters the pelvis, the uterus molds around the baby, and contractions cease. This leads to intrauterine sepsis and generalized sepsis,

or

3b. The upper segment of the uterus becomes shorter and thicker, the lower part becomes thinner and more and more stretched until it ruptures.

Either sequence leads to almost certain fetal death and possible maternal death. Thus, early recognition of a transverse lie and shoulder presentation is essential.

Describing the Presentation. In cephalic presentations the baby's head may be (1) flexed so that his chin is on his chest and the posterior occiput (O) presents (vertex presentation), (2) neither flexed nor extended (military attitude), so that the median portion of the occiput (O) presents (vertex presentation) (3) partially extended so that the forehead or frontum (F) presents (bregma or sincipital presentation), or (4) fully extended so that the face presents (face presentation) (Fig. 15–6). The chin, or mentum (M), is the point of reference in a face presentation. In the breech position the sacrum (S) is the point of reference in relation to the mother's pelvis; in a shoulder presentation it is the scapula (Sc).

Position

Position is the relationship between the presenting part and the mother's pelvis. The structure that is used as the point of reference (the occiput, the mentum, and so on) is described as being anterior (A), posterior (P), or transverse (T), and as facing the right (R) or the left (L) of the mother's pelvis.

All of the information about the position of the fetus in utero is then translated into a shorthand that in a brief form gives nurses and physicians very specific information about the position of the fetus. The components of the system of notation are summarized in Table 15–3. Figure 15–9 illustrates positions.

Table 15–3.   DESCRIBING FETAL POSITION

Right (R)	Occiput (O)	Anterior (A)
Left (L)	Sacrum (S)	Posterior (P)
	Mentum (M)	Transverse (T)
	Scapula (Sc)	

Consider the meaning of these examples.

1. LOA: the occiput, the presenting part, is facing the left anterior quadrant of the mother's pelvis (common position).

2. LOP: Here the occiput is facing the left posterior quadrant of the pelvis. This mother's labor will be longer and more difficult than that of the mother with a baby in an anterior position because the baby must rotate to a greater extent prior to delivery.

3. SA: The presentation is breech; the sacrum is the presenting part, and it faces anteriorly, i.e., the mother's pubic bone. (The presenting part does not necessarily face the right or the left; hence, only two letters may be necessary.)

4. LMT: The face is the presenting part; the chin is toward the left and midway between the anterior and posterior quadrants of the pelvis, thus transverse.

Station

The progress of the fetus through the birth canal is also described in terms of *station*. Station refers to the level of the presenting part in relation to the maternal pelvis. When the presenting part is at the level of the ischial spines, the station is zero (0). Above the ischial spines the station is -1 if the lowest segment of the presenting part is 1 cm. above the spine, -2 if 2 cm. above, and so on. Below the ischial spines the station is $+1$ when the lowest portion of the presenting part is 1 cm. below the spine, and so on.

When the station is 0, the presenting part is *engaged*. At -1 and -2, the presenting part is *fixed* but not engaged; a presenting part that is fixed is not movable. The station is $+3$ when the presenting part reaches the pelvic floor and $+4$ when the perineum is bulging (Figs. 15–10 and 15–11).

Normal Characteristics of the Fetus During Labor

Labor produces stress for the fetus. When the fetus is healthy and the labor is normal, the stress is not harmful and may even serve a useful purpose in the transition to extrauterine life.

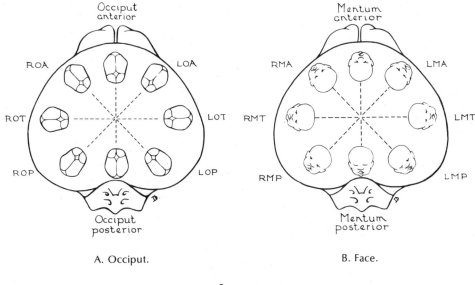

A. Occiput.

B. Face.

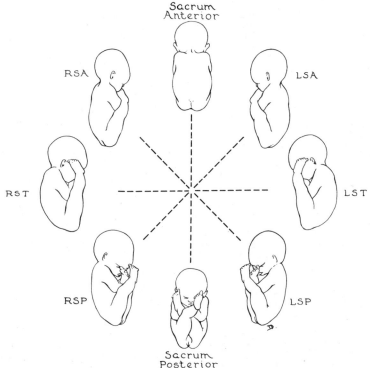

C. Breech.

Figure 15–9. Position. (From Oxorn and Foote: *Human Labor and Birth.* 3rd Edition. Englewood Cliffs, N.J., Appleton-Century-Crofts, Publishing Division of Prentice-Hall, Inc., 1975.)

How is the fetus affected during normal labor? Changes in amniotic fluid pressure have already been noted in this chapter. These changes bring pressure upon the flow of blood in the intervillous spaces and upon the fetal body. One manifestation of this stress is a brief fall in fetal heart rate that coincides with the contraction (see below). Research indicates that slight changes in fetal blood pressure also occur, although clinically fetal blood pressure is not monitored.

Physiologic Regulation of Fetal Heart Rate. Fetal heart rate is affected by several systems; recognizing this is fundamental to understanding fetal heart rate changes during labor. These systems are the parasympathetic,

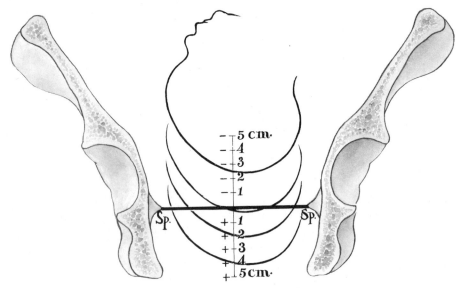

Figure 15–10. Diagrammatic presentation of the station of degree of engagement of the fetal head. The location of the forward leading edge or lowest part of the head is designated by centimeters above or below the plane of the interspinous line. (From Greenhill and Friedman: *Biological Principles and Modern Practice of Obstetrics.* Philadelphia, W. B. Saunders Co., 1974.)

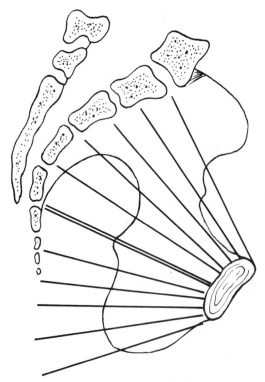

Figure 15–11. Lateral planar representation of station designations comparable to those in Figure 15–10 along the pelvic axis. Each line shows the location of the leading edge of the fetal head above or below the interspinous plane (double line). Station lines are spaced 1 cm. apart at their midpoints. (From Greenhill and Friedman: *Biological Principles and Modern Practice of Obstetrics.* Philadelphia, W. B. Saunders Co., 1974.)

sympathetic, and central nervous systems; baroreceptors and chemoreceptors; and certain hormones. Figure 15–12 and Table 15–4 summarize these systems.

Baseline fetal heart rate is the rate between contractions or between transient changes that are unrelated to contractions. The baseline rate is usually between 120 and 160 beats per minute. As in older children and adults, the intrinsic pacemaker activity leads to rhythmic contractions.

Periodic fetal heart rate patterns are brief accelerations and decelerations in rate, after which the rate returns to the baseline rate.

Uterine Contractions and the Fetus. When the uterus contracts, a vagal reflex, probably due to compression of the fetal head, may cause a brief deceleration in heart rate. The rate will not usually fall below 100, however, and will quickly return to a normal level of between 120 and 160. This pattern, and those described below, are discussed in more detail in the section on fetal monitoring in Chapter 18.

If uterine contractions interfere with the flow of blood to the fetus, hypoxia and acidosis may severely compromise the fetus. Careful monitoring of fetal heart rate in relation to uterine contractions, as well as fetal scalp sampling, is important in recognizing the presence of these abnormal conditions (see Chapter 18).

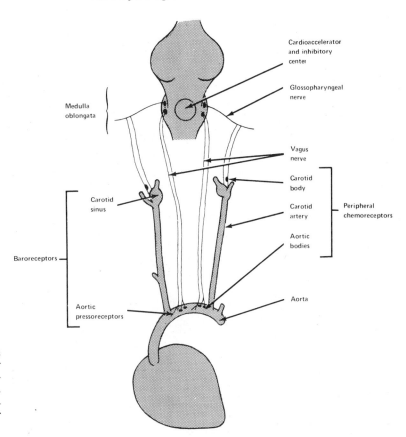

Figure 15–12. The baroreceptors and peripheral chemoreceptors and their input connections to the cardiac integrating center in the medulla oblongata. Fibers travel from this center to the heart. (From Perer: *JOGN Nursing (Supplement)*, 5:26s, 1976.)

The Stages of Labor

For convenience in communication, the process of labor is divided into four stages. These stages are briefly summarized in Table 15–5.

The First Stage

Before a baby can be delivered through the vagina, the uterine cervix must become effaced and dilated. This is the purpose of the first stage of labor.

Effacement is the process by which the cervical canal becomes shorter and thinner until it no longer is present (Fig. 15–13). Physiologically, effacement occurs because the cervical muscle fibers closest to the internal os are pulled into the lower uterine segment.

Effacement is assessed in percentages, from 0 to 100 per cent. It is not unusual for the cervix to be 50 to 60 per cent effaced as a result of Braxton Hicks contractions occurring prior to the onset of labor.

The other major process of the first stage is *dilatation* of the cervix. Dilatation is a result of uterine contractions (primarily), the hydrostatic pressure of amniotic fluid if the mem-branes are not ruptured, and the pressure of the presenting part on the cervix. At the beginning of labor, especially in the primigravida, the cervix is closed or just barely dilated (about 1 cm.). In multiparas the cervix may be dilated as much as 2 cm. (one fingertip passes through easily) before labor begins (Fig. 15–14). During the first stage of labor, the cervix dilates to an opening 10 cm. (4 inches) in diameter in order to allow the baby to pass into the vagina. Varney[28a] states that clinical expertise in assessing centimeters of dilatation can be developed not only with dilatation models but by running one's fingers around many circular objects (e.g., drinking glasses, cups, telephone dials), estimating the diameter and then measuring the object with a ruler or tape measure.

The first stage is by far the most time-consuming of the labor process. Within the first stage are three distinct phases, the *latent* phase, the *active* phase, and the *transitional* phase, diagrammed by means of Friedman's curve (Fig. 15–15).

The *latent* phase begins with the onset of regular contractions. These contractions are usually mild and are not perceived by the

Table 15–4.   SYSTEMS INFLUENCING FETAL HEAT RATE (FHR) DURING LABOR

System	Location	Relevant Function	Effect of Stimulation	Effect of Blocking	Comments
Parasympathetic nervous system—vagus (10th cranial) nerve	Originates in medulla oblongata	Supplies sinoatrial (SA) node and atrioventricular (AV) node Secretion of acetylcholine	↓ Firing SA node, therefore ↓ FHR, ↓ Atrioventricular transmission, therefore ↓ FHR Causes beat-to-beat variability	↑ FHR Eliminates beat-to-beat variability	Atropine blocks vagus by counteracting effects of acetylcholine. Even small amounts that do not increase FHR will eliminate beat-to-beat variability. Hypoxia depresses myocardial rhythm.
Sympathetic nervous system	Widely distributed in cardiac muscle	Secretion of norepinephrine	↑ FHR ↑ Strength of contraction	↓ FHR	A reserve to improve cardiac output during stress. Propranolol blocks sympathetic nerves. Blocking does not influence FHR variability.
Baroreceptors (pressure receptors)	Arch of aorta; carotid sinus (Fig. 15–12)		↑ Blood pressure (BP) causes impulses from receptors via vagus or glossopharyngeal nerve → midbrain → vagus (Fig. 15–12) ↓ FHR		

Chemoreceptors	Peripheral chemoreceptors: carotid and aortic bodies. Central chemoreceptors: medulla	Influence not well understood: Abrupt ↓ oxygen or ↑ carbon dioxide of peripheral receptors → ↓ FHR;* ↑ FHR variability. Mild ↓ oxygen or ↑ carbon dioxide → reflex tachycardia (↑ FHR). ↑ Carbon dioxide → ↑ arterial BP	
Central nervous system	Nerve impulse to and from higher brain center believed to be mediated through hypothalamus	Emotional stimuli → ↑ FHR and ↑ BP	Experimental stimulation of hypothalamus in fetal lamb → ↑ FHR
Hormonal regulation	Adrenal medulla: epinephrine, norepinephrine. Adrenal cortex: aldosterone	↑ FHR; ↑ Strength of contraction; ↑ BP; Role in fetus poorly understood	↓ FHR

*This response is opposite to that of the extrauterine infant or adult.

Table 15–5.   THE STAGES OF LABOR

Stage	Beginning	Ending	Purpose
First	Onset of regular contractions of uterus	Cervix fully dilated (10 cm.)	Effacement and dilatation
Second	Cervix fully dilated (10 cm.)	Birth of infant	Delivery of infant
Third	Complete birth of baby	Delivery of placenta	Separation and expulsion of placenta
Fourth	Expulsion of placenta	Uterus contracted, vital signs stable, lochia moderate	Prevention of uterine atony

mother as being especially painful. They may last from 15 to 30 seconds and occur every 10 to 20 minutes. The latent phase may last more than 8 hours in primigravidas and a little more than 5 hours in multigravidas.

The *active* phase begins when the cervix is fully effaced and dilatation is approximately 5 cm. Contractions are now more frequent and of longer duration and greater intensity.

Almost all mothers find the period of *transition* the most difficult in labor. Dilatation at the beginning of transition is usually 8 cm. During transition, the cervix is retracting (being retracted) over the presenting part, which is pushing into the vagina. Contractions are strong, frequent (as often as every 2 minutes), and may last as long as 70 to 80 seconds. There is always a certain amount of individual variation.

Table 15–6 summarizes the first stage of labor. Note in Table 15–6 that there is considerable difference in the length of the first stage in primigravidas and in multigravidas. There are several reasons for this difference. Once the cervix has been completely dilated, it di-

lates more easily. (If previous deliveries have been cesarean deliveries with no labor, the cervix will not dilate more easily.) Contractions in multigravidas are frequently more effective because of fundal dominance, i.e., the contraction begins in the fundus and spreads downward. Incoordination is less frequent (page 436). The pelvic floor is also more relaxed. After five births, these advantages may be counterbalanced by specific disadvantages. The uterine muscles, stretched during each pregnancy, may be less effective. The risk of complications such as abruptio placentae, placenta previa, and hemorrhage is also increased.

The Second Stage

The second stage of labor begins when the cervix is fully dilated (10 cm.). It ends with the infant's birth. During the second stage, the baby descends through the vagina and is delivered (see The Mechanism of Labor, below). The second stage may be as brief as a few minutes or as long as an hour or two.

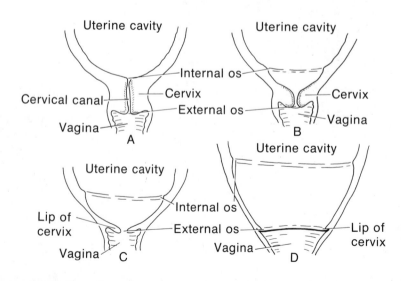

Figure 15–13. Effacement and dilatation in a primipara during labor. *A,* The cervical canal is closed; note the length of the canal. *B,* The cervix shortens, the internal os widens, and the cervical canal becomes funnel-shaped. *C,* Only a thin lip remains of cervix—effacement is complete, and dilatation is beginning. *D,* Cervical dilatation completed.

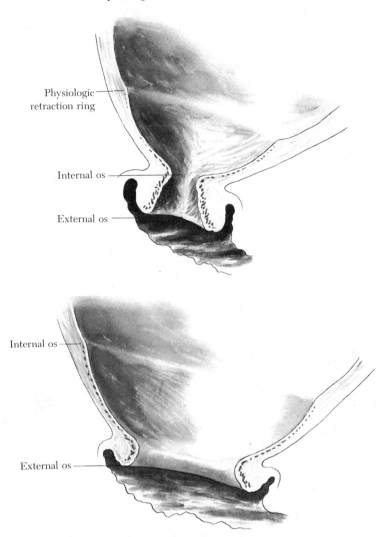

Physiologic retraction ring

Internal os

External os

Internal os

External os

Figure 15–14. Progressive effacement and dilatation of the cervix of a multipara, showing that dilatation may occur even if effacement is incomplete. (From Greenhill and Friedman: *Biological Principles and Modern Practice of Obstetrics.* Philadelphia, W. B. Saunders Co., 1974.)

Physiologic Changes

Several physiologic changes facilitate the birth of the baby:

Soft Tissue Changes. The soft tissues of the perineum hypertrophy; both blood supply and fluid content increase. These changes enable the tissues to stretch far more than they would be able to under ordinary circumstances. Changes are particularly marked in the *levator ani*, which will be markedly stretched at delivery, and in the perineal body, which changes

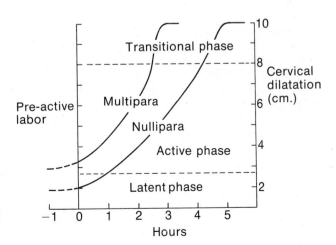

Figure 15–15. The Friedman curve diagrams the relationship between hours of active labor and cervical dilatation.

Table 15–6. THE FIRST STAGE OF LABOR

Phase	Begins	Ends	Time	Comments
Latent	Onset of regular contractions	Effacement complete Dilatation to 2–3 cm.	Primigravida— about 8½ hours	Woman usually comfortable
			Multigravida— about 5½ hours	
Active	Complete effacement Dilatation approximately 2–3 cm.	Approximately 8 cm. dilatation	Primigravida— 4 hours	Contractions more frequent, longer, and stronger
			Multigravida— 2 hours	Woman becomes increasingly restless
Transitional	Approximately 8 cm. dilatation	Cervix fully dilated	Primigravida— about 1 hour	Most difficult phase of labor for most women
			Multigravida— 10–15 minutes	

from a thick wedge-shaped tissue to a thin tissue.

Uterine Changes. The uterus becomes longer as the lower uterine segment stretches and the transverse and anteroposterior diameters shorten. As the uterus changes, the position of the fetus becomes more nearly vertical. Contractions become longer (from 50 to 90 seconds), more frequent (at 1 to 3 minute intervals), and more intense.

Increased Show. As capillaries in the cervix rupture and the membranes separate from the decidua in the lower uterine segment, the amount of bloody show increases.

Bearing Down. As the presenting part of the fetus reaches the floor of the perineum, the mother has an uncontrollable desire to bear down, adding the force of the abdominal muscles to the effect of uterine contractions.

The Mechanism of Labor

The way the fetus-passenger adapts to the maternal passage and passes through that passage is called the mechanism of labor. This mechanism consists of six movements, termed cardinal movements. Although these movements are described in sequence, many occur simultaneously, either entirely or in part. The fetus's position during each cardinal movement varies with his position at the onset of labor, but the mechanism itself is similar. Because LOA is a common position, the mechanism of labor described here is for that position. The mechanism of labor in a variety of positions is described in Oxorn and Foote's text.[22]

Mechanism of Labor in Cephalic Position. In the cephalic position the mechanism of labor involves:

1. *Descent.* Descent includes *engagement* of the head (page 417) and continues throughout the first and second stages of labor. All of the other movements are simultaneous with descent.

2. *Flexion.* As the LOA baby descends through the uterine passage, his head flexes so that his chin is on his chest. This enables the smallest diameter of the head (the suboccipitobregmatic, which is approximately 9.5 cm.) to present first. If flexion does not occur and the approximately 11.0 cm. occipitofrontal diameter presents instead, passage is far more difficult, as in a sincipital, brow, or face presentation (Fig. 15–16).

3. *Internal rotation.* Internal rotation usually occurs in the second stage of labor (i.e., after the cervix is fully dilated; see above and below) when the head reaches the pelvic floor or soon afterward. The reasons for internal rotation are three:

   a. The pelvic *inlet* is usually a transverse oval; i.e., it is slightly longer from side to side (transverse diameter) than from front to back (anteroposterior diameter).

   b. The pelvic outlet is an anteroposterior oval, being slightly longer from front to back.

   c. The fetal head is an anteroposterior oval.

Thus, the head must enter the pelvic inlet in a transverse diameter and leave the pelvis in an anteroposterior diameter. Therefore, the head must rotate; the shoulders, however, do not (Fig. 15–17). Usually the head rotates so that the occiput is anterior.

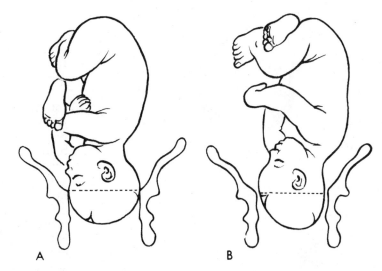

Figure 15–16. Reduction in the presenting fetal diameters as a result of flexion. The occipitofrontal diameter in a moderately deflexed sincipital presentation *(A)* is converted to the smaller suboccipitobregmatic in a well-flexed vertex presentation *(B)*. (From Greenhill and Friedman: *Biological Principles and Modern Practice of Obstetrics,* Philadelphia, W. B. Saunders Co., 1974.)

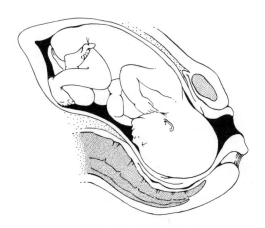

A. Lateral view.

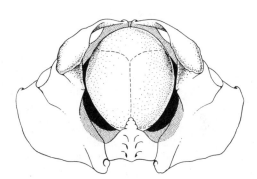

B. Vaginal view.

Figure 15–17. Internal rotation: LOA to OA. (From Oxorn and Foote: *Human Labor and Birth.* 3rd Edition. Englewood Cliffs, N.J., Appleton-Century-Crofts, Publishing Division of Prentice-Hall Inc., 1975.)

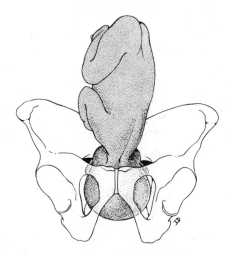

C. Anteroposterior view.

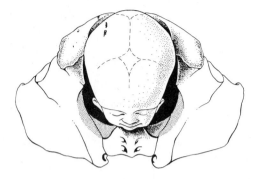

A. Vaginal view.

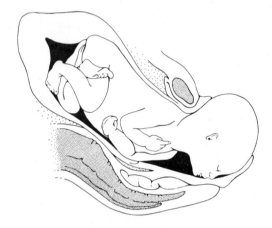

B. Lateral view.

Figure 15–18. Extension of the head: birth. (From Oxorn and Foote: *Human Labor and Birth*. 3rd Edition. Englewood Cliffs, N.J., Appleton-Century-Crofts, Publishing Division of Prentice-Hall Inc., 1975.)

4. *Extension.* As the baby reaches the pelvic floor, the combination of "push" from uterine contractions and abdominal muscles and resistance offered by the pelvic floor results in extension of the head. The perineum bulges, the head "crowns" (Fig. 15–18), and the baby is born—first the occiput, followed by the bregma, forehead, nose, mouth, and chin.

The *Ritgen maneuver* is a method of assisting the mechanism of extension and the birth of the head; its purpose is gradual delivery of the head between contractions, with minimal damage to the soft tissues (Fig. 15–19).

5. *Restitution.* Since the time of internal rotation, the neck has been twisted somewhat. After the head is born, it "restitutes" to a normal relationship with the shoulders. The baby thus returns to its original pelvic position (in this instance LOA). The head should be supported during restitution and external rotation (below).

6. *External rotation.* Just as the head rotated internally in order to pass through the pelvic outlet, so too must the shoulders. External rotation of the head is the visible evidence of internal rotation of the shoulders. The baby's position is now LOT. The anterior shoulder reaches the pelvic floor first, rotates anteriorly under the symphysis, and is born. The posterior shoulder is delivered as the mother "bears down," and the trunk and extremities follow.

Mechanism of Labor in Breech Presentation. In a breech presentation, there are mechanisms of labor for three segments of the fetus:

1. the buttocks and lower limbs.
2. the shoulders and arms.
3. the head.

If one imagines the fetus as a triangle (Fig. 15–20), with the head as the largest, most unyielding segment, the reason is easier to understand. In a cephalic presentation, the head is delivered first, and it is usually not difficult for the smaller shoulders and body to follow. In a breech presentation, each segment is larger and more difficult to deliver than the part of the fetal body that preceded it.

Consider this example of the mechanism of labor in the RSA position:

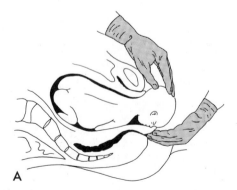
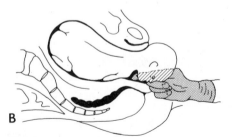

A   B

Figure 15–19. The Ritgen maneuver *(A)* facilitates birth by encouraging extension of the fetal head. If the chin lodges against the perineum, it may be extracted as in *(B)*. (After Oxorn and Foote: *Human Labor and Birth*. 3rd Edition. Englewood Cliffs, N.J., Appleton-Century-Crofts, Publishing Division of Prentice-Hall, Inc., 1975.)

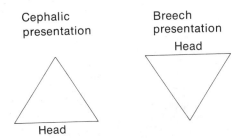

Cephalic presentation

Breech presentation

Head

Head

Figure 15–20. Breech presentation. Imagine the fetus as a triangle and the head as the largest segment. In a breech presentation, each segment is larger than the body part that precedes it.

1. *Buttocks and lower limbs. Descent* may be delayed until the cervix is dilated and the membranes ruptured. Lateral *flexion* at the waist and *internal rotation* of the hips occur. Birth occurs by *lateral* flexion, the posterior hip followed by the anterior hip.

2. *Shoulders and arms.* As the sacrum rotates (RST → RSA), the shoulders are engaged and rotate internally. The baby is lifted upward so that the posterior shoulder and arm are delivered over the perineum. The baby is then lowered, and the anterior shoulder and arm are delivered under the symphysis (Fig. 15–21).

3. *Head.* The head enters the pelvis as the posterior shoulder is born. The head *flexes* and *rotates internally* so that the occiput is under the symphysis and the back is anterior. The chin, mouth, nose, forehead, bregma, and occiput, in that order, are born over the perineum.

As in cephalic presentations, mechanisms for breech delivery in positions other than RSA vary (see Oxorn and Foote[22]).

The Third Stage

Uterine contractions begin again shortly after the baby's delivery, with a resultant retraction in the size of the uterus. The retraction decreases the area of placental attachment (Fig. 15–22), and the placenta separates from the uterine wall and is expelled through the vagina.

The lower edge of the placenta may appear first (Duncan method), or the placenta may resemble an inverted umbrella with the shiny fetal side appearing initially (Shultze method). Although the Shultze method may indicate the implantation of the placenta in the fundus and the Duncan method implantation in the uterine wall, this differentiation has no practical significance of which we are aware.

After placental separation the uterine muscles retract further, closing off the arterioles and venules that pass through the interlacing muscle fibers and controlling bleeding. If these muscles do not retract and remain retracted, hemorrhage will result.

Effect of Maternal Status on Labor and on Fetus During Labor

A number of maternal factors related to both general and reproductive health or status can influence the outcome of labor and birth. General factors include a body type that might involve possible cephalopelvic disproportion, pelvic injury, spinal deformity, a pelvic mass, tumor or invasive carcinoma, uterine surgery (including a previous cesarean delivery), anemia, and high risk conditions such as hypertension, diabetes, Rh isoimmunization, cardiac disease, or infection. Maternal reproductive

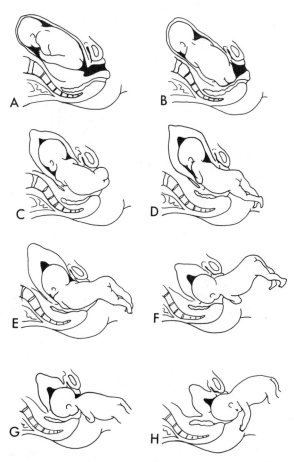

A   B

C   D

E   F

G   H

Figure 15–21. Mechanisms of labor—breech presentation (RSA). *A,* Onset of labor; *B,* descent and internal rotation of buttocks; *C,* birth of posterior buttock; *D,* feet born, shoulder engaging; *E,* descent and internal rotation of shoulders; *F,* posterior shoulder born, head enters pelvis; *G,* anterior shoulder born, head descends; and *H,* flexion and birth of head. (After Oxorn and Foote: *Human Labor and Birth,* 3rd Edition. Englewood Cliffs, N.J., Appleton-Century-Crofts, Publishing Division of Prentice Hall, Inc., 1975.)

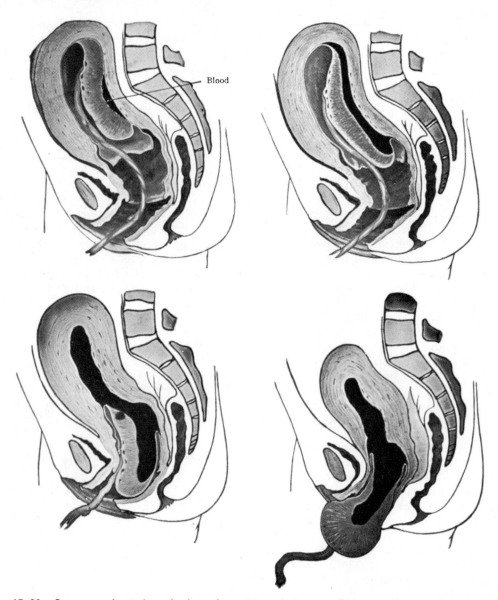

Figure 15–22. Sequence of usual mechanism of expulsion of placenta. Early central separation with formation of retroplacental hematoma shown progressing to inversion of the placenta and expulsion with fetal surface leading, followed by membranes and blood that has accumulated. (From Greenhill and Friedman: *Biological Principles and Modern Practice of Obstetrics.* Philadelphia, W. B. Saunders Co., 1974.)

factors include parity, length of gestation, antepartum hemorrhage, and rupture of the membranes prior to the onset of labor. Table 15–7 summarizes the potential effects of these conditions on labor. Many are discussed in more detail in Chapters 13 and 19. Not all of these conditions are absolute indications of problems; for example, not every woman with a short, square stature will have a pelvis too small for vaginal delivery (cephalopelvic disproportion). Many of these risk conditions will have been identified during prenatal care. Others, such as signs of infection or bleeding, may

be acute and are first noted immediately prior to or during labor.

Effects of Maternal Position During Labor

During historical times and in some traditional societies today women remain active during early labor. They maintain vertical or semivertical positions by squatting, crouching, sitting on a birthing stool, or semireclining in a hammock. In the eighteenth century, as obstetricians increasingly became the arbiters of care, first forceps and later anesthesia and

Table 15–7. EFFECTS OF MATERNAL HEALTH STATUS ON LABOR AND BIRTH

Maternal Status	Possible Effects on Labor and Birth
General	
Maternal stature: short; short broad hands and feet; shoulders wider than hips; small pelvic measurements (page 244)	Potential cephalopelvic disproportion (CPD)
Spinal deformity, e.g., kyphosis, scoliosis	Potential CPD
Spinal surgery or injury	May limit use of some anesthetic techniques (e.g., epidural anesthesia), depending on site
Pelvic fracture	Potential CPD
Pelvic mass, tumor, invasive carcinoma	Indication for cesarean delivery
Vesicovaginal fistula	Indication for cesarean delivery
Infection	
Active vaginal herpes	Indication for cesarean delivery
Systemic infection	Fetal tachycardia
	Potential infection of fetus or newborn
Hypertension	Varies with condition
Anxiety-related—increased systolic blood pressure only	
Hypertensive disease—increased systolic and diastolic blood pressure	
Diabetes	
Cardiac disease	
Anemia	
Rh isoimmunization	
Maternal hypotension	Fetus at risk of inadequate oxygenation
Maternal position	
Shock	
Drug, alcohol use	Chronic fetal distress
Previous uterine surgery, including previous cesarean delivery	Possible cesarean delivery; see Chapter 19
Antepartum hemorrhage	Possible cesarean delivery; see Chapters 13, 19
Placenta previa	
Abruptio placentae	
Length of gestation	Fetus at risk
less than 38 weeks	
more than 42 weeks	
Rupture of membranes prior to onset of labor	Risk of maternal or fetal infection increased after 24 hours
Parity	Shorter labor in multipara
	Longer labor in grand multipara
	Pendulous abdomen in grand multipara may be associated with malpresentation
Length of time since last pregnancy	Prolonged labor, increased risk of placenta previa or abruptio placentae if greater than 10 years

other technological interventions became a part of care during childbearing. The recumbent position became the prevalent one in much of Western society including, of course, the United States. The recumbent position is convenient for the health-care provider. Mauriceau, the French obstetrician who proposed the recumbent position, stated that its purpose was to facilitate management of labor by the accoucheur. It is essential now, however, to question whether it is the best position for the health of the mother and fetus.

Because the purpose of contractions is different in the first and second stages of labor, the effect of position must be examined for each stage.

The First Stage

The purpose of contractions in the first stage is effacement and dilatation of the cervix. Caldeyro-Barcia[3] reports that "if all other factors are matched, the duration of the first stage of labor is significantly shorter when the mothers were all the time in a vertical position (sitting, standing or walking) than when they were lying in bed." In one study of 91 normal primigravidas, the mean duration of the first stage from 4 cm. to 10 cm. dilatation was 147 minutes for 40 primigravidas in a vertical position and 225 minutes for 51 primigravidas lying in bed, a 36 per cent difference. Of 324 mothers (28 per cent gravida I, 30 per cent gravida II, 42 per cent gravida III or more), the mean duration for the same period (4 cm. to 10 cm. dilatation) was 135 minutes for 143 mothers in a vertical position and 180 minutes for 181 mothers lying in bed, a 25 per cent difference. The preference of 95 per cent of the women in the study for a vertical position suggests that this position is more comfortable (Diaz et al., cited by Caldeyro-Barcia[3]).

Liu[13] compared 30 women in a semiupright position with 30 women in a dorsal recumbent position. The mean intensity and frequency of contractions were increased in the semiupright women. The first stage of labor was 86 minutes shorter for the 30 women in a semiupright position. In addition, uterine relaxation between contractions was enhanced.

The first stage of labor is probably shorter in the vertical position because:

1. Contractions are more intense and more efficient, particularly in the early phase of the first stage of labor. Contractions were found to be most intense and efficient in the standing position, next in the sitting position, and least in the supine position.[17]

Roberts[25] found a lateral recumbent position to be more efficient than sitting.

2. The pressure of the fetal presenting part on the cervix aids dilatation. When the mother is in a vertical position the weight of the fetus adds 35 mm. Hg to the pressure exerted by the fetal head on the uterine cervix.[13]

3. Gold stated that when the *drive angle* (the angle between the longitudinal axis of the fetal spine and the longitudinal axis of the maternal spine) is between 60 and 80 degrees the progress of labor is better than when the drive angle is less than 45 degrees. A vertical position results in a wider drive angle.[3]

4. The fundus falls backward and rests on the sacral vertebrae when the mother is in a recumbent position. This may displace the fetal head and make entry into the pelvic inlet more difficult. When the thigh is flexed in a vertical position the abdominal wall relaxes, the fundus tilts forward, the longitudinal axis of the birth canal is straightened, and the fetal head is directed toward the pelvic inlet.[6]

The Second Stage

A vertical position for the second stage of labor has been associated with increased efficiency of expulsion in studies that span several decades (Fig. 15–23). When the mother is in a vertical position, the pelvic inlet points forward and the outlet points downward. In the squatting position, the anteroposterior diameter of the pelvic outlet is increased by as much

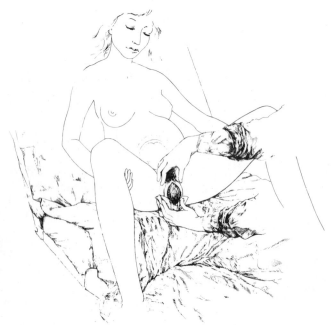

Figure 15–23. A vertical position increases the efficiency of pushing during the second stage. (Drawing provided by the Borning Corporation.)

as 2.0 cm. in some women. Flexion of the thighs against the abdomen appears to promote fetal descent and to correct unfavorable fetal positions.[25]

Intrauterine pressure achieved during the bearing down of the second stage is also related to position. Bonica[2] reported the following pressures:

Lateral position	120 mm. Hg
Supine position	125 mm. Hg
Semirecumbent position	135 mm. Hg
Sitting position	150 mm. Hg

Liu[13] reported a second stage of 34 minutes (mean) in 30 upright primigravidas; the second stage was over twice as long (74.67 minutes) in 30 primigravidas in a recumbent position. In Roberts'[25] review of several studies of the duration of labor, means ranged from 25.5 to 85 minutes for primigravidas and from 14 to 70 minutes for multigravidas.

Effects of Maternal Position on Fetus

Maternal position may affect fetal well-being through several mechanisms. Supine hypotensive syndrome has been previously discussed (page 171). The abdominal aorta may also be compressed above the bifurcation, potentially reducing blood flow through the iliac arteries.

Fetal brain mass would appear to be better protected when the mother is in a vertical position. Brain mass, because of gravity, will "sink" toward the most dependent position. When the fetus is LOA or ROA (the most common fetal positions) its brain mass will be directed toward the frontal lobes with a maternal prone or lithotomy position but toward the more developed occipital lobes with a vertical position. If the fetus is in a posterior position stress is placed on the brain stem at the foramen magnum.[14]

Maternal pulmonary ventilation appears to be improved when the mother is in a vertical position, as indicated by an increase in her pO_2 and a decrease in her pCO_2.

A maternal vertical position was also shown to decrease the number of fetal heart rate variable decelerations markedly, a fetal heart monitoring pattern that reflects compression of the umbilical cord (Chapter 18). In separate studies Flynn and Kelly[8, 9] monitored a group of women who were ambulatory during labor with a group who were recumbent. In the ambulatory group there was a virtual absence of variable decelerations; the vertical position may protect the umbilical cord from being compressed between the fetal skeleton and the

pelvis. Other differences between the two groups included shorter labors, decreased pain requiring less medication, decreased need for augmentation of labor, and improved Apgar scores.

Other Effects of Maternal Position

Mothers who are able or are allowed to assume various vertical positions have been found to take a more active role in labor and to be more interested in and responsive to their infants.[20, 21] Witek[29] found a difference in mother–infant interaction at 48 hours between mothers who delivered in a propped position compared with mothers in a recumbent position. A further advantage of the vertical position is the possibility of eye-to-eye contact between the mother and the person assisting in the delivery of the baby. Birthing chairs and birthing beds facilitate a vertical birthing position (Figs. 15–24 to 15–26).

Effect of Fetus on Labor

Certain characteristics of the fetus also have potential to affect the course of labor, including fetal size, number, and gestational age. Antepartum fetal testing (Chapter 14) may indicate

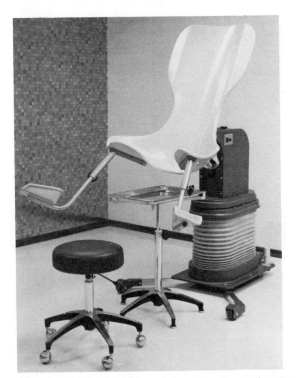

Figure 15–24. A birthing chair allows the mother to assume a physiologic, comfortable position for birth. (Photo provided by Century Manufacturing Company.)

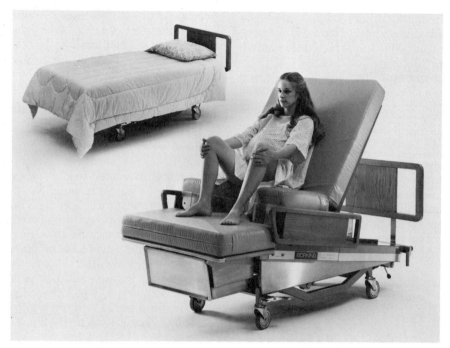

Figure 15–25. Birthing bed adjusts to allow mother to deliver baby in a vertical propped position. (Photo provided by the Borning Corporation, 1980.)

that the fetus has diminished oxygen reserves. Table 15–8 summarizes fetal characteristics that may affect labor. Many of these characteristics place the fetus in a high risk category and thus make electronic fetal monitoring a part of care when they are present (Chapter 18).

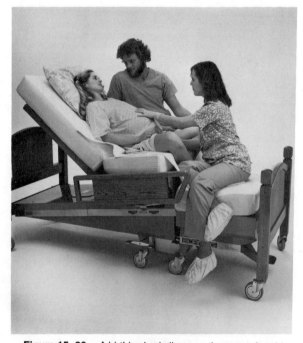

Figure 15–26. A birthing bed allows mother a comfortable position as well as allowing ease of nursing assessment. Notice the eye contact between mother and father. (Photo provided by the Borning Corporation.)

The Physiologic Basis of Pain During Labor

From ancient times pain has been associated with labor. The expression "labor pains" is familiar to nearly every woman. Is labor always painful? If so, how painful?

Pain during labor has both a physiologic and psychosocial component, as has most pain. Both factors are interwoven so closely that it is difficult to say when the physiologic component ends and the psychosocial component starts (or vice versa). The physiologic basis of pain during labor will be discussed here, whereas psychosocial factors will be discussed in Chapter 16. The adaptation of the physiologic and psychosocial concepts to nursing care during labor will be discussed in Chapter 17.

Historically, a certain degree of pain during childbirth has been considered inevitable, at least in Western society, and apparently among most of the world's peoples. The idea of pain, including labor pain, as punishment has been expressed at various times in history and still may influence our perceptions. For example, we unfortunately find on occasion that some individuals are less sympathetic to discomfort during labor when the mother is unmarried. Comments such as "she should have thought about the pain 9 months ago" or "maybe next time she'll remember what it means to have a baby before she fools around" are still heard from time to time.

Table 15–8. POSSIBLE EFFECTS OF THE FETUS ON LABOR AND BIRTH

Fetal Status	Possible Effects on Labor and Birth
Fetal size	
Large in relation to maternal pelvis	Cephalopelvic disproportion (CPD)
Small in relation to length of gestation	Fetal compromise (hypoxia) may require intervention
Gestational age	
Less than 38 weeks	Vulnerable hypoxia, birth trauma
	Breech: probable cesarean delivery
More than 42 weeks	Vertex: probable vertex delivery
	Decreased placental function
Fetal position	Labor is longer, back pain is increased when position is posterior
Fetal presentation	
Breech	Early rupture of membranes
	Longer labor
	Increased incidence of cord prolapse
	Increased incidence of cesarean delivery
Shoulder	Early rupture of membranes
	Longer labor
	Cesarean delivery
Sincipitum, brow, face	Slow progression of labor
	Cesarean delivery may be necessary
Positive contraction stress test, falling estriol levels, etc.	Fetus at risk of anoxia or distress during labor
Multiple pregnancy	At least one fetus may be breech
	Possible preterm labor
Fetal infections (TORCH group; Chapter 8)	Chronic fetal distress
Fetal congenital anomalies	Chronic fetal distress
Anomalies of the umbilical cord	Malpresentation

As prepared childbirth concepts have become widely discussed, many women have come to wonder if pain during labor is largely psychosomatic. Sometimes women feel that they have "failed" if they require any medication at all during labor or delivery.

It is important to recognize that while fear, anxiety, and tension may play a significant role in the discomfort that is felt during labor, there is also a physiologic basis for that discomfort.

Basic Physiologic Stimuli

As noted in Chapter 4, ischemia with resultant anoxia and stretching are the two basic stimuli for pain in the uterus. Pressure is a third stimulus important for pain in areas adjacent to the uterus.

Anoxia occurs during prolonged muscle contraction because the blood supply to the muscle is compromised (ischemia). The longer the contraction, the greater the ischemia and anoxia and the more intense the pain. Moreover, when the period of relaxation between contractions is too short to allow adequate oxygenation, the intensity of the pain is increased.

Stretching occurs in the cervix during effacement and dilatation. The muscles of the pelvic floor and perineum are distended during the second stage of labor. There is also traction on and stretching of the ligaments supporting the pelvic organs.

Pressure is applied to nerve ganglia adjacent to the cervix and vagina, as well as to the urethra, bladder, and rectum.

Nerve Pathways Involved in Labor

The nerves supplying the pelvis have been illustrated in Chapter 4. Two major nerve pathways carry sensory information from the pelvis; one from the uterus and cervix and the other from the perineum, vulva, and vagina.

The sympathetic pathway carries sensations from the uterus and cervix via the structures indicated here.

Uterus-cervix
↓
via sensory sympathetic nerves
↓
uterine plexus
↓
pelvic plexus
↓
hypogastric plexus
↓
aortic plexus
↓
ventral rami (T_{10}, T_{11}, T_{12})

Sensations from the perineum travel via the pudendal nerve. The pudendal nerve arises from the anterior branches of the second, third, and fourth sacral nerves, which join into a single nerve approximately 0.5 to 1.0 cm. proximal to the ischial spine. The nerve then passes through the greater sciatic foramen; crosses the sacrospinous ligament to the lesser sciatic foramen; enters the pudendal canal medial and posterior to the inferior tip of the spine; and terminates at the second, third, and fourth sacral nerves. Relief of perineal pain may be achieved by blocking the pudendal nerve pathway near the time of delivery (Chapter 17).

Relationship Between Type of Discomfort and Stage of Labor

The type of discomfort that a woman experiences will vary with the stage of labor. Table 15–9 summarizes the relationship between these two factors.

Other Physiologic Variables Influencing Discomfort

Several specific variables influence the discomfort that a mother experiences during labor.

The position of the baby makes a difference. Mothers with babies in a posterior position at the beginning of labor tend to have longer, more uncomfortable labors with discomfort centered in the lower back.

The duration of particular stages, as well as the overall duration of labor, is important. The transition stage, as noted above, is usually the

most difficult. When transition is prolonged, the labor is felt to be difficult by the mother and by those working with her.

Physiologic Effects of Labor on Maternal Systems Other Than Reproductive. Just as pregnancy affects all of a woman's body systems, so too does the process of labor. Understanding these changes is necessary for accurate assessment of a woman's status during labor.

Cardiovascular Response. *Cardiac output* steadily increases during labor. During each contraction blood is expelled from the uterus into the circulatory system, the amount being greater when the mother is in a supine position (a 15 per cent increase in cardiac output) than in the lateral position (an 8 per cent increase). At the end of the second stage of labor cardiac output has increased by 50 per cent, and increases further up to 80 per cent above prelabor values during the third stage. Pain may increase cardiac output even more. The sudden addition to the circulatory system of blood expelled from the uterus and the release of pressure on the inferior vena cava following delivery cause this marked increase in cardiac output. Gradually, cardiac output returns to nonpregnant levels by the end of the puerperium.[7]

Heart rate decreases gradually during the first stage of labor (average, 80 beats per minute) and increases during the second stage (average, 90 beats per minute). During contractions there is a further decrease in maternal pulse rate during the first stage but an increase to an average of 100 beats per minute during the pushing contractions of the second

Table 15–9.   RELATIONSHIP BETWEEN PAIN AND STAGE OF LABOR

Stage	Source of Discomfort	Pathway	Area of Pain
1	Effacement Dilatation of cervis Contraction of myometrium of uterus	Sensory sympathetic pathway → 10th, 11th, and 12th thoracic nerves and 1st lumbar nerve	Umbilical region Midsacral area Upper thighs
2	Stretching of vagina, vulva, perineum	Sensory fibers of pudendal nerves → 2nd, 3rd, and 4th sacral nerves	Perineum and surrounding structures
	Contraction of myometrium		Urge to bear down
3	Passage of placenta through cervix	Sensory sympathetic pathway → 10th, 11th and 12th thoracic nerves and 1st lumbar nerve	Umbilical region Midsacral area Upper thighs
	Contraction of myometrium		

Table 15–10. CARDIOVASCULAR CHANGES DURING LABOR AND PUERPERIUM*

Parameter	Stage of Labor			Return to Normal Values
	First Stage	*Second Stage*	*Third Stage*	
Cardiac output	Up 8–15 per cent (lateral vs. supine position)	Up by 50 per cent	Up by 80 per cent	End of puerperium
Heart rate	Down to average 80 beats per minute	Up to average 90 beats per minute; 100 beats per minute with contractions		Return to normal values 10 minutes after delivery of infant
Stroke volume	Progressive rise	Peak at delivery, then decrease to base level		Immediately following delivery
Blood pressure	Both systolic and diastolic up; higher during contractions	Systolic up 20 mm. Hg; diastolic up 15 mm. Hg		One hour following delivery
Blood volume	No significant change	Decreased (blood loss at delivery)		Decreased by 25 per cent in first hours postpartum; decrease continues until end of puerperium

*Based on Dgani and Lancet: Maternal Adjustment to Labors. *In* Iffy, L., and Kaminetzky, H. (eds.): *Principles and Practice of Obstetrics and Perinatology.* Volume 2. New York, John Wiley, 1981.

stage. Heart rate[7] returns to normal levels 10 minutes after the baby is delivered.

Stroke volume rises throughout the first stage of labor but decreases rapidly at the end of the second stage, probably because of the increase in heart rate at this time. *Blood volume* is decreased by blood loss at the time of delivery (normally about 500 ml.) and by diuresis and insensitive water loss, particularly during the first 72 hours postpartum, in which time a 25 per cent decrease occurs. Blood volume continues to decrease to prepregnancy levels throughout the puerperium.

Blood pressure increases as labor progresses both during and between contractions. By the end of the second stage of labor systolic blood pressure has risen by an average of 20 mm. Hg and diastolic blood pressure by 15 mm. Hg. Blood pressure returns to prelabor values 1 hour following delivery.

Respiratory Response. The respiratory changes of pregnancy (Chapter 7) continue through the period of labor. Respiratory rate and oxygen consumption increase with the work of labor.

A major respiratory concern in labor is the possibility of hyperventilation, either from a rapid breathing technique learned in prepared childbirth classes or from spontaneous rapid breathing as a response to effort, anxiety, and pain. During hyperventilation increased amounts of carbon dioxide are exhaled, leading to a decrease of carbon dioxide in the bloodstream and a rise in maternal pH (respiratory alkalosis). When hyperventilation ceases, baseline pH is achieved within 15 minutes.

A major concern is the effect of these maternal respiratory changes on the fetus. Several studies, in which women in labor deliberately hyperventilated for periods ranging from 5 to 18 minutes, report that fetal pCO_2 and pH increased, but that fetal oxygen levels obtained by fetal scalp sampling were not outside the normal physiologic range.[15, 19] There is some concern about the effect of hyperventilation on the fetus who is already hypoxic. It is important to recognize that if a woman hyperventilates spontaneously, she will rarely do so for the extended period of time used in the experiments.

Most women who have attended childbirth education classes have been taught to recognize signs of hyperventilation such as lightheadedness, dizziness, weakness, tingling of the fingers and around the mouth, anxiety, and, in advanced stages, cramping of fingers and tetany. To correct the problem they are instructed to breathe more slowly and to breathe into a paper bag or their cupped hands until the symptoms disappear (thus rebreathing CO_2 and correcting the respiratory alkalosis). By using these techniques more than 85 per cent of women are able to control the symptoms of hyperventilation.[5]

Many childbirth educators teach slower rates of breathing than formerly, although Cogan did not find reliable differences in the frequency or extent of hyperventilation when she compared groups of women using three breathing techniques (fast panting, 120 breaths per minute; "he" breathing, 60 to 120 breaths per minute; and slow panting, 60 breaths per minute).[5]

Acid-Base Balance. Maternal pH increases in response to hyperventilation but drops abruptly at the time of delivery owing to an increase in lactic acid, probably from the myometrium.[7] Maternal pH returns to pre-pregnancy levels the day after delivery.

Fluid Balance. Fluid is lost through insensible water loss (diaphoresis and hyperventilation) and blood loss at delivery. Oral fluid intake is restricted because of the delayed gastric emptying. If vomiting is present, body fluids are further depleted. Intravenous fluids are frequently given to laboring mothers in hospitals, although this practice is unpopular with some consumers and is not common in alternative birthing sites.

Gastrointestinal Response. Gastric emptying, which is decreased during pregnancy, virtually stops during labor. Food ingested as long as 12 hours before the onset of labor may remain in the stomach. Nausea and vomiting are not unusual, and thus the risk of aspiration is a concern.

The limiting of oral intake to clear liquid once labor has begun and the prophylactic use of antacids during the course of labor are two measures used to reduce the risk of aspiration and possible aspiration pneumonitis.

Renal Response. The combination of relaxed muscle tone of the bladder and the pressure of the baby's head on the bladder and urethra may lead to atony and distention of the bladder when as little as 100 ml. of urine is presnt. Distention is a barrier to fetal descent as well as a source of discomfort. In addition, pressure on a distended bladder may cause trauma and subsequent stases of urine and infection in the puerperium.

The activity of labor may cause some proteinuria, but usually only a trace and never more than 2 plus. A voided specimen, if contaminated by bloody show, will have protein, but it will represent the protein of the blood. A clean-catch specimen, collected carefully, should be accurate. Causes of proteinuria during labor include dehydration, exhaustion, and nutritional deficiency. Women with pre-eclampsia may also have proteinuria.

Summary

This chapter has examined the physiologic accommodation of both mother and fetus during labor. This knowledge is basic to the nursing assessment of the mother-fetus, which is discussed in Chapter 17. A knowledge of the social, cultural, and emotional correlates of labor (Chapter 16) is also a part of the nursing assessment data base.

REFERENCES

1. Atwood, R.: Parturitional Posture and Related Birth Behavior. *Acta Obstetricia et Gynecologica Scandinavica,* Supplement 57, 1976.
2. Bonica, J.: *Principles and Practice of Obstetrics Analgesia and Anesthesia.* Philadelphia, F. A. Davis, 1967.
3. Caldeyro-Barcia, R.: Physiological and Psychosocial Bases for the Modern and Humanized Management of Normal Labor. Lecture presented at International Year of the Child Commemorative International Congress, Tokyo, October, 1979.
4. Carr, K.: Obstetric Practices Which Protect Against Neonatal Morbidity: Focus on Maternal Position in Labor and Birth. *Birth and the Family Journal,* 7(4):249, 1980.
5. Cogan, R.: Pain and Hyperventilation with Fast Panting, Slow Panting and "He" Breathing During Labor. *Birth and the Family Journal,* 4(2):59, 1977.
6. Davis, J., and Renning, E.: The Birth Canal—Practical Applications. *Medical Times,* 92:75, 1964.
7. Dgani, R., and Lancet, M.: Maternal Adjustment to Labor. *In* Iffy, L., and Kaminetzky, H. (Eds.): *Principles and Practice of Obstetrics and Perinatology.* Volume 2. New York, John Wiley, 1981.
8. Flynn, A., and Kelly, J.: Continuous Fetal Monitoring in the Ambulant Patient in Labour. *British Medical Journal,* 2:842, 1976.
9. Flynn, A., and Kelly, J.: Ambulation in Labour. *British Medical Journal,* 2:591, 1978.
10. Friedman, E.: *Labor: Clinical Evaluation and Management.* New York, Appleton-Century-Crofts, 1967.
11. Greenhill, J., and Friedman, E.: *Biological Principles and Modern Practice of Obstetrics.* Philadelphia, W. B. Saunders Co., 1974.
12. Liggins, G. C.: The Foetal Role in the Initiation of Parturition in the Ewe. *In* Wolstenholme, G. E. W., and O'Connor, M. (Eds.): *Foetal Anatomy.* London, J. & A. Churchill, 1969.
13. Liu, Y.: Effects of an Upright Position During Labor. *American Journal of Nursing,* 74:2202, 1974.
14. Liu, Y.: Position During Labor and Delivery: History and Perspective. *Journal of Nurse-Midwifery,* 24(3):23, 1979.
15. Lumley, J., and Wood, C.: Effects of Changes in

Maternal Oxygen and Carbon Dioxide Tensions on the Fetus. *Clinical Anesthesia, 10*:121, 1974.

16. Martin, C., and Gingerich, B.: Factors Affecting the Fetal Heart Rate: Genesis of FHR Patterns. *JOGN Nursing, 5*(5): Suppl. 30s, 1976.

17. Mendez-Bauer, C.: Effects of Standing Position on Spontaneous Uterine Contractility and Other Aspects of Labor. *Journal of Perinatal Medicine, 3*:89, 1975.

18. Milic, A. B., and Adamsons, K.: The Relationship Between Anencephaly and Prolonged Pregnancy. *Journal of Obstetrics and Gynaecology of the British Commonwealth, 76*:102, 1969.

19. Miller, F., Petrie, R., Arce, J., et al.: Hyperventilation During Labor. *American Journal of Obstetrics and Gynecology, 120*:489, 1974.

20. Newton, N.: The Effect of Position on the Course of the Second Stage of Labor. *Surgical Forum, 7*:517, 1956.

21. Newton, N., and Newton, M.: Mother's Reactions to Their Newborn Babies. *Journal of the American Medical Association, 81*:206, 1962.

22. Oxorn, H., and Foote, W.: *Human Labor and Birth.* New York, Appleton-Century-Crofts, 1975.

23. Page, E., Villee, C., and Villee, D.: *Human Reproduction: The Core Content of Obstetrics, Gynecology and Perinatal Medicine.* 3rd Edition. Philadelphia, W. B. Saunders Co., 1981.

24. Pareri, J.: Physiological Regulation of Fetal Heart Rate. *JOGN Nursing, 5*(5):Suppl. 26s, 1976.

25. Roberts, J.: Alternative Positions for Childbirth: The Second Stage of Labor. *Journal of Nurse-Midwifery, 25*(5):13, 1980.

26. Saling, E., and Ligdas, P.: The Effect on the Fetus of Maternal Hyperventilation During Labour. *Journal of Obstetrics and Gynaecology of the British Commonwealth, 76*:877, 1969.

27. Schifri, B. S.: Fetal Heart Rate Patterns Following Epidural Anesthesia and Oxytocin Infusion During Labour. *Journal of Obstetrics and Gynaecology of the British Commonwealth, 79*:332, 1972.

28. Varney, H.: *Nurse-Midwifery.* Boston: Blackwell Scientific Publications, 1980.

29. Witek, J.: Effects of Maternal Position on Initial Interaction with the Newborn and Subsequent Maternal Behavior. Master's thesis, University of Illinois at the Medical Center, 1979.

16

Social, Cultural, and Emotional Correlates of Labor

OBJECTIVES

1. Describe changes in emotional status of the mother during labor.
2. Explain the relationship between anxiety and the course of labor.
3. Identify variables that may affect anxiety during labor.
4. Describe potential environments for labor and birth and identify advantages and disadvantages of each.

Labor and the birth of a child are universal, a part of every society. In terms of basic physiology, labor is similar for all women; the uterus contracts, the cervix is effaced and dilated, and the baby is expelled.

But the *experience* of labor differs from one society to another and also among women in an individual society. There is a physiologic basis for some differences; when the baby's position is posterior, for example, labor is usually more difficult. Physiologic differences were discussed in Chapter 15.

A significant difference lies in the *meaning of labor* for the society and for the individual mother and her family. A cross-cultural perspective is helpful in this regard. For example, one finds societies in which normal labor is largely nontraumatic, both physically and emotionally. Does this perhaps indicate that this potential may exist in other societies? Perhaps factors that contribute to a relatively easy labor can be identified.

Labor In Other Societies: Some Examples

Tafel describes a birth in a Tibetan household.

During the night Mrs. Lobzang Dandudschumo gave birth to a son. She did it outside the tent in the goat stall which had no roof but a low protective wall of earth and frozen cow dung, which kept off the worst blasts of the wind. Inside the tent it would have been a few degrees warmer, but the nomad women avoid labor in the cook rooms, for religious reasons. All night long her husband prayed with a few lamas inside the tent, to the accompaniment of kettle drums and trumpets. The temperature during the night went down to -32. The next morning the mother was already busy at the stove in the tent.[27]

McDonald notes that Tibetan peasant mothers "... work in the fields up to the time of delivery, seldom resting for more than a couple of days after the child has been born." Moreover, "The Tibetan mother goes through her time of trial practically unassisted, but she seldom has any trouble in childbirth."[19]

Among the Australian aborigines "The actual physical experience in giving birth to a child is so minimized and the social implications of the result of the birth so magnified, that the former melts away into the obscure background before the all-embracing consequences of the latter."[2]

It must be noted in this connection that childbirth among the Australians, as among many aboriginal peoples who are relatively unmixed, is a comparatively light affair for the woman, who is usually up and about her regular duties within a few hours after the delivery of the child. There is no period of confinement before the birth of the child, and there is no period of convalescence afterward, so that the actual experience of birth is by no means the traumatically impressive experience that it generally is for the white woman.[2]

Perhaps the reason that the physical experience of procreation is considered insignificant is that aboriginal beliefs about maternity regard the woman who gives birth as merely acting as a medium through whom the infant is conveyed into the proper moiety and section of the tribe. The conception, prenatal development, and birth of the child are matters completely independent of the mother in every physical sense. No association is recognized between intercourse and pregnancy. It is expected that "The physical act of intercourse between the sexes would have the effect of 'opening up' the womb of the mother, and thus, in the event of a spirit child electing to enter the particular woman it would find ingress easy and everything in order upon its arrival."[2]

The Ifaluk of the central Caroline Islands in the Pacific desire babies "...probably more than any other single thing....A couple that does not have children is greatly pitied."[3] There are no midwives among the Ifaluk. The mother delivers her own infant, and although her own mother and her mother's sister are present at the delivery, they assist only if there is some difficulty. During delivery the mother kneels on a mat, catches the baby in her arms, and holds it until the placenta is delivered. She then severs the umbilical cord with a small ocean shell.[3]

Holmberg states that there are also no midwives among the Siriono of Eastern Bolivia, nor is any assistance by friends or relatives given to women in labor under ordinary conditions.[10] When labor pains begin, the mother ties a rope above the hammock in which she will lie to deliver the infant. She loosens the hard ground beneath the hammock with a digging stick and sometimes spreads it with ashes to make it still more soft, for as the baby is born, he will slide through the strings of the hammock to the earth below. Since the hammock is only a few inches above the ground, the fall is not so great as to harm the infant, yet is sufficient to induce breathing. In the births that Holmberg witnessed, all of the infants started to breathe immediately after the shock of birth. In no instance was one slapped to give it life.

It would be a mistake to believe, however, that difficulty in labor occurs only in industrialized societies and that in a more "natural environment" birth is always uncomplicated. Even in those societies in which birth is considered a casual and easy procedure, difficulties may occur. DuBois, commenting on the people of Alor, points out that the society had chosen not to emphasize the difficulties.[9]

On the Pacific island of Bougainville, birth is considered a very painful experience; it is accompanied by anguished crying. Oliver describes this scene:

> When labor begins, the assisting women warn all boys and men to keep away from the place of birth. As labor pains increase the woman is made to sit in a low bed or log and hold onto a rope tied to an overhead beam or tree; then when birth begins she is encouraged to assist by pulling on the rope. Her mother or sister kneels behind her and massages her with heavy downward motions.[23]

The Birthing Environment: A Part of the Culture of Childbearing

As the paragraphs above indicate, the environment and the circumstances surrounding the birth of infants can vary tremendously. In the United States and in many Western European nations the majority of infants are born in hospitals. In 1935 in the United States approximately 40 per cent of deliveries occurred in hospitals; today 99 per cent are hospital births. In England approximately 50 per cent of infants were born in hospitals in 1954, but over 90 per cent were hospital births in 1974. Maternal and neonatal mortality has dramatically decreased during that period (1935–1978), and many professionals believe that hospital birth is the major factor in that decrease and that only hospitals provide the protection essential for safe delivery. However, hospital birth is probably only one of many factors responsible for the decrease; better nutrition, higher standards of living, and earlier prenatal care are probably equally as important.

Some professionals and many expectant parents believe that childbirth in hospitals has become too technologically oriented and that some of this technology is unnecessary for most mothers and families. These persons seek a more humanistic and caring environment for childbirth than they perceive in most hospitals.

Possible childbirth environments in our society currently include the traditional hospital labor/delivery suite, a birthing room (labor/delivery room) within a hospital, an alternative birthing center, which may be associated with a hospital or may be a separate facility, and the home. Each of these environments offers advantages and disadvantages in relation to a mother's health status as well as to the needs and desires of individual women and their families.

Each environment also represents a different belief system or set of values and attitudes. Those who support the idea of choice for most women believe that childbirth is an essentially normal process and that most complications are preventable. Although alternatives to traditional hospital delivery (birthing centers in hospitals, for example), are supported by some physicians, in many alternative environments nurse-midwives or lay midwives are the birth attendants. Those who believe that only hospitals are the place for birth (and frequently limiting this to the traditional labor/delivery suite within the hospital) believe that the safety of the mother and child is paramount and that safety can be guaranteed only within a hospital where an obstetrician supervises the labor and delivery of the infant.

The Traditional Hospital Labor/Delivery Suite

When either the mother or the fetus is identified as high risk because of pre-existing disease or obstetrical complications in a past or current pregnancy, access to the technologies available within hospitals is essential. Few individuals dispute this principle. However, a high risk labor should not be a reason to exclude family members during the course of the labor or birth.

Conflict arises about the best way to meet the needs of the majority of mothers (approximately 85 to 90 per cent) who will have a normal labor and birth. Should these mothers, like mothers at known risk of complications, be kept away from family and friends in an environment that may appear sterile and impersonal and over which they may feel they have little control?

Even traditional labor/delivery suites have become far more family-oriented than they were just a few years ago. The presence of fathers or other support persons in labor/delivery rooms, opportunities for bonding between infant and family in delivery rooms and recovery rooms, and encouragement of breast-feeding during the first hour after birth, are examples of family-oriented change. Moreover, in many hospitals women do have choices about the extent of certain interventions.

Nevertheless, the traditional labor/delivery environment, in comparison with other environments for birth, is usually more restrictive.

Birthing Rooms

The concept of a birthing room derives from the philosophy that birth is usually a normal physiologic event and an important experience to be shared by the expectant family. Because labor and birth may occasionally be abnormal, a family-centered environment is provided within the hospital by means of a birthing room. The environment is designed to be home-like rather than hospital-like. Walls painted a soft color, curtains, pictures, plants, and bedspreads contribute to the homelike atmosphere. Emergency equipment is kept out of clear view behind a curtain or door, quickly available but unobtrusive.

Mothers labor, deliver, and share the immediate postpartum period with their families, including the new baby, in the birthing room rather than having to be moved from a labor room to a delivery area to a recovery room. While a traditional hospital bed may be used in some birthing rooms, special birthing beds have been developed to facilitate delivery, and birthing chairs are used in some units.

The use of a single bed for labor and birth has multiple advantages. The movement of a mother from the labor to the delivery room at the end of the first stage or the beginning of the second stage breaks into the continuity of labor and the mother's concentration as well as requiring her to use her much needed energy in the transfer from bed to delivery table. The admonition to the mother "don't push, don't push" during some transports so that the baby will not be born on a stretcher can be viewed as intervention that is potentially deleterious to the baby. In addition, values such as fetal heart rate and maternal vital signs cannot be easily assessed during transport. The utilization of two beds in the labor and delivery rooms and a third bed in a recovery area involves nursing time to prepare each bed and room.

Generally there are some restrictions on the use of birthing rooms. Some birthing rooms are restricted to couples who have attended childbirth education classes, while others are not. When the mother or fetus is known to be at risk for complications during delivery (Table 16–1), a mother will be delivered in a traditional delivery room. Many analgesics and anesthetics are not used in birthing rooms because of their potential side effects (Chapter 17). Individual policies differ; paracervical

Table 16–1. CONTRAINDICATIONS TO THE USE OF BIRTHING ROOMS OR ALTERNATIVE BIRTHING SITES*

A. Pre-existing maternal disease
  1. Anemia (hemoglobin less than 9.5 g./100 ml.)
  2. Chronic hypertension
  3. Diabetes mellitus
  4. Heart disease
  5. Renal disease
  6. Pulmonary disease, including tuberculosis
  7. Psychiatric disease requiring major tranquilizer
B. Obstetrical problems
  1. Previous pregnancy
    a. Stillbirth of unknown etiology
    b. Cesarean birth (or uterine surgery)
    c. Rh isoimmunization
    d. Great multiparity (greater than 5)
    e. Infant of same gestational age with respiratory distress syndrome
  2. Current pregnancy
    a. Gestational age less than 37 weeks or greater than 42 weeks
    b. Multiple pregnancy
    c. Presentation other than vertex
    d. Pregnancy-induced hypertension
    e. Placenta previa
    f. Third trimester bleeding
    g. Membranes ruptured for longer than 24 hours
    h. Intrauterine growth retardation
    i. Suspected cephalopelvic disproportion
    j. Need for induction of labor
    k. Pelvic disease (e.g., uterine malformation, pelvic tumor, genital herpes)
    l. certain medications (e.g., lithium, magnesium)
    m. Other illness that may increase risk to mother or infant
C. Other factors
  1. Lack of prenatal care (less than three prenatal visits)
  2. Maternal age
  3. Desire of mother for anesthesia or analgesia not available in alternative site

*Each facility develops policies that may vary somewhat from this list. Some indications may be relative rather than absolute (e.g., maternal age, multiparity).

block, pudendal block, local perineal anesthesia, or small amounts of meperidine (Demerol) and tranquilizing drugs are used in some birthing rooms.

Couples who decide that they would prefer delivery in a birthing room are prepared in advance that if an emergency arises during the labor, transfer to a traditional labor or delivery room will be necessary. In one study covering 10 years of birthing room experience, 12 per cent of 1472 nulliparas and 3 per cent of 1358 multiparas were transferred. Common reasons were the need for availability of general anesthesia (although it was not always used), the need for spinal anesthesia, or presentations other than vertex.

Fetal monitoring, intravenous fluids, and other "interventions" may or may not be a part of the birthing room experience, depending on local policy or the individual needs of the mother.

In some birthing rooms a *montrice* rather than a staff nurse may care for the patient. A montrice is a nurse trained in prepared childbirth who is employed by the parents (rather than the hospital) who provides one-to-one support for the family throughout labor and delivery. The availability of a montrice solves a problem inherent in most traditional hospital environments—the loss of a supporting nurse at change of shift or because of the needs of other patients.

The use of birthing rooms, even when they are available, varies markedly from one community to another. Sumner and Phillips[26] report that the birthing room is the primary site for deliveries in Manchester, Connecticut. In contrast, in another hospital where a birthing room is available, less than 1 per cent of couples take advantage of the opportunity to use it. The active encouragement or discouragement of professionals (nurses and physicians) seems to make an important difference in utilization. Nurses and physicians trained in traditional obstetrical practices sometimes discourage women from using birthing rooms because of their own discomfort with change.

As health care costs escalate, Adkins[1] report that birthing rooms save money in terms of housekeeping costs (21 minutes for delivery), usage of linens, and usage of nursing time provides an additional incentive for this type of delivery. The reduced need for anesthesia services also reduces costs.

Alternative Birthing Centers

Alternative birthing centers (ABC's) have been developed both within hospitals and in independent out-of-hospital settings. Nurse-midwives frequently supervise labor and birth in alternative birthing centers. In 1981 there were approximately 40 to 50 ABC's in the United States. Like birthing rooms, ABC's are sites for uncomplicated deliveries and mothers at risk for complications are not admitted (Table 16–2).

The Maternity Center Association in New York and the Birth Center of Bryn Mawr are examples of a independent ABC's. Lubic describes labor and birth at the Maternity Center Association:

Table 16–2. CRITERIA FOR TRANSFER FROM BIRTHING ROOMS OR ALTERNATIVE BIRTHING SITES*

Maternal temperature greater than 38°C. (100.4°F.)
Variation from prenatal blood pressure greater than 30/15
Hemoglobin less than 9.5 g./100 ml.
Abnormalities of fetal heart rate
Prolonged labor or arrest of active labor
Prolonged second stage (greater than 1 hour in multipara, or 2 hours in nullipara)
Vaginal bleeding (differentiated from bloody show)
Any factor that requires more intensive assessment or intervention

*Each facility develops policies that may vary somewhat from this list.

When labor begins, families are encouraged to remain at home as long as they are comfortable in doing so. When they do come to the center, the mother is encouraged to be up and about with her family in the family room or garden. When the mother is admitted to one of the two labor/delivery rooms, prepared family members, including children, may accompany her. Nurse-midwives assist the mother during delivery; obstetricians are not present. No routine procedures are used. The mothers labor in a position of comfort and deliver their infants in the labor bed.

Although available, analgesia is seldom used. Oral intake of fluid is encouraged, and families bring their own food for celebrating after the birth. The healthy infant is never separated from the parents and may be cuddled and fed as they please. The pediatric examination is performed in the parents' presence.[18]

See Figures 16–1 to 16–6 for illustrations of the homelike environment provided by alternative birthing centers.

Opponents of ABC's, particularly of free-standing facilities outside of a hospital, cite the occurrence of unforeseen complications as an everpresent danger. Thiede[28] lists misdiagnosis of presenting part, unrecognized multiple gestation, cord accidents, abruption, vasa previa (exposed fetal blood vessels—i.e., outside of the Wharton's jelly), shoulder dystocia, asphyxia, and neonatal congenital anomalies as examples of complications. Thiede, an opponent of free-standing clinics but an apparent supporter of ABC's within hospitals, cites other objections:

1. Further polarization of nurse-midwives and physicians.

2. Frequent referral out of the program because conditions that develop that are not appropriate to an independent clinic, thus interrupting continuity of care.

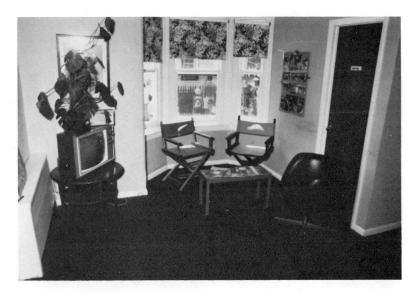

Figure 16–1. Pleasant family room with TV, magazines, and plants. Family members accompanying the mother may relax here during the hours the mother is in labor. (Courtesy of The Birth Center, Bryn Mawr, PA; photographer, David B. Miller.)

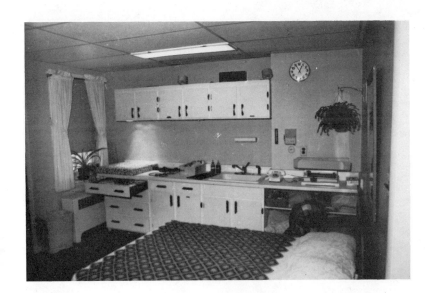

Figure 16–2. Labor and birth room in a free-standing birth center. Note that a comfortable environment is combined with easy access to equipment should increased nursing intervention become necessary (oxygen tank by side of bed, drawers and cabinets containing supplies, wall intercom and phone). A warming light at one end of the counter is for use during neonatal assessment. (Courtesy of The Birth Center, Bryn Mawr, PA; photographer, David B. Miller.)

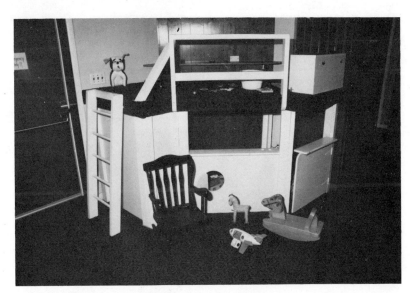

Figure 16–3. A birth center playroom for siblings who may become bored during the hours of labor and birth. (Courtesy of The Birth Center, Bryn Mawr, PA; photographer, David B. Miller.)

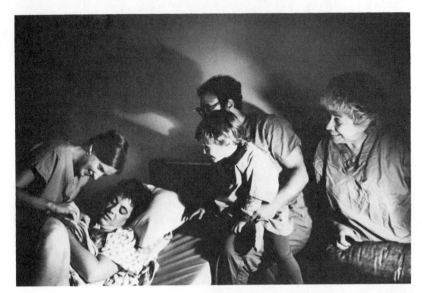

Figure 16–4. In alternative birthing centers, both within hospitals and free-standing, childbearing is a family event. Even grandmothers may participate! (Courtesy of Mariette Pathy Allen, Maternity Center Association, New York.)

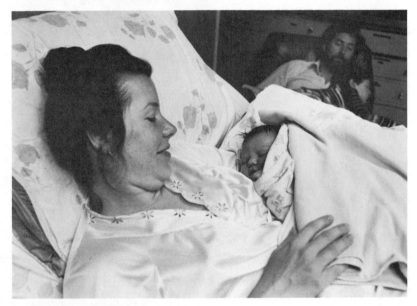

Figure 16–5. Mother and infant are not separated from each other after birth in an alternative birthing center. Note father and brother asleep on chair in background. Courtesy of Mariette Pathy Allen, Maternity Center Association, New York,)

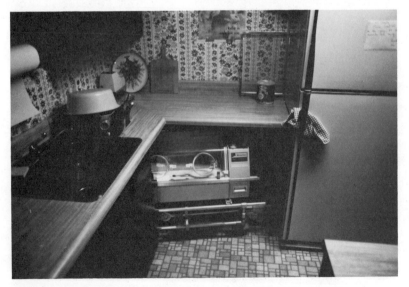

Figure 16–6. A kitchen is part of this birthing center. Families often store dishes in the refrigerator for a celebration meal after the baby is born. Note that a neonatal transport incubator is stored under the counter, providing easy access in case transport is necessary but not so obvious as to cause the family undue anxiety. (Courtesy The Birth Center, Bryn Mawr, PA; photographer, David B. Miller.)

3. Lack of opportunity for physicians in training to observe the ABC model, which might change their perspective of childbirth.

Advocates of alternative birthing sites believe that perfect safety is illusory, even in hospital settings, and that some complications may be the result of routine hospital practices. Moreover, they point out that for at least some couples who choose an ABC the choice was not between hospital and ABC but between home delivery and ABC, and thus increased safety is provided by the ABC.

Home Birth

A growing, although still very small, number of families in the United States are choosing to deliver their babies at home rather than in hospitals. To a large extent nurses and physicians have felt very negative about the home birth movement. Nurses need to be aware of the:

1. Reasons families choose home birth.
2. Potential dangers weighed against the potential advantages.
3. Possibility of compromise.
4. Role of nursing in the home birth movement.

Why Do Families Choose Home Birth?

Why do families choose a home birth (a birth that most professionals in the United States feel is potentially dangerous for mother and baby) over a hospital birth (a birth that the professionals believe is much safer)?

The parents who choose home birth are not uncaring, unconcerned mothers and fathers. Although for a minority home birth may be a part of a communal lifestyle (Chapter 5), many parents who opt for home birth are well educated and have given the issue serious consideration.

They see delivery of a baby, under most circumstances, as a natural part of family life. They object to the impersonal, often assembly line atmosphere of the hospital, and they object to the enforced separation from family and friends that often accompanies hospitalization. Most couples who choose home birth recognize that there may be risks, but they believe that there are also risks in hospital births and that with adequate precautions the level of risk can be minimal.

The cost of hospital services has been an issue for some parents. As the cost of maternity care climbs to over $2000 in many sections of the country, some couples feel financially unable to afford hospital delivery. Conversely, home delivery may be more expensive for some patients because their hospitalization insurance will not cover the costs.

Professional Reaction

Some health professionals, including certain nurses, nurse-midwives, and physicians, have been supportive of the home birth movement. Some physicians will attend home births to intervene, should the need arise. The majority of the health care community, however, has reacted with disdain. Anger has been particularly directed toward the couple who initially rejects hospital services and then seeks those services when complications arise.

Dangers versus Advantages

The greatest concern of those who oppose home birth is the danger of unexpected complications, such as prolapse of the umbilical cord or maternal hemorrhage, complications that cannot be anticipated from prenatal assessment.

The risk of complications can be lowered by endeavoring to convince mothers with a potentially greater risk of complications that even if home birth is safe for some mothers, it is not advisable for them (see box) and that even for low risk mothers all risk cannot be eliminated.

SOME CONTRAINDICATIONS TO HOME BIRTH

1. Maternal diabetes mellitus
2. Maternal heart disease
3. Maternal kidney disease
4. Any acute or chronic maternal health problem (e.g., anemia)
5. Rh incompatibility
6. Active herpes simplex virus
7. Symptoms of pre-eclampsia and/or eclampsia
8. Antepartum bleeding
9. Hydramnios
10. Maternal age less than 20 or greater than 35 years
11. Complication in previous pregnancy
12. Previous cesarean section
13. Small pelvis (cephalopelvic disproportion)
14. Abnormal presentation
15. History of large infants or increase in the size of subsequent infants
16. History of small for gestational age (SGA) babies

17. More than four previous deliveries
18. Inadequate nutrition
19. Lack of prenatal care
20. Lack of access to emergency care
21. Multiple pregnancy
22. Gestation of less than 36 weeks or greater than 42 weeks

A major argument against home birth has been that maternal and infant mortality in the United States has decreased as the number of hospital births has increased. As we compare mortality figures at the beginning of the twentieth century with corresponding figures today, this change is obvious. A number of contributing factors have changed as well. Both the general economic level of our population and the level of general education have risen. Antibiotics have been introduced. There is more awareness of nutrition, and diets are more varied. The birth rate has decreased. These factors have probably also contributed to improved outcomes.

Another comparison that is only partly relevant (because the different populations involved are not necessarily equivalent) is with certain European countries in which home birth remains popular but infant mortality is low, lower than in the United States. In the Netherlands, where infant mortality in 1973 was 11.5 per 1000 live births (compared with a rate of 17.6 in the United States), approximately 40 per cent of deliveries during that year were supervised by midwives at home.

The largest body of home birth data in the United States is that of the Frontier Nursing Service (FNS) in Kentucky. FNS nurse-midwives delivered approximately 10,000 babies in rural, predominantly substandard homes between 1925 and 1955; maternal mortality rates for white women were approximately 75 per cent lower than rates for white women in the remainder of the United States.

On the other hand, we are personally aware of infant mortality and morbidity in home births that might have been prevented by hospital delivery.

Hospital deliveries may subject mothers and infants to a different kind of risk, iatrogenic risks from oxytocics, for example. The danger of hospital-type infection is a potential hazard. Infection may be a potential hazard in home delivery as well, if proper techniques are not observed. However, given the same technique, the home is a safer place from a bacteriologic standpoint because the mother is immune to

organisms in her own home; hospital organisms, to which she may not be immune, are far more resistant.

Potential Advantages

A major advantage of home birth, frequently cited by consumers, is the opportunity to deliver their baby in a familiar and secure environment, surrounded by friends and family. There is no transfer from labor room to delivery table. The baby may be held and nursed at the mother's breast immediately after birth, an act not always permitted in the hospital setting, although probably ideal in terms of attachment behavior. The mother is not separated from her other children for a period of several days. Perhaps most significant, the mother and father take an active role in the delivery of their baby, rather than a passive "acted-upon" role.

At home the mother may be about her usual activities for a longer period of time, which often makes labor seem to be shorter. Moreover, in walking about and changing her position, uterine contractions may be more effective (as noted in Chapter 15) and less frequent. If she is less anxious because she is home, her relaxation will contribute to her comfort during labor.

Change in Emotional Status During Labor

Just as there is variation in emotional response to labor among and within societies, there is also variation as labor progresses. To what extent the reactions described below are physiologically based and to what extent they are affected by social and emotional factors (including institutional and interactional factors) is an important question for future research.

The First Stage

Early in the first stage when the mother and father (or other support person) enter the hospital, they must cope with a new environment, unfamiliar procedures, and people who are to a large extent strangers to them. The concept of culture shock (Chapter 2) is very applicable. The mother surrenders her clothes and personal belongings. It is little wonder that she may feel that she has lost her identity and been separated from her normal existence—her family and familiar surroundings.

The desire to be in familiar surroundings is one major factor cited by women who opt for home birth. All of us feel more in control when surroundings are familiar. When we are on someone else's "turf," we feel that they are in control, and when we feel we are losing control, we begin to lose self-esteem as well. As our self-esteem falls, we often become either aggressive because of our frustration or passive and dependent.

This sequence of feelings is not peculiar to labor; it affects all hospitalized patients as well as all persons at various stages of life. Much of our nursing intervention (Chapter 17) is directed toward helping the mother to cope and preventing this loss of control.

In spite of individual personality differences, the emotional characteristics of women in labor follow a pattern. When a woman first suspects she may be in labor, feelings of excitement ("It's finally happening") and some anxiety ("Will everything be OK? Will I be able to do what I planned? Will it hurt?") are common. Mothers are not usually very uncomfortable early in labor; if they come to the hospital or birthing center at this time they may pass the time by talking with the staff as well as with their family, reading magazines, or watching television.

As labor becomes more active, with contractions occurring every 3 to 5 minutes and lasting approximately a minute, most women become less outgoing. There is less small talk as they concentrate upon coping with each contraction.

By the time cervical dilation has reached 8 cm. (transition stage) some women feel out of touch with the surrounding environment. Signs of restlessness, irritability, and discouragement are some of the emotions that may be seen during transition. The frequency (every 2 minutes) and the length (70 to 90 seconds) of contractions seem overwhelming. Her body is in control; she feels out of control. A mother may say, "I'm not going to have another contraction," or "I want to go home right now," or "Don't touch me; leave me alone." Husbands or others who are with her need to know that such statements are classic transition statements; the mother should not feel guilty about what she says at this time, and family members (and nurses) should not feel hurt. Between contractions the mother in transition may feel very drowsy.

Some mothers become increasingly passive as labor progresses. They feel they cannot help themselves and make statements such as "Please help me," or "Please give me something," or "Someone help me." Other mothers are able to retain control or to regain control if it is briefly lost. Preparation for childbirth appears to be a major factor in differentiating those mothers who move toward passive dependence from those who remain active participants in their own labor.

As nurses, we need to identify ways, both through personal observations and research, in which our intervention encourages maternal behavior to be either active or passive.

The Second Stage

Following transition, many mothers are more alert and have renewed energy and excitement during the second stage. In this stage, emotions of individual mothers range from the mother who finds birth an exhilarating experience comparable to orgasm (see Sexuality, Labor, and Birth, below) to the mother who is unable to participate and sees herself as being "delivered" (recognizing that there are instances in which physiologic circumstances will not permit her active participation, discussed in Chapter 19).

The woman who is an active participant often expresses enjoyment of "pushing"; the work may be hard, but there are feelings of accomplishment, such as those that a runner or a swimmer feels after a good race.

The Third and Fourth Stages

The emotional components of the third and fourth stages are mediated by the events of the first and second stages, as well as by other factors discussed in this chapter.

Active participation usually leads to joy and heightened self-esteem for both mother and father—a "look what we did" kind of pride that is a sound basis for the completion of attachment. Lang[13] describes a feeling of elation following birth; Dick-Read[8] uses the term ecstasy; Klaus and Kennell[12] coin a term *ekstasis*.

Lang observed elation and attachment to the baby in others who observed the birth (friends and relatives present at home delivery). Klaus and Kennell suggest that in generations past, when maternal mortality was high, the attachment of observers (probably primarily women who were relatives or close friends) served the useful function of providing a substitute mother should the mother die.

Loss of self-esteem occurs if the mother or father feels that one of them behaved in an unacceptable manner. If their expectations of the labor or delivery were not fulfilled, this too will diminish self-esteem. These expectations may have been unrealistic (e.g., the mother who feels she has "failed" because she required medication) or may have been impossible because of unforeseen factors (e.g., the need for an unanticipated cesarean delivery because of difficult labor). Loss of self-esteem is particularly evident when the child is not full term or has a congenital abnormality (Chapter 28).

The psychologic work following delivery involves:

1. Recognizing the reality of the baby.
2. Integrating the birth experience into one's total life experience.
3. Furthering the attachment process.

Recognizing the Reality of the Baby. How frequently we hear immediately following the baby's birth "I can't believe he's really here" and even "Is he real?" As parents see and touch their baby, his reality, not just as a living baby but as a unique person, begins to emerge. Parents search for a characteristic that identifies him as a member of their family—a nose like his father's, dark hair like his mother's, or short little fingers like a sibling's.

Integrating the Birth Experience. During the fourth stage and again and again during the next days and weeks, the mother will talk about her labor to nearly anyone who will listen (just as patients often review a surgical experience with anyone who is available). This need to talk is an important concept, and a time must be provided for the mother to meet this need. Although friends and relatives are an important audience, a professional nurse as a listener is important as well, to reassure her that she did a good job during labor and to answer questions that she may have about her labor or delivery experience.

Furthering the Attachment Proccess. The first stages of the attachment process (planning, confirming, and accepting the pregnancy; perceiving fetal movement; and accepting the fetus as an individual) were described in Chapter 9.

Birth, followed by seeing and touching the baby, furthers attachment at the time of delivery. The concept of the fourth stage of labor as a sensitive period, during which parents and infants are bound together in complex ways, is discussed in Chapters 20 and 26.

Table 16–3. SIMILARITIES BETWEEN CHILDBIRTH AND SEXUAL EXCITEMENT*

Undisturbed, Undrugged Childbirth	Sexual Excitement and Orgasm
Breathing: During early contractions, breathing becomes deeper. Second stage of labor brings deep breathing with breath holding.	During early stages of arousal, breathing becomes faster and deeper. As orgasm approaches, breathing may be interrupted.
Vocalization: Tendency to make noises, grunts, especially in second stage of labor.	Tendency to make gasping, sucking noises as orgasm nears.
Facial expression: As birth climax approaches, the face gets an intense, strained look: observers often assume the woman is suffering great pain.	As orgasm approaches, the face gets what Kinsey et al. call a "tortured expression": mouth open, eyes glassy, muscles tense.
The uterus: The upper segment of the uterus contracts rhythmically.	The upper segment of the uterus contracts rhythmically.
The cervix: Mucus plug from opening (os) of cervix loosens.	Cervical secretion may loosen mucus plug, thus opening cervix for sperm.
Abdominal muscles: Contract periodically in second stage of labor; a strong urge to bear down develops as delivery approaches.	Abdominal muscles contract periodically during sexual excitement.
Position: Woman flat on her back, legs bent and wide apart.	Typically, the "missionary position" (woman on her back, legs wide apart).

Sexuality, Labor, and Birth

Niles Newton has suggested that labor and birth (and lactation as well) are all acts of female sexuality, closely interrelated both physiologically and psychologically.[22] At least three shared characteristics are the basis for this interrelationship.

First, labor, birth, and lactation are all influenced closely by related neurohormonal reflexes. Oxytocin is one of the substances involved, and probably one of the most significant. Second, environmental stimuli are highly important to each act. Interruption or fear of interruption, distracting sounds, and the like are inhibiting factors in the early stages of coitus, labor, and breast-feeding. Later on, as the woman becomes more involved, she becomes less aware of sensory stimuli. And third, each act is related to caretaking behavior.

Similarities between coitus and labor and delivery are summarized by Newton in Table 16–3.

Difficulty During Labor: Psychosocial Correlates

Some studies suggest a possible interrelationship between difficulties during labor and delivery and sociocultural or psychologic factors.

Davids and associates[7] predicted that women who show more signs of maladjustment during pregnancy would have more difficulties and complications in the delivery room and that women with difficult or complicated delivery would be more maladjusted than women with normal delivery.

In his study 48 women were given psychologic tests during their pregnancies. Twenty of the women were again tested postpartum. In addition, the degree of physical difficulty during each labor was classified on the basis of medical observations and records in the delivery room. Findings are tabulated in Table 16–4.

Crawford also studied relationships between anxiety and uterine dysfunction.[6] Her study

Table 16–3. SIMILARITIES BETWEEN CHILDBIRTH AND SEXUAL EXCITEMENT
(Continued)

Undisturbed, Undrugged Childbirth	Sexual Excitement and Orgasm
Central nervous system: Woman tends to become uninhibited, particularly as baby descends the birth canal. Veneers of conventional behavior disappear in later stages of labor.	Inhibitions and psychic blocks are relieved and often eliminated as orgasm nears.
Strength and flexibility: Delivery of the baby through the narrow passage requires unusual strength and body expansion.	Unusual muscular strength often develops. Many persons become capable of bending and distorting their bodies in ways they could not otherwise do.
Sensory perception: During labor the vulva becomes anesthetized with full dilation so that the woman often must be told of the emergence of the baby's head.	The whole body of the sexually aroused person becomes increasingly insensitive—even to sharp blows and severe injury.
There is a tendency to become oblivious to surroundings as delivery approaches. Amnesia develops. Suddenly, delivery complete, the woman becomes wide awake.	As orgasm approaches, there is a tendency to become oblivious to surroundings. There is loss of sensory perceptions, sometimes leading to moments of unconsciousness. After orgasm there is a sudden return of sensory acuity.
Emotional response: After birth, there is a flood of joyful emotion, which Dick-Read describes as "complete and careless ecstasy."	After coital orgasm there is a strong feeling of well-being in most persons.

*Newton: *Psychology Today,* July, 1971.

Table 16–4.   SOME DIFFERENCES BETWEEN WOMEN WITH NORMAL AND ABNORMAL DELIVERIES*

Criteria	Women with Normal Deliveries	Women with Abnormal Deliveries
Age	No significant difference in mean age	
Time in labor	Mean: 7.3 hours	Mean: 16.8 hours
I.Q.	During pregnancy: 102	During pregnancy: 101
	Postpartum: 107	Postpartum: 91
Manifest anxiety score	During pregnancy: 16.5 (range: 8–26)	During pregnancy: 23.5 (range: 14–37)
	Postpartum: 15	Postpartum: 18.5
Self-ratings		Less happy, more alienated; difference not statistically significant

*Davids, DeVault, and Talmadge: *Psychosomatic Medicine,* 23:93, 1961.

included 504 clinic patients, over half of whom were nonwhite and one-third of whom chose a Spanish questionnaire to complete rather than one in English. Her instruments were a questionnaire on symptoms of muscle tension, completed by the patient at the time of admission to the labor room; an evaluation of emotional tension made by the admitting nurse in the labor room; and data from the patient's chart.

Crawford's major hypothesis "... that women who reported more than average symptoms of muscle tension during pregnancy and demonstrated at the beginning of labor more than average physiological and behavioral signs associated with anxiety would develop physiological disturbance related to uterine dysfunction" was confirmed. The infants of these same women also had a greater tendency to develop physiologic disturbances related to hypoxia.

Rosengren questioned the relationship between the tendency to take the sick role during pregnancy (Chapter 9) and subsequent difficulty during labor and delivery.[25] In a study of 94 expectant mothers (62 clinic patients and 32 private patients) Rosengren selected two major indices as criteria of delivery room difficulty:

1. Length of labor.
2. Evidence of gross complications (e.g., the use of forceps, complications involving the cord, abnormal fetal heart rate, and so on).

The women were also divided according to two bases:

1. Women with normal labor and delivery versus those with deliveries evidencing some kind of gross abnormality.
2. Women who had taken the sick role during pregnancy versus those who did not.

Rosengren's findings in this study suggest that the "... more a woman regarded herself as 'ill' during pregnancy the greater was the likelihood of a longer period of active labor."[25]

He also found a trend toward longer labor in women of lower socioeconomic class, although not one he considered statistically significant. This might be expected in view of his previous findings that the tendency to take the sick role during pregnancy varied inversely with socioeconomic class.

Race as an independent variable in measuring the differential response to the pain experience of women in childbirth was investigated by Winsberg and Greenlick[29] in a study of 365 women (207 white; 158 black). Their findings were based on evaluations by obstetric interns and nurses in relation to cooperation, degree of pain, and response to pain. The findings indicated no difference between white and black patients of similar social class on any of the three evaluations. Age and parity were found to be the significant factors influencing response to pain.

Anxiety and Difficult Labor

The relationship between anxiety and pain has been mentioned previously. If a woman customarily responds to anxiety with sympathomimetic symptoms, learned associations result. The symptoms themselves can then "elicit and reinforce further anxiety producing a self-generating, spiraling anxiety reaction."[6]

A variety of physiologic changes are initiated by anxiety. A major response is the production of the catecholamines epinephrine and norepinephrine. Epinephrine stimulates both alpha and beta receptors; norepinephrine stimulates alpha receptors primarily. If the alpha-adrenergic receptors are stimulated there will be uterine vasoconstriction (as well as generalized vasoconstriction) and an increase in uterine muscle tone, leading to both a decrease in uterine blood supply and an increase in maternal blood supply and maternal blood pressure. If beta-adrenergic receptors are stimulated, vasodilation and relaxation of uterine muscle occur. Because the uterine vessels are already fully dilated, the dilatation of other vessels reduces the flow of blood to the uterus. Decreased uterine blood flow may cause fetal bradycardia (Chapter 18).

In separate studies Morishima et al.[20] and Myers and Myers[21] were able to produce fetal bradycardia by frightening the mother. Morishima tested both monkey mothers with no signs of placental insufficiency and those with insufficiency; when the fetus was already compromised, the fall in fetal pH and oxygenation was marked.

Lederman et al.[14, 15] found that levels of epinephrine and norepinephrine increase during labor; norepinephrine remains increased for some time following delivery. High epinephrine levels, which were correlated with maternal anxiety, led to a decrease in uterine contractions, and an increase in the duration of labor. Crawford[6] has found that Apgar scores (Chapter 20) of infants whose mothers exhibited a high degree of anxiety were lower than those of infants whose mothers exhibited less anxiety (the higher the Apgar score, the healthier the infant).

Problems in Assessment of Discomfort

One significant factor, both in cross-cultural comparisons and in comparing the experiences of women in our own society, is that it is difficult for an observer to evaluate objectively the level of discomfort experienced by another individual. This is particularly true when observer and observed do not share the same cultural heritage. As Zborowski[30] has demonstrated, people respond to discomfort in many different ways, some by "keeping a stiff upper lip," some by anguished cries, and some by silent tears. In caring for mothers during labor, as in caring for patients in many other situations, this is a basic concept of the assessment process.

Variables Affecting Anxiety During Labor

Just as anxiety appears to be a part of pregnancy for all women, so too is some degree of anxiety a common denominator of labor for most women. A number of factors influence the level of anxiety.

Customary Emotional Tone. Some individuals (men and women) are more anxious about every facet of their lives than are others. If one customarily feels positive about and in control of new situations, labor will not pose the threat that it does for the woman who feels "controlled by" and therefore helpless as she approaches an unknown experience.

Feelings About Femininity and Mothering. The birth of a baby is ultimately a feminine act. For the mother who has difficulty with her feminine identity, labor and birth may seem a difficult burden.

Attitude Toward This Pregnancy. A resented pregnancy may mean that labor is resented as well. As a mother approaches the time for delivery of a baby, it is difficult to acknowledge that she still resents the fact of being pregnant. The need to express this resentment, and the counsel that resentment of a pregnancy does not necessarily mean rejection of the baby, is a significant part of nursing intervention.

Perception of Her Mother's Childbirth Experience. A woman's perception of her mother's childbirth experience influences her anxiety level in anticipation of labor and delivery, but not her evaluation of the actual delivery.[17] It would seem, therefore, worthwhile to assess the mother's perception of her own mother's labor experience prior to the time of labor and to include that information in her record.

Intensity of Communication About Childbirth Between Mother and Daughter. Levy and McGee[17] report that the intensity of communication about childbirth between a mother and her daughter influences the daughter's feelings about childbirth (Table 16–5).

Table 16–5. EFFECT OF MATERNAL COMMUNICATION ON DAUGHTER'S EVALUATION OF HER OWN CHILDBIRTH

Communication from Mother to Daughter	Daughter's Evaluation of Her Own Childbirth
Highly favorable	Negative
Highly unfavorable	Negative
No communication	Negative
Moderate communication	Positive

Levy and McGee postulated that those women who heard only highly favorable comments were unprepared for the discomfort that may accompany labor and thus were disappointed in their experience. This concept seems important for nurses who care for prenatal patients, i.e., stressing only the positive aspects of labor may lead to frustration and a negative experience.

The mother who receives no communication may also be unprepared for the labor experience.

An intensely negative communication may be difficult to overcome, although we believe that assessment early in pregnancy of whether such communication occurred and subsequent "appropriate" intervention might be possible. (Certainly this is an area for nursing research.)

Previous Childbirth Experience. If a prior labor was long or difficult, if the infant was stillborn or died after birth, if it had a congenital anomaly, or if the experience of labor or birth was in any way unpleasant, those memories will be recalled and can affect the anxiety level in the present experience.

Presence of Risk Factors. Women who have been considered at risk throughout their pregnancies understandably approach labor and delivery with increased anxiety about their own or their infant's well-being. In addition, mothers at risk in this pregnancy may have experienced fetal or newborn death in a previous pregnancy.

Preparation for Labor. Few nurses who care for patients during labor fail to notice that preparation for labor does influence the level of anxiety for many women. The problem of raising unrealistic expectations, mentioned above and at other places in this text, along with the importance of assessment of individual needs and individualization of prenatal preparation, must guide preparation of parents for labor.

Physical Progress During Labor. Just as anxiety can influence the physical course of labor, physical factors (breech presentation, posterior position) can influence emotions. When labor is long or difficult or when there is concern for the well-being of the mother or fetus because of unusual circumstances, a heightened level of anxiety is inevitable.

Companionship During Labor: Mother and Father Together

During the past decade many couples have come to share the experience of labor and delivery. In the following chapter specific ways in which couples can work together and along

with the professional team are described. What has this experience meant to couples? Here are some responses in a study by Cook.[5]

The responses from mothers included:

"I didn't feel alone at all."

"My husband had not planned to be with me during labor and changed his mind at the last minute. Therefore his support during labor was even more meaningful."

"I could not have gone through labor without him there. He encouraged me, marked off time for me, and held my hand through it all. He was also able to help me when I forgot to breathe the correct way at particular times. He would remind me of things we learned in our course. But most of all, he was a companion; a comforter who assured me that *we* would make it" (italics mine).

"Our first child was the 'family' approach the second child was born without father in attendance, due to hospital policy. I was frantic toward the end of labor—required more medication. With the first it was a beautiful experience; the second, a horrible one."

"We have always been a close twosome. This is our first child after nearly ten years of marriage. I wouldn't think of doing anything of such great moment without him."

The responses from fathers included:

"It was the most marvelous experience of my life. Susan and I have always done everything together. When we first became pregnant, I began to feel a little left out because this was something Susan would *have* to do on her own. But Lamaze changed that! We began the course—mainly for information—and we got very excited about doing this together. I visited Susan's doctor, the hospital, and all the classes. I feel closer to Susan than ever and love our son in a way that I don't think would have been possible without Lamaze."

"I was 'in the know' at all times—no wondering what was going on in some solarium. That would've driven me crazy."

"I was benefited in a way no one can understand except a father who has witnessed the birth of his child . . . beyond definition."

"I was somewhat afraid for some reason even though I thought we were prepared. Now after going through the experience I'm glad I did because I would still wonder about it if I hadn't."

One father, who was with his wife during labor but was not allowed to be present in the delivery room said, "The time they shoved me out for delivery was the worst time of all—it seemed forever."

A father who had no prior preparation but was allowed to be with his wife during labor said, "I didn't have any preparation, and so I felt really useless, except to be there and let Jenny squeeze my hand, but it left a real impact on me. I wouldn't have it any other way than to be with her."

Not every father or every mother chooses to share the experience of labor and birth, or is able to. Cultural values, as noted earlier, are one factor that will influence individual decisions. The demands of the father's job, noninvolvement between mother and father, and occasionally (although with increasing rarity) hospital policy may separate couples. Nevertheless, for many couples, being together offers many advantages and makes labor a truly special time. When the father is not present, a friend or relative should be encouraged to be with her.

Summary

Throughout labor the physiologic process is influenced by cultural and individual emotional factors. These factors will be explored further as we examine nursing intervention during labor for normal and high risk mothers and fathers.

REFERENCES

1. Adkins, E.: All-in-One Unit Improves Patient Care in OB. *Hospital Topics, 53*:40, 1975.
2. Ashley-Montague, M.: *Coming into Being Among the Australian Aborigines*. London, George Routledge and Sons, 1937.
3. Burrows, E., and Spiro, M.: *An Atoll Culture: Ethnography of the Ifaluk in the Central Carolines*. New Haven, Human Relations Area Files, 1957.
4. Cassidy, J.: A Nurse Looks at Childbirth Anxiety. *JOGN, 3*:52, 1974.
5. Cook, M.: *Father-Participation in Childbirth: A Study Presenting its Effectiveness*. Unpublished paper, 1973.
6. Crawford, M.: Physiological and Behavioral Cues to Disturbances in Childbirth. *In* American Nursing Association: *Clinical Sessions*. New York, Appleton-Century-Crofts, 1968.
7. Davids, A., DeVault, S., and Talmadge, M.: Psychological Study of Emotional Factors in Pregnancy: A Preliminary Report. *Psychosomatic Medicine, 23*:93, 1961.
8. Dick-Read, G.: *Childbirth Without Fear*. 2nd Edition. New York, Harper & Row, 1953.
9. DuBois, C.: *The People of Alor*. Minneapolis, University of Minnesota Press, 1944.
10. Holmberg, A.: *Nomads of the Long Bow*. New York, Natural History Press, 1969.
11. Kelly, M. (ed.): *Maternity Care in Ferment: Conflicting Issues*. New York, Maternity Center Association, 1980.
12. Klaus, M., and Kennell, J.: *Maternal-Infant Bonding*. St. Louis, C. V. Mosby Co., 1976.
13. Lang, R.: Personal communication. Cited in: Klaus, M., and Kennell, J.: *Maternal-Infant Bonding*. St. Louis, C. V. Mosby Co., 1976.
14. Lederman, R., McCann, D., Work, B., et al.: Endogenous Plasma Epinephrine and Norepinephrine in Last-Trimester Pregnancy and Labor. *American Journal of Obstetrics and Gynecology, 129*:5, 1977.
15. Lederman, R., Lederman, E., Work, B., et al.: The Relationship of Maternal Anxiety, Plasma Catecholamines and Plasma Cortisol to Progress in Labor. *American Journal of Obstetrics and Gynecology, 132*:495, 1978.
16. Levinson, G., and Shnider, S.: Catecholamines: The Effects of Maternal Fear and Its Treatment on Uterine Function and Circulation. *Birth and the Family Journal, 6*(3):167, 1979.
17. Levy, J., and McGee, M.: Childbirth as Crisis: A Test of Janis's Theory of Communication and Stress Resolution. *Journal of Personality and Social Psychology, 31*:171, 1975.
18. Lubic, R.: The Childbearing Center. Maternity Center Association, New York. *In* Sumner, P., and Phillips, C.: *Birthing Rooms: Concept and Reality*. St. Louis, C. V. Mosby Co., 1981.
19. McDonald, D.: *The Land of Lama* (Human Relations Area Files). London, Seeley, Service and Company, 1929.
20. Morishima, H., Pedersen, H., and Finster, M.: The Influence of Maternal Psychological Stress on the Fetus. *American Journal of Obstetrics and Gynecology, 131*:286, 1978.
21. Myers, R., and Myers, S.: Use of Sedative Analgesic and Anesthetic Drugs During Labor and Delivery: Bane or Boon. *American Journal of Obstetrics and Gynecology, 133*:83, 1979.
22. Newton, N.: Trebly Sensuous Woman. *Psychology Today*, 68, 1971.
23. Oliver, D.: A Solomon Island Society: Kinship and Leadership Among the Siuai of Bougainville. Cambridge, Harvard University Press, 1955.
24. Rising, S.: The Fourth Stage of Labor: Family Integration. *American Journal of Nursing, 74*:870, 1974.
25. Rosengren, W.: Some Social Psychological Aspects of Delivery Room Difficulties. *Journal of Nervous and Mental Diseases, 132*:515, 1961.
26. Sumner, P., and Phillips, C.: *Birthing Rooms: Concept and Reality*. St. Louis, C. V. Mosby Co., 1981.
27. Tafel, A.: *My Tibetan Trip*. Stuttgart, Union Deutsche Vertagegesellschaft, 1914.
28. Thiede, H.: The Case for Hospital Delivery. *In* Kelly, M. (ed.): *Maternity Care in Ferment: Conflicting Issues*. New York, Maternity Center Association: 1980.
29. Winsberg, B., and Greenlick, M.: Pain Response in Negro and White Obstetrical Patients. *Journal of Health and Social Behavior, 8*:220, 1967.
30. Zborowski, M.: Cultural Components in Response to Pain. *In* Apple, D. (ed.): *Sociological Studies of Health and Sickness*. New York, McGraw Hill Book Co., 1960.

17

Caring for the Intrapartum Family

OBJECTIVES

1. Identify information to be derived from the prenatal record.
2. State specific information about the progress of labor that must be assessed by a nursing history.
3. Identify information derived from physical assessment of mother and fetus.
4. Identify information gained from vaginal examination.
5. State observations of emotional status that should be noted and recorded.
6. For each stage of labor, identify appropriate nursing assessment and intervention.
7. Describe nursing measures that may facilitate the course of labor.
8. Identify potential dangers to mother or fetus during labor.
9. Describe ways in which nurses can help mothers cope with the discomfort of labor without the use of medication.
10. Differentiate support for labor with the fetus in a posterior position from labor when the fetus is in an anterior position.
11. Identify ways in which nurses can support labor coaches.
12. Identify the major types of pharmacologic assistance given during labor, and the advantages, disadvantages, and appropriate nursing action for each.
13. Describe the process of emergency delivery.

A woman arrives at the door of the labor/delivery suite. She says she is in labor. The next hours will be among the most significant in her life and in the lives of her mate and the baby who is to be born. Our nursing care during these hours may provide the crucial difference between a physically and emotionally satisfying experience coupled with the delivery of a healthy infant or an experience long remembered with sadness and dissatisfaction. In the best of worlds, a nurse who has shared the prenatal period with the woman and her family will also be able to share labor with them.

The goals of nursing during labor are to make the occasion as safe, as comfortable, and as satisfying, physically and emotionally, as possible. In order to do this, nurses must:

1. Assess the physiologic status of the mother and fetus throughout the four stages of labor.
2. Assess the emotional status of the mother and whoever accompanies her—father, friend, or other companion—throughout the four stages of labor.
3. Plan and act to:
   a. Facilitate the course of labor.
   b. Help the mother and her companion to cope with labor.
   c. Facilitate beginning parenting in the period immediately following delivery.

Who Enters the Labor/Delivery Suite?

Until the past decade, most labor/delivery suites were closed to all but the mother and the hospital personnel who attended her. The issue of fathers in the delivery room was hotly debated.

As more couples began preparing for childbirth, pressure was placed on hospitals to allow husbands to accompany their wives to support them and participate with them in labor and delivery. In many hospitals, although not all, husbands are today welcome participants (see Fig. 17–4).

What about the woman who isn't married? What about the woman who does not wish to have her husband with her or whose husband is unable to be with her? Should every woman be able to have the companion of her choice with her? Or should she, if she chooses, come alone?

We believe the choice should be hers, and an increasing number of hospitals share this belief. And so, in this text, even though we

may use the word "husband," or "father," the same consideration should be given to anyone who accompanies the mother. Although some institutions require attendance at prenatal classes before the husband or other companion may enter the labor room, others place no prohibitions.

In a few labor settings, friends and siblings are now allowed to be present if the mother wishes.

First Contact

The mother in labor is, understandably, excited and anxious about the coming hours. Her husband or companion may be supportive or, often, even more anxious than she. Although there will be wide individual variations in the levels of anxiety, these feelings will affect even basic physiologic assessment, such as assessment of blood pressure and pulse. Our skill in enabling the mother, and her companion, to relax will benefit both her initial assessment and her entire course of labor.

Our actions as much as our words can convey interest in the individual couple. If we appear hurried and overwhelmed (and labor room nurses often *are* very rushed, with many demands made upon them), the anxiety of patients is intensified.

Without compromising the tasks essential to initial assessment, we can make each woman or couple feel welcome, make the woman feel that we will support her throughout her labor, and make this day a significant one for her or them.

Initial Assessment of the Mother

Initial assessment involves the following factors (see also Nursing Care Plan 17–1):

1. Reviewing the prenatal record.
2. Eliciting specific information from the mother about the course of this labor.
3. Assessing the physiologic status of the mother.
4. Assessing expectations of labor.
5. Assessing cultural, social, and psychological factors that are relevant to labor and birth.

Reviewing the Prenatal Record

Prenatal records, whether from a physician's office or from a clinic, should be available in the labor suite. From the moment a woman is admitted, it is essential to know if there are

Text continued on page 486

Nursing Care Plan 17–1.   Assisting A Mother In The First Stage Of Labor

NURSING GOALS:
To provide education for parents.
To maintain maternal and fetal well-being.

OBJECTIVES:
To promote comfort the mother will:
1. Know the signs of true labor.
2. Know the significance of effacement, dilatation, station.
3. Remain relaxed and in control.
4. Progress through her low risk labor. The fetus will not be compromised.
The partner will:
1. Provide physiologic and emotional support.
2. Utilize measures for maternal comfort.

ASSESSMENT	NURSING DIAGNOSIS	NURSING INTERVENTION	COMMENTS/RATIONALE
		Latent Phase	

1. Existing knowledge level of mother and partner (father or other support person)	Need for information regarding the labor process	Instruct the mother and her coach in basic anatomy and physiology:
		1. Cervix
		2. Dilatation
		3. Effacement
		4. Station
		Show chart of dilatation.
		
		Give information about true labor:
		1. Contractions:
		  a. At regular intervals
		  b. Located primarily in back
		  c. Intensified by walking
		2. Show: Usually present; note change in amount of bleeding
		3. Cervical dilatation:
		  a. Sterile vaginal examination to check dilatation and effacement.
		  b. Teach mother and partner how to time contraction—regularity and length. Encourage mother and partner to ask questions.
			Mother's knowledge level will be dependent upon paragravida, prenatal education, age, and support systems.
			
			Giving the information will help both nurse and patient to establish a nurse–patient relationship and to decrease the mother's anxiety level and that of her companion.

2. Pattern, length, and intensity of uterine contractions	Altered level of comfort due to labor	Encourage mother to walk; encourage father to be with patient during labor. Provide instruction in relaxation techniques: 1. Slow breathing 2. Progressive relaxation. Instruct mother to use slow deep breathing during contractions. No distracting conversation during contractions. Encourage mother to doze between contractions if lying down. Instruct mother to get out of bed and empty bladder every 2 hours. Keep patient clean and dry. Change linen as needed. Offer fluids to drink.	Walking during early labor has been shown to decrease the length of labor. Utilization of relaxation techniques will help patient to maintain control of her body.
3. Vital signs: Monitor blood pressure, pulse every 2 hours. Check deep tendon reflexes every 8 hours. Observe for edema at time of admission and thereafter at each voiding, if indicated. Check temperature every 2 hours.	At risk of pre-eclampsia. At risk of hypotension; secondary to position, bleeding. At risk of infection		The signs of pre-eclampsia are: 1. Increased blood pressure 2. Hyperreflexia 3. Edema 4. Proteinuria. Hypotension, increasing pulse may indicate concealed bleeding. Risk of infection increases with prolonged rupture of membranes.
4. Fetal heart tones	Potential for fetal distress during labor	Monitor fetal heart tones at least every hour. Attention should be paid to rate, regularity, and response to contractions.	Frequent auscultation of fetal heart tones will allow the nurse to identify signs of fetal distress so that appropriate nursing actions may be taken.

Continued on following page

Nursing Care Plan 17–1. Assisting A Mother In The First Stage Of Labor (*Continued*)

1. Mother's level of anxiety and discomfort

Fear and anticipation of pain

Active Phase

Encourage partner to assist labor patient. Provide time for the couple to be alone.

Utilize relaxation techniques as needed. Stroke patient's arms and legs outward from body.

Instruct patient to avoid lying flat on her back. Suggest positions of sitting, lying on side, squatting.

Provide pillows for positioning under legs and abdomen.

Offer positive reinforcement statements.

Change to somewhat faster breathing pattern, if desired.

Encourage mother to rest between contractions.

Sponge face with cool cloth.

Moisten lips.

Use effleurage, if desired.

Suggest these measure for back labor:

1. Provide firm pressure at small of back.
2. Assist into knee-hand position ("on all fours.")
3. Pelvic rock (Chapter 11).

Caution patient against hyperventilation. Instruct to cup hands over mouth and breathe, if necessary, or breathe into paper bag.

Provide emesis basin and mouthwash for nausea and vomiting.

The father's or companion's presence may help patient to be more calm. The couple can put into use any techniques they might have learned in childbirth education classes.

Lying on her back causes compression of the vena cava; hence, blood return is diminished (supine hypotensive syndrome).

Transitional Phase

1. Patient's level of discomfort, exhaustion, and apprehension	Fear and anticipation of the unknown	Reassure mother and partner about normality of sensations (apprehension, fatigue, desire to bear down).	These sensations may lead mother to experience a sense of impending doom.
		Inform couple of probable length of duration of these feelings.	Comfort measures may be provided by partner or nurse.
		Remind them that this is the transition to the time to push.	
		Assist in concentration on control of breathing pattern.	
		Cool cloth to forehead.	
		Fan mother.	
		Instruct in slightly faster and more shallow breathing, if desired.	
		Have mother blow out if she has the urge to push.	
2. Sterile vaginal examination when indicated to check for complete cervical dilatation; signs to watch for include increased amount of show, lengthening of abdominal muscles, and intense urge to bear down.	Increased potential for fetal distress	Explain to mother that she should not push or hold her breath.	Pushing before complete dilatation may result in cervical edema, resulting in a longer labor. Another possibility is trapping the anterior rim of the cervix between the symphysis pubis and the baby's head.
		Accept patient's irritability.	
		Constant presence of nurse desirable.	
3. Assess fetal heart tones.		Assess fetal heart tones every 15 minutes.	Contractions are stronger and closer together than in early labor. The head is descending further into the pelvis. The possibility therefore, for fetal distress is much greater.

Contributed by Mona B. Ketner

any factors in her history that require special physical or emotional attention. High risk factors affecting labor and delivery and the care of mothers with these conditions are discussed in Chapter 19.

Even if the current pregnancy has apparently been normal in every way, a woman who has had complications during a previous labor will have memories that come rushing back to her, both throughout the pregnancy and particularly at the time of labor. We must know about these previous experiences in order to understand her behavior during this labor. For example, a mother whose fetus died during labor in a previous pregnancy is likely to be very anxious about variations in fetal heart rate. If the present labor is progressing satisfactorily, her level of anxiety may seem inappropriate until one recognizes its true basis.

Additional essential information in the prenatal record includes the expected date of confinement (EDC) and the number of previous pregnancies and deliveries.

Eliciting Specific Information

The answers to specific questions about the course of this labor must be obtained and recorded in the woman's record.

1. When did contractions begin?
2. How often do contractions occur?
3. How long do contractions last?
4. Have the membranes (bag of waters) ruptured?
5. Has there been any bleeding?
6. When did you last eat?

If the prenatal record is not immediately available, questions about the EDC and the number of pregnancies must be asked.

Assessing the Physiologic Status

The mother usually changes into a hospital gown and is put to bed for the initial assessment. Afterward, depending on her condition and on hospital policy, she may be allowed out of bed (see below).

Evaluation of general physical status includes checking the mother's

1. Weight.
2. Vital signs (temperature, pulse, respiration, blood pressure).
3. General physical condition, including examination by a physician or a nurse-midwife, with special attention to cardiac and respiratory evaluation.
4. Blood and urine for laboratory examination.

The progress of labor is evaluated in relation to:

1. Frequency, duration, and intensity of uterine contractions (Chapter 15).
2. Vaginal examination to determine effacement and dilatation (below).

The status of the fetus is evaluated by:

1. Auscultation of fetal heart rate (page 489).
2. Abdominal palpation and vaginal examination to determine lie, presentation, and position (Chapter 15).

Vaginal Examination.   Generally, assessments of effacement and dilatation are done by vaginal examination. With a sterile glove on the examining hand, the labia are widely separated to avoid contamination, and the lubricated index and second fingers are inserted into the vagina until they touch the cervix (Fig. 17–1). By means of the vaginal examination, assessment is made of:

1. The degree of effacement.
2. The degree of dilatation.
3. Confirmation of the presenting part (as previously determined by Leopold's maneuvers).
4. Fetal position.
5. Fetal station.

Mothers are anxious for a report of the findings; the report should be given in as positive terms as possible to describe the current findings.

The importance of sterile technique cannot be overemphasized. Vaginal examination should not be done if there is fresh bleeding because this may indicate a placenta previa (Chapter 13).

Continuing Physiologic Assessment

Once baseline data are obtained, continuing physiologic assessment of the mother during the first stage of labor includes determination of:

1. Vital signs (temperature, pulse, respiration, blood pressure).
2. Frequency, duration, and intensity of contractions.
3. Progress of effacement and dialatation.

The progress of the fetus through the birth canal and the well-being of the fetus are also assessed on a continuing basis.

Assessment of Expectations of Labor

Women and their families come to labor with varying expectations. Some have no idea of what to expect, or expect only the worst. Others have very specific expectations—expecta-

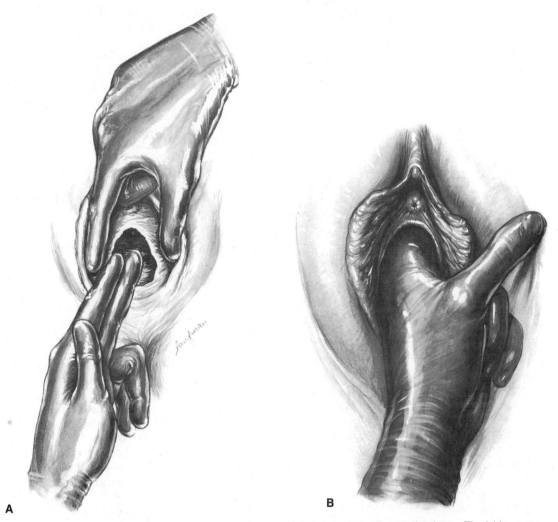

A

B

Figure 17–1. Vaginal examination. *A,* Method of making vaginal examination using sterile gloves. The labia are spread widely so that the examining fingers may be inserted without touching surrounding vulvar structures. Care must be exercised to avoid touching the anus. *B,* Vaginal examination with fingers inserted, wrist straight, and elbow sunk, to allow fingertips to point toward umbilicus. (From Greenhill and Friedman: *Biological Principles and Modern Practice of Obstetrics.* Philadelphia, W. B. Saunders Co., 1974.)

tions that may not always be fulfilled. For example, a woman who has fantasized an idealized vaginal delivery and then must have a cesarean delivery may be very disappointed.

Women who attend prenatal classes are encouraged to discuss their expectations with health-care providers in advance, but this information is not always communicated to the personnel at the labor area. Knowledge of the kind of prenatal classes attended can be a guide for nursing support during labor. A couple trained in the Bradley method will need somewhat different support from a couple trained in the Lamaze method. Nurses who care for mothers in labor should be familiar with the childbirth education classes in their community.

Table 17–1 suggests some expectations parents may have that should be assessed upon admission to the labor/delivery area. Soliciting a mother's preferences is in itself a sign of caring. Many mothers still feel that no one is really interested in their preferences and that only by making strident demands will they be able to participate actively in the decisions made on this most important day. (See also The Pregnant Patient's Bill of Rights, Appendix J.)

Assessment of Cultural, Psychological, and Social Factors

Cultural Factors. General cultural assessment was discussed in Chapter 2; cultural

Table 17–1. ASSESSING EXPECTATION OF LABOR

1. a. Have you attended prenatal classes?	YES NO
b. What type of classes did you attend?	_____
2. During labor and birth:	
a. Who would you like to be with you?	_____

   b. What are your expectations concerning*
      1. Site of labor (e.g., birthing room)
      2. Routine IV fluids
      3. Position during labor, birth
      4. Fetal monitoring
      5. Medication during labor, birth
      6. Episiotomy
      7. Breast-feeding
   c. What other expectations of labor and birth are important to you?
   d. What expectations do you have for yourself during labor and birth?
   e. What expectations do you have of your labor companion (coach) during labor and birth?
   f. What expectations do you have of me (your primary nurse) during labor and birth?
   g. What expectations do you have of our midwife or physician during labor and birth?

*Some issues, in some facilities, are not negotiable. Obviously, one cannot offer choices where they do not exist. Health status may limit choices for some women.

variables in labor and birth were discussed in Chapter 16. Although an individual woman will never fit a cultural sterotype, an awareness of her cultural background may provide clues to her expectancies of labor and delivery, the way she may react to the discomfort of contractions, her choice of and interaction with her labor companion, and other aspects of her behavior.

Psychological Factors. Mothers and fathers arrive at the labor/delivery room excited and often anxious. Some become increasingly tense and nervous during admission activities, especially those women or couples who have had no preparation for labor other than the tales of their family and acquaintances. In a totally different environment surrounded by strangers, they find themselves unable to cope.

It is not unusual for concerns other than the labor per se to be an additional source of anxiety. Perhaps the woman has not yet made plans to integrate the baby into her life. Perhaps there is difficulty with her marriage. For some women the reality of the coming baby is denied until the time of labor, when it can no longer be ignored.

If there are other children in the family, the parents may be concerned about their wellbeing at the moment, as well as their future reaction to the baby.

Couples well prepared for labor may seem confident as they begin previously practiced breathing patterns.

Emotional status should be noted in the record on admission and should be assessed and recorded on a continuing basis throughout labor.

In our observations we must not overlook the status (physical and emotional) of the father or other individual who accompanies the mother. It is often said that there are two patients to be cared for during labor, the mother and the fetus, but there are actually three. We need to be aware of the father. Is he tense? Is he fatigued? Our assessment of his needs, as well as hers, thus becomes part of the nursing care of this family.

Social Interaction. Labor and birth is a period of relatively intense social interaction of a woman with her husband or labor companion and nurses, midwife, or physician. Frequently in a hospital there are other personnel from the laboratory, anesthesia department, and a variety of support services who also interact with the mother. In a medical center, which has many student nurses and physicians, the number of persons that come in contact with the laboring couple can be overwhelming and may impair a woman's ability to relax and concentrate on coping with her labor. Assessment of social interaction must involve both an awareness of the effect of health-care providers on the mother and an assessment of the interaction between a woman and her labor companion. Assess whether the number of persons to whom the mother is exposed is fatiguing to the mother or interferes with her ability to cope; if so, the number of persons should be reduced. During the greater part of labor, the only people present should be the labor companion of the woman's choice and her primary nurse or midwife should interact quietly and supportively with her. Even in alternative birth centers, such as the one at The Farm (Tennessee), the number of attendants at birth is limited. The presence of the infant's siblings is important to some parents (Chapter 11); siblings usually come and go through the course of labor and need to be under the care of an adult other than the labor companion. Nurses need to be aware of the effects of sibling presence on the mother and on the course of her labor.

In assessing the interaction of birth companions and mothers, nurses can observe:

1. The amount of physical contact, which varies from little or none to almost continual.

2. The amount and quality of verbal interaction, which varies from little or none to almost continual.

3. The effectiveness of the companion's support, which varies from little or none to highly effective.

These observations must be interpreted in a cultural context, recognizing that both verbal and nonverbal behaviors are affected by culture.

Assessing Fetal Well-Being During Labor

The most common assessment of fetal well-being is done by observation of fetal heart rate. This assessment is necessary for all mother–fetus pairs.

As labor progresses, or fails to progress, there may be a need for further assessment: fetal scalp sampling, x-ray studies, or ultrasound examination.

Assessing Fetal Heart Rate

Heart rate is monitored intermittently by stethoscope and/or fetoscope and continuously by external or internal monitor. No one method is best under every circumstance.

Intermittent Auscultation by Stethoscope or Fetoscope

Auscultation by stethoscope or fetoscope is the traditional method of monitoring fetal heart rate and is still the most widely used. It allows the mother to be up and about between contractions and to change her position easily. It is not frightening to mothers, as monitoring devices may be. Those couples and professionals who emphasize labor as a natural physiologic process feel that intermittent monitoring is satisfactory for the large numbers of mothers with normal labors. Some mothers resent continuous monitoring not merely because it is confining but on the philosophic basis that it focuses on abnormality rather than on a normal, emotionally satisfying labor.

Intermittent monitoring does have the disadvantage of detecting only marked deviations from normal fetal heart rate. Moreover, the heart rate is often difficult to hear during a contraction, the most significant period.

The point at which fetal heart rate is best heard by fetoscope varies with the lie, presentation, and position of the fetus. Not surprisingly, tones are heard best in the area of the fetal chest or back. Figure 17–2 illustrates the approximate location of the fetal heart in several positions.

Because sound is amplified through the fetoscope via bone, it is important that pressure from the forehead of the listener holds the

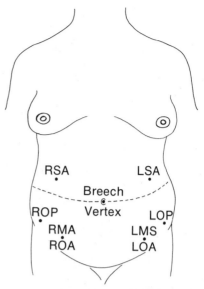

Figure 17–2. The position at which the fetal heart rate may be heard in relation to the fetal position.

fetoscope in place. If pressure is too light or too strong, it may be difficult or impossible to hear fetal heart tones. By starting with light pressure and increasing the pressure until the heart tones are heard, nurses can become skilled in this assessment.

If the fetal heart rate appears to be 70 to 80 beats per minute, check to see if this is synchronous with the mother's pulse rate. The sound of the *uterine bruit,* the passage of blood through uterine blood vessels, is sometimes mistaken for the fetal heart rate.

Blood flowing through the umbilical arteries makes a sound called the *funic souffle.* The funic souffle is synchronous with the fetal heart rate.

When listening to the fetal heart, the rate and rhythm are assessed and recorded between contractions to ascertain the baseline rate as well as the rate during a contraction. The rate may fall during the contraction but should return to the baseline within 20 to 30 seconds following the contraction.

Fetal heart rate is checked at least every 30 minutes during early labor, at least every 15 minutes during the transition phase of the first stage, and every 5 minutes at the beginning of the second stage.

In addition, fetal heart rate should be checked:

1. Following rupture of the membranes.

2. Following any intervention (e.g., expulsion of an enema, administration of medication, at the peak action time of medication).

3. Following any sudden change in the pattern of labor or any indication of complications.

Table 17–2. FACTORS AFFECTING BASELINE FETAL HEART RATE

Causes of Fetal Tachycardia (Rate > 160)	Causes of Fetal Bradycardia (Rate < 120)
Maternal hyperthermia	Fetal hypoxia (late sign)
Fetal hypoxia (early sign)	Response to vagal stimulus
Fetal sepsis	Maternal hypothermia
Maternal anxiety	Certain drugs
Fetal arrhythmia	Congenital heart block
Certain drugs	Idiopathic
Reaction to stimulus (transient)	
Idiopathic	

Continuous Monitoring of Fetal Heart Rate

Continuous monitoring of fetal heart rate (FHR) is discussed in Chapter 18.

Factors Affecting Fetal Heart Rate

Factors other than uterine contractions may affect fetal heart rate. Either bradycardia (a heart rate below 120 beats per minute) or tachycardia (a heart rate above 160 beats per minute) may occur in the baseline fetal heart rate for a number of reasons that are summarized in Table 17–2. Many of these factors are discussed in further detail in Chapter 18.

Nursing Care During the Intrapartum Period

Following the initial assessment, a plan of care for each mother is developed (Nursing Care Plan 17–1). The plan includes:

1. Facilitating the course of labor.
2. Protecting the mother and fetus.
3. Helping the mother cope with discomfort during labor.
4. Provision of human support; no mother should be left alone.
5. Provision of physical care.
6. Provision of information about the course of her labor.
7. Reassurance.

Nursing Intervention to Facilitate the Course of Labor

A number of measures may facilitate the course of labor. These include positioning the mother, avoiding a full bladder, and administering an enema.

Position

During the first stage of labor, it is not usually necessary for the mother to remain in bed (exceptions are noted below). When a woman is walking about or when she is sitting in a chair, gravity may enhance labor and make contractions more regular and efficient (Chapter 15). (Figs. 17–3 and 17–4). Walking should not be carried to the point of fatigue, however. When the mother chooses to rest in bed or when her health status requires bed rest, she should be on her side or elevated to a near-sitting position to avoid hypotensive syndrome (Chapter 15). Contraindications to walking about include:

1. Rupture of the membranes when the head is not engaged, because of the danger of *prolapse* of the umbilical cord (Chapter 19).
2. Vaginal bleeding.
3. Abnormal presentation or position.
4. Administration of sedatives or narcotics.

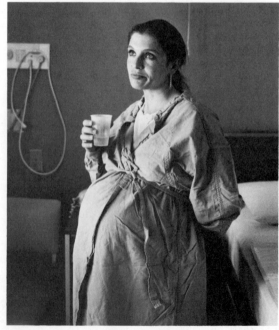

Figure 17–3. Mothers in labor may prefer to walk about or sit down during labor, which can facilitate labor and enhance contractions. Sips of water (if allowed) can alleviate the mother's dry mouth and lips. (Photograph by Suzanne Szasz.)

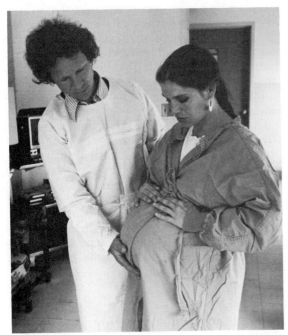

Figure 17–4. More and more hospitals today allow fathers or companions to be present during labor to provide emotional support to mothers, as this father is doing. (Photograph by Suzanne Szasz.)

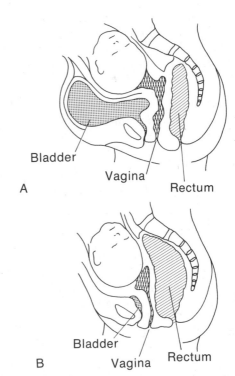

Figure 17–5. Notice how the full bladder (*A*) impedes the descent of the head. The empty bladder (*B*) is not a barrier. However, the full rectum (*B*) may be an impediment; contrast this with the empty rectum (*A*).

5. Certain maternal conditions such as heart disease.

The Urinary Bladder

Distention of the urinary bladder is not unusual during labor but it is a condition that can and must be avoided for several reasons.

A full bladder may impede the descent of the baby's head (Fig. 17–5) and also, by reflex action, may inhibit uterine contractions. The possibility of trauma and subsequent postpartum retention of urine is increased when the bladder is allowed to become distended. Moreover, a full bladder is uncomfortable for the mother. By encouraging the mother to void every 2 hours during labor, distention can usually be avoided.

Because the bladder is anterior to the lower uterine segment during labor, it is usually easy to recognize distention both visually and by palpation (Fig. 17–6).

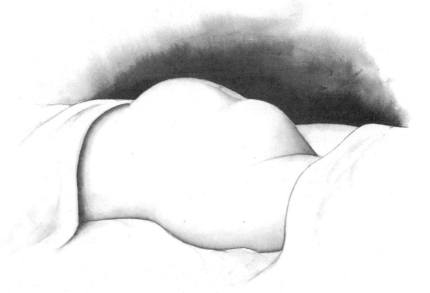

Figure 17–6. A full bladder during labor can be recognized by the characteristic soft swelling suprapubically. (From Greenhill and Friedman: *Biological Principles and Modern Practice of Obstetrics.* Philadelphia, W. B. Saunders Co., 1974.)

If distention occurs and if the mother is unable to void, catheterization may be necessary. Special precautions important in catheterizing a woman during labor include:

1. Cleansing solutions must not enter the vagina.

2. A small flexible catheter is used to minimize discomfort and trauma.

3. The catheter is inserted between contractions, when the pressure of the fetal head against the urethra is not as great.

The Administration of an Enema

Just as a full bladder may interfere with the descent of the baby's head, so also may a full rectum. For this reason, an enema may be given shortly after the mother is admitted. In addition to its cleansing effect, a warm water enema often stimulates uterine contractions.

If the mother is not admitted until labor is far advanced or if the head is well descended and pressing on the rectum, the enema is usually omitted.

During early labor, the enema may be expelled in the toilet. If small amounts of fluid continue to be expelled, it is important to take measures to avoid contaminating the vagina and vulva with fecal material.

Fetal heart rate should be checked following the expulsion of the enema.

Nursing Intervention to Protect the Mother and Fetus

In addition to the hazards of the process of labor itself, there are potential dangers in the hospital environment. Protecting women from the hazards associated with equipment and procedures is also a part of the nursing care of mothers in labor. There are potential dangers related to: (1) medications, (2) infections, and (3) electrical equipment.

Dangers of Medications

The specific side effects, such as hypotension, of certain medications are discussed later in this chapter. In general, it is important to remember that medications given for the relief of pain may make the woman drowsy. She must be protected from falling by the use of side rails and should be accompanied if she is allowed out of bed.

The danger of explosion when oxygen and gases used for anesthesia are present in labor/delivery rooms must be remembered.

Danger of Infection

Infection is a hazard to both mother and fetus. Even in excellent hospitals infection occasionally occurs, a circumstance that should be reviewed to determine the reason.

Nurses must help to develop and enforce policies that protect patients from infection. Standards for clothing, for the care of instruments and supplies, for the cleaning of rooms, and the like are helpful only if they are observed.

There is no reason to fear that fathers or other companions will be sources of infection (unless, of course, they are ill). Family members are usually eager to comply with requests about hand washing, dress, and the like—they know they are protecting their baby. Staff members are more likely to become casual.

Specific protection of the vaginal tract during preparation of the perineum, administration of enemas, and examination is described in appropriate sections.

Electrical Hazards

More electrical equipment is used in the care of laboring women than ever before. A policy that ensures frequent checking of this equipment by qualified people at designated intervals is essential. When a piece of equipment is checked, a label with the date should be attached. Only three-pronged plugs should be used. All equipment must be properly grounded. If even the slightest shock occurs, equipment should be unplugged.

Nursing Intervention to Help the Mother Cope with Discomfort

The contractions of labor are hard work and cause discomfort. Factors influencing the degree of discomfort experienced by an individual woman have been discussed in Chapters 15 and 16. Nurses intervene (1) to assist the woman in coping with general discomfort, and (2) to help her cope with the discomfort of contractions.

Coping with General Discomfort

The physiologic process of labor results in bodily changes that can add, often considerably, to a mother's discomfort. Conversely, by attending to these needs, total comfort is enhanced. This supports the mother not only physically but also emotionally because such attention demonstrates that her comfort is important to us.

Perspiration is common, as when any hard work is done, so that bathing of the face, hands, and back is comforting and relaxing. In a prolonged labor, a total bath is desirable. Gowns and clothes damp with perspiration must be changed as often as necessary.

Dryness of the lips and mouth is another discomfort during labor. In many settings, the mother is allowed nothing by mouth. In addition, the mouth-breathing techniques described in the section below contribute to dryness. Mothers who have attended childbirth preparation classes often bring lollipops, Vaseline, Chapstick, or lip gloss with them to help relieve dryness. Many women find chewing and sucking on a clean, wet washcloth refreshing. Varney[31] noted that ice chips have a drying effect and increase the discomfort of a dry mouth and lips.

Discharge from the vagina may be in the form of mucus, blood, or amniotic fluid at various stages during labor, all of which add to a feeling of discomfort. The vulva must be kept clean, with care that cleansing solutions do not enter the vagina, and gowns and linens must be changed as necessary.

Coping with the Discomfort of Contractions

There are many techniques that help mothers cope with the discomfort of labor, but they may be divided into two basic categories—coping without the use of medication and coping with the use of medication. For many women, a combination of these strategies is the most appropriate nursing intervention.

Coping without the Use of Medication

Many couples prepare for labor by attending classes in the Lamaze method, the Bradley method, or similar strategies for dealing with labor. There they acquire attitudes and tools to help them cope with labor. Unfortunately, many other women come to labor prepared with only "old wives' tales" and "horror stories". They expect the worst, and their tension makes labor far more difficult for them than it might otherwise have been.

Although prior preparation is ideal, nurses who care for women in labor can use similar strategies to make labor a more positive experience for all women.

The basics of helping a mother cope with labor involve helping her to:

1. Find a comfortable position.
2. Listen to her own voice and to the voice of whoever is coaching her during labor.
3. Focus on some object to minimize distractions from breathing patterns.
4. Adjust her breathing patterns, which vary with the stage of labor.

There is no question that the woman who has practiced these techniques prior to labor has an advantage, at least partly because she *feels* prepared. Nevertheless, good nurse coaching during labor itself can help the unprepared mother as well, in part because the close attention involved in the coaching will probably help her to be less tense and fearful.

A Comfortable Position

During early labor, sitting alternating with walking is the position of choice for many mothers. Walking is contraindicated if the membranes have ruptured and the head is not engaged (see above). We need to observe her for signs of fatigue during this period and encourage her to rest frequently. During a contraction, the woman may stand and lean forward, supported by her husband or a nurse if she is walking at the time of onset.

Another position of comfort for some mothers during part of labor is the "pelvic rock" position (Fig. 11–8).

Relaxation

Relaxation is a key to effective labor. The purpose of relaxation is to conserve energy by relaxing the other muscles of the body while the muscles of the uterus do their job. Mothers who have practiced relaxation exercises during the prenatal period (Chapter 11) will be best able to relax during labor.

Nurses can help unprepared mothers achieve some degree of relaxation. One way is to provide support for every joint—arms, legs, back, and neck. Every joint should also be bent. This support is also important for mothers who have practiced relaxing. By providing support in this way minimal energy is expended.

Nurses can also coach mothers through the relaxation process during labor. "Relax your jaw . . . relax your shoulders . . . relax your arms . . . relax your hands . . . your fingers . . ." and so on through the body is more helpful than a command to "relax," which may produce the opposite result.

Listening

All of a mother's senses are heightened during labor. She will remember for many years the sights and sounds surrounding the birth of her baby. Her heightened sensorium can be helpful is she is "tuned in" to the sound of her own voice or the voice of her coach, usually her husband or nurse. If she has been prepared to use certain techniques, she can repeat to herself, or have her coach repeat, the instructions that she has practiced.

Focusing

Each of us has had some experience in which our attention is focused so intently on one

Text continued on page 500

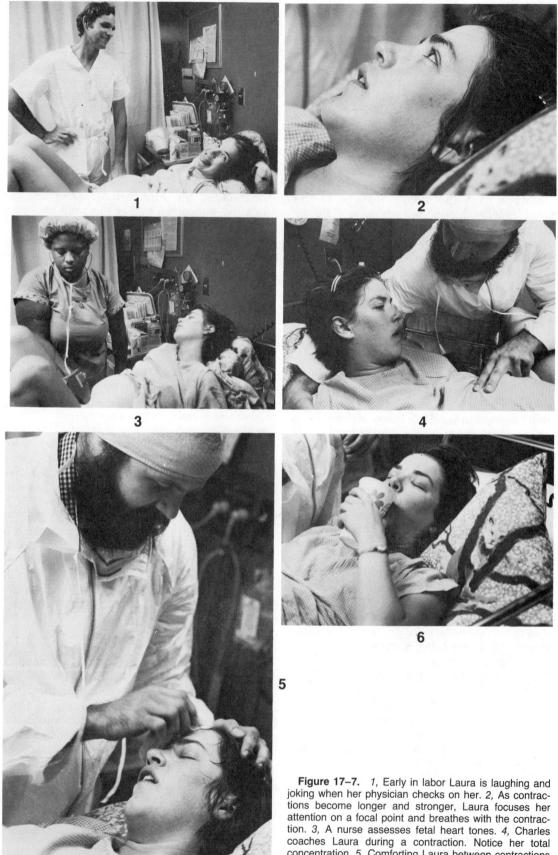

Figure 17–7. *1,* Early in labor Laura is laughing and joking when her physician checks on her. *2,* As contractions become longer and stronger, Laura focuses her attention on a focal point and breathes with the contraction. *3,* A nurse assesses fetal heart tones. *4,* Charles coaches Laura during a contraction. Notice her total concentration. *5,* Comforting Laura between contractions by wiping her forehead, *6,* . . . giving her sips of water.

Illustration continued on opposite page

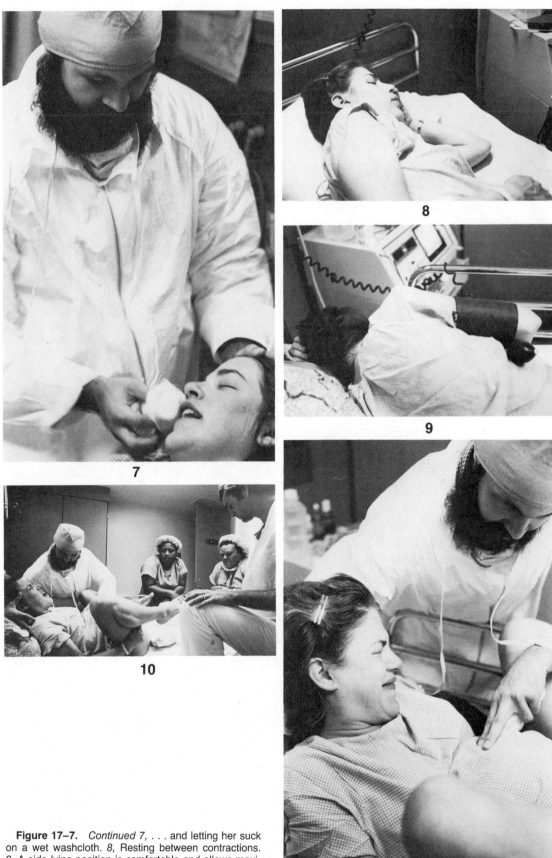

Figure 17–7. *Continued 7,* . . . and letting her suck on a wet washcloth. *8,* Resting between contractions. *9,* A side lying position is comfortable and allows maximum fetal oxygenation. *10,* Second stage: pushing with support from Charles. *11,* Pushing is hard work.

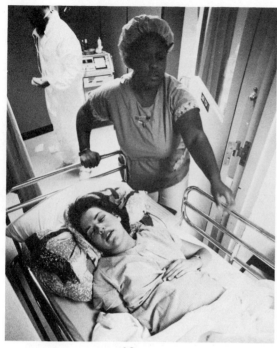

12

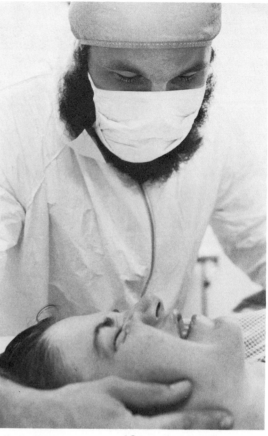

13

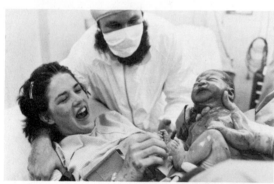

14

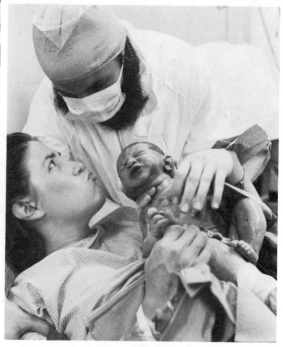

15

Figure 17–7 *Continued 12,* It's almost time! On the way to delivery room. *13,* Final pushes. *14,* It's a boy! *15,* A special time for Mom and Dad.
Illustration continued on opposite page

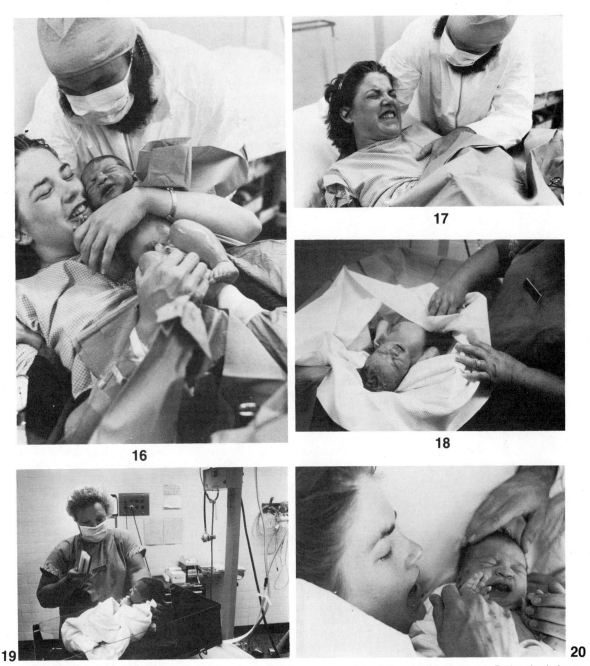

Figure I7–7 *Continued 16,* And baby makes three. *17,* One more push to deliver the placenta. *18,* Drying the baby to prevent evaporative heat loss. *19,* Baby is wrapped in a warm blanket. *20,* Back to Mom and Dad. (Photographs 1–20 courtesy of Tim Chalmers, © CMC 1982.)

Table 17–3. OVERVIEW OF NURSING CARE DURING LABOR *(Continued)*

Phase	Nursing Assessment		Nursing Action	
	Emotional	Physical	Safety	Support
		First Stage		
Latent	Excited, anxious	Contractions every 20 minutes to every 5 minutes, lasting 30–45 seconds; show	After admission, assessment of mother and fetus (see text)	Encourage relaxation, slow breathing when necessary; void every hour; clear liquids; light activity, walking; sleep if possible if it is night
			Continuing assessment of maternal vital signs, fetal heart tones (rate, location, maximum intensity), progress of labor (effacement, dilatation, station, contraction pattern—frequency, duration, intensity), maternal comfort (bladder, fatigue, emotional status, discomfort, sign of complications)	Position: vertical or side-lying throughout labor
Active	Less outgoing, increased concentration during contractions; less small talk	Contractions every 5 minutes to every 3 minutes, lasting 45–60 seconds	Continued assessment as described above; watch for signs of approach of transition	Encourage breathing with contraction; pelvic rock, counter pressure for back pain; provide for rest; encourage relaxation; encourage voiding every hour; explain progress of labor
				Comfort measures: mouth care; pillows; wet washcloth; lollipops
Transition	Restlessness, irritability, sensory overload, discouraged, weepy, sensation of drift, feeling out of touch with reality	Increased bloody show, nausea and/or vomiting, belching, hiccoughs, trembling, urge to push, drowsy between contractions	Continuing assessment as described above	Deal with one contraction at a time; breathe through urge to push; encourage rest between contractions; eye contact during contractions

Table 17–3. OVERVIEW OF NURSING CARE DURING LABOR *(Continued)*

Phase	Nursing Assessment		Nursing Action	
	Emotional	**Physical**	**Safety**	**Support**
First Stage (continued)				
				Breathe with her; massage of back and thighs. Supply any comfort measures (above) that are helpful. Support husband or coach. Explain behvior as related as related to phase of labor
Second Stage				
	Excitement; renewed energy; more alert	Contractions less intense, every 3–5 minutes, lasting 45–60 seconds; increasing pelvic pressure; perineal stretching; burning or tearing sensations as fetal head reaches pelvic floor. Baby's head anesthetizes pelvic floor by inhibiting blood supply	Assess length of second stage contraction pattern and progress through mechanisms of labor; assess fetal heart tones.	Encourage to push with pushing urge; with shoulders rounded and relaxed; jaw relaxed. Encourage relaxation of pelvic floor; encourage relaxation between contractions. Encourage light breathing and no pushing when head crowns. Supply any comfort measures (above) that are helpful.
Third Stage				
	Renewed energy; excitement of seeing, touching, holding baby	Cutting of umbilical cord. Contraction to deliver placenta usually follows in 20 minutes. May observe cord lengthening and gush of blood prior to delivery of placenta. Allowing infant to attempt to breast-feed stimulates oxytocin production, causes contraction, aids delivery of placenta, prevents hemorrhage.	Prevent neonatal heat loss; provide warmth. Suction baby's mouth if mucousy (with bulb syringe). Assess fetus, including Apgar score. Assess firmness of uterus; massage *after* placenta delivered; check placenta and membranes for completeness.	Allow parents to see, touch, hold baby. Allow mother to breast-feed if she desires. Leboyer both if desired.
Fourth Stage				
	Elation initially, later fatigue; joy of holding infant, breast-feeding, examining	Sutures if episiotomy. Oxytocin may be given to contract uterus.	Assess maternal blood pressure, pulse, fundus. Massage fundus. Have oxytocic drugs available. Continue to ensure infant warmth; observe infant for signs of distress.	Provide opportunities for family bonding. Encourage slow chest breathing and relaxation during fundal assessment and massage. Encourage Kegel exercise for perineal comfort. Encourage breast-feeding, if desired.

matter that we are oblivious to other happenings around us. We may go to a movie with a headache and focus so intently on the film that the headache is completely forgotten, only to find when we leave the theater that the headache is still there after all. An athlete may be injured early in a football or basketball game but may feel no pain until the contest is over.

During labor, focusing accomplishes the same objective—attention is diverted from the uterine contraction to some other object. Nothing is more counterproductive for the laboring mother than to lie in bed waiting for a contraction to occur, with all her attention focused on the contraction. "Here it comes . . . boy, is this awful . . . I don't think I can stand it . . . " and so on.

Mothers may focus on their husband's face or on an object in the room, such as a picture or even a doorknob. If the mother brings an object from home, we should help her place it where she wishes.

It is essential that nurses, physicians, and whoever else enters the labor room *do not interrupt* the mother who is focusing. Wait until the contraction is over. If the husband is there and if he has been prepared for labor along with his wife, he can "run interference" for her, reminding others that his wife will answer their questions when the contraction is over. Mothers who attend classes in preparation for labor may be taught to ignore questions during contractions.

Breathing Techniques

Patterned breathing is a major technique used by mothers trained in prepared childbirth classes. The patterns vary slightly, depending upon the techniques taught in a particular community. However, most employ chest breathing and/or abdominal breathing, starting at a slow rate and progressing to a more rapid rate as labor progresses.

The particular techniques described here are related to the Lamaze method. It is most important for nurses to be familiar with the types of preparation offered in their own communities so that they can be supportive of the couples they care for. There is no evidence that one type of preparation is superior to another type for all mothers, although for an individual mother it is possible that one method may be more helpful. In smaller communities, of course, alternatives may not be available.

WHY IS PATTERNED BREATHING EFFECTIVE? In Chapter 11 the relationship between tension and pain was noted (pain ╲ tension). Another facet of tension is an increase in the rate of respiration; observe your own respiratory rate the next time you feel tense and anxious.

By consciously breathing slowly, one can aid relaxation and thus effectively relieve pain due to tension. Moreover, concentration on breathing gives one control over one's emotions. A woman' is no longer helpless in the face of uncontrollable forces; she has tools that enable her to work along with her body rather than against it.

A number of breathing techniques are taught in prepared childbirth classes. Different patterns are appropriate at different stages of labor.

The Cleansing Breath. As each contraction begins, mothers are taught to take a *cleansing breath*, i.e., a deep breath that is blown out. The breath serves as a signal that a contraction is about to begin. A similar breath is taken at the end of the contraction.

Slow Chest Breathing. Slow chest breathing is usually most helpful during that stage of labor at which contractions are about 3 to 5 minutes apart and are lasting 60 seconds; the cervix will usually be about 4 cm. dilated. It is a time when normal breathing patterns are no longer adequate to help the mother cope with contractions. This pattern can be described as the type of breath you would use to "fill a bra." If the woman holds her fingers over her ribs, she will feel them spread as she breathes. The initial rate is approximately 10 breaths per minute. As contractions intensify, the rate may increase to 12 to 18 breaths per minute and still be no faster than a normal breathing pattern.

Effleurage (Chapter 11) often accompanies slow chest breathing.

Later in labor, slow chest breathing may be helpful in aiding relaxation between contractions, although other patterns are more helpful for the contraction itself.

Shallow, Light Chest Breathing. When slow breathing is no longer effective in helping a mother "keep on top of" her contractions, she may switch to a shallow, lighter breathing. This breathing should be as quiet and as low as possible; about one breath per second. Many women use shallow breathing during the active phase of the first stage, from about 6 to 7 cm. dilatation, until the beginning of transition, about 8 cm.

BREATHING DURING TRANSITION. For many women, transition (the period during which the uterus dilates from 8 to 10 cm.) is the most difficult part of labor.

A combination of light, shallow breathing with a puff, as if to blow out a candle, (at one time called pant and blow) is helpful during this period. The rate is approximately one breath per second. The pattern is breath–breath–breath–breath–puff (4:1 ratio); the ratio can be 6:1 or 8:1. As the contraction becomes more intense, there is a tendency to breathe faster and faster; the woman can briefly halve the number of breaths she takes, with two, three, or four shallow breaths and a puff at the height of the contraction, returning to the former pattern as decrement begins. As in all breathing patterns, this pattern begins with a cleansing breath and ends with a breath to blow away the contraction.

This pattern requires considerable concentration on the part of the mother and her coach. The coach may need to hold the mother's face in his (her) hands to help her concentrate.

Sometimes the mother may have an urge to push during transition. However, it is important not to push until the cervix is fully dilated. To push prematurely is not only painful but also leads to soft tissue swelling and can prolong labor. Moreover, pushing at this stage leads to fatigue in an already tired mother.

Breathing patterns do not stop the urge to push; they just help the mother refrain from adding the force of her abdominal muscles to uterine forces. Mothers need to be reassured that breathing patterns that prevent pushing do not stop the movement of the baby through the passage. Breathing patterns that prevent pushing include: (1) slow, sustained exhalation; or (2) blowing, as if blowing out candles on a birthday cake.

Watch for signs of hyperventilation (below) when these techniques are used.

HYPERVENTILATION. When breathing patterns become rapid with a longer period of expiration than inspiration, too much carbon dioxide is exhaled; this phenomenon is known as *hyperventilation*.* Hyperventilation occurs more often in women who have not been prepared for labor, but it can occur in prepared women as well. Light, quiet, even breathing is a major deterrent to hyperventilation.

The signs are lightheadedness, dizziness, tingling of the fingers, and numbness around the lips. A woman may not say anything about her symptoms, but we may see her touching her lips, as if to test them, or rubbing her hands. We should then question her about her symptoms. A later symptom is cramping of the fingers; this indicates that the woman has been hyperventilating for some time.

A simple, effective method of relieving hyperventilation is breathing into a paper bag

that is tightly sealed around the nose and chin. In this way, the woman will rebreathe her own carbon dioxide. Rebreathing should continue until symptoms disappear.

When the Fetus Is in a Posterior Position

When the fetus is in a posterior position (ROP, LOP, RSP, LSP, and so on), which may be as frequent as one in every four labors* (statistics vary from one study to another), labor is characterized by back pain that may be sufficiently intense that the discomfort of contractions seems very secondary. Back pain may also be significant in a breech presentation.

How can mothers with back pain be helped to cope with an often difficult labor? Such mothers can be assisted by providing emotional support, changing position, applying counterpressure, applying heat and cold, and encouraging conscious relaxation.

EMOTIONAL SUPPORT. When a mother realizes that her baby is in a posterior position (and she may recognize this before the position is confirmed by our examination), her first reaction may very well be, "Why me?" If her husband has been attending preparatory classes with her, he, too, may recognize that labor in a posterior position presents special needs and may share the feeling, "Why us?" We can let them know that it is all right to feel this way; they need to accept their feelings and then go on to cope with the special demands of a "back labor."

POSITION. In posterior labor, pain is centered in the lower back. The *most uncomfortable* position for a woman with posterior labor is lying on her back. With the possible exception of a brief period during which she is being examined, this woman should be off her back at all times. Why? It is the pressure of the baby's vertebral column against the mother's vertebral column that is causing the discomfort. Any position that takes the weight of the uterus off the mother's vertebrae will help. Frequent changes of position seem to be most helpful; several helpful positions are described below. The mother might assume one position for two or three contractions, then a second, then a third, and so on. For example, she may be on her left side for three contractions, assume a hand-knee position for one contraction, and then be on her right side for three contractions. She may then assume one of the sitting positions for two or three contractions. The important point for us is to be flexible

---

*Hyperventilation, of course, can occur in individuals at many times other than labor.

*Although much of labor may be in the posterior position, the baby may rotate to an anterior position prior to delivery.

enough to allow her frequent changes, as she seeks the position most comfortable for her. The best position for an individual mother is the position that feels best for her.

Sitting positions: The mother leans forward with her legs through the side rails. A pillow on the side rails will make her more comfortable. Be sure the rail is secure. Or the mother may sit in a chair, western-saddle style, or in the bed, leaning forward.

Side lying: The side-lying position allows the uterus to lie on the bed rather than on the mother's backbone. It also allows counterpressure and applications of heat or cold to be applied to the back.

Hand-knee position: The mother assumes a position on her hands and knees in bed; she arches her back up as she exhales and comes down as she inhales. Mothers can be taught to "pretend you are a donkey pulling your tail between your legs" (Fig. 11–9).

COUNTERPRESSURE. Counterpressure on the lower back can be helpful to the woman with posterior labor. Pressure can come from the heels of the husband's or the nurse's hands placed on each side of the lower spine. Even better, pressure may be obtained by using soup cans, adhesive tape cylinders, tennis balls tied in a stocking leg, or a rolling pin. The amount of pressure that feels good will vary from woman to woman, and from moment to moment in the same woman. She needs to guide her husband or nurse, saying "that's too hard," "push harder," or "that helps."

Back discomfort is almost constant during posterior labor; it does not occur only with contractions. Even if a husband is able to be with his wife, he will need periods of rest. Nurses who care for the mother will also need breaks. The bed should be at such a height that the coach (husband or nurse) does not have to bend over, a position that will lead to early fatigue and back pain for the coach. The pressure should come from the body of the coach, not the arms.

HEAT AND COLD. Warm, moist towels or ice packs, applied to the lower back, will feel comforting to many mothers. If heat is not helpful to a particular mother, try cold, and vice versa. Any time that heat is used, precautions against burning the skin are important.

The Second Stage of Labor

As the time for delivery approaches, if the mother is in a traditional hospital setting, she will be transferred to a delivery room. In other environments (Chapter 16) preparations appropriate to the individual setting are undertaken (Nursing Care Plan 17–2).

Once the cervix is fully dilated, the mother may bear down or push. Although some mothers welcome the opportunity to push, others are reluctant. Pushing may hurt; this is especially true if the baby is in a posterior position (see below). The rectal pressure that accompanies pushing makes some mothers fear they will have a bowel movement in bed, and this makes them reluctant to push. The psychologic change from a prohibition against pushing to an encouragement to push is somewhat like changing horses in midstream; it takes some getting accustomed to, especially for some couples.

The advantages of having the mother in a vertical position for pushing have been discussed in Chapter 15. Whether vertical or semihorizontal, the most effective position for pushing appears to be one in which the woman's body assumes a C shape, i.e., with chin tucked onto chest and back curved. Legs are flexed and apart. With her hands she may grasp her knees, the back of her thighs, the side rails of the bed, or handlebars on the bed for counterbalance. Elbows need to be bent in order to maintain the proper position. Straight arms and an arched rather than curved back or a head thrown back rather than tucked onto the chin will reduce the effectiveness of pushing.

Pushing efforts should be directed toward the front of the woman's body, not the back. Thus, instructions such as "bear down as if you are having a bowel movement," heard frequently in delivery rooms, are not appropriate. (Babies are born through vaginas, not rectums.) Rectal pushing may also aggravate hemorrhoids. A better instruction is "Pretend that you have a seat belt around your abdomen and try to break it with your abdominal muscles." Thus, effort will be concentrated in the abdomen. Placing one hand over the symphysis pubis and directing the mother to "push toward my hand" will also help her to push more effectively.

There is controversy about the best way to coach a mother to push during the second stage of labor. At one end of the continuum are advocates of vigorous expulsive efforts. At the other end are those who believe that spontaneous bearing down efforts are appropriate and that support persons should not encourage vigorous efforts but allow the mother to respond to her body.

The most vigorous expulsive efforts are made by taking a deep breath, after which the mother closes her glottis to hold her breath

Nursing Care Plan 17–2. Assisting a Mother in the Second Stage of Labor

NURSING GOALS:
To instruct mother in methods of pushing.
To support partner as role of coach for pushing.
To maintain fetal well-being.
OBJECTIVES:
The mother will:
1. Push effectively.
2. Give birth spontaneously.
Her partner will provide support.

ASSESSMENT	NURSING DIAGNOSIS	NURSING INTERVENTION	COMMENTS/RATIONALE
1. Patient's knowledge level of how and when to push; patient's ability to push 2. Assess progression of presenting part.	Need for education about methods of pushing Need for coach while pushing	Instruct mother in how to push effectively: Push toward vaginal opening and relax pelvic floor muscles. Use "gentle pushing" techniques. Assist mother in finding comfortable position for pushing; provide pillows for support. Instruct mother to push only with contractions. Encourage role of partner as coach. Encourage mother to relax completely between contractions. Keep mother informed of downward progress of baby. Continue to provide comfort measures as before. Transfer to delivery room when indicated, or prepare for birth in alternative setting. Continue to give directions for pushing.	Pushing using the Valsalva maneuver may cause fetal hypoxia and is not as effective as vaginal pushing. "Gentle pushing" has been shown to provide an adequate oxygen supply to the baby. Make sure patient does not push while lying flat on her back. Pushing only during contractions reinforces the work of the uterus.
3. Fetal heart tones	Greatest potential for fetal distress	Monitor fetal heart tones every 5 minutes while pushing. Monitor fetal heart tones immediately upon transferring mother to delivery table.	Pushing causes head compression; decelerations may occur. Chance for placental separation from uterus is greatly increased, especially when patient is completely dilated and transferred from one bed to another.

Contributed by Mona B. Ketner

and pushes as long as possible, taking another breath when she must. "Directed" pushing efforts may last 10 seconds or longer. One result of this method of pushing is a rise in intrathoracic pressure, initiating the following sequence (Valsalva maneuver):

Decreased intrathoracic pressure
↓
Decreased return of venous blood to the heart
↓
Decreased cardiac output
↓
Decreased maternal arterial blood pressure
↓
Decreased perfusion of placenta
↓
Decreased oxygen available to fetus
↓
Possible fetal hypoxia

Prolonged breath-holding also decreases maternal pO_2, a second factor contributing to possible fetal hypoxia. Auscultated fetal heart rate or tracing of a fetal heart rate monitor has shown deceleration following prolonged breath-holding.[8]

Caldeyro-Barcia observed the following characteristics of spontaneous bearing down efforts:

1. Spontaneous bearing down efforts usually lasted 4 to 6 seconds, a shorter period than directed efforts. The duration is shorter at the beginning and end of the contraction and increases from 0.93 to 1.87 seconds at the peak of the contraction.

2. The average number of bearing down efforts were 4 to 5 per contraction.

3. During the contraction women breathed but did not push for an average of 2 seconds between pushes.

4. The glottis was not fully closed.

Thus, a spontaneous breathing pattern during a second stage contraction might look like this: Push (4 sec.)—Rest (2 sec.)—Push (5 sec.)—Rest (2 sec.)—Push (6 sec.)—Rest (2 sec.)—Push (5 sec.)—Rest (2 sec.)—Push (4 sec.)—Rest (2 sec.)

The second stage may be longer when spontaneous pushing efforts are the only ones utilized, but this difference does not appear to affect the fetus adversely. Caldeyro-Barcia[7] found higher umbilical artery and vein pO_2 values, lower pCO_2 values, and higher pH values than those usually reported as normal.

Other advantages of a slower, more controlled second stage include slower distention of the perineal muscles, which may decrease the incidence of either lacerations or episi-

otomy; gradual, more even pressure to the fetal head; and decreased strain on the cardinal ligaments, which may protect against uterine prolapse or cystocele.

There are times when spontaneous pushing may not be effective or when there may be a need to shorten the second stage. Two different techniques of pushing, both of which result in less intrathoracic pressure and more frequent breathing than with prolonged breath-holding, are recommended. In each, the mother first takes two cleansing breaths. Then she may (1) take a deep breath, exhale partially, and then hold that breath and push, or (2) take a deep breath and exhale slowly as she pushes.

During the delivery there may be moments when the mother should not push in order to effect a slow, controlled delivery. Blowing out, as in the transition period of the first stage, will slow expulsive efforts and protect both the baby's head and the mother's perinium; "panting" will achieve the same purpose.

The delivery room is a strange environment for both the mother and father. It is often cold (in temperature). While the mother is guided onto the delivery table, the father needs to be shown where he can sit at the head of the table close beside his wife's head, so that he can talk to her and support her. Both the mother and father will need our attention during the next hour as her labor draws to a climax.

The vulva and surrounding area are cleansed with antiseptic solution, and the perineum is draped.

The area in which the baby will be received must also be warm and ready to receive the infant. All equipment for resuscitation should be available and ready for use (Chapter 23).

Perineal Lacerations

In a first degree perineal laceration, no muscles are involved. The muscles of the perineal body but not the rectal sphincter are involved in a second degree laceration. A third degree laceration extends to the rectal sphincter.

A major argument for episiotomy (below) is the prevention of perineal laceration.

Episiotomy

An *episiotomy* is an incision made in the perineum with a blunt scissors (Fig. 17–8). The vaginal opening is thus enlarged, and the likelihood of lacerations is decreased. As with many issues concerning birth, the need for episiotomy raises some controversy. In many hospitals, episiotomy is routine; others reserve episiotomy for those situations in which a perineal laceration seems likely.

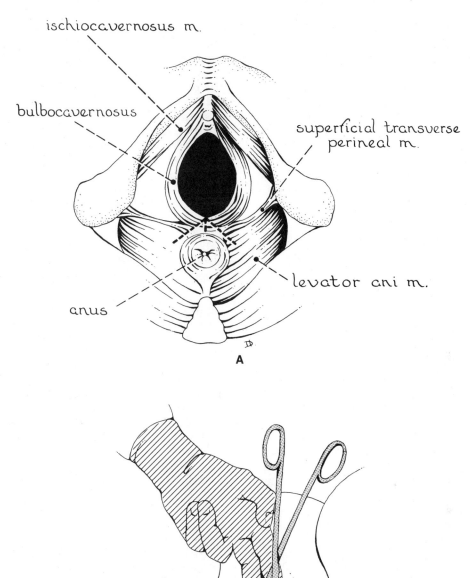

Figure 17–8. Midline episiotomy. *A,* Muscles of the pelvic floor and perineum. The sites of median and mediolateral episiotomy are shown. *B,* Incision of the midline episiotomy. (From Oxorn and Foote: *Human Labor and Birth.* 3rd Edition. Englewood Cliffs, N.J., Appleton-Century-Crofts, 1975.)

Proponents of routine episiotomy for all women in labor argue that:

1. The straight, cleanly cut episiotomy incision heals more easily than a ragged laceration.

2. A laceration may involve adjacent structures, such as the rectum or anal sphincter;

the direction of the episiotomy can be controlled.

3. Stretching and tearing of the perineum may predispose the mother to later perineal relaxation and to the possibility of cystocele or rectocele.

4. The second stage of labor is shortened.

5. The baby's head is not continually forced against the perineum.

Opponents of routine episiotomy for every woman in labor note that:

1. Laceration rates vary widely, with or without episiotomy. Most advocates of this perspective do not suggest that an episiotomy is never appropriate but that the decision can be made at the moment of crowning if laceration seems inevitable. The episiotomy may be extended by a laceration. Harris[16] reported that lacerations occurred in 22 per cent of primiparas following episiotomy. Beynon[4] noted a 13 per cent laceration extension of midline episiotomy in her own practice and reported extensions ranging from 2 to 22 per cent in the literature.

2. A second issue is protection of the pelvic floor muscles. In older studies[1, 23] evaluating both episiotomy and the use of low forceps, the condition of the pelvic floor was improved in women with episiotomy. In one recent study[24] the drug hyaluronidase was injected into the perineal body in 50 of 100 women selected randomly. The perineum was intact at delivery in 60 per cent of women receiving the drug and in 20 per cent of those who did not; at 6 weeks postpartum there was equally good pelvic support in the two groups.

Opponents of routine episiotomy believe that the prenatal and postpartum practice of Kegel exercises (Chapter 11) will improve muscle tone, thereby limiting intrapartum trauma. (Kegel exercises are also recommended for women who have an episiotomy.)

3. In preterm and other high risk deliveries in which shortening of the second stage is important for fetal or maternal well-being, episiotomy is considered important. Opponents question the necessity for a shortened second stage when the mother and fetus are healthy and the pregnancy is at term.

4. The importance of reduced pressure on the fetal head during delivery is unclear when the baby is healthy and at term. When the baby is preterm and has capillary fragility and an increased risk of cerebral hemorrhage, an episiotomy is indicated. Episiotomy is frequently necessary to facilitate delivery when birth weight is expected to be greater than 9 pounds.

5. Disadvantages of episiotomy include extension of the incision (above), increased blood loss, unsatisfactory repair, postpartum pain, and pain on intercourse. In the period immediately following birth, the repair of the episiotomy may be a distraction to the initial bonding between mother and infant.

Episiotomies are done far less frequently in Europe than in the United States. It has been suggested that one reason for the apparent necessity of episiotomy in the United States is the position in which women are placed on the delivery table (flat on their backs with legs in stirrups), which causes tension on the perineum and prevents a gradual stretching.

A technique termed "ironing out the perineum," in which the perineum is stretched, is practiced by some midwives and physicians. This technique involves a danger of separating the pelvic floor muscles, again leading to perineal relaxation.

Each mother should be evaluated individually. Although an episiotomy is probably not always indicated, it certainly would seem proper under some circumstances.

Leboyer and the Second Stage of Labor

In 1975 the French obstetrician Frederick Leboyer published *Birth without Violence,* a book largely critical of traditional methods of delivery.[20] Leboyer's concepts rapidly became a major topic of discussion among many professional and lay men and women. Leboyer feels that infants suffer emotional trauma because of the violence of birth and that this trauma will affect the personality of the infant, not only at the time of birth but later in his life as well.

Unfortunately, much of the discussion of Leboyer's work has centered on questions such as "Should the baby be immersed in warm water following delivery?" and "Should the lights in the delivery room be dimmed?" While basic ideas are overlooked. We believe that the concepts of Leboyer described below are worthy of serious consideration.

1. The process of delivery should be gentle and controlled, with unnecessary intervention eliminated.

2. The baby should be handled gently, with head, neck, and sacrum supported.

3. The baby should not be overstimulated. He should be allowed to breathe spontaneously, without painful stimuli. Moderate suctioning is preferable to vigorous suctioning; overly vigorous suctioning may lead to reflex bradycardia. Delayed cord clamping is advised. (Obviously, some babies do not breathe spontaneously and must be resuscitated, as described in Chapter 23.)

These concepts emphasize the "humanness" of the newly born infant; he is a being worthy of gentle handling. This principle is worthy of incorporation into our concept of care.

The Third Stage of Labor

The delivery of the infant ends the second stage of labor. Care is now divided between the newborn infant and the mother; adequate staff is essential to ensure that neither is overlooked (Nursing Care Plan 17–3).

The mechanics of the third stage leading to the separation of the placenta have been described in Chapter 15. Separation usually occurs from 1 to 5 minutes after the baby is delivered. Evidence of placental separation includes:

1. The protrusion of the umbilical cord from the vagina.

2. A change in the shape (more globular), consistency (firmer), and position (higher in the abdomen) of the uterus.

3. A sudden gush of blood.

The fundus is not massaged before the placenta separates. Once separation occurs, the placenta must be expelled quickly and atraumatically. The mother is encouraged to push, just as she pushed her baby out. Unlike pushing at the time of delivery, when the mother was concentrating all of her attention on birthing her baby, she is now perhaps watching her baby or listening to his cry, a hundred thoughts rushing through her mind. She needs to be coached to push effectively.

If the mother is unable to push because of anesthesia, she must be assisted in expelling the placenta:

1. The fundus is palpated to be sure that it is firm. If the uterus is not firm, it may become inverted when the placenta is expelled.

2. With one hand, exert downward pressure on the fundus; push the placenta out of the vagina.

After the placenta has separated, the fundus is massaged to facilitate contraction and thus to minimize blood loss. Accurate estimation of blood loss is essential. The average loss is approximately 250 to 300 ml.

If the placenta is not expelled, it must be manually removed. Manual removal is never a desirable situation; the risk of postpartum infection is increased and is still further increased in relation to the amount of time that elapses between birth and removal of the placenta.

The delivered placenta is always inspected; if it is not intact and fragments remain in the uterus, the chances of both postpartum hemorrhage (because the uterus cannot contract properly) and infection are heightened. Postpartum hemorrhage may be delayed for several days, occurring after the mother has returned to her home.

The Fourth Stage of Labor

The first hour following the expulsion of the placenta, often called the fourth stage of labor, is a significant one for the family. It is a time for careful observation of both mother and baby from a physiologic perspective. Equally important, it is a time when attachment is facilitated between parents and their new infant (see Nursing Care Plan 17–4).

The ideal environment during the fourth stage is a room in which mother, father, and baby can become acquainted. Mothers who have not been heavily medicated are often excited, aware, and "turned on" during the first hour after they deliver. Fathers are eager to be with the mother and baby. The baby of an unmedicated mother is usually alert and looking about for the first 30 to 45 minutes of life. If put to breast, he will suck, stimulating the secretion of oxytocin, which is the body's physiologic mechanism for contracting the uterus. Just the sight of her baby and the sound of his cry will also stimulate the mother's uterine contractions, through the mediation of the sympathetic nervous system.

Thus, if we consider maternal and infant behavior and physiology, the practices of some hospitals in the United States appear designed in direct contradiction to the needs of infants and their parents.

These practices, as in the other stages of labor, evolved largely during the era of administering general anesthesia during birth. The first hour after birth, like the period following surgery, was one of recovery from anesthesia. The mother, asleep, was not aware of her baby. The baby slept as well. Immediate instillation of silver nitrate into his eyes for prophylaxis against ophthalmia neonatorum (Chapter 20) made the quiet, alert look of today's baby virtually unknown.

Perhaps the ideal situation is having both mother and baby together in a recovery bed with a warmer over the entire bed. Lacking such a warmer, the mother and baby can still be warmed with blankets; the heat of the mother's body also warms the baby. Adequately warmed, the mother and baby can touch skin-to-skin, whether the mother chooses to breast-feed or not (the significance of touch is discussed in Chapter 21). The father

Text continued on page 512

Nursing Care Plan 17–3.   Assisting a Mother in the Third Stage of Labor

NURSING GOALS:
To perform immediate nursing assessment of newborn infant.
To maintain thermoregulation of the newborn.
To promote maternal–paternal–infant attachment.
To continue to act as coach for pushing.

OBJECTIVES:
The mother will:
1. Begin interaction with her newborn by being able to see, stroke, and hold her newborn.
2. Deliver her placenta spontaneously.
Her partner will:
1. Begin interaction with the infant by being able to see, stroke, and hold his newborn.
2. Continue to provide support to mother.
The infant will:
1. Sustain respirations after spontaneous initiation.
2. Remain warm in the extrauterine environment.

ASSESSMENT	NURSING DIAGNOSIS	NURSING INTERVENTION	COMMENTS/RATIONALE
1. Infant's general physical status	Potential for cold stress and respiratory distress immediately after birth	Perform Apgar score at 1 minute and 5 minutes.	Some cold stress is inevitable at birth and immediately thereafter.
		Assess body systems by observation and auscultation.	Thermoregulation is of paramount importance at this time. The infant loses a large percentage of body heat from his head.
		Check the number of umbilical cord vessels.	The presence of only two umbilical cord vessels may indicate kidney or other congenital anomalies.
		Monitor airway and breathing. Observe for grunting, retracting, and nasal flaring.	
		Provide warmth with radiant heat and warm blanket.	
		Prevent further heat loss by placing cap on infant's head.	
2. Immediate family interaction	Need for parental attachment	Encourage mother to see and hold infant immediately.	The parents may stroke infant with fingertips as first interaction.

	Enable parents to explore infant. Allow for skin-to-skin contact. Place baby on mother's abdomen.	These first minutes of family interaction are permanent impressions for the parents. The baby is alert.
	Assist mother with breast-feeding on delivery table, if desired.	Problems of attachment may be identified by the nurse.
	Encourage father to hold infant.	
3. Placenta's readiness to separate; ability of uterus to immediately contract	Observe for the signs of placental separation: 1. Uterus rises upward in the abdomen. 2. Umbilical cord protrudes 3 inches or more out of the vagina. 3. Uterus changes to a globular shape and becomes firmer. 4. Sudden trickle or spurt of blood.	These signs are sometimes apparent within 1 minute after delivery of the infant and usually within 5 minutes.
Potential for fragmented placenta delivery	Instruct mother to push in order to expel the placenta.	
Potential for boggy uterus, leading to excessive amount of lochia	Placental expression, gentle downward pressure on the fundus to allow the placenta to glide gently out of the vagina may be needed if the patient's pushing fails to deliver the placenta.	Expression should be done only when the uterus is hard; otherwise inversion of the uterus is a possibility.
	Inspect placenta to make sure it is intact.	If a fragment of the placenta is left in the uterus, there may be subsequent hemorrhage.
	Massage fundus after delivery of placenta. Check tendency toward uterine atony. Express clots as necessary. Administer oxytocin (Pitocin) after delivery of placenta.	

Contributed by Mona B. Ketner

Nursing Care Plan 17–4.   Assisting a Mother in the Fourth Stage of Labor

NURSING GOALS:
To prevent postpartum hemorrhage.
To promote parent–infant attachment.
To promote rest and comfort for the mother.

OBJECTIVES:
The mother will:
1. Relate appropriately to her newborn infant.
2. Recover without excessive vaginal bleeding.
3. Know the need for fundal massage.
4. Be able to massage her own fundus.
5. Remain warm and comfortable.

ASSESSMENT	NURSING DIAGNOSIS	NURSING INTERVENTION	COMMENTS/RATIONALE
Assess blood pressure, pulse, and respirations every 15 minutes for 1 hour.	Potential for postpartum hemorrhage	Explain reason and process of postpartum assessments.	Signs of shock include lowered blood pressure, rapid and weak pulse, and cool clammy skin.
Check temperature and dryness of skin.		Massage fundus in gentle circular motion if boggy. Express any clots.	Relaxation of the uterus is a major cause of postpartum hemorrhage.
Check fundus every 15 minutes for 1 hour.		Catheterize patient if she is unable to void after other nursing measures are used.	A full bladder may displace the uterus to one side and cause a boggy fundus, resulting in increased bleeding.
Check amount and consistency of lochia every 15 minutes.			
Assess bladder for distention.			
2. Assess patient for risk factors associated with postpartum hemorrhage: a. Older age b. High parity		Instruct mother about the importance of uterine massage. Teach her how to massage her own fundus. Encourage her to use re-	

c. Rapid labor
d. Prolonged first and second stages of labor
e. Extremely large infant
f. Multiple birth

laxation and breathing techniques as in the first stage of labor (slow, relaxed breathing) during fundal massage.

3. Patient's degree of fatigue and exhaustion

Need for comfort and rest

Offer patient a complete bed bath. — Bath is refreshing and may enable patient to rest more fully.

Wipe perineum from front to back. Instruct patient in washing from front to back. — This front-to-back direction helps to decrease the possibility of vaginal and urinary tract infections.

Offer fluids to drink. Reposition patient as needed. Provide dry, clean gown and warm blankets. — Chilling accompanied by shaking often occurs in the early period following delivery. Warm blankets help to control shaking.

Provide quiet environment for rest; encourage patient to rest.

Apply ice pack to perineum if patient had episiotomy. — Ice will help prevent swelling.

4. Family interaction

Need for parental attachment

Continue with interventions from third stage of labor.

Provide more time for new family unit to be alone for bonding. — The infant is alert and awake with open eyes during the first hour after delivery.

Delay eye prophylaxis until baby is in nursery. — Eye prophylaxis performed immediately after birth has been shown to decrease eye movement in the infant.

Explain to parents the importance and significance of the first hours past birth with regard to the family bond.

Contributed by Mona B. Ketner

is with them, and the attachments of parents to baby and baby to parents begins.

Principal nursing goals for this period include:

1. Comfort for each member of the family.
2. Careful assessment of the mother.
3. Careful assessment of the baby.
4. Facilitation of attachment.

The assessment and immediate care of the baby is described in Chapter 20; the facilitation of attachment is discussed in Chapter 26.

Comfort

The father's comfort is enhanced by a comfortable chair beside the mother's bed, and often by a chance to go to the bathroom or have something to eat. A father who feels faint during or following delivery may be reacting to hunger rather than to excitement.

A smooth, dry bed for the mother, a frequent change of perineal pads, a blanket because she may feel chilled all over or complain of cold feet—these are measures that provide comfort and thereby enhance bonding. If there is perineal discomfort, the application of an ice pack is frequently valuable in reducing edema and in providing relief.

Maternal Physiologic Assessment and Intervention

The major maternal danger during the fourth stage is postpartum hemorrhage. Thus, immediate physiologic assessment is directed toward those aspects that evaluate blood loss.

1. Is the fundus firm?
2. Where is the fundus in relation to the umbilicus?
3. Is there evidence of a perineal hematoma?
4. Does either maternal pulse (rapid, thready) or maternal blood pressure (falling) indicate abnormal bleeding?
5. Is the bladder full?

The Fundus. The uterus continues to contract and relax during the hour following delivery. When the uterus relaxes, bleeding from the vessels at the placental site occurs until thrombi form. Thus, it is important that the uterus be in a state of contraction.

The role of endogenous oxytocin (i.e., oxytocin produced in the mother's body) has been mentioned. Synthetic oxytocin is usually given to the mother following delivery in the form of Pitocin, Methergine, or Ergotrate.

The firmness of the fundus is assessed every 15 minutes during the first hour (more frequently if the uterus does not remain contracted). Each time before the fundus is

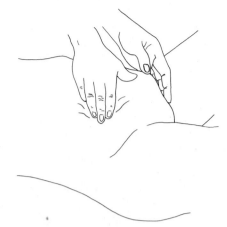

Figure 17–9. Fundal massage, external view. While the left hand supports the bottom of the uterus, the right hand palpates the fundus and massages.

checked, the mother should be addressed, and if she is dozing, she should be alerted, with a statement such as, "Mrs. Yancy, I need to check your uterus to be sure it is firm." We need to recognize that this is not a comfortable procedure for the mother and to let her know that we realize this.

With the mother's legs flexed, the fundus is palpated by cupping one hand above the uterus and the other below (Figs. 17–9 and 17–10). The fundus should be felt in the midline at approximately the level of the umbilicus. The fundus is usually higher in multigravidas because the uterine muscles have been more stretched; factors such as polyhydramnios, multiple pregnancy, and a number of others

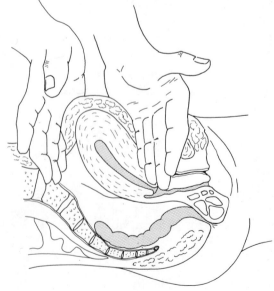

Figure 17–10. Fundal massage, internal view. As in Figure 17–9, the left hand supports the uterus while the right hand palpates the fundus.

will also affect uterine size and thus the position of the fundus after birth. If the fundus is not firm, it is gently massaged until it becomes firm.

The presence of blood and clots in the uterus is a barrier to contraction. Clots and blood are expressed by applying pressure for approximately 5 seconds, resting, and then reapplying pressure until all clots are removed. Hands are positioned for the expression of clots as they are for the assessment of the fundus.

The same factors that affect the position of the fundus after delivery also predispose the mother to uterine *atony*, i.e., a lack of tone in the uterine muscles that makes it more difficult for them to remain contracted. In addition to hydramnios and multiple pregnancy, uterine atony or hypotonicity also is possible:

1. In any pregnancy in which the baby is large.
2. When labor has been very rapid or prolonged.
3. When the mother has pre-eclampsia or eclampsia.
4. When the mother had general anesthesia.
5. When the mother is a multipara.

The Perineum. Vaginal discharge following delivery is called *lochia*. The characteristics of lochia, which change during the days following birth, are described in Chapter 25. During the fourth stage of labor, lochia is red (*rubra*) in color and contains blood, membrane fragments, decidua, lanugo, and vernix. Bright red blood in the lochia indicates fresh bleeding; this is *not* the expected color and requires immediate assessment to determine the source and intervention to control it. Lochia will smell like fresh blood, but it should not be foul smelling; foul-smelling lochia or mucus in the discharge indicates sepsis in the mother and potentially in the baby as well.

Lochia is partially absorbed by perineal pads; a record of the number of pads used, the degree to which they are saturated, and a description of clots provides an indication of excessive bleeding. When the pad is checked, the mother must be turned on her side so that lochia that may have pooled beneath the sacrum is not overlooked.

When the pad is checked, the perineum and surrounding skin should be gently washed; dried lochia is most uncomfortable.

Hematoma. Not only the amount and color of the lochia but also the condition of the perineum itself should be assessed. The complaint of intense pain when the pad touches the perineum may indicate a hematoma, the result of tearing of a blood vessel and subsequent bleeding into the loose connective tissue.

The skin over the area of hemorrhage is bluish-black. As bleeding continues, the hematoma may distend the perineum and dislocate the anus, rectum, and vagina. These subsequent symptoms are not usually evident until several hours after delivery, when pain may be reported in the vagina, rectum, or legs as well as in the perineum. However, early detection during the fourth stage may prevent a more extensive problem.

Aside from the intense discomfort, a hematoma may predispose to infection and, if bleeding is extensive, to anemia. Large hematomas are evacuated through the vaginal mucosa; the vaginal canal is then packed for 12 hours to assure hemostasis. Transfusion and antibiotics may be utilized if indicated. A small hematoma may be allowed to absorb; the mother should be carefully observed for signs of local or generalized infection.

A mother with intense pain is going to need particular help in enjoying her baby; this problem is discussed in Chapter 28.

Pulse and Blood Pressure. Usually blood pressure returns to normal prenatal levels shortly after delivery. Pulse rates are frequently somewhat slower than before pregnancy during the first 7 to 10 postpartum days.

Blood pressure and pulse are assessed every 15 minutes during the first hour, principally to ascertain excessive bleeding. However, changes in blood pressure and pulse may not occur until bleeding is already excessive; they are only one parameter by which bleeding is judged. When bleeding is so excessive that changes occur, a *rapid, thready pulse* usually precedes a drop in blood pressure. Thus, one cannot assume that an increase in pulse rate is insignificant if blood pressure remains normal.

Factors that may contribute to an elevated blood pressure during the fourth stage include excitement and certain medications, especially Ergotrate. Blood pressure is also affected by circadian rhythm (the 24-hour biologic cycle), being highest in the late afternoon and lowest in the middle of the night.

Sedation given during labor and certain types of anesthesia (caudal anesthesia, for example, or a saddle block) may lead to maternal hypotension in the hour following delivery.

The Urinary Bladder. A full urinary bladder inhibits contraction of the uterus and thus predisposes the mother to postpartum hemorrhage, both during the fourth stage and in the hours that follow.

Nursing evaluation of the fullness of the bladder is important because the effect of anesthesia may interfere with the mother's recognition of her need to void. A full bladder is felt above the symphysis pubis and below the fundus, which may be displaced upward and away from the midline.

Pharmacologic Support During Labor and Birth

In many instances, prenatal preparation reduces the need for medication during labor, but it does not necessarily eliminate that need. Even if every mother were ideally prepared, the circumstances of labor vary, pain thresholds vary, and a variety of needs make the use of medication a valuable help for some women. No women should be made to feel that she has "failed" because her medication was asked for or given.

Nurses have many responsibilities in relation to analgesia and anesthesia during labor. A thorough knowledge of each medication, the reason it is given, the advantages and disadvantages in relation to the mother and baby, and the progress of labor is essential both for the antepartal nurse who prepares couples for delivery and for the nurse who cares for families during labor. The nurse in the labor room must also recognize signs that indicate the presence of complications related to medications and must know how to quickly alleviate problems that may arise. Each type of analgesia or anesthesia is associated with specific areas of nursing support.

Any medication used for analgesia or anesthesia during labor should be judged by the following criteria:

1. Neither the mother nor the baby should be endangered.
2. The efficiency of uterine contractions should not be decreased.
3. The woman should continue to be able to participate in her labor.
4. The method for giving the medication should be simple enough to avoid complications in administration.

It is apparent from Tables 17–4 and 17–5 that no medication currently used meets all of these criteria. Great care is essential when any medication is used.

Medications given during labor can be classified into six groups:

1. Sedatives and tranquilizers, which relieve apprehension and thus aid relaxation.
2. Amnesics, which erase the memory of pain.
3. Regional analgesics, which interrupt pain pathways.

4. General analgesics, which increase the tolerance of pain by approximately 50 per cent.
5. Local or regional anesthetics.
6. General anesthetics, which prevent perception of pain in the central nervous system (CNS).

Each group necessitates special care for the woman who receives one or more medications.

Effects of Analgesia or Anesthesia on the Fetus and Newborn

In evaluating the potential effects of medications given to mothers during labor and birth on the fetus and newborn, a number of factors need to be taken into account. These factors involve not only the properties of the drug itself and the route of administration but also individual characteristics of both the mother and the fetus or newborn.

Placental Transfer. Drug-related factors in placental transfer include fat solubility, molecular weight, degree of ionization, and protein binding. Drugs with a molecular weight of less than 600 cross the placenta easily; the placenta is relatively impermeable to drugs with a molecular weight greater than 1000. Highly charged molecules cross poorly, fat-soluble substances cross easily, and drugs highly bound to protein cross poorly.

Other factors that affect placental transfer include uteroplacental blood flow, pH in maternal and fetal blood, the surface area of the placenta, and the thickness of placental membranes.

Drug Metabolism, Absorption, Distribution, and Excretion. Many drugs given to the mother must be metabolized by the immature fetal or neonatal liver. The fetus may be slow to inactivate a drug. In addition, metabolites of a drug that may have no effect in adults may affect the fetus.

Effects of a drug will depend on the fetal organs or tissues that absorb the drug and the organs involved in excretion (kidneys, liver, or lungs).

Inherent Properties of the Drug. Some drugs are inherently more potent than others.

Other Maternal or Fetal Factors. Maternal factors, including hypertension or hypotension, and cardiac or respiratory depression, may increase the depressant action of drugs because they may cause depression of the fetus in themselves. Depressing drugs act synergistically in an already compromised fetus to produce newborn depression. A preterm fetus or newborn is more easily depressed by drugs than a fetus at term.

Sedatives

Barbiturates such as secobarbital, pentobarbital, and phenobarbital are the principal sedatives used in labor. For the woman in early labor who is very tense and anxious, sedatives are given to promote relaxation. They do not have any pain-relieving action, but they do reduce the amount of analgesia needed when they are given in combination with analgesics.

When a mother is admitted with rupture of the membranes but without contractions, or when she has been in labor for a number of hours but contractions are weak and irregular, sedation may be given to allow her to nap. Mothers who have prepared for labor may resist this idea. However, we can explain that following a rest not only are contractions frequently more effective but she will be better able to work with her contractions when she has slept. The assurance that we will awaken her, if she does not awaken when regular contractions begin, is important.

Disadvantages. Sedatives may slow and prolong labor. In most women when pain is present, and in some women at any time, sedatives may have the opposite effect from that desired; the mother may become restless and even delirious rather than relaxed. Nausea, vomiting, and decreased blood pressure may occur.

Barbiturates may cause marked respiratory distress in the newborn and drowsiness for 24 to 48 hours following birth because these drugs are metabolized more slowly by the infant than by the adult. Aside from the physiologic effect on the infant, the significance in terms of parent–infant interactions must be considered. For these reasons, barbiturates are never given when delivery is imminent. They are particularly dangerous in preterm deliveries.

Nursing Support. One factor concerning the effect of medication given during labor is the woman's expectation of the effect. Thus when a sedative or any mediciation is given, a comment such as, "This medicine will help you rest between contractions," or whatever statement is appropriate, will actually help her to rest between contractions. It is also important to tell her how she is likely to feel, and when. For example, "You will begin to feel drowsy in a few minutes."

Once medication for sedation has been given, the room should be semidarkened and as quiet as possible. Certainly, the father, friend, or coach can remain with the mother, but they should understand the purpose of the medication and allow her to rest. Nursing assessment can be planned to allow periods of rest.

Tranquilizers

A variety of tranquilizing drugs (Table 17–4) may be given during early labor. Like sedatives, they are used chiefly during early labor to relieve apprehension. Because they potentiate the action of both barbiturates and analgesics, the doses of these other types of medications are reduced by half when they are given along with a tranquilizer.

Disadvantages. Both maternal hypotension and a delay in the onset of respirations in the infant are possible when tranquilizers are given. Tranquilizers are considered dangerous in preterm labor.

Nursing Support. The supportive care given a mother receiving barbiturate sedation is equally applicable to the mother receiving a tranquilizer.

Amnesics

Hyoscine (scopolamine) was formerly used as an amnesic. However, it is rarely used today. Women are no less aware of pain when it occurs but have no memory of pain afterward. They frequently sleep between contractions but are very restless and excited during the contraction. Because of this, women given scopolamine should not be left unattended. When used, scopolamine is given in conjunction with an analgesic to minimize restlessness during contractions.

Analgesics

Meperidine (Demerol) and Stadol are the analgesics used most frequently during labor; morphine sulfate and alphaprodine (Nisentil) are also used on occasion.

Demerol does not offer immediate or complete relief of pain. Within a few minutes, pain will be less sharp, but maximum effectiveness is not achieved for 60 to 90 minutes. At this point the woman's pain threshold will be increased by approximately 50 per cent. Effects last for 2 to 3 hours.

Disadvantages. Hypotension is the most serious side effect of Demerol. Other side effects may include facial flushing, dryness of the mouth, diaphoresis, decreased urinary output, and nausea and vomiting. Morphine may also cause facial flushing and oral dryness.

The biggest disadvantage of analgesia is respiratory depression in the infant. The degree of depression is related to the amount given, the time that the drug is given in relation to delivery, the infant's weight and gestational age, and the degree of trauma at

Table 17–4. PHARMACOLOGIC RELIEF OF PAIN DURING LABOR

Classification	Medication or Method	Standard Dose	Placental Transfer	Duration of Action (hours)	Effect on Labor	Effect on Mother	Effect on Fetus
Sedative	Phenobarbital (Nembutal)	to 100 mg. IM, 50 mg. IV	Rapid*	4–6	Large amounts impair uterine activity and prolong labor	CNS depressant Mother lethargic and sleepy Nausea, vomiting, decrease in blood pressure possible	Respiratory distress Drowsiness for 24–48 hours
	Secobarbital (Seconal)	to 100 mg. PO, 50 mg. IV	Rapid	4–6			
	Phenobarbital (Luminal)	15–30 mg. IV, PO	Rapid	12–14			
Tranquilizer	Diazepam (Valium)	2, 5, or 10 mg. IV, IM, PO	Rapid	1–1.5 (IV) 2–3 (IM)	No recognized effect	Relief of apprehension, drowsiness, confusion May cause maternal hypotension	May cause delay in onset of respirations
	Promazine (Sparine)	25 mg. IM, PO	Rapid	3–4			
	Chlorpromazine (Thorazine)	25 mg. IM, PO	Rapid	6–8			
	Promethazine (Phenergan)	25–50 mg. IM, PO	Rapid	6–8			
	Hydroxyzine (Vistaril)	75–100 mg. IM, PO	(?)	(?)			
	Propiomazine (Largon)	10–20 mg. IM, PO	Rapid	3		Woman may become excited and delirious	
Amnesic	Hyoscine (Scopolamine)	0.25–0.60 mg.	Rapid	3–4		Dryness of mouth and throat	
Analgesic	Meperidine (Demerol)	25–100 mg. IM, every 3–4 hours	Rapid	2–3	Minimal effect on contractions Relaxation may speed dilatation of cervix	Good analgesia; becomes most effective in 60–90 minutes; lasts 2–3 hours Side effects: facial flushing, dryness of mouth, decreased urinary output, diaphoresis, hypotension, nausea and vomiting	May cause serious respiratory depression if given 2–3 hours before delivery Minimal respiratory depression if given less than 1 hour before delivery
	Morphine sulfate	8–15 mg. IM	Rapid	3–4	Varies: may weaken or stop contractions May lead to more efficient contractions in irritable uterus	CNS depressant Mother lethargic and sleepy Side effects: facial flushing, dryness of mouth	May cause serious respiratory distress Peak action 1.5 hours after IM administration Administration within 3 hours of birth dangerous

Type	Agent	Dosage	Onset*	Duration (hrs)	Effect on labor	Side effects	Respiratory/fetal effects
Inhalant	Alphaprodine (Nisentil)	20–40 mg. IM, IV		1½–2	No apparent effect on labor	Side effects: euphoria, sedation, dizziness, nausea	Respiratory depression
	Self-administered by hand-held mask: Methoxyflurane (Penthrane), Trichloroethylene (Trilene)		Rapid			Analgesia during first stage of labor (may be used for analgesia or anesthesia during second stage). Too much Penthrane can cause maternal hypotension; slow and/or shallow respirations; too much Trilene can cause irregular pulse and rapid respirations; patient may experience numbness and/or dizziness.	Possible hypoxia. Possible CNS depression
Regional anesthetic	Paracervical block, Pudendal block	10 ml. on each side			Not predictable	Almost immediate relief (3–5 minutes) of pain of approximately 1–2 hours' duration; may need to be repeated	Fetal bradycardia in 20–30 per cent; in 5 per cent, bradycardia below 100
	Mepivacaine (Carbocaine), Lidocaine (Xylocaine), Bupivacaine (Marcaine)		Slower than lidocaine, mepivacaine		Some labors appear shortened; some appear inhibited	Transient numbness of lower extremities, maternal tachycardia, dizziness, euphoria, anxiety, hypotension reported	Bupivacaine metabolizes most quickly
Conduction anesthetic	Caudal, Epidural, Procaine (Novocain)			Short	May slow labor if given too early or in too large a dose (obliterates bearing down reflex in second stage)	Begins to relieve pain in 5–10 minutes; effects last 45–60 minutes. Potential hypotension; nausea, pallor, lightheadedness, abnormal vital signs are indications	Hypotension may lead to fetal hypoxia. Behavioral differences in newborn in first days following delivery; vary with drug
	Dibucaine (Nupercaine)			Long			
	Lidocaine (Xylocaine)			Intermediate			
	Tetracaine (Pontocaine)			Long			
	Mepivacaine (Carbocaine), Bupivacaine (Marcaine)			Intermediate			

*Rapid: <2 minutes IV; <5 minutes IM

Table 17–5. GASES USED IN OBSTETRIC ANESTHESIA

Gas	Advantages	Disadvantages
Ether	Good muscle relaxation Does not interact with oxytocics Wide margin of safety	Flammable Takes effect slowly Causes nausea and vomiting Irritates respiratory tract
Methoxyflurane (Penthrane)	Nonflammable Nonirritating to respiratory tract	Too high a level leads to: 1. maternal hypotension 2. infant respiratory depression 3. maternal renal failure
Nitrous oxide (N_2O) and oxygen	Light anesthesia 25 per cent N_2O can be eliminated from baby by ventilation after birth	High concentrations (above 75 per cent N_2O) compromise oxygenation
Cyclopropane	Used chiefly in operative delivery	Highly explosive; not used intermittently for this reason

the time of delivery. These drugs should not be given 2 to 3 hours prior to delivery. The danger is particularly great in preterm delivery. Demerol given intramuscularly (IM) within an hour of delivery does not appear to affect the initiation of breathing, but many clinicians avoid Demerol at this time.

As little as 50 mg. of Demerol has been demonstrated to affect the infant's behavior during the first days of life, which in turn may affect interaction between parent and infant.

Naloxone hydrochloride (Narcan), 0.01 mg. per kg. of baby's weight, is the narcotic antagonist currently used to mitigate depression from narcotics. Given IM it begins to be effective in 2 to 3 minutes, acting by competing with the narcotic at binding sites. When naloxone is given, nurses who care for the baby following delivery must be informed; as the drug is metabolized, the baby may again become depressed.

The narcotic antagonists formerly used, nalorphine (Nalline) and levallorphan tartrate (Lorfan), reversed narcotic-induced respiratory depression in many instances but contributed to respiratory depression from other causes.

Nursing Support. Continuing assessment of both mother and fetus and reduction of environmental stimuli as described above are major areas of nursing support.

Self-Administered Inhalant Analgesia

Methoxyflurane (Penthrane) and trichloroethylene (Trilene) are administered as analgesics during the first stage of labor via a mask that the mother holds in her hand.

Disadvantages. These medications are potent anesthetics; they are sometimes given for anesthesia during the second stage of labor. For this reason, no one but the mother must hold the mask (see Nursing Support, below). Too much Penthrane can cause maternal hypotension and slow, shallow respirations. Too much Trilene can cause an irregular pulse and rapid respirations. Potential problems for the fetus or infant are hypoxia and central nervous system depression.

Nursing Support. A women receiving inhalation analgesia needs constant nursing supervision. As long as she holds the mask herself and does not prop the hand that is holding it, the mask will fall away if she loses consciousness. However, if anyone else holds the mask for her, she may become anesthetized. Vital signs are assessed frequently. Because Penthrane persists in the body between contractions, the dial on the inhaler may need to be adjusted downward after a period of use.

Any liquid remaining in the inhaler at the end of the day must be discarded; leftover medication may decompose.

Regional Anesthesia: Paracervical Nerve Block

A paracervical nerve block involves the administration of a local anesthetic into the pelvic plexus, those nerves located in the paracervical tissue that supply the uterus, vagina, bladder, and rectum. Five to 10 ml. of solution is injected on each side, at 3 o'clock and 9 o'clock or at 4 o'clock and 8 o'clock (Fig. 17–11). Because the pudendal nerve is not blocked, the perineum is not anesthetized.

Paracervical blocking is usual at from 4 to

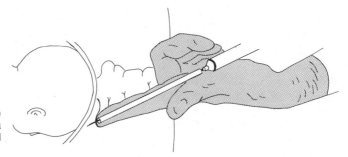

Figure 17–11. Paracervical nerve block. The needle is introduced through a guide in the vagina into the mucosa for 6 to 12 mm. If there is no blood return, anesthetic solution in injected.

6 cm. cervical dilatation. Relief of pain is almost immediate and lasts from 1 to 2 hours. When the block ceases to be effective, the return of pain is rapid. Depending on the progress of labor, the paracervical block may be repeated. When the fetal head reaches station +2 and when cervical dilatation reaches 8 cm., paracervical blocking becomes technically more difficult.

Disadvantages. Paracervical blocking is used only when the fetus is assessed to be healthy. In approximately 20 to 30 per cent of patients, there is transient fetal bradycardia; in 5 per cent the fetal heart rate drops below 100, possibly due to the depressant effect of the local anesthetic on the fetal myocardium. A paracervical block is not administered if delivery is expected within 30 minutes.

The effect on labor varies; labor appears to be inhibited in some women, while in others it appears to be shortened.

Maternal reactions may include hypotension, numbness of the lower extremities, tachycardia, dizziness, and euphoria.

Nursing Support. Fetal heart rate must be monitored very closely until it is stable; a fetal heart rate monitor is important if bradycardia is noted.

The mother's reaction to the anesthetic is also evaluated frequently.

Regional Anesthesia: Pudendal Nerve Block

A pudendal nerve block involves the administration of a local anesthetic into the pudendal nerves on the right and left of the perineum (Figs. 17–12 and 17–13). The pudendal block anesthetizes only the perineum, relaxing perineal muscles and anesthetizing the area for episiotomy, delivery, and episiotomy repair. The pudendal nerve is blocked after dilatation is complete; the mother will usually be positioned for delivery. The mother can expect to feel pressure during the delivery even though she does not feel pain. Occasionally, a pudendal block fails to give relief of pain.

Disadvantages. Unless medication is injected into the pudendal artery by mistake, pudendal nerve block is safe for both mother and infant.

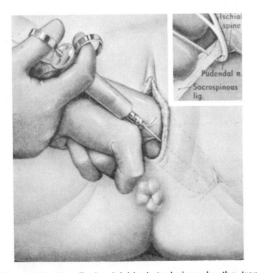

Figure 17–12. Pudendal block technique by the transvaginal approach, showing relationship of pudendal nerve to the ischial spine and sacrospinous ligament (inset) and the method by which the needle is guided by the fingers in the vagina and advanced through the sacrospinous ligament to block the nerve. (From Bonica: *Principles and Practice of Obstetrical Analgesia and Anesthesia.* Philadelphia, F. A. Davis Co., 1967.)

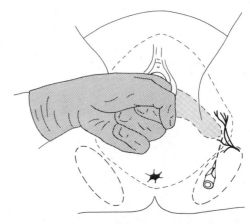

Figure 17–13. Blocking the pudendal nerve through the perineum (percutaneous transperineal pudendal nerve block). (After Oxorn and Foote: *Human Labor and Birth,* 3rd Edition. Englewood Cliffs, N.J., Appleton-Century-Crofts, 1975.)

Nursing Support. Because the mother is usually draped for delivery at the time that the pudendal nerve is blocked, she may be anxious about what she cannot see. The idea of a needle through the perineum or vagina is not necessarily reassuring. We should explain how the injection will help and how she will feel. There may be some discomfort as the medication is injected; this will be brief.

Fetal heart rate and maternal vital signs are monitored each minute for 15 minutes following pudendal nerve block and then every 5 minutes until stable.

Peridural Anesthesia: Caudal and Lumbar Epidural

Peridural anesthesia involves the injection of an anesthetic into the extradural space. The anesthetic *does not* penetrate the dura or the spinal cord. There is no "spinal headache" because the basis of such headaches is the leaking of cerebrospinal fluid through the puncture hole in the dura. Only if the dura is accidentally penetrated should there be a problem of headache after peridural infiltration.

Peridural anesthesia may be administered into the caudal space within the sacrum or into the epidural space at the second, third, or fourth lumbar interspace (Fig. 17–14). A single injection may be made, or, frequently, a catheter may be threaded through the needle into the space to allow a continuous injection of medicine over a period of hours for anesthesia during both labor and delivery. Lumbar epidural anesthesia is the type most frequently used in many areas of the United States today.

Anesthesia is achieved because nerves supplying both the uterus and the perineum pass through the peridural space and are anesthetized by the solution that has been injected. Loss of sensation occurs in 5 to 30 minutes with caudal infiltration and in 5 to 10 minutes with epidural infiltration. Vasodilatation of the legs, which the mother reports as a "warm feeling," is usually the first sign that the block is effective. Anesthesia is effective for 45 minutes to an hour.

Caudal anesthesia is ineffective in about 15 per cent of the women to whom it is administered; the failure rate for lumbar epidural anesthesia is approximately 1.5 to 2 per cent.

Disadvantages. Started too early, peridural anesthesia may slow the course of labor; administration is therefore delayed until the cervix is more than 4 cm. dilated.

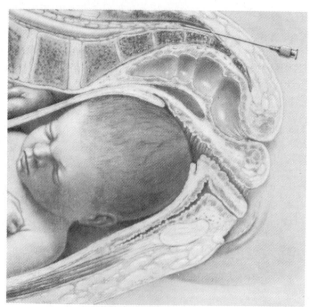

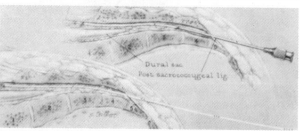

Figure 17–14. Continuous caudal block anesthesia technique, showing needle in sacral canal (top), with plastic catheter threaded through it (middle) and with needle withdrawn (bottom), leaving the catheter in place for purposes of administering anesthetic solution. (From Bonica: *Principles and Practice of Obstetrical Analgesia and Anesthesia.* Philadelphia, F. A. Davis Co., 1967.)

The major disadvantage is the possibility of severe maternal hypotension and resultant decreased blood flow to the fetus. Hypotension occurs because the interruption of sympathetic vasomotor innervation leads to decreased peripheral resistance and a decrease in venous return to the heart. Schifrin[26a] found that nearly 25 per cent of women who were given peridural anesthesia showed fetal heart rate patterns characteristic of uteroplacental insufficiency. The incidence of decreased uterine blood flow rose to 72 per cent when the woman was hypotensive. Because of this, constant monitoring of both the mother's vital signs and the fetal heart rate (preferably with a continuous fetal heart rate monitor) is essential.

The obliteration of both uterine and perineal sensations means that the mother does not have a desire to push during the second stage. The second stage may be lengthened, and forceps may be required for delivery. Coaching can alert her to the presence of a contraction and can encourage her to push at the most effective time.

Conduction anesthesia (both peridural and spinal, to be described below) interferes with the ability of the woman to void; frequent bladder observation and sometimes catheterization are necessary.

Infection is a potential hazard in any injection. Peridural anesthesia is not attempted if there is any evidence of infection at the puncture site. Excellent aseptic technique is essential in handling all equipment used for the injection of medication. Once contracted, infections of the epidural space are difficult to combat.

Nursing Support. Before the injection occurs, the mother needs to know how she will feel—her legs will feel weak and may shake briefly. This loss of control is frightening to some mothers if it is not anticipated.

It has already been emphasized that a nurse must remain with the mother to monitor her closely. If she complains of a metallic taste in her mouth, of dizziness or ringing in her ears, or appears confused or excited, it is possible that the anesthetic has entered the circulatory system through the epidural vessels.

Signs of hypotension that require immediate intervention include dizziness, pallor, nausea, and a change in vital signs in the mother and late decelerations (see below) in the fetus. Turn the mother to her left side and provide intravenous fluids and oxygen.

Following delivery, the mother who has had peridural anesthesia may be dizzy the first time she sits up in bed. She should be prepared for this feeling so that she will not try to get up when she is alone.

Spinal Anesthesia

With the exception of low spinal anesthesia (see Saddle Block, below), spinal anesthesia is rarely used for vaginal delivery. Spinal infiltration is frequently used, however, for cesarean delivery. A local anesthetic is injected through the dura into the subarachnoid space at the level of the third or fourth lumbar interspace.

Disadvantages. As is true with other types of conduction anesthesia, hypotension is a potential problem. When hypotension occurs, uterine contractility is also diminished.

Because the dura is punctured, postspinal headache is possible. The mother will usually remain flat on her back for a period of time following delivery, a position that requires some planning in order to facilitate early interaction between the mother and baby.

Nursing Support. Nursing support is similar to that for a mother with an epidural anesthetic, in terms of hypotension.

Oxygen is given to the mother to maintain a good level of oxygenation at the level of the placenta. An intravenous infusion is started if intravenous medication should be necessary.

Saddle Block (Low Spinal Anesthesia)

Injection of medication into the conus of the dural sac anesthetizes the area that would come in contact with a saddle when riding a horse, hence the term "saddle block."

A saddle block is given only when delivery is imminent; anesthesia of the perineum lasts for approximately 1 hour.

Disadvantages. The mother must sit for the injection of medication when a saddle block is used so that the medication will gravitate downward. At a time just prior to delivery, when the saddle block is instituted, this is a most difficult position, requiring not only physical assistance but a great deal of emotional encouragement and support. The mother remains sitting for approximately 30 seconds following infiltration and then is placed on her back with her neck flexed.

A saddle block has no apparent effects on the mother or fetus except that the mother with a saddle block may occasionally have a postspinal headache.

Nursing Support. Nursing support for the mother with a saddle block is the same as for mothers with other types of conduction anesthesia (epidural, spinal).

The Effect of Local and Regional Anesthesia on the Newborn Infant's Behavior. Although it has been recognized that various modes of analgesia or anesthesia affect the newborn infant's respiration, less attention has been paid to other possible effects of anesthesia. Studies by Standley and associates[30] and by Scanlon and associates[26] have noted differences in behavior.

Standley's group evaluated 60 first-born, healthy infants, 48 to 72 hours old, born to white, middle class mothers who had medically uneventful pregnancies and deliveries. Mothers had received commonly used analgesics (chiefly Demerol with Phenergan or Vistaril); anesthetic agents such as lidocaine, tetracaine, or mepivacaine via saddle block (42 of the 52 women receiving anesthesia); pudendal block; paracervical block; and so forth. Babies of mothers receiving anesthesia demonstrated decreased motor maturity and greater irritability when tested.

Scanlon's group tested 41 newborn infants during the first 8 hours of life. The 28 infants whose mothers had received continuous lumbar epidural blocks showed significantly lower scores on tests of muscle strength and tone and less vigorous rooting behavior (but no differences in sucking behavior).

Because the baby's early behavior is felt to be a significant factor in the early relationship between parents and infants (Chapter 20), this difference may prove to be an important one. It is also necessary to discover if there are differences at later periods, 1 week or 1 month, for example. Techniques for behavioral assessment (Chapter 21) have increased our capability of evaluating the effect of anesthesia on the newborn infant.

General Inhalation Anesthesia

General anesthesia is infrequently used for uncomplicated vaginal delivery today; the most common use is in an acute obstetric emergency.

Much of the care given to all mothers during labor is directed toward the possibility that the mother may require a general inhalation anesthetic. She is allowed nothing by mouth (NPO), to prevent possible vomiting and aspiration. Antacids are frequently given so that if she does vomit and aspirate, the aspirate will be less acid. Nurses in the United States do not always realize that the practice of keeping women NPO during labor is by no means universal.

When inhalants are given to produce anesthesia (rather than analgesia), tracheal intubation is essential (below). Suction apparatus must be available and an intravenous infusion running.

One of several gases may be used. Each has specific advantages and disadvantages (Table 17–5).

Nursing Support. As with any patient who receives general anesthesia, vomiting is a danger for the mother in labor. She also presents special problems:

1. Unlike the surgical patient, she may have eaten a large meal shortly before she came to the hospital.

2. Stomach emptying is delayed during labor and may cease entirely. Thus, even if several hours have elapsed since she last ate, the potential for aspiration is still present.

Both during and after delivery, the woman who receives general anesthesia must be protected from aspiration.

In addition, the nursing assessment and support given to all patients who receive general anesthesia is also important for the mother.

A major disadvantage of general anesthesia is the barrier it raises to early maternal–infant interaction, as discussed below.

Transcutaneous Electrical Nerve Stimulation

Transcutaneous electrical nerve stimulation (TNS) has been described since the time of Socrates, but only recently has this technique been used to manage clinical pain in a large number of acute and chronic conditions.[32] Use of TNS in obstetrics is still rare in comparison with other techniques but appears to be free of complications.[2]

The physiologic basis of the efficacy of TNS is derived from the spinal gate-control hypothesis of Melzack-Wall. Electrical stimulation of non-nociceptive afferent fibers attempts to modify nociceptive afferent input from the pain stimuli.

Augustinsson[2] describes the use of TNS for obstetrical pain relief in 147 women. Two pairs of electrodes were taped to the gravida's back at levels corresponding to the afferent pathways for pain to the spinal cord, Th_{10}–L_1 during the first stage and S_2–S_4 during the second stage (Fig. 17–15). Low intensity stimulation was given continuously; the mother could initiate high intensity stimulation when she felt it necessary. During the second stage, sacral stimulation was usually given at high intensity at all times, and 98 patients received pudendal blocks in addition. Four patients had epidural block anesthesia. TNS was helpful in back pain, a finding also reported by Shealy and Maurer.[28] Of the 147 women treated, 65 (44 per cent) considered pain relief by TNS to

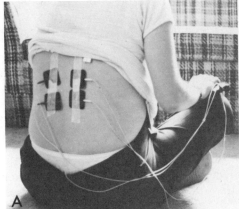
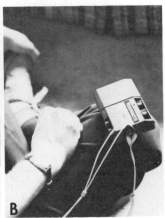

Figure 17–15. *A,* The electrodes from the transcutaneous electrical nerve stimulator (TNS) are taped to the gravida's back at T_{10} to L_1 during the first stage of labor. *B,* The gravida is able to control the intensity of stimulation by adjusting the control mechanism.

be good to very good, 65 (44 per cent) experienced a moderate effect, and 17 (12 per cent) considered TNS to have no effect. No complications occurred.

Hypnosis

Women who have been prepared to use hypnosis in labor may enter a state of deep relaxation in response to a cue from the hypnotist. The woman will not be unconscious, but she should be disturbed as little as possible. She will probably be numb from her abdomen to her knees. Hypnosis does not relieve all discomfort in all hypnotized women, but it usually lessens or eliminates the need for medication. Because hypnotism is not a shared experience between a woman and her husband, it has limited appeal for many women.

Nursing Support of the Husband or Coach

Labor is hard work for the parturient; it is also hard work for her husband or whoever supports her during labor. The more nurses can facilitate that support, the better the childbearing experience for both persons. (Because the birth companion will not always be a husband, we will refer to that person as a coach in this discussion.)

Coaches, like mothers, frequently work hard during labor. They may rub the mother's back, apply counterpressure, bathe her face, breathe with her, encourage her verbally, and so on. As contractions become more frequent, the coach may be busy every minute. While the mother is resting between contractions, her coach may be rinsing out a washcloth.

A nurse may suggest that the coach have a bathroom and refreshment break periodically, assuring him that the mother will not be left alone. Depending on the length of labor, a break at least every 2 hours is advisable.

Before transition approaches, a final rest period will give him energy for transition and the second stage.

Just as coaches reassure mothers that they are doing well, nurses can reassure both. Frequently, this is a brand new experience for the coach, and he is just as anxious as the mother. In addition, helping the coach to use good body mechanics when he leans over to rub the mother's back or wipe her face will decrease his fatigue. Particularly during transition, when the mother may seem unappreciative and the coach must say and do the same things over and over again, the nurse's support is very important.

Coaches and mothers interact with varying degrees of closeness. Physical contact between them may be limited, moderate, or continual. Individual personality differences and social and cultural differences will affect the interaction during labor. Since interaction during labor and birth reflects, to a large extent, a couple's customary mode of interaction, nurses must be sensitive to the way they can support the needs of individual families rather than expect a family to conform to an idealized image of a couple in labor.

Rarely, a coach will appear to be affecting a mother in a negative way; this is a difficult situation for the nursing staff and must be considered on an individual basis. At times the presence of the coach may be important to the mother even if we perceive the situation as less than desirable.

Emergency Delivery by the Nurse

Occasionally, a nurse finds herself caring for a mother for whom delivery is imminent, but there is no nurse-midwife or physician available. The mother may be in the hospital, but labor has progressed so rapidly that no one is prepared. Or she may be at home or in a public place.

It is not surprising that the mother and whoever is with her may be anxious to the point of near panic. We may feel equally anxious, but a major task for us is to assure her that most mothers can birth their babies with a minimum of difficulty. Nurse and parents work as a team with continuing communication.

The strict asepsis of the delivery room may not be possible outside of the hospital, but clean hands and a clean delivery area, covered with newspapers or clean linen of some type (towels, sheets), are usually possible.

1. The head will probably be crowning; encourage the mother to pant and *gently* control the progress of the head, particularly at the height of the contraction. Do not attempt to hold the head back. If possible, the head should be delivered between contractions to protect the baby's brain and the mother's perineum.

2. If the membranes have not ruptured when the head is delivered, rupture them immediately so the infant will not aspirate amniotic fluid when he breathes.

3. As the head is delivered, support it with one hand while you wipe away any blood or mucus on the face with the other.

4. In approximately 25 per cent of deliveries, one or more loops of cord are around the baby's neck. As soon as the head is delivered, feel around the neck to see if there are any loops of cord. A cord loosely wrapped about the neck may be slipped over the baby's head. If it is wrapped tightly, it will have to be clamped in two places and cut.

5. At the next contraction, help direct the anterior shoulder under the symphysis pubis with very gentle downward pressure on the side of the head. Supporting the baby, allow the birth of the posterior shoulder. The remainder of the body will follow easily.

6. Hold the baby so that the mucus will drain from his respiratory tract. Be sure there is no traction on the cord. The baby should cry; gently rubbing his back will help to stimulate that cry.

7. Dry the baby and place him on his mother's abdomen. Both of these acts help to keep him warm, which is vital (Chapter 20). He should be covered and positioned so that his head is dependent to facilitate further drainage of mucus.

8. The cord need not be cut right away. Cutting the cord with a dirty instrument is never the proper procedure. This is obviously not a problem if the emergency delivery occurs in a labor room or somewhere else in the hospital but could be a major problem in a car

or a shopping center. Once the cord has stopped pulsating, it can be tied but left intact until the mother and baby can be taken to a hospital or until sterile equipment is available.

9. When it is apparent that the placenta has separated, ask the mother to bear down with the next contraction to deliver the placenta.

10. Putting the baby to breast following the delivery of the placenta stimulates the production of oxytocin, which in turn causes uterine contraction and prevents postpartum hemorrhage. As with all mothers, watch closely for postpartum hemorrhage. Massage the fundus if the uterus relaxes.

11. If the mother is not in the hospital, she and the baby should be transported to a hospital for further evaluation and care.

Planned Home Delivery

Home delivery is discussed in Chapter 16. A nurse who is participating in a planned home delivery (as opposed to an emergency home delivery) must be aware of the legal implications in her particular state.

In a planned home delivery, sterile equipment will usually have been prepared. Some plan in the event of an emergency for either the mother or the baby should be decided upon well in advance of the time of delivery.

The Experience of Labor and Birth

Every labor, every birth, is unique. This should not be surprising. Every mother and every newborn is different from every other. The following accounts of labors are written by women in their own words.

My first contraction came at 5:00 A.M.; it woke me. My water must have broken simultaneously. The bed was wet. My husband said, "It's time" because blood had come with the water. I had my second contraction 5 minutes later and the third 3 minutes later. My husband called the doctor, who responded, "Bring her on in." The next contractions were from 1 to 2 minutes apart. Thank goodness, we lived near the hospital. My goody bag and suitcase had been packed for weeks. My husband had to take me down the steps and put me in the car. When we got to the hospital (5:30 A.M.) I couldn't walk. He brought the wheelchair to the car. After a vaginal check the nurse told me, "Mrs. C., you're fully dilated. We're just waiting for the doctor . . . along with . . . don't push, don't push." What would I have done if I didn't know how to breathe. (6:10 A.M.). The doctor arrived. My husband, who had been with me all the time (excluding registration), dressed along with the doctor, as they rolled me down the hall. It was a quick prep. I wanted to push so bad that I'd forget to breathe. My husband reminded me. At 6:20 A.M. my 6 pound, 8 ounce baby girl was born with 10 fingers, 10 toes, and strong lungs.

About 4:00 A.M. I started feeling some strong period cramps and then the membrane plug broke (about 6:00 A.M.). Then some very intense contractions started, but they were so inconsistent that we were not sure about going to the hospital, and then about 9:00 A.M. we decided that something was odd, so we left for the hospital about 9:50. When Dr. B. checked me I was already at 7 [cm.]. They started my IV and shaved me, and we were going to the labor [room] (where my husband was waiting), when my water broke, and the baby's head was right there. I never got the epidural, and I went from 7 to 10 [cm.] in 25 minutes, so they hurried me to the delivery room. They told my husband to get his greens on, and while he was dressing she was born. It was so fast that they couldn't wait for my husband to finish dressing. They had just enough time to make the episiotomy and she was here. I went all natural, and I'm very glad. My husband came in just after, so he got to weigh her and all the other stuff. We really enjoyed these moments together.

Well, we had a girl—6 pounds, 14 ounces, 20 inches, and she's beautiful.

Very long preliminary labor started 2:00 A.M. Friday. Went to clinic at 10:00 A.M. The doctor said I was 3 cm. dilated and to go on to the hospital after a while. I waited all day at a friend's house. The contractions continued to come at 5- to 8-minute intervals, though somewhat closer together when I walked around.

We finally decided to go to the hospital at around 6:00 P.M. I was checked at 2 cm. less than that morning. Well, I should have known then what to expect. As time went on, I was checked at 5 cm., then 3 cm., then 7 cm., then 5 cm. A bit discouraging, to say the least!

Saturday morning, after nothing much had changed, and after a bit of sleep induced by a shot of morphine and a Seconol, Dr. F. suggested using Pitocin to speed things up. They regulated my contractions to 2½ to 3 minutes apart; they were stronger, but the *real* change came when sometime during the afternoon the doctor broke my water, and they installed an interior fetal monitor.

I might say at this point that the best position for me during all but transition was sitting cross-legged. My husband rubbed my back—the nurses kept wanting me to try lying on my side, but it hurt my back too much.

During transition I began to be tired and didn't think I could make it—I didn't recognize the stage. It had taken me so long, I guess I didn't dare hope the end was in sight. Finally, they said I could push even though there was still a rim on my cervix. Well, within 3 or 4 pushes, the baby's head was visible! The doctor had been told when they said I

could push, but he didn't come until 20 or so minutes after the baby's head was visible. I had a hard time waiting—ended up going from the birthing room into the delivery room, so that I could get some nitrous oxide. It was easier to wait then but after 10 minutes or so I just didn't care what anyone said, I was going to have that baby then and there!

So they got a resident to come to deliver the baby, but just as he was getting ready to do the episiotomy, my doctor walked in to do it. The baby was delivered post-haste; I remember looking at him lying on the table getting his eyedrops.

My husband was *very* supportive during the entire labor and delivery. He only had one queasy moment when he saw the doctor start the episiotomy. The nurses took care of him, though, and after 30 seconds or so he was fine.

We are glad we attended Lamaze classes and will use psychoprophylaxis in the future if we have another child. Thank you!

My labor began about 3:30 A.M. May 4. My contractions were bearable at approximately 7 minutes apart. I stayed at home until around 5:15 A.M., when they narrowed down to 5 minutes. I arrived at the hospital at 5:40 A.M. My contractions drifted back to 10 minutes apart and stayed that way until around 11:00 A.M. The contractions began getting stronger and closer, but dilatation was not progressing. Pitocin was used after the membranes were ruptured around lunchtime. This brought the baby down. Our baby was very large and posterior, and this made labor much longer and difficult. After the baby began to crown he rotated on his own. Delivery occurred at 3:13 P.M. He was a forceps delivery, weighing in at 9 pounds, 13½ ounces. He was 22 inches long, head 14½ inches, chest 14½ inches. Labor was 12 hours long.

Contractions began at 5:00 A.M., Wednesday, September 10, and were 5 minutes apart by 10:30 A.M. Went to hospital when I was 3 cm. dilated. Labored all day. At 5:30 P.M. still only 3 to 4 cm. dilated. Frustrating! Slow breathing O.K. all day—5 minutes apart—until 5:30, when I vomited. After that, contractions picked up—2 minutes apart. At this point, Ah-hees not helpful, but blowing out was— "Blow contraction away." Contractions painful and very hard to relax. Decided at 8 cm. to have epidural for relief (at 8:30 P.M.). I wanted to *enjoy* the delivery and felt I was at the point of not even thinking about the baby. Let epidural wear off so I could feel to push. Pushed beginning at 11:00 P.M. (was catheterized first). Went to delivery room around midnight. The doctor asked if I wanted help pushing or wanted to have forceps—wanted to push. K. was born 12:10 A.M. Thursday (had episiotomy). I bled a lot during labor, so they did a sonogram to be sure it wasn't placenta previa; decided it probably was a lacerated cervix.

The day of delivery I felt tired but had a desire to want to clean house and get groceries. I started spotting about 2:30 P.M. and felt pressure but no pain. About 6:00 P.M. I started feeling a cramp in my lower stomach. It would be about 5 minutes apart for two or three times, then about 15 or 20 minutes apart. Very irregular. Left for hospital about 8:30 P.M. Pains getting more regular, about 5 minutes apart all the time. Checked in at hospital. Starting using slow breathing about 10:30 (didn't need any breathing methods before this time; pain not that severe). Used slow breathing method all through delivery. Water broke about 12 midnight. Used blowing method to help keep from pushing, and slow breathing. Baby born at 12:44 A.M. It was a very exciting and rewarding experience for me and my husband.

When she was born she was very alert and seemed very aware of what was going on.

The doctors said I had a meconium stain, but it didn't affect the baby at all.

Summary

The number of hours of contact between parents and nurse during labor may be equal to or greater than the number of hours of contact during the entire prenatal period.

Nurses have much to offer families during these hours. By our careful assessment of the mother and fetus or infant, by planning and intervention that provides physical and emotional comfort and support, and by continuing evaluation of the care we give, we do provide the significant difference in childbearing for parents and their babies.

REFERENCES

1. Aldrich, A., and Watson, P.: Analysis of End-Results of Labor in Primiparas After Spontaneous Versus Prophylactic Methods of Delivery. *American Journal of Obstetrics and Gynecology, 30*:554, 1935.
2. Augustinsson, L., Bohlen, P., Bundsen, P., et al.: Pain Relief During Delivery by Transcutaneous Electrical Nerve Stimulation. *Pain, 4*:59, 1977.
3. Barnes, A.: Prophylaxis in Labor and Delivery. *New England Journal of Medicine, 294*:1235, 1976.
4. Beynon, C.: Midline Episiotomy as a Routine Procedure. *Journal of Obstetrics and Gynecology of the British Commonwealth, 81*:126, 1974.
5. Bing, E.: *Six Practical Lessons for an Easier Childbirth.* New York, Bantam Books, 1969.
6. Caldeyro-Barcia, R., Noriega-Guerra, L., Cibils, L., et al.: Effect of Position Changes on the Intensity and Frequency of Uterine Contractions During Labor. *American Journal of Obstetrics and Gynecology, 80*:285, 1960.
7. Caldeyro-Barcia, R.: *Intrapartum Fetal Monitoring.* Presentation at the 2nd Memorial Ignatz Semmelweis Seminar, Cherry Hill, New Jersey, September, 1976.
8. Caldeyro-Barcia, R.: *Physiological and Psychological Bases for the Modern and Humanized Management of Normal Labor.* Lecture presented at International Year of the Child Commemorative International Congress, Tokyo, October, 1979.
9. Chabon, I.: *Awake and Aware.* New York, Dell Publishing Company, 1966.
10. Cogan, R., and Edmunds, E.: The Unkindest Cut? *Contemporary Ob/Gyn, 9*, 1977.
11. Eiger, M., and Olds, S.: *The Complete Book of Breastfeeding.* New York, Bantam Books, 1973.
12. Ericson, A.: *Medications Used During Labor and Birth.* Minneapolis, International Childbirth Education Association, 1977.
13. Ewy, E., and Ewy, G.: *Preparation for Childbirth.* New York, New American Library, 1972.
14. Grad, R. K., and Woodside, J.: Obstetrical Analgesics and Anesthesia: Methods of Relief for the Patient in Labor. *American Journal of Nursing, 77*:242, 1977.
15. Greenhill, J., and Friedman, E.: *Biological Principles and Modern Practice of Obstetrics.* Philadelphia, W. B. Saunders Co., 1974.
16. Harris, R.: An Evaluation of the Median Episiotomy. *American Journal of Obstetrics and Gynecology, 106*:660, 1970.

17. Huprich, P.: Assisting the Couple Through a Lamaze Labor and Delivery. *MCN, 2*:245, 1977.
18. Karmel, M.: *Thank You, Dr. Lamaze.* Philadelphia, J. B. Lippincott Co., 1959.
19. Lamaze, F.: *Painless Childbirth: The Lamaze Method.* New York, Pocket Books, 1972.
20. Leboyer, F.: *Birth Without Violence.* New York, Knopf-Random House, 1975.
21. Melzack, R., and Wall, P.: Pain Mechanism: A New Theory. *Science, 150*:971, 1965.
22. Miller, F. C., Petrue, R. H., Arce, J., et al.: Hyperventilation During Labor. *American Journal of Obstetrics and Gynecology, 120*:489, 1974.
23. Nugent, F.: The Primiparous Perineum After Forceps Delivery: A Follow-up Comparison of Results with and without Episiotomy. *American Journal of Obstetrics and Gynecology, 30*:249, 1935.
24. O'Leary, J., and Erez, S.: Hyaluronidase as an Adjuvant to Episiotomy. *Obstetrics and Gynecology, 26*:66, 1965.
25. Page, E., Villee, C., and Villee, D.: *Human Reproduction. The Core Content of Obstetrics, Gynecology and Perinatal Medicine.* 2nd Edition. Philadelphia, W. B. Saunders Co., 1981.
26. Scanlon, J., Brown, W., Weiss, J., et al.: Neurobehavioral Responses of Newborn Infants After Maternal Epidural Anesthesia. *Anesthesiology, 40*:121, 1974.
26a. Schifrin, B.: Fetal Heart Rate Monitoring During Labor. *Journal of the American Medical Association, 221*:992, 1972.
27. Scott, J. R., and Rose, N. B.: The Effect of Lamaze Preparation on Labor and Delivery. *New England Journal of Medicine, 294*:1205, 1976.
28. Shealy, C., and Maurer, D.: Transcutaneous Nerve Stimulation for the Control of Pain. *Surgical Neurology, 2*:45, 1974.
29. Standley, K., and Nicholson, J.: Observing the Childbirth Environment: A Research Model. *Birth and the Family Journal, 7*(1):15, 1980.
30. Standley, K., Soule, A., Copano, S., et al.: Local-Regional Anesthesia during Childbirth: Effect on Newborn Behaviors. *Science, 186*:634, 1974.
31. Varney, H.: *Nurse-Midwifery.* Boston, Blackwell Scientific Publications, 1980.
32. Woolf, C.: Transcutaneous Electrical Nerve Stimulation and the Reaction to Experimental Pain in Human Subjects. *Pain, 7*:115, 1979.

18

Electronic Fetal Heart Rate Monitoring

OBJECTIVES

1. Define:
   a. baseline fetal heart rate
   b. baseline fetal heart rate variability
   c. beat-to-beat variability
   d. fetal tachycardia
   e. fetal bradycardia
   f. early deceleration
   g. late deceleration
   h. variable deceleration
   i. prolonged deceleration
   j. tachysystole
   k. tetanic contraction
   l. basal tone
   m. waveform
2. Describe various ways of monitoring fetal heart rate and uterine contractions, indicating advantages and disadvantages of each.
3. Describe the significance of acceleration and deceleration patterns; indicate the nursing action appropriate to each.
4. Relate information obtained from electronic fetal heart rate monitoring to the physiology of fetal heart rate changes described in Chapter 15.
5. Identify possible relationships between medications given to the mother during labor and birth and fetal monitor tracings.
6. Describe the purpose and process of fetal scalp sampling.
7. Describe ways in which nurses can support mothers during electronic fetal monitoring.
8. Identify information that should be recorded on the monitoring strip.
9. Identify and discuss controversial issues related to electronic fetal monitoring.

Electronic fetal heart rate monitoring is used in from 60 to 70 per cent of all labors today. The incidence of electronic fetal monitoring varies with the birthing environment; the greatest use occurs in traditional labor/delivery units.

Initially, intrapartum fetal heart rate monitoring was a technique reserved for women considered at high risk for fetal distress during labor. A major impetus for the increased use of monitoring has been a strong desire to decrease perinatal mortality and morbidity, coupled with the recognition that some women who are at low risk during the prenatal period develop high risk conditions during the course of labor.

The controversy surrounding fetal heart rate monitoring centers on its use in low risk mothers. Few argue with the need and value of monitoring in mothers with maternal, placental, or fetal factors that have been identified as risks. Some professionals, both nurses and physicians, feel that it is desirable to monitor every mother during labor. Others feel that although monitoring offers obvious advantages for certain mothers—those who have recognized high risk conditions, those who show evidence of fetal distress, and perhaps all those who are primigravidas—there is no need to monitor all mothers.

For although the advantages of monitoring are obvious (the nurse or physician is continually aware of the pattern of fetal heart rate and uterine contractions, and thus variations from normal are readily recognized), there also are potential disadvantages (see Areas of Controversy, below).

For some couples, and for some nurses, the *idea* of fetal monitoring conflicts with the idea of birth as a natural process.

Dulock and Herron[7] interviewed 71 women (36 primigravidas and 35 multiparas) concerning their knowledge of and attitudes toward fetal monitoring. In their group, only 21 per cent of the women came to labor without a prior knowledge of monitoring. Childbirth classes were the source of information for 38 per cent, the prenatal clinic for 14 per cent, and an antenatal tour of the maternity unit for 11 per cent. Previous labor experience, friends, or the media were the resource for 16 per cent. Thus for 63 per cent, health professionals were the source of information, underscoring the importance of our own attitude in the formation of mothers' attitudes.

The authors then asked the women about their initial feelings concerning monitoring, both before and after an explanation was

Table 18–1. PREDELIVERY REACTIONS TO FHR MONITORING AMONG 71 WOMEN BEFORE AND AFTER EXPLANATION OF MONITORING*

	Before		After	
	No.	**%**	**No.**	**%**
Curious	28	39	15	21
Fearful	14	20	10	14
Secure	6	8	23	32
Intrusive	3	5	3	5
Impersonal	2	3	1	2
No response	18	25	19	26

*Dulock and Herron: *JOGN*, 5 (Suppl.) 69s, September–October, 1976.

given. Their results are summarized in Table 18–1.

Thirty-one of the 71 women initially interviewed by Dulock and Herron were monitored during delivery and were subsequently interviewed on the second or third postpartum day. Seventy-seven per cent (24 women) made some positive comments. Monitoring was helpful to these women in:

1. Anticipating a contraction and thus beginning controlled breathing and relaxation techniques early.

2. Knowing when the peak of the contraction had passed.

3. Coordinating "pushing" with the peak of the contraction during the second stage.

4. Feeling secure that the baby's heart was beating.

5. Feeling that should something "go wrong" it would be noted immediately.

Seventy per cent (22) of the 31 women made some negative comments (obviously most women had some positive and some negative feelings). Negative comments centered on:

1. The discomfort and immobility of external belts.

2. The discomfort and feeling of "invasion" in the insertion of the internal monitor.

Total postdelivery response was reported as positive by 85 per cent; of these same 31 women, only 39 per cent had felt positively about monitoring before delivery. The common experience of the women who felt neutral about monitoring following delivery was a long, difficult labor or an unexpected cesarean delivery. No woman in this group reported feeling negative about monitoring following delivery (Table 18–2).

Although we cannot generalize on the basis of such a small sample, this study both points the way for future studies and suggests that:

Table 18–2. COMPARISON OF BASIC ATTITUDES TOWARD MONITORING PRE- AND POSTDELIVERY AMONG 31 WOMEN WHOSE LABORS WERE MONITORED*

	Predelivery		Postdelivery	
	No.	**%**	**No.**	**%**
Positive	12	39	26	85
Neutral	9	29	5	15
Negative	3	10	0	0
No comment	7	22	0	0

*Dulock and Herron: *JOGN*, 5 (Suppl.) 70s, September–October, 1976.

1. The nurse's own attitudes are important.
2. Explanations are important.
3. The mother's attitudes following delivery are more positive than their attitudes prior to delivery.

Nursing Support During Continuous (Electronic) Fetal Monitoring

Ideal nursing support for mothers who are to be monitored begins in the prenatal period with discussion of the use of monitors and, if possible, the opportunity to see and touch the monitor and perhaps see a demonstration of external monitoring.

When a mother enters a labor environment in which a monitor may be used, nurses need to assess her prior knowledge of the use of the electronic fetal monitor and then explain in simple terms the practice within that particular setting. Because practices vary from one setting to another, this explanation is particularly important (Nursing Care Plan 18–1). For example, if a mother believes that electronic fetal monitoring is used only when high risk conditions exist, but the facility in which she labors monitors all mothers initially as a screening procedure, the experience of monitoring could be unnecessarily frightening.

Physical care of the mother who is being monitored includes helping the mother find a comfortable position and helping her to change position as she desires. The skin under the belts and transducers of external monitors may become irritated. The external monitor should be moved frequently and the skin condition assessed. Powder or cornstarch under the belt (not the transducer) may alleviate irritation. The recent development of a monitoring system that allows the mother to be ambulatory or to assume a variety of positions should aid maternal comfort as well as allow her to assume positions advantageous to the course of labor (Chapter 15).

The insertion of the fetal scalp electrode in the internal monitoring system is of concern to many parents. Showing them the very small size of the electrode and explaining that it will be attached only to soft, loose tissue (not the baby's brain, as some parents fear) is frequently reassuring. Explain that the internal catheter (which measures uterine contractions) will be lying within the uterus next to the baby.

Mothers who must be monitored can make use of all of the positive aspects mentioned by Dulock and Herron (above). Although it is not usually as helpful for the mother to watch the monitor, her labor companion can note when a contraction is beginning and when the acme is past and thus help her to relax and cope with the contraction.

Methods of Continuous Fetal Monitoring

Four methods of continuous fetal heart rate monitoring are phonocardiogram, abdominal wall electrocardiogram, Doppler ultrasound, and scalp electrode (Table 18–3). The first three methods are indirect, i.e., the fetus is monitored through the abdominal wall. In the fourth method, an electrode is attached directly to the fetal scalp; this is possible only after the membranes have ruptured.

Phonocardiogram

The *phonocardiogram* is a microphone that picks up the fetal heart sounds. However, it also picks up other sounds, including any sounds that the mother makes when she moves. These sounds make the noise level impractical for labor. The phonocardiogram is valuable in evaluating the fetus prior to labor, however.

If the fetal heart rate is very slow, it may be doubled by phonocardiogram; a very rapid rate may be halved. This is because no fetal monitor currently available can count rates slower than 30 to 60 beats per minute or more rapid than 240 to 250 beats per minute.

Abdominal Wall Electrocardiogram

An *abdominal wall electrocardiogram* is recorded with electrodes placed on the mother's

Nursing Care Plan 18–1. Caring for a Woman in Labor With the Fetal Heart Monitor

NURSING GOAL:
To monitor labor pattern and fetal heart rate.

OBJECTIVES:
The mother will:
1. Know the reason for the use of the monitor.
2. Be comfortable while the monitor is in use.
3. Be well-informed in case of fetal distress.

ASSESSMENT	POTENTIAL NURSING DIAGNOSIS	NURSING INTERVENTION	COMMENTS/RATIONALE
1. Risk factors for potential fetal distress	Need for fetal monitoring due to prematurity, postmaturity, toxemia, prolonged rupture of membranes, fetal bradycardia or tachycardia, meconium staining, irregular labor pattern, Pitocin induction or augmentation, history of fetal demise, etc.	Determine need for fetal heart monitor based on nursing diagnosis.	The fetal heart monitor has two purposes: 1. To monitor labor pattern. 2. To monitor fetal heart rate, especially in response to uterine contractions.
2. Assess potential prior knowledge of fetal heart rate monitoring	Need for additional information	Explain purpose and mechanics of monitor to patient and partner; apply monitor.	Fathers often use the monitor to help with timing of contractions.
3. Assess mother's comfort	Need for comfort measures	Assist mother to side-lying position. Adjust monitor belts to comfortable positions.	
4. Assess FHR contraction pattern and interpret tracings:			
a. Assess baseline fetal heart rate (FHR)	Normal: 120–160 bpm; Baseline tachycardia; Baseline bradycardia	Intervention based on cause (Table 18–5).	
b. Assess beat-to-beat variability (BBV)	BBV present; BBV absent; BBV absent with FHR abnormality (see below)	Intervention as discussed in text.	
c. Assess relationship of FHR to uterine contraction	Acceleration; No change and BBV; Deceleration (Table 18–4)	No intervention required. Intervention as discussed in text	
d. Assess basal resting uterine tone (amniotic fluid pressure)	Normal: less than 10 mm. Hg; Hypertonus: greater than 12 mm. Hg		
e. Assess uterine tone (amniotic fluid pressure) during contractions	Normal: 20–50 mm. Hg; Hyperactive: greater than 50 mm. Hg		
f. Assess frequency and length of contractions	Hyperactive labor: contractions more often than every 2 minutes; Tetanic contractions: contraction longer than 90 seconds	Frequently due to oxytocin infusion. Stop oxytocin; infuse D_5W (see text and Chapter 19).	

Assessment	Observations	Intervention	Rationale
g. Assess shape (waveform) of contraction	Uniform waveform; early and late decelerations Variable waveform: variable decelerations	Intervention based on pattern.	
h. Tracings: Early decelerations Variable decelerations Late decelerations Tachycardia Bradycardia		For early decelerations: Continue to observe fetal heart rate. Inform patient of decelerations and their significance. For variable decelerations: 1. Try different position changes—on left side, right side, knee-chest. 2. Continue to monitor fetal heart rate. 3. Inform patient of the decelerations, reasons for actions. 4. Inform physician. For late decelerations: 1. Turn to left side. Begin nasal oxygen at 4 liters per minute. 2. Increase the rate of the IV fluids. Continue to monitor. 3. Inform patient of decelerations, reasons for actions. 4. Inform physician. For persistent tachycardia: 1. Check the patient's temperature. Increase IV fluid rate. Begin nasal oxygen at 4 liters per minute. 2. Inform patient of tachycardia, reasons for actions. 3. Inform physician. For persistent bradycardia: 1. Increase IV fluid rate. Try different position changes as in variable decelerations. 2. Begin nasal oxygen at 4 liters per minute. 3. Inform patient of bradycardia, reason for actions. 4. Inform physician. 5. Note all position changes and medications on the monitor strip.	Early decelerations are a result of head compression. Variable decelerations are a result of cord compression. Late decelerations are a result of uteroplacental insufficiency. An increased maternal temperature will result in fetal tachycardia. Bradycardia may be the result of cord compression, sudden severe drop in maternal blood pressure, or similar factors. However, some infants normally maintain a low fetal heart rate baseline of 100 to 120. The fetal heart rate is responsive to these actions; the response will be seen on the monitor strip.

Contributed by Mona B. Ketner.

Table 18–3. METHODS FOR CONTINUOUS MONITORING OF FETAL HEART RATE

Indirect/Direct	Method	Description	When Used	Advantages	Disadvantages
Indirect	Phonocardiogram	Microphone	Antepartum	Noninvasive	Picks up many sounds; too noisy for labor Very slow rate may be doubled* Very fast rate may be halved*
Indirect	Abdominal wall electrocardiogram	Electrocardiogram	Antepartum Labor	Noninvasive	Picks up fetal and maternal QRS complex* Limited success early third trimester May count maternal rate
Indirect	Doppler ultrasound	Ultrahigh frequency sound waves "bounced" off moving heart or valves	Antepartum Labor	Noninvasive Satisfactory in 90–95 per cent of laboring patients	1–3 beats/minute variability in rate Very slow rates may be doubled* Very high rates may be halved* Transducer may be uncomfortable Mother's position changes limited Constant repositioning necessary May count maternal rate
Direct	Fetal electrode	Electrode on fetal scalp detects fetal QRS	Labor	Most reliable Many noise signals filtered out Usually better tolerated by the mother Mother may change positions more easily	Invasive; membranes must be ruptured Cervix must be 1–2 cm. dilated Presenting part must be accessible

*Monitors currently available cannot count rates less than 30–60 beats/minute or greater than 210–250 beats/minute.

abdomen. Both the maternal QRS complex and P waves and the fetal QRS complex are recorded. Usually the maternal QRS complex is larger and can be identified. Each brand of abdominal electrocardiogram monitor offers solutions for separating maternal and fetal patterns; more solutions will undoubtedly become available in the years to come, because no totally satisfactory answer has yet been found.

Doppler Ultrasound

The principle of ultrasound was described in Chapter 14. When used to monitor the fetal heart, ultrasound waves are "bounced off" the walls of the moving heart or heart valves. Because two sets of heart valves are moving at different times (the bicuspid and the tricuspid valves), the system is designed so that once the movement of one valve is detected, the system will not respond for a specific period of time. Understanding this is important because:

1. If the fetal heart rate is very rapid, every beat may not be detected.

2. If the fetal heart rate is very slow, the movement of both valves may be indicated as beats on the monitor, thus doubling the rate.

Because monitors vary in the range of their response, the nurse must know the specifics of the particular instrument used in the practice setting.

Direct Fetal Scalp Electrode

The most reliable technique for measuring fetal heart rate is a stainless steel spiral electrode that is inserted into the fetal scalp after the membranes have ruptured (either spontaneously or artificially). The electrical signal detected is the QRS complex, which denotes the passage of an electrical impulse through the heart. The machine computes the fetal heart rate on the basis of the time interval between each QRS complex.

Monitoring Uterine Contractions

The monitoring of fetal heart rate alone is not sufficient. What is particularly significant is the relationship between fetal heart rate and uterine contractions. Like fetal heart rate, uterine contractions can be monitored externally or internally.

The External Tocotransducer

The external tocotransducer converts the force of each uterine contraction into an elec-

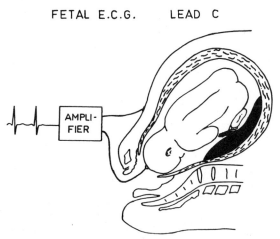

Figure 18–1. The placement of an electrode on the fetal scalp and a transcervical catheter to measure amniotic fluid pressure. (From Willis: *The Canadian Nurse,* Dec., 1970.)

trical signal that may then be displayed on a strip of paper. External monitoring is useful only in indicating the timing of contractions, not their intensity. In order to function properly, the external tocotransducer must be moved as the mother's position is changed. External monitoring is also less comfortable for the patient.

Internal Measurement of Intrauterine Pressure

Changes in intrauterine pressure can be measured by inserting a small, open-ended plastic catheter that is filled with fluid through the cervix into the uterus. The catheter is attached to a strain gauge that sends out an electrical signal reflecting the pressure placed against it (Fig. 18–1). Through this internal system, one can monitor not only rate but baseline tone and intensity of contractions. This capability is particularly important if oxytocin is used to stimulate contractions (see below).

When using internal monitoring, remember that:

1. Any break in the system, such as an air bubble, a leak, or a meconium plug will impair accuracy.

2. The height of the strain gauge must match the height of the catheter tip.

Terms Describing Fetal Heart Rate and Uterine Contractions

A number of terms are used to describe fetal heart rate and uterine contractions.

Baseline fetal heart rate is the rate between contractions or between transient changes unrelated to contractions.

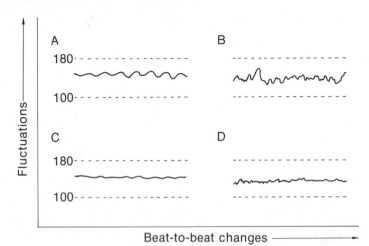

Figure 18–2. Fetal heart rate variability. *A,* Normal changes in rhythm; decreased beat-to-beat variability. *B,* Normal changes in rhythm and beat-to-beat variability. *C,* Decreased changes in rhythm and beat-to-beat variability. *D,* Decreased changes in rhythm; normal beat-to-beat variability. (After Yeh, Forsythe, and Hon: *Obstetrics and Gynecology, 41*:355, 1973.)

Baseline fetal heart rate variability refers to fluctuations in the baseline fetal heart rate (Fig. 18–2). Short-term variability occurs between successive pairs of heart beats. Long-term variability is related to fetal activity and averages 5 to 15 beats per minute when the fetus is active but may be suppressed when the fetus is asleep. Depressed variability due to sleep should not last longer than 15 minutes. The absence of short-term, beat-to-beat variability indicates a need for immediate future evaluation of the fetus. It may be drug-related (narcotics, barbiturates, tranquilizers, anesthetics, atropine, or scopolamine) or due to fetal hypoxia and acidosis. A smooth baseline may precede the late decelerations described below as an indication of fetal hypoxia.

In small, premature infants absence of baseline variability reflects immaturity of the cardiac control mechanisms.

Exaggerated variability (more than 25 beats per minute) is frequently a sign of hypoxic stress; it may precede beat-to-beat arrhythmia and fetal bradycardia.

Fetal tachycardia is a fetal heart rate greater than 160 beats per minute. Prematurity, maternal fever, mild or chronic hypoxia, intrauterine fetal infection, maternal anxiety, fetal activity, and drugs such as atropine, scopolamine, isoxsuprine (Vasodilan), and ritodrine are potential causes of fetal tachycardia.

Fetal bradycardia is a fetal heart rate of less than 120 beats per minute. Hypoxia, maternal hypothermia, arrhythmias of the fetal heart, and drugs, including agents used for local anesthesia, are potential causes of fetal bradycardia. Fetal bradycardia does not always indicate severe fetal distress, but it should always be investigated.

Deceleration patterns, seen on the fetal monitoring strip, indicate the way in which fetal heart rate slows in a characteristic manner in response to certain stimuli. The timing and configuration of the deceleration in relation to

the uterine contraction indicate certain factors about the fetus.

Acceleration patterns involve fetal heart rate acceleration above the baseline.

Tachysystole describes uterine contractions that are too frequent. The normal frequency for uterine contractions during active labor is one every 2.5 to 5 minutes. Contractions occurring more frequently than every 2 minutes (hyperactive labor, Chapter 15) indicate tachysystole.

A *tetanic contraction* is a sustained, continuous contraction that lasts longer than 90 seconds. Tetanic contractions are frequently due to oxytocin administration (Chapter 19).

Basal tone or *resting tone* is the pressure within the resting uterus between contractions. It can be measured only during internal monitoring. Resting tone is usually 5 to 10 torr; it is frequently elevated when the mother is receiving oxytocin. When the mother changes positions the resting tone on the monitor recording is altered, but this is frequently due to a change in the relationship of the tip of the catheter used in internal monitoring to the pressure transducer. To obtain an accurate reading, the catheter tip and the pressure transducer must be on the same level. Flushing the catheter to ensure potency and recalibration will also indicate whether uterine tone is accurate or the result of an artifact of the monitoring system.

Waveform refers to the recorded shape of the uterine contraction. It may be uniform (symmetrical) or variable. Early and late decelerations are usually uniform; variable decelerations have a variable waveform.

The Relationship between Fetal Heart Rate and Uterine Contractions

Deceleration patterns may be early, late, or variable. Some major characteristics of each

Table 18–4. DECELERATION PATTERNS

Relation of Fetal Heart Rate to Uterine Contractions

Type of Deceleration	Configuration	Onset	Low Point	Return to Baseline	Comments	Mechanism
Early	U-shaped	Early in contraction cycle	Corresponds to peak of contraction	By end of contraction	The stronger the contraction, the greater the fetal heart rate; slowing rarely below 110–120 beats/minute. Occur in vertex presentation only. Appear after 6–7 cm. cervical dilatation	Compression of fetal head (see text)
Late	U-shaped	20–30 seconds or more after onset of contraction	After peak of contraction	After end of contraction	Degree of fetal heart rate slowing reflects intensity of contraction	Fetal hypoxia (see text)
Variable	Irregular	Variable relation of fetal heart rate to uterine contraction	Variable relation of fetal heart rate to uterine contraction	Variable relation of fetal heart rate to uterine	Variable in every aspect including magnitude and occurrence with successive contractions	Umbilical cord compression
Prolonged	Wide U-shaped	Variable relation of fetal heart rate to uterine contraction		Variable relation of fetal heart rate to uterine	Cannot predict when or whether deceleration will end	Maternal hypotension. Uterine hyperactivity. Paracervical block. Umbilical cord compression

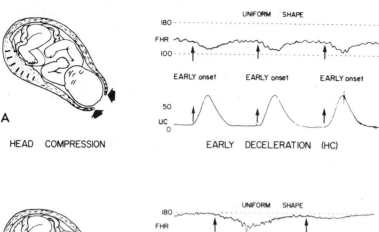

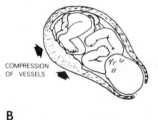

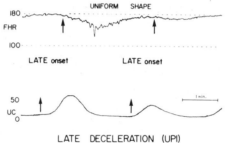

Figure 18–3. Patterns of fetal bradycardia. *A,* Early deceleration due to head compression (HC). UC is the tracing of uterine contraction. This is also known as a Type I dip. *B,* Late deceleration due to uteroplacental insufficiency (UPI). This is also known as a Type II dip. *C,* Variable deceleration due to cord compression (CC). (From Hon: *An Atlas of Fetal Heart Rate Patterns.* New Haven, Conn., Harty Press, Inc., 1968.)

type are summarized in Table 18–4 and Figure 18–3.

Early Deceleration. Compression of the descending fetal head during a uterine contraction elevates fetal intracranial pressure and thereby reduces the flow of blood to the fetal brain. Chemoreceptors in the brain are stimulated, and by reflex action fetal heart rate is slowed. This is the physiologic basis of early deceleration.

Although this sequence might appear threatening to the fetus, the transient hypoxia is apparently well tolerated by the fetus. Thus, early decelerations are, in our present state of knowledge, benign.

Late Deceleration. When the flow of blood from the mother to the placenta is compromised and fetal pO_2 falls to 20 mm. Hg (normal is approximately 30 mm. Hg), fetal heart rate slows. The drop does not occur immediately at the time that the contraction begins. Rather it is progressive, dropping as the pressure of the

uterine contraction increases and as the fetal oxygen stores (oxygen bound to fetal hemoglobin) decrease. Return to normal occurs following the contraction, as the flow of blood to the uterus increases.

Late decelerations and no beat-to-beat variability usually occur when the fetus is *chronically* asphyxiated and acidotic, resulting from chronic pathology involving the placenta or maternal–fetal exchange. One might expect such a pattern in some mothers with hypertensive disease, for example. The depressed fetal heart rate is due to the effect of hypoxia on the fetal myocardium.

Late decelerations with normal beat-to-beat variability and a normal baseline fetal heart rate usually indicate *acute* compromise of maternal–fetal exchange. The heart rate slows because of a reflex triggered by stimulation of the chemoreceptors within the brain, as in early deceleration. Because the stimulus is acute, intervention (e.g., administering oxygen, turning the mother to her side, see below) may often relieve this second cause of late deceleration.

Examples of the cause of late decelerations include maternal hypotension and uterine hyperactivity.

Often both chronic and acute conditions exist simultaneously. Careful evaluation will suggest which is the more significant at a particular moment in an individual woman's labor and thus the type of intervention most appropriate.

Variable Deceleration. Variable decelerations are also principally reflex in origin. Umbilical cord compression results in a lack of oxygen in the fetal blood from compression of the umbilical vein and in fetal hypertension from compression of the umbilical arteries. Baroreceptors are activated by the former and chemoreceptors by the latter; as a result, the vagus nerve is stimulated, and the fetal heart rate slows. The pattern is probably variable because the degree of cord compression changes from one contraction to another; cord compression may also occur between contractions.

Variable decelerations indicate fetal distress when (1) beat-to-beat variability is decreasing or (2) baseline fetal heart rate is increasing.

Prolonged Deceleration. *Prolonged decelerations* are always a cause for concern; they may be due to maternal hypotension or to uterine hyperactivity or may follow a paracervical block. Nursing intervention includes administration of oxygen, maternal position change, and displacement of the uterus. Unless the cause is readily identified and corrected, delivery is indicated.

Acceleration Patterns. Acceleration in fetal heart rate above the baseline level between contractions usually indicates fetal wellbeing. Tactile stimulation, such as that during an examination, may cause fetal heart rate acceleration, as may the touch of the uterine lining during a contraction.

Acceleration may be a sign of danger when it occurs late in the contraction cycle and when beat-to-beat variability has been lost. This acceleration pattern may be a forerunner of a late deceleration pattern.

Recognition of Patterns. The recognition of fetal heart rate patterns is not always as straightforward as the examples described above. The reason may lie in the system itself (placement of the monitor or interference, for example) or in multiple factors affecting the fetal heart rate. Individuals with equal experience may interpret a pattern differently, just as some electrocardiogram (EKG) patterns in adults may be interpreted in more than one way. Nurses who care for laboring patients must constantly assess, improve, and evaluate their skills in this area.

Assessment of Uterine Contractions

The fact that intrauterine pressure can only be measured using an internal monitor has been noted previously. Clinical correlates of amniotic fluid pressure are found in Table 18–5.

Certain abnormal variations in labor patterns are defined in relation to amniotic fluid pressure:

1. *Hypertonus*: resting pressure from 12 to 30 or more mm. Hg. Resting pressures above 30 mm. Hg are dangerous to the fetus because oxygen exchange in the intervillous space is compromised.

2. *Hyperactive labor*: contractions that exceed 50 mm. Hg or that occur more frequently than every 2 minutes, or both. Again, the fetus is compromised because there is inadequate time for oxygenation in the intervillous space.

3. *Hypoactive labor*: contractions with an intensity of less than 30 mm. Hg or more than 5 minutes apart, or both. When labor is hypoactive, there is little progress, and labor is likely to be prolonged.

Table 18–5. CLINICAL CORRELATES OF AMNIOTIC FLUID PRESSURE

Amniotic Fluid Pressure (mm. Hg)	Clinical Correlates
10	Normal tonus
20	Contraction felt by abdominal palpation
25	Woman perceives "pain"; considerable individual variation
50	Height of contraction

Charting on the Monitor Tracing

As the discussion in this and previous chapters indicates, fetal heart monitor tracings are interpreted not in a vacuum but in relation to a variety of factors. Factors that should be noted on the monitor tracing itself to aid interpretation include:

1. Dilatation
2. Station
3. Maternal vital signs
4. Medications and treatments given to the mother, including oxygen and analgesia
5. Changes in maternal position
6. Meconium in amniotic fluid
7. Fetal scalp pH
8. Discontinuance of tracing to change paper, during transit, etc.
9. Any occurrence that may affect the tracing or the fetus (e.g., maternal shivering, a maternal seizure, pushing)

Maternal Medications, Fetal Heart Rate, and Uterine Contractions

A number of medications given to the mother will produce variations in the tracings of both fetal heart rate and uterine contractions. Proper interpretation of a tracing requires an appreciation of the effects of medications. Whenever a medication is given, the time, name, dose, and route should be recorded on the tracing itself.

Drugs Affecting Variability. Drugs with an atropinelike action, sedatives, tranquilizers (especially diazepam), narcotics, parasympathetic blocking agents, and magnesium sulfate may cause a loss of beat-to-beat variability. Exaggerated beat-to-beat variability may also occur following the administration of local anesthetic drugs (e.g., paracervical block, epidural block). Exaggerated variability is frequently a sign of hypoxic stress; beat-to-beat arrhythmia and bradycardia may follow.

Drugs Affecting Fetal Heart Rate. Drugs given to the mother that inhibit the transmission of the vagal response to the fetal SA node can cause fetal tachycardia; atropine is an example.

Bradycardia is related to increased vagal stimulation; sympathetic blocking agents such as the local anesthetics used in epidural and paracervical anesthesia may produce bradycardia.

Drugs Affecting Uterine Contractions. The major drug affecting uterine contractions is oxytocin (Chapter 19). When a mother is receiving oxytocin, careful attention must be given to the frequency, duration, and intensity of contractions and the basal resting uterine tone.

Drugs Indirectly Affecting the Fetus. Drugs that cause hypotension in the mother (antihypertensive agents such as Apresoline; local anesthetic agents and techniques) may indirectly affect the fetus; maternal hypotension decreases uterine blood flow, leading to potential fetal hypoxia, and the FHR tracing will show late decelerations.

Intervention When FHR Pattern Is Abnormal

If the assessment indicates an abnormality in the fetal heart rate pattern (late decelerations, loss of variability), the following actions are indicated:

1. Explain what is happening and reassure the mother and her companion.
2. If oxytocin is infusing, stop the Pitocin drip and switch immediately to a dextrose and water solution that is piggybacked into intravenous line (see Uterotonic Agents, in Chapter 19).
3. Turn mother to left side.
4. Check monitor functioning.
5. Rule out prolapse of the umbilical cord (Chapter 19).
6. Begin maternal oxygen.
7. Assess possible causes: maternal hypotension, abruptio placentae, tachysystole, tetanic contractions, drugs, maternal anemia.
8. Be prepared to determine fetal scalp pH (below).
9. Be prepared for a possible cesarean delivery.

Areas of Controversy

A basic argument of those who oppose the general use of electronic fetal monitoring is the concept that childbirth is a normal experience for most women; fetal monitoring is viewed as one of several examples of interference with birth, a natural process. One specific way in which monitoring may interfere with a "natural" labor is confinement of the mother to a bed. Since vertical positions, standing, walking, and sitting have been shown to facilitate labor by increasing contractions and since the rate of cervical dilatation is associated with less pain (Chapter 15), confining a mother to bed with a monitor may indeed affect the course of her labor, although that effect may not be evident in statistics of perinatal morbidity and mortality.

Table 18–6.   RATES OF CESAREAN DELIVERY IN PATIENTS WITH AND WITHOUT ELECTRONIC FETAL MONITORING

Study	Patients Without EFM (no.)	Patients With EFM (no.)	CSR Without EFM (%)	CSR With EFM (%)
Haverkamp, 1976	241 (HR)	242 (HR)	6.6	16.5
Haverkamp, 1978	232 (HR)	233 (HR)	5.6	17.6
		230 (HR)*		11.0
Renou, 1976	175 (HR)	169 (HR)	14.0	20.0
Kelso, 1978	253 (LR)	251 (LR)	4.4	9.5

EFM, electronic fetal monitoring
CSR, cesarean delivery rate
HR, high risk patients
LR, low risk patients
*With fetal scalp sampling.

The two belts required by the external monitor can interfere with the coping techniques couples have learned, specifically effleurage (light stroking of the abdomen) and back rubs. Just the presence of the belts, which must fit snugly if monitoring is to be effective, is irritating to some women.

One potential disadvantage of electronic fetal monitoring is the way the monitor is used. If nurses walk into the room and look at the monitor but not at the mother (and father), the monitor can be a barrier to good care rather than a way of enhancing care. This, of course, is a disadvantage over which nurses have control. Monitors *do not* reduce the number of nurses required to care for mothers in labor, although they may change the way in which nurses use their time (more time for coaching and support; less time for auscultation of fetal heart rate). Fathers, too, sometimes become so entranced with watching the monitor that they forget their coaching role.

Several objections are related specifically to internal (direct) fetal monitoring. Technically, direct monitoring is generally considered more reliable. However, direct monitoring requires rupture of the amniotic sac. Spontaneous rupture of the membranes occurs at 9 cm. or more in 85 per cent of women studied by Diaz.[5] Caldeyro-Barcia[4] has suggested that intact membranes allow the pressure of the uterine contraction to be evenly distributed to all parts

of the fetus. He believes that early rupture may be a factor in traumatic brain damage.

Fetal scalp abscess is an occasional complication at the site of fetal electrode attachment, but several studies, including a prospective study by Okada et al.,[22] have found that the abscesses are usually small, the infection is generally mild, requiring only topical treatment, and only very rarely is hospitalization prolonged. Nevertheless, for the occasional baby who is more seriously affected it is important to ask if the risk is worth the benefit.

Because the rate of *cesarean births* has more than doubled in the United States between 1968 and 1976 (Chapter 19), the same time period in which fetal monitoring has become increasingly widespread, the question naturally arises: has fetal monitoring been the cause of the rise in cesarean birth? A number of studies have attempted to answer that question. In Table 18–6, comparison is made between cesarean birth rates in women who were not monitored and women who were. In Table 18–7, the comparison is between the rate of cesarean delivery before and after the introduction of electronic fetal monitoring. Questions that must be asked include the following:

1. Are the groups being compared comparable?

2. Is the increase in the cesarean rate due to more cesarean deliveries for fetal distress? Increase in the cesarean rate because the baby

Table 18–7.   CESAREAN BIRTH RATES BEFORE AND AFTER THE INTRODUCTION OF ELECTRONIC FETAL MONITORING

Study	Before EFM (%)	Year	After EFM (%)	Year
Koh, 1975	6.4	1971	12.5	1973
Lee and Baggish, 1976	7.3	1969-1971	10.4	1972-1974
Gabert and Stenchever, 1977	3.2	1970	10.5*	1975
Hughey, 1977	2.6	1968, 1969	6.9*	1974-1975

EFM, electronic fetal monitoring
*Primary cesarean delivery.

is a breech presentation or might require a midforceps delivery, both changes that have occurred during the same period of time, cannot be attributed to fetal monitoring.

In Kilso's research,[16] no increase in cesarean deliveries due to fetal distress was shown, but in two Haverkamp studies[11, 12] there was a difference. However, the difference in rates for monitored and unmonitored groups appears to be primarily due to differences in the characteristics of women in the groups. When these differences are controlled, the association between monitoring and cesarean birth is negligible in the population study.[2]

Two studies report a decrease in cesarean delivery because some potentially high risk mothers who at one time would have routinely been delivered by the cesarean route (the diabetic mother, for example) may now be monitored and delivered vaginally.[3, 15]

The cost of electronic fetal monitoring versus the possible benefits in a low risk population have also been questioned. The estimated cost of electronic fetal monitoring per delivery was $30 to $60 in 1978. For those who argue that fetal monitoring results in an increase in cesarean birth rate, there are additional costs. The prevention of cerebral palsy or mental retardation in a *single* individual has been estimated to save over $170,000, the lifetime cost of maintaining and rehabilitating a severely handicapped child and adult.[6] One might consider the cost of a lifetime of income lost, in addition, and the family grief that cannot be measured in dollars. We do not at this time know what the impact of fetal monitoring on mental retardation might be, but the issues must be raised before data can be gathered.

Fetal Scalp Blood Sampling

Fetal bradycardia or a pattern of late deceleration or variable decelerations that do not respond to treatment indicates possible fetal distress. At the first indication of fetal distress, fetal scalp sampling is usually indicated. One reason is that although a "good" fetal heart rate pattern usually indicates a healthy fetus, a pattern of variable or late decelerations is not as reliable. In addition, the information from a series of fetal scalp samples is more valuable than the data from a single sample.

Laboratory values vary somewhat from one institution to another. A fetal scalp pH value of 7.25 or above is usually considered within normal limits. Values from 7.20 to 7.24 indicate a need for continuing assessment, while two or more values below 7.20 may indicate a need for immediate intervention.

The technique itself involves puncture of the fetal scalp (or buttocks) with a microscalpel that is inserted through a conical endoscope (Fig. 18–4). Following the collection of blood in a heparinized glass capillary tube, pressure is applied to the puncture site with a sponge throughout the next two contractions. The site is then observed during a third contraction; if no bleeding occurs, the endoscope is removed.

Continuing fetal distress that is not rapidly alleviated is an indication for medical intervention. Nurses are often the first to detect such distress and have a significant responsibility in communicating the exact nature of the distress to a physician immediately. A record of that communication should be in the mother's record for legal purposes. The impor-

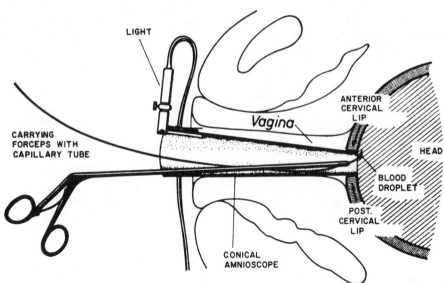

Figure 18–4. Diagram showing method of obtaining a fetal blood sample. (From Willis: *The Canadian Nurse*, Dec., 1970.)

tance of both the communication and the record cannot be overemphasized.

Summary

Electronic fetal heart rate monitoring is an important tool in fetal assessment in many labors. Nurses who care for mothers during labor and birth in most settings must be knowledgeable about the use of fetal monitors and the nursing skills that can enhance the care of mothers who are monitored. Always, however, the primary focus of our attention should be on the mother and her labor companion rather than on the monitor alone.

REFERENCES

1. Afriat, C., and Schifrin, B.: Sources of error in fetal heart rate monitoring. *JOGN, 5*:11, 1976.
2. *Antenatal Diagnosis*: Report of a consensus development conference. Bethesda, National Institutes of Health, 1979.
3. Beard, R., Edinger, P., and Sabanda, J.: Effects of routine intrapartum monitoring on clinical practice. *Contributions to Gynecology and Obstetrics, 3*:14, 1977.
4. Caldeyro-Barcia, R.: Some consequences of obstetrical interference. *Birth Family Journal, 3*(2):34, 1975.
5. Caldeyro-Barcia, R.: The influence of maternal position on time of spontaneous rupture of the membranes, progress of labor, and fetal head compression. *Birth Family Journal, 6*(1):7, 1979.
6. Conley, R.: *The Economics of Mental Retardation.* Baltimore, Johns Hopkins University Press, 1973.
7. Dulock, H., and Herron, M.: Women's response to fetal monitoring. *JOGN, 5*:68s, 1976.
8. Gabert, H., and Stenchever, M.: The results of a five-year study of continuous fetal monitoring on an obstetric service. *Obstetrics and Gynecology 50*:275, 1977.
9. Goodlin, R.: Fetal monitoring. *In* Iffy, L., and Kaminetzky, H. (eds.): *Principles and Practice of Obstetrics and Perinatology,* Vol. II. New York, John Wiley, 1981.
10. Gray, J.: Nursing care for monitored women in labor. *American Journal of Nursing, 78*:2104, 1978.
11. Haverkamp, A., Thompson, H., McFee, J., et al.: The evaluation of continuous fetal heart rate monitoring in high-risk pregnancy. *American Journal of Obstetrics and Gynecology, 125*:310, 1976.
12. Haverkamp, A., Orleans, M., et al.: A controlled trial of the differential effects of intrapartum fetal monitoring. *American Journal of Obstetrics and Gynecology, 134*:399. 1979.
13. Hon, E.: *An Introduction to Fetal Heart Rate Monitoring,* 2nd edition. Los Angeles, University of Southern California School of Medicine. Copyrighted by the author, 1975.
14. Hughey, M., La Pata, R., McElin, T., et al.: The effect of fetal monitoring on the incidence of cesarean section. *Obstetrics and Gynecology, 49*:513, 1977.
15. Kelly, V., and Kulkarni, D.: Experiences with fetal monitoring in a community hospital. *Obstetrics and Gynecology, 41*:818, 1973.
16. Kilso, I., Parsons, R., Lawrence, G., et al.: An assessment of continuous fetal heart rate monitoring in labor: a randomized trial. *American Journal of Obstetrics and Gynecology, 131*:520, 1978.
17. Koh, K., Greves, D., Yung, S., et al.: Experience with fetal monitoring in a university teaching hospital. *Canadian Medical Association Journal, 112*:455, 1975.
18. Langhorne, F.: The fetal monitor: Friend or foe? *MCN, 1*:313, 1976.
19. Lee, W., and Baggish, M.: The effect of unselected intrapartum fetal monitoring. *Obstetrics and Gynecology, 47*:516, 1976.
20. Lowensohn, R. I.: Instrumentation for fetal heart rate monitoring. *JOGN, 5*:75, 1976.
21. Martin, C., and Gingerich, B.: Factors affecting the fetal heart rate: Genesis of FHR patterns. *JOGN, 5*:305, 1976.
22. Okada, D., Chow, A., and Bruce, U.: Neonatal scalp abscess and fetal monitoring: factors associated with infections. *American Journal of Obstetrics and Gynecology, 129*:185, 1977.
23. Parer, J.: Physiological regulation of fetal heart rate. *JOGN, 5*:265, 1976.
24. Paul, R., and Petrie, R.: *Fetal Intensive Care.* Wallingford, Conn.: Corometrics Medical Systems, Inc., 1979.
25. Renou, P., Chang, A., Anderson, I., et al.: Controlled trial of fetal intensive care. *American Journal of Obstetrics and Gynecology, 126*:470, 1976.
26. Schifrin, B.: Fetal heart rate monitoring during labor. *Journal of the American Medical Association, 221*:992, 1972.
27. Wiley, J.: The nurse's legal responsibility in obstetric monitoring. *JOGN, 5*:77s, 1976.
28. Yeh, S., Forsythe, A., and Hon, E.: Qualification of the fetal heart beat-to-beat interval differences. *Obstetrics and Gynecology, 41*:355, 1973.

19

Variations in Labor

OBJECTIVES

1. Define:
   a. induction
   b. amniotomy
   c. oxytocic agents (uterotonic agents)
   d. dystocia
   e. cephalopelvic disproportion (CPD)
2. Describe how emotional support is given for parents when labor varies from their expectation.
3. Identify nursing responsibilities in caring for a mother receiving an oxytocic agent.
4. Describe assessment of abnormal patterns of labor. Indicate nursing interventions that may be of value.
5. Differentiate the use of low forceps and midforceps. Explain how nurses can utilize this information to help parents.
6. Identify the major reasons for cesarean delivery.
7. Describe nursing support for couples when a cesarean delivery is necessary.
8. Identify tocolytic agents used to arrest premature labor; describe the action and side effects of each.
9. Describe special problems for infants and parents in delivery in a multiple gestation pregnancy.
10. Describe nursing assessment needed to identify
    a. rupture of the uterus
    b. prolapse of the umbilical cord
    c. amniotic fluid embolism
    Indicate appropriate nursing intervention for each.
11. Describe the modification of nursing intervention during labor when the mother has each of the following:
    a. pre-eclampsia or eclampsia
    b. diabetes mellitus
    c. heart disease

For many reasons, the course of labor may vary from the pattern described in Chapters 15 and 17. Some variations, such as those of presentation, have already been discussed.

Variations are related to:

1. A need to induce labor for specific reasons.

2. Failure of labor to progress.

3. Contractions that are too strong or too frequent.

4. Recognition of fetal distress.

5. Preterm labor.

6. Multiple gestation.

7. Emergencies that occur during the course of labor.

8. The needs of individual patients (the mother with heart disease, for example).

Supporting Parents When Labor Varies

When the course of labor varies from what parents expect, it is understandable that the anxiety that all parents feel to some extent is compounded.

Nurses can help all parents during the prenatal period by emphasizing that there are many possible variations in labor and that by no means are all of them life-threatening or damaging to their baby.

Some high risk labors are anticipated as when the mother has diabetes or pregnancy-induced hypertension, for example. Plans may be made for labor and birth at a tertiary center that may be miles from the mother's home. She may be admitted to the center in advance of labor, lengthening her period of separation from family and familiar surroundings. Culture shock, previously mentioned as a problem for many women in a labor environment, is intensified in the high technology, crisis-oriented environment in which most high risk mothers labor and deliver. Attention to her individual needs for comfort as well as safety, encouraging the support of husband or other family members, and the availability of a primary nurse in whom she can develop trust are even more important for the high risk mother.

Mothers (and fathers) react in varying ways to the technology associated with a high risk birth. For some who did not anticipate any problems in their labor, the need for devices such as the fetal monitor can be very disappointing. Others find that the opportunity to determine that their fetus is doing well is reassuring.

When the unforeseen occurs during the course of labor, the mother and her companion should be told what is happening. No matter what we have to tell them, suspecting that something is not as it should be (and they will suspect this) and not being told the truth will make them even more anxious.

Although no mother should labor alone, the mother with a difficult labor is particularly in need of constant support. When staffing does not permit continuing attention to every mother (an unfortunate reality in most labor rooms), this mother has priority, not only for physiologic reasons but also because of her special emotional needs. High risk parents have a particularly strong need to feel the staff is competent to care for them, no matter what may happen.

Keeping the mother continually informed will usually eliminate the necessity for abruptly presenting her with a dramatic change of plans—a sudden cesarean delivery, for example, which may cause total panic. Of course, there are instances in which sudden change occurs for which no one was prepared, such as a marked change in fetal heart rate. Nurse and physician must act rapidly to deal with the physical emergency, but at the same time the mother and her companion must also be informed.

When fathers were first allowed in labor rooms in increasing numbers in the late 1960's and the early 1970's, there were many questions about "what will we do with the father if there is some unexpected change in the mother's condition?" Nurses and physicians, barely comfortable with fathers during labor under the best of circumstances, often felt they could not cope with their presence during emergencies.

In many labor rooms, the atmosphere has changed. There is a recognition that fathers not only are able to cope with the unexpected but can help support the mother during an emergency or change of course in a way that professionals never could.

Obviously, this is not true for all fathers under all circumstances. Nor are all nurses or physicians as yet comfortable with parents in every situation. But the idea that fathers must immediately leave when complications are suspected is no longer practiced as a hard and fast rule.

Uterotonic Agents and the Induction of Labor

Uterotonic agents stimulate the contractile activity of uterine muscle. Oxytocin, prostaglandins, and ergot alkaloids are uterotonic agents used in the care of childbearing women. Prostaglandins are used principally to induce abortion (Chapter 30); ergot alkaloids (ergonovine or methylergonovine) are used in the postpartum period (Chapter 27). The focus in this chapter will be on oxytocin.

Oxytocin is synthesized in the paraventricular nuclei and probably also in the supraoptic nuclei of the hypothalamus and transported to the pituitary gland (once thought to be the site of production), from which it is released directly into the bloodstream. Both stimulation of the nipple and dilatation of the cervix and vagina will cause the release of oxytocin by initiating the firing of neurons in the nuclei of the hypothalamus. The role of endogenous oxytocin (i.e., oxytocin synthesized within the woman's own body) in the initiation of labor was discussed in Chapter 15.

Exogenous synthetic oxytocin is used to *induce* labor (i.e., initiate labor) and also to augment labor when uterine contractions are ineffective (see Nursing Care Plan 19–1).

The Induction of Labor. Labor may be induced for a variety of medical indications and is occasionally induced for "social" indications. The practice of inducing labor for the convenience of either patient or physician (social indications) is condemned by many, but, although far less frequent now than even a few years ago, it continues to exist. Two major disadvantages of an elective induction for social reasons are the delivery of a preterm infant because the gestational age was incorrectly assessed and the failure of the labor to progress, often resulting in a cesarean delivery that may not have been necessary. Bernstine[4] states, "Oxytocin stimulation should not be used for the elective induction of labor for patient or physician convenience."

Induction may be indicated for the health of the mother or the fetus in the following instances: (1) pre-eclampsia or other hypertensive or renal problems of the mother; (2) intrauterine growth retardation of the fetus; (3) postmaturity (gestation greater than 42 weeks); (4) diabetes mellitus or severe Rh isoimmunization in the mother; (5) rupture of membranes in the absence of uterine contractions; (6) initiation of labor following fetal death.

Induction of labor is contraindicated in women with multiple pregnancies or any other condition in which the uterus is overdistended because of the increased risk of uterine rupture. Others at increased risk of rupture are women with uterine scars, women over 35 years of age, and grand multiparas. Any of these conditions is a contraindication to induction.

The Augmentation of Labor. Uterine dystocia and nursing interventions to alleviate it are discussed below. If cephalopelvic disproportion has been ruled out as the reason for dystocia and the pelvis is sufficiently large for vaginal delivery, synthetic oxytocin (Pitocin) may be given to stimulate uterine contraction. Once uterine contractions have been established, progress usually occurs within 2 hours. If not, the woman should be re-evaluated because there may be previously undetected cephalopelvic disproportion.

Caring for Women Receiving Oxytocin

Oxytocin is a potentially dangerous medication; uterine rupture, hyperstimulation of the uterus with resultant decrease in fetal oxygenation, and abruption of the placenta have occurred when the administration of oxytocin is not carefully controlled.

Oxytocin should be administered only when nurses who are knowledgeable about the care of mothers receiving oxytocin can be in constant attendance. There is great individual variability in the response of women to oxytocin; there is no way to predict in advance how sensitive an individual uterus will be.

Oxytocin should be administered intravenously using an infusion pump to ensure constant flow. A "piggyback" set-up, with 5 per cent dextrose in water in one line and the oxytocin in 1000 ml. of 5 per cent dextrose in water in the other line, is utilized. The dextrose solution should be attached close to the site of needle insertion in the woman's own arm so that if it is necessary to discontinue the oxytocin solution, glucose can be given immediately and no additional oxytocin that might be in the line will be infused.

Electronic fetal heart rate monitoring is appropriate for mothers receiving oxytocin in order to provide continuous assessment of both uterine contractions and fetal heart rate. Baseline observation for 30 minutes prior to the initiation of the oxytocin is important. It is possible to assess contractions and fetal heart tones without a monitor, but when oxytocin is used the continuous assessment provided by the fetal heart rate monitor is desirable.

Initially, a low dose of oxytocin is given, and uterine response is assessed. The dose may be increased after 15 to 30 minutes if contractions do not occur and there are no side effects. The ideal response is a moderate to strong contrac-

Nursing Care Plan 19–1. Management of Labor Induced or Augmented with Oxytocin

NURSING GOAL:
To establish a regular labor pattern.

OBJECTIVES:
The mother will:
1. Experience regular uterine contractions.
2. Have contractions no closer than every 3 minutes.
3. Know the reason for induction/augmentation of labor.

ASSESSMENT	POTENTIAL NURSING DIAGNOSIS	NURSING INTERVENTION	COMMENTS/RATIONALE
1. Presence or absence of a regular labor pattern	Need for labor induction or augmentation due to postmaturity, pregnancy-induced hypertension, prolonged rupture of membranes, failure to progress, among other factors	Place fetal heart monitor on mother.	The monitor will show an accurate picture with regard to both labor pattern and fetal heart rate.
		Establish mainline IV therapy.	The exact amount of oxytocin is easily regulated by an infusion pump. The IV containing the oxytocin must be piggybacked at the nearest port so that it can be discontinued immediately in case of overstimulation and tetanic uterine contractions.
		Explain procedure and its reasons to patient.	
		Inform her that the contractions will become regular and hard fairly quickly.	
		Inject 10 units of oxytocin into 1000 ml. of IV fluid. Place the tubing in an infusion pump.	
2. After oxytocin is initiated, assess: a. Blood pressure b. Pulse c. Respirations d. Fetal heart tones e. Frequency, duration, intensity of contractions f. Pattern on FHR monitor Assess every 15 minutes for 1 hour, then every 30 minutes if stable.		Piggyback the IV fluid containing oxytocin into the mainline IV at the port nearest the vein puncture site.	Contractions should not be any closer than every 3 minutes or exceed 90 seconds in duration because of compromised oxygen supply to fetus.
		Begin oxytocin at ordered rate.	
		Increase oxytocin by prescribed amount every 15 minutes until contractions are established at intervals of every 3 minutes.	Contractions can become uncomfortable more quickly with augmented labor.
		Discontinue oxytocin if contractions are more than 90 seconds' duration or occur more than every 3 minutes, or if there are signs of fetal distress.	If mother is using a breathing technique, she may need to use a more complex technique to cope with augmented contractions.
		Assist patient with breathing and comfort measures to cope with strength of contractions.	Hang mainline IV at the same level as the IV containing oxytocin.
		Maintain contractions at regular established intervals.	Decrease the rate of the mainline IV as the rate of oxytocin is increased in order to avoid fluid overload.
		Oxytocin may be decreased as the patient's labor mechanisms take over.	
3. Signs of fluid overload: a. Headache b. Vomiting		Monitor patient's IV intake. Limit total hourly IV intake to 150 ml.	

Contributed by Mona B. Ketner.

tion lasting 45 to 60 seconds and recurring every 2 to 3 minutes. Between contractions the uterus should be completely relaxed.

In addition to the continuous assessment of contractions and fetal heart rate, maternal blood pressure and pulse should be assessed prior to administration of the oxytocin and every 15 to 30 minutes thereafter. Large amounts of oxytocin may relax the smooth muscle of the blood vessels, causing hypotension with subsequent tachycardia and increased cardiac output. Oxytocin also has a weak antidiuretic effect, which can result in water intoxication if large volumes of intravenous fluid are given. Intake and output should be carefully recorded.

The oxytocin intravenous drip is discontinued if signs of fetal distress, hyperstimulation, or other side effects occur. Occasionally signs of hyperstimulation occur after the dosage is increased, and these may be relieved if the dosage is returned to the previous level.

Since the half-life of oxytocin is approximately 3 minutes, the amount in the blood drops rapidly when the infusion is discontinued. (This is the reason that intramuscular oxytocin is not used; circulating oxytocin would be replenished by oxytocin in the muscles.)

Amniotomy

Amniotomy, the artificial rupture of the membranes, is sometimes used to initiate labor. However, labor does not always follow, and fetal infection becomes a risk, particularly if the membranes are ruptured more than 24 hours before delivery.

There are specific risks associated with amniotomy. When fetal membranes are intact, the pressure of the contracting uterus is transmitted equally throughout the uterus. (Pascal's principle states that whenever the pressure of a confined liquid is increased or diminished at any point, the change in pres-

sure is equally transmitted through the entire liquid.) This protects the fetal head and the umbilical cord from pressure or compression. Caldeyro-Barcia[10] reported on the increased incidence of cerebral damage when membranes are ruptured early in labor, a finding not yet confirmed by subsequent research.

Infection, if labor progresses slowly, is a possible complication. The incidence of infection in mother and baby when membranes have been ruptured more than 24 hours is markedly increased.

If amniotomy is performed before the fetal presenting part is in the cervix, prolapse of the umbilical cord may occur.

Slow Progression of Labor

The phrase failure of labor to progress is frequently used to describe labor in which the pattern varies from that of the Friedman curve (Fig. 19–1). However, such a phrase has a negative connotation, and we suggest the substitution of "slow progression" and will use that phrase in this discussion. (Refer to Chapter 15 to review the meaning of latent, active, and transitional labor.)

Labor does not always progress in the manner described in Chapter 15. *Dystocia* is the term used to describe difficult labor. Dystocia may be due to a problem of powers, passage, or passenger (Table 19–1) or a problem in the interrelationship of one or more of these factors.

Assessing Slow Progression of Labor

Continuing assessment of a woman's progress during labor is the basis by which slow progression is recognized. Table 19–2 summarizes certain specific criteria that are useful in determining whether the course of labor is normal.

The Friedman curve (described in Chapter 15) is a simple method of recognizing abnormal

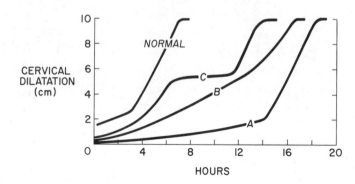

Figure 19–1. Major aberrant labor patterns. *A*, Prolonged latent phase; *B*, protracted active phase; and *C*, secondary arrest of dilatation. (From Page, Villee, and Villee: *Human Reproduction: The Core Content of Obstetrics, Gynecology and Perinatal Medicine.* 2nd Edition. Philadelphia, W. B. Saunders Co., 1976. Modified from Friedman.)

Table 19–1. DYSTOCIA IN LABOR

Problem Area	Basis	Intervention
Powers	Dysfunctional contractions	Rest, possibly with sedation Possible oxytocin
Passage	Cephalopelvic disproportion (CPD)	Cesarean section
Passenger	Abnormal presentation Abnormal fetal development	Varies with specific cause

patterns of labor. By plotting an individual woman's progress, patterns that vary from the norm may more quickly be recognized.

Prolongation of the Latent Phase. Line A in Figure 19–1 illustrates prolongation of the latent phase. Some reasons for prolongation of this phase include analgesia (too much, too soon), ineffective contractions, and a cervix that is not in an appropriate state for dilatation (an "unripe" cervix).

Nursing intervention can generally eliminate the need for analgesic medications too early in labor. Prenatal preparation for childbirth is generally very helpful, but even when this preparation is lacking the labor room nurse can use techniques described in Chapter 15 to help women relax and cope with their contractions. Mothers who do not live far from the hospital and who have intact membranes often elect to spend the latent phase of labor at home in familiar surroundings rather than come to the hospital or birthing center.

Ineffective contractions may be due to anatomic or physiologic factors, such as the position of the mother, or psychological factors, such as anxiety. The relationship of maternal position and maternal anxiety to labor has been previously discussed (Chapters 15 and 16).

Allowing the mother to rest by giving her a sedative or a narcotic will usually result in: (1) cessation of contractions (indicating false labor) or (2) more effective contractions and active labor after the rest period. Should neither occur, oxytocin may be given.

Prolonged Active Phase. The prolongation of the active phase of labor may be primary, in that the entire course of labor is prolonged, or it may occur as a secondary arrest in a labor previously progressing in a normal fashion.

Primary dysfunctional labor is due to fetal malposition, cephalopelvic disproportion (CPD), or inefficient myometrial contractions, in that order. Excessive sedation or conduction anesthesia may cause a *secondary arrest* of labor; fetal malposition and CPD are also causes of secondary arrest.

The treatment of secondary arrest depends upon discovering the cause. Inefficient myome-

trial activity may be helped by rest and later by administering oxytocin. Cesarean delivery will be necessary if CPD is the diagnosis (see below).

Intervention When the Progress of Labor Is Slow

Based on an understanding of the physiologic and psychologic factors that may impede the progress of labor, the following interventions may help many mothers:

1. Changes in position may help. Walking, sitting, and lying on one's side all appear to enhance the effectiveness of contractions. Mothers should not labor lying on their backs.

2. Help the mother to relax. A warm shower, the presence of a support person, and the removal of stressful persons are helpful. In some instances medication may be necessary, *after* other remedies have been utilized.

3. A full bladder can be an obstacle to delivery and may inhibit uterine action. Mothers should void every hour.

4. Endogenous oxytocin, produced by nipple stimulation, may be helpful; for some mothers exogenous oxytocin (e.g., Pitocin) may be necessary (see below).

5. When other measures are ineffective, a cesarean delivery may be necessary (see below).

Operative Procedures

Medical intervention in difficult labor often involves operative procedures. The most common operative procedures are the use of forceps and cesarean delivery.

The Use of Forceps. In their desire for a "natural" birth, some mothers fear the use of forceps in the delivery of their baby. Carefully and correctly used, forceps can assist in the safe delivery of a baby.

Most commonly, forceps are applied after the fetal head is crowning; this is called a *low forceps* or *outlet forceps* delivery (Fig. 19–2). The use of outlet forceps is usually elective, i.e., the physician chooses to use forceps to better control the delivery, to protect the fetal

Table 19-2. A COMPARISON OF NORMAL AND ABNORMAL PATTERNS DURING LABOR

	Type of Pattern	Assessment Criteria	Possible Cause
Normal	Friedman curve	Duration: <20 hours primipara <14 hours multipara	

Hypoactive	Prolonged latent phase
	Prolonged acceleration phase
		Duration:
		  >20 hours primipara
		  >14 hours multipara
			False labor
			Dysfunctional contractions
			Unprepared cervix
			Sedation given too early

	Prolonged active phase	Dilatation:
		  <1.2 cm./hr. primipara
		  <1.5 cm./hr. multipara
		    or
		No progress over a 2 hour period
			Fetal malposition
			CPD
			Inefficient activity of uterine
			  muscles

	Prolonged deceleration Slow descent of fetal head	>3 hours primipara >1 hour multipara <1 cm./hr. primipara <2 cm./hr. multipara No descent	Abnormal descent through the pelvis Fetal malposition Possible CPD

Hyperactive	Tetanic contractions	Uterus does not relax between
		  contractions
			Mechanical obstruction to descent,
			  including pathologic retraction
			  ring
			Overstimulation with oxytocics

	Precipitate labor	Dilatation > 5 cm./hr.	Hyperactive contractions
	Precipitate delivery	Unusually short second stage	
Irregular	Irregular contractions	Intensity varies Duration varies No pattern	Etiology unclear

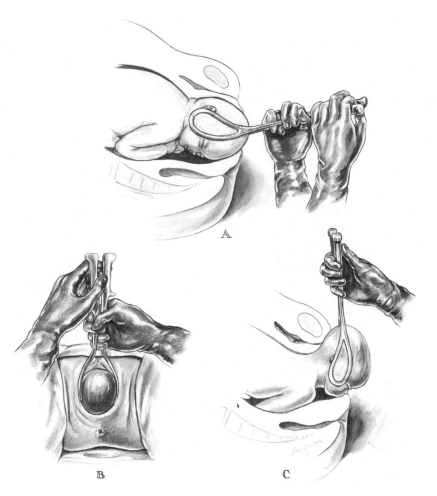

Figure 19–2. Low forceps delivery. *A,* The forceps are in place; the handles are separated with the left index finger and thumb; the pull is forward and downward with combined forces. *B,* Traction is continued, but with partial elevation of the head; the handles are separated to avoid compression of the fetal head. *C,* The head is delivered by further extension over the perineum. (From Greenhill and Friedman: *Biological Principles and Modern Practice of Obstetrics.* Philadelphia, W. B. Saunders Co., 1974.)

head from "battering" against the perineum, and to minimize trauma to the perineal tissue.

A *midforceps* delivery, when the head is engaged but has not yet reached the perineal floor, is usually done for a specific reason. That reason may be maternal (inability of the mother to push because of conduction anesthesia, insufficient uterine activity, eclampsia, heart disease, or exhaustion, for example) or fetal (fetal bradycardia, meconium in the amniotic fluid, or fetal malposition, for example).

In all deliveries utilizing forceps the operator must be highly skilled (nurses do not apply forceps and most nurse-midwives do not apply forceps).

1. Forceps are not used when there is cephalopelvic disproportion

2. The head must be engaged before forceps can be applied

3. The cervix must be completely effaced and dilated

4. The exact presentation and position of the fetus must be known

5. The presentation must be cephalic

6. The membranes must be ruptured and

7. The bladder must be empty before forceps can be applied

Anesthesia is given to the mother for a midforceps delivery in order to assure perineal relaxation.

Explanations to the mother, such as "the forceps will help guide the baby's head through the birth canal," are essential. Some mothers may wonder at the time about "forceps marks" on the baby and need to be reassured that they will be only temporary.

The Use of a Vacuum Extractor. An alternative to the use of forceps is the vacuum extractor. Modern techniques of vacuum extraction are credited to Malstrom in 1954, although the principle was attempted by Younge in the early eighteenth century and by Simpson and others in the nineteenth century. Early studies in the 1960's reported a high incidence of fetal complications, but more recent studies have suggested a lower rate of severe fetal complications with vacuum extraction than with forceps.[16] Vacuum extractors may thus become more popular in the United States in the coming years.

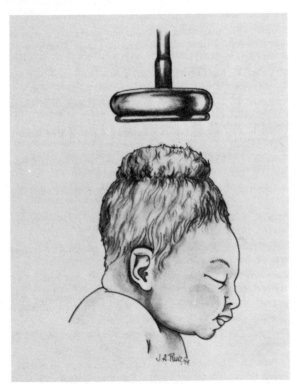

Figure 19–3. Virtually all infants delivered by vacuum extraction have a chignon or caput. This small suction knob is innocuous and will greatly diminish in size within a few hours after birth. (From Iffy, and Kaminetzky: *Principles and Practice of Obstetrics and Perinatology,* Volume 2. New York, John Wiley, 1981.)

The vacuum extractor consists of disk-shaped cups (available in three sizes), a traction chain, pieces of tubing that connect to the traction chain, a vacuum pump, and a vacuum trap bottle. Following delivery, the extractor is washed in cold water and autoclaved. Rubber tubing usually needs to be replaced two to three times a year.

The cup is placed over the posterior fontanel, with the sagittal suture pointing to the center of the cup. A vacuum is then created by electrical pump; the slowly increasing negative pressure of the vacuum creates a large caput succedaneum that fills the cup (Fig. 19–3) over a period of 6 to 8 minutes. When fetal distress requires rapid delivery, the vacuum may be created within a minute by increasing negative pressure more rapidly.

Vacuum extraction is utilized when the mother needs assistance in the second stage of labor. This may occur when the fetal occiput persists in a posterior position, in multiple births, or when maternal illness requires a shortened second stage.

Several advantages of vacuum extraction in comparison with forceps delivery have been noted. No lateral pelvic space is required to attach the vacuum extractor, in contrast to forceps, so that vaginal lacerations are infrequent. Injury to the mother's bladder, vagina, uterus, and bowel is reduced. Because the procedure is not painful for the mother, little or no anesthesia is required. The mother is able to push with her contractions. In twin deliveries, vacuum extraction is reported to facilitate greatly the delivery of the second twin, and may even be life-saving.[3] When the fetal occiput remains posterior or transverse, traction applied by the vacuum extractor will usually allow the fetus to rotate on his own; no attempt is made to rotate the head manually. The traction force exerted by forceps was found to be 40 per cent greater than the force of the vacuum extractor.[26a]

A major disadvantage of vacuum extraction is the development of the chignon, or caput. Usually the caput is markedly diminished within a few hours after delivery, but it may last from 5 to 7 days. Long-term follow-up has not revealed any neurologic defect.[24, 35] Other types of possible scalp trauma include cephalhematoma (Chapter 21), scalp necrosis, and ulceration. Subgaleal hematoma, in which bleeding occurs between the galea and the vault of the skull, is a rare complication. Subgaleal hematoma may also occur in spontaneous delivery or forceps delivery. The use of the vacuum extractor is controversial in preterm deliveries because of the increased possibility of bleeding. Previous fetal scalp sampling and the attachment of a fetal electrode may lead to bleeding if the vacuum extractor is attached.

Both maternal and infant complications are increased if vacuum extraction is attempted through a cervix that is not fully dilated. Other contraindications include cephalopelvic disproportion, a face, brow, or breech presentation, a head that is not engaged, and unruptured membranes.

As vacuum extraction becomes more widespread, nurses must be prepared to discuss the advantages, disadvantages, and contraindications with families.

Cesarean Birth

A cesarean birth is an operative procedure in which an infant is delivered through an incision in the abdominal and uterine walls. *Primary* cesarean birth describes a woman's first cesarean birth; subsequent cesarean births are commonly termed *repeat* cesarean births. The term cesarean section has been used for many years, but many nurses (and others) are now using terms such as cesarean delivery, cesarean childbirth, and cesarean birth to emphasize the birth experience rather than an operative procedure. The cesarean birth rate in the United States tripled during the 1970's, from 5.5 per cent in 1970 to 15.2 per cent in 1978. The increase has occurred in all parts of the country. Although cesarean birth rates are slightly lower in Canada and lower still in many European nations, an increase has occurred there also. Because of the precipitous rise in cesarean births, the National Institutes of Health organized a Consensus Development Conference in 1980. The 19-member task force included 1 nurse-midwife, 12 physicians, 1 representative of a consumer advocacy group (C-Sec., Inc.), a psychologist, a sociologist, an attorney, an economist, and a health researcher. The results of this study are likely to be widely discussed during the next several years. The central issues were:

1. Why and how have cesarean delivery rates changed in the United States and elsewhere, and how have these changes affected pregnancy outcome?

2. What is the evidence that cesarean delivery improves the outcome of various complications of pregnancy?

3. What are the medical and psychological effects of cesarean delivery on the mother, infant, and family?

4. What economic factors are related to the rising cesarean rate?

5. What legal and ethical considerations are involved in decisions on cesarean delivery?*

Indications for Cesarean Birth

Table 19–3 shows the major anatomic or physiologic factors that have had the greatest effect on the cesarean birth rate. Each will be discussed in detail.

---

*A single copy of the full report of the Task Force, containing a description and analysis of the literature, may be obtained at no cost from the Office of Research Reporting, NIHCD, Building 31, Room 2A34, 9000 Rockville Pike, Bethesda, Md. 20205. Shearer,[33] the task force member representing C-Sec., describes the process and her views of the report.

Dystocia has been discussed earlier in this chapter along with nursing interventions that may facilitate labor and thereby avoid the need for cesarean birth. Since approximately one-third of all cesarean births are due to dystocia, intervention to relieve the causes of dystocia may be significant in reducing the incidence of cesarean birth.

The Consensus Development Task Force recommended that "in the absence of fetal distress, management of dysfunctional labor may include such measures as patient rest, hydration, ambulation, sedation, and use of oxytocin, prior to considering cesarean birth." They also suggest peer review within hospitals, examination of the efficacy of methods for assessing the progress of labor, and research clarifying the factors which affect the progress of labor including the efforts of emotional support, ambulation, rest, sedation, and oxytocin stimulation.

Repeat Cesarean Births. The widely held belief of "once a cesarean, always a cesarean" is being questioned. Because nearly one-third of all cesarean births are repeat cesareans, the question deserves careful review. Repeat cesareans are not routine in England and many European nations; they occur only when there is a valid indication. For example, if the previous cesarean delivery was due to placenta previa, a cesarean birth for the present pregnancy may not be indicated. However, if the mother's pelvis is small and the infant is large (CPD), then a second cesarean birth is appropriate.

The Consensus Development report states, "Based on maternal and neonatal mortality rates, the practice of routine repeat cesarean birth is open to question." Bottoms et al.[8] suggested that, using a selective approach, "between 30 and 60 per cent of patients can have vaginal deliveries" after cesarean birth. Criteria used in the selection of mothers include:

1. Desire for a vaginal birth.

2. Absence of the indication for the prior cesarean birth.

3. Uncomplicated pregnancy.

Table 19–3. INDICATIONS FOR CESAREAN BIRTH

Indication	Per Cent of all Cesareans (1978)	Per Cent Contribution to Rise in Rate
Dystocia	31	30
Repeat cesarean	31	25–30
Breech presentation	12	10–15
Fetal distress	5	10–15

Cesarean Childbirth: National Institutes of Health Consensus Development Conference Summary. Bethesda, Office of Research Reporting, NIHCD, 1981.

4. A low segment transverse uterine incision.

5. Vertex presentation.

6. Normal course of labor.

Vaginal delivery prior to the cesarean birth is considered a favorable although not an absolutely essential criterion.

The type of uterine incision used in the previous cesarean delivery is particularly important. The practice of repeat cesarean delivery began in the United States in the early 1900's to avoid uterine rupture during labor. At that time, almost all cesarean incisions were of the "classic" type—a vertical incision in the body of the uterus. A subsequent cesarean birth is still considered necessary for mothers who have had classic, inverted T, or low vertical uterine incisions, or in whom there is no documentation of the site and type of incision.

The Consensus Development report suggests a trial of labor and delivery for women who have had a previous low segment transverse cesarean birth "in hospitals with appropriate facilities, services, and staff for prompt emergency cesarean birth." These mothers should not, in our opinion, consider out-of-hospital delivery. If a hospital does not have the appropriate facilities, the mother should be told this in advance of labor and given information and the opportunity to choose a hospital that does.

Breech Presentation. Nationally, the proportion of breech presentations delivered by cesarean rose from 11.6 per cent in 1970 to 60.1 per cent in 1978, accounting for approximately 10 to 15 per cent of the overall rise in the cesarean birth rate. The relationship between cesarean birth and improvement in the mortality and morbidity of the newborn varies with the infant's birth weight and gestational age, the type of breech presentation (Chapter 15), maternal pelvic size, and other congenital anomalies. More data must be collected in well-designed studies on both vaginal and cesarean deliveries of infants with breech presentation. The Consensus Development report recommended that vaginal delivery of a term infant with breech presentation should remain an obstetric choice when:

1. The anticipated weight of the infant is less than 8 pounds (3600 grams) but greater than 5 pounds 8 ounces (2500 grams).

2. The dimensions and shape of the pelvis are normal (Chapter 10).

3. The presentation is frank breech without a hyperextended head.

4. The delivery is to be conducted by a physician experienced in vaginal breech delivery. This last condition may become increasingly difficult to meet because obstetric residents trained in some centers have little or no experience in vaginal breech delivery.

A prenatal postural exercise that *may* result in a baby turning from a breech to a vertex presentation is described in Chapter 11. *External version,* in which a qualified practitioner places hands on the woman's abdomen and, using firm gentle pressure, shifts the baby to a head-down position, is far less common now in the United States than formerly.[14, 31] Risks include the possibility of premature labor and problems with the placenta or umbilical cord. A cesarean delivery is considered safer by many practitioners. Previous cesarean birth or uterine surgery, active labor, rupture of membranes, and engagement of the presenting part are contraindications.

Fetal Distress. Approximately 5 per cent of cesarean births are attributed to fetal distress. Fetal distress is generally first detected through electronic fetal monitoring. Because electronic fetal monitoring (EFM) became widely used during the same decade that cesarean birth rates increased so dramatically, some observers have associated EFM with this rise. A number of studies[18, 19, 22, 29, 32] have shown an increase in the cesarean birth rate in comparison with those in whom fetal heart rate is auscultated. Crude cesarean birth rates are higher in EFM mothers, but comparability of the two populations (the monitored vs. the auscultated mothers) and interpretation of statistics have resulted in continued controversy.

In Neutra's 1979 study,[29] in which statistical techniques were used to control for a number of potentially confusing variables, cesarean birth rates were found to be higher for unmonitored mothers in one subgroup (nulliparas with malpresentation), higher for monitored mothers in two subgroups (multiparas, multiparas with arrested labor), and not significantly different in five groups.

One relationship between EFM and the cesarean birth rate that does not seem to have been explored is an indirect one. The positive effect of moving about during labor, changing positions, and lying on one's side have been previously noted. Continuous EFM restricts ambulation and may also restrict change of position. Perhaps some cesarean births attributed to dystocia may be related to the secondary effects of EFM.

If there is a relationship between EFM and an increased cesarean rate, is it due to the possible overdiagnosis of fetal distress? In many hospitals, fetal scalp blood pH determination is utilized when fetal distress is noted prior to the decision for cesarean delivery; this practice is strongly recommended (Chapter 18).

Other Health Factors Related to Cesarean Birth

In addition to the four categories described, other indications for cesarean birth include placenta previa; abruptio placentae; herpes II virus infection of the vulva, vagina, or both; prolapse of the umbilical cord; and severe maternal hypertension. Maternal diabetes was previously considered to be a common indication for cesarean birth, but with better maternal prenatal care, diabetic mothers do not have such large babies or the other problems, such as maternal hypertension and poor placental perfusion, associated with diabetes. Thus, in some hospitals today, more diabetic mothers are able to have vaginal deliveries. The mother of an infant with erythroblastosis fetalis may have a cesarean delivery if the baby appears to be in trouble.

Social and Demographic Factors

In addition to the anatomic and physiologic factors just described, social and demographic changes may also be important in the rising incidence of cesarean births.

1. There is an increase in the number of primiparous births and in births to women over 30 years old. Women in this age group are more likely to have cesarean births; the cesarean birth rate for mothers over 30 was 20 per cent in 1978.[30]

2. Cesarean birth rates vary with the type of hospital. In 1978 in the National Hospital Discharge Survey, the cesarean birth rate was 16.4 per cent for private hospitals, 15.8 per cent for voluntary nonprofit hospitals, and 13.1 per cent for state government hospitals.[30]

3. Women who receive maternity care from physicians who primarily practice gynecology are more likely to have a cesarean birth than women who receive care from those who practice primarily obstetrics[29a] or from family practitioners or midwives. This may reflect patterns of referral of high risk mothers with complications of labor or delivery, or it may reflect differences in philosophy or training. The finding that rates for cesarean births are significantly higher in hospitals with more than 500 beds than in hospitals with fewer than 100 beds may be related to the physicians practicing in these hospitals.

4. The current malpractice climate in the United States was the reason most frequently given by physicians for the increase in cesareans.[25] They expressed the fear that if a cesarean delivery is not performed under a variety of circumstances and the infant is "less than perfect," the parent will sue the physician. Although this issue is questionable from a philosophical point of view, one can sympathize with the physician who must make a decision in regard to a particular situation.

5. It is unclear to what extent economic factors are related to the rise in cesarean rates. A cesarean delivery takes less time than the close surveillance of labor, which makes it less costly to the physician. Moreover, the physician usually receives a higher fee for less time. In areas where hospital beds are plentiful, increased cesarean births mean fewer empty beds because of longer hospital stays. Cesarean birth is, however, more costly to the individual patient and to third-party insurers (and thus to all who have health insurance or pay taxes).

Types of Cesarean Birth

Low Segment Cesarean Incision. A low segment cesarean incision is the most common type of abdominal delivery today. The incision is made in the lower part of the uterus, behind the bladder (Fig. 19–4). There is less hemorrhage because the incision is in an area of thin fibrous tissue. Fewer abdominal adhesions result from a low incision than from the other cesarean procedures.

Classic Cesarean Incision. In the classic procedure, a midline incision is made in the abdomen between the umbilicus and the symphysis pubis. The baby is grasped by his feet and delivered through an opening in the uterus approximately 11 cm. long. Because the incision traverses the thick uterine muscle, there is a greater possibility of hemorrhage, of poorer healing and possible rupture, and of postoperative adhesions to the bowel and therefore of obstruction. Nurses caring for women following cesarean birth must know the type of procedure used in order to make pertinent observations.

Under certain circumstances, such as a placenta previa (Chapter 13), a classic incision may be preferred by the obstetrician.

Cesarean Hysterectomy. In cesarean hysterectomy, the uterus is removed after the delivery of the baby. Possible reasons include uterine tumors, uterine rupture, and uncontrollable bleeding following delivery.

Nursing Care and Support During and Following a Cesarean Delivery

The decision for cesarean delivery and the operative procedure itself are medical decisions in which neither nurse nor parent have

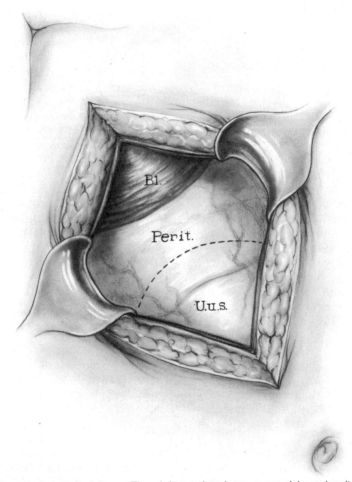

Figure 19–4. Low segment Cesarean delivery. The abdomen has been exposed by a longitudinal incision, and the operative field is exposed. The dotted line shows the intended elliptical incision in the loose pubocervical peritoneum. *Bl.,* bladder, *Perit.,* peritoneum; and *U.u.s.,* upper uterine segment. The patient is oriented here so that her head is down and to the right. (From Greenhill and Friedman: *Biological Principles and Modern Practice of Obstetrics.* Philadelphia, W. B. Saunders Co., 1974.)

a major role. However, the nursing role in other aspects of care for these mothers and their families is *significant* (see Nursing Care Plans 19–2 and 19–3).

Consider the couple who have prepared for childbirth through reading, attendance at classes for expectant parents, or discussion with friends. The moment of birth has come to have special meaning for many such couples. They may have heard glowing descriptions of the joy of "pushing" their baby out and of the exhilaration of the moment of birth. When they find that they will not have this experience, it is not surprising that some parents express a feeling of disappointment and loss, *if* they are given the opportunity to express that disappointment. They may feel "abnormal," different from other couples.

To compound their feelings of loss and abnormality, their baby may be treated differ-ently. Because the incidence of respiratory distress is higher in infants delivered abdominally (Chapter 23) and because fetal distress, maternal diabetes, pre-eclampsia, or some other condition affecting the fetus may have necessitated the procedure, infants delivered by cesarean are frequently placed in special care nurseries and separated from their parents for a longer period than are babies delivered vaginally. Thus hospital policies related to abdominal delivery may be a barrier to important early contact.

If the cesarean delivery is an elective procedure, preoperative preparation is similar to that for abdominal surgery. In addition to the physical preparation of the mother, the baby's heart rate should be checked. Time must be found to allow both parents to ask questions and to express their feelings about abdominal delivery.

Immediate physical postoperative care is again similar to that of postoperative abdominal surgery care. Assessing the fundus is difficult because of abdominal dressings and tenderness, so particularly careful attention must be paid to other signs that indicate bleeding, such as blood pressure and pulse rate. If the mother is awake (i.e., if she has had spinal or epidural anesthesia), she should have an early opportunity to see, touch, and hold her infant (Fig. 19–5 *G, H*).

Special infant needs will be related to specific problems, such as an infant with transient tachypnea, an infant of a diabetic mother, and so on (Chapter 23).

The Experience of Cesarean Birth

Naomi was 24, married, and expecting her first child. She attended prepared childbirth classes with her husband because she wanted to be awake and participate in her baby's delivery, and because she believed that Lamaze techniques would help her have a faster, more comfortable labor and delivery. Naomi described her labor and delivery experience as follows (see Fig. 19–5 *A–H* for photographs of cesarean birth)

I had my first contraction about 8:00 Sunday evening, April 6th. The contractions were about 60 seconds long and 10 minutes apart. I noticed some bloody show when I went to the bathroom. By 10:00 the contractions were about 5 minutes apart, so we left for the hospital. At the hospital I was examined and found that I was only 2 cm. dilated. Things stayed about the same all night. The doctor examined me about 8:30 A.M. I was 3 cm. dilated. He wanted to break my water, but I asked him not to. I don't think it's good for the baby. By 10:30 I was only 4 cm. dilated and having a harder time keeping up with the contractions. The nurse convinced me that breaking my water wouldn't hurt the baby and that it would help speed things up. I wasn't sure I could handle the harder, faster contractions, but I figured they'd get that way eventually. I might as well go ahead before I got even more tired. The doctor broke my water around 11:45 A.M., and the contractions came about 3 minutes apart and 90 seconds long. They were very painful. My husband really helped me hang on with my breathing. I had a lot of trouble with my legs shaking between contractions. I decided to try some Demerol to help me relax. What a disaster! I think the doctor gave me too much. I was much better off when the stuff wore off. I kept falling asleep between contractions, and my husband had a hard time getting me to concentrate on my breathing during contractions. By 3:00 P.M. I was 5 cm dilated. The doctor decided to have a pelvimetry done. That was rough. The contractions were *really* painful. They decided the baby's head was too big to fit through, so we got ready for cesarean section. I had a hard time deciding between general anesthesia and an epidural. I wanted my husband with me, so I decided on the epidural. It was really easier than I expected. They had me ready by 4:00 P.M. Charlie was born at 4:14 P.M. My husband got to hold him in the delivery room. We also got to keep him with us in the recovery room. I got him to nurse a little bit. I came home Saturday, the 12th. I think the C-section was a breeze, and I'm not afraid to have another baby the same way. I hope we can have another baby at _____ Hospital. They really took good care of us. They treated me like a person, not an object.

The film we saw on C-sections in our Lamaze class helped me decide on the epidural anesthesia. I'm glad we took the classes. They helped us a lot. I think I would have been too afraid to have an epidural had I not seen the film on it. It let us know what to expect.

The Mother with Premature Labor

The major cause of neonatal death is birth of the infant before 37 weeks—a preterm or premature birth. In more than 60 per cent of spontaneous preterm labors, it is not possible to determine the reason for the premature contractions. However, a large number of maternal and fetal conditions have been associated with preterm labor (see Nursing Care Plan 19–4).

Prenatal assessment should identify women with these conditions, and close attention should be given to their prenatal care. Even with excellent prenatal care not every mother with preterm labor can be identified; in one series 38 per cent of mothers with preterm labor had no identifiable risk factor.[13]

Factors associated with premature labor are not necessarily causes per se. For example, although preterm labor occurs more frequently in adolescent mothers, it is likely that lack of prenatal care and socioeconomic status rather than age are responsible (Chapter 29).

Some mothers who are considered at very high risk for premature labor (e.g., mothers with a history of preterm births) may spend much of their pregnancy at bed rest (on their left side for maximum placental perfusion). For most mothers, intervention begins with the recognition of premature labor.

Recognizing premature labor is not always a simple matter; a woman may be experiencing Braxton-Hicks contractions. Yet if intervention is delayed too long, it may not be possible

Text continued on page 560

Nursing Care Plan 19–2. Assisting the Mother Having Planned Cesarean Delivery

Immediate Preoperative Phase

NURSING GOALS:
To promote education.
To prepare mother and family for her surgery, both emotionally and physically.

OBJECTIVES:
The patient will:
1. Understand the procedures involved in a cesarean delivery.
2. Be physically and psychologically prepared for her surgery.
3. Accept the reasons for cesarean delivery.

ASSESSMENT	POTENTIAL NURSING DIAGNOSIS	NURSING INTERVENTION	COMMENTS/RATIONALE
1. Existing knowledge level of mother regarding her surgery and postoperative course; this depends upon parity, previous cesarean birth, childbirth education classes, and the mother's medical conditions.	Mother's lack of knowledge about her upcoming surgical experience.	Inform mother of reasons for the cesarean delivery and procedures involved. Family's lack of knowlege about cesarean delivery Instruct mother about need for turning, coughing, and deep breathing postoperatively. Encourage questions from mother and father; allow time for discussion, including father.	Reinforcing previous teaching may help to decrease the mother's anxiety level just prior to surgery. The father is made to feel a part of the abdominal delivery if he is included in discussions of what is going to happen; he may better support the mother if well-informed.
2. Emotional status: mother's perception and family's perception of cesarean delivery, verbal expressions of adequacy or inadequacy, disappointment, concern over body image	Fear. Potential alterations in self-concept	Listen; clarify concerns; have father available as long as possible; encourage father to be with mother during delivery. Provide reassurance. Ascertain mother's degree of disappointment, concern over body image.	Interaction with others will reduce the mother's feelings of isolation and make her feel more "normal." Slight concerns and worries now may lead to extreme problems in the postoperative phase.
3. Mother's degree of physical preparation for cesarean delivery	Potential for physical complications during surgery and postoperatively	Shave abdomen; insert indwelling catheter for drainage; position mother on left side.	The numerous hairs on the abdomen harbor bacteria. Keeping the bladder empty during surgery decreases the possibility of accidental perforation. Lateral position promotes venous return.

Immediate Postoperative Phase

NURSING GOALS: To promote optimum recovery.
To prevent postpartum hemorrhage.
To promote bonding.

OBJECTIVES: The mother will:
1. Relate appropriately to her newborn infant (partner will be included in bonding process).
2. Recover without excessive vaginal or abdominal bleeding.
3. Know the need for fundal massage.
4. Be able to massage her own fundus.
5. Remain warm and comfortable.

ASSESSMENT	POTENTIAL NURSING DIAGNOSIS	NURSING INTERVENTION	COMMENTS/RATIONALE
1. Vital signs and contractility of uterus	Potential for postpartum hemorrhage	Proceed with interventions from the fourth stage of labor. Maintain intravenous flow rate. Massage fundus after administration of pain medication to ensure comfort. Encourage mother to use techniques of coping (focusing, breathing). Monitor amount of bleeding on abdominal dressing. Monitor patency of indwelling catheter to bladder.	Vital signs may vary owing to medications or anesthetic agents. Fundal massage is painful for the mother and may be neglected, but its importance cannot be overlooked. If the catheter does not drain properly, the bladder may fill with urine and displace the uterus to the side.
2. Level of discomfort due to surgery; patient's complaints of pain, restlessness	Pain	Administer pain medications as patient's needs dictate. Monitor drug dose if the mother is breast-feeding her infant. Position patient for comfort; support incision for coughing and deep breathing. Provide quiet environment for rest; provide clean gown and linens. Offer warm blanket.	Many analgesic agents are passed into the mother's breast milk.
3. Family interaction; mother's and father's reactions to infant; mother's and father's interaction between each other	Need for maternal–infant attachment	Proceed with interventions from the fourth stage of labor; maintain patient comfort; provide early opportunities for interaction. If infant requires nursery care because of illness, keep parents informed of progress. Discuss feelings about cesarean delivery and mother's self-image.	Interaction may be delayed owing to recovery from anesthesia and mother's pain. Another reason for delay may be transportation of the baby to the nursery immediately after birth because of illness.

Contributed by Mona B. Ketner.

Nursing Care Plan 19–3.   Assisting the Mother Having an Unplanned Cesarean Delivery

Immediate Preoperative Phase

NURSING GOALS:
To prepare mother for her surgery immediately—both emotionally and physically
To educate mother and family quickly regarding the surgical procedure.
OBJECTIVES:
The mother will:
1. Know the reason for the immediate cesarean delivery.
2. Experience quick physical preparation for the surgery.

ASSESSMENT	POTENTIAL NURSING DIAGNOSIS	NURSING INTERVENTION	COMMENTS/RATIONALE
1. Medical reason for emergency cesarean delivery: ruptured uterus, amniotic fluid embolism, umbilical cord prolapse, fetal distress 2. Existing knowledge level of mother (See NCP 19–2, No. 1)	Need to prepare mother quickly physically and emotionally for unplanned cesarean delivery	Inform mother and father of medical reasons and necessity for cesarean delivery. Answer questions quickly and honestly. Stay with mother; perform procedures while answering questions and reassuring mother.	Mother and father will be very anxious; quick explanations must be given owing to the emergency situation.
3. Emotional status of mother (See NCP 19–2, No. 2) 4. Mother's lack of physical preparation for the procedure (See NCP 19–2, No. 3)		Observe for feelings of failure at not having a vaginal delivery.	The need for an emergency cesarean may lead mother and father to feel that they did something wrong or that they failed in some way.

Immediate Postoperative Phase

NURSING GOALS:
To promote optimum recovery.
To prevent postpartum hemorrhage
To promote bonding.

OBJECTIVES:
The mother will:
1. Relate appropriately to her newborn infant (partner will be included in bonding process).
2. Recover without excessive vaginal or abdominal bleeding.
3. Know the need for fundal massage.
4. Be able to massage her own fundus.
5. Remain warm and comfortable.

ASSESSMENT	POTENTIAL NURSING DIAGNOSIS	NURSING INTERVENTION	COMMENTS/RATIONALE
See Nursing Care Plan 19–2			Pain and fatigue levels may be more intense due to possible long labor, failed forceps delivery before cesarean delivery.
			Emergency cesarean may lead to feelings of inadequacy or failure.
		Reinforce quick preoperative explanations; answer all questions regarding cesarean delivery.	Allow time for questions, exploration of feelings; more time is available for explanations and teaching during the recovery period.

Contributed by Mona B. Ketner.

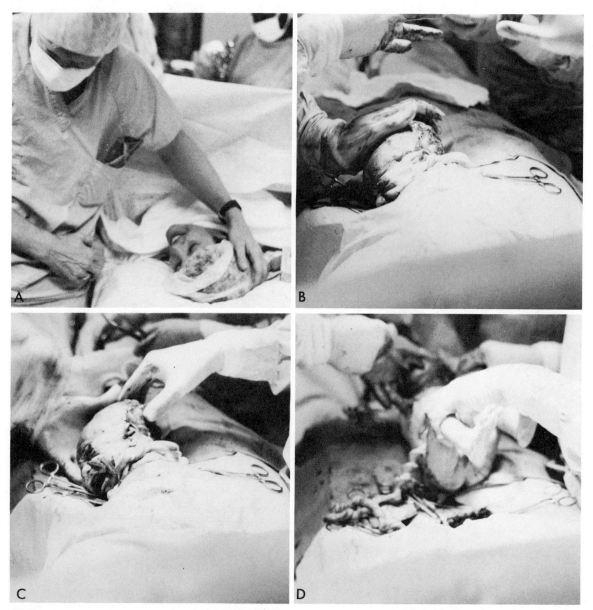

Figure 19–5. *A,* Mom and Dad are together as cesarean delivery begins. Epidural anesthesia allows Mom to be awake throughout delivery. *B,* Baby's head is delivered through the incision. . . *C,* the shoulders are delivered. . .*D,*. . . and the second stage is completed as the rest of the baby emerges.

Illustration continued on opposite page

to stop a true labor. By custom, premature labor is diagnosed when contractions occur no more than 10 minutes apart or two or more times in 15 minutes and last 30 seconds or longer. Cervical changes are carefully assessed, using as little cervical manipulation as possible, to avoid both infection and increase in uterine activity. Gravidas need to understand the importance of contacting their health-care provider should contractions occur at any point during pregnancy. Women need to know how to time contractions and the interval between contractions (Chapter 15).

The decision to intervene to arrest premature labor depends on maternal, fetal, and uteroplacental factors. In general, maternal contraindications involve serious maternal disease (e.g., uncontrolled diabetes, uncontrolled hypertension, severe cardiovascular renal disease). Fetal contraindications include fetal distress, serious anomalies, growth retardation, and fetal death. Abruption of the placenta, intrauterine infection, and advanced labor (cervical dilatation greater than 8 cm.) are further contraindications to labor suppression. Other factors, considered relative contrain-

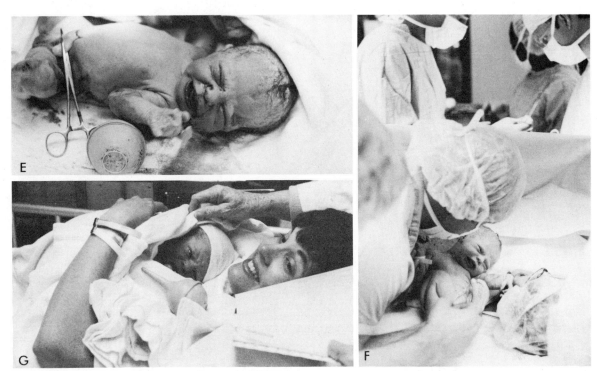

Figure 19–5 *Continued E,* It's a girl! *F,* Mom and Dad meet their daughter while the surgical team completes the cesarean delivery. *G,* With a stocking cap and blanket to prevent heat loss, Mom and Baby, along with Dad, are on their way to the recovery room.

dications to the arrest of labor, depend upon both the length of gestation and the availability of appropriately intensive nursing care to permit monitoring of both mother and fetus. Relative contraindications include less severe forms of maternal and fetal disease, premature rupture of the membranes, placenta previa at less than 35 weeks' gestation with little bleeding, erythroblastosis, and cervical dilatation between 4 and 8 cm. Because each institution will generally determine the criteria that for them represent absolute and relative contraindications, criteria for intervention will vary somewhat from one locality to another.

From a positive perspective, labor inhibition is generally utilized when the fetus is alive and between 20 and 35 weeks' gestational age, when the mother is in labor, and when there are no contraindications.

Caring for the Mother in Preterm Labor

A mother who believes she is in premature labor needs care in a hospital that has adequate nursing staff to provide closely supervised care of both mother and fetus, the capability of assessing fetal maturity, and access to neonatal resuscitation and intensive care should labor continue and a preterm infant deliver.

Initial assessment of the mother includes basic information about her health and obstetrical history and evaluation of her uterine contractions and cervix. A fetal monitor is helpful in the assessment of contractions; true contractions will appear round and smooth on the monitor. The length and frequency of contractions can also be easily assessed with the fetal monitor.

Assessment of the fetus focuses on fetal size, fetal maturity, and the presence of fetal distress. Prenatal history, ultrasound, amniocentesis to determine the L/S ratio, and fetal heart rate monitoring are all utilized. If the fetus is mature (generally defined as having an L/S ratio of greater than 2 to 1), arrest of labor is unnecessary.

Mothers and families are understandably highly anxious when they suspect premature labor. They are frequently both emotionally and physically unprepared for the labor process, and have very unrealistic fears of long-term illness or death for their infant. A primary nurse who can remain with each mother throughout the process of assessment and intervention can offer much needed support.

Bed rest (lateral position always) combined with adequate hydration, either orally or intravenously, is the initial intervention. When the mother lies on her side, the blood supply

Text continued on 567

Nursing Care Plan 19–4. Prevention and Management of Premature Labor

NURSING GOALS:
To prevent the birth of a preterm infant by preventing premature labor.

OBJECTIVES:
1. All women receive prenatal instruction, which includes recognition of signs of preterm labor.
2. The woman at risk of preterm labor is identified and receives appropriate prenatal supervision.
3. Premature labor is recognized and treated.
4. Side effects of tocolytic drugs are identified and treated immediately.

ASSESSMENT	POTENTIAL NURSING DIAGNOSIS	NURSING INTERVENTION	COMMENTS/RATIONALE

Identify woman at risk for premature labor:
 	
1. *Maternal factors*
  Low socioeconomic status
  Adolescent pregnancy
  Single marital status
  Primiparity
  Anemia
  Smoking
  Narcotic addiction
  Previous preterm birth
  Repeated induced abortion
  Chronic hypertensive vascular disease
  Severe pre-eclampsia
  Infection
    Urinary tract infection
    Amnionitis
    Syphilis
    Hepatitis
    Febrile illness
  Traumatic accidents
  Maternal weight less than 50 kg. (110 lbs.)
	At risk for premature labor	Provide frequent prenatal supervision in ambulatory setting and through home visits by community health nurse. Provide continuing nutritional assessment and intervention.
		
		Screen for urinary tract infection (UTI) on a continuing basis and treat UTI promptly. (See Nursing Care Plan 13–8.)
		
		Provide education to all pregnant women (with special attention to women at risk).
		
		1. Subtle symptoms of preterm labor.
		  a. Menstrual-like cramps
		  b. Low backache
		  c. Pelvic pressure
		  d. Change in vaginal discharge (character or amount)
		  e. Diarrhea
		  f. Increase or change in any of above signs
			One previous preterm birth is associated with a 25–50 per cent risk of subsequent preterm birth.
			
			Creasy and Herron[12a] recommend weekly prenatal visits for women at risk.
			
			Supplement teaching with written material.
			
			This system is based on the work of Creasy and Herron[12a] and Herron, Katz and Creasy.[19a]
			
			During weekly visits, cervical assessment for position, consistency, effacement and dilatation, and assessment of station is performed beginning at 24–26 weeks.

2. *Uterine factors*
   Uterine overdistention
   Multiple pregnancy
   Polyhydramnios
   Intrauterine device (IUD) left in place
   Multiple abortions
   Premature rupture of membranes
   Congenital uterine anomalies
   Incompetent cervix
3. *Fetal or Placental factors*
   Placenta previa
   Abruptio placentae
   Genetic abnormalities
   Fetal death
   Reduction in uterine blood

Identification of cervical changes (see Comments column) may be a part of assessment by nurse-midwife, nurse practitioner, or physician. If cervical changes are noted, external electronic monitoring for 1–2 hours to detect uterine contractions is suggested.

Identify early signs of premature labor:

1. Gestational age 20–37 weeks
2. Contractions less than 10 minutes apart, or 2 or more times in 15 minutes, or 8 in 60 minutes
3. Contractions last 30 seconds or longer
4. Cervical changes: beginning of dilatation or effacement

Assessment following hospitalization:

1. Maternal assessment
   a. Health history
   b. Reproductive history
   c. Fetal monitoring to document frequency and duration of uterine contractions

Possible premature labor

Premature labor

2. Teach women to differentiate contracted and relaxed uterus. Women are asked to monitor themselves twice each day and at any time the above symptoms occur.
3. Refer women with increased uterine activity to hospital.

Gravida is hospitalized.
Bed rest in lateral position.
Provide fluids (oral, intravenous).

Tocolytic drugs may be used to inhibit uterine contractions (see below and Figures 19–6 and 19–7).

In lateral position blood flow to uterus improves, muscle ischemia diminishes, contractions may stop.

Hydration improves perfusion, lowers ischemia, and may inhibit oxytocin.

Continued on following page

Nursing Care Plan 19–4.   Prevention and Management of Premature Labor (*Continued*)

ASSESSMENT	POTENTIAL NURSING DIAGNOSIS	NURSING INTERVENTION	COMMENTS/RATIONALE

2. Fetal assessment
  a. Size
  b. Maturity (L/S ratio, etc.)
  c. Status (heart rate, signs of fetal distress from fetal monitoring)
	Immature fetus
	
	Fetal distress		

3. Maternal and family reaction to premature labor	Maternal anxiety Family anxiety Guilt related to possibility of actions may have caused premature labor.	Encourage parents to verbalize concerns, express feelings.	
Identify women who should not receive tocolytic therapy.		Review maternal records, health history, and physical assessment to prevent inappropriate administration of tocolytic agents.	
1. Premature rupture of membranes 2. Cervical dilatation greater than 4 cm 3. Fetal demise 4. Congenital anomaly incompatible with life 5. Severe hemorrhage 6. Alcoholism, liver disease, diabetes (ethanol) 7. Maternal cardiovascular disease (Beta-adrenergic receptor stimulants)			

Nursing Care Related to Specific Tocolytic Agents

Assessment	Intervention	Rationale
Ethanol Identify signs of inebriation (slurred speech, disorientation, nausea and vomiting, crying)		
Signs of inebriation secondary to ethanol administration	Provide safety for mother during and following ethanol administration.	
	Explain reason for maternal behavior to women and family prior to treatment; remind family during treatment of reason for behavior.	
At risk for aspiration pneumonites	Antacids, antiemetics given	Ethanol may cause nausea. Ethanol promotes gastric secretion.
At risk for hypoglycemia	Glucose (oral or IV) given to protect against hypoglycemia	Ethanol inhibits glyconeogenesis.
Identify signs of dehydration: 1. Decreased urinary output 2. Poor skin turgor 3. Hypotension 4. Tachycardia 5. Elevated temperature		
At risk for dehydration	Provide adequate fluid intake to prevent dehydration during and following ethanol therapy.	
At risk for fetal central nervous system depression	Use nursing techniques such as relaxation and breathing to minimize need for narcotics during labor.	The combination of alcohol and narcotics may lead to severe central nervous system depression.
Identify neonatal distress in infant of mother who has received ethanol: 1. Preterm infant (Nursing Care Plan 23–2) 2. Blood glucose 3. Blood gases 4. Signs of intoxication a. Lethargy b. Apnea c. Abnormal reflexes		
At risk for hypoglycemia At risk for acidosis At risk for intoxication	See Nursing Care Plan 23–2.	
	Provide supportive care (neutral thermal environment, oxygen and ventilation as necessary, fluid with glucose, electolytes).	
Beta-Adrenergic Receptor Stimulants: Isoxsuprine (Vasodilan) Ritodrine hydrochloride (Yutopar) Terbutaline (Brethine)	See Table 19–5 for dosage, specific side effects of individual drugs.	

Continued on following page

Nursing Care Plan 19–4.   Prevention and Management of Premature Labor (*Continued*)

ASSESSMENT	POTENTIAL NURSING DIAGNOSIS	NURSING INTERVENTION	COMMENTS/RATIONALE
Assess effectiveness of medication:			
1. Electronic fetal monitoring (EFM) to identify absence of contractions	At risk for continued preterm labor.	Explain reasons for monitoring. Teach women the feeling of a relaxed uterus.	
2. Uterus relaxed by palpation			
Identify side effects:			
1. Hypotension and tachycardia. Assess vital signs every minute until they begin to stabilize, then every 3 minutes until stable, then every 15 to 30 minutes following initial administration and each time the level of drugs is changed.	Decreased blood pressure, increased heart rate secondary to tocolytic drug	Maintain blood pressure at 90/60 or greater. Provide intravenous hydration.	
		Encourage side-lying position to minimize supine hypotension.	
2. Hypervolemia: monitor intake/output			
3. Complaint of substernal pain.	Substernal pain secondary to increased force of heart contractions related to tocolytic drug		
4. Blood glucose: identify hyperglycemia	Hyperglycemia secondary to glucogenolysis	Assess blood glucose in infant.	
	Risk of infant hypoglycemia		
5. Monitor fetal heart rate (EFM)	At risk for fetal tachycardia secondary to drug	See Nursing Care Plan 18–1.	
	At risk for fetal bradycardia secondary to maternal hypotension		
6. Monitor serum potassium	At risk for hypokalemia	Potassium will be added to fluids to correct electrolyte imbalance.	
After contractions have ceased	Need for information about maintenance of oral tocolytic therapy	Explain significance of maintaining correct dosage of tocolytic drug following discharge from hospital.	
	Need for information about appropriate action if contractions return	Explain need to contact health-care provider at first indication of labor (above).	

Table 19–4. EFFECTIVENESS OF INTERVENTION STRATEGIES IN PREMATURE LABOR

Method	Effectiveness (Per Cent)
Bed rest, lateral recumbent position	40–70
Ethanol	65–70
Beta-adrenergic receptor stimulants	60–90

to the uterus improves. Because ischemic muscle contracts, this improvement in blood supply may stop contractions. Rapid hydration, by expanding blood volume, may also improve perfusion and, in addition, may inhibit oxytocin release by a mechanism within the distended left auricle of the heart.[5] For some women, rest and hydration will be the only treatment needed (Table 19–4).

If uterine contractions continue and cervical changes are present, myometrial tocolytic drugs may be used to stop contractions. Because these drugs are most effective in early labor, careful nursing assessment of each woman's status is essential. When contractions are more frequent than two in 15 minutes and cervical changes are present, administration of a tocolytic agent is started soon after admission assessment.

Tocolytic Treatment. Drugs that inhibit uterine contractions are called myometrial tocolytic agents. There are four major drugs or groups of drugs:

1. Progestogens.
2. Antioxytocic agents.
3. Beta-sympathomimetic drugs.
4. Magnesium sulfate.

Progestogens. *Endogenous progestogens,* such as progesterone, function to maintain pregnancy by preventing uterine contractions. Progestogens have not been found effective in arresting labor once it has started but may prevent or delay preterm labor in women at risk.[21] Progestogens have been implicated in the masculinization of the female fetus if they are taken by the mother early in pregnancy; there is no evidence that this is a problem later in pregnancy at the time a tocolytic agent would be used. In Johnson's study no adverse neonatal effects were found.

Antioxytocic Agents. Oxytocin is a hormone that has a major influence on uterine contractions. An antioxytocin may either prevent oxytocin release or block the action of oxytocin on the myometrium.

Ethanol inhibits the release of oxytocin; it does not appear to exert a direct effect on myometrial contractility. Ethanol may also improve uterine blood flow (thereby reducing contractions) and inhibit prostaglandin formation (prostaglandins are a factor in uterine contractions). An initial loading dose of 7.5 to 15 ml./kg. of body weight is given IV for 2 hours, followed by a maintenance dose of 1.5 ml./kg. The infusion is continued for 6 hours after contractions have stopped. Reloading may be necessary. If labor occurs for a third time within a 72-hour period, further treatment with alcohol is considered of little value.

Ethanol treatment is unpleasant for the mother and her family. The ethanol concentration in the blood is in the range of 150 ± 45 mg./dl., the upper limit for intoxication.[7] The mother may exhibit any of the signs of inebriation—slurred speech, disorientation, nausea, and vomiting, crying, and the like. All of this must be explained to both the woman and her family prior to the initiation of treatment; reminders during treatment that her behavior is due to ethanol are also important. Antacids and antiemetics are given as a protection from aspiration pneumonitis, a potential problem because of nausea and because ethanol promotes gastric secretion. Glucose is given to protect against hypoglycemia, which may result from the inhibition of glyconeogenesis by ethanol. The possibility of hypoglycemia is reduced by intravenous dextrose and by encouraging oral intake. Because ethanol causes diuresis through the inhibition of antidiuretic hormone (ADH) from the posterior pituitary, women must be observed for possible dehydration. Careful intake and output records and assessment of signs of dehydration (decreased output, poor skin turgor, decreased blood pressure, increased temperature, and heart rate) are essential. Adequate fluid intake is important after ethanol therapy is discontinued to prevent dehydration at that time.

Should ethanol therapy fail to inhibit labor, drugs that potentiate the action of alcohol (narcotics, sedatives, antihistamines) should be avoided during labor. Nursing support using relaxation and breathing techniques is far more appropriate than drugs that may result in severe central nervous system depression in the newborn. Even without the addition of other drugs, preparation for special newborn care from the moment of birth is important for an infant who is both preterm and may be depressed by ethanol. Infants are assessed for hypoglycemia, acidosis, and signs of intoxication (including lethargy, apnea, and abnormal reflexes).

Ethanol therapy is not used in women with a history of alcoholism or uncompensated liver

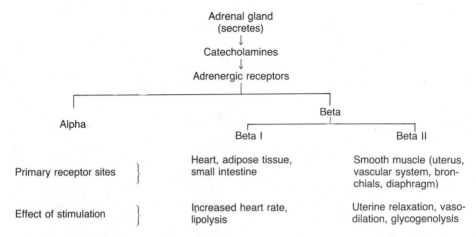

Figure 19–6. The relationship between the adrenal gland, adrenergic receptors, and beta-adrenergic receptor stimulants.

disease, and rarely in mothers with diabetes. With the advent of the beta-adrenergic receptor stimulants (below), ethanol is used far less frequently than in the past decade.

Beta-Adrenergic Receptor Stimulants. It has been recognized since 1948 that the action of catecholamines on beta-adrenergic receptors in smooth muscle, including smooth muscle of the uterus, causes relaxation (Fig. 19–6). Several beta-II adrenergic receptor stimulants are currently in use for the inhibition of premature labor. The most widely used in the United States at this time are isoxsuprine (Vasodilan), ritodrine hydrochloride (Youtopar), and terbutaline (Brethine). Although the effects of each drug are generally similar, nurses must also recognize how the specific effects of each

differ (Fig. 19–7). Initial therapy with each drug is usually intravenous using an infusion pump and a "piggyback" set-up. Subsequently, the mother may receive parenteral therapy with isoxsuprine and terbutaline, and oral maintenance with all three drugs. Oral medication may begin prior to discontinuing the IV. The dosages of all drugs are carefully evaluated in relation to uterine contractions, maternal pulse and heart rate, and fetal heart rate. As more experience is gained using these drugs to inhibit premature labor, dosage recommendations may change. None of the drugs has been shown to be effective prior to 20 weeks' gestation and should not be used before this time.

Nursing care is directed toward:

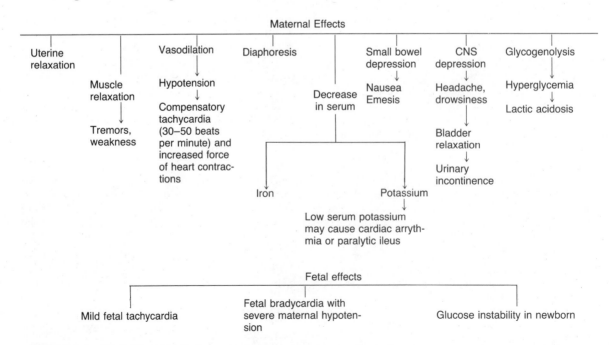

Figure 19–7. Maternal and fetal effects of beta-adrenergic receptor stimulants.

Table 19–5.   BETA-ADRENERGIC RECEPTOR STIMULANTS

Drug	Isoxsuprine	Ritodrine	Terbutaline
Regimen:			
IV Initial dose	0.25–0.5 mg./min.	0.05 mg./min.	10 mg./min. or bolus 0.25 mg.
Maximum dose	1.0 mg./min.	0.3 mg./min.	10–80 mg./min.
Maintain (time)	60–90 min. to 12–14 hr.	12 hr.	1 hr., then decrease to lowest effective dose
Parenteral	5–20 mg. IM every 3–6 hr. for 1–2 days		0.25 mg. sub four times a day to every 4 hr., for 3 days
Oral therapy	5–20 mg. every 3–6 hr.	5–10 mg. every 4–6 hr. up to 15–20 mg. every 6 hr.	2.5–5 mg.
Total length of treatment	Until moderate physical activity resumed	Until 37–38 weeks' gestation	Until 36 weeks
Maternal side effects (see also Fig. 19–7 for general side effects)	Hypotension, tachycardia (with or without hypotension), chest pain Acidosis in diabetic mother Maternal pulmonary edema, adult RDS Decreased serum iron, potassium	Tachycardia Chest pain (higher heart force) Hyperglycemia Maternal pulmonary edema, adult RDS Decreased serum iron, potassium	Tachycardia Chest pain (higher heart force) Tremors Palpitations Dizziness Maternal pulmonary edema, adult RDS
Fetal side effects	Fetal tachycardia Hypoglycemia	Fetal tachycardia Hypoglycemia	Fetal tachycardia Hypoglycemia
Comments		More specific beta-II receptor stimulator than isoxsuprine	Selective beta-II receptor stimulator

1. Assessing the effectiveness of the medication.

2. Preventing deleterious side effects.

3. Reassuring the mother and family by making the mother as comfortable as possible and interpreting the sensations she may be feeling as a result of the medication to her and her family.

The effectiveness of the medication is assessed through electronic fetal monitoring and through palpation of the relaxed uterus. Side effects vary markedly from one woman to another. *Hypotension* secondary to vasodilation and tachycardia are assessed by blood pressure and pulse measurements every minute until they begin to stabilize, then every 3 minutes until stable. Once stable, vital signs are recorded every 15 to 30 minutes. Each time the level of drugs is changed, the assessment regimen is repeated. Blood pressure is maintained at 90/60 or greater. Immediate hydration with 500 to 1000 ml. of intravenous fluid is usual; intake and output must be carefully monitored to prevent overhydration. Pulmonary edema has been reported as a side effect of these drugs.[2] A side-lying position and the use of hypertonic or isotonic IV solutions may minimize hypotension.

Maternal tachycardia, which is usually a compensatory reaction to hypotension, may increase from 30 to 50 beats per minute or greater. If either hypotension or tachycardia exceeds the parameters established for an individual woman, the drug is discontinued and supportive intervention, including the Trendelenberg position (with the mother lying on her side), is begun. The increased force of heart contractions causes some women to complain of substernal pain.

Assessment of serum glucose levels monitors potential hyperglycemia due to glycogenolysis. Physiologic saline, administered through the intravenous line, may prevent serious hyperglycemia.[7] When the mother has hyperglycemia, subsequent hypoglycemia in the infant following birth must be assessed carefully, just as it is in the infant of a diabetic mother.

Fetal heart rate is continually monitored. Fetal tachycardia as a direct result of the drug, and fetal bradycardia as a response to maternal hypotension and subsequent decreased placental perfusion and oxygenation, are both possible.

Serum potassium is assessed periodically and appropriate correction made. The side effects of beta-adrenergic receptor stimulants cause them to be contraindicated in women with heart disease and relatively contraindicated in women with hypertension, thyroid disease, or diabetes mellitus.

Magnesium Sulfate. Although magnesium sulfate ($MgSO_4$) does not yet have FDA approval as a tocolytic agent, it is being used experimentally for that purpose in some tertiary centers. Its side effects and nursing precautions are discussed in Chapter 13.

Follow-up. Once premature labor has been halted, the mother is gradually shifted to oral maintenance therapy. She must understand the importance of maintaining the correct dosage and also the importance of rehospitalization should contractions begin again. The care she receives during a first hospitalization may be an important factor in her willingness to undergo subsequent tocolysis. Her feeling that she is welcome at the hospital and that she and her baby are very important to the staff cannot be overlooked.

Any mother who has had premature labor in one pregnancy is at risk for this condition during a subsequent gestation. She should know that should she become pregnant again she should seek early prenatal care from a practitioner who is able to provide comprehensive services for the prevention of prematurity.

When Premature Labor Cannot Be Stopped

If it is at all possible, the mother should be admitted to a medical center that is equipped to care for a preterm baby. Transporting a fetus in utero presents far fewer hazards than transporting an immature infant. Moreover, there are real advantages to having both mother and baby in the same hospital to facilitate bonding. Admittedly, that choice is not always available.

The delivery of a preterm infant must be even more gentle than a delivery at term. The cranial bones are poorly calcified and offer little protection to the brain; the danger of cerebral hemorrhage resulting in death or brain damage is a very real one. A large episiotomy and very careful use of forceps are attempts to prevent injury to the baby's brain.

Little or no analgesia is used in order to prevent respiratory depression. Techniques of relaxation and breathing described in previous chapters are often very helpful to mothers during premature labor.

Because the baby may need resuscitation at birth and other medical attention and because he is at risk of hypothermia (Chapter 23), it is rarely possible for the mother and father to hold their baby during the time following birth. If at all possible, and especially if the baby is to be transferred to another hospital, they should have the opportunity to see and touch him. In addition, they must be kept aware of his condition and taken to the nursery to see him as soon as possible (see also Chapters 23 and 28).

Labor Following Prolonged Pregnancy

A prolonged pregnancy is one that exceeds 42 completed weeks' gestation. From 5 to 15 per cent of all pregnancies are prolonged. Very young mothers and mothers over 35 appear to have a higher incidence of prolonged pregnancy.

The reason for prolonged pregnancy in most instances is unclear. Many pregnancies suspected to be prolonged may actually be a result of a mistake in dating. In infants with anencephaly, the absence of an intact pituitary-adrenal axis in the fetus is believed to be important, but these infants account for only a small part of prolonged pregnancies.

The majority of infants born following a prolonged pregnancy have continued to grow. However, about 20 to 40 per cent of infants who are "postmature" reflect varying degrees of decreased placental perfusion and thus decreased intrauterine nutrition (see Chapter 23 for infant characteristics).

Intrapartum risk factors in postterm pregnancies include intrapartum fetal distress, meconium-stained amniotic fluid, and increased fetal size (macrosomia). Uteroplacental insufficiency may cause oligohydramnios, subsequent umbilical cord compression, and the possibility of meconium passage and meconium aspiration.

Although some practitioners argue for intervention after 42 weeks' gestation, the relatively frequent inaccuracy of gestational dating leads others to prefer fetal assessment. Nonstress tests, twice weekly contraction stress tests to detect late decelerations (uteroplacental insufficiency) and variable decelerations (cord compression), ultrasound to detect oligohydramnios, and estriol and human placental lactogen measures are the techniques most commonly used. Expectant parents need frequent reassurance during the period past their expected date of delivery. If the expected date of delivery (EDC) was presented early in pregnancy as an approximate time period it will be easier for them to accept variability later. Freeman[15] reported a study of 679 postdate women surveyed with contraction stress tests in which there were no perinatal deaths and no greater neonatal morbidity than in a control group of 500 women at term. Additional data of this type could help to reassure women with prolonged pregnancies that with surveillance their fetus is not in jeopardy.

Labor In A Multiple Gestation Pregnancy

Just as the antepartal period may be complicated when there is more than one fetus (Chapter 14), so too may labor. Twins often deliver prior to term, thus presenting the same problems of labor and premature delivery as those described above. The second twin, and the second and subsequent infants in other multiple deliveries, is particularly at risk.

The delivery of the first twin is similar to that of other preterm infants. The presentation and condition of the second infant is then evaluated; he may be delivered shortly after the first baby, or a period of time may elapse before the second twin is ready for delivery. The presenting part may change several times before it is finally engaged and delivered.

Friedman and Little[14a] report that second twins born between 2½ and 15 minutes after the first twin fared best; mortality rates tripled if delivery was either sooner or later.

This is a most difficult time for parents. The first infant may be in poor condition, requiring resuscitation. The wait for the delivery of the second twin may seem far longer than the actual time involved. It is a time of "not knowing," which is always hard to cope with. Sometimes the professional staff is so involved in delivery and resuscitation that the anxious parents are overlooked. They need to know what is happening.

Not every multiple birth is equally hazardous. Recently, our intensive care nursery was notified that a mother with twins and a second mother with triplets were expected to deliver within 2 or 3 hours. We prepared for five admissions, but all of the triplets were healthy babies close to 5 pounds in weight who were able to be cared for in the full-term nursery and were discharged along with their mother when they were 4 days old. Only the preterm twins required intensive care.

The mother who delivers more than one infant usually has an overdistended uterus and is at risk of developing postpartum hemorrhage. Very careful observation during the fourth stage of labor and after she returns to the postpartal unit is essential.

Labor and Birth in Mothers Over 35 Years of Age

Kessler[23] reports that the spontaneous onset of labor is less frequent in primiparas over 35 in comparison with both younger primiparas and older multiparas. There was no significant difference, however, between the latter groups. As a result of decreased spontaneous labor in these women there is an increase in induced labor.[6, 23, 28]

Very little information is available concerning the progress of labor in women over 35 years old. Cohen and his colleagues[12] examined the effects of age in 6248 parturients; they found that the active phase of labor and the descent of the head was more likely to be prolonged in women over 35 who were nulliparas than in younger women; this was not true of multiparas. The difference was not related to analgesia, anesthesia, or CPD. The authors speculated that perhaps the myometrium became less efficient, although there is no current physiologic evidence to support this theory. A prolonged active phase may lead to a decision for cesarean birth; the incidence of cesarean birth is increased in women over 35, as is the incidence of vacuum extraction and forceps delivery.

Although the few available studies vary, most report no significant increase in maternal mortality in older mothers. Perinatal mortality (mortality of the fetus or newborn) is frequently increased in older primiparas.[20, 23]

The incidence of postpartum complications is unclear; an increased risk of postpartum hemorrhage and retained placenta has been suggested.

Coping With Emergencies During the Four Stages of Labor

Rupture of the Uterus

When labor does not progress for any of a variety of reasons mentioned in this chapter or when contractions are very intense, usually because of oxytocin infusion, rupture of the uterus may occur. Frequently, the baby is seriously damaged or dies; maternal mortality is from 5 to 10 per cent (see Nursing Care Plan 19–5).

Uterine rupture is usually sudden, accompanied by a sharp abdominal pain. The mother has symptoms of shock. Both uterine contractions and fetal heart tones cease. Hemorrhage may occur into the peritoneal cavity rather than into the vagina.

Nursing Care Plan 19–5.   Management of the Mother with Ruptured Uterus

NURSING GOAL:
To maintain maternal and fetal well-being.
OBJECTIVES:
The mother will:
1. Know the implications of a ruptured uterus.
2. Be prepared for an immediate cesarean delivery.
Her partner and family will be informed on maternal and fetal status.

ASSESSMENT	POTENTIAL NURSING DIAGNOSIS	NURSING INTERVENTION	COMMENTS/RATIONALE
1. Risk factors associated with ruptured uterus: a. Previous cesarean delivery b. Obstetric trauma c. Mismanagement of oxytocin induction	At risk for uterine rupture	Careful administration of oxytocin (Nursing Care Plan 19–1) Attention to warning signs	
2. Warning signs of impending uterine rupture: a. Restlessness, anxiety from strong uterine contractions b. No labor progress c. Presence of lower uterine segment ballooning out and a retraction ring, along with tenderness above the symphysis	Need to prepare mother for emergency cesarean delivery due to ruptured uterus	Carefully assess mother; do not leave alone. Notify physician.	

3. Signs and symptoms of ruptured uterus:
   a. Excruciating pain
   b. Cessation of uterine contractions
   c. Vaginal hemorrhage

Alert physician of signs, symptoms of ruptured uterus.
Immediately proceed with interventions for unplanned cesarean delivery (Nursing Care Plan 19–3).
Initiate oxygen therapy by face shield at 6–8 liters/minute.
Monitor blood pressure, pulse, respirations, and fetal heart rate.

Position mother on left side until delivery.
Observe for signs of shock.
Inform mother and father of significance of ruptured uterus and reasons for quick nursing actions.
Be prepared (equipment and personnel) to resuscitate newborn (Nursing Care Plan 23–1).

If a ruptured uterus is not detected for a long period, peritonitis may occur.
If a ruptured uterus is not treated, shock and death may result.
The mother and father will be frightened. More detailed explanations may be given during the recovery period.

Following delivery
Assess as high risk cesarean birth (Nursing Care Plan 19–2)

Assess hemoglobin, hematocrit (potential for significant blood loss)

Ascertain if hysterectomy performed

Nursing Care Plan 19–2
Grief related to hysterectomy

Nursing Care Plan 19–2

Answer questions, encourage verbalization of feelings about hysterectomy as well as cause of uterine rupture.

Contributed by Mona B. Ketner

Immediate recognition and intervention are essential; immediate hysterectomy is usually the course taken.

Prevention, by careful evaluation of the mother throughout labor, and intervention, when labor fails to progress, can avert most instances of rupture of the uterus.

Complications of the Placenta

The two most common complications involving the placenta, placenta previa and abruption of the placenta, have been discussed in Chapter 13.

Several variations in placental development may cause intrapartum or postpartum problems. Careful examination of the placenta following delivery is essential for identification of these problems and the prevention of potential complications.

A *succenturiate placenta* has one or more accessory lobes of fetal origin. If the accessory lobe (or lobes) separates from the main body of the placenta and is retained within the uterus, the uterus cannot contract firmly, and serious postpartum hemorrhage is possible. Intrauterine fetal hemorrhage may also occur; the fetus will be pale and cyanotic with a weak pulse, tachycardia, and tachypnea. Inspection of the placenta may reveal that blood vessels are torn at the margin.

In a *circumvallate placenta* (Fig. 19–8) a double layer of amnion and chorion forms a whitish ring that covers varying amounts of the fetal side of the placenta, leaving the central portion exposed. Prior to birth a circumvallate placenta may cause placental abruption, prematurity, or fetal death. Maternal hemorrhage at the time of or following placental separation may occur because of abnormalities during the separation process.

In a *battledore placenta* the cord is inserted at or near the placental margin. The risk of cord compression, rupture of the umbilical vessels, and preterm delivery is increased.

A *placenta accreta* is attached so closely to the myometrium that separation is difficult and there is a possibility of hemorrhage. The extent of placenta accreta varies from contact of the villi with, but no penetration of, the endometrium (placenta accreta vera), to penetration of the myometrium (placenta increta) or penetration through the myometrium to the adjacent structures (placenta percreta). Placenta accreta vera is most common, placenta percreta least common. Frequently, small areas of the placenta rather than the entire surface are involved, and those fragments of placenta are retained when the placenta is delivered.

It is theorized that a defective endometrium may be the cause; placenta accreta is frequently associated with placenta previa (where implantation is low) and with previous cesarean deliveries in which scar tissue is present.

Again, inspection of the placenta to ascer-

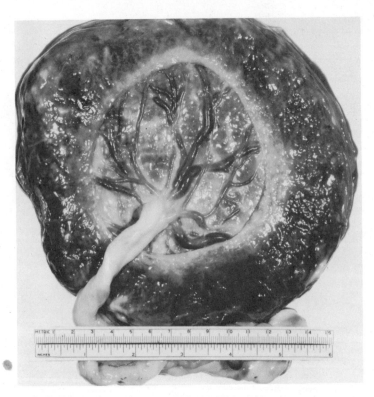

Figure 19–8. Circumvallate placenta (From Page, Villee, and Villee: *Human Reproduction,* 3rd Edition. Philadelphia, W. B. Saunders Co., 1981.)

tain whether fragments are missing is essential. Frequently, hysterectomy is required to control bleeding.

A large number of placental infarcts or evidence of calcification may indicate compromised fetal nutrition and gas exchange prior to delivery. Infants should be observed carefully, particularly for signs of hypoglycemia.

Prolapse of the Umbilical Cord

When the umbilical cord is at the level of the presenting part or below the presenting part, the cord is said to be *prolapsed* (Fig. 19–9). This is a serious complication because pressure on the cord prevents the fetus from receiving oxygen and can cause serious brain damage or death if intervention is not rapid and successful (see Nursing Care Plan 19–6). If the cord prolapses outside of the vagina, umbilical vessels may constrict, also compromising fetal oxygen supply.

The risk of a prolapsed cord is higher under certain circumstances:

1. The membranes rupture before the presenting part is engaged.
2. The presentation is breech or transverse.
3. The infant is preterm.
4. The pregnancy is a multiple gestation.
5. Hydramnios is present.

A prolapse of the cord most commonly occurs following rupture of the membranes. For this reason the mother and fetus are carefully assessed at that time. Observe the mother for protrusion of the cord from the vagina (seen sometimes but not always), meconium staining of the amniotic fluid, or the passage of meconium. (If the presentation is breech, meconium does not necessarily indicate fetal distress.)

Fetal heart rate changes and variable decelerations on the fetal heart monitor are fetal indications of cord prolapse and compression.

Nursing Intervention. The goal of nursing intervention is to relieve pressure on the cord. At the same time, it is necessary to calm and support the mother so that she can cooperate in her own care. This mother must have constant nursing attendance; a second nurse must find the physician if one is not present in the delivery room.

Pressure on the cord is relieved by elevating the mother's hips on a pillow or by helping the mother to assume a knee-chest position (Figs. 19–10 and 19–11). Oxygen is given by mask to the mother in order to provide the highest possible level to the fetus. If the cord is protruding, it should be kept moist with sterile saline. Delivery should be as quick as possible by cesarean.

Should a mother experience a prolapsed cord

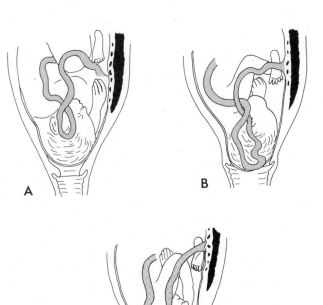

Figure 19–9. Prolapse of the umbilical cord. *A,* Occult prolapse. Because the membranes are unruptured, there is little pressure on the cord. *B,* Forelying cord. There may be pressure on the cord. *C,* Prolapsed cord with a high risk of cord compression.

Nursing Care Plan 19–6. Management of the Mother with Prolapsed Umbilical Cord

NURSING GOAL:
To maintain fetal well-being.
OBJECTIVES:
The mother will:
1. Know the significance of prolapsed umbilical cord.
2. Experience preparation for emergency delivery of the baby.

ASSESSMENT	POTENTIAL NURSING DIAGNOSIS	NURSING INTERVENTION	COMMENTS/RATIONALE
1. Observe for predisposing factors: breech or shoulder presentation, transverse lie, rupture of membranes, multiple gestation, small fetus, long cord, polyhydramnios. Identify prolapsed cord.	At risk for prolapsed cord related to (specific reason). Need to prepare mother for immediate delivery due to prolapsed umbilical cord.	Relieve pressure of presenting part on cord manually by leaving gloved fingers in vagina continuously until delivery.	This is a life-saving measure for the fetus in order to maintain fetal circulation.
2. Check cord for pulsation. Continuously monitor fetal heart tones; observe for decelerations.	Fetus at risk related to prolapsed umbilical cord	Notify physician. Proceed with interventions for unplanned cesarean delivery. Have mother assume knee-chest position or adjust bed to Trendelenburg position.	If the cord does not pulsate this may indicate fetal death. Fetal distress is common due to pressure on the cord. Cesarean delivery is the treatment of choice prior to complete cervical dilatation. The force of gravity may help to relieve cord compression.
		Wrap the cord in sterile saline soaks if the cord prolapses out of the introitus. Do not push cord back into uterus. Inform mother of the danger of umbilical cord prolapse and reason for nursing actions.	Wrapping the cord helps to decrease the chance of uterine infections. Pushing the cord back could traumatize the cord.

Contributed by Mona B. Ketner

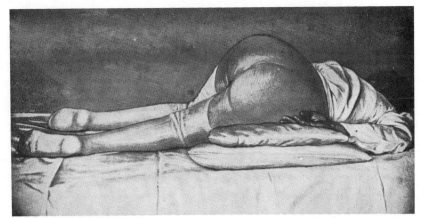

Figure 19–10. One approach to managing the prolapsed cord is the elevated Sim's position, whereby the pelvis is raised on pillows above the level of the uterine fundus. (From Greenhill and Friedman: *Biological Principles and Modern Practice of Obstetrics.* Philadelphia, W. B. Saunders Co., 1974.)

when she is not in the hospital (usually at the time of rupture of the membranes), she must be hospitalized as quickly as possible. In a car or ambulance, the same principles of care apply:

1. Elevate hips.
2. Give oxygen if available.
3. Apply a moist covering to the cord.

Amniotic Fluid Embolism

If amniotic fluid enters the mother's circulatory system, an embolus may form in the arterioles or capillaries of the pulmonary circulation, resulting in fetal and maternal death (see Nursing Care Plan 19–7).

The mother receiving oxytocin who has rapid, intense contractions is most at risk; hence the careful monitoring of the mother receiving oxytocin is important. (This has been emphasized previously but can hardly be overstressed.) A multipara with a large fetus is also at increased risk.

How does the amniotic fluid enter the mother's circulation? Potential pathways include:

1. Rupture of the membranes into the upper uterine segment, with entry through the site of the placenta.
2. Partial separation of the placenta, which exposes blood vessels in the myometrium.
3. Rupture of the uterus.
4. Entry through the endocervical veins.

When these conditions occur, very strong contractions may force amniotic fluid into the circulation. The mother will quickly become dyspneic and cyanotic. Immediate intervention is aimed at relieving respiratory distress by administration of oxygen and change of position and summoning assistance.

A side effect of amniotic fluid embolism is disseminated intravascular coagulation (DIC) (Chapter 13), related to the thromboplastic properties of amniotic fluid. Thus, the mother must be constantly evaluated for symptoms of hemorrhage and shock.

To be in labor and to suddenly find that you are unable to breathe is understandably overwhelming for the mother and whoever is with her. They should never be left alone for both physiologic and supportive reasons.

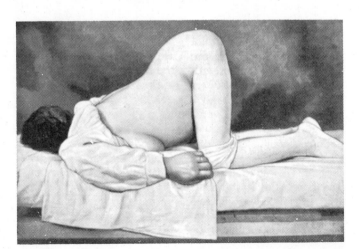

Figure 19–11. A useful method of displacing the head out of the pelvis to relieve cord compression by placing the patient in the knee-chest position. (From Greenhill and Friedman: *Biological Principles and Modern Practice of Obstetrics.* Philadelphia, W. B. Saunders Co., 1974.)

Nursing Care Plan 19–7. Management of the Mother with Amniotic Fluid Embolism

NURSING GOAL:
To maintain maternal and fetal homeostasis.

OBJECTIVES:
The mother will:
1. Know the significance of amniotic fluid embolism.
2. Experience preparation of immediate delivery of her baby; her partner and family will be informed of maternal and fetal status.

ASSESSMENT	POTENTIAL NURSING DIAGNOSIS	NURSING INTERVENTION	COMMENTS/RATIONALE
1. Presence of risk factors associated with amniotic fluid embolism: difficult and rapid labor, oxytocin induction, artificial rupture of membranes, placental separation, cervical tears.	At risk of amniotic fluid embolism Need to maintain maternal vital signs at minimal level to maintain life past delivery	Alert physician of signs of amniotic fluid embolism. Proceed with interventions for unplanned cesarean delivery (Nursing Care Plan 19–3). Initiate oxygen therapy by face shield at 6–8 liters/minute.	Amniotic fluid embolism may occur during or after a difficult and rapid labor. Fluid may leak into the chorionic plate and enter maternal circulation with rupture of membranes, uterine rupture, and placental separation.
2. Presence of signs of amniotic fluid embolism: chest pain, dyspnea, tachycardia, cyanosis, hemorrhage.	Need to prepare mother for immediate cesarean delivery or forceps delivery due to embolism.	Monitor blood pressure, pulse, respirations, and fetal heart tones. Monitor amount of vaginal bleeding. Observe for signs of shock. Position on left side until delivery. Constant presence of nurse important. Prepare for blood transfusion and insertion of a CVP line. Prepare for fibrinogen replacement. Inform mother and father of the significance of amniotic fluid embolism and the reasons for nursing actions. Be prepared (equipment and personnel) to resuscitate newborn (Nursing Care Plan 23–1).	Maternal mortality is very high. Immediate nursing care is essential if the mother's life is to be saved. DIC may result in acute hemorrhage. Fluid overload could occur. Maternal venous return is optimal while on left side; mother and father will be apprehensive and they will need reassurance; additional explanations may be given during the recovery period after delivery.

Contributed by Mona B. Ketner.

Maternal Conditions Requiring Modification of Care During Labor

Care during labor is modified for mothers with particular problems. The most common conditions are pre-eclampsia (or pregnancy-induced hypertension) diabetes, and heart disease.

The Mother with Pregnancy-Induced Hypertension

When a mother has severe pregnancy-induced hypertension (Chapter 13), her care is directed toward (1) improving her condition, and (2) determining the maturity and condition of the fetus.

The aim of her care is to control the manifestations of her disease until the fetus shows evidence of being sufficiently mature for extrauterine existence (Chapter 14).

Once the fetus is believed to be mature, labor is induced by amniotomy and oxytocin infusion (see above). Mother and fetus are carefully monitored, and should be watched especially for symptoms of pre-eclampsia–eclampsia in the mother and for fetal distress. The fetus is at risk because the blood supply to the placenta is often compromised.

The mother who has been receiving magnesium sulfate prior to labor will continue to receive the medication during labor and into the postpartum period. All of the precautions discussed in Chapter 13 continue to apply.

Induction is not always possible. It may have been attempted and failed. The cervix may not appear to be ready ("ripe"). For these and other reasons, cesarean delivery may be necessary.

Regardless of the type of delivery, there is the possibility of a high risk infant; adequate personnel and equipment must be ready to care for a sick baby.

Following delivery, the mother with eclampsia continues to need especially careful observation. Because of the reduced circulating blood volume that is characteristic of pregnancy-induced hypertension, blood loss following delivery must be kept at a minimum. Frequent assessment, fundal massage, and an empty bladder facilitate this goal.

Blood pressure and urine output must be interpreted together. If blood pressure decreases and urine output increases, the disease process is resolving. If both blood pressure and urine output decrease, hemorrhage must be suspected. Increased or unchanged blood pressure indicates that the disease process continues. The mother is at risk of seizures until she has started to diurese, which may be as late as 48 hours after the birth of her baby. If she remains in an obstetric intensive care unit and if her baby is in an intensive care nursery, it may be difficult to provide contact between mother and baby. Any action that can promote her attachment—a Polaroid picture of her baby or a careful description of his condition and care—is very important.

Once diuresis occurs, blood pressure usually returns to prepregnancy levels, edema disappears, and the mother is no longer at risk.

The Mother with Diabetes

Labor and Delivery. The last 3 to 4 weeks of pregnancy are particularly hazardous to the fetus of a diabetic mother; mortality is high, possibly because of inadequate placental function.

When the fetus is judged mature on the basis of the tests described in Chapter 13, or when his status is obviously deteriorating, he is delivered. Formerly, a large number of babies of diabetic mothers were delivered by cesarean; today, in some facilities, diabetic mothers may labor with careful monitoring of the fetus. Regular insulin and intravenous glucose are given to the mother on the day of delivery, when she is allowed nothing by mouth. Maternal glucose levels are assessed every 30 minutes; the level is kept between 60 and 100 mg./dl.[26] Insulin is discontinued at the time of delivery. If the mother is allowed to become hyperglycemic, the newborn is at increased risk of hypoglycemia (see Infants of Diabetic Mothers, Chapter 23).

Perinatal mortality statistics suggest that no diabetic mother should be allowed to continue her pregnancy beyond the expected date of delivery.

Following Delivery. When the placenta is delivered, a major source of insulin antagonism is removed very suddenly from the mother's body. Insulin needs drop dramatically; less insulin may be required than prior to pregnancy. Some mothers require no insulin during the first 24 to 48 hours after delivery. The mother will need both close monitoring of her serum glucose and support during this period of reregulation of her diet and insulin.

Because her baby may be in an intensive care nursery during the first hours and perhaps days after birth (Chapter 23), she will also need supportive nursing care to help her deal with her fears and other feelings about the baby (Chapter 28).

About 6 to 9 months following delivery, insulin requirements will probably be at prepregnancy levels. This means that long-term follow-up will be necessary for mothers with diabetes. The single check-up at 4 to 6 weeks is not appropriate. Contraceptive instruction prior to discharge from the hospital is also important; a pregnancy immediately following delivery would not be advisable.

The Mother with Heart Disease

The impact of labor on the maternal cardiovascular system (Chapter 15) makes labor a time of risk for women with heart disease. Cardiac output, stroke volume, and blood pressure increase; heart rate initially decreases and then increases.

Mothers with heart disease are normally delivered vaginally. Cesarean delivery is performed only if there is an obstetric reason, such as cephalopelvic disproportion. Cardiac disease per se is not an indication for cesarean delivery.

During labor, as during pregnancy, the goal is to decrease cardiac load. The amount of work done by the woman herself is minimized. This mother labors in the semi-Fowler's position and at times on her side. Supine hypotensive syndrome (Chapter 7) is particularly dangerous for her, so she should never lie flat on her back.

Several specific measures are important in protecting the mother with heart disease during labor. This mother should be very closely supervised, not just by mechanical monitoring, although this will probably be a part of her care, but also by close nursing observation. Her vital signs, particularly pulse, respirations, and blood pressure, must be checked and recorded more frequently than those of an apparently healthy mother.

If she is receiving intravenous fluids, the rate is closely monitored to prevent fluid overload and subsequent congestive failure. Should heart failure occur, the treatment is medical: morphine, oxygen by mask, intravenous digitalis, and a diuretic such as furosemide (Lasix).

Every effort is made to reduce the levels of anxiety and of pain, which may in themselves lead to heart failure. Although this should be the goal for every mother, special effort must be made for the mother with cardiac disease. Continuous caudal or epidural anesthesia may be used for this purpose; spinal anesthesia is not used for mothers with cardiac disease because of the effect on the cardiovascular system (Chapter 17).

Antibiotics may be given to prevent the possibility of endocarditis.

The mother with heart disease should not "push" during the second stage. Frequently she is anesthetized to prevent pushing. If there is no progress after 30 to 60 minutes, the delivery may be assisted with forceps.

The position for delivery is the semi-Fowler's position, with the legs supported at the level of the heart or below.

During the third stage of labor (1) fluid moves from the extravascular space to the vascular tree, and (2) blood from the lower extremities flows unobstructed toward the heart with the emptying of the uterus and the removal of pressure on the vena cava. Thus during the third and fourth stages mothers must be observed very carefully for signs of heart failure.

SUMMARY

Mothers with a labor that varies from normal need both emotional support to help them cope with the unexpected variations and the anxiety and fear that accompany the unknown and careful, knowledgeable attention to the physiologic aspects of their care. Families must not be excluded in the care of these mothers.

REFERENCES

1. Abdul-Karim, R., and Beydoun, S.: Premature Labor. *In* Iffy, L., and Kaminetzky, H. (eds.): *Principles and Practice of Obstetrics and Perinatology.* New York, John Wiley, 1981.
2. Adverse Reactions from Treating Premature Labor with Beta Agonists. *FDA Drug Bulletin,* 11(2):13, 1981.
3. Baggish, M.: Vacuum Extraction. *In* Iffy, L., and Kaminetzky, H. (eds.): *Principles and Practice of Obstetrics and Perinatology,* Volume 2. New York, John Wiley, 1981.
4. Bernstine, R.: Uterotonic Agents. *In* Iffy, L., and Kaminetzky, H. (eds.): *Principles and Practice of Obstetrics and Perinatology,* Volume 2. New York, John Wiley, 1981.
5. Bieniarz, J., Burd, L., Motew, M., et al.: Inhibition of Uterine Contractility in Labor. *American Journal of Obstetrics and Gynecology,* 111:874, 1971.
6. Biggs, J.: Pregnancy at 40 Years and Over. *Medical Journal of Australia,* 1:542, 1973.
7. Bills, B.: Nursing Considerations: Administering Labor-Suppressing Medications. *MCN,* 5:(4):252, 1980.
8. Bottoms, S., Mortimer, G., and Sokol, R.: The Increase in the Cesarean Birth Rate. *New England Journal of Medicine,* 302:559, 1980.

9. Bottoms, S., and Sokol, R.: Mechanisms and Conduct of Labor. *In* Iffy, L., and Kaminetzky, H. (eds.): *Principles and Practice of Obstetrics and Perinatology.* New York, John Wiley, 1981.

10. Caldeyro-Barcia, R.: Intrapartum Fetal Monitoring. Presentation at the 2nd Memorial Ignatz Semmelweis Seminar, Cherry Hill, New Jersey, September 1976.

11. *Cesarean Childbirth.* National Institutes of Health Consensus Development Conference. Bethesda, Md., Office of Research Reporting, NIHCD, 1981.

12. Cohen, W., Newman, L., and Friedman, E.: Risk of Labor Abnormalities with Advancing Age. *Obstetrics and Gynecology, 55*:414, 1980.

12a. Creasey, R., and Herron, M.: Prevention of Preterm Birth. *Seminars in Perinatology, 5*:295, 1981.

13. D'Angelo, L., and Sokol, R.: Prematurity: Recognizing Patients at Risk. *Perinatal Care, 2*:16, 1978.

14. Fall, O.: External Cephalic Version in Breech Presentation Under Tocolysis. *Obstetrics and Gynecology, 53*:713, 1979.

14a. Friedman, E. A., and Little, W. A.: An Evaluation of the Management of Twin Delivery. *Bulletin of Sloane Hospital, 4*:39, 1958.

15. Frieman, R., Garite, T., and Modanlow, H.: Postdate Pregnancy: Utilization of Contraction Stress Testing for Primary Fetal Surveillance. *American Journal of Obstetrics and Gynecology, 140*:128, 1981.

16. Gries, J., Bieniarz, J., and Scommenga, A.: Comparison of Maternal and Fetal Effects of Vacuum Extraction with Forceps or Cesarean Deliveries. *Obstetrics and Gynecology, 57*:571, 1981.

17. Haddad, H., and Lundy, L.: Changing Indications for Cesarean Section: a 38 Year Experience at a Community Hospital. *Obstetrics and Gynecology, 51*:133, 1978.

18. Haverkamp, A., Thompson, H., McFee, J., et al.: The Evaluation of Continuous Fetal Heart Rate Monitoring in High Risk Pregnancy. *American Journal of Obstetrics and Gynecology 125*:310, 1976.

19. Haverkamp, A., Orleans, M., Langendoerfer, S., et al.: A Controlled Trial of the Differential Effects of Intrapartum Fetal Monitoring. *American Journal of Obstetrics and Gynecology, 134*:399, 1979.

19a. Herron, M., Katz, M., and Creasy, R.: Evaluation of a Preterm Birth Prevention Program: Preliminary Report. *Obstetrics and Gynecology 59*:452, 1982.

20. Horger, G., and Smythe, A.: Pregnancy in Women Over Forty. *Obstetrics and Gynecology, 49*:257, 1977.

21. Johnson, J., Austin, K., Jones, G., et al.: Efficacy of 17 α Hydroxyprogesterone Coproate in the Prevention of Premature Labor. *New England Journal of Medicine, 293*:675, 1975.

22. Kelso, I., Parsons, R., Lawrence, G., et al.: An Assessment of Continuous Fetal Heart Rate Monitoring in Labor: A Randomized Trial. *American Journal of Obstetrics and Gynecology, 131*:526, 1978.

23. Kesslor, I., Lancet, M., Borenstein, R., et al.: The Problem of the Older Primipara. *Obstetrics and Gynecology, 56*:165, 1980.

24. Malmstrom, T.: Vacuum Extractor: Indications and Results. *Acta Obstetricia et Gynecologica Scandinavica 43*:Suppl. 1, 1964.

25. Marieskind, H. *An Evaluation of Caesarean Section in the United States.* Washington, D.C., Office of the Assistant Secretary for Planning and Evaluation/Health, 1979.

26. Mintz, D., Skyler, J., and Chez, R.: Diabetes Mellitus and Pregnancy. *Diabetes Care, 1*:Jan./Feb., 1978.

26a. Kelly, J.: Use of the Vacuum Extractor for Delivery. *Contemporary Ob/Gyn,* Dec., 1973.

27. Moore, D., Bingham, P., and Keesling, O.: Nursing Care of the Pregnant Woman with Diabetes Mellitus. *JOGN Nursing, 10*(3):188, 1981.

28. Morrison, T.: The Elderly Primigravida. *American Journal of Obstetrics and Gynecology, 121*:465, 1975.

29. Neutra, R., Greenland, S., and Friedman, E.: The Effects of Monitoring on Cesarean Section Rates. Cited in *Antenatal Diagnosis,* III: *Predictors of Intrapartum Fetal Distress.* Bethesda, Md.: National Institutes of Health, 1979.

29a. Pearson, J.: Review of Practice Shows "Surprising" Rise in Cesareans. *Ob/Gyn News, 14*:1, 1979.

30. Placek, P., and Taffel, S.: Trends in Cesarean Section Rates for the United States, 1970–1978. *Public Health Reports, 95*(6):540, 1980.

31. Ranney, B.: The Gentle Art of External Cephalic Version. *American Journal of Obstetrics and Gynecology, 116*:239, 1973.

32. Renou, P., Chang, A., Anderson, J., et al.: Controlled Trial of Fetal Intensive Care. *American Journal of Obstetrics and Gynecology, 126*:470, 1976.

33. Shearer, E.: NIH Consensus Development Task Force on Cesarean Childbirth: The Process and the Result. *Birth and the Family Journal, 8*(1):25, 1981.

34. Wheeler, L., and Jones, M.: Pregnancy-Induced Hypertension. *JOGN Nursing, 10*(3):212, 1981.

35. Zachau-Christiansen, and Villumsen, A.: Follow-up Study of Children Delivered by Vacuum Extraction and by Forceps. *Acta Obstetricia et Gynecologica Scandinavica 43*: Suppl. 7, 1964.

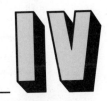

The Newborn Infant

20

Transition to Extrauterine Life

OBJECTIVES

1. Define:
   a. surfactant
   b. foramen ovale
   c. ductus arteriosus
   d. ductus venosus
   e. thermoneutral environment
   f. ophthalmia neonatorum
   g. Apgar score
2. Identify nursing goals during the infant's transition to extrauterine life.
3. Identify three distinct periods during the transition; describe the physiologic characteristics of each and signs of possible illness.
4. Describe the differences in physiologic function between the fetus and the newborn infant in regard to the following:
   a. respiratory system
   b. circulatory system
   c. renal function
   d. hepatic function
   e. blood
   f. acid-base balance
   g. glucose metabolism
5. Identify mechanisms of heat loss in infants. Explain how the infant attempts to maintain warmth and how nursing intervention facilitates this maintenance.
6. Explain why thermoregulation is essential to the newborn. Identify normal temperature limits and environmental temperature for healthy term infants.
7. Identify the stimuli that are important to the establishment of respirations. Describe nursing action to facilitate respirations.
8. Explain the reason for and methods of prophylaxis of ophthalmia neonatorum. Discuss how the timing of prophylaxis can facilitate bonding.

Objectives continued on page 585

9. Name the components of the Apgar score and the scoring for each. Explain the interpretation of an individual Apgar score.
10. Explain why assessment of gestational age is important. Identify physical and neurologic characteristics utilized in assessment of gestational age.
11. Explain the importance of comparing gestational age with body and head size.
12. Identify the components of an initial physical assessment immediately following birth.
13. Describe procedures to ensure the accurate identification of each newborn.
14. Explain the concept of a critical period. Describe the ways in which nurses can facilitate initial bonding while meeting the physiologic needs of the baby.
15. Describe current recommendations for care of the newborn skin and umbilical cord.

Probably no other 24-hour period in an individual's history is as momentous as the first. Even mere survival is significant; approximately half of the neonatal deaths (i.e., deaths during the first 28 days of life) occur within these first 24 hours, primarily, but not entirely, due to prematurity.

Consider the changes that the newborn must face. Externally his environment could hardly be more different. Formerly warm, dark, and totally liquid, it is now chilly, filled with glaring light, and dry. Strange sounds, sights, touches, and tastes surround him.

Changes in his internal environment are equally dramatic. He must, almost instantly, convert to a different mode of respiration and circulation. Blood vessels carrying blood high in oxygen content prior to birth will now carry blood with lower oxygen content. Liver and kidney functions alter, and a number of metabolic processes must reorganize for the new way of life.

Also significant are the beginning relationships between the baby and his parents that develop during the first day.

Nursing Goals

There are three basic goals of nursing care during these first 24 hours:
1. To use careful observation to detect any sign or behavior that indicates abnormality. Since changes in newborn infants occur in a

very short period of time, their detection depends upon the nurses who are with the baby.
2. To meet the basic physiologic needs of the baby, achieved through the interaction of parents and nurses.
3. To facilitate the relationship between the baby and his parents.

Each goal is equally important, and we plan to achieve them simultaneously (see Nursing Care Plan 20–1). Even in a life-threatening situation, for example, when an infant and his parents may need to be separated, we can facilitate their relationship by our own relationship with his mother and father (Chapter 28).

In order to achieve these goals, nurses must know:
1. What the newborn is like during the first 24 hours of transition.
2. What physiologic changes normally take place.
3. What his immediate needs are and how they can best be met.
4. What the significance of parent–infant contact is during the first 24 hours and how we can best facilitate it.

Specific Periods during the Transition

Close observation shows that both the vital signs and the clinical appearance of a newly born baby vary within the first 24 hours. The initial transition includes an immediate period of reactivity, an interval during which the
Text continued on page 591

Nursing Care Plan 20–1. Healthy Newborn: Care During Transition to Extrauterine Life (First 24 Hours of Life)

NURSING GOALS:
To provide an environment that allows the newborn a smooth transition from intrauterine to extrauterine life.
To identify variations in health status of the newborn.
To facilitate interaction between parents and their newborn infant and identify problems in attachment.
To provide prophylaxis for ophthalmia neonatorum and hemorrhagic disease of the newborn.

OBJECTIVES: During the first 24 hours of life the newborn:
1. Receives a thorough physical assessment.
2. Begins feeding.
3. Receives eye prophylaxis and vitamin K prophylaxis.
4. Has opportunities to interact with his parents to facilitate attachment.

ASSESSMENT	POTENTIAL NURSING DIAGNOSIS	NURSING INTERVENTION	COMMENTS/RATIONALE
Identify any factors in maternal history that may predispose newborn to physical or interactional disorders:	At risk for neonatal disorder related to (specific factor; for example, lag in attachment is related to lack of prenatal attachment behavior; erythroblastosis is related to maternal blood type).	Based on specific identified needs	Prenatal and intrapartum record (or summary) must be available to nurses who care for newborn infant and family.
1. Physiologic risk factors			
2. Social risk factors			
3. Emotional risk factors			
Immediate assessment:			
1. Assess newborn at 1 and 5 minutes by assigning an Apgar score.		Clear mucus from mouth and nose prior to respiratory effort.	
2. Note respiratory effort.		If resuscitation is necessary, see Nursing Care Plan 23–1.	
3. Check umbilical cord for two arteries and vein; assess bleeding from clamped cord.		Dry infant.	
4. Note any obvious anomalies (e.g., gastroschisis, meningocele). Assess skin, cry, head, motor activity, Moro reflex (Chapter 21).		Place infant with head dependent on mother's abdomen, preferably next to her skin, in bed under warmer where parents can see him, or wrap the baby in warm blanket for parents to hold. Place stockinette cap on head.	
5. Weigh and measure infant.		Apply cord clamp; be sure there is no bleeding.	
6. Note parents' reactions to infant (nonverbal behaviors and verbal comments).		Assist mother, partner in seeing and touching infant.	

7. Continue to assess infant's physiologic and behavioral responses during initial interaction with parents.

Identify infant (e.g., matching namebands for mother and infant) before infant leaves birth room.

Provide opportunity for initial breast-feeding if this is desired by mother. If infant does not suckle immediately, reassure mother that this is not unusual.

If mother is Rh negative or if need for umbilical vessel catheterization is suspected, leave cord 2–3 inches long.

Within the first 2 hours:
1. Complete physical assessment as described in Chapter 21.

Risk related to specific alteration in health.

Related to specific assessment. See Nursing Care Plans in Chapters 23 and 24 for care of infants with specific alterations in health.

Areas to be included in the newborn assessment:
a. General appearance (activity, cry, muscle tone, posture, symmetry, reflexes)
b. Skin color (cyanosis, pallor, jaundice, meconium staining)
c. Skin (rash, petechiae, ecchymosis, desquamation)
d. Head (molding, caput succedaneum, cephalhematoma, anterior and posterior fontanels, sutures, condition at site of internal fetal monitor if one used)
e. Eyes (shape, placement, drainage, conjunctival hemorrhage)
f. Nose (patency, bridge, flaring of nares)
g. Mouth (shape, fusion of palate)
h. Neck (length, masses)
i. Heart and lungs (see Vital signs, below)

Continued on following page

Nursing Care Plan 20–1. Healthy Newborn: Care During Transition to Extrauterine Life (First 24 Hours of Life) *(Continued)*

ASSESSMENT	POTENTIAL NURSING DIAGNOSIS	NURSING INTERVENTION	COMMENTS/RATIONALE
j. Abdomen (masses, number of cord vessels, umbilical hernia, kidney, bladder if palpable, liver, spleen)			
k. Genitalia (descent of testes, scrotal rugae; relationship of size of labia)			
l. Anus (patency, location, rectal fissure)			
m. Extremities (peripheral pulses, abnormal position of foot, subluxation/dislocation of hips, number of digits, clavicles)			
n. Spine (curvature, defects)			
2. Assess gestational age. Compare gestational age with length, weight, head and chest circumferences to identify infant as AGA, SGA or LGA.	Risk of specific complications related to (preterm, postterm, SGA, LGA)	See specific nursing care plans in Chapter 23.	
3. Assess vital signs: a. Initial rectal temperature, then subsequent axillary temperature—at least every hour until stable, then every 4 hours for 24 hours	Hypothermia Hyperthermia Temperature instability	Provide thermoneutral environment. Minimize heat loss with stockinette cap. No bath should be given before infant's temperature has stabilized at a skin temperature of at least 97.6° F.	Newborns have poor thermoregulation
b. Heart rate initially and apical every 4 hours for 24 hours; note murmurs, irregular rhythm	Tachycardia >160 bpm Bradycardia <100 bpm		
c. Respirations: note rate and signs of respiratory distress (grunting, retracting, nasal flaring, cyanosis; see Nursing Care Plan 23-4).	Irregular respiration common Tachypnea >60 per min Periods of apnea	Provide 1. Eye prophylaxis for ophthalmia neonatorum (AgNO₃ or penicillin drugs)	Tachycardia and tachypnea can be a sign of respiratory problems and/or hypoglycemia

Assessment	Intervention	Rationale
4. Note initial voiding. Note urinary stream in male infant.	Failure to void within 24–48 hours	Failure to void may indicate urinary tract obstruction or shock.
5. Note initial stool (meconium)	Failure to stool within 24–48 hours	Absence of meconium stool may indicate intestinal obstruction, meconium ileus and/or plug.
6. Blood glucose assessment (routine assessment of blood glucose in every infant is controversial)	Hypoglycemia	
7. Assess parent-infant interactions during feeding:		
a. Mother's comfort on feeding infant	Need for assistance during first feedings	Provide early feeding for all infants. Assist mother in choice of feeding (Nursing Care Plans 22-2 and 26-5).
b. Father's comfort in feeding if bottle-fed	Need for information about infant feeding	See Nursing Care Plans 22-2 and 26-5.
c. Early care-giving activities of the parents	Need for assistance in care-giving	
	Need for information about care-giving	Explain options available to mother (e.g., rooming in).
		Encourage mother to care for infant as her health status permits.
Continuing assessment of attachment behaviors:		A mother who has had a long difficult labor or cesarean delivery may not be ready to participate in care-taking immediately.
1. Nonverbal behaviors (holding, en face, cuddling, kisses, smiles)	Lag in attachment (when positive behaviors do not occur)	Show ways of holding, cuddling.
2. Positive verbal comments (uses terms of affection, calls infant by name, sees family resemblance in infant, perceives infant as attractive, responsive).		Make positive comments about infant.
		Provide opportunities for as much interaction with infant as mother's health allows.
3. Mother expresses positive feelings toward baby's father.		
(See also Nursing Care Plan 22-1.)		

2. Prophylaxis for hemorrhagic disease of the newborn (vitamin K injection)

Refer for further evaluation.

Refer for further evaluation.

Table 20–1. THE TRANSITION TO EXTRAUTERINE LIFE IN THE HEALTHY TERM NEWBORN

	Initial Period of Reactivity (First 15 to 30 Minutes)	Period of Relative Inactivity (30 Minutes to 2 Hours)	Second Period of Reactivity (2 to 6 Hours)
Respirations	Irregular; peak at 60–90 per minute; transient rales; grunting, nasal flaring, thoracic retractions; sternal retractions not unusual; brief apnea	Respiratory rate declines: periods of rapid respirations with dyspnea; shallow, synchronous breathing with barreling of chest	Brief periods of rapid respirations; periods of irregular respirations with apneic pauses
Heart rate	Tachycardia; mean peak 180 beats per minute at 3 minutes	Heart rate declines; 120–140 beats per minute	Labile; wide swings from bradycardia to tachycardia
Color	Brief cyanosis; acrocyanosis	Color improves; flushing when crying	Abrupt color changes
Body temperature	Drops	Low	Begins to rise
Bowel sounds	Absent initially; present after 15 minutes	Present	Bowel cleared of meconium
Oral mucus	May be visible	Small amounts watery mucus	Prominent; may have gagging and vomiting
Activity	Alert, exploratory, intensely active	Sleeps; quiet activity	More responsive
Response to stimuli	Vigorous	Relatively unresponsive to external and internal stimuli	
Signs of possible illness	Rapid, shallow breathing; signs of cerebral hemorrhage: twitching, apnea, full fontanel, opisthotonos	Signs of respiratory distress: grunting, tachypnea	Persistence of subnormal temperature; hypoglycemia; apnea, cyanosis; lethargy

baby is relatively unresponsive and inactive, and then a more active period again. The transition usually is complete in the healthy full-term newborn by about 6 hours of age.

The initial period of reactivity lasts for approximately 15 to 30 minutes after birth and is characterized by activity in many body systems. The heart beats rapidly, muscle tone is increased, and the baby is alert and exploring. He may have tremors of his extremities or chin and sudden outcries that stop as suddenly as they began. He sucks, swallows, grimaces, and moves his head from side to side.

If the mother has not been anesthetized, the baby is generally alert during this period and will look at his mother and father attentively. This period seems designed by nature for the attachment of parents and baby. Then, for approximately an hour and a half, he becomes much more quiet and relatively unresponsive. His color improves as his muscle tone returns to normal. Heart and respiratory rates decline. Both external and internal stimuli bring little response.

A second period of activity completes the transition. Specific differences in these three periods are compared in Table 20–1. By comparing the activities of healthy infants with these norms, nurses can come to recognize more readily what is usual and unusual during this significant time.

Physiologic Changes

The physiologic functioning of the infant differs from that of the fetus in several important respects.

Respiratory Changes

At approximately 24 weeks' gestation, alveolar cells begin to produce *surfactant,* a lipid substance essential in preventing alveolar collapse after birth. By 26 to 28 weeks, pulmonary alveoli proliferate, and capillaries multiply in very close proximity to them, two additional antecedents necessary for postdelivery respiration.

Throughout fetal life, the lungs are filled with lung fluid, which keeps them partially expanded so that it will not be as difficult for them to expand at the time of delivery.* What happens to this fluid? In a vertex delivery the pressure of the birth canal on the fetal thorax literally "squeezes" part of the fluid from the lungs and out through the baby's nose and

---

*Consider how much easier it is to blow up a balloon that has been previously filled with water or air than a brand new one that has never been expanded.

mouth. The remaining fluid is picked up by the blood vessels and lymphatics surrounding the lungs, a process greatly facilitated by the changes in pulmonary vasculature described below (see next section on circulatory changes).

When the baby is delivered in a presentation other than vertex, by cesarean delivery or by breech presentation, for example, this fluid is not as easily expelled from the lungs. The lungs are stiff, and the baby breathes rapidly for several days, a condition termed *transient tachypnea* of the newborn (page 623).

A combination of factors appears to cause the baby to take his first breath (below). Within 10 minutes after birth the volume of air remaining in the lungs at the end of expiration is the same as it is at 5 days of age. Vital capacity reaches values proportional to those of an adult within 8 to 12 hours after birth.

Circulatory Changes

Fetal circulation is illustrated in Figure 20–1. The establishment and maintenance of good respiration influence the changes that occur in the cardiovascular system at the time of birth (Fig. 20–2). Within moments following delivery:

1. Oxygen enters the lungs, and pulmonary alveoli expand.

2. The oxygen lowers resistance in the pulmonary vessels, allowing blood to flow more freely to and from the lungs. (In the fetus, no more than 10 per cent of the total circulating blood flowed through the lungs.)

3. Pressure in the right atrium decreases because of the increased flow of blood to the lungs.

4. Pressure in the left atrium increases because of the increased flow of blood from the lungs.

5. With oxygenation, the ductus arteriosus begins to constrict, becoming functionally closed during the first 24 hours. (If the PaO_2 is low or becomes low during the first days of life, the ductus arteriosus has the capacity to remain open or to reopen.)

6. The umbilical vessels, already clamped in the delivery process, contract.

7. As pressure in the left side of the heart begins to exceed that in the right side (due to the activation of pulmonary circulation described above), the valve of the foramen ovale becomes "plastered" against the septum secundum, thus functionally closing the foramen ovale.

Although functional changes in circulation take place very shortly after birth, structural

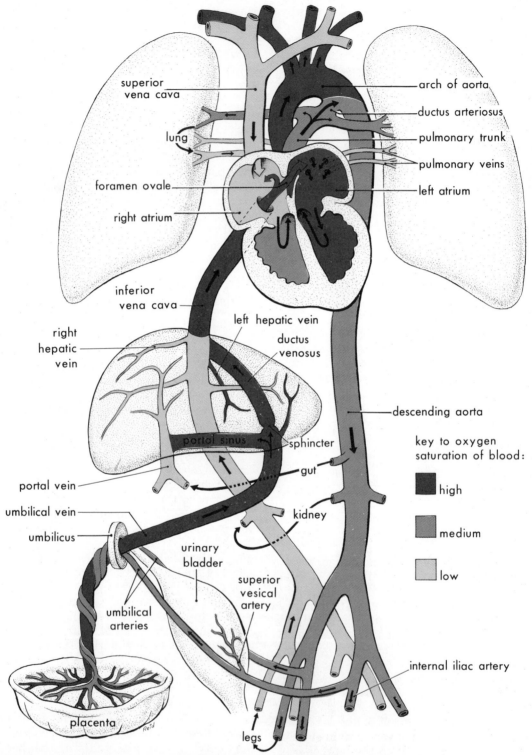

Figure 20–1. A simplified scheme of the fetal circulation. The darkened areas indicate the oxygen saturation of the blood and the arrows show the course of the fetal circulation. The organs are not drawn to scale. (From Moore: *The Developing Human: Clinically Oriented Embryology.* 2nd Edition. Philadelphia, W. B. Saunders Co., 1977.)

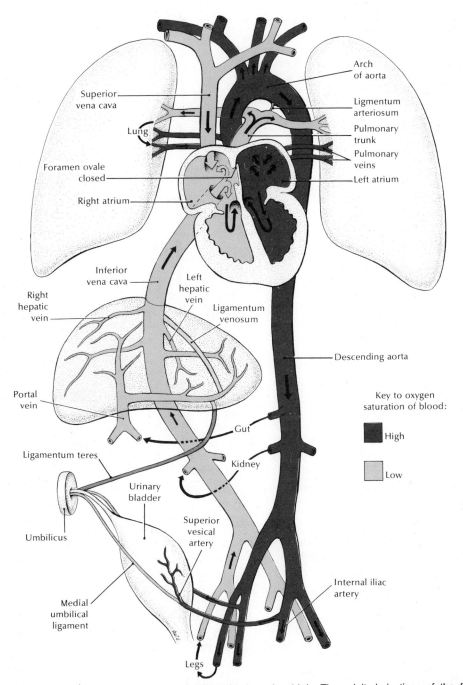

Figure 20–2. A simplified representation of the circulation after birth. The adult derivatives of the fetal vessels and structures that become nonfunctional at birth are also shown. The arrows indicate the course of the neonatal circulation. The organs are not drawn to scale. (From Moore: *The Developing Human: Clinically Oriented Embryology.* 2nd Edition. Philadelphia, W. B. Saunders Co., 1977.)

changes occur over a period of many months (Table 20–2).

Changes in Kidney Function

Prior to birth the kidney is apparently not essential to life, although it forms urine that becomes part of the amniotic fluid from about the twelfth gestational week. Even a fetus with total renal agenesis may exist intact, because the placenta carries on the necessary regulatory functions. At birth, however, the kidney must immediately begin to function; the infant totally lacking kidneys cannot survive.

Just as pulmonary vascular resistance decreases, allowing more blood to flow to and

Table 20–2.   STRUCTURAL CHANGES FROM FETAL TO INFANT CIRCULATION*

Structures in Fetal Circulation	Approx. Time of Anatomic Obliteration	Resulting Structures
Foramen ovale	1 year	Fossa ovalis
Ductus arteriosus	1 month	Ligamentum arteriosum
Ductus venosus	2 months	Ligamentum venosum of the liver
Umbilical arteries	2–3 months	Distal portion: lateral umbilical ligaments
		Proximal portion: internal iliac arteries, which function throughout life
Umbilical vein	2–3 months	Ligamentum teres of the liver

*From Moore: *The Newborn and the Nurse.* Philadelphia, W. B. Saunders Co., 1972.

from the lungs, so also does the vascular resistance of the renal vessels decrease, allowing increased blood flow to the kidneys with a marked improvement in kidney function within a few days.

Kidney function, however, remains immature for many months. The glomerular filtration rate is low, a factor particularly significant in the sick baby because the excretion of drugs by the kidney is limited. Acid-base balance is labile because the bicarbonate threshold is low. (In adults no bicarbonate is spilled into the urine until serum levels reach 24 to 26 milliequivalents per liter [mEq./L]; term newborns lose bicarbonate when serum levels reach 21 to 22 mEq./L and preterm babies at levels of 19 to 20 mEq./L.) Newly born infants also retain hydrogen ion, another factor in acid-base metabolism. Because the loop of Henle is short, newborns have a limited ability to concentrate their urine.

Changes in Liver Function

In the fetus the liver is the chief organ of blood formation from the third to the sixth months and continues to produce some cells into the first postnatal week.

Some functions that were handled by the placenta during fetal life must now be undertaken by the liver, such as the excretion of bilirubin. Placental excretion of bilirubin seems to explain why there is usually a minimal rise of serum bilirubin levels in cord blood in newborn infants with erythroblastosis (Chapter 24) but a rapid increase within a few hours after birth.

Glucuronyl transferase, the enzyme necessary for the conversion of indirect bilirubin to water-soluble direct bilirubin that can then be excreted by the kidneys, is less active during the first days of life. Thus even the small degree of hemolysis that normally occurs in the newborn can cause a pronounced degree of hyperbilirubinemia and subsequent jaundice.

Prothrombin and blood clotting Factors VII (proconvertin), IX (plasma thromboplastin component), and X (Stuart-Prower) are synthesized in the liver. The prothrombin level is low in cord blood. Prothrombin time, which measures the activity of Factors VII and X,* may be within a normal range or low at birth but will become most prolonged at 3 to 4 days of life and will continue at abnormally prolonged levels for 2 to 3 additional days. About 75 per cent of term infants and an even greater number of preterm infants show this drop in clotting factors. These changes are related to the inability of the baby to synthesize and utilize vitamin K; this means that these infants have a greater risk of hemorrhage than infants who have no drop in clotting factors.

In most nurseries 1.0 mg. of vitamin K is given to every newborn shortly after birth. This practice has virtually eliminated hemorrhagic disease of the newborn. Larger amounts of vitamin K do not enhance its therapeutic value; moreover, larger doses predispose the baby to hyperbilirubinemia and kernicterus. Giving vitamin K to the mother during labor rather than to the baby has been found to be less dependable. Natural vitamin K preparations (e.g., AquaMephyton, Konakion) act more rapidly than synthetic preparations (e.g., Hykinone, Synkamin) and are considered a better choice for that reason.

Infants of low gestational age have an even more limited ability to synthesize clotting fac-

---

*Factor V (proaccelerin) is also measured in prothrombin times, but is at normal levels in the newborn.

tors, even in the presence of large amounts of vitamin K.

Changes in the Blood

By the sixth month of fetal life the bone marrow has become the chief site of blood formation. At the time of birth it is highly active, with most of the marrow space involved in red cell production. This means that there is little marrow reserve to increase red cell production if any excess hemolysis occurs. As mentioned above, the liver may continue to produce red blood cells during the first week of life because of this lack of marrow reserve; the spleen is an additional site of extramedullary hematopoiesis.

Hemoconcentration appears to be a major characteristic of the first hours of life. Hemoglobin concentration rises by as much as 17 to 20 per cent during the first 2 hours, then drops slightly, but still remains elevated until some time between the first and third weeks. Hemoglobin levels in the term newborn range from 17 to 22 grams per 100 ml. and from 15 to 17 grams per 100 ml. in the preterm baby. Decreasing hemoglobin levels during the first week indicate red cell destruction or blood loss. Hematocrit values also rise abruptly during the first hours of life and then decline slowly; values at 1 week of age are close to values in cord blood (57 to 58 per cent for term newborns; 45 to 55 per cent for preterm infants) (Appendix A).

Red blood cells increase during the first hours, so that the level of cells is more than 500,000 per cu. mm. higher than the level of cells in cord blood. The red blood cells of the newborn infant are usually larger than those of an older infant; by the end of the second month cells are close to adult size in infants born at term. Most studies seem to indicate that the lifespan of red blood cells of term infants is the same or only slightly shorter than that of a normal adult, while that of preterm infants is definitely shorter. There is no universal agreement about this, however.

A small increase in the white cell count likewise occurs at the time of birth, possibly also due to hemoconcentration. Following this initial peak, the white cell count drops, and leukocytes become markedly less efficient at phagocytosis after the first 24 hours and throughout the first month. One study reports the mean number of leukocytes as 18,000 at birth, 12,200 at 7 days, and 11,400 at 14 days.[1] (See also Appendix A.) This decrease in number and activity of leukocytes is one factor in the newborn's lowered resistance to infection (Chapter 22). White cell counts vary widely from infant to infant and even within the same infant from day to day for no apparent reason. Thus a single elevated white cell count is of little value; two or more tests are needed when sepsis is suspected.

When comparing blood values during the first hours and days of life, it is important to remember that capillary samples, usually obtained from the heel or toe, have higher concentrations than venous samples. It is believed that this is because of the relatively sluggish circulation in the peripheral blood vessels, which in turn leads to transudation of the plasma. Warming the area by wrapping it with a warm towel for a few minutes before the sample is obtained and also discarding the first few drops of the sample minimize these differences. Even then, capillary samples should not be compared with venous or arterial samples.

Acid-Base Balance

All newborn infants are to some degree acidotic at the time of birth. In infants with normal lungs and ventilation, the acidosis corrects itself within the first hour (Table 20–3). Infants who have had a period of apnea or a delay in the onset of respirations will be more acidotic, with pH values falling below 7.0.

Values will vary according to the site from which the sample was obtained. There is considerably less oxygen and slightly more carbon dioxide in venous blood. If the sample is obtained from a heel stick and the heel is not warmed adequately, the blood obtained may be venous blood. The pH and pCO_2 values will vary slightly, but the pO_2 of venous blood is normally 40 mm. Hg while the pO_2 of arterial

Table 20–3. NEONATAL ACID-BASE BALANCE

	pH	pO_2	pCO_2	HCO$_3$ (Bicarbonate)
Cord blood	7.2	16–32*	60–70	23
Arterial blood at 1 hour	7.32	90–100	35–40	20

*Values vary considerably, even in vigorous newborns, from as low as 0 to as high as 96 mm. Hg in a number of studies. Mean pO_2, if from cord blood, varied from 16 to 32 mm. Hg in several reports.

blood is normally 90 to 100 mm. Hg. Thus in high risk babies who need close monitoring an umbilical artery catheter is usually inserted shortly after delivery (Chapter 23).

Metabolic Changes

Because plasma glucose and calcium are regulated by the placenta during fetal life, even a healthy newborn shows immaturity in glucose and calcium metabolism during his first days. It is from 1 to 2 weeks before homeostasis is obtained. Metabolism may be severely taxed in babies who are preterm, who develop postnatal illness, or who are infants of diabetic mothers or mothers with hyperparathyroidism. (See Hypoglycemia and Hypocalcemia [Chapter 23].)

The Delivery Room: Meeting Immediate Needs

In the moments following birth the baby needs both warmth and established respirations. An initial physical assessment must be made. He should be protected from ophthalmia neonatorum and must also be properly identified. Parents should have some opportunity to see and hold their child.

The Need for Warmth

The temperature of the newborn infant at the moment prior to delivery is about ¾ of a degree higher than that of his mother. The need of the newborn baby for warmth is an immediate priority. We place it ahead of the establishment of respirations in this text (although for practical purposes attention to the two is virtually simultaneous) because when resuscitation is necessary, body temperature must be maintained during any attempt at resuscitation, or these efforts will be hampered.

The Baby's Attempts to Maintain Warmth. Delivery rooms in the United States are usually cold, chilly places—about 15 degrees colder than the environmental temperature in the uterus. For those who are wrapped in sterile gowns and working under hot lights, this is comfortable. But for even a normal newborn infant, wet with amniotic fluid and naked, this cold is highly undesirable. (Who among us enjoys walking into an air-conditioned room directly from a swimming pool?) A term baby can compensate for a certain amount of cold stress because of stores of glucose and brown fat. For a baby prior to term, stress from cold can truly be the difference between life and death.

The chief reason why cold is so threatening is that cold increases oxygen consumption.* The baby becomes unable to meet his oxygen needs from room air and switches to anaerobic metabolism, causing an accumulation of lactate with the subsequent development of metabolic acidosis. Chilling may also lead to vasoconstriction and, in turn, to tissue hypoxia, and may result in an earlier predisposition to kernicterus (Chapter 23).

Energy expenditure is also increased. A newborn infant can lose as many as 200 calories per kilogram per minute in the delivery room through four separate mechanisms: evaporation, convection, radiation, and conduction. If we realize that an adult who is fully able to compensate for heat loss generates only 90 calories per kilogram per minute, we can appreciate how severe this heat loss is.

Like the older child or adult, the baby does attempt to maintain his body temperature by retaining and producing heat. *Vasoconstriction* is the principal means of heat retention. Vasoconstriction is more difficult for those babies whose mothers have been treated with magnesium sulfate for pregnancy-induced hypertension. *Insulation,* a significant means of heat conservation in older individuals, is limited in a newborn because of both the small amount of subcutaneous fat and the large surface area in relation to body weight. (The surface area to body mass ratio is also important in fluid balance.) The smaller the infant, the more deficient his insulation: infants weighing less than 2500 grams have virtually no subcutaneous fat. *Assumption of the fetal position* is a further attempt to conserve heat.

Heat production in newborns is accomplished principally by increasing the metabolic rate, thus causing the increase in oxygen consumption. This is termed *nonshivering thermogenesis,* in contrast to the shivering thermogenesis of older humans.

Brown fat, which accounts for approximately 2 to 6 per cent of the total body weight in term babies, is one of two energy sources required for increasing this metabolic rate (glucose is the other). Brown fat is found chiefly at the base of the neck, in the mediastinum, and surrounding the kidneys. When temperature receptors perceive cold, norepinephrine acts upon brown fat to release free fatty acids as energy sources for increased metabolism.

Meeting the Needs of the Baby for Warmth. Ideally, a baby should be placed in

---

*Knowing that hypothermia is used in surgery to reduce oxygen consumption, the question quite naturally is why chilling should increase oxygen consumption in the baby. The distinction must be made between the true, deep hypothermia in a controlled situation, which lowers the metabolic rate, and chilling, which increases metabolism.

a *thermoneutral environment* as quickly as possible after birth. A thermoneutral environment is one that enables the baby to maintain a body temperature of 36.5°C. (97.7°F.), plus or minus 0.5°C., with the minimum use of energy. The younger and smaller a baby, the higher the thermoneutral environment must be. Older, larger newborns have a wider tolerance of cold than smaller infants, but not the tolerance of a baby 1 to 2 months old.

Every delivery room should be equipped with a means of warming the baby without restricting the care that is given to him. Both the warmer and the blanket in which the baby is to be wrapped should be heated in anticipation of the delivery so that the baby is immediately placed in a warm environment. In this way heat loss by radiation and conduction is minimized. Without such warming, the baby would radiate heat in an attempt to raise the temperature of the entire delivery room— rather like trying to raise the temperature of an entire building with a single fireplace.

Conductive heat loss is eliminated by laying the baby on a warm, dry towel or blanket. The single act of drying the baby reduces heat loss from evaporation by 50 per cent. By avoiding the possibility that a current of cool air might blow across the baby, convective heat loss is also controlled.

In our justifiable concern for keeping the baby warm, it is easy to overlook the desire and need for parents to touch and hold their baby immediately following birth. In addition,

an increasing number of mothers are asking to breast-feed at this time. Celeste Phillips, a California nurse, has done some interesting research in this area that is discussed on page 612.[27]

One final note on warming: *hyperthermia*, as well as hypothermia, also increases oxygen consumption and thereby compromises the baby. Hyperthermia occurs far less often in our cold delivery rooms; it is more a possibility in a nursery in which the room or incubator temperature is not well regulated or in which the infants are placed too near sunshine or heating ducts (Fig. 20–3).

The Establishment of Respirations

What causes the newborn to take his first breath? Multiple stimuli—thermal, tactile, chemical, and reflex—are probably all important. *Thermal* stimulation is inevitable; the contrast between the 37°C. temperature of the uterus and the roughly 23°C. temperature of the average delivery room provides more than the needed difference. Further chilling, as discussed above, is highly undesirable.

Tactile stimuli should be gentle; the traditional "spank" is neither necessary nor advisable. The handling of the baby that is involved in the delivery process will usually be adequate. A light flick to the soles of the feet may be an additional help.

How *chemical* stimulation affects the initiation of breathing is unclear. As already men-

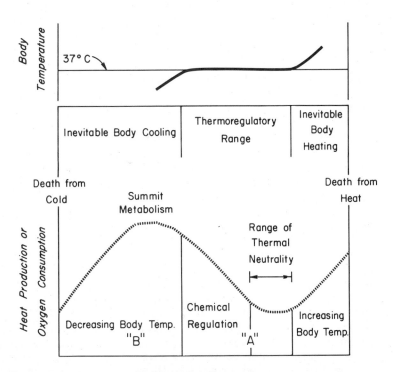

Figure 20–3. Effect ot environmental temperature on oxygen consumption and body temperature. (From Klaus and Fanaroff: *Care of the High-Risk Neonate.* Philadelphia, W. B. Saunders Co., 1973. Adapted from Merenstein and Blackmon.)

tioned, the infant is normally acidotic at birth; acid-base balance is restored within the first hour of life.

Reflex stimulation may be due to receptors in the airway. Their location and their role in the initiation of respiration is not clear.

The initial force necessary to aerate the lungs for the first breath is 10 to 20 times greater than that needed for the second and subsequent breaths, an important factor if resuscitation is necessary.

Facilitating the Establishment of Respirations. For over 90 per cent of newborns, clearing fluid and mucus from the air passages by gentle suction with a bulb syringe and gravity is all that is necessary to facilitate respirations. The baby is placed in the warmer or on the mother's abdomen in a *head down* position, preferably on his side, so that any additional fluid can drain from his respiratory tract and will not be aspirated. Resuscitation of those infants who do not breathe spontaneously is discussed in Chapter 23.

Prevention of Ophthalmia Neonatorum

Prior to the use of silver nitrate prophylaxis, 25 per cent of the children in schools for the blind in the United States were blind because of ophthalmia neonatorum, a gonococcal infection of the eye contracted during labor and delivery by direct contact with gonococcal organisms in the cervix. Occasionally the infection occurs during the first days of life, possibly by contamination from the mother's fingers.

The occurrence of ophthalmia neonatorum dropped dramatically both in the United States and in Europe as Credé prophylaxis with silver nitrate, and later antibiotic prophylaxis to a lesser extent, became legally mandatory in many areas. However, as the worldwide incidence of gonorrhea has increased to epidemic levels, so too has the incidence of ophthalmia neonatorum.

Prophylactic Eye Care (Table 20–4). In addition to gonococcal ophthalmia neonatorum, chlamydial ophthalmia neonatorium (Chapter 21) must be considered. Silver nitrate, long utilized to prevent gonococcal ophthalmia neonatorum, is not effective against chlamydial infections.

Parents who feel that immediate postnatal eye contact with their infants is important in the bonding process are concerned about the interference of any eye prophylaxis, either silver nitrate or antibiotic ointment, with the infant's vision or with the appearance of the infant. This concern is addressed in recommendation No. 3 below.

The American Academy of Pediatrics recommends:

Table 20–4. PROPHYLACTIC EYE CARE*

Silver nitrate
1. Carefully clean eyelids and surrounding skin with sterile cotton, which may be moistened with sterile water.
2. Gently open baby's eyelid and instill two (2) drops of silver nitrate on the conjunctival sac. Allow the silver nitrate to run across the whole conjunctival sac. Carefully manipulate lids to insure spread of the drops. Repeat in the other eye. Use two (2) ampules, one for each eye.
3. After one minute, gently wipe excess silver nitrate from eyelids and surrounding skin with sterile water. *Do not irrigate eyes.*

Ophthalmic ointment (erythromycin or tetracycline)
1. Carefully clean eyelids and surrounding skin with sterile cotton, which may be moistened with sterile water. *Do not irrigate eyes.*
2. Gently open baby's eyelids and place a thin line of ointment, at least ½ inch (1–2 cm.), along the junction of the bulbar and palpebral conjunctiva of the lower lid. Try to cover the whole lower conjunctival area. Carefully manipulate lids to insure spread of the ointment. *Be careful not to touch the eyelid or eyeball with the tip of the tube.* Repeat in other eye. Use one tube per baby.
3. After one minute, gently wipe excess ointment from eyelids and surrounding skin with sterile water. *Do not irrigate eyes.*

*National Society to Prevent Blindness, Committee on Ophthalmia Neonatorum, April, 1981.

1. A 1 per cent silver nitrate solution in single-dose ampules or single-use tubes of an ophthalmic ointment containing 1 per cent tetracycline or 0.5 per cent erythromycin are effective and acceptable regimens for the prophylaxis of gonococcal ophthalmia neonatorum.

2. None of the agents used for prophylaxis should be flushed from the eye following instillation. Critical studies have not evaluated the efficacy of silver nitrate prophylaxis with and without flushing, but anecdotal reports suggest that flushing may reduce the efficacy of the drug. In addition, flushing probably does not reduce the incidence of chemical conjunctivitis.

3. Prophylactic measures should be taken shortly after birth. No studies have evaluated the effectiveness of delayed prophylaxis. Some authors suggest that prophylaxis may be administered more effectively in the nursery than in the delivery room. Although definitive data are not available, delaying prophylaxis

for up to 1 hour after birth probably will not affect the efficacy of the drug used and should facilitate initial maternal–infant attachment. Hospitals in which prophylaxis is delayed should establish a check system to ensure that all infants are treated.

4. Infants born by cesarean delivery should also receive prophylaxis against gonococcal ophthalmia. Although gonococcal infection is usually transmitted during passage through the birth canal, ascending infection also occurs. However, the precise risk of gonococcal infection in untreated infants born by cesarean delivery has not been determined.

5. Most infants born to mothers with clinically apparent gonorrhea are protected from gonococcal ophthalmia with current modes of prophylaxis. However, an occasional case of gonorrheal ophthalmia may occur in such infants.

Prophylaxis does not always prevent gonococcal infections. There are a number of possible reasons why this is so, several of which are directly related to nursing care.

The medication may have been inadvertently overlooked. Perhaps the baby was in severe distress and was rushed immediately to an intensive care nursery, with total attention being focused on life-saving procedures. Or perhaps the mother needed unusual attention from delivery room personnel. In each obstetric-neonatal system there must be checks against overlooking such an important facet of care.

In addition to those factors related to the procedure itself, prophylaxis may fail because the disease has become established before birth, by premature rupture of the maternal membranes, or was acquired by the baby subsequent to prophylaxis, by contamination from the hands of the mother or hospital personnel. Silver nitrate will not prevent other types of newborn conjunctivitis caused by other infectious agents.

Recognition of the symptoms of ophthalmia neonatorum and its treatment are discussed in Chapter 21.

Immediate Physical Assessment

Immediate physical assessment of the newborn at the time of delivery includes Apgar scoring at 1 and 5 minutes after birth, estimation of the state of maturity, and a screening examination for congenital anomalies and neonatal disease.

Apgar Scoring

Apgar scoring has been termed an "instant physical." It is valuable because it quickly assesses cardiopulmonary and neurologic function and also communicates a picture of the baby's condition, not only to those present at the time of delivery but also to those who will care for the baby in the days that follow. Moreover, researchers in years to come can understand from an accurate Apgar rating a great deal about the baby's condition in those first minutes of life.

Apgar scoring should be done at 1 and 5 minutes after birth. These scores are considered useful for different purposes. The 1-minute score indicates the condition of the baby at birth. The 5-minute score reflects both birth status and the care given in the first minutes of life. Thus the 5-minute score is a better indicator of long-term health and chance of survival. In a national review of Apgar scores, Querec[28] found that scores at 5 minutes were improved over 1-minute scores. The most favorable Apgar scores occurred in infants who weighed between 2501 and 4500 grams and who had mothers who were 20 to 34 years old, married, had received prenatal care, and had high educational attainment.

The method of scoring is summarized in Table 20–5. Although all items scored are

Table 20–5. THE APGAR SCORING METHOD*

Sign	0	1	2
Heart rate	Absent	Below 100	Over 100
Respiratory effort	Absent	Minimal; weak cry	Good; strong cry
Muscle tone	Limp	Some flexion of extremities	Active motion; extremities well flexed
Reflex irritability (response to stimulation on sole of foot)	No response	Grimace	Cry
Color	Blue or pale	Body pink; extremities blue	Pink

*From Apgar: *Anesthesia and Analgesia,* 32:260, 1953. Apgar, et al.: *J. American Medical Association,* 168:1985, 1958.

numerically equivalent, a score of 9 obtained because the heart rate is less than 100 beats per minute is obviously more significant than a score of 9 obtained because the extremities are blue, the latter occurring in about 85 per cent of normal, healthy newborns. However, because low scores in heart rate and respiratory effort are usually accompanied by low scores in other areas as well, such problems in evaluation of total scores usually do not arise.

A baby with an Apgar score of 0 to 2 is severely asphyxiated; a score of 3 to 6 represents mild to moderate asphyxia. Infants with scores of 7, 8, 9, or 10 rarely need resuscitation and have low rates of mortality and morbidity.

The Components of Apgar Scoring. *Heart rate* is the most important of the five signs. If a slow heart rate (less than 100 beats per minute) can be corrected, respirations will probably follow. (A heart rate greater than 170 beats per minute may also indicate moderate asphyxia, although it is not a part of Apgar scoring and is not as significant as the severe asphyxia related to bradycardia.) Heart rate is most accurately obtained by using a stethoscope. The rate can be visually observed at the junction of the umbilical cord and the skin. Score 2 points for heart rates over 100 beats per minute, 1 point for those under 100 beats per minute, and 0 for the absence of heart rate on auscultation.

Respiratory effort is second in importance. Untreated apnea leads to respiratory and metabolic acidosis and death if successful intervention does not occur. Vigorous respirations score 2 points; irregular and ineffective (but present) respirations score 1 point; and apnea scores 0.

Muscle tone in the just-born baby means good motion of all extremities and active flexion of arms and legs with resistance to extension. Such behavior scores 2 points. Less tone scores 1 point, while a limp, flaccid baby receives a score of 0.

Reflex irritability refers to some form of stimulation. After pharyngeal suction, the tip of the catheter is placed just inside the nares. If the baby coughs or sneezes, the score is 2 points, with 1 point for a grimace, and 0 for no response. When there is a delay in clamping the umbilical cord, this procedure has been found unsatisfactory, and the flicking of the sole of a foot may be substituted, with a score of 2 points for a cry in response, 1 point for a grimace, and 0 for no response.[4]

Color is the most obvious and least significant of the Apgar criteria. Only 15 per cent of infants are pink all over at 1 minute and thus score 2 points; more common is the pink baby with blue hands and feet who scores 1 point.

A baby totally blue or pale scores 0. Because blue hands and feet are so common in newborns, some neonatologists feel that an Apgar rating of 10 is an unlikely finding.

Estimation of Gestational Age

The gestational age of a baby is the number of completed weeks that have elapsed from the first day of his mother's last normal menstrual period to the time of birth. Accurate estimation of gestational age is important in planning the care for each newborn that best meets his needs. Until relatively recently, maternal history, obstetric evaluation, and the weight of the newborn baby have been the principal criteria for estimating the gestational age of an infant. But many mothers are unsure of menstrual dates or have irregular periods. Some have first trimester bleeding, which may be mistaken for a period. The obstetric evaluation of the height of the fundus is only a rough estimate of gestational age, because it assumes normal fetal growth. When mothers receive no prenatal care, parameters such as the height of the fundus and fetal heart tones are obviously not available. The baby's weight can be misleading, as some babies weigh less than might be expected for their age while others are large in size yet deliver before term.

A *term* infant has a gestational age of from 38 weeks to 41 weeks, 6 days. An infant born prior to 38 weeks is called preterm; an infant of 42 or more weeks' gestation is called postterm. When estimated gestational age is compared with birth weight, preterm, term, and postterm babies are classified as small for gestational age (SGA), appropriate for gestational age (AGA), or large for gestational age (LGA). SGA infants may be intrauterine growth retarded (IGR). These concepts are discussed more fully below.

Because babies within every combination of age and weight have particular characteristics and needs during the first 24 hours, as well as later, an immediate assessment of age is highly important. In more and more nurseries, nurses are assuming this responsibility.

The accurate assessment of gestational age is based upon the fact that a number of physical characteristics and neurologic signs vary with the gestational age of the baby. However, it has been recognized that estimating age on the basis of one or two characteristics (ear cartilage and breast tissue, for example) is not sufficiently accurate because of individual variations. But when a number of criteria are scored, the total score is a reasonably reliable index of the infant's gestational age. Criteria from Farr and colleagues' scoring of physical characteristics[9] and from Dubowitz and colleagues' neuromuscular assessment[8] are shown in Table 20–6 and Figure 20–4, with the scoring chart represented in Figure 20–5 and described below.

Scoring should be done as soon as possible after birth. Skin criteria are not accurate after 24 hours; if assessment is delayed beyond that time a more accurate estimate is obtained by eliminating the external criteria and doubling the neurologic score. Scoring can usually be done regardless of the baby's state, i.e., awake or asleep, hungry or recently fed, and so on.

External Physical Characteristics. The lower the gestational age, the thinner the infant's *skin* will be. Because of the thinness of the skin, blood vessels are closer to the surface in the preterm infant (Fig. 20–6). Veins and venules are distinctly seen, particularly on the abdomen, and the skin is much redder than in the term baby. With each successive week the skin becomes thicker and paler and abdominal veins are less clearly seen.

Prior to 28 weeks, *lanugo*, a fine, downy hair, covers the entire body. In each subsequent week until term, some of the lanugo disappears, first from the face and later from other areas of the body. At term it is slight, if present at all.

Transverse creases on the sole of the infant's foot are absent prior to 32 weeks. From 32 to 36 weeks, approximately, the creases are found only on the anterior one-third of the foot; two-thirds of the foot are covered by 38 weeks. By 40 weeks the entire sole is a series of complex crisscrosses (Fig. 20–7).

There is usually no *breast nodule* before 33 weeks. Until 36 weeks the nodule will usually be no larger than 3 mm.; at term the nodule is from 4 to 10 mm., surrounded by a full areolar area.

Because ear cartilage is not developed before 36 weeks, the pinna of the ear is flat and stays folded. Term babies have a firm ear that recoils when rolled flat (Figs. 20–8 and 20–9).

In both males and females the genitals con-

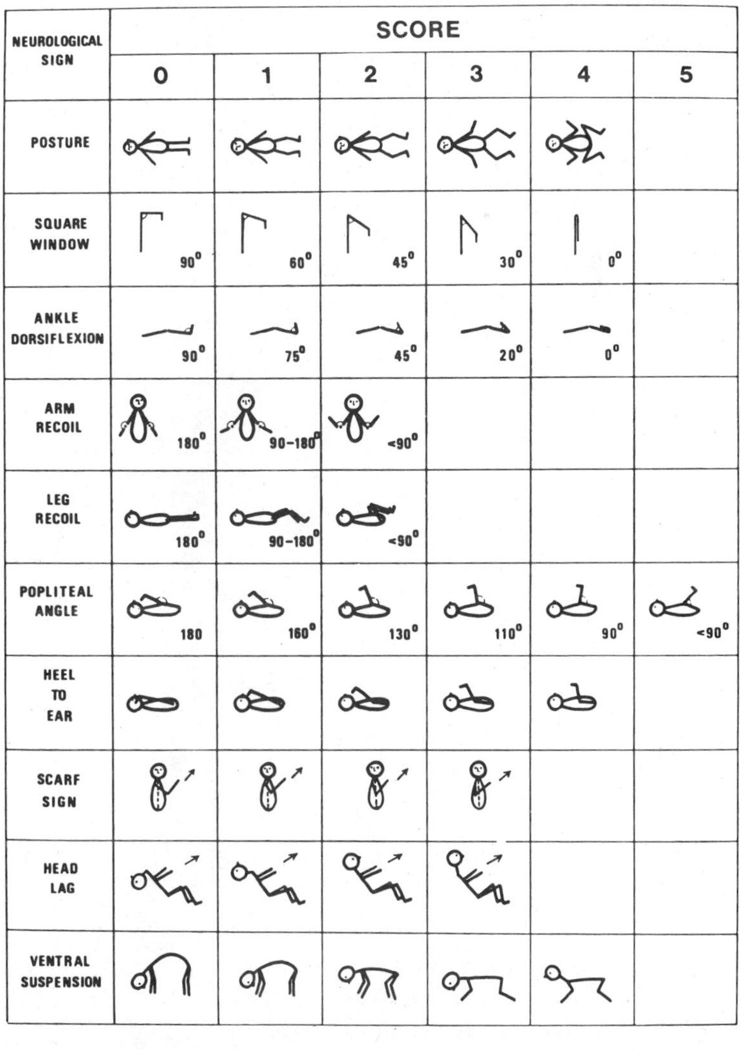

Figure 20–4. Scoring system for neurologic criteria. (From Dubowitz, Dubowitz, and Goldberg: *Journal of Pediatrics*, 77:1, 1970.)

Table 20–6. SCORING SYSTEM OF EXTERNAL PHYSICAL CHARACTERISTICS*

External Sign	Score†				
	0	1	2	3	4
Edema	Obvious edema of hands and feet; pitting over tibia	No obvious edema of hands and feet; pitting over tibia	No edema		
Skin texture	Very thin, gelatinous	Thin and smooth	Smooth; medium thickness. Rash or superficial peeling	Slight thickening. Superficial cracking and peeling, especially of hands and feet	Thick and parchment-like; superficial or deep cracking
Skin color	Dark red	Uniformly pink	Pale pink; variable over body	Pale; only pink over ears, lips, palms, or soles	
Skin opacity (trunk)	Numerous veins and venules clearly seen, especially over abdomen	Veins and tributaries seen	A few large vessels clearly seen over abdomen	A few large vessels seen indistinctly over abdomen	No blood vessels seen
Lanugo (over back)	No lanugo	Abundant; long and thick over whole back	Hair thinning especially over lower back	Small amount of lanugo and bald areas	At least ½ of back devoid of lanugo
Plantar creases	No skin creases	Faint red marks over anterior half of sole	Definite red marks over > anterior ½; indentations over < anterior ⅓	Indentations over > anterior ⅓	Definite deep indentations over > anterior ⅓

Nipple formation	Nipple barely visible; no areola	Nipple well defined; areola smooth and flat, diameter < 0.75 cm.	Areola stippled, edge not raised, diameter < 0.75 cm.	Areola stippled, edge raised, diameter > 0.75 cm.
Breast size	No breast tissue palpable	Breast tissue on one or both sides, < 0.5 cm. diameter	Breast tissue both sides; one or both 0.5 to 1.0 cm.	Breast tissue both sides; one or both > 1 cm.
Ear form	Pinna flat and shapeless, little or no incurving of edge	Incurving of part of edge of pinna	Partial incurving whole of upper pinna	Well-defined incurving whole of upper pinna
Ear firmness	Pinna soft, easily folded, no recoil	Pinna soft, easily folded, slow recoil	Cartilage to edge of pinna, but soft in places, ready recoil	Pinna firm, cartilage to edge; instant recoil
Genitals: Male	Neither testis in scrotum	At least one testis high in scrotum	At least one testis right down	
Genitals: Female (with hips ½ abducted)	Labia majora widely separated, labia minora protruding	Labia majora almost cover labia minora	Labia majora completely cover labia minora	

*Adapted by Dubowitz, Dubowitz, and Goldberg: J. Pediatrics, 77:1, 1970 from Farr, Mitchell, Neligan, et al.: Developmental Medicine and Child Neurology, 8:507, 1966.
†If score differs on two sides, take the mean.

Score   Units

	0	1	2	3	4	5	6	7	8	9
0						26.0	26.0	26.5	26.5	27.0
10	27.0	27.5	27.5	28.0	28.0	28.5	29.0	29.0	29.5	29.5
20	30.0	30.0	30.5	30.5	31.0	31.0	31.5	31.5	32.0	32.0
30	32.5	33.0	33.0	33.5	33.5	34.0	34.0	34.5	34.5	35.0
40	35.0	35.5	35.5	36.0	36.0	36.5	36.5	37.0	37.5	37.5
50	38.0	38.0	38.5	38.5	39.0	39.0	39.5	39.5	40.0	40.0
60	40.5	40.5	41.0	41.0	41.5	42.0	42.0	42.5	42.5	43.0
70	43.0									

Figure 20–5. To determine gestational age in weeks, take score from examination, find on chart, and read off value in weeks. For example, for a score of 44, find 40 in the far left column. Then read across to the column headed by 4. The gestational age is 36.0 weeks. (From Dubowitz, Dubowitz, and Goldberg: *Journal of Pediatrics,* 77:1, 1970.)

tinue to develop during the last weeks of gestation. Prior to 28 weeks the testes are undescended, and no rugae are present on the scrotum. From 28 to 36 weeks the testes normally are descending and are found first high in the inguinal canal and subsequently lower in the canal. Rugae also develop during these weeks, so that by approximately 36 weeks the testes are in the scrotum, which has well-developed rugae. Testes remain undescended in approximately 3 per cent of term infants, illustrating why no one criterion is adequate in determining gestational age.

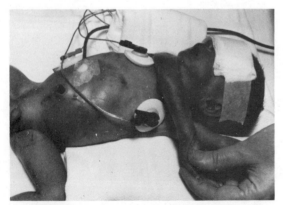

Figure 20–6. Thin skin in the premature newborn as demonstrated by blood vessels showing through above and to the right of the navel. Note also scarf sign.

In female infants the relative size of the labia majora and labia minora changes as the fetus becomes more mature. Before 28 weeks the clitoris and labia minora are prominent. In the weeks that follow, the labia majora grow, covering the labia minora by 36 to 38 weeks (Figs. 20–10 to 20–12).

Signs of Neuromuscular Maturity. Muscle tone is flaccid at 28 weeks, accounting for many of the criteria associated with neuromuscular maturity. *Posture* should be observed with the baby lying quietly on his back. Flexor muscle tone increases as the baby approaches term and is strong in an infant of 40 weeks' gestation (Figs. 20–13 to 20–17).

The *square window* refers to the angle at the wrist when the infant's hand is flexed (Fig. 20–18). The examiner's thumb is placed on the dorsal aspect of the baby's hand, with the examiner's index and third fingers on the dorsal aspect of the baby's forearm. As the baby increases in gestational age, the angle at the wrist decreases to 0.

Like the wrist joint evaluated in the square window, the *ankle dorsiflexion* (Fig. 20–19) evaluates the flexibility of the joints. Early in gestation the joints are relatively stiff; they become more relaxed closer to term, an accommodation that allows the larger infant to mold himself into the small space available to him within the uterus.

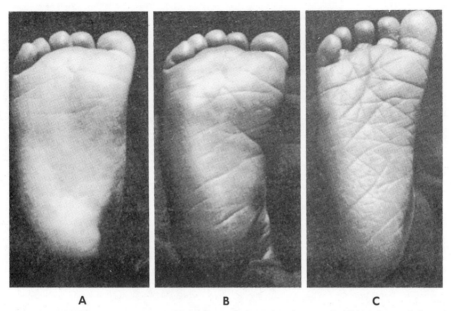

A   **B**   **C**

Figure 20–7. Plantar aspect of the foot in infants of varying gestional ages. *A,* Thirty-six weeks' gestation. Note the transverse creases on the anterior third only. *B,* Thirty-eight weeks' gestation. Note that the transverse creases extend to the heel. *C,* Forty weeks' gestation. Note transverse crease over entirety of sole, and additional wrinkling. (From Klaus and Fanaroff: *Care of the High-Risk Neonate.* Philadelphia, W. B. Saunders Co., 1973.)

Arm recoil is measured with the baby lying supine. The arms are extended by pulling on the hands. The angle of the elbow is measured after the release of the hands.

Leg recoil is also measured with the baby supine. The hips and knees are fully flexed for 5 seconds, then extended by traction on the feet, and then released.

The *popliteal* angle is also measured with

the infant supine and the pelvis flat on the examining table. The baby's thigh is held in the knee-chest position by the examiner's left index finger and thumb. The leg is then extended by gentle pressure applied behind the ankle from the examiner's right index finger, and the popliteal angle is measured.

Assessment using the *scarf sign* is based on the position of the elbow when the baby's hand

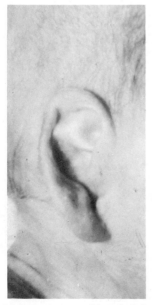

Figure 20–8. Immature ear. (From Lubchenco: *The High Risk Infant.* Philadelphia, W. B. Saunders Co., 1976.)

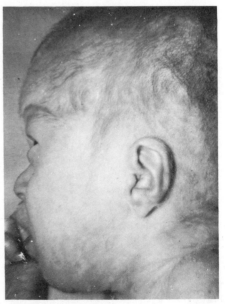

Figure 20–9. Mature ear at term. (From Lubchenco: *The High Risk Infant.* Philadelphia, W. B. Saunders Co., 1976.)

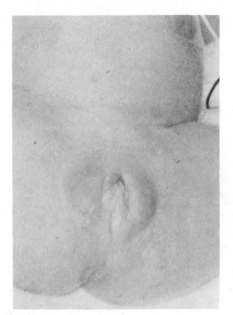

Figure 20–10. Very immature female genitalia, 28 weeks' gestation. (From Lubchenco: *The High Risk Infant.* Philadelphia, W. B. Saunders Co., 1976.)

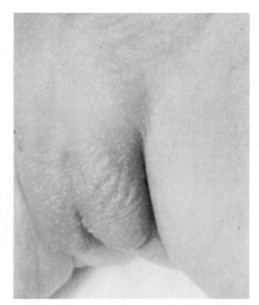

Figure 20–12. Term female genitalia. (From Lubchenco: *The High Risk Infant.* Philadelphia, W. B. Saunders Co., 1976.)

is drawn across his body to the other shoulder, as far as it will go without resistance.

In the *heel-to-ear maneuver* the baby's foot is drawn toward his head, and the distance from his foot to his ear is assessed. The knee is left free; it will fall alongside the abdomen.

Head lag is measured with the infant supine. Grasp each forearm just above the wrist and

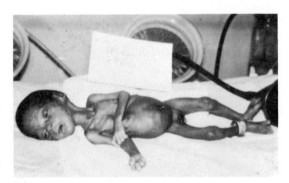

Figure 20–13. Hypotonia, less than 28 weeks. (From Lubchenco: *The High Risk Infant.* Philadelphia, W. B. Saunders Co., 1976.)

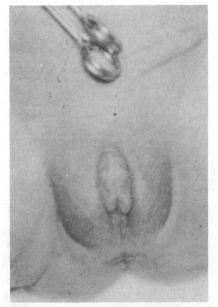

Figure 20–11. Immature female genitalia, 35 weeks' gestation. (From Lubchenco: *The High Risk Infant.* Philadelphia, W. B. Saunders Co., 1976.)

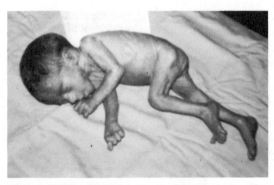

Figure 20–14. Beginning hip flexion, 32 weeks. (From Lubchenco: *The High Risk Infant.* Philadelphia, W. B. Saunders Co., 1976.)

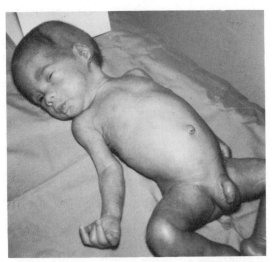

Figure 20–15. Froglike position, extended arms, 34 weeks. (From Lubchenco: *The High Risk Infant.* Philadelphia, W. B. Saunders Co., 1976.)

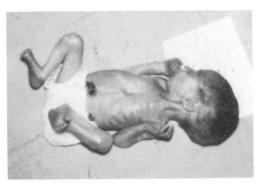

Figure 20–17. Tight flexion, all extremities, 38 to 40 weeks. (From Lubchenco: *The High Risk Infant.* Philadelphia, W. B. Saunders Co., 1976.)

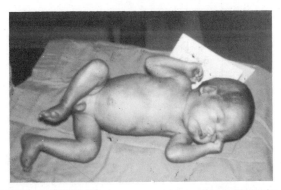

Figure 20–16. Flexion, arms and legs, loose, 36 weeks. (From Lubchenco: *The High Risk Infant.* Philadelphia, W. B. Saunders Co., 1976.)

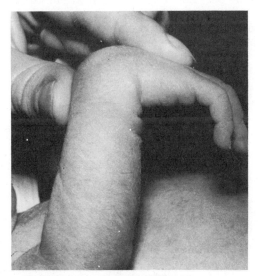

Figure 20–18. Technique for square window. (From Dubowitz, Dubowitz, and Goldberg: *Journal of Pediatrics,* 77:1, 1970.)

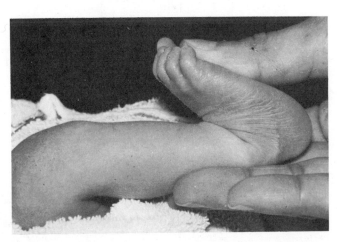

Figure 20–19. Technique for dorsiflexion of foot. (From Dubowitz, Dubowitz, and Goldberg: *Journal of Pediatrics,* 77:1, 1970.)

gently pull the baby to a sitting position. To what extent does he support his head? This is a measure of active muscle tone, which increases with gestational age.

The position of the infant when he is held in *ventral suspension* is another measure of active tone. Hold the baby with his chest in the palm of your hand. Muscle tone increases with gestational age.

Comparing Gestational Age and Body Measurements

Either before or after gestational age is ascertained, the baby is weighed, and length and head circumference are measured. Using the Colorado Growth Charts (Fig. 20–20), the baby's measurements can then be compared with the norms of the chart. (Although the Denver norms may not be totally accurate for all parts of the country—babies born at sea level are somewhat larger—they are considered the best standard of reference currently available.)

If length, weight, and head circumference are all below the tenth percentile* on the Colorado Growth Charts, the baby is considered both small for gestational age and intrauterine growth retarded. The insult to these babies probably occurred early in pregnancy, perhaps caused by an early viral illness. The long-term prognosis for normal development of these babies is usually poor.

When length and weight are less than the tenth percentile for the baby's gestational age, but head size is normal (approximately the fiftieth percentile), the baby's growth was probably affected during the third trimester. Common causes are maternal toxemia, hypertension, long-term malnutrition in the mother, and maternal vascular disease. These babies are small for gestational age and are more at risk than babies who are appropriate for ges-

---

*Tenth percentile means that 90 per cent of the babies of that gestational age are larger.

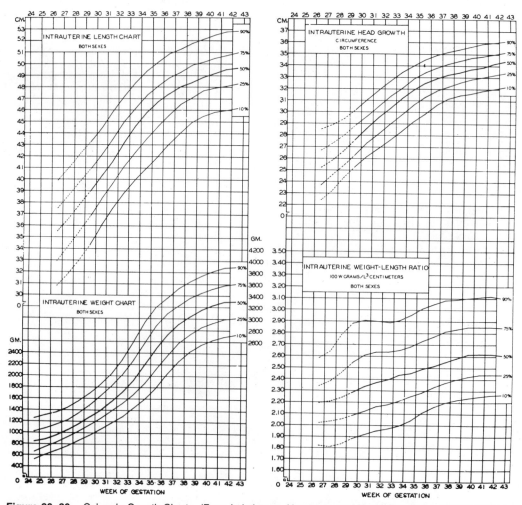

Figure 20–20. Colorado Growth Charts. (From Lubchenco, Hansman, and Boyd: *Pediatrics, 37:*403, 1966.)

Table 20–7. INITIAL ASSESSMENT

	Within Normal Limits	Needs Further Investigation
Skin	Covered with vernix	Absence of vernix
	Acrocyanosis, perioral cyanosis	Generalized cyanosis
	Petechiae of head and neck-breech presentation	Generalized petechiae Pallor Meconium staining
Cry	Lusty	Weak or absent
Head	Molding	Tense or rigid anterior fontanel
Respirations		Dyspnea
		Subcostal, substernal retractions
Cord	Two arteries, one vein	Single umbilical artery
	Unstained	Stained
Motor activity	Symmetrical	
Moro reflex	Present	Absent
	Symmetrical	Absent on one side

tational age, but they usually have a brighter future than those infants with intrauterine growth retardation.

Babies whose weight, length, and head circumference fall between the tenth and ninetieth percentiles are appropriate for gestational age. At every age these infants have a better chance for survival than babies of the same age who are either SGA or LGA infants.

A baby with measurements above the ninetieth percentile is large for gestational age. The special problems of infants in each of these groups are discussed in Chapter 23.

Physical Screening

In addition to Apgar scoring, measurement, and estimation of gestational age, additional physical screening is also important in planning the baby's care. Although some variations from normal are obvious (a meningocele, for example), others are more subtle and may be overlooked if each baby is not evaluated systematically. The scope of this brief screening is summarized in Table 20–7 and is discussed in detail in Chapter 21 in relation to the more extensive examination of the baby in the nursery.

In addition to the baby, the placenta should also be examined, as described in Chapter 17.

Identification

Before either mother or baby leaves the delivery room, the baby must be identified. Identification bands for mother and infant, with matching numbers as well as names, are one means of identification. The bands should include the name of the mother and the sex of the baby and should be checked each time the baby is removed from his crib or taken from the nursery, as well as at the time of discharge.

Footprinting is another widely used means of identification, but unless it is done properly, it is worthless. In a study by the Chicago Board of Health, policemen who were accustomed to interpreting fingerprints found that 98 per cent of the footprints submitted by Chicago hospitals were valueless and could not be used as a means of identification. However, 2 minutes of instruction to the hospital personnel responsible for taking footprints produced prints from which positive identification could be made in 99 per cent of the cases.[12]

Thompson and colleagues[34a] found that even experienced nurses (including one trained by a police dermatologist) produced footprints that were technically inadequate for identification purposes in 89 of 100 instances. Of the 11 rated technically acceptable, only 1 had all the points necessary for purposes of identification in a court of law. Moreover, when two sets of footprints of 20 preterm infants were obtained, one at birth and one 4 to 8 weeks later, not a single set could be matched by a police dermatologist.

Thompson estimates the cost of a single footprint at 50 cents and the annual cost in the United States (if 60 per cent of infants are footprinted) at a million dollars, and suggests that other methods of identification are more appropriate. A number of hospitals have discontinued footprinting newborns in recent years.

In a computer search of the legal literature, the authors found no instance in which an infant footprint was utilized in court for identification purposes.

If footprints are made, the following steps are suggested:

1. Use a disposable footprinter ink plate and a smooth, high gloss paper.
2. Wipe the baby's foot immediately after birth so that the vernix will not dry on it. This will make the foot easier to clean when the footprint is made.
3. Before making the print be sure the baby's foot is clean and dry. Cleaning should be gentle, so that the skin of the baby's foot will not peel.
4. Be sure that there is not too much ink on the pad.
5. Flex the baby's knee so that his leg is close to his body; grasp the ankle between the thumb and middle finger, with the index finger pressing on the upper surface of the foot just behind the baby's toes to prevent the toes from curling.
6. Press the footprinter firmly to the baby's foot.
7. Touch the baby's foot gently to the footprint chart, which should be attached to a hard surface such as a clipboard. Place the heel on the paper first and "walk" the foot gently onto the chart with a heel-to-toe motion. Then lift the foot off the chart; do not slide it off. The foot should not be rolled back and forth, either on the inking pad or on the footprint chart. It is particularly important to get a good impression of the ball of the foot, since the best identification can be made from the friction ridges in that area.
8. Before the baby leaves the delivery room, check the print for legible friction ridges, preferably with a magnifying glass. If the ridges are not clear, take another print.

After a satisfactory print is made, the excess ink is wiped from the baby's foot. Commonly, the mother's fingerprints are placed on the same sheet as the baby's footprint. As in every other aspect of newborn care, it is most important that the baby not be chilled during the process.

An alternate means of identification has been suggested by Shepard,[31, 32] which involves writing a name or code on the infant's chest with a pen or pencil treated with silver nitrate. The method is rapid and can easily be carried out under the warming cradle. The silver nitrate leaves an indelible tattoo that lasts for 3 to 4 weeks and eventually disappears completely.

The Baby and His Parents

The baby born in many American delivery rooms today becomes an instant occupant of a highly technical world. At times even his father is excluded from his world or is only tolerated as an unnecessary onlooker. Sometimes his mother may get only the briefest glimpse before her new baby becomes "the property" of nurses and hospital regulations. Because many parents questioned practices that separate them from their infants during the first moments and days of life, these practices changed markedly during the 1970's.

The Concept of a Critical Period

The concept of birth as a critical period in the development of a mother–infant bond suggests that later maternal behavior is highly dependent upon what happens in the period immediately following delivery. The validity of this concept has been demonstrated in a number of animal species, such as goats, sheep, cattle, mice, rats, and monkeys. Subsequent mothering behavior is disturbed when mothers and their young are separated shortly after birth. Similar periods of separation several days later do not have the same influence on the mother's behavior.

We do not know for certain that a similar critical period exists for human infants. It has been well documented that more extensive separation, such as the separation that a preterm baby may have from his mother for a period of weeks, does apparently interfere with mothering (Chapter 28). Moreover, Klaus and Kennell[20] have demonstrated in a group of 14 mothers that those with extended early contact with their infants showed an increased level of caretaking and mothering. Behavior of these mothers, compared with a control group, continued to differ when the babies were a year old and again at 2 years after birth. These studies suggest that it may very well be that the time a mother and father spend with their baby in the first hour or so after delivery may have some significance for that baby's long-range development.

In addition to the effect of early interaction on behavior, there may be physiologic advantages as well. Brodish[5] compared normal term newborns who were with their mothers in the postpartum recovery room with those who were not. All of the infants were formula-fed. The infants with early interaction took more formula and lost less weight than the group that did not have early bonding. Of course, the early interaction may have influenced maternal feeding behavior rather than infant response.

One important factor during this period may be the particular characteristics of the infant during this first hour. When a healthy infant is not influenced by medications given to his mother, he is alert to both sights and sounds. He will frequently gaze intently into the faces of his parents, follow their movements with his eyes, listen to the sound of their voices,

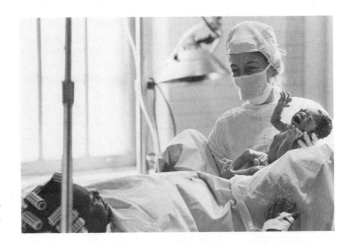

Figure 20–21. Need to see. Nurse-midwife showing infant to mother. (Photograph courtesy of S. Szasz.)

and respond to their touch by cuddling, quieting, and "embracing." It is hard to overestimate the power of this infant response on parents. One mother stated, "He was lying in the warmer beside me while the episiotomy was being 'stitched-up.' He began to cry and I spoke to him, and he immediately quieted and started looking for me." Even as she described the event weeks later it was obvious that this was a "magical moment" for her.

Although most research has concentrated on mothers, one study done in Sweden[22] suggests that fathers who had extended contact with their newborn sons and daughters were more likely to interact with them as they grew older.

The Process of Attachment

In Chapter 9 prenatal factors in attachment (planning, confirming, and accepting the pregnancy, fetal movement, and accepting the fetus as an individual) were discussed. The attachment process continues to develop with the birth of the baby, seeing, touching, and giving him care. Kang[18] notes that the events surrounding delivery can provide an atmosphere that enhances attachment. The unique characteristics of the infant, along with the parent's sense of excitement in the culmination of the hard work of labor, combine to produce moments that are ideal in furthering attachment.

Hearing the baby cry, seeing and touching him, holding the baby close to one's own body, and breast-feeding are behaviors that encourage attachment. Rubin[30] has described the initial touching process: the mother first touches her baby with the tips of her fingers, then massages the baby with the palms of her hands, and then enfolds the infant in her arms.

Support for the mother from the baby's father or companion during labor and birth

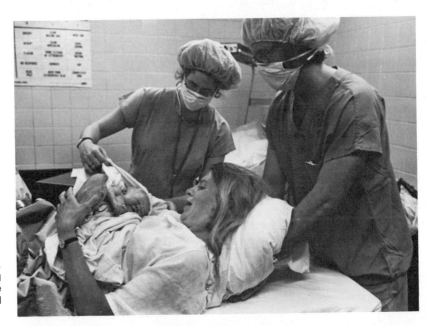

Figure 20–22. Need to touch. Note that father is actually helping to hold the mother up to see the baby. Note Apgar chart on wall and large clamp.

coupled with support from nurses and other care-givers creates an environment for attachment. Conversely, the lack of support may result in angry feelings that interfere with attachment.

If the mother is heavily medicated at the time of birth, or if labor has been particularly difficult and she is in pain or exhausted, her focus may be on herself rather than on her baby. If either mother or baby is ill, the opportunity to spend time together may be reduced or bypassed at this time immediately after delivery. When the baby requires special care, we can support the parents by our honesty about the baby's problems. Frequent communication with the parents about his progress, descriptions of his physical characteristics, and acceptance of their grief and other feelings will help them at this time of crisis (see Chapter 28).

Nursing Actions that Enhance Attachment. From the moment a mother and father (or other companion) enter the labor and birth environment, the support they feel will be a factor in their attachment to their infant. In keeping them fully informed throughout labor, in providing comfort as well as safety (Chapter 17), nurses create an atmosphere that enhances the attachment process.

Following the baby's birth, the opportunity to spend time holding, caressing, talking to, and gazing at their infant is a basic need of parents. Some new parents may be afraid they will hurt or drop the baby; others may touch him very tentatively. Statements such as, "Your baby likes you to stroke him," or "She likes to hear the sound of your voice" can encourage parents' interaction. Parents may ask, "Can my baby really see me" or "Can my baby really hear my voice," and they can be reassured that babies indeed are able to see and hear. (See Chapter 21 for a discussion of the baby's sensory capabilities.)

When the baby is less responsive, parents need assurance that each baby is unique and that some babies are more sleepy than others following birth. The specific reason for an individual baby's behavior should always be assessed in the context of a total examination (Chapter 21). Medication given to the mother is frequently a cause of a sleepy, less alert baby. A baby who is chilled may also be less active.

Mothers who plan to breast-feed will often want to begin breast feeding during the initial bonding period. Oxytocin, released when the breast is suckled (Chapter 26), causes the smooth muscle of the uterus to contract and aids in the prevention of postpartum hemorrhage.

Early initiation of breast feeding also ensures the rapid drainage of the colostrum that is in the duct system of the mother's breast and allows the milk to move through the ducts to the milk reservoirs as it forms. Colostrum received in early sucking aids the peristalsis and passage of the meconium that is in the baby's intestinal tract at the time of birth. Some infants will "latch on" to the breast immediately; others will nuzzle and lick but will not really suck well in these first hours. Nurses need to reassure mothers of infants in this second group that this behavior is normal and that it provides nipple stimulation just as the sucking does. If mothers become overly tense and anxious during the initial breast feeding experience, their feelings of anxiety may be a barrier to subsequent attempts at feeding.

Not every mother or couple wishes or is ready to participate in the kinds of experiences described here. A mother who is groggy from medication or anesthesia will probably be unable to hold her baby. Heavy medication also interferes with early breast-feeding, not only because of the mother's level of consciousness but also because the baby may suck poorly owing to the effects of drugs that have crossed the placenta prior to delivery.

During the period of initial attachment, nurses should be sensitive to other needs of both the mother and the baby. Of particular concern is the need of the baby for warmth. Phillips[27] found that term newborns who were well dried (to prevent heat loss from evaporation) and covered (to prevent heat loss from convection) could be held by their mothers on the delivery table for 15 minutes without significant loss of body temperature. All of the 115 infants in the study weighed over 5 pounds, had 1-minute Apgar scores of 7 or higher, and were delivered vaginally. Neither mother nor baby had any major complications.

The infants' temperatures were recorded at both 5 and 15 minutes after delivery. As shown in Figure 20–23, at 5 minutes after delivery the mother-held babies had higher temperatures than those babies in heated beds. Temperatures of the mother-held infants dropped more at 15 minutes than those of the babies in the heated cribs but remained well above 97.0°F. (36.1°C.).

An interesting additional finding that infants' temperatures dropped more in delivery rooms heated to 72.0°F. (22.0°C.) than in delivery rooms at 75.0°F. (24.0°C.) indicates that further study of optimum delivery room temperature might be useful.

When nursing assessment or intervention is necessary, explanations of the reason for the

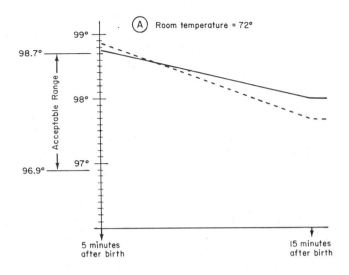

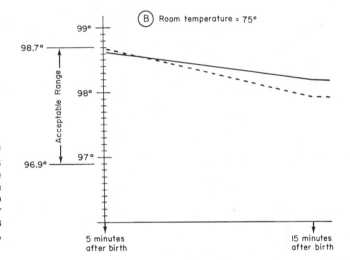

Figure 20–23. *A,* Mean rectal temperature (°F) of 51 newborns put into heated beds (———) and of 33 newborns given to their mothers to hold (------) while room temperature was maintained at 72° F. *B,* Mean rectal temperatures (°F) of 14 newborns put into heated beds (———) and of 17 newborns given to their mothers to hold (------) while room temperature was maintained at 75° F. (From Phillips: *JOGN, 3:*11, 1974.)

action and minimal interference with parent–infant interaction supports attachment.

Assessment of Parent–Infant Interaction

The period immediately following birth is so busy with meeting the physical needs of mothers and infants and facilitating bonding that the assessment and recording of parent–infant interaction, except in cases of extreme behavior, may be neglected. Recognizing that many variables, social and individual, influence behavior, and that attachment develops at different rates in different individuals, it is nevertheless helpful for nurses to assess and record information such as:

1. How the mother looks (sad, happy, apathetic, disappointed, angry, exhausted, frightened)
2. What the mother says (to the baby, to the father or others present; use of the baby's name)
3. What the mother does (eye contact, cuddling, touching, examining, kissing, hugging)

Positive signs of attachment can be assessed from the mother's record and from conversation with the parents during labor as well as following birth. The prenatal record should indicate if the pregnancy was planned, if the mother received prenatal care, and if she attended prenatal classes. Anecdotal records may indicate evidence of the mother's acceptance of the pregnancy and plans for the baby. The availability of support persons can be assessed. Indications of attachment in the period immediately following birth include positive realistic comments about the baby (attractiveness, eyes, hair, cuddliness, and so on), the use of affectionate terms, acceptance of the baby's sex, and behaviors such as reaching out, touching, holding, hugging, smiling, kissing. Seeing family characteristics in the baby is a positive sign, as is the expression of affection toward the baby's father or other family members present.

Behaviors at the time of delivery that *may* indicate future problems in parent–infant interaction include:

1. Passive, ambivalent, or rejecting behavior
2. Focusing of attention on self rather than on the baby
3. Refusal or reluctance to hold the baby
4. Hostility to the father
5. Verbal expressions of hostility or disparaging remarks about the baby
6. Remarks indicating disappointment over sex or physical characteristics[14]

It is important to recognize that many mothers who display some of these behaviors immediately following delivery may do so because of their own discomfort or exhaustion. Not every mother or father instantly falls in love with their baby. One mother of two daughters remarked about the birth of her third daughter instead of a son, "I could hardly look at her for two days." For her, attachment came slowly, but it did come.

For all parents, and particularly when attachment seems problematic, nurses can help to facilitate the process.

Continuing Physiologic Needs

At some time in the hour following his birth, the baby will be transferred either to a central nursery or perhaps to a room with his mother. As already noted, during the first hour or so most babies sleep. Physiologically they begin to stabilize. Nursing responsibilities include monitoring and maintaining temperature and administering vitamin K to prevent hemorrhage, as discussed above. Skin and cord care are important nursing functions during the transition period. Protection from infection, an immediate and continuing need, is discussed in Chapter 22.

Monitoring and Maintaining Body Temperature

Taking the initial body temperature rectally shortly after birth accomplishes the dual purpose of checking for an imperforate anus and for temperature. Subsequent temperature checks may be taken in the axilla to eliminate the danger of irritating and/or perforating the rectum. Some hospitals prefer that all temperatures be axillary, including the initial one. An axillary temperature of 96.0°F. (35.5°C.) to 99.0°F. (37.2°C.) is considered within normal limits, although a temperature above 96.8°F.

(37.0°C.) is desirable. Heavier infants tend to have higher body temperatures.

The need for a thermoneutral environment continues in the hours and days that follow birth. During the first hours a term newborn who is healthy will probably maintain temperature adequately with blankets and perhaps a hot water bottle, the latter filled halfway at a temperature of 105°F. (checked by thermometer at each filling). Air should be expressed from the hot water bag, and the bag should be completely covered and placed outside the blanket in which the baby is wrapped. Radiant warmers have replaced hot water bottles in many nurseries. A baby under a warmer should not be clothed. In both instances the infant's temperature should be rechecked frequently.

A nursery temperature of approximately 75.0°F. (24.0°C.) is considered adequate for the term baby to maintain temperature. (See Chapter 23 for variations in preterm and postterm infants.)

Initial and Subsequent Skin Care

In 1953 Wolfenstein pointed out that many infant and child care practices follow trends that are as much or more related to the belief that new ideas are better than old ones as they are to new scientific knowledge.[35] As a basis for her study, she examined the widely distributed government publication *Infant Care* for its advice on common matters such as breastfeeding, toilet training, and thumb sucking.

The skin care that is given to new infants is one aspect of nursery care that in many ways appears to follow somewhat cyclic trends. Recognizing that such cycles, or swings of a pendulum, may occur is not merely a curious and interesting sidelight of nursing care. Awareness of such trends should (ideally) make us more perceptive in our evaluation of new ideas. Then perhaps we will be able to balance the tendency of some to reject new ideas simply because they are new with the equally strong predilection of others to see all new ideas as better than old ways.

Much of the advice given student nurses and mothers in the first decade of the twentieth century, a time of home delivery and no central heating, was not a great deal different from our ideas today.

...We must remember that the newborn baby is a very tender object, exceedingly susceptible to the influence of cold, and with a very delicate skin. Indeed, in the case of children weakly at birth the physician often forbids any washing whatever until the vitality has increased. In giving a bath it is consequently necessary to guard most carefully against draughts. The doors and windows must be closed, and the child should be protected still further by placing a folding screen around the nurse's chair and the tub, and by doing the bathing before a fire unless the weather be very hot.

The washing and drying should be done thoroughly, rapidly, and yet with the greatest gentleness. . . .[15]

It was considered important to remove the vernix caseosa, and oil was used for that purpose.

The new-born baby is more or less covered with a whitish, waxy substance which must be removed entirely, especially from all the folds and hollows of the body such as the armpits, hollows of the knees, groins, and ears, as otherwise irritation of the skin is apt to be set up. As the cleansing is not easily accomplished by ordinary washing, it is necessary first to rub the skin all over with olive oil or with purified white vaseline. This is much better than lard unless the latter has been carefully freed from salt by washing. . . .[15]

We may be amused by some of the 1907 statements, but has our practice changed all that much? For example,

The first washing of the baby is the business of the monthly nurse, and the mother has no share in it.[15]

An initial oil bath was still advised nearly half a century later in an obstetric nursing text.

The baby's first bath is usually an oil bath to remove the vernix caseosa. This also prevents unnecessary evaporation from the skin and chilling of the body. The oil (sweet oil, mineral oil or some special preparation used by the hospital) for this purpose should be poured into a container which is placed in hot water and allowed to stand until it is thoroughly warm. The nurse should apply the oil gently but rapidly all over the parts where the baby has much vernix. . . In some hospitals this initial oil bath is followed by a soap-and-water bath with only the daily oil bath thereafter. In others the initial oil bath is followed by the daily soap-and-water bath. In still others the bath is omitted altogether until the day of discharge, at which time a soap-and-water bath is given.[36]

Subsequently, questions arose about the possible value of the vernix as a barrier to infection, and for a time it was recommended that the vernix be left undisturbed.

In 1963 Gluck and Wood advised that the bathing of all infants in the nursery with a hexachlorophene preparation each day would virtually eliminate staphylococcal infections.[13] This practice spread widely in the United States. However, in late 1971 warnings were issued by the Food and Drug Administration after both animal and human studies demonstrated absorption of hexachlorophene into the bloodstream. Most hospitals discontinued the use of hexachlorophene for infant bathing, although they continued to use it for personnel handwashing. During this period it was felt that the vernix might encourage infection, and it was thoroughly removed.

Current Recommendations for Skin Care

In 1975 the American Academy of Pediatrics made the following recommendations for the skin care of newborns. These recommendations have been endorsed by the executive board of the American College of Obstetricians and Gynecologists.

1. Cleansing of the newly born infant's skin should be delayed until the infant's temperature has stabilized after the cold stress of delivery.

2. Cotton sponges (not gauze) soaked with sterile water are used to remove blood from the face and head and meconium from the perianal area. As an alternative, a mild nonmedicated soap can be used, with careful water rinsing. Potential bacterial contamination of bar and liquid soaps should be remembered.

3. The remainder of the skin should be untouched unless grossly soiled. There is evidence to indicate that the vernix caseosa may serve a protective function, some evidence to indicate that it has no effect, and no evidence to indicate that it is harmful.

4. For the remainder of the infant's stay in the hospital nursery, the buttocks and perianal region should be cleansed with sterile water and cotton. As an alternative, a mild soap with water rinsing may be used as required at diaper changes and more often as indicated.

Such a regimen, termed dry skin care, is felt to diminish skin trauma and to avoid the risk of exposing newborn babies to agents with known or unknown side effects.

Cord Care

Because the stump of the umbilical cord is a potential portal of entry for septic organisms, observation and care of the cord is an important nursing responsibility. No single method of cord care has been proved to totally eliminate colonization and disease. Alchol, iodophor preparations, and triple dye are probably the three substances used most frequently, either alone or in combination. Mothers are instructed to continue cord care at home until the stump drops off, which may be as early as 5 to 7 days or as late as 2 weeks after delivery.

Summary

In this chapter the major changes of the transition to extrauterine life have been discussed. Immediate needs were considered, together with the ways in which nursing can best meet those needs in the light of our current knowledge. In the chapter that follows we will examine the term newborn more closely in order to differentiate appearance and behavior that are within the range of normal from appearance and behavior that need special attention.

REFERENCES

1. Altman, P. L., and Dittmer, D. S.: *Blood and Other Body Fluids.* Washington, D.C., Federation of American Societies for Experimental Biology, 1961.
2. American Academy of Pediatrics: Prophylaxis and Treatment of Neonatal Gonococcal Infections. *Pediatrics,* 65:1047, 1980.
3. Apgar, V.: Proposal for a New Method of Evaluation of the Newborn Infant. *Anesthesia and Analgesia,* 32:260, 1953.
4. Apgar, V., Holaday, D. A., James, L. S., et al.: Evaluation of the Newborn Infant: Second Report. *Journal of the American Medical Association,* 168:1985, 1958.
5. Brodish, M. S.: The Relationship of Early Bonding to Initial Infant Feeding Patterns in Bottle-Fed Newborns. *JOGN,* 11(4):248, 1982.
6. Dargassies, S.: Neurological Maturation of the Premature Infant of 28 to 41 Weeks' Gestational Age. *In* Falkner, F. (ed.): *Human Development,* Philadelphia, W. B. Saunders Co., 1966.
7. Dubowitz, L. M. S., and Dubowitz, V.: Assessment of Gestational Age. *Nursing Mirror,* Aug. 13, 1971.
8. Dubowitz, L. M. S., Dubowitz, V., and Goldberg, C.: Clinical Assessment of Gestational Age in the Newborn Infant. *Journal of Pediatrics,* 77:1, 1970.
9. Farr, V., Kerridge, D. F., and Mitchell, R. G.: The Value of Some External Characteristics in the Assessment of Gestational Age at Birth. *Developmental Medicine and Child Neurology,* 8:657, 1966.
10. Farr, V., Mitchell, R. G., Neligan, G. A., et al.: The Definition of Some External Characteristics Used in the Assessment of Gestational Age in the Newborn Infant. *Developmental Medicine and Child Neurology,* 8:507, 1966.
11. Fisher, D., and Behrman, R.: Resuscitation of the Newborn Infant. *In* Klaus, M. H., and Fanaroff, A. A. (eds.): *Care of the High Risk Neonate.* Philadelphia, W. B. Saunders Co., 1973.
12. Gleason, D.: Footprinting for Identification of Infants. *Pediatrics,* 44:302, 1969.
13. Gluck, L., and Wood, H. F.: Staphylococcal Colonization in Newborn Infants With and Without Antiseptic Skin Care. *New England Journal of Medicine,* 268:1265, 1963.
14. Gray, J., Cutler, C., Dean, J., et al.: Perinatal Assessment of Mother-Baby Interaction. *In* Helfer, R., and Kempe, C. (eds.): *Child Abuse and Neglect.* Cambridge, Mass., Bollinger, 1976.
15. Griffith, J. P.: *The Care of the Baby: A Manual for Mothers and Nurses.* Philadelphia: W. B. Saunders Co., 1907.
16. *Hospital Care of Newborn Infants.* Evanston, Ill., American Academy of Pediatrics, 1974.
17. Johnson, R. W.: The Case of the Nearly Mixed-up Babies. *RN,* Oct. 1974.
18. Kang, R.: Parent-Infant Attachment. *In* Duxbury, M., and Carroll, P. (eds.): *Early Parent-Infant Relationships.* White Plains, N.Y., National Foundation/March of Dimes, 1978.
19. Klaus, M. H., and Fanaroff, A. A. (eds.): *Care of the High Risk Neonate.* Philadelphia, W. B. Saunders Co., 1973.
20. Klaus, M., and Kennell, J.: *Maternal-Infant Bonding.* St. Louis, The C. V. Mosby Co., 1976.
21. Klaus, M., Jerauld, R., Kreger, N., et al.: Maternal attachment: importance of the first post-partum days. *New England Journal of Medicine,* 286:460, 1972.
22. Lind, J.: Personal communication cited in Klaus, M., and Kennell, J.: *Maternal-Infant Bonding.* St. Louis, The C. V. Mosby Co., 1976.
23. Lubchenco, L. O.: Assessment of Gestational Age and Development at Birth. *Pediatric Clinics of North America,* 17:125, 1970.
24. Moya, F., and Lehr, D.: Drug Therapy. *In* Abramson, H. (ed.): *Resuscitation of the Newborn Infant.* St. Louis, The C. V. Mosby Co., 1966.
25. National Society to Prevent Blindness: *Prevention and Treatment of Ophthalmia Neonatorum.* National Society to Prevent Blindness, 1981.
26. Oski, F., and Naiman, J.: *Hematologic Problems in the Newborn.* 2nd Edition. Philadelphia, W. B. Saunders Co., 1972.
27. Phillips, C. R.: Neonatal Heat Loss in Heated Cribs vs. Mothers' Arms. *JOGN,* 3(6):11, 1974.
28. Querec, L.: Apgar Score in the United States, 1978. *Monthly Vital Statistics Report,* 30(1):Suppl., May 6, 1981. (Public Health Service Pub. No. 81-1120.)
29. Ringler, N., Kennell, J., Jarvella, R., et al.: Mother to infant speech at two years—effects of early postnatal contact. *Journal of Pediatrics,* 86:141, 1975.
30. Rubin, R.: Maternal Touch. *Nursing Outlook* 9:828, 1963.
31. Shepard, K. S.: *Care of the Well Baby.* Philadelphia, J. B. Lippincott Co., 1968.
32. Shepard, K. S.: Further on Footprinting. *Pediatrics,* 43:639, 1969.
33. Statement of the Committee on Fetus and Newborn, American Academy of Pediatrics: Skin Care of Newborns, *Pediatrics,* 54:December, 1974.
34. Sweet, A. Y.: Classification of the Low-Birth-Weight Infant. *In* Klaus, M. H., and Fanaroff, A. A. (eds.): *Care of the High Risk Neonate.* Philadelphia, W. B. Saunders Co., 1973.
34a. Thompson, J., Clark, D., Salisbury, B., and Cahill, J.: Footprinting the newborn infant: not cost-effective. *Journal of Pediatrics,* 99:797, 1981.
35. Wolfenstein, M.: Trends in Infant Care. *American Journal of Orthopsychiatry,* 33:120, 1953.
36. Zabriskie, L., and Eastman, N.: *Nurses Handbook of Obstetrics.* Philadelphia, J. B. Lippincott Co., 1952.

21

The Term Newborn: Physical and Behavioral Assessment _____

OBJECTIVES

1. Define:
   a. dextrocardia
   b. Moro reflex
   c. tonic neck reflex
   d. rooting reflex
   e. ophthalmia neonatorum
   f. lanugo
   g. vernix caseosa
   h. milia
   i. erythema toxicum
   j. caput succedaneum
   k. cephalhematoma
   l. microcephalus
   m. hydrocephalus
   n. talipes equinovarus
   o. talipes calcaneovalgus
   p. syndactyly
   q. polydactyly
   r. anencephalus
   s. fontanel
   t. micrognathia
   u. omphalocele
   v. gastroschisis
   w. hypospadias
   x. epispadias
   y. adrenogenital syndrome

2. Identify the states of consciousness in the newborn infant. Describe factors influencing each state.
3. State the range of normal in the following neonatal vital signs: temperature, heart rate, respiration.
4. State the mean weight, length, and head and chest circumference in term newborns.
5. Explain the cause of weight loss in the first days of life. State the average amount of loss.
6. Identify the major reflexes present in newborn; describe the manner of eliciting each reflex and the significance of an absent or abnormal response.
7. Describe the infant's sensory capability.
8. Describe normal and abnormal characteristics for each of the following: skin, skin color, head, eyes, ears, mouth and jaw, trunk, genitalia, extremities, vomiting, stools, urine, behavior.
9. Describe the purpose of an assessment of interactional behavior.

As nurses, we need to be thoroughly familiar with the normal variations in a newborn infant's appearance and behavior for two equally important reasons. First, because the condition of a newborn changes rapidly, nurses are usually the first to suspect that some change may be outside the range of normal and in need of special attention. Moreover, parents most frequently query nurses about their baby. Mothers and fathers often have an unrealistic image of how their baby will look—an image that more closely resembles a child of several months than a just-born infant. And so to many parents a "molded" head looks misshapen, and *milia* (tiny cysts) may seem to be blemishes on their baby's skin. Our explanation and reassurance can help them accept their baby as he is at this time in his life, laying a foundation for the acceptance of each subsequent stage of development in its turn.

Observation of the newborn is a unique skill and one that can be learned. Although babies are limited to nonverbal communication, their signal system, once understood, tells a great deal about them. The position in which they lie in their bassinet, the color of their skin, their cry, and the way they root and suck—these signs and many others indicate health or illness.

The characteristics described in this chapter are for term newborns; characteristics of preterm and postterm infants are described in Chapter 23.

Types of Assessment

Newborn infants may be assessed by a variety of parameters, each designed to give specific kinds of information. The *Apgar score* and the *assessment of gestational age* was described in Chapter 20.

A *general physical* assessment is a part of each baby's care. An initial assessment is made following delivery. Daily assessments are also essential because of the rapid changes a baby undergoes during the first days after birth. An assessment of interactive behavior has been developed by Brazelton.[3]

State

State is a concept that describes a way of being. Characteristics that commonly occur together, including activity, breathing patterns, eye movements, and response to stimuli, differentiate one state from another. Both physiologic and behavioral assessment of newborns must be interpreted within the context of state. For example, heart and respiratory rates will vary from state to state; in charting these parameters state should be recorded if interpretation of these rates is to be accurate. Other physiologic factors that vary with state are blood flow, muscle tone, and electroencephalographic (EEG) pattern. The feeding patterns of an infant who spends much time in the active alert and crying states will probably vary from those of an infant who sleeps a great deal. As adults, we recognize that not only does our sleep state vary from our waking state but also we may even be in a variety of states when awake. At one time we may be very alert, with our attention intently focused on a specific matter, while at other times our minds may wander. Some adults train themselves or are trained to achieve certain states, such as the state of conscious relaxation that is a part of childbirth education for some women.

Weiss, in a paper published in 1934,[32] was the first to recognize that infants are also able to manifest a variety of states. Prechtl,[29] Wolff,[33, 34] and Brazelton[4] have studied states in infants. Following Brazelton, six such states are described.

Sleep States

State 1: Deep Sleep. The baby is sleeping deeply. His eyes are closed, and there are no eye movements. At regular intervals, however, one may observe "startle" or jerky movements. Breathing is smooth and regular. It is difficult to arouse the baby for feeding or other interaction (Fig. 21–1).

State 2: Light Sleep. The baby is sleeping lightly; his lids are closed, but rapid eye movements (REM) can be observed. Respirations are irregular; there are occasional sucking movements. Random movements, startles, smiles, and "fussy" sounds can be observed.

Light sleep is the major sleep pattern of term newborns (accounting for approximately 60 per cent of the sleep time). Term infants sleep in cycles of approximately 50 to 80 minutes; within the cycle 35 to 60 minutes will be spent in light sleep and 15 to 20 minutes in deep sleep.[25] Sleep cycles in preterm infants are not as well organized, even after they reach 40 weeks of age.[9] An external stimulus may produce either no change in state or a change to deep sleep or to a drowsy state.

Waking States

State 3: Drowsy. The baby's eyes may be opened or closed but they appear dull and glazed. Activity is variable; facial movement may or may not be present. Breathing is commonly irregular during both light sleep and drowsy states. Visual stimuli such as a face or auditory stimuli such as a voice may arouse

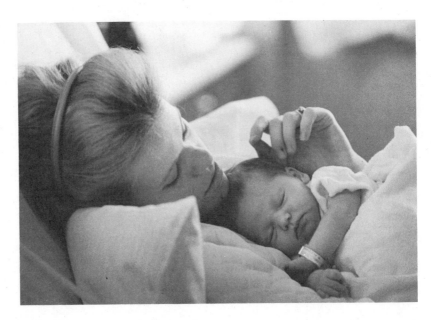

Figure 21–1. The deep sleep state. (Photograph by Suzanne Szasz.)

the infant to the quiet alert state. Reactions to stimuli may be slow.

State 4: Quiet Alert. The baby has a bright-eyed look as he focuses his attention on sights or sounds with little general activity (Fig. 21–2). In the first hours after birth infants are commonly in a prolonged quiet alert state if not affected by medications given to the mother. The quiet alert infant who gazes at his parents with a bright-eyed look has a marked effect on them. They make statements such as "He's really looking at me" and "She looks as though she knows us." A quiet alert response in an infant can be elicited in various ways, such as holding the infant in an upright position (e.g., at one's shoulder as if burping him), talking to him, or providing a visual stimulus or an object for sucking.

State 5: Active Alert. The baby is awake and very active; his arms and legs are moving. Breathing is irregular. "Fussy" describes this state well; stimuli such as hunger, noise, and too much handling disturb the baby easily. Some infants are able to console themselves quite readily and return to a less active state; others require more frequent intervention from care-givers (see below).

State 6: Crying. The baby is crying intensely; it is difficult to catch his attention with visual and auditory stimuli. The eyes may be open or closed, breathing is irregular, and activity is very marked. There are changes in skin color. As in the active alert state, some infants can console themselves or are easily consoled by others, whereas other infants are far more difficult to quiet.

Factors Affecting State. State is related to both external and internal environments. Room temperature, for example, has been shown to be related to the amount of time an infant spends in quiet sleep. In a study by Parmalee, and associates,[28] newborns were found to spend 32 per cent of their day in quiet sleep at 30°C. (86°F.), 46 per cent at 31°C. (89°F.), and 55 per cent at 34°C. (93°F.). In a very early study Weiss[32] found that infants were more active under minimal light than under moderate light. In the dark, background noise affected activity.

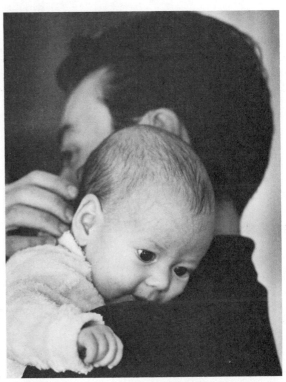

Figure 21–2. The quiet alert state. (Photograph by Suzanne Szasz.)

Table 21–1. ASSESSMENT OF NEWBORN STATES

	Deep Sleep	Light Sleep	Drowsy	Quite Alert	Active Alert	Crying
Activity	Still, occasional startle	Quiet, some body movement	Variable	Quiet	Active; may be fussy	Active; crying
Breathing pattern	Smooth, regular	Regular	Irregular	Regular	Irregular	Very irregular
Eye movement	None	Rapid eye movement (REM)	Lids heavy; eyes may open and close	Bright-eyed alert, intent gaze	Open, less bright-eyed	Open or tightly closed
Facial movement	Occasional sucking; no other movement	Occasional smiles, fussy sounds	Occasional movement	Bright, alert look	Active facial movement	Grimaces
Level of response	Response to intense stimuli only; difficult to arouse baby	Increased response to external and internal stimuli	Response may be slow	Focus on stimuli in environment	Sensitive to stimuli (e.g., hunger, fatigue, discomfort)	Very sensitive to unpleasant stimuli

Brackbill and colleagues[2] found that infants slept more and cried less in a prone position than in a supine position. Total body restraint (swaddling) will often induce sleep states, although partial swaddling is associated with active alert or crying states.[29] Korner[19] demonstrated that when a crying infant is lifted and held to the care-giver's shoulder with his head supported he becomes alert and begins to scan the environment (Fig. 21–2). Positions that induce the next greatest amount of visual alertness are horizontal movement and sitting up.

Gestational age, neurologic damage, and drug addiction (heroin or methadone) in the infant's mother are examples of factors that cause sleep states to vary from the patterns described in healthy full term newborns. In term infants hunger usually induces an awake state; hunger does not awaken preterm infants, however.[28]

Sex differences were recognized to affect state by Korner.[19] Male infants were found to startle more frequently in all states, whereas female infants smiled reflexively more often and showed more rhythmic mouthing.

Assessing State. In assessing state, the following characteristics should be noted: activity, breathing pattern, eye movements, facial movements, and level of response. Table 21–1 summarizes the relationship between these characteristics and the six newborn states.

The transition from one state to another can also be assessed. In some babies state changes progress smoothly; the baby, for example, wakens slowly from deep sleep to light sleep to drowsy, and then to quiet alert or active alert. Other babies make very rapid state changes. They may move directly from a sleep state to crying. An infant who spends little time in the middle states, such as the quiet alert state, will have a different kind of interaction with care-givers than one who has periods of quiet alert behavior.

Physical Assessment

It is important to develop a systematic approach to the physical assessment of the newborn. Before touching the infant, observe his general characteristics: muscle tone, posture, movement (unilateral or bilateral), the presence of obvious edema, and any startles or tremors (see below).

Because undressing the baby frequently causes him to cry and crying elevates his heart rate and makes auscultation of the heart, lungs, and bowel sounds difficult, many examiners prefer to evaluate these signs before

undressing the baby. The remainder of the physical assessment can then be completed with the infant undressed. The environment should be in the infant's thermoneutral range so that he will not be stressed by cold (Chapter 20). Many nurses conduct a physical assessment in the presence of parents; the assessment provides a marvelous opportunity to acquaint parents with their baby's characteristics and to answer their questions.

VITAL SIGNS IN NEWBORNS

Within Normal Limits

Temperature
  Temperature: 97.4–98.6°F. (36.3–37.0°C.); mean: 98.0°F. (36.7°C.)
Heart
  Heart rate: 90 to 180 beats per minute (average: 120 to 140)
Respirations
  Respiratory rate: 30 to 60 respirations per minute (average: 40)
Bilateral breath sounds
  Transient tachypnea of the newborn
  Diaphragmatic and abdominal breathing
Blood Pressure
  Blood pressure: systolic: 70–75 mm. Hg; diastolic: 30–40 mm. Hg

In Need of Special Attention

Temperature
  Wide variation in temperature (greater than 2°F.) from one reading to the next
Heart
  Weak pulse
  Absence of femoral pulses
  Heart sounds on the right side of the chest
  Tachycardia
  Gallop rhythm
  Indistinct heart sounds
  Cardiomegaly
  Active precordium
Respirations
  Intercostal retractions; retractions of the xiphoid
  Grunting on expiration
  Flared nostrils
  Rales
  Ronchi
  Paradoxical breathing
  Cyanosis
  Tachypnea

Vital Signs in Newborns

Temperature

Body temperature in newborns is measured in the axilla for 2 to 3 minutes. As noted in

Chapter 20, frequent taking of rectal temperatures can harm the rectal mucosa. It seems preferable for mothers to use the axilla also if they need to check the baby's temperature at home during his first weeks.

Infant temperatures normally range from approximately 97.4°F. (36.3°C.) to 98.6°F. (37.0°C.). The problems associated with a temperature that is too low were discussed in Chapter 20. An elevated temperature in a newborn is not necessarily a sign of infection as it often is in an older child; it is just as likely to indicate a reaction to a room that is too warm, too much clothing or too many covers, or dehydration. In babies who are not fed or who do not feed well, dehydration is not uncommon on the second or third day of life. With adequate hydration, temperatures become normal.

Instability of temperature, with temperature swings of more than 2°F. from one reading to the next or subnormal temperatures, is often the first sign of illness in a baby. Here again, however, changes in environmental temperature may be the culprit. For example, if the baby is in such a position in the nursery that the sun shines on his bed for part of the day, his temperature may rise and then fall as the sun moves on.

Heart Rate

Heart rate should be checked routinely even in healthy term newborns after the initial transition period, at approximately 8-hour intervals during the first few days of life, and of course it is always evaluated in the initial physical assessment.

Heart rate fluctuates markedly during the transition period (Chapter 20). Following transition, the infant's state affects heart rate; the rate may fall to 100 beats per minute or below during periods of very deep sleep and may rise as high as 180 beats per minute during active crying. Therefore, the infant's state should be noted on the chart if state is felt to be the reason for a heart rate that falls outside the range of normal. Tachycardia in the resting infant is frequently an early sign of heart failure.

Heart rate is auscultated at the apex and counted for 60 seconds. Heart sounds should be most audible on the left side of the chest between the sternum and the nipple at the third or fourth intercostal space. Heart sounds orginating on the right side of the chest may be due to *dextrocardia,* not an immediate threat in itself, or to a *diaphragmatic hernia,* a condition in which a portion of the abdominal organs enters the thoracic cavity through a defect in the diaphragm. The defect is usually, but not always, on the left. In a baby with a diaphragmatic hernia, the heart is pushed to the right, the left lung may not expand, and the baby is often in severe respiratory distress. A diaphragmatic hernia is a true surgical emergency. Prompt recognition is very important.

Pneumothorax (air in the pleural cavity) is another life-threatening cause of heart sounds heard on the right (Chapter 23).

First and second heart sounds should be heard distinctly. In newborns, the first and second heart sounds are of equal intensity. Possible causes of poorly heard heart sounds are pneumothorax (air in the pleural cavity), pneumomediastinum (air in the mediastinum, the space in the midchest between the pleura), and heart failure. Three heart sounds (with the same rhythm as the spoken word "Tennessee") constitute a gallop rhythm and are a sign of heart failure.

Listen for heart sounds at the right and left axillae. Heart sounds are normally not heard at the right axilla.

Cardiomegaly (cardiac enlargement) may be suspected on physical examination because of the location of heart sounds and can be confirmed by chest x-ray, echocardiogram, and electrocardiogram. Infants of diabetic mothers and infants with erythroblastosis may have cardiomegaly at birth. Cardiac enlargement several days following birth may be due to heart failure.

Activity of the precordium (i.e., a visible heartbeat in the area of the chest over the heart) must be evaluated in relation to the size of the baby. The precordium may appear active in a thin preterm baby because of the absence of subcutaneous tissue. An active precordium in an infant who is not thin suggests the possibility of a congenital heart defect.

Cardiac assessment also includes the evaluation of femoral and dorsalis pedis pulsations. Femoral pulses are difficult to palpate in some infants. If a dorsalis pedis pulsation is present, femoral pulsation is also present. Absence of pulsation suggests the possibility of coarctation of the aorta (Chapter 24) because of diminished blood supply to the lower extremities. A bounding femoral or dorsalis pedis pulsation suggests a patent ductus arteriosus (Chapter 23).

Heart murmurs heard during the first days of life, when no other symptoms of heart disease are present, are often benign and will disappear; the absence of a murmur in a baby with other symptoms of heart disease is considered serious (Chapter 24). The presence of a murmer is always noted on the chart.

Respiration

Normal respiration in newborn infants differs from respiration in older infants and adults in several distinct ways. The difference is even more marked in preterm infants. One of the more obvious of these differences is rate. Respiratory rate should always be measured when the baby is quiet. If cardiac rate and temperature are evaluated at the same time as respiration, respiratory rate should be measured first because the baby may become active or may cry when the thermometer is inserted or when he is touched with the stethoscope. Average respiratory rate during the first 2 weeks of life is approximately 40 respirations per minute, although apparently healthy babies may show momentary extremes ranging from 20 to 100 respirations per minute under normal resting conditions. The infant's position has been shown to affect respiratory rates very slightly. More important than the rate at any given moment is the trend in rate over a period of time.

The increased respiratory rate in infants compared with the rate in older persons is due to the infant's metabolic need to move much more air per minute in proportion to his body weight because of his proportionally larger area of skin surface.

In most hospitals, the rate of respiration is not routinely checked in new infants. Such a check during the first 6 hours, once each hour for low risk infants and once each 30 minutes for high risk infants (Chapter 23), is a helpful screening procedure. Rates over 60 respirations per minute or rates that show an increasing trend merit further investigation. In addition to checking rate, it is important to listen for good breath sounds on both sides.

Although respiratory rates in *transient tachypnea of the newborn* may exceed the usual range of normal, the condition is not considered pathologic. Transient tachypnea may follow cesarean delivery or delivery involving breech presentation. Air exchange is usually good in transient tachypnea. The baby's problem is that he must be fed carefully to avoid aspiration during these first days. When respirations are continually faster than 60 breaths per minute, alternate routes of feeding should be considered. Transient tachypnea is differentiated from more serious respiratory problems in that there are no retractions, cyanosis, or respiratory grunts, nor are the blood gases abnormal.

Neonatal breathing is diaphragmatic and abdominal; movement of the chest and abdomen should be synchronized. A lag on inspiration or alternating "seesaw" movements of the chest and abdomen (paradoxical breathing) are signs of respiratory distress (Fig. 21–3).

If intercostal muscles are being used to any extent or if retractions are visible in the xiphoid area, there is respiratory distress. A respiratory grunt is another sign of respiratory distress. The grunt occurs when the baby closes his glottis to slow down expiration, nature's way of compensating for a low carbon dioxide. Although marked nasal flaring indicates respiratory distress, occasional flaring is seen in many newborns.

Respiratory rates below 30 or very shallow respirations may reflect analgesia (particu-

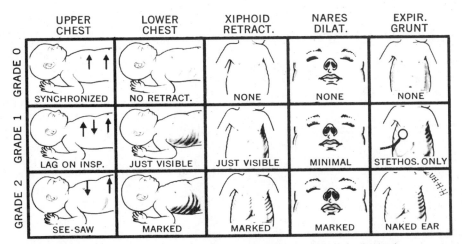

Figure 21–3. This index is designed to provide a continued evaluation of the infant's respiratory status. An index of respiratory distress is determined by grading each of five arbitary criteria: chest lag, intercostal refraction, xiphoid retraction, nares dilation, and expiratory grunt. The "retraction score" is computed by adding the values (0, 1, or 2) assigned to each factor that best describes the infant's manifestation at the time of a single observation. A score of 0 indicates no respiratory distress; a score of 10 indicates severe respiratory distress. (From Silverman and Anderson: *Pediatrics, 17*:1, 1956.)

larly Demerol) given to the mother during labor. The baby of a toxemic mother who received large amounts of magnesium sulfate prior to delivery may have rapid, shallow respirations due to hypermagnesemia.

Breath sounds should be heard bilaterally. Rales are noncontinuous sounds produced by moisture in the air passages. Fine rales, which originate in the small distal bronchioles, may be present in the first hours after birth before all the lung fluid has been absorbed. Fine rales sound like the fizzling of a carbonated drink or the roll of a piece of hair between your fingers near your ear. Rales are heard during inspiration and may be most apparent at the end of a deep inspiration. If rales continue, lung disease such as respiratory distress syndrome or pneumonia may be suspected (Chapter 23).

Rhonchi are continuous sounds caused by the movement of air through passages narrowed by secretions, swelling, or other obstruction. In newborns, rhonchi may indicate aspiration. Rhonchi are heard on both inspiration and expiration.

In assessing and describing respirations, specific points should always be noted. To report only that an infant is having respiratory distress is not adequate. It is essential to describe the signs and symptoms. Is nasal flaring present? Is there a respiratory grunt? Are retractions present? Are they intercostal (between the ribs), subcostal (at the lower margin of the ribs), or sternal (beneath the sternum)? Is there paradoxical breathing? What is the respiratory rate? Is the baby cyanotic? Is cyanosis subtle and localized, limited perhaps to the nailbed, the area around the mouth, or the mucous membranes of the mouth, or is it generalized?

Blood Pressure

Blood pressure is not routinely checked on the healthy term neonate in most nurseries. Blood pressure monitoring of sick infants is discussed in Chapter 23.

SIZE

Mean weight: 6.2–9.1 pounds (approximately 2800–4115 grams)

Mean length: 18.8–21.0 inches (47.6–53.3 cm.)

Head circumference: 13–14 inches (33–35.5 cm.)

Chest circumference: 12–13 inches (30.5–33.0 cm.)

Size

Weight

Ninety-five per cent of term infants weigh between 5.5 pounds (2.5 kg.) and 10 pounds (4.6 kg.). The mean is approximately 7.5 pounds for boys and 7.4 pounds for girls. Non-white babies tend to weigh slightly less than white infants of the same gestational age. The various reasons for birth weights that fall outside these ranges and the special problems entailed in the care of these babies are discussed in Chapter 23.

All babies lose some of their birth weight during the first days of life. The loss averages about 7 per cent of initial weight, with the range normally falling between 5 and 10 per cent. Why this loss of weight? The passage of meconium from the intestines is one factor. A second is the consumption of fat, protein, glycogen, and glucose in the production of energy by the baby. The third reason is a loss of more fluid from the body, both in urine and in insensible water loss, than is taken in. Since water constitutes approximately 35 per cent of body weight at the time of birth, the baby is not harmed by negative water balance within normal limits.

Weight gain begins from 3 to 5 days after birth; most infants have attained their birth weight by the time they are 10 days old. Birth weight normally doubles at 4 to 5 months and triples by the baby's first birthday.

Length

The average length of a term infant is 20 inches (50.8 cm.); the mean for girls is slightly less than that for boys. Measuring length is somewhat difficult because of the strong tendency of the baby's legs to flex; however, accuracy is important. If the baby is placed so that the top of his head is parallel with the end of the mattress and if a mark is placed at the point to which his heels reach, the distance, rather than the squirmy baby, can be measured. The significance of an error of just 1 inch is clear when we realize that a baby measuring 20 inches is at the fiftieth percentile, whereas a baby measuring 19 inches is very close to the tenth percentile. Length increases about 4 inches (10 cm.) during the first 3 months, 2 additional inches (5 cm.) by 6 months, and a total of 10 to 12 inches (25 to 30 cm.) during the first year.

Head and Chest Circumference

Head circumference is measured at the level of the occiput and the supraorbital ridges. At birth it is approximately 13 to 14 inches (33 to 35.5 cm.). The size of the head is even less affected by intrauterine growth retardation than is length, so here again percentile tables can be useful in evaluating what has happened to the baby in utero.

An accurate record of head circumference at birth is also important in evaluating head growth. The head should increase about 2 inches during the first 4 months and a total of 4 inches during the first year. If head circumference is above the ninety-seventh percentile at birth and continues to exceed normal measurements, or if it remains below the third percentile, medical evaluation is necessary.

Chest circumference, measured at the level of the nipples, is approximately 1 inch smaller than head circumference, about 12 to 13 inches (30.5 to 33.0 cm.) at birth. The chest grows slightly more rapidly than the head in the first months. In babies whose head and chest size are above the fiftieth percentile, chest size may exceed head size by 6 months of age. In small infants (below the tenth percentile), head size remains larger until 15 to 18 months of age. If the head measurement exceeds that of the chest by more than 1 inch (2.5 cm) at 3 months or, at the other extreme, if the head is smaller than the chest in the early months, medical evaluation of the baby is important.

NEUROMUSCULAR DEVELOPMENT

Within Normal Limits

Strong flexor muscle tone
Symmetrical posture and movement
Brief tremors or twitching

In Need of Special Attention

Hypotonicity or hypertonicity
Lack of movement on one or both sides
Weak, random movements
Prolonged tremors or convulsions

Neuromuscular Development

Normally a term newborn assumes a characteristic pattern. When lying on his abdomen, his knees are drawn up, raising his pelvis. On his back he rolls to one side or the other. Whatever his position, his arms and legs are strongly flexed and his alignment is basically symmetrical. These two characteristics—symmetry and flexion—are significant indicators

of normality. However, certain exceptions, related to the mode of delivery, are not considered abnormal. The baby born in the breech position with his legs extended will usually continue to have extended legs during the newborn period. Babies who present face first during delivery lie in a position resembling *opisthotonos,* an arched position of the body. Unlike the baby with true opisthotonos, these infants have normal muscle tone.

Both "floppiness" (hypotonicity) and rigidity (hypertonicity) in a term baby are abnormal findings. (By contrast, preterm infants have far less muscle tone, the degree of the tone being a strong indicator of gestational age; see Chapter 20). A variety of central nervous system problems, neuromuscular and connective tissue disorders, infection, dehydration, and other types of illness may be the cause of both hypotonicity and hypertonicity.

A fractured clavicle or an injury to the brachial plexus is a common reason for lack of movement on one or both sides. With these conditions the *Moro reflex* (p. 630) will also be unilateral. Both of these conditions are treated as soon as they are discovered.

The arm and shoulder of a baby with a fractured clavicle are immobilized, usually with a stockinette bandage that holds the arm against the chest with the hand across the chest. Fractures of the clavicle heal with no deformity. Occasionally the clavicle may be fractured without the loss of movement; a knot felt along the clavicle from 3 to 4 days to about 1 week after birth is the only symptom. The knot, or callus, is gradually absorbed.

Injury to the nerve fibers of the brachial plexus may occur during delivery if there is traction on the head during the delivery of the shoulder. Such an injury can lead to paralysis of part of the arm or even of the entire arm. Most common is Erb-Duchenne paralysis of the upper arm resulting from injury to the fifth and sixth cervical nerves. The affected arm lies immobile at the baby's side (Fig. 21–4). Treatment involves positioning of the arm and physical therapy. Even during bathing and dressing the baby, the arm should be positioned at shoulder level. This means that the mother, in order to feel confident, must have the opportunity to care for her infant while they are both in the hospital (Chapter 28). The degree of nerve injury is the principal factor in recovery. If nerves are intact, muscle function will generally return in a few months. If the nerve fibers are lacerated, neuroplasty may bring about partial recovery.

Although brief tremors or twitchings are not unusual in normal newborns, they must be differentiated from somewhat more prolonged

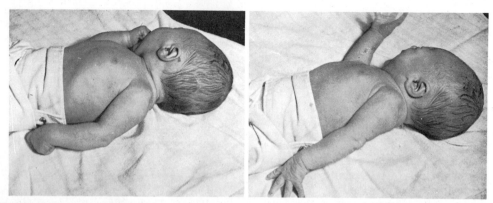

Figure 21–4. Brachial palsy of the left arm (asymmetrical Moro reflex). (From Nelson, Vaughan, and McKay: *Textbook of Pediatrics,* 9th Edition. Philadelphia, W. B. Saunders Co., 1969.)

tremors and from seizures, which may indicate a variety of pathologic conditions such as hypoglycemia, hypocalcemia, infection, or neurologic damage (Chapter 24).

Because of the immaturity of the newborn infant's cerebrum, seizure behavior is different from that of an older child or adult. Neonatal seizures may consist of no more than chewing or swallowing movements, deviation of the eyes, rigidity or flaccidity, or pallor or flushing. Rarely will the classic grand mal, petit mal, or jacksonian types of seizure be seen.

During a seizure a baby must be watched carefully for any sign of regurgitation. Charting should include the duration of seizure activity, the time at which it occurred, and the areas of the body involved. The baby's behavior and cry before and after the seizure should be recorded.

Neonatal seizures do not automatically suggest permanent brain damage. In one study by Rose and Lombroso[30a] it was found that newborns with seizures but with a *normal EEG* had an 86 per cent chance of normal development at the age of 4 years.

Reflexes

Evaluation of reflexes in the term infant is important in recognizing neurologic abnormalities and such problems as brachial plexus injury or fracture of the clavicle. In the preterm baby reflex evaluation is an additional help in estimating gestational age (Chapter 20). As the baby matures and becomes able to respond in other ways, newborn reflexes disappear. Persistence of these reflexes beyond the time at which they should no longer normally be present suggests central nervous system pathology.

Table 21–2 and Figures 21–5 to 21–8 summarize information about major reflexes of newborn infants.

The Senses

An interest in the newborn's sensory system is not a matter merely of academic curiosity. Our understanding of how the baby perceives the world influences our behavior toward him and his needs.

Touch

Of all the senses, touch appears to be the most significant in the infant's first weeks of life. A term newborn has approximately 25,000 square cm. of skin surface, by far the largest organ system in the body. Through his skin—his fingertips, his lips, and his total body—he first experiences the world and becomes aware of it. Cutaneous stimulation has been shown to be absolutely essential for life in a variety of animal species. Other studies suggest that it may be equally significant in the relationship between human parents and their babies. Many of the baby's reflexes are related to touch. The rooting reflex is elicited by touching his cheek; the grasp reflex is elicited by touching the palm. A crying baby may frequently be consoled by placing one's hand on his chest or abdomen.

Vision

Like the brain, the eye achieves a greater proportion of total growth before birth than does the rest of the body. Newborns see most acutely objects that are 8 to 12 inches from their eyes; this is the distance from the mother's face when the infant is at the breast or the distance from the care-giver's face when the baby is rocked in the arms or when he is being bottle-fed. Faces, particularly eyes with their sparkle and movement, seem to be especially interesting to infants. The baby's face brightens and his body becomes quiet as he gazes intently (Fig. 21–9). Patterns are gazed at twice as long as plain colors.[12] Varied figures are preferred to plainer figures.[18] Red and yellow seem to be preferred colors.

Most infants will not only gaze at a stimulus but follow it as well. Greenman[17] found that 26 per cent of 127 infants followed a 4-inch red ring during the period in which they were in the delivery room. Between ½ hour and 12 hours of age, 56 per cent of the infants followed the ring, and 76 per cent of them followed it by 48 hours of age. Goren and associates[16] demonstrated that at birth a newborn will follow an ungarbled representation of the human face for 180 degrees but will follow a scrambled presentation for only 60 degrees.

A newborn is also sensitive to light; he will not open his eyes when a bright light is shining in his face. Because eye-to-eye contact is important for parents as well as babies, the environment should be one in which the lighting is somewhat subdued.

Visual attention plays an important part in parent–child interaction. Listen to mothers when a sleeping baby is brought to them. "I've never seen his eyes," they tell you in disappointment. "When will he open them?" Visual attention from their baby gives obvious pleasure to both parents, who will then hold and cuddle him to get more visual attention.

Korner and Grobstein[22] suggest still another relationship between maternal attention and visual alertness. They found that when a baby cried and was picked up and placed on the shoulder, the infant not only ceased crying but frequently became alert and began to scan the environment. Thus it appears that the baby who is picked up frequently has many more opportunities to scan his world. What this might mean in terms of infant learning we can only imagine at this time.

Consider the Aivilik Eskimo infant, who during his early months sees the world from every possible angle while strapped to his mother's back. Aivilik adults demonstrate superior mechanical ability, repairing equipment that American mechanics have abandoned in despair. The Aivilik need not turn a book "properly" to look at an illustration; such is his visual orientation that he sees the picture right side up even if it is held in a horizontal or upside down position.[5] The possible correlation of these adult characteristics with the care and visual experiences received during early infancy is a promising area for future research. Do other infants who spend much of their early months on their mothers' backs have similar abilities? Will the increasing practice of "backpacking" American infants change their visual-spatial orientation?

Hearing

Infants have shown not only that they are able to attend to sound and turn their heads toward the sound of a voice but also that they can discriminate between highly similar speech sounds such as "ba" and "pa" as early as 24 hours after birth.[7a]

By 3 days of age, even with less than 12 hours of contact, healthy term infants can distinguish their mother's voice from that of another woman and show a preference for the voice of their mother. DeCasper and Fifer[7] played tape recordings to infants of mothers reading a Dr. Seuss book and strangers reading the same book to infants. The infants could produce the voice they liked best by varying their sucking on a pacifier. It took only minutes for the infants to learn to keep their mother's voice on the recording; when the type of sucking required was changed, the babies changed their sucking in order to continue to hear their mother's voice.

Differences in sound frequency lead to differences in behavior. Newborns appear to be alert to and attend to female voices more readily than to male voices, probably because of the higher pitch. Many adults, male and female, use a falsetto voice when talking to newborns, and this in turn is rewarded by the attention of the infant.

State also appears to be a factor in the behavioral response of newborns to sound frequencies. Babies respond more to high frequencies when they are awake and more to low frequencies when they are drowsy or in a state of light (REM) sleep. Low frequencies have a soothing effect and also elicit gross motor activity.[10] Could this different response to the frequencies of male and female voices be a partial basis for the different response of infants to male and female care-givers?

Loud noises lead to startles; the absence of startles in the first days of life should lead to further evaluation of the infant's hearing.

Newborns respond differently to patterned speech than to a constant auditory stimulus. These differences can be demonstrated in heart and EEG changes as well as by observation of the infant's behavior, such as initiation or cessation of crying, dilation of the pupils, or turning the head, which characterize the response to a patterned stimulus. In addition to this response to patterned speech, Condon and Sander[6] have shown that infants move rhythmically in response to speech more fre-

Table 21–2. NEONATAL REFLEXES*

Reflex	Manner of Elicitation	Gestational Age when Present Consistently	Age when Disappears	Comments
Moro	A hand clap or slap on the mattress. The baby should respond with extension of the trunk and extension and abduction of the limbs, followed by flexion and adduction of the limbs (as if to embrace).	32 weeks	From 1 to 3 or 4 months	A sudden noise or motion may also elicit response. Consistent absence suggests brain damage. Absence on one side may indicate brain damage, fractured clavicle, or injury to brachial plexus.
Tonic neck	When the baby is supine and the head is turned to one side, the arm and leg the baby is facing extend while the opposite arm and leg flex in a "fencing" position.	Incomplete at birth in normal term infant; often more definite in leg than arm	During the first 6 months, although a partial response may remain until second or third year	If persistent asymmetry and a full response are easily obtained, a cerebral lesion is suggested.
Stepping	When held erect and body supported under the arms with soles flat on table top and trunk inclined forward, baby takes regular, alternating steps.	May tiptoe at 32 weeks; heel-to-toe motion at 40 weeks	6 weeks	Failure to step on several occasions suggests neurological abnormality; stepping with only one foot indicates a unilateral problem.
Neck righting	When head turned to one side, trunk will follow.	34 to 36 weeks	Continues to develop	Other righting reflexes develop as baby grows older.
Placing	When held erect with dorsum of foot drawn against underedge of table top, foot is lifted and placed atop table.	35 weeks	6 weeks	Failure to place or unilateral placing suggests neurological abnormality, as does persistent extension or scissoring of legs.

Reflex	How Elicited	Development	Disappears	Comments
Palmar grasp	Pressing the examiner's finger into the baby's metacarpophalangeal groove causes the baby to grasp the finger.	Finger grasp is present as early as 28 weeks, but it is approximately 36 weeks before the baby can lift himself off the mattress	4 to 6 months	Examiner uses other fingers to help baby grasp.
Plantar grasp	Pressure on the plantar surface of the foot causes flexion of the toes.	After 36 weeks	8 to 15 months	
Traction response	After baby grasps hands of examiner, baby pulled to sitting position; baby will flex elbows and support head.		Persists	
Rooting	Stroking the upper or lower lip or the side of the cheek causes the baby to turn his mouth and face toward the stimulus and open his mouth.	Fairly good by 32 weeks; complete at 34 weeks	3 to 4 months when baby awake; 7 to 8 months when baby asleep	May be difficult to elicit immediately after feeding. Utilize both rooting and sucking reflexes when putting baby to breast or offering bottle.
Sucking	Stroking the lips produces sucking.	Excellent by 34 weeks; reasonably strong at 32 weeks	12 months; diminishes at 3 to 4 months	May be difficult to elicit in recently fed baby; weak or absent in baby with brain damage.
Swallowing	Place object on back of tongue.	34 to 36 weeks	Persists	

*From Moore: *Newborn, Family and Nurse,* 2nd Edition. Philadelphia, W. B. Saunders Co., 1981.

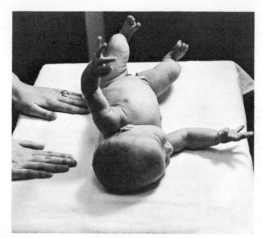

Figure 21–5. Moro reflex. (From Davis and Rubin: *De Lee's Obstetrics for Nurses.* 18th Edition. Philadelphia, W. B. Saunders Co., 1966.)

quently than to disconnected vowel sounds or to a tapping noise.

Since the human voice is the most readily available patterned auditory stimulus, it seems that, just as the human face is the optimum visual stimulus, the human voice is the optimum auditory stimulus. Parents who talk and sing to their babies are, therefore, providing them with important stimulation.

Taste

In early fetal life the taste buds are distributed throughout the mouth and throat, but prior to term they begin to disappear from all areas but the tongue. Research evidence indicates that newborns can discriminate not only between sweet and nonsweet substances but also between similar tastes, preferring sucrose (which is sweeter) to glucose.[11] This ability is present in infants as young as 1 to 3 days of

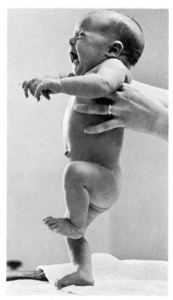

Figure 21–7. Stepping reflex. (From Davis and Rubin: *De Lee's Obstetrics for Nurses.* 18th Edition. Philadelphia, W. B. Saunders Co., 1966.)

age, suggesting that it is innate rather than learned by experience, although these preferences may be altered by experience.

There is some evidence that female infants may be more responsive to sweet tastes. Nisbett and Gurwitz[27] found that females were more responsive to a sweetened formula and increased their consumption of it significantly compared with males. This finding may be related to other studies that suggest a heightened oral sensitivity in females.[20]

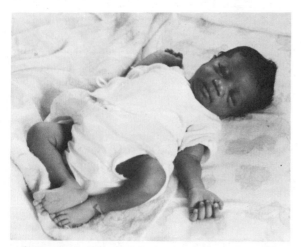

Figure 21–6. The tonic neck reflex in a week old baby.

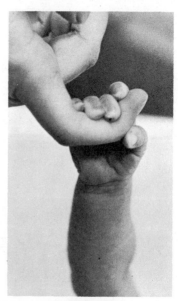

Figure 21–8. Grasp reflex. (From Davis and Rubin: *De Lee's Obstetrics for Nurses.* 18th Edition. Philadelphia, W. B. Saunders Co., 1966.)

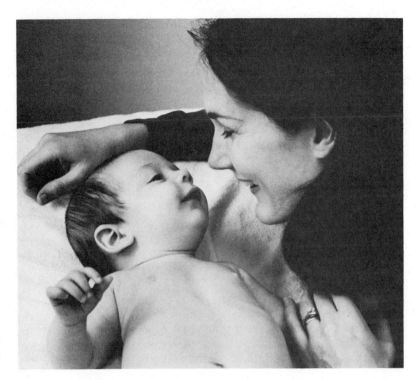

Figure 21–9. The infant gazes intently at the mother. (Photograph by Suzanne Szasz.)

Smell

A sense of smell—that is, a response to olfactory stimuli—is present at birth and appears to increase over the next several days. Macfarlane,[26] using gauze that he placed inside the mother's bra and the bra of another mother to soak up milk between breast-feedings, was able to show that although the infant did not discriminate between the pads at 2 days of age, by six days he turned more frequently toward his own mother's pad; and by 10 days this effect was even more striking.

Engen et al.,[11a] using anise oil, asafetida, acetic acid, and phenyl alcohol, showed that babies could differentiate two smells.

SKIN

Within Normal Limits

Lanugo
Vernix caseosa
Milia
Mongolian spots
Erythema toxicum
"Stork's beak mark"

In Need of Special Attention

Impetigo
Cracked or peeling skin
Hemangiomas

Skin

The softness of newborn skin is emphasized in advertisements for a variety of cosmetic preparations. In the first day or so after birth, however, sensitive infant skin does not often resemble that of the baby of television or magazine illustrations. Mothers and fathers can be disappointed if we don't help them understand what is normal during the first week or so of life.

Both the fine downy hair called lanugo and vernix caseosa have been discussed in the preceding chapter. Vernix, which is a mixture of water and oil and contains sebum, skin cells, and other materials, protects fetal skin from maceration by amniotic fluid prior to delivery.

Milia are tiny cysts frequently found across the bridge of the nose or on the chin. They disappear without treatment within a few weeks after birth (Fig. 21–10).

Mongolian spots, seen most commonly on the sacrum or buttocks of some black babies, may appear at first glance to be bruises. They also disappear spontaneously within a few weeks to several months.

Differentiation of the lesions of the very common *erythema toxicum* (also called urticaria neonatorum or "flea-bite rash," although fleas are in no way involved) from that of the far more serious *impetigo* (Fig. 21–11) is highly important. From 30 to 70 per cent of normal

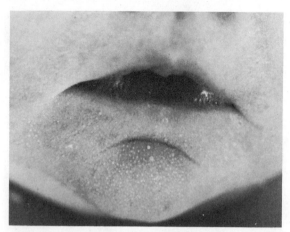

Figure 21–10. Milia are tiny sebaceous cysts commonly found on the chin or across the bridge of the nose. Milia disappear within a few weeks after birth.

requires treatment, impetigo is a bacterial infection (caused by group A beta-hemolytic streptococci or by *Staphylococcus aureus*) that can lead to a generalized infection, always serious in a newborn. The pustular vesicles rupture, producing a thick, moist, yellow crust that must be soaked off, and antibiotic ointment must be applied to the area. Everyone who comes in contact with the baby must wash very carefully to avoid infecting other infants in the nursery. Special care must also be taken with the baby's linen and other items involved in his care.

Cracked or peeling skin may be seen in the baby who is small for gestational age or in the post-term infant.

"Birth Marks"

Any large, discolored area of the skin, even when it is not a threat to the baby's physical well-being, is highly distressing to the baby's parents because it is so obvious. To the extent that birth markings affect the way parents feel about their baby and the way in which they treat him, they can have far-reaching significance.

At first glance a "stork's beak mark" may

term infants will develop toxic erythema, but it is rare in preterm babies. Although most commonly occurring during the first 4 days of life, the rash may be seen at any time during the initial 2 weeks. Papules appear on the first day, look worse on the second, and are often entirely gone within 72 hours. The baby's trunk and diaper area are usually affected.

Unlike toxic erythema, which almost never

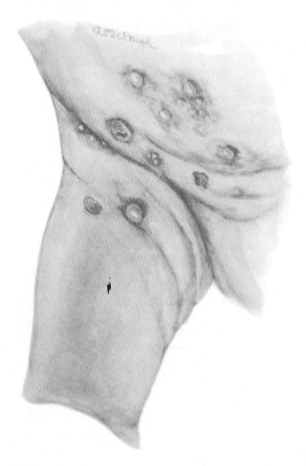

Figure 21–11. Impetigo of the newborn. (From Davis and Rubin: *De Lee's Obstetrics for Nurses.* 18th Edition. Philadelphia, W. B. Saunders Co., 1966.)

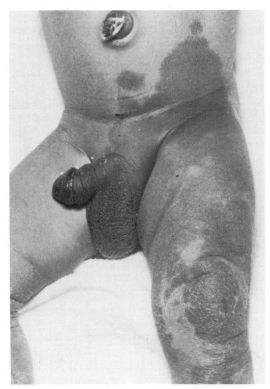

Figure 21–12. A port wine stain does not fade. If it occurs on face or arms it can be covered with a cosmetic preparation.

appear to be a nevus flammeus or a port wine stain (see at left). However, the affected area, which is usually on the occiput, the eyelids, or the glabella (the smooth space between the eyebrows above the nose), blanches on pressure and is often lighter in color than a nevus flammeus or a port wine stain. These marks disappear completely before the end of the first year.

A port wine stain is a flat, purple or dark red lesion, consisting of mature capillaries, which is present at birth (Fig. 21–12). Port wine hemangiomas located above the bridge of the nose tend to fade; others do not, but since they are level with the surface of the skin, they can be covered with a cosmetic preparation such as Covermark.

Strawberry hemangiomas (nevus vasculosus) are elevated areas consisting of immature capillaries and endothelial cells. They may be present at birth or may appear during the first 2 weeks following birth, and continue to enlarge for 6 months to a year. After the baby's first birthday they begin to regress, the process of involution taking as long as 10 years (Fig. 21–13). One-half to three-fourths of strawberry hemangiomas disappear by the time the child is 7 years old, leaving virtually no physical

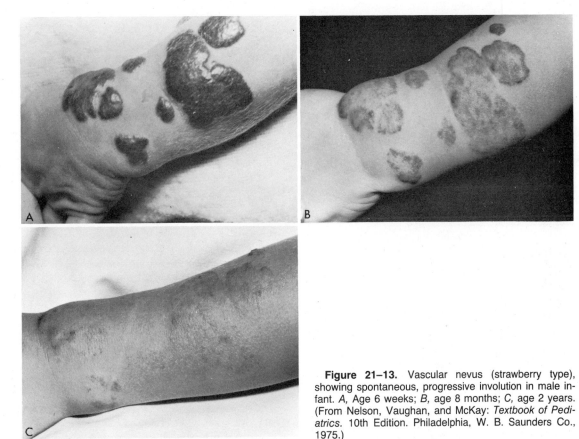

Figure 21–13. Vascular nevus (strawberry type), showing spontaneous, progressive involution in male infant. *A,* Age 6 weeks; *B,* age 8 months; *C,* age 2 years. (From Nelson, Vaughan, and McKay: *Textbook of Pediatrics.* 10th Edition. Philadelphia, W. B. Saunders Co., 1975.)

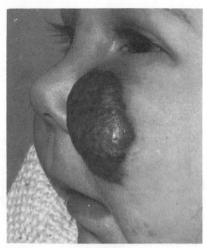

Figure 21–14. A cavernous hemangioma. (From Moschella, Pillsbury, and Hurley: *Dermatology*. Philadelphia, W. B. Saunders Co., 1975.)

evidence that they ever existed. The end result seems to be better if the hemangioma is untreated unless it interferes with normal functioning because of its location. Helping parents to accept both their child and the concept that no treatment is the best treatment is a major challenge. A series of illustrations showing regression of similar marks in other children may help parents through the years of waiting.

A third type of lesion, the cavernous hemangioma, consists of dilated vascular spaces with thick walls that are lined with endothelium (Fig. 21–14). The overlying skin is not involved. Enlargement may precede regression, which occurs only in some instances.

SKIN COLOR

Within Normal Limits

Red
Cyanosis of the lips, fingernails, toenails, hands, and feet (acrocyanosis)
Cyanosis of the presenting part
Jaundice after 36 to 48 hours
Harlequin sign

In Need of Special Attention

Pale or gray color
Generalized cyanosis
Jaundice during the first 24 hours
Mottled skin

Skin Color

The very red color of a just-born baby's skin is due to both the high concentration of red

blood cells in the vessels and the thin layer of subcutaneous fat that causes the blood vessels to be closer to the surface of the skin.

Artificial lighting in a hospital nursery may make it difficult to evaluate slight changes in a baby's color. A periodic check of the baby's color in natural light coming from a window helps to detect these changes. If hospital nurseries are painted a cream color, observation of color changes is easier.

Cyanosis

It is not unusual for a newborn infant to have localized cyanosis caused by either immature peripheral circulation in the lips, hands, and feet, or by stasis, which tends to produce cyanosis in the part presenting at delivery. (Stasis leads to cyanosis because the very slow passage of blood through the tissues causes an increased amount of oxygen to be released from hemoglobin.)

Generalized cyanosis, however, is a cause for concern. Sometimes generalized cyanosis is so slight that the baby must be compared with an infant who has obviously good color in order to detect its presence. Such a comparison is needed when the baby has other symptoms of respiratory distress and the possibility of cyanosis is raised. In babies with dark skin, cyanosis can often be best observed in the mucosal lining of the mouth.

The relationship between cyanosis and crying is an important observation. The baby may be cyanotic except when he cries vigorously and thereby raises his intake of oxygen. The baby with atelectasis is one such example. Other babies may become cyanotic when they cry, a sign that is indicative of the more persistent cyanosis associated with some types of congenital heart disease.

Cyanosis related to apnea usually can be terminated by provoking the baby to cry, by gently flicking either the soles of his feet or his buttocks.

Cyanosis is one of a number of nonspecific signs associated with hypoglycemia and hypocalcemia, both of which occur particularly often in the infants of diabetic mothers.

Babies with bilateral *choanal atresia* (occlusion of the posterior nares by either bone or membrane) will be cyanotic because infants are obligate nose breathers; they breathe through their mouth only with great difficulty. Diagnosis is made by holding a wisp of cotton in front of each nostril; the air movements of respiration can then be readily observed.

Babies with choanal atresia require surgery. Until surgery is arranged, they can breathe through their mouth if a nipple with a large hole in it is taped in place, or an airway is inserted.

Sudden cyanosis and apnea in a baby who apparently has been doing well may be due to excessive, thick mucus obstructing the upper respiratory tract. For this reason a bulb syringe should be kept in each baby's bed, and a suction machine with a supply of catheters should be available for nasal suction. Lowering the baby's head will aid in draining the mucus, a technique that can easily be shown to mothers. Once the obstructing mucus is removed, the baby becomes pink and immediately resumes respirations.

Damage to the central nervous system, either because of developmental abnormalities or because of trauma during delivery, is another cause of cyanosis. This baby is likely to have very irregular breathing and may have some other signs of central nervous system damage, such as a high-pitched cry, muscle tone that is either very floppy or rigid, or the absence of a Moro reflex. As is true of infants who are cyanotic because of respiratory distress, crying and oxygen tend to improve color.

Babies who are cyanotic because of cardiac anomalies are rarely helped by oxygen and generally appear to become worse when they cry. At first these newborns may be only briefly pale or cyanotic during feeding or following an injection. Babies who have markedly decreased cardiac output or heart failure will have arms and legs (not just hands and feet) that are cool to the touch. Babies who are pink in the upper half of their body but cyanotic in the lower trunk and legs probably have a patent ductus arteriosus, which causes blood to be shunted from right to left through the ductus (i.e., returning to the body without going to the lungs to be perfused with oxygen). (See also Chapters 23 and 24).

Pallor

Pallor may be due to anemia, hemorrhage, hemolysis of red blood cells, or shock. Loss of blood may have occurred through fetal–maternal transfusion before the cord was clamped. Sometimes when twins share a single placenta, there is a transfusion from one twin to the other. If there is no visible source of external hemorrhage, such as from the umbilical cord, a pale baby must be watched for signs of internal bleeding in the vomitus or stool. Babies with intracranial damage are often pale because of shock. Gray color is also associated with infection and with chloramphenicol intoxication. Either pallor or cyanosis confined to one extremity is a sign of interference with local circulation.

Jaundice

About 40 to 60 per cent of term infants (and a higher percentage of preterm babies) are jaundiced on the second to third day of life. Because there is no discernible pathologic reason for this jaundice, such as a hemolytic anemia or sepsis, the jaundice is termed physiologic, which is perhaps a misnomer since it obviously does not occur in every infant.

By definition, jaundice that is termed physiologic never occurs during the first 24 hours, does not cause levels of indirect bilirubin that rise above 10 to 12 mg. per 100 ml., and rarely lasts past the first week of life, the exception occurring occasionally in breast-fed infants.

The yellow color of the jaundice in these babies, as in individuals of any age, is due to high levels of bilirubin; the source of bilirubin is the breakdown of red blood cells.

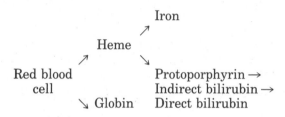

Both globin, which is a protein, and iron are reused by the body. Indirect (unconjugated) bilirubin is fat-soluble; it is transported in plasma bound to albumin. In the liver, fat-soluble bilirubin is conjugated mainly with glucuronic acid in a reaction in which the catalyst is the enzyme glucuronyl transferase. Once conjugated, bilirubin is water-soluble; conjugated (direct) bilirubin passes into the duodenum as a component of bile and is excreted in the stool. However, in newborn infants much of the bilirubin found in the meconium is unconjugated and can be reabsorbed from the gut. This unconjugated bilirubin contributes to an increased level of bilirubin in newborns.

There is no general agreement about the cause of physiologic jaundice. Production of bilirubin by the newborn (at rates of 6 to 8 mg. per kg. per 24 hours) is approximately two and one half times that of an adult, at least partly owing to the fact that the lifespan of red blood cells in newborns is 90 days, compared with the 120-day lifespan of adult erythrocytes. Less blood goes to the liver in some infants because the ductus venosus remains open, and thus some blood that would otherwise circulate in the liver does not do so.

A deficiency of glucuronyl transferase has been considered a factor in neonatal jaundice, but this has been questioned by one study.[8] The decreased amount of Y and Z' carrier proteins in the cells of the liver is now considered a more likely answer.

As long as the bilirubin remains within the circulatory system, no jaundice is visible because the red of the hemoglobin obscures the yellow of the bilirubin. But when the indirect bilirubin level rises above 7 mg. per 100 ml. in term infants, bilirubin moves outside the vascular space and is then visible. It often takes higher levels of bilirubin to bring about visible jaundice in low birth weight babies because the capillary bed lies closer to the skin surface since there is less subcutaneous fat. The red of the hemoglobin is thus reflected on the skin surface, obscuring the yellow of the jaundice. Jaundice can be visualized, however, by blanching the skin with the thumb.

Treatment is rarely necessary for physiologic jaundice in an otherwise healthy baby. There is serious danger of kernicterus (Chapter 23) in an infant whose level of indirect bilirubin rises to 20 mg. per 100 ml. or more, but in physiologic jaundice (by definition) bilirubin levels do not exceed 12 mg. per 100 ml. and are usually lower. Phototherapy is used occasionally to treat the baby with physiologic jaundice, but since its chief use is with babies of low birth weight, this treatment is discussed in Chapter 23. Jaundice other than physiologic is also discussed in Chapter 24.

Jaundice and Breast Milk. In some breast-fed infants there is a pattern of jaundice that begins on the third day of life and continues to rise, peaking at 7 to 10 days in treated infants and as late as 15 days in untreated infants. Indirect bilirubin values may range from 10 to 27 mg per 100 ml. True breast milk jaundice is estimated to occur in less than 1 in 200 breast-fed infants.[15]

The cause of breast-milk jaundice is a metabolite in the milk of some mothers (5 beta-pregnane-3 alpha, 20 beta-diol, a breakdown product of progesterone and an isomer of pregnanediol) that inhibits glucuronyl transferase (above) and thus prevents the conjugation of bilirubin.

Not every instance of jaundice in the infant of a mother who is breast-feeding is breast-milk jaundice. Unfortunately, there is no easy way to differentiate the causes of jaundice; every infant must be considered carefully on an individual basis. If the mother has breast-fed a previous infant and that baby was jaundiced, the possibility of breast milk jaundice in the present baby is likely; 70 per cent of previous children will also have had breast milk jaundice. Jaundice in a previous infant who was bottle-fed suggests that other factors as well as breast milk jaundice should be considered.

Lawrence[24] suggests the following regimen to establish the diagnosis of breast milk jaundice and to treat the problem:

1. When the indirect bilirubin level in the infant is above 15 mg per 100 ml. for more than 24 hours, obtain a bilirubin determination 2 hours after a breast-feeding and then discontinue breast-feeding for at least 12 hours. Formula is substituted for breast milk during this period. The mother empties her breasts by pump or manual expression (Chapter 26) to maintain her milk supply.

2. Measure the infant's bilirubin level after 12 hours without breast milk. If the bilirubin level has dropped by 2 mg per 100 ml., breast-feeding can be resumed. If the bilirubin level has not dropped by this amount, the period of formula feeding is extended. If bilirubin continues to rise in the absence of breast-feeding, the cause is not breast-feeding. Breast-feeding is resumed and other causes are sought.

3. After breast-feeding is resumed, there may be a slight increase in bilirubin levels followed by a slow and steady decrease. Rarely will the increase be so great that breast-feeding must again be discontinued. Bilirubin is assessed at 10 and 14 days after birth in the clinic or office. Rarely, high levels of bilirubin persist over a period of weeks; in such cases, breast-feeding must be discontinued.

Mothers are frequently disappointed when they must discontinue breast-feeding, even briefly, because of jaundice. The fact that a substance in their own milk is causing a problem for their baby makes the situation even more distressing. Explanations by the nurse about the reason for the interruption in breast-feeding, reassurance that the problem is only temporary, and a willingness to listen to each mother's feelings and concerns will help her cope with this difficult period.

The Head

Because the head is the most obvious of all the body areas, head contour is a particular source of concern to many parents. Those variations that most concern mothers and fathers are likely to be the more common ones, which are usually within normal limits. We must be aware of other variations that suggest possible illness.

THE HEAD
Within Normal Limits
A large head in proportion to the rest of the body

Anterior fontanel; diamond-shaped; approximately 2 to 3 cm. wide

Posterior fontanel: triangular; approximately 0 to 1 cm. wide

Molding
Craniotabes
Caput succedaneum
Cephalhematoma

In Need of Special Attention

Microcephalus
Hydrocephalus
Anencephalus
Fontanels that are depressed or bulging

A newborn's head is large in proportion to the rest of his body, about one-third the size it will be when he reaches adulthood. His brain weighs approximately 400 grams; it will be more than doubled, weighing 1000 grams, by his first birthday.

The measurement of head circumference has already been described. Head circumference is measured during the initial examination in the nursery, not only to identify present abnormalities but to record a baseline measurement for the evaluation of future growth. Although head measurement is not the only indication of conditions such as hydrocephalus and microcephalus, it is one valuable factor in the assessment of head growth and in the early identification of problems. *Hydrocephalus,* in which an excessive amount of cerebrospinal fluid leads to rapid head growth, may be present at birth or may even by predicted during antenatal examination. More commonly, it is recognized in the early weeks and months of life. *Microcephalus* occurs when brain growth is arrested and the skull does not grow. Possible causes include infection, injury, and genetic maternal irradiation during early pregnancy.

If the anterior end of the neural tube fails to close (Chapter 7), the cranial vault will be mainly absent, a condition termed *anencephalus.* An anencephalic baby will not survive for long, although rarely he will live for days or even weeks. Our concern for these families is to help them cope with a devastating experience (Chapter 28).

The *fontanels,* especially the anterior fontanel (because of its larger size), have been the basis for folk beliefs for many generations. Some mothers are still afraid to touch the baby's head; we see babies who are a few weeks old with varying degrees of skin problems because the mother has not shampooed the baby's head for fear of damaging his brain. We need to anticipate such a possibility by explaining the function of the open fontanel both as protection of the head during delivery by allowing for molding (see below) and as a provision for further brain growth over the next 18 months. Reassurance that the brain is well protected by the tough membrane that covers it and needs no special handling and encouragement to wash the baby's head at each bath are also important.

A closed anterior fontanel is usually related to microcephaly and is a matter of serious concern. The posterior fontanel, however, may be closed in a normal newborn. Both a *bulging fontanel,* which may indicate intracranial hemorrhage or infection, and a *depressed fontanel,* which indicates dehydration, are abnormal. The fontanels should be inspected each day when the baby is bathed.

Molding describes the process by which the bones of the head accommodate themselves to the pelvic outlet in order to facilitate delivery. The baby's head may look misshapen to the parents, but we can assure them that it will be well rounded within a few days (Fig. 21–15).

Craniotabes refers to the softening of localized areas in the cranial bones. These areas are easily indented by the pressure of a fingertip, but resume their shape when the pressure is removed. The cause of craniotabes is unknown, and there is no treatment. Although the condition may persist for a number of months, it eventually disappears completely.

A *caput succedaneum* is edema of the superficial tissues that overlie the bone of the part of the head presenting first during delivery. It is caused by the pressure of the cervix on the tissues involved, the cervix acting as a tourniquet with resultant venous congestion, edema, and extravasation of blood. There may be some discoloration of the skin. A caput succedaneum presents no physical problem to the baby but may be a source of worry to the parents. It is visible immediately after birth and is usually absorbed within a few days (Fig. 21–16 *C, D*).

Another common condition in newborns, *cephalhematoma,* takes several weeks or even months to be completely resolved. In a cephalhematoma blood collects between a cranial bone and the overlying periosteum (Fig. 21–16*A, B*). Consequently, the cephalhematoma is confined to areas between suture lines, although a baby may have more than one cephalhematoma. By contrast, a caput succedaneum, because only the soft tissue is involved, crosses suture lines. Neither a caput nor a cephalhematoma requires treatment; the fluid is never aspirated. To do so would risk infection.

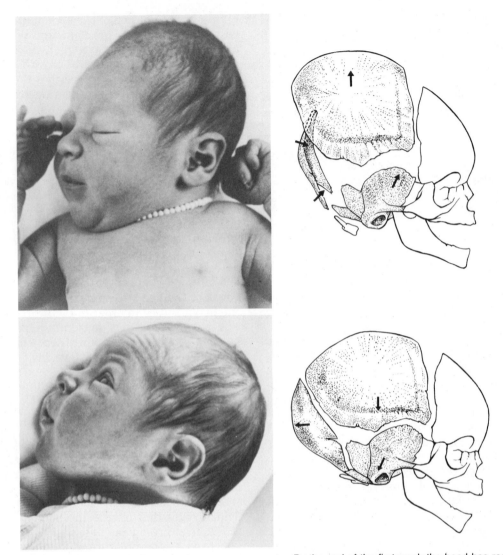

Figure 21–15. Molding during birth causes temporary asymmetry. By the end of the first week the head has regained its normal shape.

Eyes

Eye-to-eye contact is one of the significant steps in bonding a mother and father to their infant. Although neonates tend to keep their eyes shut rather tightly during the first days of life, it is important that we, as well as the parents, have an opportunity to observe them. Tilting the head gently backward may cause the baby to open his eyes. Never try to force the lids apart with the fingertips.

EYES

Within Normal Limits

Transient strabismus
Subconjunctival hemorrhage
Swelling and watery discharge following the administration of silver nitrate (chemical conjunctivitis)
Swelling following forceps delivery
Brushfield's spots
Visual reflexes present
Doll's eye movements
Strabismus
Ability to follow an object

In Need of Special Attention

Constant and fixed strabismus
Discharge beginning after the first 24 hours or lasting more than 3 days
Purulent discharge
Opacity of the pupil
Large cornea; corneas of unequal size
Epicanthic folds in non-oriental babies
Brushfield's spots
Stagnant tears
Hypertelorism

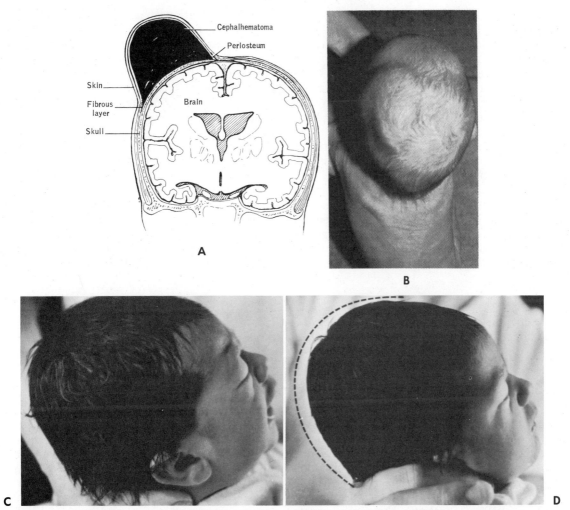

Figure 21–16. Cephalhematoma and caput succedaneum. *A,* The collection of blood lies between the periosteum and the skull bone. *B,* Typical limitation of cephalhematoma by clearly visible coronal, sagittal, and lambdoid sutures. *C,* Edema of the scalp in caput succedaneum. *D,* Reduction of edema. (From Moll: *Atlas of Pediatric Diseases.* Philadelphia, W. B. Saunders Co., 1976.)

The gray-blue color of a newborn baby's eyes is actually an absence of pigmentation, which will develop throughout the first year. Eye color is usually distinguishable by 3 months. Although the lacrimal gland is small, it is capable of producing tears. The absence of tears is not unusual in the first weeks of life, however. Stagnant tears that may flow down the baby's cheek may indicate a blocked tear duct. Because mucus cannot be washed away, it may appear as creases or a film over the eyeball. Massage over the tear duct will frequently open the duct in a few days. If the duct fails to open, a lacrimal probe may be used by a physician to alleviate the problem.

Because convergence of the eyes is not fully developed until about 3 months, newborns at times appear "cross-eyed," a matter of some concern to their parents. This apparent strabismus is normal and transient; it is 3 to 4 months before eye movements are consistently coordinated. However, constant strabismus, even in these early weeks, needs medical evaluation.

Another transient characteristic, *doll's eye movement,* may be apparent during the first 10 days of life. When the infant's head is turned, the eyes may remain in their original position instead of turning with the head.

Visual reflexes are the principal means of assessing vision in newborns. Pupils should constrict in response to light (pupillary reflex); if there is no pupillary reflex by 3 weeks of age it is possible that the infant is blind. Newborns blink in response to bright light; therefore, eyes should be examined in subdued light.

The red reflex is elicited by examination with an ophthalmoscope set at 0 diopter; the pupil is viewed from a distance of 10 inches.

Normally, the fundus reflects a red or orange color. If the light pathway is interrupted, as it is with an opacity in the cornea, the anterior chamber, or the lens, there will be a white or a partial red reflex.

As noted in the prior discussion of states, in the quiet alert state newborns will follow an object that is moving either vertically or horizontally. A human face is a preferred visual object; a visual stimulus combined with an auditory stimulus is more compelling than a visual stimulus alone.

A red ring around the cornea, or a small patch of red, indicates subconjunctival hemorrhage, which is due to changes in vascular pressure during delivery. The hemorrhage absorbs in 2 to 3 weeks without treatment and apparently without complication.

Conjunctivitis

Prophylaxis against ophthalmia neonatorum (infection of the newborn's eyes caused by *gonococci*), and inclusion conjunctivitis (caused by *Chlamydia trachomatis*), has already been discussed (Chapter 20). Although preventive treatment radically reduces the incidence of these conditions, it does not entirely eliminate the possibility that they may occur. Recognition of ophthalmia neonatorum and inclusion conjunctivitis is further complicated by the fact that the earliest symptoms, conjunctivitis and a watery discharge, resemble a reaction to the silver nitrate that is given for prevention. Drug-related conjunctivitis, however, rarely lasts longer than 24 hours; any conjunctivitis that lasts longer than 3 days is considered due to infection.

Because of an incubation period of 1 to 3 days, conjunctivitis due to ophthalmia neonatorum will occur at a later period of time than that related to silver nitrate administration and will be followed in approximately 24 hours first by a watery discharge and subsequently by a thick purulent exudate. The cornea becomes dull and ulcerates rapidly. A gelatinous exudate appears in the anterior chamber of the eye. This exudate is under great pressure; everyone who handles the baby should do so carefully and should protect his or her own eyes.

Once ophthalmia neonatorum is suspected, samples of the exudate are examined. Because the disease progresses rapidly to ocular perforation and blindness, parenteral penicillin therapy is begun as soon as the causative organism is identified as being gram positive (the group in which the gonorrhea bacteria belong). A single large dose (150,000 units of aqueous penicillin) is given, because peak blood level rather than total dose is the critical factor. Local treatment includes saline eyewashes and topical antibiotics. Great care is taken to protect the uninvolved eye; it may be taped shut.

Response to treatment is usually dramatic. The baby is significantly improved within 24 hours and is no longer considered infective. Treatment continues, however, for 2 to 5 days. If there is no response within 24 to 48 hours, the possibility of a resistant organism is considered.

Silver nitrate prophylaxis is not effective in preventing *Chlamydia* infections; erythromycin or tetracycline is used instead. Chlamydial ophthalmia neonatorum is treated with oral erythromycin, 30 to 50 mg. per kg. of body weight per day, divided into four doses, for 2 weeks.

Congenital Disorders

An opaque pupil indicates *congenital cataract* (Fig. 21–17), a condition that may, but does not always, cause major visual problems. Surgery is the treatment if there is significant visual difficulty that cannot be corrected by glasses, but results are often not as satisfactory as those in adult cataract surgery. When maternal rubella is the cause (and this is the most frequent cause), surgery should be delayed until after the second birthday to avoid activating the virus.

A baby with an unusually large cornea (the corneas may be of unequal size) is likely to have congenital glaucoma, a condition that requires immediate treatment if the baby's vision is not to be permanently damaged. The cornea may also be hazy or cloudy. Confirmation of glaucoma is made by measuring intraocular tension. The treatment is immediate surgery.

A fold of skin across the inner angle of the eye (*epicanthic fold*) is normal in Oriental babies and is not necessarily abnormal in other infants. But since epicanthic folds in non-Oriental babies are sometimes associated with Down's syndrome and certain other congenital abnormalities, they should be noted on the baby's record for proper follow-up.

Brushfield's spots (white spots scattered through the circumference of the iris) may occur in infants with Down's syndrome (Chapter 3) but also occur in normal infants.

If the distance between the inner canthi exceeds 3 cm., the term *hypertelorism* is used to describe the condition. Hypertelorism occurs in a number of syndromes and may be associated with congenital anomalies or mental retardation.

attention to the sound of a voice. A crying infant is frequently quieted by someone talking to him; in the quiet alert state an infant may turn to search for a voice. When a sudden noise is introduced, such as the ringing of a bell or a hand clap 12 inches from the baby's ear, he will often respond with a startle or blink. Since this acoustical reflex is difficult to elicit, neither the presence nor the absence of a response is considered an absolute indication of either hearing or deafness but is interpreted within the context of total behavior.

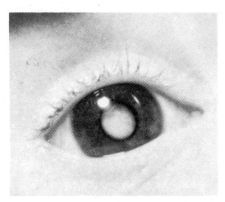

Figure 21–17. Congenital cataract. The opaque lens stands out sharply. (From the collection of Dr. Arnall Patz. *In* Schaffer and Avery: *Diseases of the Newborn.* 4th Edition. Philadelphia, W. B. Saunders Co., 1977.)

EARS

Within Normal Limits

Upper part of ear on a plane with angle of eye
Response to sound

In Need of Special Attention

Low-set ears
Absence of response to sound
Sinus tracts
Preauricular skin tags

Ears

The normal position of the newborn's ears is with the upper part on the same plane as the angle of the eye. Ears that are set lower may be associated with a congenital renal disorder or an autosomal chromosomal abnormality (Fig. 21–18). Sinus tracts in front of the ears and preauricular skin tags should be noted.

Many infants demonstrate that they pay

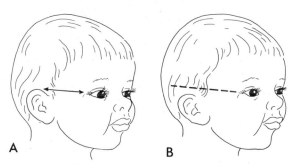

Figure 21–18. The normal position of the newborn's ears (*A*) contrasted with low set ears (*B*).

MOUTH AND JAWS

Within Normal Limits

Sucking pads
Epithelial "pearls"
Labial tubercle
Large tongue with short frenulum
Some mucus

Need of Special Attention

Cleft lip and palate
Thrush
Excessive frothy mucus
Corners of the mouth that don't move when the baby cries
Micrognathia

Mouth and Jaws

The mouth of a newly born baby is uniquely designed for its principal function—sucking. Stimulating the baby to cry will make him open his mouth so that the inside can be inspected. Note the pads of fat in the cheeks (sucking pads) that prevent collapse of the cheeks, which would make sucking difficult. Occasionally a newborn will already have one or more teeth; these teeth are usually pulled to facilitate sucking.

Epithelial "pearls" (also called Epstein's pearls and Bohn's nodules) are raised white areas of epithelial cells that are not infrequently found on the hard palate or gums. They present no problem (except possible concern to the parents) and will shortly disappear (Fig. 21–19). Epithelial pearls should not be confused with thrush (see below).

The labial tubercle is also of occasional concern to parents because it looks like a blister and is frequently termed a "sucking blister." It occurs in the center of the upper lip, is of no known significance, and needs no care.

For a day or so after birth, some babies have

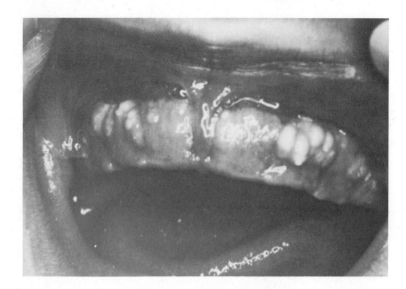

Figure 21–19. Epstein's pearls are sometimes mistaken for teeth. Firm white or gray nodules, they cause no problems and disappear within a few weeks.

a fairly large amount of mucus, which can usually be aspirated with a bulb syringe. Continued excessive mucus that is frothy, as if the baby were "blowing bubbles," suggests a *tracheoesophageal fistula.* This calls for an immediate examination of the baby, during which an attempt is made to pass a catheter through the esophagus into the stomach. If the catheter curls up or will not pass, the baby must not be fed until further testing is done.

Although a cleft lip and a large cleft of the hard and soft palate are immediately visible, smaller clefts may not be noticed unless care is taken to inspect each baby's mouth for evidence (Fig. 21–20). Even small clefts are important; the baby is at higher risk of infection, speech may be affected, and proper dentition is made difficult.

Monilia (Thrush)

Thrush, an infection caused by the fungus *Candida albicans,* is unfortunately common in some nurseries. Numerous small white and gray patches on the tongue and in the mouth (Fig. 21–21) are the indications of thrush. In addition to distinguishing thrush from epithelial patches, we must also not mistake milk curds for thrush. Thrush can be differentiated by gently wiping away the patches with a cotton-tipped applicator. Beneath plaques of thrush the mucosa will be raw and bleeding.

Babies with thrush will usually be poor eaters. Although there are many other more serious reasons for failure of a baby to feed well—heart defects, infection, and central nervous system damage, for example—any

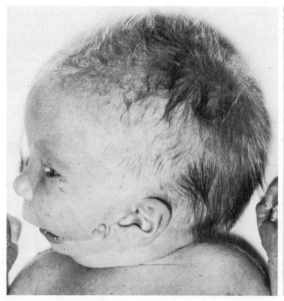
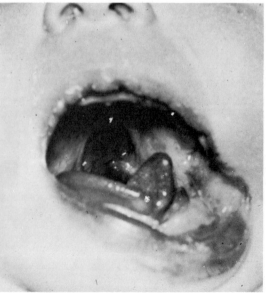

Figure 21–20. Large midline cleft in the posterior half of the palate. (From the files of Harriet Lane Home. *In* Schaffer and Avery: *Diseases of the Newborn.* 4th Edition. Philadelphia, W. B. Saunders Co., 1977.)

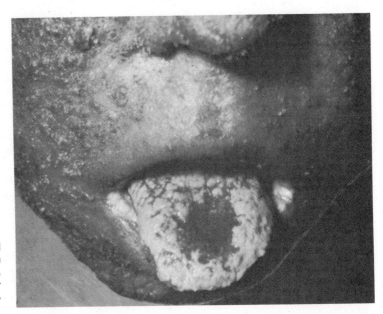

Figure 21–21. Numerous small white and gray patches on the tongue and palate are an indication of thrush. (From Pillsbury, Shelley, and Kligman: *A Manual of Cutaneous Medicine.* Philadelphia, W. B. Saunders Co., 1961.)

baby who is eating poorly should be given a thorough examination of the mouth. Babies receiving oral antibiotics are particularly susceptible. Most healthy newborns who acquire thrush do so in the delivery process, being infected by *Candida* in the mother's vagina.

Treatment usually includes the administration of a nystatin solution orally every 6 hours. Milk is rinsed from the mouth with water before treatment is started, and the solution is administered slowly and gently so that it will be widely distributed throughout the oral cavity before it is swallowed. Individual lesions are sometimes painted with a 1 per cent solution of aqueous gentian violet. Excess amounts of gentian violet should not be used because the solution may be irritating if the baby swallows it. After gentian violet is used, the baby should be placed face downward so that saliva containing the solution will drain out of the mouth. A paste of sodium bicarbonate can be used to remove gentian violet stains from clothing and bedding. Treatment is continued for 14 days even though all visible evidence of thrush is gone to ensure that the fungus itself is eradicated.

Candida albicans can also be present in the stool and the diaper area may become infected with a bright-red rash. Rarely, the entire skin surface becomes infected.

All linen and equipment used by a baby with thrush must be carefully handled to prevent spread of the infection to others. Thorough hand washing by mothers and staff after each interaction with the baby is essential. If the mother is breast-feeding, nystatin ointment is applied to both the nipple and the areola after each feeding to prevent reinfection of the baby and breakdown of nipple tissue. With proper treatment, thrush is not an indication for the cessation of breast-feeding.

Limited Facial Movement

Movement on one side of the face only when the baby cries is due to injury to a facial nerve, either because of pressure in utero or injury during delivery. When the baby cries, the mouth is drawn to that side (Fig. 21–22). Occasionally such paralysis is congenital and unrelated to trauma. Outcome depends upon the extent of the injury to the nerve fibers. If the nerves are only slightly injured, improvement usually occurs within a few weeks without treatment. If the nerve fibers have been torn and paralysis persists, neuroplasty may be necessary. If the baby is unable to close his

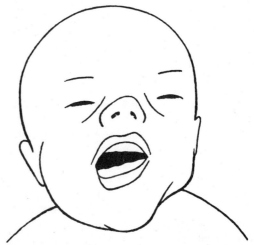

Figure 21–22. Intrauterine pressure or obstetrical trauma may result in limited facial movement for several weeks or even months before spontaneous recovery occurs.

eye on the affected side, eye care is also essential.

An abnormally small jaw, *micrognathia,* may cause respiratory distress because the tongue falls back into the pharynx. This can be partially relieved by keeping the baby on his stomach so that the tongue falls forward. Sometimes the tongue is temporarily sutured in place until the jaw grows. Many babies with micrognathia have a cleft palate as well.

TRUNK

Within Normal Limits

Breast engorgement
Bluish-white umbilical cord
Cutis navel
Granulation tissue in navel
Abdomen moderately protuberant
Liver and kidneys palpable
Bowel sounds

In Need of Special Attention

Knot on clavicle
Bleeding from or around the cord
Yellow discoloration of the cord at the time of birth
Exudate at the cord site
Cord with one artery and one vein
Distended, "shiny" abdomen
Scaphoid abdomen
Umbilical hernia
Mass in the abdomen
Absence of abdominal musculature
Curvature or absence of vertebrae

Trunk

A knot on the clavicle indicates a fracture, which will heal without difficulty.

Breast engorgement is often a concern to a mother when she examines her baby. During pregnancy, maternal hormones cross the placenta and enter the fetal circulation. By the time of birth, the infant's breasts may be enlarged and may even secrete fluid resembling colostrum or milk, referred to as "witch's milk" by some mothers. The enlargement lasts from a few days to as long as several weeks. Mothers need to know that this enlargement is perfectly normal. The breasts should not be handled other than in routine bathing. No attempt should ever be made to express the fluid in the breasts; to do so is to risk mastitis.

The Umbilical Area and Cord

The umbilical area and cord also cause many parental questions. Bluish-white at birth, the

cord begins to dry right away and usually separates in 6 to 8 days, with the umbilicus healing in about 2 weeks. Because mothers and their term babies often stay in the hospital only 3 to 4 days, and many times even less, cord care quickly becomes the mother's responsibility. It is generally recommended that the cord and the umbilicus be cleaned each day with a cotton ball dipped in alcohol and that submerging the baby's body in his bathtub be delayed until after the area has healed.

The cord should be checked initially for the presence of a single umbilical artery; normally there are two arteries and one vein. The single artery occurs in about 1 per cent of all newborns, more frequently in white infants. For some reason the single artery is associated with an increased incidence of various congenital anomalies and with higher perinatal mortality. It is probably a part of a complex of malformations rather than the cause of those malformations. For those infants with a single artery who survive the perinatal period, there is no apparent difference in mortality and morbidity (other than a higher incidence of hernia), an important fact for reassuring parents about this infant and for future genetic counseling.

Yellow discoloration of the cord at the time of birth is an indication of hemolytic disease; these babies need careful observation and evaluation (Chapter 24). Exudate around the cord usually signifies infection, although a baby may have an umbilical infection serious enough to cause generalized sepsis with no local signs at all. A weeping cord should be cleaned with alcohol several times a day. Cord bleeding may be due to inadequate tying, or it may be a symptom of a bleeding disorder.

Cutis navel describes an umbilical cord that projects beyond the skin. It looks at first glance as if the baby might have an umbilical hernia, but a hernia can be returned to the abdomen while a cutis navel cannot. In addition, hernias become more pronounced when the baby cries. No special treatment of cutis navel is required; the navel will slowly invaginate.

Umbilical hernia is more common in black newborns than in infants of other races. The hernia is due to a weakness or imperfect closure of the umbilical ring. Most umbilical hernias that occur in small infants disappear spontaneously by the baby's first birthday. Possibly because there is no general agreement on how, or even if, umbilical hernias should be treated, "folk" remedies abound. A silver dollar may be found strapped to the baby's abdomen when he comes for a check-up, or various forms of binders may be wrapped around him. Studies have produced conflicting evidence about the value of "strapping" the

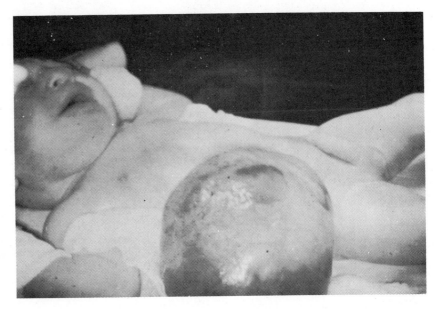

Figure 21-23. Large omphalocele. Note covering of the sac and its relationship to the umbilicus, which extrudes from the lower portion. (From Schaffer and Avery: *Diseases of the Newborn.* 4th Edition. Philadelphia, W. B. Saunders Co., 1977.)

hernia. Surgery is usually avoided unless the hernia persists until the child is 3 to 5 years old or unless it creates problems for the baby or becomes progressively larger after the baby is a year old.

Abdominal Wall Defects

A central defect in the peritoneal, muscular, and ectodermal layers of the abdominal wall is termed an *omphalocele*. The defect is covered by a translucent membrane that covers both bowel and solid viscera (Fig. 21-23). An omphalocele may vary in size from a small hernia to a huge mass that contains all the abdominal viscera.

Gastroschisis differs from an omphalocele in that the abdominal wall is developed but a defect remains at the base of the umbilical stalk.

Prior to surgery, every effort is made to keep the viscera sterile by covering them with moist sterile saline sponges or gauze and sterile plastic. The viscera are only partially replaced during initial surgery; an envelope is created over the remainder, a little more bowel being returned to the abdomen each day in order to keep respiratory distress at a minimum. An alternative procedure involves suturing the skin over the abdominal contents and deferring their return to the abdomen until both baby and abdomen have grown larger.

When the abdominal muscles are absent, the abdomen has a wrinkled appearance from which the term *prune-belly syndrome* is derived. Infants with this disorder, 95 per cent of whom are male, may have a number of associated defects for which they must be carefully observed. The associated defects may include undescended testicles, intestinal malrotation, imperforate anus, dilated and tortuous ureters, hydronephrotic kidneys, and a dilated hypertrophied bladder. Prognosis is related to the degree of gastrointestinal obstruction and the extent of the renal problems. An abdominal binder may be applied to provide support. Surgery to relieve the back pressure of urine on the kidneys is performed in some infants.

Abdominal Distention

Although the abdomen is moderately protuberant in all babies, a distended abdomen, which may appear shiny because the skin is stretched, is definitely abnormal. An overly distended abdomen may be related to several conditions. An infant with the type of tracheoesophageal fistula in which there is an opening between the trachea and the stomach will become distended from the continual entry of air. Distention is also an early sign of infection. Congenital obstructions of the gastrointestinal tract and congenital megacolon are also conditions causing distention in newborns. It is important to know whether distention is increasing or decreasing. Marking the area of the distention with a waxed pencil makes this easier to detect.

The opposite of distention, a scaphoid abdomen, suggests the possibility of a diaphragmatic hernia (Chapter 24).

Visible peristaltic waves may move from left to right, as in pyloric stenosis (seen usually in the 2 to 4 week old infant rather than immediately after birth) or from right to left, as in small bowel obstruction. Most prominent during and after feeding, peristaltic waves may be more easily visualized by focusing a light on the baby's abdomen while he is being fed.

Abdominal Palpation and Auscultation

Abdominal muscles must be relaxed for the abdomen to be palpated. Relaxation is aided by flexing the infant's knees toward the abdomen or by holding the infant semierect with one hand while palpating the abdomen with the other. The liver is usually felt 2 to 3 cm. below the right costal margin. The tip of the spleen may not be palpable until the end of the first week. Kidneys are palpated by placing one hand beneath the infant's flank and the other below the costal margin and pressing them together. Both kidneys should be palpable. The tip of the left kidney and the lower half of the right kidney should be felt approximately 1 to 2 cm. above the umbilicus. Any solid mass in the abdomen that can be palpated is abnormal.

Bowel Sounds

Bowel sounds should be present within a few hours after birth. Bowel sounds heard in the thoracic cavity may indicate diaphragmatic hernia; however, it is not unusual for bowel sounds to be transmitted to the pleural cavity. There is no pathologic condition in 20 to 25 per cent of newborns in whom bowel sounds cannot be heard during the neonatal period.

Assessment of the Back

The vertebrae should be palpated for defects in the closure of the vertebral canal (spina bifida occulta) and for abnormal curvature of the spine. When the meninges protrude through the bony defect, the resultant *meningocele* or *myelomeningocele* is obvious (Chapter 24).

GENITALIA

Within Normal Limits: Female

Red and swollen
Vaginal discharge
Vaginal bleeding
Hymenal tag

Within Normal Limits: Male

Scrotal swelling

In Need of Special Attention

Excessive vaginal bleeding
Undescended testicles in a term baby
Hypospadias, epispadias
Ambiguous genitalia

Genitalia

Edema of the genitalia is not uncommon in either male or female babies. It is especially noticeable in babies delivered from the breech position. Such edema disappears within a few days.

A vaginal discharge of thick, white mucus is passed by all baby girls in the first week of life. Occasionally the mucus is blood tinged about the third or fourth day, staining the diaper. This pseudomenstruation, like breast engorgement described previously, is due to the influence of maternal hormones and their withdrawal. Excessive vaginal bleeding is not normal; it may be due to a blood coagulation defect.

A hymenal or vaginal tag may be distressing to the mother, but it will drop off within a few weeks.

Undescended Testicles

Normally, testicles descend into the scrotum in the eighth month of fetal life. The descent of both testes should be assessed by palpation. It is possible that a baby boy with undescended testicles is of a younger gestational age than originally suspected. Gestational age should be evaluated as described in Chapter 20.

Hypospadias and Epispadias

Hypospadias is a condition in which the urethra opens on the ventral surface of the penis (Fig. 21–24). Surgical correction is usually made by the time the boy is 2 years old and should always be made before he starts school, so that he will be able to urinate in the same way as the other boys in his class. These babies should *not* be circumcised because the foreskin is used in the surgical repair.

Epispadias is the opening of the urethra on the dorsal aspect of the penis. Epispadias is far less common than hypospadias and is also surgically corrected.

Ambiguous Genitalia

When the genitalia do not appear to be clearly male or female further investigation is required. Adrenogenital syndrome (congenital adrenal hyperplasia), a genetic recessive defect in which one of several enzymes necessary to the production of adrenal steroids is deficient, may be the reason. Because the adrenals are unable to produce large amounts of cortisol, increased quantitites of androgens, precursors of cortisol production, are present. Internal

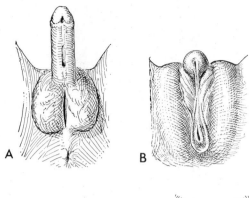

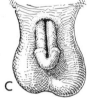

Figure 21–24. Anomalies of the human genitalia. *A,* Hypospadias, showing in one drawing a composite of the different locations. *B,* Hypospadias of a severe degree in a false male hermaphrodite. *C,* Epispadias. (From Arey: *Developmental Anatomy: A Textbook and Laboratory Manual of Embryology.* Revised 7th Edition. Philadelphia, W. B. Saunders Co., 1974.)

genitalia are not usually affected because the malfunction begins in the twelfth week of life after the internal structures have developed.

In 90 per cent of infants with congenital adrenal hyperplasia the defect is a deficiency of 21-hydroxylase; several other enzymes are involved in the remaining 10 per cent. In 70 per cent of these infants, the defect is varying or incomplete. Female infants may be affected only mildly; for example, there may be a slight enlargement of the clitoris, or the labia may be fused and a penis may be present. Male infants usually appear normal at birth or have an enlarged penis.

In the 30 per cent of severely affected infants the condition also results in aldosterone deficiency, with associated failure to thrive, hyponatremia, hyperkalemia, and eventually vascular collapse and death. This is called the "salt-losing" form of the disease. It is necessary, therefore, to recognize these infants early in life not only for a proper assignment of sex but also, in some instances, to preserve life. Unfortunately, the external signs in males are usually not as evident, and the baby may become severely ill before the condition is recognized. Diagnosis is made by laboratory evaluations of metabolites in urine and plasma. Treatment is the lifelong provision of cortisone and of a mineralocorticoid preparation to ensure adequate growth. Girls require surgery if labial fusion exists and occasionally more extensive vaginoplasty.

Ambiguous genitalia may also result from

hormones given to the mother during pregnancy (see Chapter 8).

If we consider that the first question parents ask about their new infant is generally whether it is a boy or a girl, we can appreciate how devastating the presence of ambiguous genitalia is to parents. The baby's chromosomal sex should be determined as quickly as possible, and the parents should be given information, support, and reassurance. Fortunately, the long-term prognosis for normal reproductive function and psychosocial development is excellent in infants with 21-hydroxylase deficiency, and the more severe, salt-losing form of the disease is controlled by doses of cortisone.

THE EXTREMITIES

Within Normal Limits

Flexion of arms and legs
Extension of legs in a baby born in breech position

In Need of Special Attention

Abnormal position or posture of an extremity
Polydactyly
Syndactyly
Single transverse palmar crease (simian crease)
Talipes equinovarus
Talipes calcaneovalgus
Inability to abduct thigh

The Extremities

The flexed position of the baby's arms and legs has already been mentioned. Ordinarily extension of the extremities is abnormal, but it is not unusual in a baby born in the breech presentation to have his legs extended.

Abnormal positioning of an arm may be due to brachial injury or to a fractured clavicle, discussed above, or, rarely, to a fractured humerus.

An extra finger or toe, polydactyly (Fig. 21–25), or webbing of the fingers or toes, syndactyly (Fig. 21–26), may be a familial trait or may be associated with other anomalies. When the extra finger or toe is little more than a skin tag, it may be tied off shortly after birth. When surgery is indicated, it is usually delayed for 2 to 3 years in polydactyly and even longer in syndactyly.

A single transverse crease in the palm of

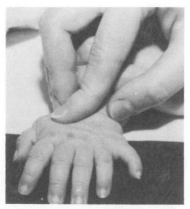

Figure 21–25. Polydactyly, showing a supernumerary finger. (From Swenson: *Pediatric Surgery.* 1958. Courtesy of Appleton-Century-Crofts, Publishing Division of Prentice-Hall, Inc., Englewood Cliffs, N.J.)

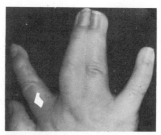

Figure 21–26. Syndactyly involving webbing of the third and fourth fingers. (From Swenson: *Pediatric Surgery.* 1958. Courtesy of Appleton-Century-Crofts, Publishing Division of Prentice-Hall Inc., Englewood Cliffs, N.J.)

the hand (simian crease) is often associated with Down's syndrome but also occurs in normal, healthy babies.

About 95 per cent of clubfoot deformities are *talipes equinovarus* (Fig. 21–27), in which the foot is turned downward and inward (medially), somewhat like the hoof of a horse (hence the name). The force required to return the foot to normal position gives some indication of the severity of the problem. When treatment is started even before the baby is discharged from the nursery, good results are likely. Such treatment usually involves a series of casts that gradually change the position of the foot until it is overcorrected. In *talipes calcaneovalgus* (Fig. 21–28), the foot is flexed and deviates laterally. Often passive exercise is the only treatment required, although casts may also be used.

Inability to Abduct Thigh

Early recognition of *congenital hip dysplasia,* a condition in which the acetabulum is shallow and incompletely ossified, is very important for successful treatment. With the baby lying on his back, the thighs are flexed, one at a time, outward and then downward to touch the table or bed (Fig. 21–29). When one thigh does not abduct easily, the diagnosis is quite probable. Other indications include a consistent sharp click heard on the affected side during abduction and higher on extra creases observed on the buttock of the affected side when the baby is lying prone. (See also Chapter 24.)

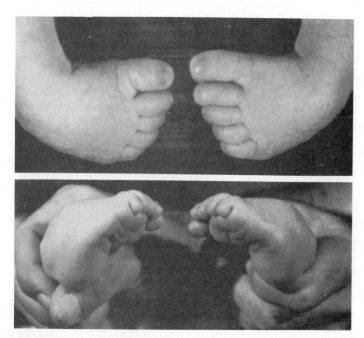

Figure 21–27. Congenital clubfeet. (From Miller: *Journal of Pediatrics, 51*:527, 1957.)

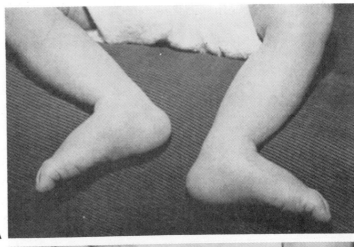

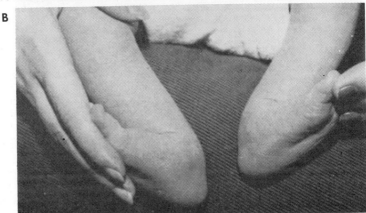

Figure 21–28. Calcaneovalgus deformity. *A,* Feet at rest. *B,* Same feet under test. (From Miller: *Journal of Pediatrics, 51:*527, 1957.)

intracranial pressure. After the first day, vomiting may still be related to these causes, but it can also be a sign of many other conditions, including septicemia, overfeeding, pyloric stenosis, milk allergy, and adrenal insufficiency.

Blood in the vomitus of a breast-fed baby, unless copious, very possibly originates from fissures in the mother's nipple. Maternal blood swallowed during delivery is also a common

---

VOMITING

Within Normal Limits

Mild regurgitation

In Need of Special Attention

Persistent vomiting
Bloody emesis
Bile-stained emesis
Projectile vomiting

Vomiting

Mild regurgitation is not at all unusual in newborns and is due principally to two factors, swallowed air and a certain amount of immaturity of the cardiac sphincter.

Vomiting is quite another matter. Vomiting that occurs shortly after birth or within the first 24 hours is likely to be due to obstruction of the upper digestive tract or to increased

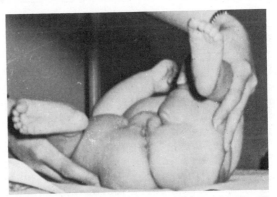

Figure 21–29. Infant with subluxation of left hip. The nurse is able to abduct the right thigh down to the level of the table, but not the left. (From Pray: *Pediatrics,* 9:94, 1952.)

cause of blood appearing in the vomitus of the newborn in the first 2 or 3 days of life. An *Abt test* differentiates maternal blood from fetal blood, based on the fact that fetal hemoglobin is much more alkali-resistant than adult-type hemoglobin.

Bloody emesis accompanied by marked abdominal distention and sudden distress may indicate gastric perforation.

Dark green vomitus indicates an obstruction of the gastrointestinal tract (Chapter 24).

Whether or not vomiting is projectile is always a significant observation. Projectile vomiting in the first week is often related to intestinal obstruction; beginning in the second week the cause may be pyloric stenosis.

STOOLS

Within Normal Limits

Meconium stools for 3 to 4 days
Transitional stools: greenish brown to yellow
Stools that vary with type of feeding.
Breast-fed baby—has from one to six golden to mustard stools in 24 hours; bottle-fed baby has pale yellow, more regular, more formed stools than stools of breast-fed baby
Darkened stools in the baby receiving iron
Faint purple stools in the baby treated with gentian violet
Bright green stools in the baby under phototherapy lights (Chapter 24)

In Need of Special Attention

Failure to stool within 48 hours
Meconium stool but no feces
Thick, puttylike meconium
Small, puttylike stool
Diarrhea
Bloody stools

Stools

The consistency, color, and odor of stools are all important in evaluating a baby's general condition. Because color changes can occur shortly after defecation, evaluation has to be made right away if it is to have meaning.

Stool consistency and color vary during the first days according to both age and type of feeding. The first stools are of *meconium,* an odorless, viscid material that is dark green to black in color. Meconium stools may last from 3 to 4 days.

Meconium stools are followed by greenish-

brown to yellow transitional stools. In breast-fed infants, the next stools will be golden to mustard colored. Stools of breast-fed infants may be more frequent initially than those of bottle-fed infants; at home, however, some breast-fed infants may normally have no stool for several days. The stools of bottle-fed babies are pale yellow in color. They tend to be more formed and more regular than those of breast-fed infants.

No stool passed with 48 hours after delivery usually suggests intestinal obstruction. If meconium is passed initially, but then no feces are passed, the obstruction is in the ileum. Thick, puttylike meconium is the initial symptom of meconium ileus, the neonatal symptom of cystic fibrosis. A small, puttylike stool may be due to stenosis or to atresia somewhere in the bowel.

Diarrhea

Diarrhea is a somewhat nonspecific symptom in newborns. It may simply be the result of overfeeding, although "starvation stools" are probably a more common cause. Some babies will have diarrhea from formulas that will have no adverse effects on other infants. Diarrhea due to enteric infection (Chapter 22) can spread rapidly through a nursery if the ill baby is not immediately isolated.

Aside from the danger of sepsis, diarrhea is extremely serious in newborns because of the baby's very labile water balance. The extent of water loss can be estimated by measuring the water margin around the stool if the baby has not voided in the diaper. Because infant stools are acid and the intestinal membranes of newborns are delicate, bloody diarrhea is not as unusual at this age as it is in older patients.

A baby may also have flecks of blood in his stool from an anal fissure. A stool with either bright red or old blood is usually a sign of intestinal bleeding. As with blood in the vomitus, a distinction must be made between fetal and maternal blood.

URINE

Within Normal Limits

Peach-colored crystals

In Need of Special Attention

Failure to void
Bloody urine

Urine

The peach-colored discoloration of the diaper of a newborn is due to crystals of uric acid, which are not pathologic at this age.

It is exceedingly important that the occurrence of voiding be noted on the baby's chart during his hospitalization. Failure to void may be due to decreased production of urine or to a mechanical obstruction to voiding. The most common cause of failure to void in the newborn period is dehydration; babies who are small for gestational age are particularly susceptible. Other causes of decreased urine production include hypotension, severe asphyxia, and renal anomalies such as the absence of one or both kidneys or polycystic kidneys.

It is not unusual for an infant to fail to void in the first 12 hours following birth He may not void until the second or even the third day, depending upon his fluid intake, the environmental temperature, and the condition of his digestive and nervous systems.

Bloody urine suggests renal injury. The cause may be birth asphyxia, renal vein thrombosis, or an infection.

Edema

It is not always easy to recognize generalized edema in a newborn. Normally a baby should have very fine wrinkles over the knuckles of his hands and feet. If these wrinkles are not evident, generalized edema may be present. Severe generalized edema may be present. Severe generalized edema at the time of birth may indicate erythroblastosis fetalis heart failure because of congenital heart disease, or electrolyte imbalance. Firm, sustained pressure is necessary to demonstrate pitting edema in a newborn because of the limited amount of subcutaneous tissue.

On the other hand, edema of the presenting part is not unusual or a cause for concern. Some preterm babies have a transient edema for no discernible reason. Although infants of diabetic mothers may appear edematous, their excess weight is due to fat rather than to accumulated fluid.

Metabolic Problems: Phenylketonuria and Hypothyroidism

In addition to those conditions that can be detected by physical assessment, screening of infants for phenylketonuria (PKU) and hypothyroidism is a part of neonatal evaluation. Screening for PKU is required by law in many states; mass screening for hypothyroidism was first reported in 1973. Fortunately, the same specimen of capillary blood, obtained by heel stick and transferred to filter paper, can be used in both tests.

Phenylketonuria

PKU is an autosomal recessive disease (Chapter 3) in which phenylalanine, an amino acid, accumulates because of an error in metabolism. Undetected, this accumulation leads to irreversible mental retardation in affected infants. In the United States, PKU occurs approximately once in 14,000 births.

Because concentrations of phenylalanine may not rise sufficiently to be detected in the first days of life, testing should be deferred until the third to sixth day or until dietary protein has been ingested for 24 to 48 hours. When mothers and infants stay in the hospital for a shorter time than usual, alternative plans for performing a screening test are necessary. When mothers are breast-feeding, breast milk (not colostrum) must have been taken for 24 hours. A screening test made on a home visit can provide an opportunity for a community health nurse to assess and teach the family as well as to screen for PKU.

If the initial screening test is negative (i.e., no phenylalanine is present) the test should be repeated within 2 to 4 weeks after birth. The most common reason for an initial negative test is an inadequate blood sample. Blood sampling is only the preliminary step in recognition of PKU; phenylalanine is found in urine and blood in other conditions as well.

The treatment of PKU is dietary. Phenylalanine is restricted in the diet by substituting Lofenalac for milk (with a small amount of cow's milk added to provide the phenylalanine added for growth). Later, strained foods low in protein are added to the diet.

Dietary treatment is monitored by regular blood testing (daily during the first week, weekly until the baby is 2 months old, twice a month from 2 months to 1 year, and monthly after that) and urine testing (daily during the first month, twice weekly until the baby is 6 months old, weekly until his first birthday, and twice a month from that time on). The reason for this constant monitoring—which parents must understand—is that although a normal dietary level of phenylalanine will cause mental retardation, a diet too low in this essential amino acid will not meet the baby's growth requirements. Dietary treatment initiated in the first 3 months of life will prevent or minimize mental retardation. Controversy exists over how long a special diet should be continued; continuation through adolescence is frequently recommended. If a woman with PKU plans to become pregnant, a low phenylalanine diet should be started several months prior to conception. The risk of producing a mentally retarded infant is very high if the mother remains on a general diet during pregnancy.

Hypothyroidism

Congenital hypothyroidism is far more common than PKU; the incidence of thyroid dysgenesis, the most common cause of congenital hypothyroidism, is estimated at 1 in 6000. The etiology is unknown; rarely is more than one member of a family affected.

Without detection and treatment many affected infants die of respiratory disease or infection or survive to become mentally deficient dwarfs. If treatment (replacement therapy with thyroid hormone) is started by 6 weeks of age, normal development can be expected.

Fisher et al.[13] reported that in screening 1,046,362 infants, 277 were found to have hypothyroidism (an incidence of 1 in 3684 births). Only 8 of the 277 had clinical signs of hypothyroidism in the first 1 to 2 months. One may suppose that none of these 269 infants would have received early treatment if screening had not been available.

hours in each 24-hour period. Listening to the cries of infants will enable us to become more skilled in recognizing an abnormal cry, such as the high-pitched, shrill cry or the excessive, irritable crying of the baby with an infection or brain damage or the baby of a drug-addicted mother. A total absence of crying also suggests brain damage. If the crying sounds very hoarse, there may be partial paralysis of the vocal cords. Crying because of hunger will usually be accompanied by rooting and sucking. Even a tiny baby may also cry because of a desire to be held. Such a desire is really a need; *babies truly need to be touched and held.* Meeting such a need is no way "spoiling" a baby. Excellent nursing care involves being able to recognize that need, just as we now recognize the need for feeding, and taking the baby to his mother for "loving" or, if this is not possible at a particular moment, taking time to hold the baby ourselves. (See also Consolability, p. 654.)

A shrill, high-pitched cry suggests some type of central nervous system damage, such as hemorrhage or infection. A shrill cry may also be the first sign of kernicterus (Chapter 23). If you cringe when the baby cries, there is probably something wrong.

A hoarse cry is usually related to congenital laryngeal malformation or to an injury of the larynx during birth. A laryngoscopic examination is usually necessary to determine the exact cause, which may range from a mild problem that requires no treatment to a life-threatening condition.

BEHAVIOR

Within Normal Limits

Strong, vigorous cry
General alertness and responsiveness
Spontaneous activity
Sleeps 65 to 70 per cent of the time

In Need of Special Attention

Shrill or hoarse cry
Absence of a cry
Hyperirritability
"Sleepy" baby

Behavior

The crying of a healthy term infant is strong and vigorous; he may cry for as much as 2

Sleep

The concept of sleep *states* was discussed at the beginning of this chapter. Careful observation indicates that newborns do not sleep as much as we may have believed at one time. Even during the first 3 days of life, a healthy term infant may be awake for brief periods that total 7 to 8 hours, roughly 30 per cent of the 24-hour span. Part of the waking time will be spent in crying (state 6), as noted above. From 2 to 3 hours will be feeding time. Periods of light sleep (state 2) will be interspersed with times when the baby is alert and responsive (state 4).

Many parents seem to expect their baby to sleep most of the time. Unless they are aware that a certain amount of wakefulness, sometimes accompanied by fussiness, is normal, they may feel that something is wrong. Although extreme hyperirritability in an infant is abnormal, the drowsy, "sleepy" baby who is rarely awake needs to be evaluated as well.

Assessment of Interactional Behavior

It is frequently stated that each newborn infant is an individual. Yet to a large extent we persist in treating infants as if they were all alike.

A Neonatal Behavioral Assessment Scale[4] (developed by Brazelton[4]) emphasizes the individual personality of each newborn. It is not possible to assess an intact newborn infant using the Brazelton scale and ever again to believe that all newborns are all alike or that newborns function on a subcortical, reflex level. During the months in utero, the personality has been shaped, but until now there has not been a systematic way to evaluate personality.

The items evaluated in the Brazelton assessment are listed in Table 21–3. A detailed description of each item and the scoring of the response are beyond the scope of this book. The assessment process is described in detail in *Clinics in Developmental Medicine*, No. 50,[4] and in a series of three films (see Appendix H).

Brazelton emphasizes that repeated assessments are of far more value than a single assessment.

Table 21–3. THE BRAZELTON ASSESSMENT*

Environment: Quiet, semidarkened room; temperature of room 72°–80°F.

Infant: Asleep, covered, dressed, midway between feeding

Observe for 2 minutes—note state
Response decrement to flashlight
Response decrement to rattle
Response decrement to bell
Uncover infant; note reaction
Response decrement to light pinprick
Speed of state change
Test ankle clonus, foot grasp, Babinski response
Undress infant
Pull to sit
Standing
Walking
Placing
Incurvation
Body tone when held across hand
Crawling—prone responses
Pick up and hold
Glabella reflex
Spin
Orientation (inanimate and animate); visual, auditory, and visual and auditory
Cloth on face
Tonic neck response
Moro response

*Adapted from Brazelton: *Clinics in Developmental Medicine. No. 50.* Philadelphia, J. B. Lippincott Co., 1973.

Because the total assessment takes approximately 30 minutes, there are few, if any, nurseries that can screen every baby using the Brazelton scale.

However, we would like to describe several ways in which items of the Brazelton scale are of value in better understanding the baby and in helping his parents to understand him better.

Response Decrement to Inanimate Visual and Auditory Stimuli. A flashlight, a rattle, and a bell are used as stimuli. When a baby is first presented with a stimulus, such as a light flashing in his eyes, he responds with a grimace and with body movements; perhaps he awakens. But as the stimulus is presented again and again, he normally begins to ignore it and eventually has little or no response. This process, called habituation, is one measure of central nervous system integration. The baby who consistently fails to habituate to stimuli should have careful follow-up during the neonatal and postnatal periods. His failure may be related to a transient problem, such as a high level of medication that crossed the placenta during labor, or to a more serious central nervous system problem.

These responses are measured in sleep state 1, 2, or 3, described at the beginning of this chapter.

Orientation Response to Visual and Auditory Stimuli. Most infants will focus their attention on a bright red ball and follow it briefly when they are in the quiet alert state (state 4) or will shift their eyes and turn their head toward the sound of a rattle or bell in state 4 or 5.

Even more entrancing to most babies is the human face, which the baby may follow from right to left and up and down. When the examiner moves her face from the baby's line of sight and talks to him from one side in soft, continuous, high-pitched tones, many babies will become alert, turn their head toward the stimulus, and search for the sound with their eyes.

Demonstrating this behavior to parents is one way of helping them recognize their baby's capabilities. Many parents believe that playing with a newborn baby—talking to him or looking at him—either will spoil him or is a game that is fun for them but means little to the baby because he can't see or hear. As they see us interact with their baby and begin to interact with him themselves, and as he responds to them, both bonding and a pattern of caretaking that will provide for sensory stimulation are facilitated.

Cuddliness. Infants respond in various

ways to being held. In the Brazelton assessment, cuddliness is assessed with the infant held against the examiner's chest (see Fig. 21–1) or on the examiner's shoulder (state 4 or 5).

Some babies resist being held; they stiffen or thrash or push away. Others are passive, neither resisting nor participating. Still others relax and mold themselves to the body of the holder, nestling the head in her (his) arm. If held to the shoulder, a cuddly baby molds to the holder's body and nestles his head against the holder's shoulder.

The baby who is *consistently* irritable when held and never "cuddles" may be brain damaged. However, normal infants vary markedly in how cuddly they are. Schaeffer and Emerson[31] followed 37 mother–infant pairs throughout the first 18 months of the infants' lives. Nine babies were evaluated as noncuddlers, 19 as cuddlers, and 9 as intermediate between the other two groups. Cuddlers enjoyed, accepted, and even sought physical contact. Noncuddlers were highly intolerant of physical restraint; they were active and restless. The noncuddlers tended to have accelerated motor development, while the cuddlers were more placid, slept more, and formed earlier and more intense attachments.

It is interesting that Schaeffer and Emerson found no consistent differences in mother–child interaction between cuddlers and noncuddlers, suggesting that the baby's behavior was indeed an expression of his personality. They also suggest that cuddlers may be more affected by a lack of physical contact than noncuddlers, and thus this kind of deprivation will affect some infants more than others.

From the standpoint of anticipatory guidance, helping parents assess the relative cuddliness or noncuddliness of their baby could be significant. Some parents feel that they must be doing something wrong if their baby does not cuddle to them. They can feel rejected. They need to know that there is a wide range of variability in perfectly normal babies.

Consolability.   When the baby is actively crying (state 6), how easily is he consoled? A few babies may be consoled by face alone, or by seeing a face and hearing a voice. Others require (in progressive order) a hand on their abdomen, restraint of one or both arms, holding, rocking, dressing, and a pacifier or finger to suck.

What kind of intervention is most soothing to neonates? Korner and Thoman[23] explored the efficacy of body contact in comparison with vestibular stimulation (i.e., picking the baby up and moving him). They found that vestibular stimulation was more effective, both in soothing the infant and in bringing him to an alert state, than was body contact and suggest that such stimulation is often overlooked with the prevailing emphasis on the importance of body contact.

Self-Consolation.   Infants console themselves in a variety of ways—by attempting to place a hand in the mouth, by sucking a fist or the tongue, or sometimes by gazing at an object or listening to a sound. Here again, normal infants vary considerably in their ability. These differences can make a marked difference in the way the new baby adjusts during the first weeks of life—both in how much he is able to comfort himself and to what extent his mother, father, or others must intervene to console him. Korner[19] also suggests that the strength of the oral drive and the baby's ability to comfort himself may also influence the intensity with which weaning is experienced.

Part of becoming acquainted with a baby is the recognition of the way in which an individual baby responds to various kinds of soothing. In one small study of 35 neonates who were 2 to 3 days old, Birns and her coworkers found that babies who were easily soothed by one stimulus were easily soothed by all stimuli, while others were difficult to soothe in any manner. It is not hard to imagine how mothers of those babies easily soothed may begin to feel competent rather quickly, while the mother of a baby who cries a great deal, no matter what she does, may begin to doubt her ability to ever become a good mother. Just why some babies are difficult to console (other than those who are brain damaged or ill) is not clear. Freedman and Freedman[14] compared 24 Chinese-American neonates with 24 European-American newborns. Although there was no significant difference in the amount of crying in the two groups of babies, the Chinese infants stopped crying in a "dramatically immediate" period of time when they were picked up.

Behavioral Assessment and Nursing Practice and Research

One need not systematically assess each baby by using a Brazelton scale to utilize the concept of behavior assessment in practice. Each time a baby is picked up, his cuddliness may be assessed. His response to face and voice can be noted when he is alert. His ability to console or quiet himself is usually apparent. All of these cues can help us guide his parents in recognizing their baby's individuality and needs as distinct from the needs of other babies (including any siblings) and as distinct from their own needs and ideas of how a baby should be nurtured. Brazelton's book *Infants and Mothers*[3] describes infant individuality in an "average" baby, a "quiet" baby, and an "active" baby as they develop during the first year of life. This book is written for parents (parents with a high school education or greater); we recommend it to many families.

The potential value of newborn behavioral assessment in nursing research seems almost unlimited. Some examples, from other researchers, have been indicated above. Brazelton assessments have indicated differences in the behavior of infants receiving certain local-regional anesthetics (Chapter 17). Systematic cross-cultural evaluations are also possible.

Summary

Newborns individually and as a group are unique. What is normal in terms of appearance and behavior at this special time of life differs in many ways from the norms of any other period.

Because the newborn infant's condition can change so rapidly, nurses are the primary observers of each baby's condition. A combination of knowledge and experience ensures good care for each baby in our nurseries.

REFERENCES

1. Birns, B., Blank, M., and Bridger, W.: The Effectiveness of Various Soothing Techniques on Human Neonates. *Psychosomatic Medicine, 28*:316, 1966.
2. Braekbill, Y., Douthitt, T., and West, H.: Neonatal Posture: Psychophysiological Events. *Neuropaediatrie, 4*:145, 1973.
3. Brazelton, T. B.: *Infants and Mothers: Differences in Development.* New York, Dell Publishing Co., 1969.
4. Brazelton, T. B.: Neonatal Behavioral Assessment Scale. *Clinics in Developmental Medicine, 50*:1973.
5. Carpenter, E.: Space Concepts of Aivilik Eskimos. *Explorations Five,* June, 1955.
6. Condon, W., and Sander, L.: Synchrony Demonstrated Between Movements of the Neonate and Adult Speech. *Child Development, 45*:456, 1974.
7. DeCasper, A., and Fifer, W.: Of Human Bonding: Newborns Prefer Their Mothers' Voices. *Science, 208*:1174, 1980.
7a. DeCasper, A., Butterfield, E., and Cairns, G.: The role of contingency relations in speech discrimination by newborns. Paper presented at the Fourth Biennial Conference of Human Development, Nashville, Tennessee, April 1976.
8. DiToro, R., Lupi, L., and Ansanelli, V.: Glucuronation of the Liver in Premature Babies. *Nature, 219*:265, 1968.
9. Dreyfus-Brisac, C.: Organization of Sleep in Prematures: Implications for Caregiving. In Lewis, M., and Rosenblum, L. (eds.): *The Effect of the Infant on its Caregiver.* New York, John Wiley, 1974.
10. Eisenberg, R.: *Auditory Competence in Early Life: The Roots of Communicative Behavior.* Baltimore, University Park Press, 1976.
11. Engen, T., and Lipsitt, L.: Ability of Newborn Infants to Discriminate Sapid Substances. *Developmental Psychology, 10*:741, 1974.
11a. Engen, E., Lipsitt, L., and Kaye, H.: Olfactory response and adaptations in the human neonate. *Journal of Comparative Physiologic Psychology, 56*:73, 1963.
12. Fantz, R. L.: Pattern Vision in Newborn Infants. *Science, 140*:296, 1963.
13. Fisher, D., Dussault, M., Foley, T., et al.: Screening for Congenital Hypothyroidism: Results of Screening One Million North American Infants. *Journal of Pediatrics, 94*:700, 1979.
14. Freedman, N. C., and Freedman, D. G.: Behavioral Differences Between Chinese-American and European-American Newborns. *Nature, 244*:1227, 1969.
15. Gartner, L., and Lee, K.: Jaundice and Liver Disease. In Behrman, R., Driscoll, J., and Seeds, A. (eds.): *Neonatal-Perinatal Medicine,* 2nd Edition. St. Louis, C. V. Mosby Co., 1977.
16. Goren, C., Sarty, M., and Wu, P.: Visual Following and Pattern Discrimination of Face-like Stimuli by Newborn Infants. *Pediatrics, 56*:544, 1975.
17. Greenman, G. W.: Visual Behavior of Newborn Infants. In Solnit, A. J., and Provence, S. A. (eds.): *Modern Perspectives in Child Development.* New York, International University Press, 1963.
18. Hershenson, M. R., Munsinger, H., Kessen, W., et al.: Preference for Shapes of Intermediate Variability in the Newborn Human. *Science, 147*:630, February 5, 1965.
19. Korner, A.: Individual Differences at Birth: Implications for Early Experience and Later Development. *American Journal of Orthopsychiatry, 41*:608, 1971.
20. Korner, A.: The Effect of the Infant's State, Level of Arousal, Sex and Ontogenic Stage of the Caregiver. In Lewis, M., and Rosenblum, L. (eds.): *The Effect of the Infant on Its Caregiver.* New York, John Wiley, 1974.
21. Korner, A.: State as Variable, as Obstacle, and as Mediator of Stimulation in Infant Research. *Merrill-Palmer Quarterly, 18*:77, 1972.
22. Korner, A., and Grobstein, R.: Visual Alertness as Related to Soothing in Neonates: Implications for Maternal Stimulation and Early Deprivation. *Child Development, 37*:867, 1968.
23. Korner, A., and Thoman, E.: Visual Alertness in Neonates as Evoked by Maternal Care. *Journal of Experimental Child Psychology, 10*:67, 1970.
24. Lawrence, R.: *Breastfeeding: A Guide for the Medical Profession.* New York, C. V. Mosby Co., 1980.
25. Lenard, H.: Sleep Studies in Infancy: Facts, Concepts, and Significance. *Acta Paediatrica Scandinavica, 59*:572, 1970.

26. Macfarlane, A.: *The Psychology of Childbirth.* Cambridge, Mass.: Harvard University Press, 1977.

27. Nisbett, R., and Gurwitz, S.: Weight, Sex and the Eating Behavior of Human Newborns. *Journal of Comparative Physiological Psychology, 73*:245, 1970.

28. Parmalee, A., Brueck, K., and Brueck, M.: Activity and Inactivity Cycles During the Sleep of Premature Children Exposed to Neutral Temperatures. *Biology of the Neonate 4*:317, 1962.

29. Prechtl, H.: The Behavioral States of the Newborn Infant (A Review). *Brain Research, 76*:185, 1974.

30. *Prevention and Treatment of Ophthalmia Neonatorum.* New York, National Society to Prevent Blindness, 1981.

30a. Rose, A., and Lombroso, C.: Neonatal Seizure States: A Study of Clinical, Pathological and Electroencephalographic Features in 137 Full-term Babies with a Long-Term Follow-Up. *Pediatrics, 45*:404, 1970.

31. Schaeffer, H., and Emerson, P.: Patterns of Response to Physical Contact in Early Human Development. *Journal of Child Psychology and Psychiatry, 5*:1, 1964.

32. Weiss, L.: Differential Variations in the Amount of Activity of Newborn Infants Under Continuous Light and Sound Stimulation. *University of Iowa Studies of Child Welfare, 9*:9, 1934.

33. Wolff, P.: Observations on Newborn Infants. *Psychosomatic Medicine, 21*:110, 1959.

34. Wolff, P.: The Causes, Controls, and Organization of Behavior in the Neonate. *Psychological Issues, 5*: Monograph 17, 1966.

22

The Term Newborn: Needs and Responses to Needs

OBJECTIVES

1. Describe how the needs for warmth and cleanliness are met in healthy term newborns.
2. Explain why the need for water is proportionately greater in newborns than in older infants and children.
3. Describe the needs of infants for calories, protein, carbohydrates, fat, vitamins, and minerals. Explain how these needs are met by both breast milk and formulas.
4. Discuss specific ways in which nurses can facilitate both breast- and bottle-feeding.
5. Describe the effects of nutritional deprivation in the early weeks of life.
6. Identify cellular and immunologic factors important in resistance to infection. Explain how resistance differs in newborns when compared with older persons.
7. Specify portals of entry for infectious agents in newborns that do not exist in older persons.
8. Identify factors contributing to the risk of infection in newborn infants.
9. Describe nursing action to protect newborns from infection.
10. Discuss arguments for and against routine circumcision. Identify infants in whom circumcision is contraindicated. Describe care of an infant following circumcision.
11. Identify topics to be included in the education of parents. Describe specific content for each topic.

What does the newborn baby need—not just to sustain life in the first days and weeks—but to build a foundation for growing both biologically and emotionally in the months and years that follow?

It is impossible to separate biologic needs from emotional needs. For example, food intake is an obvious biologic need—a certain quantity of fluid, carbohydrate, protein, and so on is required. But studies demonstrate that merely providing the proper nutrients is not sufficient: babies appear to have a real need for being held and touched while they are being fed.

What are the newborn's needs? How can they best be met? How do we communicate this information to his parents? This chapter will explore needs of infants relating to nutrition, warmth, cleanliness, protection from infection, the process of circumcision, and the need of parents to learn about caring for their infant after discharge. The needs associated with parenting and the ways that we can guide parents in meeting the emotional needs of their babies will be discussed in Chapter 26.

The nursing response to these needs at times involves giving direct care to the baby, but frequently it is the parents who are responsible for immediate care. In the 1980's, healthy term infants spend much or all of their day with their parents and a limited time in a central nursery. As a consequence, nursing actions are becoming increasingly supportive and educative to the parents and less directly involved with interaction with the infant. Because parents and healthy infants leave the birthing site within hours to a very few days following birth, new strategies must be developed to assist families during these first days (see Education for Parenting, below).

The Need for Warmth

The significance of warmth for each newborn infant from the moment of birth was emphasized in Chapter 20. Once the transition period is over, term newborns who are healthy usually have no difficulty maintaining satisfactory body temperature in the hospital. But what happens when the baby goes home? Commonly, babies are overdressed and overwrapped at home and are too warm rather than too cool. Mothers and grandmothers mistakenly interpret the cool hands and feet that are common to newborns (because of their immature peripheral circulation) as a sign that the baby is chilled and needs additional clothing and wrapping. Thus babies return for pe-

riodic check-ups on a midsummer's day wrapped like a polar Eskimo, and even in the winter newborns may show signs of heat rash (see also Education for Parenting, below).

The Need for Bathing

Bathing as a part of nursery care has been discussed in Chapter 20. Our concern here is what we teach mothers about bathing. In many hospitals the "baby-bath demonstration" is the central focus of teaching. Perhaps we make it seem too important at times. We certainly miss the point if we so emphasize a certain procedure that as a result mothers feel more inadequate rather than more knowledgeable.

Bathing serves three main purposes. The obvious one is cleanliness, important in protection from both infection and irritation. A second purpose is the opportunity for observation. We have already noted that the initial bath in the hospital gives us a chance to carefully observe many of the baby's characteristics. Subsequent bathing, both in the hospital and at home, may alert the mother to the first signs of eczema or heat rash or to any one of a multitude of signs that do not seem quite normal (see Nursing Care Plan 22–1).

Perhaps the most important purpose of all is the opportunity that bathing provides for interaction between mother or father and baby. Although a tiny baby does not particularly seem to enjoy bath time and appears happiest at the end, when he is out of the water and snugly wrapped in a warm towel, before many weeks bath time can become a real pleasure for everyone involved.

We need to teach mothers how to bathe their babies in a manner that is as uncomplicated as possible. Few mothers have someone to help them once they go home from the hospital, only 3 or 4 days following delivery. Baby nurses who work in homes, once common, are practically nonexistent. Grandmothers may live hundreds of miles away, and many are busy with their own lives. Neither of these changes is necessarily bad. The presence of someone who seems to know "everything" about babies can make young parents feel inadequate.

No elaborate equipment is needed for bathing the baby. A kitchen sink with a counter beside it serves well. Or a plastic dishpan makes an excellent tub if a separate container is preferred. Provide a mild soap, washcloth, and towel. Cotton balls and alcohol are necessary to cleanse the umbilicus during the first 2 weeks. If a circumcision is not healed, Vase-

Text continued on page 667

Nursing Care Plan 22–1. Healthy Newborn: Care After Transition to Extrauterine Life

NURSING GOALS:
To provide an environment that meets the physiologic, social, and emotional needs of the infant.

OBJECTIVES:

1. Physiologic assessment continues on a daily basis during hospitalization and in the home or ambulatory setting following hospitalization.
2. Parents are able to meet their infants' needs for cleanliness, sleep, nutrition, circumcision care (if appropriate), and protection from infection.
3. Feeding is consistent with infant needs and parental wishes; parents are comfortable about their ability to feed infant.
4. Parents identify unique characteristics of their infant and develop coping skills suitable to those characteristics.
5. Parents demonstrate positive signs of attachment to their infant.
6. Parents have realistic expectations of early infant development.
7. Siblings accept the new baby without feeling threatened about loss of parental love.
8. Screening tests are performed as mandated by state laws (PKU, hypothyroidism, galactosemia).
9. Parents understand the need for infant health supervision, including immunization, and know how to obtain care.
10. Parents recognize signs of neonatal illness and know how to obtain health care quickly when illness is suspected.

ASSESSMENT	POTENTIAL NURSING DIAGNOSIS	NURSING INTERVENTION	COMMENTS/RATIONALE
Physiologic assessment	Based on assessment		
1. Follow-up finding in initial assessment (e.g., resolution of molding, cephalhematoma, caput succedaneum, skin rashes)			
2. Identify changes in any system (e.g., appearance of jaundice on second or third day)	Infant at risk for hyperbilirubinemia	Lab test of direct and indirect bilirubin may be ordered. Phototherapy may be required (see Nursing Care Plan 23–8).	
3. Weigh daily in hospital. Weigh at 2 weeks of age; assess mother's plan for follow-up care.		Avoid chilling infant during weighing. (Nursery scales should be checked for accuracy each month.)	Weight loss does not generally exceed 10 per cent. Birth weight should be regained by 10–14 days.
4. Frequency of voiding			
5. Changes in stooling	Parents need information about normal voiding and stooling patterns.	Wipe buttocks with water or soap and water as needed after stooling. Explain stooling patterns to parents: meconium; transition; yellow loose stools in breast-fed infants; more formed stools in bottle-fed infants.	Mothers may interpret stools of breast-fed infants as diarrhea if proper explanation is not provided.
6. Vital signs: axillary temperature every 8 hours if stable after 24 hours, pulse, respirations	Parents need to learn how to assess infant temperature.	Teach parents to use thermometer.	Thermometer should always be held during use.

Continued on following page

Nursing Care Plan 22–1. Healthy Newborn: Care After Transition to Extrauterine Life *(Continued)*

ASSESSMENT	POTENTIAL NURSING DIAGNOSIS	NURSING INTERVENTION	COMMENTS/RATIONALE
Screening tests 1. PKU	Parents need information about screening test.	Explain reason for testing to parents. Infants must have ingested milk for at least 24 hours prior to testing; if there is a discharge prior to this time, explain to parents and arrange for testing (by community health nurse on home visit or have infant brought to ambulatory care center).	These tests are not required in all states.
2. Hypothyroidism		Test for hypothyroidism utilizes same specimen as test for PKU.	
3. Galactosemia		Galactosemia test also requires milk intake prior to testing. If parents refuse test ask them to sign statement to that effect; remind them that testing can be done at future time if they change their minds. Infant is at risk of brain damage in interim if disorder exists.	
Circumcision Care 1. Assess parent's knowledge of circumcision prior to procedure.	Parents need information about circumcision.	Provide information about circumcision; explain that circumcision is a matter of individual choice. Prepare infant for circumcision (using restraint such as circumcision tray). Ensure that infant remains warm during procedure. Ensure comfort during and following procedure.	There are no medical indications for routine circumcision; the procedure cannot be considered an essential component of health care.[1] It is preferable not to perform circumcision at the time of delivery.
2. Following circumcision note: a. Bleeding b. Voiding c. Cleanliness of incised area d. Absence of odor or discharge		Protect circumcision with Vaseline gauze for at least 24 hours. Infant may be more comfortable on back or side for 24–48 hours. Explain circumcision care to parents, including signs that should be reported to health-care provider.	Circumcision is frequently performed shortly before discharge; parents must know how to assess circumcision.

Parents' understanding of infant needs; ability to care for infant

1. Cleanliness

Parents need information about infant development and care.

Parents need opportunity to practice skills involved in infant care.

1. Cleanliness.
   a. Parents should have opportunity to bathe infant in hospital.
   b. At home, suggest sponge bath until cord drops off; infant may then have tub bath. Wash head daily when giving bath. Powder and lotion are unnecessary and may cause irritation in some infants.
   c. Diaper rash: expose diaper area to air (diaper under baby). Some babies cannot tolerate moisture-proof pants or diapers. Baby powder with cornstarch will intensify rash caused by fungus. If exposure to air does not improve rash, parent should contact health-care provider. Heat lamp (25 watts, 24 inches from baby) and ointment may be suggested.
   d. Genital hygiene
      (1) Girls: labia should be gently separated.
      (2) Boys
          1. Uncircumcised: prepuce should be gently retracted if possible and penis washed.
          2. Circumcised: following healing penis should be washed as part of daily bath.

Daily tub bath not essential if sponge bath is given and diaper area cleaned at each change. This knowledge reassures parents in first weeks as mother is recovering.

Desitin ointment and A & D ointment are available without prescription.

Prepuce is not fully retractable in most newborns; parents should know this is normal.

2. Clothing

2. Clothing
   a. Parents should become comfortable with dressing, diapering baby prior to discharge.
   b. Discuss dressing infant at home: diaper and shirt are frequently all that is needed. Avoid overdressing. Launder infant clothes in mild soap; rinse well.

Continued on following page

Nursing Care Plan 22–1. Healthy Newborn: Care After Transition to Extrauterine Life *(Continued)*

ASSESSMENT	POTENTIAL NURSING DIAGNOSIS	NURSING INTERVENTION	COMMENTS/RATIONALE
3. Sleep-wake cycle; crying		3. Sleep-wake cycle; crying a. Infant will be awake about 6–7 hours intermittently throughout day, but there is considerable individual variation. b. Most infants have a "fussy period" each day during the first 3 months of life when they are difficult to comfort. Inability to comfort does not indicate parental inadequacy. Coping may include rocking, riding in stroller, singing, talking. Provide telephone number of resource when parents feel they are unable to cope with crying.	Prompt response to crying may decrease crying in later months. Parents need to know that some infants are more active, cry more; some are more quiet (Chapter 21).
4. Nutrition a. Weight gain (see above, No. 3) b. Diaper wet at each feeding		4. Nutrition. See Nursing Care Plans 26–5 for breast-feeding and 22–2 for bottle-feeding.	
5. Infant safety		5. Safety. Provide safety information. Always test *bath* water *just before* placing baby in it (bath water can burn). Clean toxic substances from floor cabinets. Lock medicine cabinets. Be sure crib slats are sufficiently close together so infant's head cannot fit between slats. Use a padded bumper on the crib. (A dresser drawer, with firm padding, is a good bed.)	

Be sure that lead-free paint is used not only in baby's room, toys, and furniture, but also throughout the home.

Use an approved infant car seat every time the baby is in an automobile.

Consider safety in toy purchases. Be sure that toys have no small parts that can come off and be swallowed or inhaled.

Caution parents to NEVER:

a. Leave baby alone even for a moment (he can move and might fall).

b. Leave baby in or near water (e.g., tub)

c. Leave baby near a portable table heater or vaporizer, wall heater, grilled floor heater, radiator, electric outlet, or connected appliance cord, lamps, or windows.

d. Use pillows or thin plastic mattress covers.

e. Allow a passenger in an automobile to hold baby in lap.

6. Protection from infection

a. Teach parents to wash their hands prior to giving care to infant in the hospital or birth center and at home. All health care personnel must observe this practice not only to protect infant but also to provide model behavior for parents.

b. Protect infant from persons with infection: colds, diarrhea, vomiting, skin lesion, herpetic infection, communicable disease.

6. Protection from infection

Continued on following page

Nursing Care Plan 22–1. Healthy Newborn: Care After Transition to Extrauterine Life (Continued)

ASSESSMENT	POTENTIAL NURSING DIAGNOSIS	NURSING INTERVENTION	COMMENTS/RATIONALE
Assessment of attachment			
1. Identify signs of prenatal attachment (examine prenatal record)	Lag in prenatal attachment related to		
a. Pregnancy planned	a. Unplanned pregnancy		
b. Early prenatal care	b. Lack of prenatal care		
c. Attended prenatal classes	c. Lack of prenatal education		
d. "Nesting" behavior; planned for infant needs, considered names.	d. Absence of nesting behavior		
e. Supporting from baby's father or others	e. Lack of support system		
2. Identify prenatal complications that may affect attachment	Unwanted pregnancy		
a. Unwanted pregnancy			
b. Considered abortion			
3. Identify intrapartal signs of attachment (examine intrapartal record)			
a. Verbal and nonverbal behavior (admires infant; touching, holding infant, etc.)			
4. Identify complication of labor that may have interfered with attachment	Lag in attachment related to		
a. Long difficult labor	a. Long difficult labor		
b. Maternal complications that prevented early bonding	b. Maternal complications		
c. Neonatal complications that prevented early bonding	c. Neonatal complications		
5. Identify parental attachment behaviors in postpartum period	Lag in attachment (when these behaviors do not occur)	Provide opportunities for all mothers and fathers to spend prolonged periods of time with infant through rooming-in. Encourage their participation in all aspects of infant care.	
a. Positive verbal behavior (terms of affection, calls infant by name, sees family resemblance in infant, perceives infant as attractive, responsive)			
b. Positive nonverbal behavior (hugs, kisses, smiles, etc.)		Help parents discover the unique characteristics of their infant: how	

c. Expresses positive feelings toward baby's father
d. Verbalizes enjoyment in caring for infant
e. Verbalizes recognition of infant's unique characteristics
f. Responds appropriately to infant's states (e.g., does not try to waken and feed baby who is sound asleep, calms fussy baby, talks to baby in quiet alert state)
g. Exhibits signs of self-esteem

		she or he likes to be consoled, positions preferred for eating, burping, holding, etc.
		Help parents recognize the cues by which their baby makes needs known. Explain that they will become increasingly proficient in this.
		Comment positively about baby's positive attributes.
		Praise parents for care-giving efforts to increase their sense of competence as parents.
		Refer to community health nurse and other health-care provider to further assess and facilitate attachment after delivery when indicated.

7. Identify infant characteristics that contribute to attachment
a. Term infant
b. No physical abnormalities
c. Preferred sex
d. Feeds well (rooting, sucking, burping)
e. Consolable
f. Cuddles
g. Periods in quiet alert state
h. Smooth transition from one state to another

Lag in attachment (when infant does not meet one or more criteria).

Allow additional time for attachment as needed and refer for continuing assessment and intervention as indicated.

Marked lag in attachment may necessitate prolonged hospital stay.

When infant lacks positive characteristics, additional time may be necessary for attachment to occur.

Identify response of siblings
1. Verbal comments of parents, siblings
2. Inquire about siblings' preparation for birth of baby
3. Observe interaction of siblings, infant, and parents

Parents need information about sibling reactions to newborn and ways in which parents can help siblings cope.

Anxiety of parents or siblings as related to newborn infant.

Provide opportunities for parents, siblings to verbalize concerns about reaction to new infant.

Provide opportunities for sibling visits in hospital or birthing center.

Suggest resources to parents to use in explaining birth to siblings.

Encourage parents to consider a variety of ways to help siblings continue to feel special (see also Chapter 11).

Continued on following page

Nursing Care Plan 22–1.   Healthy Newborn: Care After Transition to Extrauterine Life   *(Continued)*

ASSESSMENT	POTENTIAL NURSING DIAGNOSIS	NURSING INTERVENTION	COMMENTS/RATIONALE
Assess parents' understanding of early infant development	Parents need information about early infant development.	Describe and demonstrate infant's sensory and motor capabilities.	
	Parents need information about resources for early infant development.	Describe expected developmental changes during first weeks, emphasizing individual variation.	
		Provide resources: pamphlets, books, telephone numbers, information about groups or classes for new parents.	
Plans for continuing health supervision for infant	Parents need information about infant health supervision: sources, costs, when to seek health care for infant.	Provide information about sources of infant health supervision in community, including costs, hours of availability.	Assessment at 2 weeks allows practitioner to ensure that birth weight is regained, answer questions.
		Explain need for early supervision.	Recommended immunization schedule: diphtheria-pertussis-tetanus (DPT) at 2, 4, and 6 months; polio at 2 and 4 months
		Explain need for immunization.	
Ability to recognize illness in infant	Parents need information about signs of neonatal illness.	Provide written information about signs of neonatal illness. 1. Loss of appetite 2. Vomiting or diarrhea 3. Lack of energy (lethargy) 4. Difficulty in breathing 5. Sunken eyes or fontanel or full, tight fontanel 6. Drainage from umbilical area 7. White patches in mouth (thrush) 8. Looks sick	
		Provide information about contacting health-care provider when illness is suspected.	
		Teach use of thermometer (see above); explain that absence of temperature elevation (fever) does not mean infant is not sick.	

Table 22–1 BABY'S BATH AT HOME

Sponge Bath	Complete Bath
1. Gather equipment, including baby's clean clothes, so that you won't have to leave the baby once the bath begins.	
2. Fill basin, sink, or tub with water that feels comfortable to your elbow. (Hands accustomed to hot water used in dishwashing are not as good indicators as sensitive elbow skin.)	
3. Wash each eye from the nose outward, using a clean section of washcloth for the second eye. Do not wash across the bridge of the nose; infection, if present, could be transferred.	
4. Soap the baby's head with bath soap. Holding the baby securely in a football position, rinse the head with water. Dry with a towel.*	
5. Wash the baby's face with soap; rinse and dry.	
6. Soap trunk, arms, and legs with hands; turn baby to abdomen to wash back. Wash genital area last.†	
7. Rinse with washcloth and clear water, rinsing genital area last.	7. Immerse baby in tub for rinsing.
8. Pat baby dry. Check to be sure that creases, such as the neck folds and inguinal area, are dry and clean.	
9. Clean the area around the umbilicus with alcohol until it is healed, at about 2 weeks of age.	9. Cleaning umbilical area no longer required.
10. Dress the baby, and brush his hair.	

*Because of the open fontanel, many mothers are afraid to wash the baby's head, and subsequent scalp infections are not uncommon at check-up time. This therefore becomes an important part of teaching.

†In girls, the labia are gently separated, and the genitalia are cleansed from front to back. In boys, the folds of the scrotum are cleansed; the foreskin is not retracted. A Vaseline dressing covers the penis during the first 24 hours following circumcision. Soap will be irritating to the circumcision area for several days; the area is best rinsed with clear water until it heals. Normally the circumcision will be healed earlier than the umbilicus and thus prior to the time the baby has a tub bath.

line and gauze pads will protect the penis if the diaper appears to be rubbing, and certainly this is necessary during the first 24 hours at home. (Some babies are circumcised shortly before discharge.) Baby powder is really not necessary and probably not advisable. For those mothers who feel they are neglecting their babies unless they powder them, cornstarch is an acceptable substitute. It should be used only on the baby's bottom.

Until the baby's umbilicus is healed, a sponge bath is suggested. Immersing the baby might risk infection through the umbilical portal of entry.

A basic regimen for infant bathing is described in Table 22–1. Mothers, and fathers too, should have as many opportunities to bathe their baby in the hospital as possible. A second bath in the evening will not harm the baby if the father would like such an opportunity. Parents don't gain confidence by watching nurses bathe babies, either by observing through the nursery window or in a classroom or even at the mother's bedside. Our "efficiency" and expertise may only overwhelm them, making them feel even less adequate. Parents gain confidence by caring for their own baby *as much as possible,* and our responsibility is to give them as much opportunity as they desire. This is possible even in hospitals that do not formally practice rooming-in. Instead of bringing the baby to his mother dressed and "bundled" in the morning, the baby can be brought to his mother's room for his bath.

Bath time could just as easily be in the evening as in the morning. It might vary from family to family, depending on individual needs and desires. This kind of flexibility is valuable not only during the brief hospital period, but perhaps even more important, it conveys to parents a "permission" to be flexible and adaptive in baby care at home. Some previous generations of mothers thought, and some mothers still feel, that a daily bath before the 10 A.M. feeding is a binding rule. The "to the minute scheduling" of some maternity units may reinforce this kind of rigidity. Mothers should know that babies may be bathed at a time that best fits the schedule of both parents and infants. For example, nearly every baby has a "fussy" period during his first weeks, a time when he is neither hungry nor sleepy but seems at somewhat of a loss as to what he wants—probably some companionship and loving. The time of day varies from one baby to another but is remarkably consistent in an individual infant. In many instances this time is a good one for bathing.

There will also be some days when a bath seems more than a mother can manage, particularly when she is still recovering from pregnancy and delivery. Mothers need to know that an occasional missed bath is all right too. A sponge bath can be substituted for a tub bath—just a quick wipe with the washcloth to be sure that there is no milk in the neck folds and that the baby's bottom is well washed.

The Need for Nutrition

If animal mothers could listen and reflect upon the many discussions and arguments of humans about the subject of infant nutrition, they would probably be amused. Feeding their young must seem a simple matter. But because we are reasoning beings who are as influenced by our culture as by our biologic heritage, issues concerning infant feeding have become complex and need thorough review.

We are coming to recognize the lifelong significance of feeding during the first weeks and months of life. Not only is undernutrition a real hazard during the time of rapid brain and body growth, but overnutrition during infancy may contribute to adult obesity and to all the problems associated with obesity. Moreover, the emotional context in which food is offered probably has long-term meaning.

The Nutritional Needs of the Baby

As a biologic organism, an infant needs water, protein, carbohydrate, fat, vitamins, and minerals, just as we all do, although proportionately his needs will vary from ours. The discussion in this section describes the requirements of normal, term newborns. The nutritional needs of preterm infants and others with special problems are discussed in Chapter 23.

A baby's diet must enable him to grow and meet his needs for energy. By the analysis of data from several sources, Fomon has demonstrated that in the baby's first 4 months of life (during which most babies double their birth weight) nearly one-third of caloric intake is used for growth.[19] During the subsequent 8 months of the first year, both growth rate and the percentage of calories required for growth decline appreciably (Table 22-2). By the time a baby is 2 to 3 years old, only 1 per cent of his caloric intake is used for growth; the remainder is required to meet the energy needs of a very active toddler.

The Need for Water

The need of a newborn baby for water is proportionately higher than that of an older child or an adult for several reasons:

1. The percentage of water in relation to total body mass is greater than at any other period of life, a total of 70 to 75 per cent. About 30 to 35 per cent of total body weight in the newborn is extracellular water, compared with 25 per cent in the older infant and an average of 20 per cent in the adult. Because of this, the infant has proportionately less fluid reserve. Loss of fluid or lack of intake will deplete his extracellular fluid very rapidly. In a 24-hour period an infant replaces about 50 per cent of his extracellular water; by contrast an adult replaces only 14 per cent of his extracellular water in the same period. A large part of the difference in weight between a newborn and an older infant disappears by the time the baby is 10 days old, because the loss of the excess extracellular water accounts for much of the weight loss that occurs during the first days of life.

2. The larger surface area of the newborn in relation to his body mass means a higher ratio of water loss through evaporation, the rate of loss per kilogram being twice that of an adult. Thus the newborn's fluid balance is much more susceptible to environmental temperature and humidity. Water loss can be very high in a high temperature–low humidity environment, both in the hospital or at home.

3. Metabolic rates are higher in newborn infants. A newborn produces 45 to 50 calories

Table 22-2. WEIGHT GAIN AND CALORIES USED FOR GROWTH DURING THE FIRST YEAR

	0-4 Months	4-12 Months
Percent calories used for growth	32.8	7.4
Approximate weight gain (kg.)	3.5	3.5
Approximate weight gain (pounds)	7.7	7.7

per kg. of body weight every 24 hours. The basal metabolic level for adults during the same period is from 25 to 30 calories per kg. Since metabolism uses water, a higher rate of metabolism utilizes a proportionately greater quantity of water.

4. The kidneys of a newborn have about half the concentrating ability of the kidneys of a normal adult. Although this is quite adequate for the baby's needs under normal conditions, newborn kidneys are less able to conserve fluid if the baby is stressed. In an older person, scanty urine is a fairly reliable sign of dehydration, but because of this limited ability to conserve water, newborns may not have decreased urinary output until they are severely dehydrated. Normally, higher levels of phosphate and potassium in the blood of newborns are also related to renal immaturity.

How much fluid does a newborn need? Age, weight, and environmental temperature all influence fluid needs in healthy term infants. In preterm or sick newborns water needs are further modified. Term infants require approximately 140 to 160 ml. of water per kg. of body weight by the third to fourth day following birth (average, 150 ml. per kg.). For a baby weighing 3500 grams (3.5 kg., 7 pounds 11 ounces) we would calculate:

150 ml. $\times$ 3.5 kg. = 525 ml. per day

525 ml. $\div$ 6 feedings = approximately 88 ml. per feeding, or about 3 ounces

525 ml. $\div$ 8 feedings = approximately 66 ml. per feeding, or about 2 ounces

It is not unusual for babies to have an increased intake at some feedings and a decreased intake at others. In healthy term infants undue concern with the exact amount of formula ingested at each feeding can be more harmful than helpful.

An advantage of breast-feeding is the inability to measure the exact intake; the baby is allowed to set his own pace. Formula-fed infants should be allowed to set their own pace as well. It is only when there is marked variation from the norm over several feedings that the cause of the abnormality needs to be investigated. Possible reasons may be illness in the baby, improper feeding techniques (e.g., the mother may be holding the bottle so that the nipple is not filled with milk), or a mother's difficulty in interpreting her baby's signals of hunger and fullness.

Unless the baby seems particularly thirsty or his surroundings are so hot and dry that his insensible water loss is very high, additional water is not necessary, although he may certainly have some if he wants it. Some infants seem to like occasional water, while many others are uninterested.

The Need for Calories

How many calories does an infant need for energy and for growth? For the healthy term infant, 110 calories per kg. of body weight per 24 hours is recommended.

Consider what this means for a baby weighing 3 kg. (6.6 pounds) in the second week of life. During the first 2 weeks the average need would be approximately 330 calories per day (110 calories per kg. $\times$ 3 kg.). Most term newborns receive formulas containing 20 calories per kg. Thus the baby would need about 17 ounces of formula during a 24-hour period. If divided among six feedings, this would mean slightly less than 3 ounces per feeding.

Although it is important to be aware of caloric needs, it is also important not to be so fascinated with numbers that our view of infant feeding becomes highly rigid. As noted above, one of the possible advantages of breast-feeding is that we do not know just how much milk a baby takes during a particular feeding or during a particular day. When the baby appears satisfied, he is allowed to stop eating. The bottle-fed baby should have the same privilege, assuming he is a normal, healthy infant. Consistent failure to feed well, if adequate time is allowed at a feeding, may indicate illness. It is, for example, often an early sign of congenital heart disease (Chapter 24).

We know that bottle-fed infants gain weight more rapidly than breast-fed babies (Fig. 22–1). At one time this was thought to represent an advantage of formula-feeding over breast-feeding, but recent concerns about infant feeding and adult obesity have forced us to reconsider this supposition. It is believed that a high caloric intake during the first weeks and months of life leads to cellular mitosis in the fat cells. The result is an increased number of fat cells and consequent hyperplasia of fat tissue. Once these fat cells are present, the possibility of fat cell hyperplasia, with subsequent hypertrophy, may be continuously present. Even if the fat cells "shrink" during a weight reduction program, they continue to be present in fatty tissue with the potential to hypertrophy again.

Are formula-fed infants overfed? Weight gains far in excess of the gains of a healthy, breast-fed baby could be considered excessive and could present potential problems for the obese baby in later years.

The Need for Protein

Considering the rapid rate of growth during a baby's first year, it should not be surprising that protein is highly important in newborn nutrition. A dietary intake of approximately 9

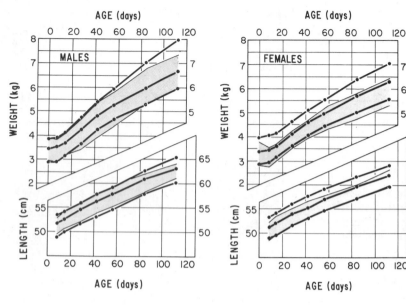

Figure 22–1. Comparison of weight gain and length. Heavy lines indicate formula-fed infants and shaded areas cover values for breast-fed infants. (From Fomon et al.: *Acta Paediatrica Scandinavica* (Suppl. 223), 1971.)

grams of protein per day is necessary to provide for growth and to cover protein losses from the skin and in the urine. Recommended intakes are usually calculated at the slightly higher level of 14 grams per day during the first month, 15 grams per day for the second month, and 16 grams per day from the fourth month through the remainder of the first year. (Although infants in the later months of the first year need an increased amount of protein for maintenance, their rate of growth decreases, and thus their overall protein need remains stable.)

The principal protein in human milk is lactalbumin; casein is the primary protein in cow milk. Lactalbumin contains a higher percentage of essential amino acids. Casein in raw, unprocessed cow milk is a tough, rubbery substance that tends to make the cow milk curd difficult to digest. However, modern processing softens the curd and eliminates the major cause of its indigestibility.

Mothers with limited incomes sometimes try to stretch formula by making it more dilute and by offering sugar water at some feedings, obviously compromising protein as well as other nutrients. Our role in such instances is not to chastise but to help mothers understand the importance of proper feeding and especially to help them provide the milk their infants need for adequate growth.

The Need for Carbohydrate

Thirty-seven per cent of the calories in human milk come from carbohydrate. In commercially prepared formulas the percentage of carbohydrate varies from 32 to 51 per cent, with the majority of preparations falling in the 40 to 45 per cent range. When the proportion of calories from carbohydrate in a formula is too low (below 20 per cent), babies are not able to tolerate the high levels of protein and fat that would then make up their formula. If carbohydrate is in excess of 50 per cent, the baby may have loose stools because of his inability to hydrolyze disaccharides, resulting in impaired growth and development.

The carbohydrate of milk is lactose. The lactose content of human milk is proportionately higher than that of milk of any other species. Babies with galactosemia, an autosomal recessive disorder, lack the enzyme (galactose-1-phosphate uridyltransferase) that is necessary to metabolize lactose. They must be fed nonmilk formulas.

The Need for Fat

Free fatty acids are now considered the most important source of energy for the young infant. Studies in rats indicate that when fat intake is too low, cerebral function is affected. This is important because myelinization of the human brain takes place over the first 3 years of life.

A formula providing 1 per cent of the caloric intake from two of the essential fatty acids, linoleic acid and arachidonic acid, is apparently sufficient for healthy development. But such a formula would be so high in protein that the renal solute load (see below) would be excessive, and the carbohydrate would be so high that diarrhea would result. Those formulas that derive 30 to 35 per cent of their calories from fat are generally the most acceptable.

Although the fat content of cow milk is

higher than that of human milk, the proportion of fatty acids varies. Fat is the main source of calories in human milk. The fat of human milk is more easily digested than the fat of cow milk. In addition, human milk contains the enzyme lipase, essential to the digestion of fats. Because of lipase, large proportions of free fatty acids become available to the baby even before digestion can begin in the intestine.

Skim milk has no place in infant diet and is not advised for children under the age of 2 years. There are three major reasons for this:

1. The calories in skim milk appear to be inadequate to meet needs for growth and energy. Body stores of fat are used to fulfill energy requirements. As fat stores are depleted, any illness that interferes with food intake could then become life-threatening.

2. Protein intake is very high in skim milk diets.

3. Essential fatty acids may be inadequate in skim milk diets.

The Need for Vitamins

The need for vitamins is met somewhat differently in breast-fed babies than in babies receiving formulas.

Human milk satisfies all of the baby's vitamin requirements except for that of vitamin D, *if the mother's vitamin intake is adequate.* Adequate maternal intake is particularly important in relation to vitamin C, which must be included in the mother's diet each day. The vitamin C content of human milk is in the range of 40 mg. per liter. The vitamin D content of breast milk is less than 100 I.U. per quart, about one-fourth the recommended daily intake, and thus supplementation is necessary.

Cow milk is deficient in both vitamin C and vitamin D. Levels of B vitamins are probably adequate. The folic acid content, although apparently sufficient for infants weighing more than 2500 grams (5.5 pounds), may be inadequate for low birth weight babies. Limited folic acid intake leads to megaloblastic anemia, so called because the primordial erythrocyte does not mature past the megaloblastic stage, by a process outlined in the following diagram.

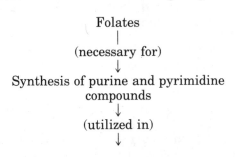

Folates
|
(necessary for)
↓
Synthesis of purine and pyrimidine
compounds
↓
(utilized in)
↓

Formation of nucleoproteins
|
(necessary for)
↓
Maturation of primordial erythrocytes (precursors of mature red blood cells)

Megaloblastic anemia is sometimes masked in infancy because of the more common iron deficiency anemia.

Hypervitaminosis A, rather than a vitamin A deficiency, is a more likely risk for babies on many formulas. About 600 I.U. of vitamin A per day is considered an adequate intake; many commercial formulas contain from 1500 to more than 2700 I.U. of vitamin A per liter. Babies receiving skim milk formulas and those with chronic steatorrhea (fatty stools) do need to receive supplementary vitamin A in a water-miscible preparation.

The possibility of toxicity from excessive vitamin D has been suggested but is unproven at this time. In the United States, evaporated milk, most commercial formulas, and most fresh whole milk is fortified at the level of 400 I.U. of vitamin D per quart, the recommended daily intake. If the formula contains less than this amount or if, as noted above, the baby is breast-fed, supplementation will be necessary.

Relatively little is known about the role of vitamin E in newborn nutrition, although there is some indication that a vitamin E–dependent anemia may exist in some preterm babies.

The importance of vitamin K was discussed in Chapter 20. The vitamin K content of cow milk is generally higher than that of human milk. By the second week of life, the healthy baby's intestinal flora will have developed sufficiently to supply all of the baby's needs for vitamin K. In the interim a single injection of vitamin K is given to the baby to prevent possible hemorrhage.

Obviously, the need for vitamin supplementation is highly individualized. In some commercial formulas, vitamins are included in the preparations themselves. Often these formulas are prescribed to protect the baby, on the theory that even the best mothers may forget to give extra vitamins at least part of the time. The cost of "complete" formulas is higher than standard formulas, however, which may present problems for some families. There is also a difference in the cost of dry preparations, which the mother mixes with water, in comparison with the same but higher priced formula that is already mixed. Mothers are often not aware of this; in our daily practice we find mothers on the verge of destitution feeding their infants the more expensive ready-to-use products. By keeping ourselves up to date on the relative costs of the formulas prescribed in our communities and by teaching mothers to prepare the less costly milk products, we can make a real contribution to infant nutrition.

The Need for Minerals

A number of minerals play a role in newborn nutrition, but the need for most of them is apparently met with little difficulty. The most frequent exception to this is iron. Studies have shown that the incidence of iron deficiency anemia (defined as a hemoglobin concentration of 10 grams per 100 ml. or less) ranges from 25 to 76 per cent in infants over 6 months of age from economically deprived areas and from 1 to 2 per cent in babies from more affluent families.

Iron requirements during the first year of life equal the difference between the level of iron at birth and the amount of iron required for growth and hemoglobin production between birth and the first birthday. Twins and premature and low birth weight infants accumulate limited stores of iron in utero, as do babies of iron-deficient mothers. Bleeding after birth, from the cord or circumcision or internally, and clamping of the umbilical cord before pulsation has stopped are additional factors in depleting iron stores.

Formulas fortified with iron or supplemental iron (ferrous sulfate drops) are given to most formula-fed infants. Ferrous sulfate drops are best absorbed when given between meals, although the small doses that are given for the prevention of iron deficiency anemia (1 mg. per kg. per day) are believed to result in adequate absorption. Gastrointestional distress is rare at this dosage level. Because of the risk of accidental poisoning in siblings, no more than 1 month's supply of ferrous sulfate should be kept in the house.

Term infants whose mothers had adequate iron intake during pregnancy will have a store of iron sufficient for the first 3 to 4 months, after which time iron must be added to the diet. If cereals fortified with iron are offered by age 4 to 6 months and continue to be used throughout the first year, the occurrence of iron deficiency anemia can be reduced considerably. The *term* baby most at risk of developing iron deficiency anemia (that is, the baby whose mother was herself anemic) is often the baby whose mother can least afford the baby meat and egg yolk and tends to switch him from the more expensive, iron-fortified cereals as soon as possible. This baby may also receive less well-baby care and hemoglobin monitoring.

Although breast milk contains iron in small quantities (approximately 1 mg. per liter), there is evidence that breast milk facilitates the absorption of iron. Saarinen, Siimes, and Dallman[56] found that term infants absorbed an average of 49 per cent of a trace dose of extrinsic iron administered during breast-feeding in contrast to about 10 per cent absorbed from cow milk. Several possible reasons for this difference exist. Iron absorption appears to be increased when protein is lower,[30] when lactose is increased,[1] when phosphorus, which decreases iron absorption, is lower,[53] and when vitamin C content is high. Breast milk meets all of these qualifications. An additional factor contributing to the rarity of iron deficiency anemia in breast-fed infants may be the absence of the microscopic amount of blood loss into the gastrointestinal tract that is found in bottle-fed infants.[42a] Although further research is necessary, breast milk does appear to play a more significant role in meeting iron needs during the first year of life than might be expected from the level of iron it contains.

Calcium absorption and metabolism are more efficient with human milk consumption, largely eliminating the risk of hypocalcemia in the breast-fed neonate. Not only the total amount of calcium present but also the ratio of calcium to phosphorus is significant. When phosphorus levels increase in the blood, calcium is eliminated. Pure cow milk, given to newborns, may overload the body with phosphorus and lead to hypocalcemia.

Some research suggests that high levels of *sodium chloride* ingested during the early months may lead to adult hypertension.

Fluoride is considered the most effective dietary deterrent of tooth decay currently available. If formula is made with fluoridated water, fluoride intake should be adequate. Because of the low fluoride content of breast milk, fluoride supplementation of 0.25 to 0.50 mg. per day is frequently recommended.[19, 65]

Renal Solute Load

Renal solute load refers to the amount of urea and electrolytes excreted in the urine. If a preparation with a high concentration of solutes is ingested, increased water must be excreted to eliminate the waste products of that preparation.

The renal solute load of cow milk, even when it is diluted with water and carbohydrate, is considerably higher than that of human milk. The renal solute load of commercially prepared formulas varies. In the healthy term infant renal solute load is of limited concern, but it becomes important if the baby has a high level of insensitive water loss (due to fever, for example) or lives in a hot environment.

Meeting Nutritional Needs: Infant Feeding

Breast-feeding is recommended for all healthy term infants and vigorous preterm infants.[1] Nevertheless, the decision as to how she will feed her baby should be made by the mother, after discussion with her husband (an important consideration sometimes overlooked). Our role, as nurses, is to support the family's decision, whatever it may be, and to help prepare parents to feed their baby in the manner they have selected. It is just as inappropriate to "force" breast-feeding on the mother who, for whatever reason, does not wish to do so as it is to fail to help the mother who truly desires to breast-feed.

Factors Influencing a Mother's Decision to Breast-Feed

The incidence of initial breast-feeding is increasing in the United States, as is the duration of breast-feeding (Table 22–3). This increase reverses a trend that began following World War I in which bottle-feeding was preferred by many women and encouraged by many health professionals as "more scientific."

A number of variables appear to influence the choice of breast-feeding, although they will not necessarily predict the choice of an individual woman. In general, a woman appears more likely to choose breast-feeding if she herself was breast-fed as an infant and if she is married and is supported in her decision by her husband, has a higher level of education and income, has had a previous successful breast-feeding experience, and receives support from her peers and from health-care personnel. Single mothers, mothers who smoke, mothers who have had health complications during pregnancy, and mothers who work outside the home are less likely to choose breast-feeding.[57]

Nurses obviously cannot influence some of these variables (such as whether a mother was breast-fed herself when she was an infant or the years of education a mother has completed), but special support and encouragement given during the prenatal period to mothers who are less likely to breast-feed may encourage some of them to consider this option.

Prenatal nutritional education, such as that offered by the WIC (Women, Infants' and Children's) Program does encourage breast-feeding in addition to offering continued education, encouragement, and incentives in the postnatal months. The WIC program is designed for women of limited income; families with higher incomes should have access to the same information and encouragement.

Differences in Breast Milk and Formula

Some major differences between breast milk and formulas have been discussed in the preceding section. An additional difference is the role of colostrum and breast milk in maintaining resistance to infection. Traditionally, it has been recognized that breast-fed babies have a lower incidence of infection than those who are bottle-fed. To some extent this may be attributed to a lack of contamination of the milk itself, but this is not the only factor.

Colostrum, the fluid in the breasts prior to delivery and during the first 24 to 72 hours postpartum, contains very high levels of immunoglobulin (IgA), which offers protection against *Escherichia coli,* one of the major newborn pathogens. When mothers have a high level of antibody to poliomyelitis, some transfer of immunity has been found in their babies. Antibodies for mumps, vaccinia, influenza, and Japanese B encephalitis have also been found in human milk, but it is not known to what extent these antibodies protect the baby.

The intestinal flora (another factor in maintaining resistance to infection) of the breast-fed baby differs from the flora of the bottle-fed baby. The flora of the breast-fed baby has been

Table 22–3. PERCENTAGE OF INFANTS BREAST-FED AT VARYING AGES IN 1971 AND 1978*

Age of Infant	1971	1978	Percentage of Change (1971–1978)	Seven-year ARG†
1 week	24.7	46.6	21.9	9.5
2 months	13.9	34.9	21.0	14.1
3 to 4 months	8.2	26.8	18.6	18.4
5 to 6 months	5.5	20.5	15.0	20.7

*From Moore: *Newborn, Family and Nurse.* 2nd Edition. Philadelphia, W. B. Saunders Co., 1981. Developed from data in Martinez and Nalezienski: *Pediatrics, 64:*686, 1979.

†ARG = average annual rate of gain.

Table 22–4. IMMUNOLOGICAL FACTORS IN HUMAN MILK*

Factor	Function (in vitro)	Effects of Heating*
Lactoferrin	Inhibits growth of organisms, e.g., *E. coli* and *Candida albicans*, by chelating metabolically active iron	Two-thirds destroyed by pasteurization
Lysozyme	Acts with IgA and complement to destroy *E. coli*	Activity reduced 97 per cent by boiling for 15 minutes
Complement (C3, C4)	Enhances chemotaxis and phagocytosis by WBCs	Destroyed by pasteurization
Secretory IgA and other immunoglobulins	Contain antibodies to many common bacterial and viral pathogens including polio virus types 1, 2, and 3, *E. coli, Salmonella,* and *Shigella*	Destroyed by boiling; 0–30 per cent loss with pasteurization
Growth factor *Lactobacillus bifidus*	*L. bifidus* produces organic acids that lower pH of feces and impede colonization by *E. coli* and other pathogens	Stable to boiling
Antistaphylococcal factor	Inhibits staphylococci	Not known
Lactoperoxidase	Kills streptococci	Not known; presumably destroyed by boiling
Leukocytes Macrophages (80–90 per cent of leukocytes) monocytic phagocytes	Highly phagocytic Produce lysozyme, C3, C4	Destroyed by pasteurization; also destroyed by freezing
Lymphocytes (10% + of leukocytes)	Produce secretory IgA antibodies, interferon	
B$_{12}$ and folic acid–binding proteins	May interfere with the growth of microorganisms depending on folic acid or vitamin B$_{12}$	
Lipids (unsaturated fatty acids)	Active against *S. aureus* and multiple viruses including herpes simplex	Stable after boiling for 30 minutes

*From Moore: *Newborn, Family and Nurse.* 2nd Edition. Philadelphia, W. B. Saunders Co., 1981. After Welsh and May: *J Pediatr 1:*94, 1979.

shown to protect against certain organisms in addition to those protected against by the flora of the bottle-fed baby.

Other antimicrobial factors found in human breast milk are summarized in Table 22–4. The effects of heating are noted because breast milk is sometimes collected in milk banks and pasteurized.

Helping the Mother Who Chooses to Breast-feed

In contemporary Western society it is highly unrealistic to suppose that mothers who wish to breast-feed will automatically be able to do so. In tribal villages and in traditional societies, and in the Western world of several generations ago, many women lived close to one another in extended families. Consequently, a girl grew to adulthood with many opportunities to observe mothers and infants together and could thus learn about breast-feeding gradually through the years. But few mothers in the Western world today have such opportunities. Many have never seen an infant fed at breast. Female relatives are usually fewer in number and are often separated by many miles.

Assistance in breast-feeding—advice, counsel, and emotional support—comes chiefly from two groups. The first is composed of professionals—nurses and physicians. The second is made up of mothers who have themselves successfully breast-fed. The latter group provides assistance through a more formal structure such as the La Leche League or informally as neighbors and friends. Perspectives about breast-feeding vary somewhat between these two groups. Knafl,[39] in a small study that is part of a larger investigation, reports that in the second group both La Leche literature and mothers stress breast-feeding as an integral part of total mothering. Factors such as convenience and nutritional superiority appear less important, although not necessarily unimportant, to this group. However, the nurses whom Knafl interviewed (the staff from two hospitals and the nurse faculty from a university school) thought of breast-feeding in terms of better nutrition and temporary immunity for the baby and maternal convenience and health after discharge from the hospital. Only 8 of 19 nurses (42.1 per cent) mentioned mother–infant interaction as a benefit.

Knafl's findings support our own observations and what we hear in discussions with nurses. Some mothers have intense feelings about breast-feeding that are not shared by staff members. The staff may feel hostile to-ward these mothers for their "unrealistic expectations." The mother, in turn, may feel that staff members have more concern for "routine" than for mothers and their infants. Such tension is detrimental to successful breast-feeding (see below) and can be a long-lasting source of disappointment to mothers.

Dealing with such conflict or potential conflict is as much a nursing responsibility as is the physical care of mothers and babies. Joint meetings between mothers, La Leche leaders, and staff nurses and physicians can afford an opportunity to deal with specific points of conflict, such as breast-feeding in the delivery room, feeding on demand, and supplemental feedings between times at breast. Nurses might attend La Leche meetings, not to espouse their own point of view, but to better understand the feelings of breast-feeding mothers and to show their genuine concern for these feelings.

Even with open communication, there will be occasional problems between individual mothers and staff. But if these conflicts can be recognized as individual idiosyncracies rather than as a reason to label all breast-feeding mothers as "fanatics," they can be resolved in helpful ways. The goal of both professionals and volunteers is the same—the start of an interaction between mother and baby that is emotionally and physically sound.

Support for the mother who chooses breast-feeding should begin in the prenatal period, as soon as the decision to breast-feed is made. Following delivery, previous learning can be reinforced and supplemented. (See Chapters 25 and 26 for further discussions of breast-feeding, including the techniques of breast-feeding.)

Helping the Mother Who Chooses to Bottle-feed

Because more mothers in the United States bottle-feed than breast-feed, because "failure to thrive" in the early weeks of life is often related to poor feeding technique, and because inadequate nutrition in the first months following birth may compromise the baby's long-term potential, our nursing role in helping mothers who choose to bottle-feed is significant (see Nursing Care Plan 22–2). It is no more realistic to expect a mother to "instinctively" know how to bottle-feed her baby than it is to expect a mother to intuitively know how to breast-feed. The mother who plans to bottle-feed needs to know how to prepare feedings and when, how much, and how to feed her baby.

Nursing Care Plan 22–2.   Helping the Formula-Feeding Mother

NURSING GOALS:
To provide parents who choose to bottle-feed their infant with the knowledge and skills necessary for successful feeding.

OBJECTIVES:
1. Identify prior infant-feeding experience and prenatal education about infant feeding.
2. Assist parents during early feeding experiences.
3. Identify problems perceived by parents.

ASSESSMENT	POTENTIAL NURSING DIAGNOSIS	NURSING INTERVENTION	COMMENTS/RATIONALE
1. Prior experience in infant feeding	Lack of experience in infant feeding	Provide support during early infant-feeding experiences.	
a. Prenatal preparation: Assess information provided (1) Content (2) Source	Lack of prenatal education related to formula-feeding	Provide information about: 1. Formula preparation 2. Cost of types of preparations of prescribed formula	Written information to which parents can refer at home should supplement oral teaching.
2. Observe infant feeding. Note:	Need for information about formula-feeding	3. Amount of formula to be offered at each feeding (approximately 3 ounces after 24–48 hours)	
a. Way in which infant is held: "en face" position	Need for assistance in formula-feeding	4. Frequency of feeding: meaning of demand feeding	
b. Way in which bottle is held: milk fills nipple at all times		5. Average length of feeding: 20–30 minutes	
c. Length of feeding time		6. Adjustment of feeding practices as appropriate to infant needs:	
d. Characteristics of infant feeding (e.g., slow eater with frequent pauses, rapid gulper)			

e. Parent's adjustment of feeding in response to infant cues
f. Parent's interaction with infant during feeding (e.g., talks to infant)

3. Assess understanding of bottle-feeding during first year.

Need for information about bottle-feeding during first year

a. Patience with infant who feeds slowly
b. Softer nipple with larger holes for infant who tires easily; firmer nipple with smaller holes for infant who "gulps" and chokes
c. More frequent feedings for infant who takes only small amounts at a feeding

Demonstrate positions for burping.

Describe stool of bottle-fed infant: light yellow, sour, irritating to skin. Explain importance of thorough cleansing of skin after each stool.

Provide information about:
1. Continuation of formula throughout first year
2. Postponement of other foods for 4–6 months
3. Prevention of "bottle mouth" by giving nothing but water if bedtime bottle is used
4. Prevention or reduction of otitis media by avoidance of "propped" bottles and giving only clear water if bedtime bottle is used

Boiling for 5–10 minutes will soften firm nipples.

Formula Preparation

The preparation of formulas has been greatly simplified in recent years. Some of the simplifications, such as ready-to-feed formula and disposable bottles, add considerable expense to infant care, with only a very small advantage in ease of preparation and saving of time.

In the simplest method of formula preparation, the *single bottle method,* each bottle is prepared individually at the time it is used. Bottles, caps, and nipples are washed in hot, soapy water and are rinsed thoroughly. Tap water is mixed with either a powder or a concentrated liquid formula preparation. When there is any question about the safety of the water supply, the water should be boiled for 5 minutes prior to use. Some pediatricians would prefer that all water be boiled during the first months of life.

When the single bottle method is used, the bottle should be given to the baby immediately after preparation. It will not need to be warmed, since the water used is at room temperature. Even cold formula is not harmful to babies, although some may not care for it. Any formula that remains in the bottle after a feeding must be discarded. Following feeding, the bottle and nipple are rinsed in cold water, so that they will be easier to clean later.

The single bottle method eliminates a great deal of relatively costly equipment that also takes up space in small kitchens. No refrigeration is required, other than that for a single can of concentrated formula, and none at all is necessary if a powder preparation is used. This method is also valuable for the breast-feeding mother when she needs a supplementary feeding.

A second method still in use is *terminal sterilization.* A day's supply of bottles is prepared; the bottles are placed in a large pan in 3 to 4 inches of water and are sterilized for 25 minutes, with timing started when the water boils. The pan is cooled until it can be comfortably touched; the bottles are then refrigerated until feeding time. Many mothers warm these refrigerated bottles before feeding the baby, but this is not essential.

A third method, the *aseptic method,* involves boiling both equipment and ingredients and then combining them under aseptic technique. Prepared bottles are then refrigerated. The aseptic method is little used in the United States today, as newer, less time-consuming methods have proved to be safe.

Formula preparation involves not only cleanliness but also proper combination of the necessary ingredients. Mothers on limited budgets may try to "stretch" expensive milk products by adding more water than called for. Or, misunderstanding directions, they may not add sufficient water, giving the baby a very highly concentrated preparation as a result. Nurses must help mothers understand not only how to prepare formula but also why accuracy is important in measuring ingredients.

When to Feed

Lactation is facilitated when breast-fed babies are fed "on demand," that is, when they are awake and show they are hungry by rooting and sucking. Bottle-fed babies also need to be fed when they are hungry. The length of time between feedings will vary. At first many babies seem to want to eat every 3 hours, even though in the majority of hospitals that do not have rooming-in, babies may be allowed to eat only every 4 hours. Hospital rigidity may convey the impression to new mothers that the every-4-hour schedule is the only "right" way to feed an infant, an unfortunate idea. There may be one period during the day when a baby will wait as long as 5 hours, interspersed between shorter intervals. When a baby seems consistently hungry less than 3 hours after each feeding, he probably needs to be offered more formula. By the time a baby is a few weeks old, he will probably have developed a pattern of feeding and sleeping that is fairly consistent from day to day.

How Much Formula?

In the review of fluid and caloric needs earlier in this chapter, it was noted that six feedings of approximately 3 ounces would meet the requirements of a baby weighing 6.5 pounds. Offering 3-ounce feedings after 24 to 48 hours of age is a good beginning. Amounts are increased as the baby shows that he is still hungry when the bottle is finished (wide awake, sucking, and searching for more). Twenty-four hour intake should not exceed 1 quart, however.

Mothers should know that babies' appetites vary from one feeding to the next, so that they will not become overly concerned when the baby takes less formula. Consistent failure to feed well, however, is often a first sign of illness.

Techniques of Bottle-Feeding

The bottle-feeding mother, like the breast-feeding mother, needs to be comfortable and relaxed before she begins to feed her baby. Feeding will take from 20 to 30 minutes (many

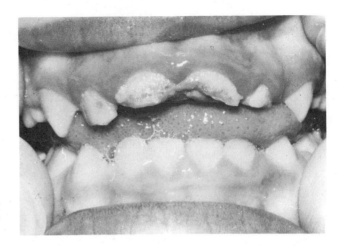

Figure 22–2. The difference in the upper and lower incisors is characteristic of bottle caries. (From Trippie and Jennings: *Keep Abreast Journal*, 3(2):114, 1978.)

mothers don't realize that this much time is necessary), and the mother may tire before her baby has finished if she is dangling on the side of her bed or perched on the edge of a chair.

Encouraging the mother to wash her hands before she holds and feeds her baby during the time that she is in the hospital may help to establish a habit that will carry over when she is home.

No one, not even a tiny baby, can swallow well lying flat on his back; the baby should be held in a semi-erect position (see Complications of Bottle-Feeding, below). The bottle is held so that the nipple is filled with milk. The baby needs frequent opportunities to "burp" at least once in midfeeding and again at the end of feeding (below).

Parents who are bottle-feeding must be encouraged to hold their babies throughout each feeding. Skin-to-skin contact is possible and important for these mothers and their babies, just as it is for mothers and their breast-fed babies.

One advantage of bottle-feeding is the opportunity it gives fathers to have an important role in caring for their baby.

At least once or twice during the mother's hospital stay, we can talk with her while she is feeding the baby in order to observe the process and also to answer questions that arise during feeding that she may forget later. Plans for subsequent teaching and referral are based on observations made at this time.

Complications of Bottle-Feeding

The prevention of two potential complications of bottle-feeding, otitis media (an infection of the middle ear) and nursing bottle syndrome, is a part of the education of mothers who bottle-feed.

If the baby is allowed to nurse lying flat on his back, milk may be regurgitated into the

eustachian tube. In infants the eustachian tube is straight rather than curved as it is in older children and adults, so that infection arising in the eustachian tube easily spreads to the ear. Beauregard[5] found that 85 per cent of a group of bottle-fed infants with otitis media fed while their bottles were propped, whereas only 8 per cent of a matched group who did not have otitis media fed while their bottles were propped.

Nursing bottle syndrome, also called *bottle caries* or *bottle mouth,* is a type of tooth decay that occurs in approximately 1 per cent of children who take a bottle of milk, juice, or carbohydrate-containing liquid* to bed with them at naptime or bedtime.[66] A particular pattern of tooth decay results, affecting the maxillary incisors most severely. Other affected teeth are the maxillary first primary molars, the maxillary primary cuspids, and the mandibular first primary molars (Figs. 22–2 and 22–3).

The infant who takes a bottle to bed usually lies down with the nipple held against his palate. His tongue protects the lower (mandibular) incisors. As he becomes sleepy and swallows less frequently the carbohydrate-containing liquid pools around the teeth, and acid formation begins. Caries are usually first seen when the baby is 10 to 12 months old.

A baby should not be allowed to take a bottle to bed that holds any liquid other than clear water. Checking an infant's mouth at each health check-up and querying parents about feeding practices is also important because caries develop long before children normally have their first dental visit (at about 3 years of age).

Approximately one child in every five will have some form of allergic disease by the age of 20. Allergies account for one-third of all visits to pediatricians' offices, one-third of all days lost from school, and one-third of all

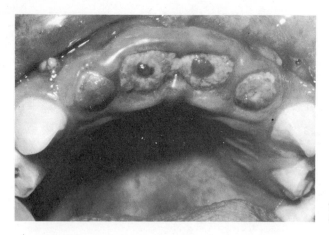

Figure 22–3. This child's teeth are so badly destroyed that they will have to be removed surgically. (From Trippie and Jennings: *Keep Abreast Journal,* 3(2):114, 1978.)

chronic disease in children under 17. Glaser[28] proposed that the abandonment of breast-feeding has been a major factor in the substantial increase in allergic problems that has occurred in this century. Because a family history of allergy is an important factor in the subsequent development of allergy, it has been suggested that during the first 6 months after birth, a time when infants are particularly susceptible to sensitization, no cow milk formula be given to infants who are at risk of developing allergy (i.e., infants with a strong family history of allergy).[42a]

Care Following Feeding

Whether infants are fed at breast or by bottle, they swallow air along with their milk. Following feeding, a baby needs to be "bubbled" or "burped." This may be effectively accomplished in several ways. The traditional posture of holding the baby against the mother's shoulder and gently rubbing his back is certainly satisfactory (Fig. 22–4). An alternate method is to hold the baby in a sitting position, supporting his head and chest with one hand and gently rubbing his back with the other.

Some babies do not easily bring up an air bubble. Efforts to make the baby burp should not be so vigorous that a sleeping baby is awakened, since sleep after feeding is a normal physiologic pattern.

Because it is normal for the baby to sleep after feeding, his care should be planned so that baths and other care are given prior to feeding rather than afterward.

Nurses have long assumed that a prone or right-sided position was most appropriate following feedings. Blumenthal et al.[7] found no difference in the time needed for the stomach to empty in relation to the baby's position; most stomach contents were emptied within 20 minutes. However, other advantages of a prone position have been noted: decreased dia-

per rash,[37] decreased likelihood of aspiration,[33] enhanced sleep,[8] and, in preterm infants, enhanced respiratory function.[43]

Nutritional Deprivation during the First Weeks of Life

What happens when nutrition is not adequate during the newborn period? Obvious effects may be inadequate growth in length and failure to gain weight. It is strongly suspected that nutritional deficiency may affect the central nervous system as well. The effects of nutritional deficiencies on the central nerv-

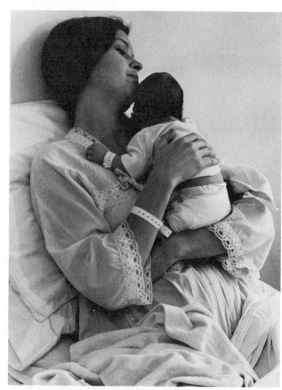

Figure 22–4. A mother burping her infant in a traditional posture. (Photograph by Suzanne Szasz.)

ous systems of very young animals have been demonstrated in a succession of studies over nearly 50 years. Rats with inadequate caloric intake during the period of most rapid postnatal brain growth exhibited marked retardation.[60] Severe undernutrition has been shown to influence the chemical composition of the brains of infant pigs, so that their brains resemble those of considerably younger pigs.[19]

Even more important than a lack of calories is a lack of protein. A number of animal studies have examined protein deficiency in the presence of adequate caloric intake. In a London study, weanling rats, piglets, and puppies born of well-nourished mothers were fed diets adequate in calories but severely deficient in protein. The animals showed signs of degenerative changes in their nerve cells. Electroencephalograms (EEGs) were abnormal; one researcher noted certain resemblances between the EEGs of pigs in the study and those of children with kwashiorkor, a condition involving severe protein deficiency.[45]

The animal studies showed that the time at which nutritional restriction occurs is significant. Food restriction prior to weaning was associated with permanent changes in the size and chemical composition of the brains in rats. Food restriction for an equal period of time, but imposed at the time of weaning, also led to brain alterations, but these later alterations disappeared during a subsequent period of adequate nutrition.[69]

Evidence from another study supports this concept. Abnormalities in the myelination of the nervous systems of rats, brought about by undernutrition from the period after weaning (age 3 weeks) until 11 weeks of age, were corrected by normal diet between 11 and 19 weeks of age.[19]

Lack of specific vitamins and minerals also led to deformities in the animals studied.

In human infants rapid development of the brain occurs after birth. Head circumference increases from approximately 34 cm. at birth to 46 cm. by the first birthday and then at a rate of roughly 0.5 cm. each succeeding year until the adult size of 52 cm. is reached. Similarly, the weight of the brain, about 400 grams at birth, more than doubles during the first year, to 1000 grams, and continues to grow for many years. Brain mass increases until about 25 years of age.

In addition to these changes in size, a major change in brain structure occurs during the first years of life. At birth, the infant brain contains most of the 10 billion neurons that it will have during the individual's lifetime. But neurons are packed very densely in the small infant skull. The neurons enlarge and the connecting links between them increase in number and complexity very rapidly until 4 years of age and then more slowly until 12 years of age. Because of this, it is believed that when nutritional deficiencies, particularly protein deficiencies, are severe enough to limit height and weight gains during the first years of life, brain development and the related motor, language, and adaptive behaviors are also likely to be affected. The earlier the period of deprivation, the more serious the consequences. In studies of children with kwashiorkor, rates of progress in behavioral development were related to the age at which the children were admitted to the hospital. Relatively little progress was made by children who had kwashiorkor at the age of 3 to 6 months; there was better development in children who were 15 to 29 months old at the time they were admitted. Children who were 37 to 41 months of age at the time of admission demonstrated the best rate of behavior development.[19]

Maternal Deprivation or Undernutrition?

Whitten and associates have proposed that undernutrition may not always be recognized for what it is.[71] Studies in the 1940's suggested that emotional deprivation in an infant or young child could be directly responsible for the child's failure to grow and thrive.[24, 61, 63] Whitten et al. point out that none of these psychologic studies determined the babies' caloric intakes. Their own study involved 13 maternally deprived infants, 11 of whom gained weight at an accelerated rate when they were fed adequately in a hospital environment that deliberately simulated their home situations (i.e., they were confined in windowless rooms and were neither talked to or smiled at nor held for feeding). The two babies who did not gain remained anorectic. Both of them had a history of repeated attempts by the mother to force-feed them. It was reported that one father, reacting to his baby's poor intake, had tried to "ram a hamburger down the infant's throat."

In a second group of seven infants, all seven gained rapidly in their own homes when they were fed an adequate diet in the presence of a public health nurse acting as an observer. Whitten et al. believe that there was no improvement in home environment that could account for the increase in weight. For example, one infant, who was visited 42 times by the nurse (3 times a day for 14 days), was found alone in a crib in a back room on every occasion. Forty-one times the baby was returned to the back room before the nurse left. Yet during the 14-day period the baby gained 26 ounces.

A second infant gained 22 ounces during an 8-day feeding program in spite of the fact that during that period his family was evicted for nonpayment of rent and he had been physically abused by his father.

When the mothers were questioned prior to the period of the observed feedings, most of them claimed that their babies ate adequately. During supervised home feedings, however, some mothers began to realize that their babies actually had been underfed.

There is no question that maternal deprivation can seriously affect the development of an infant or child. We suggest here, however, that inadequate knowledge of nutritional needs also is a factor in "failure to thrive."

The Need for Protection from Infection

In centuries gone by, and in parts of the world today, infection claimed and still claims the lives of many, many newborns. One of the major advances of modern maternity care has been the reduction of deaths by infection, a highly significant achievement. But in reducing infection we have often erected barriers to a comfortable relationship between parents and their babies. In meeting one need, protection from infection, an equally important one— the need of parents to become acquainted with their baby and to hold and care for him—and the need of their baby for that care was frequently compromised. Because of this, the issue of infection in newborn infants needs to be examined carefully, so that we plan nursing care based on *all* the needs of the infant and his family. The discussion below relates chiefly to the apparently healthy term infant. The prevention of infection in the newborns with special kinds of problems is discussed in Chapters 23 and 24.

Why Are Newborns Prone to Infection?

The body's response to infection is both cellular and immunologic. In both types of response, newborns differ from older children and adults.

Cellular Factors.   White blood cells and lymphocytes are the cells that enable all of us to resist infection. The white blood cells important in newborn resistance are the polymorphonuclear leukocytes (called polys) and the monocytes (called macrophages when they are in tissue).

The action of polys in newborns (and even more so in preterm infants) is not as efficient as it is in older children and adults. This is because in order to ingest bacteria the poly must first travel to the site of the infection, a process dependent upon complements C3 and C5. Newborns have only 50 per cent of the C3 and C5 complement of older individuals. Like polys, monocytes also participate in the phagocytosis of bacteria. In addition, monocytes play a role in the initiation of antibody formation.

Lymphocytes produce antibody and govern cell-mediated immunity; they function adequately in newborns. However, because there has normally been no previous contact with an antigen (bacteria), there is no pre-existing antibody.

Immunologic Factors.   A second response of the body to infection involves immunoglobulins, which are synthesized by plasma cells and which react specifically with the antigens that stimulate their formation. Immunoglobulins are classified into five groups: IgG, IgM, IgA, IgD, and IgE.

IgG crosses the placental barrier, and the baby will thus be passively immune to certain infections (e.g., diphtheria, tetanus, measles, rubella, mumps, and diseases caused by certain group A streptococci) *if* his mother is immune to them. Because much of the IgG crosses the placenta during the third trimester, IgG levels are lower in preterm infants. The preterm baby partially compensates by producing IgG more rapidly than the term baby following delivery. Note that pertussis is not among the diseases against which the infant is protected; pertussis immunization is usually started at 4 to 6 weeks following delivery to give the baby protection.

IgM is the first immunoglobulin made by the baby after birth; it does not cross the placenta (the molecule is too large). If IgM is found in cord blood, intrauterine infection is suspected. The absence of IgM does not rule out infection, however. Since the immunoglobulins against gram-negative bacteria are chiefly IgM molecules, their presence in cord blood *may* be an indication of gram-negative sepsis in the newborn.

IgA is the primary immunoglobulin of colostrum. The IgA of colostrum is somewhat different from the IgA in blood; it is more stable against oral acids. IgA is the immunoglobulin for gram-negative rods such as *E. coli*, which probably explains the protection against *E. coli* diarrhea afforded by breast milk.

Little is known about IgD at this time. IgE

is the antibody involved in allergic reactions and is not presently believed to be significant during the newborn period.

Potential Portals of Entry

A third factor in the increased risk of infection in newborns is the relatively large number of potential portals of entry: the umbilical vessels, circumcisions, and skin breaks from forceps, for example. Delicate infant skin breaks down easily. Low gestational age and many types of congenital anomalies increase the risk of infection still further (Chapter 23).

Newborn Defense Mechanisms

The newborn is not totally defenseless against infection. In addition to the mechanisms described above, he has certain unique characteristics.

Gastric acid levels in the baby are very high on the first day of life. This is probably protective in that the baby may swallow gram-negative organisms at the time of the first breath; however, the organisms may be destroyed by the high level of acid. Gastric acid levels drop on the second day, when colostrum with its protective immunoglobulin is available to the infant, one more example of the physiologic interaction between mother and baby.

Shortly after delivery the baby begins to develop intestinal flora. This bacterial flora, commonly alpha-hemolytic streptococci, protects the baby from invasion by pathogenic bacteria. If the baby is given antibiotics for some reason, the normal flora is destroyed, allowing the invasion of more virulent bacteria.

Infants at Increased Risk of Infection

Both maternal and neonatal factors (Table 22–5) increase the risk that an infant may become infected. These factors should be assessed in each infant and their presence noted on the infant's chart. Although infection does not always occur when one of these factors is present, awareness of their presence can facilitate early recognition of neonatal infection.

Prevention of Infection

Proper handwashing is the most important single factor in protecting newborn infants from infection. Brushes for scrubbing, particularly scrubbing for several minutes, have been found to be neither necessary nor desirable in the nursery. Hands and arms (to the elbows) should be washed with a hexachloro-

Table 22–5. MATERNAL AND NEONATAL FACTORS THAT INCREASE THE RISK OF INFECTION

Maternal Factors
  Rupture of membranes for more than 24 hours prior to birth
  Fever or other signs of infection in the mother during the week prior to birth
  Foul-smelling or purulent amniotic bleeding
  Prolonged labor
  Excessive manipulation during labor
  Infectious disease in the mother: syphilis, gonorrhea, tuberculosis, rubella, vaccinia, polio, salmonellosis

Fetal Factors
  Preterm birth
  Need for resuscitation following birth
  Insertion of equipment (e.g., endotracheal tube, umbilical artery catheter)
  Frequent blood sampling, exchange transfusions
  Presence of congenital anomalies (e.g., esophageal atresia, omphalocele, gastroschisis, exstrophy of bladder, myelomeningocele)

phene or iodophor preparation for 2 to 3 minutes on entering the nursery and rewashed for a shorter period of time if any equipment considered "contaminated" is touched. Contaminated surfaces include pens and pencils, telephones, charts—anything that is not specifically designed for the baby. Touching one's face or nose also contaminates one's hands. Hands should, of course, be washed after caring for one baby before touching another infant or any equipment belonging to another infant.

Because iodophor preparations are active against both gram-negative and gram-positive organisms, they are considered superior to hexachlorophene preparations, which are active against only gram-positive bacteria. Some individuals, however, are sensitive to the iodophor preparations, so it is recommended that both be available. The containers for handwashing preparations must be sterilized at regular intervals.

Mothers and fathers should wash their hands well each time they hold their baby, a pattern that not only helps to prevent infection in the hospital but suggests an important habit for baby care at home.

Neither parents not personnel should care for a baby if they have an infectious illness—a fever of undetermined origin, a cold, vomiting or diarrhea, an open skin lesion, a herpes infection, or a communicable disease. If a mother must be isolated from her baby because of infection, it is a major part of our nursing responsibility to maintain other contacts between the family and their infant, such as frequent opportunities to see the baby and to talk with us about him.

Visitors other than the father (who should not really be considered a visitor) and possibly other children in the family do not seem necessary on obstetric units. Limiting visitors not only reduces the chance of infection but also gives the mother more time for rest and for her baby.

Babies must also be protected from other babies with infections by isolating the affected infant.

Proper care of the furnishings and equipment and of the nursery itself is still another way of preventing newborn infection. Any equipment that becomes wet during use must be cleaned and sterilized each 24 hours. Special attention is also important for areas such as sinks and sink drains, which are continually wet, and for floors, walls, windowsills, and countertops.

Each individual baby's unit should be thoroughly cleaned before a new infant is admitted. This cleaning includes the walls of the unit and the drawers and shelves, as well as the baby's mattress and bassinet. Some institutions use a disposable bassinet of heavy cardboard with its own mattress, which the mother may then take home with her at the time of discharge and use as a baby bed during the first weeks of life.

The physical set-up of the nursery may help to prevent infection. An ideal arrangement is that of small, multiple nurseries of four to six infants to which no new infants are admitted until all previous babies are discharged and the entire nursery is cleaned. Such a system is called a "cohort" system.

Since the baby will spend at least part of each day in his mother's room, this room must also be scrupulously clean for the protection of both baby and mother. Coats and packages should never be placed on the mother's bed, nor should visitors be allowed to sit on the bed. A diaper placed between the baby and the bedclothes is an added protection. Wrapping the baby in a blanket and discouraging the mother from unwrapping him is not justified as a prevention against infection. Most mothers will ignore such prescriptions in their very natural and necessary desire to inspect their baby.

Rooming-in and Infection

The original rationale for the separation of mothers and babies in hospitals, in an era when infant mortality was far higher than it is today, was the protection of the baby from infection. It is legitimate to wonder if putting mothers and babies back together for either part or all of the day, as in rooming-in (Chapter 26) might lead to an increased incidence of infection. More than 20 years of experience have not shown this to be a problem. The precautions of careful handwashing and eliminating contact with individuals who have infections are, as discussed above, important in rooming-in.

Circumcision

Circumcision, the surgical excision of the prepuce (foreskin) of the penis, is a practice at least 7000 years old and is widely performed in the United States today. The routine practice of circumcision has been questioned in the past decade, however. In 1971 the Committee on Fetus and Newborn of the American Academy of Pediatrics stated that there are no valid medical indications for circumcision in the neonatal period. The data were reviewed in 1975, and no basis was found for changing the statement.[15]

For some parents, the wish to circumcise is related to religious beliefs; circumcision is a religious rite for Jewish and Moslem families, for example. Other families may seek information about the advantages and disadvantages of circumcision.

Proponents of circumcision argue that (1) circumcision is a factor in the prevention of carcinoma of the penis and prostate in males and of the cervix in females, (2) circumcision is prophylactic against a number of diseases, including herpes genitalis, (3) hygiene is facilitated, and (4) the absence of circumcision may make a boy feel different from his peers. Opponents argue that the studies linking cancer and the absence of circumcision are invalid for a variety of methodologic reasons. Terris, Wilson, and Nelson[64] found no significant difference in the circumcision status of marital partners of 1148 women with histologically confirmed cases of cancer of the cervix and an equal number of women matched as controls.

In comparing the incidence of carcinoma of the penis in white male populations in temperate zones in the United States and Scandinavia, no difference was found in the rate (1:100,000) for circumcised and uncircumcised males. The incidence of cancer of the penis is higher (9:100,000) among uncircumcised males in the tropics.[27] Ravich[55] suggested that carcinoma of the prostate is higher in circumcised males. Studies from diverse cultures indicate that when hygiene is good, carcinoma of the penis is rare; if hygiene is poor, circumcision appears to offer little protection.[29]

As to the ease in retracting the foreskin for purposes of hygiene in infant boys, the prepuce, still developing at birth, is normally nonretractable. Of 100 newborns, only 4 had a fully retractable prepuce; in 54 the glans could be uncovered to reveal the external meatus, whereas even the tip of the glans could not be uncovered in the remaining 42. Separation of the prepuce from the glans usually occurs between 9 months and 3 years. Gairdner[25] suggests that during the years the child is incontinent the prepuce protects the glans from infection due to wet diapers.

Balanitis, infection of the foreskin, occurs only in uncircumcised males and requires staged surgical correction. Balanitis was common among uncircumcised American soldiers stationed in desert areas during World War II because of sand under the foreskin, a factor that may have influenced an increased incidence of circumcision in the decades that followed.

Opponents of circumcision are particularly concerned with the pain involved in the procedure. They emphasize that we do not know what the long-term effects of this pain and stress may be. An anesthetic is rarely used because it is believed that the infant will have no memory of the pain. Kirya and Werthmann[38] suggest that a penile dorsal nerve block with 1 per cent lidocaine without epinephrine virtually abolishes pain from circumcision, as evidenced by the infant's quiet alert state after the initial infiltration of the medication. No complications or untoward effects of lidocaine were present in 52 infants, nor were any other complications of circumcision observed. Because the infant no longer was distressed, parents were allowed to witness the circumcision.

Opponents of routine circumcision are also concerned about complications. Hemorrhage, sufficient to require intervention to stop bleeding, and infection are the most commonly reported complications; hemorrhage was more than twice as common as infection in one study.[27] Infection was more frequent when a Plastibell method was used. Less frequent complications include penile edema, urinary retention, and, rarely, denudation or sloughing of the penis. Urinary retention is assessed by charting the first voiding after the procedure is completed.

Certain infants should not be circumcised in the neonatal period. Absolute contraindications include infants with hypospadias (because the foreskin is needed for surgical repair), infants who possibly have a bleeding problem, infants with congenital anomalies or illness, and premature infants. If the parents of a premature infant desire circumcision, the procedure is deferred until the baby weighs at least 2500 grams (5.5 pounds).

Circumcision should never be performed in the delivery room immediately following birth for several reasons. Certainly it is unjustified to perform a painful procedure on an infant during a time that should be devoted to allowing parents to become acquainted with their new infant. Moreover, cold stress caused by the temperature of the delivery room is a hazard. The fact that a neonatal anomaly or illness is a contraindication to circumcision and that such a condition may not be readily apparent in the delivery room is an additional reason for delaying the procedure until the infant is at least 12 to 24 hours old, is stable, and has had a complete physical examination.

Although some parents will have discussed the advantages and disadvantages of circumcision with a nurse, midwife, childbirth educator, or physician prior to the time of birth, others will not have considered the question. In raising the question in childbirth education courses, I find that some mothers do not know the meaning of the word circumcision. In one study, over half the women questioned did not know whether their husbands were circumcised.[63] In other surveys the proportion of women who did not know their husband's circumcision status varied from 5 to 10 per cent in private practice to approximately 35 per cent in clinic populations.

Thus, if parents are to make informed decisions, a discussion of circumcision should be part of prenatal and postpartum education. Before asking parents what decision they have made, nurses should ask them if circumcision has been discussed with them and should assess their knowledge. Further education can be provided if it is necessary.

Following circumcision, a sterile gauze bandage saturated with Vaseline is applied and then changed at each diaper change for the first few days. This promotes comfort and helps to control bleeding. The infant may be more comfortable on his side or back while the circumcision is healing (see Nursing Care Plan 22–1).

Because infants are frequently discharged on the day they are circumcised, the care of the circumcision area and signs of complications should be discussed with the parents.

In addition, the need for lifelong penile hygiene must be discussed with the parents of both circumcised and uncircumcised infants. In the uncircumcised infant, the foreskin is retracted gently, if possible, and the penis washed as part of daily hygiene. As the boy grows and becomes responsible for his own care, he is reminded about penile hygiene just as he is reminded about washing behind his ears.

Education for Parenting

The goal of parent education is the provision of information that will help mothers and fathers understand the unique characteristics, capabilities, and needs of their own newborn infant and thus be better able to care for him. To achieve this goal, a variety of strategies is necessary.

For many parents, specific parenting education begins in prenatal childbirth classes, but not all parents attend these classes. Rooming-in experiences following birth offer excellent opportunities for mothers and fathers to start to care for their babies while support persons who can answer questions are close at hand. Some parents leave the birthing site too quickly to utilize rooming-in, however, and others may elect not to have rooming-in or, in some instances, may not be offered the opportunity. In some communities public health nurses make one or more home visits to every family with a new infant. Some nurses who practice in collaboration with physicians also make home visits. Nurse-midwives who deliver infants may continue to serve as resources to new parents during the first week of the baby's life. A telephone call from the hospital nursing staff to the home a few days after discharge provides an opportunity for questions from parents as well as some assessment by the nurse. Dean and coworkers[16] describe individual teaching sessions in the hospital in which parents are guided by a nurse in getting to know their own infant. They found that these 20-minute sessions decreased parental anxiety; decreased anxiety, in turn, may enhance attachment as well as facilitate learning.

What information is important for parents? The answers to the following questions frequently asked by parents can serve as a guide in planning for their educational needs.

1. What are our baby's current characteristics and capabilities?

Table 22–6. SELECTED BOOKS FOR PARENTS ABOUT INFANTS AND PARENT–INFANT RELATIONSHIPS

Barr, E.: *Teenage Pregnancy: A New Beginning.* Albuquerque, New Futures, 1900. Includes information about baby care as well as pregnancy and family planning. Written for teenagers.

Brazelton, T. B.: *Infants and Mothers: Differences in Development.* New York, Dell Publishing Co., 1969. Follows the development of three babies, a quiet baby, an average baby, and an active baby, through the first year, emphasizing their unique characteristics. For parents with high school education or beyond and professionals. Available in paperback.

Brenner, E.: *A New Baby! A New Life!* New York, McGraw-Hill Book Co., 1973. Simple, easy-to-read text and lovely drawings make this book valuable for all parents. Paperback.

Caplan, F.: *The First Twelve Months of Life.* New York, Bantam Books, 1978. Excellent information for parents educated beyond high school and professionals; nurses will need to adapt information for other parents. Based on research done at the Princeton Center for Infancy and Early Childhood. Available in paperback.

Frailberg, S.: *The Magic Years.* New York, Scribner's, 1968. Parent-child relationships for parents with high school education or beyond.

Johnson & Johnson: *Infant Development Guide.* Sommerville, N.J., 1978. Beautifully illustrated, comprehensive book. Shows fathers as active participants in child care. Editorial advisory board includes Kathryn Barnard, Professor of Nursing at Washington School of Nursing. Hardback.

Koschnick, K.: *Having a Baby.* Syracuse, N.Y., New Readers Press, 1979. Written at a fourth to fifth grade reading level, this book is valuable for mothers who would be unwilling or unable to read more complex material. Includes infant as well as prenatal care. Paperback.

Parke, R.: *Fathers.* Cambridge, Mass., Harvard University Press, 1981. Examines the role of fathers in infant/child development; describes research. College educated parents and professionals. Paperback.

Sutherland, J. (ed.): *Child Care.* Van Nuys, Calif.: Sutherland Learning Associates, 1979. Good information; easily readable, well illustrated. Refers only to doctor as health care provider, which is unfortunate. Paperback.

White, B.: *The First Three Years of Life.* New York, Avon Books, 1975. Excellent information for parents educated beyond high school and professionals; nurses will need to adapt information for other parents. Based on research done at Harvard University. Available in paperback.

2. How will our baby develop over the next few weeks?

3. How can we best meet our baby's physical needs?

4. What are our baby's emotional needs?

5. How can we keep our baby healthy?

6. How will we know if our baby is sick?

As an adjunct to verbal instruction provided directly, written information is important. A lot of things have happened to new parents very quickly; it will take time to absorb all of this new information. Some parents will consult books for further information or reinforcement of what has been discussed with them; for other parents the material we provide will be their only written reference. In addition to the books listed in Table 22–6, useful written materials are frequently available from state departments of health and agricultural extension services.

What Are Our Baby's Current Characteristics and Capabilities? Physical characteristics, sensory capabilities, and the unique behavior of their infant can be explored with parents. The presence of the baby during this discussion is most important. Parents can ask such questions as "What is that lump on his head?" as they inquire about a cephalhematoma or "Why are his breasts swollen?" The baby's ability to follow an object with his eyes, to turn toward the sound of a voice, to console himself and to be consoled are much more meaningful when parents can observe this behavior in their own infant. Exploration of each baby's characteristics is equally feasible in a hospital, birthing center, or home.

How Will Our Baby Develop Over the Next Few Weeks? The first weeks of life encompass a period of rapid physical, social, and developmental change. Parents can expect their infant to:

1. Regain birth weight by approximately 10 days.

2. Tremble and startle less frequently.

3. Decrease feedings from 7 or 8 to 5 or 6 per day.

4. Have fewer bowel movements (varies with type of feeding).

5. Sleep longer at each nap.

6. Have longer periods of alertness.

7. Become somewhat more predictable.

8. Enjoy seeing faces, kicking legs.

9. Make cooing noises, hand-to-mouth movements.

10. Become quiet at the sound of the human voice.

Babies give more positive feedback to parents each week as the brief periods of alertness lengthen. The baby's excitement when Mom, Dad, or siblings come into the room, his increasing ability to quiet to the sound of a familiar voice, his cooing sounds and his ability to make eye contact, the decrease in crying time—all these behaviors increase the pleasure of being a parent. By helping parents to anticipate and watch for signs of their baby's development, nurses can further the parents' appreciation of and interaction with him.

The importance of talking to the baby from the beginning can be stressed. Although many parents do this automatically, others believe that talking is silly when a baby cannot understand. Yet this early verbalization appears to be important in the later development of speech.

In addition to helping parents understand their infant, an overview of his expected development in the first weeks can help parents cope with the feeling that the baby will forever consume all their time and energy. Parents need reassurance that a cycle will become increasingly evident in which the baby awakens when he is hungry, cries, is fed, has a period of alertness after feeding, and then becomes drowsy and sleeps again.

How Can We Best Meet Our Baby's Physical Needs? Information about bathing, feeding, and other aspects of physical care has been presented in this chapter. Another physical need is the need for safety.

A number of the recommendations in Table 22–7 have been voiced for years. The recognition of the importance of infant car seats is somewhat more recent. When infants (and children) are not restrained, both the likelihood of accident and the likelihood of injury in an accident increase. Accidents increase because the infant diverts the driver's attention. In one study, 31 per cent of the accidents were caused by an unrestrained infant or child falling.[31] The same researchers found that 24 collisions in a 4-year period were due to improperly used restraints. Injuries increase because the child is not protected.

For newborns and infants weighing less than 15 to 20 pounds, a tub-shaped carrier that cradles the baby in a semi-erect position is advised. Infant carriers should always *face the rear* of the car so that the force from a crash is distributed over the infant's back. The carrier is secured to the seat using an adult seat belt. Although the rear seat of the car is the ideal location for an infant carrier, many parents when driving alone are uncomfortable if they cannot see the baby; placing the carrier in the front seat, facing toward the rear, is considered acceptable.

Infants should be placed in an approved

Table 22–7.   INFANT CAR SAFETY SEATS*

	Manufacturer	Safety Seat Name	Comments
Infant Carriers **Weight Range:** **Birth to 17–20 lbs.** **Height Range:** **Birth to 26 in.**	*Century*	Trav-L-Ette	Recommended in center front or center rear for increased side protection
	General Motors	Ford Infant Carrier Infant Love Seat Mopar Infant Safety Carrier	Ford, General Motors, and Chrysler infant carriers are identical, but retailed as different brands. Minor changes between pre and post 1981 models
	Questor	Dyn-O-Mite Dyn-O-Mite #441	Use only in seating position where seat belt buckle rests more than 1 inch from plastic belt guide on carrier
Infant Carriers Which Convert to Toddler Seats **Weight Range:** **Birth to 40–43 lbs.** **Height Range:** **Birth to 40–43 inches**	*Century*	Century 100	5 point harness, push button buckle, elevated, no tether
		Century 200	2 shoulder straps attached to lower body shield, push button buckle, elevated, no tether
		Century 300	5 point harness with table-like shield, push button buckle, elevated, no tether
		Trav-L-Guard	5 point harness, elevated, no tether
	Collier-Keyworth/ Bobby Mac	2 in 1 Car Seat 3 in 1 Car Seat	5 point harness for infant plus body shield for toddler, no tether, 3 in 1 has high chair attachment
		Champion Car Seat Champion 3 in 1 Car Seat	3 point harness for infant plus body shield for toddler, no tether, 3 in 1 has high chair attachment
		Deluxe Car Seat	5 point harness for infant plus body shield for toddler, no tether
		Deluxe II Car Seat	3 point harness for infant plus attached swing-down shield for toddler, no tether
		Super Car Seat	5 point harness for infant and toddler. Elevated, top tether strap required
	Cosco/Peterson	Safe and Easy 13-203 Safe and Easy 13-313 Safe and Easy 13-314 Safe and Easy 313A	5 point harness, push button buckle, single point harness adjustment, elevated, 13-203 requires top tether strap but others do not, check model numbers carefully when making selection
		Safe-T-Seat 78	5 point harness, elevated, push button buckle, top tether strap required if manufactured before 1980
		Safe-T-Seat 78A	5 point harness, elevated, push button buckle, no tether
		Safe-T-Shield 81A	3 point push button buckle, harness for infant, attached swing-down shield for toddler, elevated, no tether

Table 22–7. INFANT CAR SAFETY SEATS* *(Continued)*

Manufacturer	Safety Seat Name	Comments
International/ Teddy Tot	Astroseat VI Astroseat #9120* Astroseat #9121*	5 point harness, elevated, no tether. (Also available: Models #9120A and #9121A with push button buckle.)
Kolcraft	Hi Rider	5 point harness for infant plus shield for toddler, elevated, no tether, requires long seat belt for toddler position
Questor/Kantwet	Care Seat #986 Care Seat #988 Care Seat #989 One-Step #401	5 point harness, elevated, top tether strap optional but recommended 5 point harness, elevated, no tether 2 shoulder straps attached to lower body shield, elevated, top tether strap required
Strolee	Wee Care #597S* Wee Care #597SF* Wee Care #598*	5 point harness, elevated, top tether strap required, recommended for use by infants only if manufactured after April, 1980
	Wee Care #597A	5 point harness, push button buckle, elevated, top tether strap required
	Wee Care #599* Wee Care #599SF* Wee Care #599V*	5 point harness threaded through spring-loaded arm rest/shield, push button buckle, elevated, top tether strap required
Welsh	Travel Tot #367* Travel Tot #368* Travel Tot #369*	5 point harness, adjusts to four heights for toddler, no tether, some assembly required

*This list was prepared by the University of North Carolina Highway Safety Research Center in 1981. Similar lists may be available in other states. As new types of seats become available nurses should look for information about tests of the seats in simulated crash situations.

restraint (Table 22–7) for their very first automobile ride (i.e., when they leave the hospital or birthing center for their first trip home). Thus, nurses caring for mothers and infants following birth should discuss the importance of car seats with parents. Infant seats are perceived as an unnecessary expense by many parents, particularly those with limited resources. In some communities, there are programs through which infant car seats are loaned to families at little or no expense. Garage sales and second-hand shops may also be less expensive sources of car seats. Parents are urged to take a list of approved seats with them when shopping and to inspect second-hand seats for signs of damage.

Proper *environmental temperature* is a physical need that has been previously discussed in relation to the hospital. At home some

parents (and many grandparents) have a tendency to keep babies too warm. An environmental temperature of 68° to 72°F. is fine. At night, the temperature can be as low as 65°F.

Babies can go outdoors at any time after they return home. In summer weather, it is necessary to take some care to protect them from sunburn.

Many parents have questions about the baby's clothing—how much and what kind. Babies need no more clothing than adults in the same environmental temperature. Just a diaper or a diaper and a cotton shirt is sufficient if the parents are wearing shorts. If the parents need a sweater, the baby probably does also.

New babies need very few clothes—shirts, diapers, and two or three cotton gowns are really sufficient. Babies grow so rapidly during the first weeks and months that clothes are

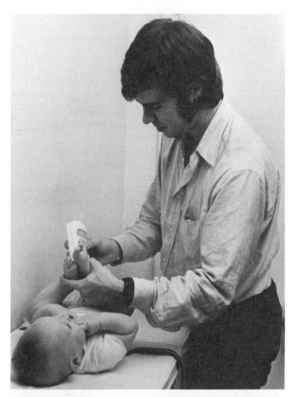

Figure 22–5. A father diapering the infant. (Photograph by Suzanne Szasz.)

quickly outgrown. It makes sense to use the money for items of long-term value such as a good crib mattress that can be used for several years.

Plastic pants and disposable diapers with plastic coverings cannot be tolerated by some babies. When infants have a tendency to develop diaper rash, discontinuing the use of plastic pants is one of the first changes in routine that parents can make. Some babies will be able to wear waterproof pants during the day when diapers are changed frequently but need to avoid them at night (Fig. 27–5).

Although booties, socks, and little shoes may be cute, babies are better off without any foot covering. Parents should know that it is normal for a baby's hands and feet to be slightly cooler than his trunk.

How Can We Best Meet Our Baby's Emotional Needs? The infant's development of trust is the primary task of the first year. Trust develops when an infant's basic needs are met in a consistent way. Because infants differ, the best way to meet needs will also differ. Some babies will need more holding and rocking, whereas other babies will be best served by less stimulation.

One of the major concerns of parents is what to do when their baby cries. Crying is the baby's way of communicating a need or distress, and parents need to respond to these cries during the early weeks and months of life. There appears to be no danger of "spoiling" during the first weeks; indeed, prompt response early in life seems to lead to less subsequent crying.[6] Yet it is hard to convince parents of this. When parents in childbirth education classes are asked to respond to the statement, "It's OK to pick up a baby when he or she cries," most parents disagree or are undecided. In some classes only one or two parents will agree that it is all right to pick up the crying baby; fathers agree more frequently than mothers.

After the birth of the infant discussion with parents about their response to crying and other behaviors can focus on the particular and unique needs of their infant as they come to know him.

How Can We Keep Our Baby Healthy? How Can We Know if Our Baby Is Sick? Health care education for new parents includes preventive care, the recognition of illness, and knowing what to do if the baby appears ill.

Where will the baby receive health care? From a nurse practitioner or physician? In a private office or a public clinic? Some parents have thought carefully about this aspect of baby care but others have not. Some parents may need additional information about the options available to them. Many infants, even infants with high risk conditions, have no "health care home," receive few or none of the necessary immunizations, and may be rarely if ever seen by a professional during the first year. When parents have made no plans, a referral to a public health nursing service can provide continuity of care. Even when parents have made a plan for continuing health care, they may not utilize that plan in the first weeks following birth. Many day-to-day questions about feeding, crying, bowel movements, rashes, and the like may seem too trivial for a call to a clinic or office yet may be a source of worry to the parents. In some hospitals, a nurse may call the mother several days after discharge to give her the opportunity to ask questions. Home visits in both the public and private sectors are available in many communities.

Preventive health care includes many aspects of care that have already been described (e.g., nutrition, bottle mouth caries, safety) or will be in subsequent chapters. The importance of immunization should be emphasized; the fact that immunization is important for their baby is a more effective way of getting the parents' cooperation than are reasons of epidemiology (e.g., the prevention of disease in the population).

How do parents recognize that their baby is ill? Every mother and father should be taught how to take their baby's temperature before they leave the hospital. They should also know that they ought to take the baby's temperature before calling the clinic or office if they think the baby is sick. The physician will want to know whether the temperature is elevated. Other clues to illness include:

1. Loss of appetite.
2. Vomiting or diarrhea.
3. Lack of energy (lethargy).
4. Difficult breathing.
5. Sunken eyes or fontanel or full fontanel.
6. Drainage from the umbilical area.

7. White patches in mouth (thrush).
8. Nonspecific symptoms (looks sick).

Parents should have the telephone numbers of their health-care provider and the hospital emergency room handy. A good place to put the number is on the bottom of the telephone. Families without telephones should know the location of the nearest one that they can use.

Summary

Nurses act to meet the needs of newborns directly, through the education of parents, and by facilitating parent–infant interaction in hospitals, in birthing centers, and in the community.

REFERENCES

1. American Academy of Pediatrics: *Standards and Recommendations for Hospital Care of Newborn Infants.* 6th Edition. Evanston, Illinois, American Academy of Pediatrics, 1974.
2. Amine, E., Hegstead, D.: Effect of Dietary Carbohydrates and Fats on Inorganic Iron Absorption. *Journal of Agricultural Food Chemistry, 23*:204, 1975.
3. Applebaum, R. M.: The Modern Management of Successful Breast Feeding. *Pediatric Clinics of North America, 17*:203, 1970.
4. Barr, E.: Teenage Pregnancy, A New Beginning. Albuquerque, New Futures, 1980.
5. Beauregard, W.: Positional Otitis Media. *Journal of Pediatrics, 79*:294, 1971.
6. Bell, S., and Ainsworth, M.: Infant Crying and Maternal Responsiveness. *Child Development, 43*:1171, 1972.
7. Blumenthal, I., Ebel, A., and Pildes, R.: Effect of Posture on the Pattern of Stomach Emptying in the Newborn. *Pediatrics, 63*:532, 1979.
8. Brackbill, Y., Douthitt, T., and West, H.: Psychophysiologic Effects in the Neonate of Prone Versus Supine Placement. *Journal of Pediatrics, 82*:82, 1973.
9. Brazelton, T. B.: *Infants and Mothers: Differences in Development.* New York, Dell Publishing Co., 1969.
10. Brazelton, T. B.: Neonatal Behavioral Assessment Scale. *Clinics in Developmental Medicine, 50*: 1973.
11. Brazelton, T. B.: *Does the Neonate Shape His Environment?* (Perinatal Reprint Series). White Plains, N.Y., National Foundation/March of Dimes, 1974.
12. Brenner, E.: *A New Baby: A New Life.* New York, McGraw-Hill Book Co., 1973.
13. Brown, J., and Helper, R.: Stimulation—A Corollary to Physical Care. *American Journal of Nursing, 76*:578, 1976.
14. Caplan, F.: *The First Twelve Months of Life.* New York, Bantam, 1978.
15. Committee on Fetus and Newborn: Report of the Ad Hoc Task Force on Circumcision. *Pediatrics, 56*:610, 1975.
16. Dean, P., Morgan, P., and Towle, J.: Making Baby's Acquaintance: A Unique Attachment Strategy. *MCN, 7*:37, 1982.
17. Eid, E. E.: Follow-up Study of Physical Growth of Children Who Had Excessive Weight Gain in the First Six Months of Life. *British Medical Journal, 2*:74, 1970.
18. Fantz, R.: Pattern Vision in Newborn Infants. *Science, 140*:296, 1963.
19. Fomon, S. J.: *Infant Nutrition.* 2nd Edition. Philadelphia, W. B. Saunders Co., 1974.
20. Fomon, S. J.: What Are Infants Fed in the United States? *Pediatrics, 56*:350, 1975.
21. Fomon, S. J., and Anderson, T. (eds.): *Practices of Low Income Families in Feeding Infants and Small Children.* Washington, D.C., MCH Service, U.S. Department of Health, Education and Welfare, 1972.
22. Fomon, S. J., Filer, L. J., Thomas, L. N., et al.: Growth and Serum Chemical Values of Normal Breastfed Infants. *Acta Paediatrica Scandinavica,* Suppl. *202,* 1970.
23. Frailberg, S.: *The Magic Years.* New York, Scribner's, 1968.
24. Fried, R., and Mayer, M.: Socio-emotional Factors Accounting for Growth Failure in Children Living in an Institution. *Journal of Pediatrics, 33*:444, 1948.
25. Gairdner, D.: The Fate of the Foreskin: A Study of Circumcision. *British Medical Journal, 1*:433, 1949.
26. Gartner, L., and Lee, K.: Jaundice and Liver Disease. In Behrman, R., et al. (eds.): *Neonatal-Perinatal Medicine: Diseases of the Fetus and Infant.* 2nd Edition. St. Louis, C. V. Mosby Co., 1977.
27. Gee, W., and Ansell, J.: Neonatal Circumcision: A Ten-Year Overview. *Pediatrics, 58*:824, 1976.
28. Glaser, J.: The Dietary Prophylaxis of Allergic Disease in Infancy. *Journal of Asthma Research, 3*:199, 1966.
29. Grimes, D.: Routine Circumcision of the Newborn Infant: A Reappraisal. *American Journal of Obstetrics and Gynecology, 130*:125, 1978.
30. Gross, S.: The Relationship Between Milk Protein and Iron Content on Hematologic Values in Infancy. *Journal of Pediatrics, 73*:521, 1968.

31. Hall, W., and Council, F.: Warning: In Cars Children May be Hazardous to Their Parents' Health. American Association for Automotive Medicine, *Proceedings,* October 7-9, 1980.

32. Hammar, S. L., Campbell, M., Campbell, V., et al.: An Interdisciplinary Study of Adolescent Obesity. *Journal of Pediatrics, 80:*373, 1972.

33. Hewitt, V.: Effect of Posture on the Presence of Fat in Tracheal Aspirate in Neonates. *Australian Paediatric Journal, 12:*267, 1976.

34. Johnson and Johnson: *Infant Development Guide.* Sommerville, N. J., 1978.

35. Johnson, N.: Breast-Feeding at One Hour of Age. *MCN, 1:*12, 1976.

36. Kanaaneh, H.: Detrimental Effects of Bottle Feeding. *New England Journal of Medicine, 286:*791, 1972.

37. Kietal, H., Cohn, R., and Harnish, D.: Diaper Rash, Self-Inflicted Excoriations and Crying in Full-Term Newborn Infants Kept in the Prone or Supine Position. *Journal of Pediatrics, 57:*571, 1960.

38. Kirya, C., and Werthmann, M.: Neonatal Circumcision and Penile Dorsal Nerve Block—A Painless Procedure. *Journal of Pediatrics, 92:*998, 1978.

39. Knafl, K.: Conflicting Perspectives on Breast Feeding. *American Journal of Nursing, 74:*1848, 1974.

40. Korner, A.: Individual Differences at Birth: Implications for Early Experience and Later Development. *American Journal of Orthopsychiatry, 41:*608, 1971.

41. Korner, A., and Thoman, E.: Visual Alertness in Neonates as Evoked by Maternal Care. *Journal of Experimental Child Psychology, 10:*67, 1970.

42. Koschnick, K.: Having a Baby. Syracuse, N.Y.: New Readers Press, 1979.

42a. Lawrence, R.: *Breastfeeding: A Guide for the Medical Profession.* New York: C. V. Mosby Co., 1980.

43. Martin, R., Herrell, N., Rubin, D., et al.: Effect of Supine and Prone Positions on Arterial Oxygen Tension in the Preterm Infant. *Pediatrics, 63:*528, 1979.

44. Naismith, D.: Bottle Feeding Makes Fat Mamas—and Fat Babies, Too. *Medical Opinion, 3:*38, 1974.

45. Nelson, G., and Dean, R.: The Electroencephalogram in African Children: Effects of Kwashiorkor and a Note on the Newborn. *Bulletin of the World Health Organization, 21:*799, 1959.

46. Newton, M., and Newton, N.: The Normal Course and Management of Lactation. *Child and Family, 9:*102, 1970.

47. Newton, N.: Decline of Breast Feeding, 1: Psychological Implications. *Nursing Times,* September 22, p. 1267, 1967a.

48. Newton, N.: Decline of Breast Feeding, 2: Social Aspects of Breast Feeding. *Nursing Times,* September 29, p. 1320, 1967b.

49. Newton, N.: Decline of Breast Feeding, 3: Psychophysical Regulating Mechanisms. *Nursing Times,* October 6, p. 1346, 1967c.

50. Newton, N.: Trebly Sensuous Woman. *Psychology Today, 5:*68, 1971.

51. Newton, N., and Newton, M.: Psychological Aspects of Lactation. *New England Journal of Medicine, 277:*1179, 1967.

52. Parke, R.: *Fathers.* Cambridge, Mass.: Harvard University Press, 1981.

53. Peters, T., Apt, L., and Ross, J.: Effects of Phosphates Upon Iron Absorption Studies in Normal Human Subjects and in an Experimental Model Using Dialysis. *Gastroenterology, 61:*315, 1971.

54. Ravelli, G., Stein, Z., and Susser, M.: Obesity in Young Men after Famine Exposure in Utero and Early Infancy. *New England Journal of Medicine, 295:*349, 1976.

55. Ravich, A.: Role of Circumcision in Cancer Prevention. *Acta Urologica Japonica, 11:*76, 1965.

56. Saarinen, U., Siimes, M., and Dallman, P.: Iron Absorption in Infants: High Bioavailability of Breast Milk Iron as Indicated by the Extrinsic Tag Method of Iron Absorption and by the Concentration of Serum Ferritin. *Journal of Pediatrics, 91:*36, 1977.

57. Sauls, H.: Potential Effect of Demographic and Other Variables in Studies Comparing Morbidity of Breast-Fed and Bottle-Fed Infants. *Pediatrics, 64:*523, 1979.

58. Schaeffer, H., and Emerson, P.: Patterns of Response to Physical Contact in Early Human Development. *Journal of Child Psychology and Psychiatry, 5:*1, 1964.

59. Schmidt, M. H.: Superiority of Breast Feeding: Fact or Fancy. *American Journal of Nursing, 70:*1488, 1970.

60. Scrimshaw, N.: Infant Malnutrition and Adult Learning. *Saturday Review, 16:*64, 1968.

61. Spitz, R.: Hospitalism: An Inquiry into the Genesis of Psychiatric Conditions in Early Childhood. *Psychoanalytic Study of the Child, 1:*53, 1945.

62. Sutherland, J. (ed.): *Child Care.* Van Nuys, California: Sutherland Luminary Associates, 1979.

63. Talbot, N. B.: Dwarfism in Healthy Children: Its Possible Relation to Emotional, Nutritional and Endocrine Disturbances. *New England Journal of Medicine, 236:*783, 1947.

63a. Terris, M., and Oalmann, M.: Carcinoma of the cervix, an epidemiologic study. *Journal of the American Medical Association, 174:*1847, 1960.

64. Terris, M., Wilson, F., and Nelson, J.: Relation of Circumcision to Cancer of the Cervix. *American Journal of Obstetrics and Gynecology, 117:*1056, 1973.

65. Thompson, D.: Breast Milk and Dental Caries: The Question of Fluoride. *Keep Abreast Journal, 3:*108, 1978.

66. Trippie, R., and Jennings, R.: Nursing Bottle Syndrome. *Texas Medicine, 73:*47, 1977.

67. Tronick, E., and Brazelton, T. B.: Clinical Uses of the Brazelton Neonatal Behavioral Assessment. *In* Friedlander, B. Z., et al. (eds.): *Exceptional Infant, 3: Assessment and Intervention.* New York, Brunner/Mazel, 1975.

68. Wenick, M.: Malnutrition and Brain Development. *Journal of Pediatrics, 74:*667, 1969.

69. Wenick, M., and Noble, A.: Cellular Response During Malnutrition at Various Ages. *Journal of Nutrition, 89:*300, 1966.

70. White, B.: *The First Three Years of Life.* New York, Avon Books, 1975.

71. Whitten, C., Pettit, M., and Fischhoff, J.: Evidence That Growth Failure from Maternal Deprivation Is Secondary to Undereating. *Journal of the American Medical Association, 209:*1675, 1969.

23

Caring for the Newborn with Special Problems: Problems Related to Resuscitation, Gestational Age, and Weight

6. Explain why thermoregulation is of particular concern in preterm infants. Identify nursing actions that ensure that infants will remain in a thermoneutral environment.
7. Describe the pathophysiology of the respiratory distress syndrome. Explain why RDS is a major source of concern in preterm infants.
8. Discuss the ways in which nutritional needs of preterm infants may be met.
9. Identify the danger of hyperbilirubinemia. Explain why preterm infants are at particular risk. Identify nursing responsibilities in the treatment of hyperbilirubinemia.
10. Discuss why preterm infants are particularly susceptible to infection. Describe the signs of neonatal sepsis and nursing actions needed for the care of infants with sepsis.
11. Discuss ways in which nurses can meet the sensory needs of preterm infants.
12. Describe the important issues in discharge planning for preterm infants.
13. Identify the unique characteristics and needs and the appropriate nursing interaction when infants are postterm, small for gestational age, and large for gestational age.

No area of maternal and child health has changed or continues to change more rapidly than that involving the care of high risk newborn infants, those babies who differ from "normal" because of their gestational age, their weight, or because of some congenital or acquired abnormality. Care of these babies involves careful attention to physiologic, emotional, and developmental needs. It should take place in a nursery that involves parents in planning and giving care and should be provided by personnel who are as sensitive to the needs of these parents as they are to the needs of high risk babies.

A general textbook concerned with the care of mothers and infants cannot cover in detail all that a nurse needs to know in order to give highly specialized intensive care to newborns. An understanding of the complexity of that care, however, can help nurses who work with parents in many phases of child bearing better appreciate the needs of both families and infants. We have chosen in this chapter to look at those concepts of high risk care that we feel should be a part of the basic knowledge of nurses who care for mothers and infants. These concepts include:

1. A philosophy of care for high risk newborns.
2. Early recognition of the baby who is at risk.

3. Resuscitation of the baby who fails to breathe spontaneously.
4. Identification and care of the most common problems occurring during the first days of life.

Chapter 24 discusses the needs of infants with selected congenital anomalies. Chapter 28 discusses the needs of parents of high risk babies and the ways in which we can help them cope with those needs.

A Philosophy of Care

As technology has enabled us to sustain life at an earlier gestational age—first at 36 weeks, then at 34 weeks, and now at even less than 28 weeks—there has been a growing concern about the quality of the life that is given to the tiny babies who survive these first weeks. Parents, nurses, other health-care providers, legislators (who make decisions about health-care funding), and the public (who pay much of the cost through taxes and insurance premiums) ask whether the infants who survive will be developmentally and neurologically normal.

When Lubchenco and her associates studied infants weighing less than 1500 grams who were born in the years 1949 to 1953, when intensive care nurseries as we know them today had not yet been developed,[38] they found that over half of these low birth weight babies had some central nervous system impairment and scored less than 90 (considered the lower limit of normal) on intelligence tests. Others, although of average intelligence, were clumsy and had poor hand-to-eye coordination and other perceptual motor problems, indicating a failure of central integration. Sixty-six per cent had retrolental fibroplasia (RLF) (see below). In a study published 9 years later, Peacock and Hirara[45] followed infants weighing less than 1500 grams for 4 years or longer. Of 56 infants, 46 (82 per cent) were considered developmentally and neurologically normal at age 4. A number of other studies report similar findings. However, because follow-up to age 4 is not sufficient to reveal the presence of learning disabilities or minimal brain dysfunction, concern still remains. Nevertheless, it does appear that good care is contributing not only to an increased number of surviving infants but also to the increased survival of healthy children and adults.

Central Nervous System Development

If a major goal of high risk newborn care is an intact central nervous system, knowledge of central nervous system development in utero and in the period following birth is a foundation for such care.

Neuronal development peaks at 12 to 18 weeks of gestational age (Fig. 23–1). Insults during the period of rapid neuronal development lead to a decreased number of neurons and to mental retardation, which is often severe. Examples of such insults are viral diseases (rubella, cytomegalic inclusion disease) and radiation. Nothing that we now know

reverses the effects of these insults; they must be prevented.

The cerebellum reaches its peak of development during the first days after birth. If the baby fails to receive cerebellar nutrition (oxygen, glucose, maintenance of acid-base balance) in the first days following birth, problems in cerebellar development will result in perceptual motor difficulty. The child may be clumsy and lacking in fine coordination, even though his intelligence may be normal.

The cells of the brain stem and of the cerebral cortex grow more slowly than those of the cerebellum, developing during the months and years following birth. Their development depends upon continued support during these months rather than on support for a period of a few critical days. Thus a child may be intelligent (a function mediated by the cerebral cortex) and still have perceptual motor difficulty (which is mediated by the cerebellum).

A great deal of the myelinization of the neurons also takes place following birth. Myelin is a cholesterol substance that acts as "insulation" for the neurons. Without myelinization, when neurons "fire," messages go off in all directions. Thus a newborn, who normally has incomplete myelinization, reacts to a stimulus with his whole body. As a child grows older, his movements normally become less general and more specific, and he is able to accomplish finer coordination. If myelinization remains incomplete, this finer coordination is never achieved.

How can we use this knowledge of central nervous system development to plan better care for mothers and babies? First, it seems obvious that we must have a concept of care that embraces the entire perinatal period, beginning at conception and not merely at birth.

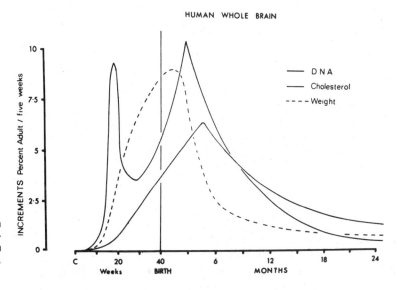

Figure 23–1. DNA accumulation is an indication of cell number (neurons). Cholesterol content measures the deposition of myelin. (From Räihä: *Pediatrics*, 53:147, 1974.)

This care begins with the early recognition of the mother who has a potential for delivering a high risk baby, together with the assurance that she receives the kind of care she needs (Chapter 13).

Recognition of the Baby at Risk

A baby is considered at high risk because of gestational age (less than 37 weeks or more than 42 weeks) and/or because of weight (less than 2500 grams). Obviously, within these parameters there are varying degrees of risk; the prognosis for a baby weighing more than 2000 grams is far different than for a baby weighing less than 1250 grams, other factors being equal (such as the presence of congenital malformations and so on). Babies may also be at high risk because of congenital malformations, birth injury, sepsis, respiratory distress, metabolic disorders, or hematologic problems. Many high risk newborns have two or more simultaneous problems. Many preterm babies have respiratory distress, hypoglycemia, hyperbilirubinemia, and sepsis, for example.

Signs of difficulty may be obvious immediately following birth, or they may not appear for several hours or days. Still other types of difficulty may not appear for weeks or months (some types of congenital heart defects, for example). In certain genetic disorders, although the potential is present at the time of birth, the disease itself may not appear until later in life. Examples are Huntington's chorea and certain muscular dystrophies.

The Baby at Risk in the Delivery Room: Failure to Breathe Spontaneously

Resuscitation of the newborn baby who does not breathe spontaneously is a major emergency. Not only do we hope to save the infant's life, but we also hope to prevent brain damage (which may manifest itself in major problems such as seizures, cerebral palsy, and developmental retardation, as well as in learning disorders and other more subtle difficulties).

The goal of resuscitation is a healthy baby who retains his maximum potential for growth and development. This goal is accomplished by:

1. Providing oxygen and removing carbon dioxide.
2. Providing alkali for buffering the excess acid that is produced during anaerobic metabolism.

Table 23–1. RESUSCITATION

A = Airway
B = Breathing
C = Circulation
D = Drugs
E = Environmental temperature

3. Maintaining circulation.
4. Providing drugs if necessary.
5. Maintaining a thermoneutral environment (Table 23–1).

What is the role of the nurse in the resuscitation of a distressed newborn? In many hospitals the attending physician is responsible for both the mother and the newborn infant in distress. Obviously, in these hospitals the delivery room nurse must also be highly knowledgeable about newborn resuscitation, because the physician's attention is necessarily divided. In some hospitals, the delivery room nurse is *the individual responsible* for a distressed newborn.

The ideal situation is one in which two or three persons can devote their undivided attention to an infant requiring resuscitation, and an additional nurse is available to support the parents. When one considers what it must be like for a mother, lying on the delivery table, aware that she has not heard her baby's cry, aware from seeing worried faces that something is amiss, it is not hard to imagine that a major nursing responsibility is support for the mother, and for the father or other family member as well. Unfortunately, in the hurry of the average delivery, this is the responsibility that seems most often overlooked.

If regionalization of maternity care (Chapter 31) brings a majority of mothers whose babies are at risk to adequately equipped and staffed centers for delivery, this ideal may be achieved. In the meantime we must be prepared to give the very best care within the framework of our current practice.

Anticipating the Need for Resuscitation

While the need for resuscitation may occur at any birth, the risk of birth asphyxia is increased in certain circumstances. When the mother has a high risk condition during the prenatal or intrapartum period (Chapters 13 and 19), when there is an abnormality of the placenta or umbilical cord (Chapter 19), or when the fetus is compromised because of gestational age of less than 37 weeks or more than 42 weeks, infection, erythroblastosis, or intrauterine distress (fetal tachycardia, bradycardia, or the passage of meconium), the likelihood of a need for resuscitation is increased.

When Does an Infant Need Resuscitation?

Apgar scoring (Chapter 20) is a rapid assessment technique that can be used to identify infants in need of resuscitation. Infants with an Apgar score of 6 or less may need resuscitation. Infants with scores of from 0 to 3 will probably need vigorous resuscitation. Resuscitation may be necessary after the baby is in the nursery because of respiratory or cardiac depression.

Preparation of Equipment for Resuscitation

Before *every* delivery, equipment for resuscitation of the baby should be ready. Not every instance of respiratory distress can be anticipated from the maternal history or from the course of labor. Basic equipment includes:

1. A bulb syringe for suctioning.
2. A DeLee glass bulb with catheter for aspiration of mucus.
3. Newborn and premature airways.
4. A laryngoscope with small blades (size 0 and size 1).
5. Small endotracheal tubes with obturators (sizes 12 to 18 F [2.5 to 4.0 mm.]).
6. A resuscitation bag capable of delivering 100 per cent oxygen with the proper adapters to connect it to the endotracheal tubes or mask; infant face masks in varying sizes.
7. Oxygen and suction equipment, including various sizes of catheters (sizes 5 to 10F).
8. Syringes and needles.
9. Umbilical vessel catheters.
10. Drugs, including sodium bicarbonate, 10 per cent dextrose in water, epinephrine 1:10,000, and narcotic antagonists.
11. Stethoscope.
12. Adhesive tape, tincture of benzoin.

Resuscitation Technique

The baby's head should be slightly dependent and turned to the side to facilitate drainage of the fluid in the trachea. This fluid, which amounts to approximately 30 ml. per kg. of body weight, is not amniotic fluid but arises from the alveolar cells.

Airway. The airway must be cleared. Suctioning with a bulb syringe may be all that is necessary. A longer suction catheter may stimulate the vocal cords and lead to laryngospasm, with subsequent apnea and cyanosis. Be sure that the baby's tongue is not obstructing his airway. Pulling the baby's chin forward and up will relieve obstruction by the tongue. A small airway may also be useful.

When the baby is delivered through thick, "pea soup" meconium, *meconium aspiration syndrome,* that is, the aspiration of meconium into the lungs, may occur. The baby's mouth and nose are suctioned before the shoulders are delivered, if possible. Following birth an endotracheal tube is inserted, and the trachea is suctioned before the first breath forces the meconium further into the respiratory tree. Today, many physicians feel that the baby with thin, watery meconium in the amniotic fluid does not require endotracheal intubation and suction.

Breathing. Tactile stimulation, such as gently rubbing the infant's back (Perez maneuver), drying him with a towel, or gentle suction may initiate respiration. Vigorous stimulation, such as back slapping or immersion in cold water, is more dangerous than helpful.

These steps will be all that is necessary for many babies. If the infant still fails to breathe, oxygen may be given by bag and mask at the rate of 30 to 40 breaths per minute. The mask must fit tightly over the baby's nose and mouth. If the mask is working properly, one can observe the baby's chest rise and fall during ventilation and can hear oxygen entering the lungs with a stethoscope. During initial resuscitation 100 per cent oxygen is given; 100 per cent oxygen is not believed to be toxic during this short period.

Prior to the first breath the wet internal surfaces of the lungs adhere to one another in much the same manner as wet glass slides adhere to each other in the laboratory. Therefore, the first breath requires more pressure than subsequent breaths, from 40 to 100 cm. of water pressure. The initial puff of air, when it reaches the larynx, often stimulates the baby to breathe and may be all that is necessary. If further ventilation is required, the pressure should be from 25 to 45 cm. of water pressure.

A baby with primary apnea* or one who is gasping when resuscitation begins, and infants with Apgar scores of 3 to 6 will usually respond within 15 to 20 seconds to suction and oxygen by face mask (Table 23–2).

Mouth-to-mouth breathing is an alternative if bag and mask ventilation is not possible. This method uses only the amount of air in the breather's mouth, not the total volume of air in the lungs, again to avoid overexpansion. Oxygen may flow from a tube into the blower's mouth to increase the oxygen concentration of air blown into the baby's lungs.

If heart rate does not increase immediately, intubation will be necessary. When the baby is totally unresponsive at birth (the rag doll, Apgar 1 baby), intubation is generally the

---

*Primary apnea is defined as apnea during which spontaneous respirations can be induced by appropriate sensory stimuli; secondary apnea is apnea in which respirations cannot be induced by sensory stimuli.[15a]

Table 23–2.   RESUSCITATION IN RELATION TO APGAR SCORING

Apgar Score	Level of Asphyxia	Probable Treatment
0–2	Considered asphyxiated until proven otherwise	Intubation
3–6	Mild to moderate	Suction; oxygen by bag and mask
7–10		Rarely will need resuscitation

initial step. Immediate intubation is also recommended for the baby born through septic amniotic fluid and for the baby delivered in the vertex position through "pea-soup" meconium. If these babies are treated by bag and mask ventilation before they are intubated and suctioned, meconium or septic fluid will be forced into their lungs. A stillborn baby who, by accurate fetal monitoring, has been known to be dead for less than 10 minutes prior to delivery may also be immediately intubated. Brain damage would be too severe to resusci-

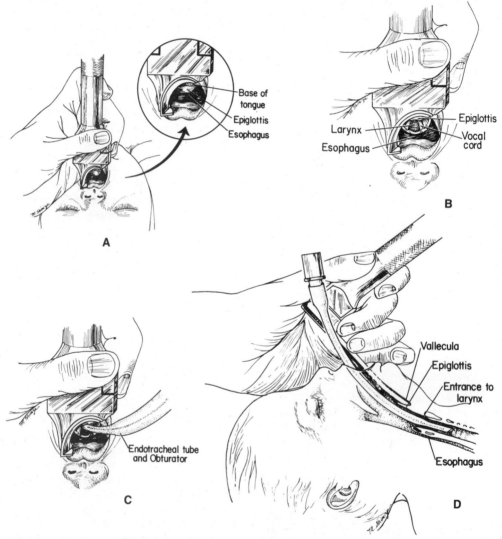

Figure 23–2.   Technique of endotracheal intubation. The Miller blade should be inserted near the midline and moved to the left side of the mouth, gently deflecting the tongue. As it is advanced, the base of the tongue and epiglottis are visualized. The blade should be advanced in the same plane of movement into the vallecula (see *D*); as the blade is gently raised, the epiglottis swings anteriorly, revealing the opening of the larynx. If secretions or meconium are noted, gentle suctioning should be done before insertion of the endotracheal tube. On certain occasions when the epiglottis is not adequately raised, the blade tip may be placed posterior to the epiglottis, which can then be gently raised to expose the vocal cords. The endotracheal tube is advanced from the right corner of the mouth and inserted while maintaining direct visualization. The laryngoscope blade is then carefully withdrawn while the position of the tube is maintained by the right hand on the infant's face. Note the tip of the blade in the vallecula. (From Klaus and Fanaroff: *Care of the High-Risk Neonate.* 2nd Edition. Philadelphia, W. B. Saunders Co., 1979.)

tate a baby dead for a longer period. Infants with a sunken abdomen (possible diaphragmatic hernia, Chapter 24) are also intubated.

The baby's head is slightly extended, and a laryngoscope is inserted by someone *experienced* in its use (Fig. 23–2). Mucus and blood are quickly aspirated. Prolonged suction not only wastes time but may cause reflex bradycardia. An endotracheal tube is inserted, and mouth-to-tube or bag-to-tube ventilation is begun. The baby's inspiratory phase should be slightly less than half the time of the ventilation cycle, so that adequate time is allowed for passive expiration. As in other forms of resuscitation, the baby's chest should be monitored by observation and auscultation. A stethoscope is used to listen for the entry of air into the stomach also, which will indicate that the endotracheal tube is in the esophagus.

Pulmonary infection is a risk in both mouth-to-mouth and mouth-to-tube resuscitation; pneumothorax and pneumomediastinum can occur from too vigorous ventilation by any route.

The heavy use of narcotics during labor, so popular only a few years ago, has now decreased markedly in most delivery rooms. Morphine and meperidine (Demerol) are still used, however. Much of the respiratory depression caused by morphine and Demerol can be overcome by the use of naloxone (Narcan), which acts by competing with the narcotics at receptor sites. Narcan is given intramuscularly in a dose of 0.01 mg. per kg. The nursery personnel *must be told* that the baby has received Narcan, because the baby may have respiratory depression again in the hours following delivery and may require an additional dose.

Accurate records of treatment of the baby must be kept.

Circulation. The clearing of the airway and the initiation of breathing should take less than 1 minute. If the infant is still cyanotic 60 to 90 seconds after birth, the cause may be low cardiac output, a cyanotic congenital heart disease, or a lung abnormality. Polycythemia is an uncommon but possible cause; in polycythemia there is an excessive number of red blood cells, and the baby is unable to oxygenate all of them.

If the heart rate remains less than 50 beats per minute after 30 seconds of ventilation, cardiac massage is needed (Fig. 23–3). The thumbs should be on the middle third of the baby's sternum; pressing on the lower third may cause laceration of the liver. The rate of cardiac massage is approximately 100 chest compressions per minute, slower than a baby's normal rate of 130 to 150 beats per minute to allow the heart to refill so that the cardiac output will be adequate. If cardiac massage is

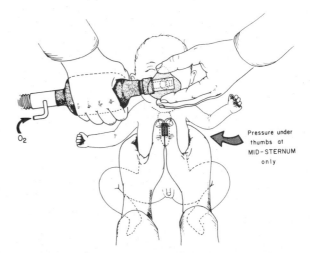

Figure 23–3. External cardiac massage. The correct position for the thumb is on the sternum with the fingertips on the back. External cardiac massage may be terminated once a rhythmical heartbeat is documented. (From Todres, I. D., and Rogers, M. C.: Methods of external cardiac massage in the newborn infant. *Journal of Pediatrics*, 86:781, 1975.)

given at a rate of 100 chest compressions per minute and ventilation occurs at a rate of 30 to 40 breaths per minute, the ratio will be 3:1. Massage is discontinued briefly each 30 seconds to check for a spontaneous heartbeat, and is stopped once a rhythmic beat occurs.

Drugs. If the baby does not respond satisfactorily to ventilation and cardiac massage, the use of drugs may be necessary. The narcotic antagonist naloxone has already been discussed as a cause of respiratory depression in the infant. Emergency medications are used less frequently than previously because it is now recognized that the drugs themselves may be dangerous for the infant. However, if they are used properly in appropriate dosages, they can also be life-saving. Table 23–3 describes the most frequently used emergency drugs.

Sodium bicarbonate ($NaHCO_3$) is given so frequently that nurses need to be thoroughly familiar with its use. Sodium bicarbonate is given to combat acidosis. *Respiratory acidosis* occurs because the baby is unable to eliminate carbon dioxide. In addition, a baby who is not breathing converts from the aerobic metabolism of glucose (i.e., metabolism using oxygen) to anaerobic metabolism (i.e., metabolism without oxygen). Lactate accumulates during anaerobic metabolism, and the baby quickly develops metabolic acidosis. If the acidosis is purely respiratory, sodium bicarbonate is of no value and is in fact harmful. This is because $NaHCO_3$ breaks down to sodium plus water plus carbon dioxide, thereby increasing the level of carbon dioxide in the baby's system. In the absence of blood gas values in the moments immediately following birth, it is

Table 23–3.   DRUGS AND BLOOD PRODUCTS FOR NEONATAL RESUSCITATION EMERGENCIES*

Drugs	Dosage and Rate	Reason for Administration	Comments
Sodium bicarbonate (NaHCO₃) (1 mEq = 1 ml) Diluted 1:1 (Sterile H₂O)	2 to 3 mEq/kg IV; over 1 to 2 min	Metabolic acidosis	Baby must be ventilated during administration
Epinephrine (1:1000) Dilute 1:10,000 (NaCl)	0.1 to 0.5 mg/kg IV	Heart rate falling or below 50 bpm in spite of resuscitation	May be given in cardiac muscle
Calcium gluconate Dilute 1:1 (after every third dose NaHCO₃)	100 mg/kg slow IV	Replace calcium depleted during asphyxia	Calcium and bicarbonate cannot be mixed in infusion solutions; causes bradycardia if injected too rapidly; cardiac massage should accompany epinephrine
Atropine sulfate	0.01 mg/kg IV	Severe bradycardia	Observe for later distress
Naloxone (Narcan)	0.01 mg/kg IV/IM	Reverse narcotic depression	
Albumin (may mix 1:1 with NaCl or NaHCO₃)	1.0 g/kg IV	}	
Fresh frozen plasma	10 to 20 ml/kg IV	} Circulatory support	O negative blood is used in emergencies
Packed RBC	10 to 20 mg/kg IV		
Whole blood	10 to 20 ml/kg IV	}	
Glucose (10%)	2 ml/kg for first 5 minutes	Necessary for metabolism	During the first day, continue glucose at 80 mg/kg/day; follow with blood glucose determinations.

*From Moore: *Newborn, Family and Nurse.* 2nd Edition. Philadelphia, W. B. Saunders Company, 1981.

assumed that delayed respiration also results in metabolic acidosis, and sodium bicarbonate is therefore given. However, *the baby must be continuously ventilated* by either bag and mask or bag and endotracheal tube to prevent the accumulation of carbon dioxide.

The initial dose of $NaHCO_3$ is 2 to 3 mEq. per kg. of body weight given intravenously. As soon as blood gas values are available, the dosage can be calculated as follows:

mEq = weight of baby in kilograms $\times$ 0.3 $\times$ base deficient (desired bicarbonate level − actual bicarbonate level)

For example:

Weight of baby = 3000 grams (3 kg.)
Bicarbonate level (blood gas) = 16
Desired level (blood gas) = 21
Base deficit = 5 (21 − 16)
    $3 \times 0.3 \times 5 = 4.5$ mEq.

The prepared dose is diluted 1:1 with sterile water and given slowly through an umbilical vein catheter (no faster than 1 mEq. per kg. per minute).

The possible role of sodium bicarbonate in intracranial hemorrhage in premature infants makes it imperative to use this agent only in severe life-threatening metabolic acidosis and then in appropriate doses. (See also Problems of Acid-Base Balance, below.)

Environmental Temperature. The critical need for warmth has already been noted in Chapter 20. It is crucial that the baby's need for warmth be met during resuscitation or other efforts may be compromised. The environment should allow the baby to maintain an axillary temperature of 97.6°F. (36.5°C.). This is the thermoneutral temperature (i.e., the temperature at which the least amount of oxygen is required by the baby).

The environmental temperature required to keep the baby's temperature at this level will vary with the size of the baby. Failure to maintain a thermoneutral environment increases the baby's need for oxygen, leading to the anaerobic metabolism described above.

How Long Can the Neonate Tolerate Asphyxia?

In adults asphyxia of 4 minutes or longer leads to irreversible brain damage. The length of time a just-born infant can tolerate asphyxia is unknown, but apparently it is a somewhat longer period. This is probably due to a lower metabolic rate in certain key areas, such as the brain, and to higher stores of glycogen per kilogram of body weight (in comparison with adults), which can be converted to glucose for anaerobic metabolism.

Maintenance of circulation is important in assisting the baby's survival of asphyxia, in part because it may help to distribute the lactate resulting from anaerobic metabolism to tissues with a lower hydrogen ion concentration.

If hypoxia continues, these protective mechanisms will be overcome, and brain damage and death will result.

Physiologic Response Following Asphyxia

Possible physiologic responses to asphyxia involve many systems. The extent of involvement will vary from one baby to another, depending upon the severity of the asphyxia, gestational age of the baby, and other individual factors. There is an accumulation of both carbon dioxide and lactic acid, as noted above. It may be several hours following resuscitation before acidosis is completely resolved. Acidosis may lead to other complications, including constriction of pulmonary blood vessels and hypotension. When the pulmonary vasculature is constricted, fetal circulation patterns may persist, and oxygenation is compromised further.

The mobilization of glycogen, which protects the baby's brain and heart during resuscitation efforts may result in hypoglycemia in the hours that follow. Infants may also have hypocalcemia, perhaps secondary to bicarbonate therapy, as well as sodium or potassium imbalance.

Hypoxia may cause kidney damage, with involvement of both tubules and glomeruli. Signs of renal damage include initial oliguria or anuria followed by diuresis, hematuria, or proteinuria, or a combination of these.

Hypoxia may damage the intestinal tract, causing decreased intestinal motility and, several days later, symptoms of necrotizing enterocolitis (NEC) (see below).

Care of an Infant Following Resuscitation

When a baby has required more than the briefest resuscitation, special care is important in the hours that follow until the baby's stability is ensured. The possible physiologic responses just described are the basis for this care, and continuous assessment to detect early signs of complications is the focus of care (see Nursing Care Plan 23–1). Nursing interventions listed in Nursing Care Plan 23–1 are discussed in specific sections later in the chapter. Infants who have required resuscitation may need to be transported to a perinatal center for subsequent care (Chapter 24).

Nursing Care Plan 23–1.   Resuscitation of the Newborn Infant

NURSING GOALS: To provide rapid, appropriate resuscitation that not only will preserve life but will result in an infant who retains maximum potential for growth and development.

OBJECTIVES:
1. At the completion of resuscitation, measurements of the following functions will be within the range of normal:
   a. respiratory rate and pattern (spontaneous or assisted)
   b. heart rate
   c. color
   d. activity
   e. blood pressure
   f. acid-base balance
   g. temperature
2. Problems associated with resuscitation in the early neonatal period will be identified and corrected.
3. Iatrogenic complications will be avoided.
4. Parents will be informed and supported during the resuscitation procedures.

ASSESSMENT	POTENTIAL NURSING DIAGNOSIS	NURSING INTERVENTION	COMMENTS/RATIONALE
1. Identify the need for resuscitation prior to delivery.*	At risk of neonatal depression	Be prepared to resuscitate; have extra personnel available.	Need for resuscitation is increased in these infants.
a. Prenatal factors			
(1) Pregnancy-induced hypertension			
(2) Rh sensitization			
(3) Severe maternal health problem, including diabetes mellitus			
(4) Preterm or post-term labor			
(5) Multiple gestation			
(6) Fetus SGA or LGA			
(7) Falling estriol levels			
(8) Immature L/S ratio			
b. Intrapartal factors			
(1) Diagnosis of fetal distress by fetal monitor			
(2) Abnormal presentation			
(3) Meconium-stained amniotic fluid			
(4) Foul-smelling amniotic fluid			
(5) Vaginal bleeding			
(6) Prolapsed cord			
2. Identify newborn needing resuscitation.		Be prepared to resuscitate; have extra personnel available.	
(1) Heart rate less than 100 beats per minute			
(2) Cyanosis		Perform Apgar scoring (Chapter 20).	
(3) Limp			

(4) Apgar score of 6 or less, at 1+ or 5 minutes
(5) No respirations or evidence of increased respiratory effort
3. Assess effects of resuscitation efforts. If heart rate is less than 50 beats after 30 seconds of ventilation, begin cardiac massage. Failure to respond indicates need for drugs.

Resuscitation procedure:
1. Ensure thermoneutral environment
2. Clear airway
3. Provide tactile stimulation

If infant fails to breathe:
4. Provide oxygen
   a. Bag and mask
   b. Bag and endotracheal tube
   c. Rate: should be 30–40 breaths per minute
5. Cardiac massage
   a. Rate: should be 100 beats per minute
   b. Ratio of heart beat to breaths should be 3:1
   c. Place thumbs over midthird of baby's stomach
6. Drugs (see Table 23–3)

4. Identify potential problems of resuscitated infant in early neonatal period.

Cardiac assessment
Heart rate (measure by cardiac monitor)
   Bradycardia
   Tachycardia
Heart murmur
Cyanosis
Blood pressure

Administer oxygen.
Digitalis given per physician order.
Correct acidosis.

Provide volume expansion by giving IV fluids.

Hypoxia
Possible congestive heart failure; shock. Persistence of fetal circulatory patterns may occur owing to hypoxia; hypotension may be due to shock.

Respiratory assessment
Tachycardia
Cyanosis
Grunting
Nasal flaring
Other signs of respiratory distress

Respiratory therapy
(See specific discussions in text regarding levels and types of respiratory intervention.)

Respiratory distress syndrome
Aspiration
Pneumothorax

*Approximately half of infants requiring resuscitation cannot be identified prior to birth.

Continued on following page

Nursing Care Plan 23–2.   Care of Preterm Infant *(Continued)*

ASSESSMENT	POTENTIAL NURSING DIAGNOSIS	NURSING INTERVENTION	COMMENTS/RATIONALE
Renal assessment Anuria Oliguria Low specific gravity Hematuria Proteinuria		Measure intake and output carefully. Assess specific gravity of urine, hematuria, proteinuria; weigh infant twice in 12–24 hours. Restrict intake of fluid and electrolytes (see text).	Hypoxic damage to kidneys
Metabolic assessment Hypoglycemia (Dextrostix) Hypocalcemia Acidosis (blood gas assessment) Alkalosis (rare) Blood gas assessment		Give IV glucose. Give IV calcium. Therapy based on cause (see text); correct iatrogenic causes.	Glycogen may be depleted during hypoxia. Lactic acidosis may result from anaerobic metabolism. *Respiratory causes of alkalosis:* tachypnea, too rapid assisted ventilation *Metabolic causes of alkalosis:* excess $NaHCO_3$
Electrolytes			Sodium, potassium altered during hypoxia
Gastrointestinal assessment Ileus: observe for first meconium stool. Signs of NEC Abdominal distention Blood in stools (Hematest) Delayed stomach emptying		P.O. intake: small amounts as ordered; specific formula Frequently given by gavage Measure residual in stomach prior to feeding.	NEC caused by hypoxic damage to gastrointestinal tract.
Central nervous system assessment Identify signs of lethargy. Seizures Determine cause (Dextrostix, calcium level).	Seizures due to specific alteration in body function	Intervene to correct glucose or calcium deficit.	Hypoxic damage to brain can cause seizures. Seizures can be secondary to hypoglycemia, hypocalcemia.
Sepsis Multiple signs, frequently nonspecific; septic "work-up" (see text)		Antibiotic therapy (see text)	Stress plus interventions (e.g., intubation, umbilical catheterization) increase the risk of sepsis.

Weight and Gestational Age as Factors in High Risk

Until recently, infants were classified as full-term or "premature" largely on the basis of whether they weighed more or less than 2500 grams (5 pounds, 8 ounces) at birth. Such designations are still used in the statistics of many nations. As noted in Chapter 20, it is now considered more useful to group infants as postterm (greater than 42 weeks' gestational age), term (38 to 41 weeks, 6 days' gestational age) and preterm (less than 38 weeks' gestational age). Postterm, term, and preterm infants may be small for gestational age (SGA), appropriate for gestational age (AGA), or large for gestational age (LGA). The criteria for placing infants in one of these categories are described in Chapter 20.

Infants of 37 to 38 weeks' gestation, sometimes referred to as "borderline prematures," frequently receive care in a nursery for term infants. Yet these infants may still have mild temperature instability and may feed slowly and become jaundiced. If delivered by cesarean section, approximately 8 per cent will develop respiratory distress syndrome (RDS). Thus, they too require special attention; their needs may be overlooked if nursing observations are not thorough.

Unique Characteristics of Preterm Infants

In comparison with most parents' image of what a new baby should look like (often based on magazine pictures of 6-month old babies), the "premie" falls far short of expectations. In addition to the obvious differences in weight and proportion, the head of this born-too-early baby is large and his body is scrawny. He may be badly bruised because of the extreme fragility of his capillary vessels. Such an appearance can be a disappointment to some parents in the first days after birth—a feeling they may voice or keep to themselves depending on their personalities and how comfortable they feel with the nurses and doctors who care for them.

Many of the characteristics of preterm infants form the basis for assessment of gestational age as described in Chapter 20 (see also Nursing Care Plan 23–2). Preterm infants have less flexor muscle tone than infants born at term, so their extremities are frequently extended rather than flexed. The skin is thin, with visible blood vessels; even infants as old as 34 weeks' gestational age have relatively little subcutaneous fat because that layer is chiefly deposited in the 4 weeks prior to term. Because the preterm infant's skin is so thin, insensible water loss is increased.

The lack of subcutaneous fat is important in planning care of the preterm infant. Energy is stored in the body as glycogen and fat. Because the fat and glycogen stores of a preterm baby are practically nonexistent, they will be quickly depleted; the baby will rapidly become hypoglycemic if a source of glucose is not provided.

Thermoregulation in the infant is increasingly affected as the weight of the baby decreases because the ratio of surface area to body mass increases (see section on Thermoregulation, below).

The thin skin of preterm infants is easily broken in the course of everyday care through the use of tape, urine bags, and other devices that come in contact with the baby's skin. Great care must be taken to protect the baby's skin because breaks serve as portals for infection (as well as causing discomfort for the baby). Small amounts of "paper tape" can be used instead of regular adhesive tape. Diapers can be weighed to measure output to avoid using urine collection bags, and in most cases a urine specimen can be extracted from the diaper with a syringe. Solvents are available to facilitate the removal of adhesive tape.

The more premature the baby, the larger will be his head in proportion to his body because of the cephalocaudal progression of development. *Lanugo* is abundant on the body of a premature infant. Genitalia are less well developed in premature infants than in term infants. Testes do not descend until the eighth month of fetal life. The labia majora do not cover the labia minora until term approaches.

Respiratory Development and Function

Of all the differences between preterm and term infants, none is more significant than the development of the respiratory tract. This is the crucial difference between viability and nonviability in a preterm infant. Prior to 26 to 28 weeks' gestation, there is limited development of the alveoli (the tiny air sacs at the terminal ends of the respiratory system through which oxygen and carbon dioxide are exchanged) and the alveolar capillaries. Within the alveoli there are two types of cells—type I cells, which give structure to the alveolus, and type II cells, which produce several compounds collectively termed *surfactant*. The most abundant of the surfactant compounds, accounting for 50 to 70 per cent of surfactant, is *lecithin*. It is the function of

Text continued on page 713

Nursing Care Plan 23-2.   Care of Preterm Infant

NURSING GOALS: To provide care for the infant of less than 37 weeks' gestation that will meet his unique needs.
To facilitate attachment between parents and their preterm infant.

OBJECTIVES: As a result of nursing care given the infant:

1. Unique risk factors in addition to prematurity will be identified.
2. Thermoneutral environment will be maintained.
3. Respirations will be initiated and maintained.
4. Fluid and electrolyte balance will be maintained.
5. Adequate nutrition will be provided in a manner commensurate with gestational age and health status.
6. Infection will be prevented; if not prevented, signs of sepsis will be recognized early and appropriate treatment provided.
7. Kidney and bowel function will be maintained.
8. Cardiac function will be maintained.
9. Neuromuscular deformity will be prevented.
10. Appropriate levels of sensory stimulation will be provided.
11. Iatrogenic complications will be prevented.

Parents will:

1. Express appropriate feelings related to their infant's condition.
2. Show evidence of attachment to their infant.
3. Demonstrate ability to care for their infant.
4. Integrate the baby into the family, or
5. Grieve for their infant who dies.

ASSESSMENT	POTENTIAL NURSING DIAGNOSIS	NURSING INTERVENTION	COMMENTS/RATIONALE
1. Identify risk factors from maternal history.	Infant at risk of complications related to preterm birth and (specific medication given to mother or specific complication)		
a. Preterm birth may be spontaneous or induced because of maternal illness. b. Medications given mother		Supportive care is given as indicated in this Nursing Care Plan.	
(1) Betamethasone			Betamethasone *decreases* risk of RDS. Betamethasone accelerates fetal lung maturation.
(2) Magnesium sulfate (Assess infant for respiratory depression, neuromuscular depression)	At risk of respiratory and/or neuromuscular depression related to maternal MgSO$_4$	Intervene to correct respiratory depression or neuromuscular depression.	MgSO$_4$ is related to neuromuscular depression.

Assessment	Nursing Diagnosis	Nursing Intervention	Rationale
(3) Analgesics and anesthetics used during labor (see Chapter 17 for specific effects); respiratory depression may be increased in preterm infants.	At risk of respiratory depression related to maternal medication (specific)	Administration of naloxone hydrochloride (Narcan) 0.01 mg. per kg.	As naloxone is metabolized, further respiratory depression may occur and dose may need to be repeated.
c. Complications of labor or birth (1) Fetal distress (2) Asphyxia at birth (Apgar score) (3) Breech delivery (4) Cesarean delivery (5) Meconium staining d. Maternal complications (1) Maternal diabetes (2) Pregnancy-induced hypertension (3) Maternal hemorrhage (4) Maternal infection (5) Prolonged rupture of membranes	At risk of complications related to preterm birth and (specific problem)	Nursing intervention needed in addition to care related to prematurity. Must consider infant's needs in relation to specific complications (e.g., increased risk of hypoglycemia in infant of diabetic mother, increased risk of respiratory distress in infant following cesarean birth, increased risk of sepsis in infant following prolonged [>24 hours] rupture of membranes).	
2. Environmental temperature; infant's temperature	At risk for cold stress	Provide thermoneutral environment (see Nursing Care Plan 23–3).	Cold stress precipitates or enhances many alterations in health status in preterm infants.
3. Gestational age relationship of gestational age to weight, length, and head circumference	Preterm infant Small for gestational age (SGA) Appropriate for gestational age Large for gestational age (LGA)	See Chapter 20 for appropriate classification if small or large for gestational age in addition to care related to preterm status. (See also Nursing Care Plans 23–12 and 23–13.)	
4. Respiratory effort a. Rate b. Pattern (symmetrical, paradoxical) c. Breath sounds (bilateral) d. Nasal flaring e. Grunting f. Retractions (describe)	At risk for respiratory distress related to immature respiratory function	Provide thermoneutral environment. Position for optimal respiratory effort; change position frequently to facilitate drainage. Suction mucus as necessary; suction mouth before nose to utilize respiratory monitor. Plan care to avoid fatigue.	
5. Color a. Cyanosis (circumoral, acrocyanosis, general) b. Plethora c. Pallor d. Relationship to activity		Specific nursing care is related to mode of respiratory support: room air, oxygen hood, CPAP, ventilator (see Nursing Care Plan 23–4).	

Continued on following page

Nursing Care Plan 23–2.   Care of Preterm Infant (Continued)

ASSESSMENT	POTENTIAL NURSING DIAGNOSIS	NURSING INTERVENTION	COMMENTS/RATIONALE
6. Apnea of prematurity a. Accompanying bradycardia b. Color change c. Change in muscle tone d. Infant's temperature	At risk for apnea related to prematurity (infants less than 30–32 weeks' gestation)	Apnea of prematurity 1. Provide prompt tactile stimulation. 2. Provide oxygen if condition not relieved (no greater than 30 to 40 per cent). 3. Correct possible causes. 4. If theophylline is ordered, assess heart rate prior to each dose; dose may be withheld if heart rate is more than 180 beats per minute.	
7. Need for fluid and electrolytes (see Nursing Care Plan 23–6)	At risk for dehydration At risk for fluid overload At risk for electrolyte imbalance	Administer fluids as ordered to maintain balance.	
8. Nutritional needs (see Nursing Care Plan 23–6)	At risk for inadequate nutrition	Provide adequte nutrition for growth. Minimize caloric expenditure; provide thermoneutral environment; plan timing of intervention to allow periods of rest. See Nursing Care Plan 23–6 for specific nutritional intervention.	

9. Infection
 a. Measures for prevention of infection:
  (1) Review nursery policies and adherence to policies frequently, paying particular attention to handwashing.
  (2) Take cultures of nursery and equipment on a random periodic basis to determine effectiveness of procedures.
	At risk for sepsis because of immaturity
	
	At risk for sepsis because of intervention
		1. Insist on careful handwashing by all personnel prior to touching infant or equipment.
		2. Maintain a clean environment.
		
		3. Maintain cleanliness or sterility of all equipment as appropriate.
		4. Prohibit infant care by persons with infectious disease.
		
		See Nursing Care Plan 23–9 for care of infant following infection.	

b. Note early signs of sepsis (see also Nursing Care Plan 23–9).
   (1) Specific behavior change (e.g., lethargy, change in feeding behavior)
   (2) Hypotension (systolic blood pressure 30 mm. Hg)
   (3) Apnea, retractions, other signs of respiratory distress
   (4) Vomiting, abdominal distention
   (5) Pallor
   (6) Temperature instability
   (7) Glucose intolerance
   (8) Metabolic acidosis
   (9) Hyperbilirubinemia
   (10) Changes on CBC, differentiated WBC

10. CNS damage

a. Assess glucose, calcium levels in blood on continuing basis.

At risk of CNS damage due to hypocalcemia

Provide intravenous glucose and/or early feeding to prevent hypoglycemia. Glucose levels should be maintained between 40 and 100 mg./dl.

Give calcium replacement if calcium is less than 7 mg./dl.

Hypoglycemia and hypoxia are major causes of neonatal brain damage.

b. Assess infant for signs of hypoxia. Blood gases or PaO_2 provides most accurate assessment.

At risk of CNS damage due to hypoxia

Give oxygen to maintain PaO_2 between 50 and 80 mm. Hg. Ensure patent airway.

c. Increased intracranial pressure (evident by bulging fontanel, widened sutures, rapid increase in daily head circumference)

Help parents understand reason for additional testing (e.g., CAT scan, CNS tap).

Seizures in the neonatal period, particularly those of metabolic origin, are not necessarily forerunners of a lifelong seizure disorder.

d. Seizure activity
   (1) Abnormal eye movements
   (2) Abnormal mouthing movements
   (3) Apnea
   (4) Abnormal movements (clonic, tonic, localized)

Continued on following page

Nursing Care Plan 23–2.   Care of Preterm Infant *(Continued)*

ASSESSMENT	POTENTIAL NURSING DIAGNOSIS	NURSING INTERVENTION	COMMENTS/RATIONALE

e. Alteration in muscle tone
  (1) Hypertonic
  (2) Hypotonic
f. Alteration in reflexes
  (1) Absent
  (2) Hyporeflexia
  (3) Difficult to elicit
  (4) Hyperreflexia
  (5) Asymmetrical			

11. Renal function a. Urine output (weigh diapers) b. Urine specific gravity	Decreased urine output Increased urine concentration	Ensure adequate balance of fluid intake, considering additional insensitive loss of infant under radiant warm or phototherapy lights.	
12. Bowel function a. Frequency and characteristics of bowel movements; relationship to infant's age	Decreased bowel function	Infant may need glycerin suppository to stimulate defecation. Cut small piece from suppository; mold before inserting in rectum.	
b. Abdominal distention	Diarrhea	Abdominal distention may indicate NEC.	
c. Occult blood in stool (hematest, Abt test to differentiate from maternal blood)	At risk for gastrointestinal bleeding	If blood in stool, suspect NEC, notify physician.	
13. Cardiac function Electronic heart rate monitoring pulse	Bradycardia related to hypoxia, hypothermia	Correct underlying cause.	
Auditory assessment of: a. Cardiac rate b. Cardiac rhythm c. Presence of murmurs d. Bradycardia or tachycardia in relation to interventions	Bradycardia related to (e.g., insertion of gauge tube, secondary to apnea)	Provide thermoneutral environment.	
e. Relationship of apnea and bradycardia (apnea preceding bradycardia)			
14. Identify symptoms related to decreased blood volume. a. Carefully record all blood withdrawn for testing.	At risk for decreased blood volume	May require blood replacement.	Total blood volume approximately 85 ml. per kg.

b. Pallor
c. Hypotension (systolic blood pressure less than 30 mm. Hg)
d. Hematocrit less than 35 per cent

15. Identify potential for neuromuscular deformity.
    a. Posture
    b. Muscle tone
    c. Symmetry

16. Identify need for sensory stimulation.
    a. Infant's response to stimulation (attends to stimuli, becomes quiet)

    b. Signs of overstimulation
       (1) Color change
       (2) Disorganized motor activity
       (3) Unstable cardiac, respiratory rates
       (4) Decreased PaO_2
       (5) Apnea, bradycardia

17. Parent–infant attachment (see Nursing Care Plans 22–1, 28–1)

At risk of neuromuscular deformity

Change position frequently.
Position for correct body alignment.

Need for increased stimulation
Need for decreased stimulation

Provide stimulation (see text):
1. Visual (faces, cutouts, mobiles properly placed)
2. Tactile
3. Kinesthetic
4. Auditory

Inappropriate stimulation.
Need of parents for information and modeling about their role in stimulation.

Protect from overstimulation:
1. Avoid sudden stimuli.
2. Provide for periods of sleep.
3. Help develop sleep-wake rhythm with periods of diminished light.

Lag in parent–infant attachment
Parents need knowledge about infant; need opportunity to care for infant; need opportunity to express feelings.

Promote attachment:
Make positive statements about infant's progress.
Encourage parents to touch, hold infant, participate in care as infant's condition allows.
Explain all treatment and infant's condition on a continuing basis.
Provide continuing opportunity for questions.
Provide continuing opportunity for expression of concerns, feelings.
Encourage sibling visits; discuss reactions of siblings with parents.
Refer to appropriate resource for counseling about financial concerns.

Continued on following page

Nursing Care Plan 23–2. Care of Preterm Infant *(Continued)*

ASSESSMENT	POTENTIAL NURSING DIAGNOSIS	NURSING INTERVENTION	COMMENTS/RATIONALE
18. Readiness of infant and parents for discharge (see Nursing Care Plan 23–10).	Infant unready for discharge because of (specific cause)	Prepare parents for discharge (see Nursing Care Plan 23–10).	
Assess home environment by community health nurse home visit prior to infant discharge.	Parents unready for infant discharge because of (specific cause)	Hospital nurse: contact community health nurse well in advance of discharge so that home environment can be assessed.	
	Home environment unready for discharge because of (specific cause)	Community health nurse should assess home, report to hospital.	
19. Continuing assessment following discharge		Provide knowledge and/or skill based on assessment.	
a. Physical assessment: infant gaining approximately 1 ounce per day; no physical problems noted	Inadequate infant growth	If infant's growth is inadequate observe feeding practices; note number of feedings per day, amount (formula) or time (breast).	
b. Parenting: parents becoming increasingly skilled in infant care, including interactive behavior and provision of stimulation.	Specific problem (e.g., diaper rash, feeding problems) Need for help in (specific skill, e.g., feeding, bathing) Inadequate stimulation	Provide opportunities for questions and expression of feelings about parents' relationship to infant or to one another.	
c. Attachment: parent's comments and behaviors indicate attachment (observe parent–infant interaction at home or during ambulatory care visit).	Excessive stimulation Inappropriate stimulation Lag in attachment	Help parents to appreciate infant's unique characteristics. Model appropriate stimulation techniques; talking, rocking, "en face," stroking.	
d. Infant development is appropriate when allowance is made for number of weeks of prematurity.	Delayed infant development	Provide information about infant development adjusted for prematurity.	
e. Infant is brought to office or clinic for health care appointments, immunizations, etc.	Failure to keep appointments		
f. Assess family relationships, particularly mother–father relationship and sibling reactions; "normality" restored following crisis of preterm birth.	Family stress related to crisis of prematurity	Refer family for counseling for major family problems.	

lecithin and other surfactant compounds to prevent the collapse of the alveoli on expiration. When surfactant production is inadequate, respiratory distress syndrome (RDS) results.

Generally, the surfactant system is mature at about 36 to 37 weeks' gestational age. Because corticosteroids appear to hasten maturation, intrauterine stress such as pre-eclampsia (which involves increased maternal corticosteroid production) may lead to earlier maturation. In the form of *betamethasone*, corticosteroids may be given to mothers 24 hours prior to delivery to hasten lung maturity if preterm birth appears inevitable. When corticosteroid production is decreased, as it is in a mother with diabetes mellitus (see below), lung maturity is frequently delayed beyond 37 weeks.

Preterm infants differ from term infants in their breathing patterns; respirations are more irregular in preterm infants, and there is periodic apnea. Both the relative weakness of the respiratory muscles and the decreased rigidity of the thoracic cage lead to hypoventilation, which results in the retention of carbon dioxide and subsequent acidosis.

Fatigue of the respiratory muscles is increased in preterm infants because of the small percentage of type I muscle fibers in the diaphragm that resist fatigue. Although adult diaphragms are composed of 50 per cent type I fibers and diaphragms in term infants have 25 per cent type I fibers, the diaphragms of preterm infants may have less than 10 per cent. The result is fatigue, slowed respirations, and apnea.[43]

Response to hypoxia also varies. Rather than responding to hypoxia with increased ventilation, the preterm infant may become further depressed, particularly if he is also hypothermic. The preterm infant seems to be less sensitive to increased levels of carbon dioxide when he is also hypothermic.

Respiratory complications may also arise because of the weak cough and gag reflexes of preterm babies, which increase the possibility of aspiration.

Gastrointestinal Development and Function

Gastrointestinal motility is decreased in preterm infants; stools may be infrequent, resulting in abdominal distention. Glycerin suppositories will usually stimulate defecation. For a small preterm infant, a small piece of a suppository can be shaped in the nurse's warm hands before insertion.

The sucking and swallowing reflexes of the baby born before 34 weeks' gestation are not sufficiently coordinated to allow direct feeding from breast or bottle; alternative feeding methods are necessary. In addition, the immature digestive system of the preterm baby makes certain dietary adjustments necessary. Not only must the types of carbohydrate, fat, and protein given be adapted to the special needs of the preterm baby, but factors such as renal solute load must also be considered (see below).

Liver Development and Function

The liver of a preterm infant is relatively less mature than that of a term infant; this increases the likelihood of hyperbilirubinemia. Great care must be taken when drugs that must be excreted through the liver are administered.

When the liver is immature, it has a decreased ability to conjugate bilirubin (i.e., to convert indirect bilirubin to direct bilirubin). This is one factor in the increased incidence of hyperbilirubinemia in preterm infants. Another factor that may be equally or more significant is the decreased number of Y and Z carrier proteins in the liver cells, to which bilirubin must bind in the conjugation process. If the level of protein is low (as when blood volume is decreased) or if other substances are competing for binding sites (as when the baby is acidotic or receiving certain drugs), there is a danger of development of kernicterus (even though total bilirubin levels may not be excessively high) because of the higher level of unconjugated bilirubin that is free to enter the brain cells.

An increased susceptibility to bruising in preterm infants, which leads to increased red blood cell destruction, and delayed feeding, which may allow reabsorption of bilirubin from the meconium in the intestines, also increase the risk of hyperbilirubinemia. In addition, any condition that leads to lower levels of albumin in the infant, such as decreased blood volume, decreases the ability of bilirubin to bind to albumin and thus allows greater circulation of unconjugated bilirubin.

For all these reasons, serum bilirubin is monitored closely in preterm infants. The treatment of hyperbilirubinemia is discussed later in this chapter.

Cardiovascular Development and Function

The transition from fetal to adult circulation, described in Chapter 20, is sensitive to the increased level of oxygen that occurs in the baby's circulatory system following his initial respiration. When oxygen levels are low, the fetal circulation pattern may persist;

particularly frequent in the small preterm infant is a persistent patent (open) ductus arteriosus (PDA) or an intermittent PDA. A distinct murmur caused by the rush of blood through the PDA can be heard on auscultation and should be assessed along with the baby's vital signs. If the ductus arteriosus remains open, the baby's condition will usually deteriorate (see page 746).

Renal Development and Function

Because of a reduced blood supply to the kidney, glomerular filtration rate is also decreased, and thus preterm infants are more likely to retain fluid and to excrete drugs poorly than are term infants. Moreover, when blood pressure is low, kidney perfusion and therefore urinary output will be diminished. When body water is low, however, the kidneys are not able to concentrate urine to conserve water, and the baby may become easily dehydrated.

Within the renal tubules themselves both reduced absorption and reduced secretion may occur. Reduced absorption of glucose and amino acids means that glucose and protein may be spilled into the urine at lower serum levels than in more mature infants or older children. Metabolic acidosis is more likely because of the decreased ability to retain bicarbonate. Reduced secretion in the tubules, like reduced glomerular filtration rate, limits drug clearance. The doses of medication given to preterm infants are very small, but they may accumulate in the body nevertheless.

In infants with a gestational age of less than 29 to 30 weeks, abnormal fluid retention with pedal edema and, later, more generalized edema may occur. Pulmonary congestion may follow.

Immunologic Competence

Immunologic competence refers to the ability of an organism to resist infection. Immunologic competence involves cellular factors such as white blood cells, factors that enhance the ability of white blood cells to destroy bacteria, and immunoglobins such as IgG, IgM, and IgA. For a variety of reasons white blood cells function less effectively in preterm infants. Moreover, IgG, which crosses the placenta and provides the newborn with immunity against certain infections to which his mother is immune (e.g., diphtheria, measles, tetanus), is present in limited amounts because transplacental passage occurs primarily in the third trimester. IgA, the primary immunoglobin of colostrum, is not available to the baby who does not receive breast milk (many preterm babies do not).

Neurologic Development and Function

Neurologic development is one of the criteria for the assessment of gestational age described in Chapter 20. A preterm infant is relatively immature neurologically, but as he increases in gestational age, neurologic maturation can be observed.

Although a very premature infant sleeps most of the time, by 28 weeks the baby should respond to touch or to a noxious stimulus such as a pin prick, and should become quiet after soothing. Before 32 weeks, response to a light (blink, constriction of pupils) may not occur. Preterm infants will not usually be able to follow objects with their eyes. Infants older than 28 weeks respond to loud noises with a startle.

Reflexes are present at varying stages. The Moro reflex is usually absent before 28 weeks, involves lateral extension of the upper extremities only from 28 to 33 weeks, and becomes complete after 33 to 34 weeks. As noted in the discussion of the gastrointestinal tract, sucking and swallowing functions, although present, are not sufficiently coordinated until about 34 weeks. The rooting reflex may be observed after 32 weeks. By 32 weeks the palm grasp becomes strong, and most infants will have a good cry.

Thermoregulation

Basic problems of thermoregulation for newborns are discussed in Chapter 20. These problems are magnified in preterm infants because they are less able to produce heat, less able to conserve heat, and at a greater risk of heat loss than a full-term infant (who is in turn at greater risk than an older infant or child).

Heat Production. There are three basic mechanisms of heat production in humans—shivering thermogenesis, nonshivering thermogenesis, and voluntary muscle activity. Nonshivering thermogenesis is the principal means of heat production in the newborn.

Nonshivering thermogenesis occurs when norepinephrine stimulates the metabolism of brown fat. Brown fat, which accounts for 2 to 6 per cent of the body weight in newborns, contains fat vacuoles, mitochondria, and an abundant blood and sympathetic nerve supply. Most brown fat is found between the scapulae at the base of the neck, surrounding the kidneys and adrenal glands, and in the mediastinum. Oxygen is required to metabolize brown fat for energy.

Preterm infants may be compromised in heat production in one or more of the following ways:

1. Because brown fat accumulates more rapidly in the third trimester, preterm infants have decreased amounts of brown fat, as do infants who are small for gestational age.

2. Norepinephrine (noradrenalin) release may be decreased in preterm infants.

3. Because oxygen is required for the metabolism of brown fat, infants who have been or who are hypoxic have a diminished capacity for heat production. Infants with decreased perfusion will also be limited in their ability to transport oxygen to the necessary areas of heat production.

4. Reduced caloric intake decreases the number of calories available for thermogenesis.

Heat Conservation. Newborns do make some attempts to conserve heat. A term newborn may assume a flexed position, which diminishes exposed surface area. Preterm infants, however, have difficulty conserving heat by changing body posture. Peripheral vasoconstriction is a second mechanism of heat conservation.

Heat Loss. Not only is heat production limited in preterm newborns, but heat loss is increased. It is by reducing heat loss that nursing care makes a particularly significant contribution (see Nursing Care Plan 23–3). Heat loss occurs when heat flows from the interior of the body to the surface (internal gradient) and from the body surface to the environment (external gradient). Preterm infants, because of diminished subcutaneous fat and thin skin, are at increased risk of loss through the internal gradient. Skin temperature is generally about 0.5°C. lower than internal temperature, so that heat is constantly flowing from the body interior to the surface.

Heat loss to the environment occurs when the environmental temperature is lower than the baby's thermoneutral environment (i.e., the environmental temperature at which the baby utilizes the least amount of oxygen; Chapter 20). Table 23–4 shows the relationship between weight, age, and thermoneutral temperature.

Heat loss occurs through conduction, convection, evaporation, and radiation. Nursing intervention to protect infants from each type of heat loss is described in Table 23–5 and Nursing Care Plan 23–3.

Providing a Thermoneutral Environment. A thermoneutral environment for preterm infants is provided either by a radiant warmer over the baby's bed or by an incubator. An overhead warmer provides radiant heat through infrared heat rays that are absorbed by the skin and warm the peripheral blood; heat is transferred to deep structures by conduction and the circulation of peripheral blood. Whereas some warmers produce continuous heat and can be controlled only manually, others offer the option of Infant Servo-Control (ISC), just as some incubators do.

The use of a radiant warmer without a Servo-Control can be dangerous. Hyperthermia and even burns may occur when output is high. Low output may produce heat insufficient to prevent hypothermia. The skin sensor of the Infant Servo-Control should be covered with gauze or a folded piece of tape to insulate the sensor from the heat of the warmer, which can interfere with its proper functioning. There must be nothing else between the probe and the heating element of the warmer. Even bending over the baby to give care may interpose the care-giver's head and shoulders between the probe and the warmer, thus interfering with its function. Care in placing the baby in the bed beneath the warmer is important; not all of his bed will be warmed by the rays. The baby may be on his abdomen, side, or back, but the sensor probe must always be applied to the skin surface nearest the warmer, never beneath the baby's body. Like the thermostat of a furnace, the warmer turns on when the baby's own temperature falls below the desired level of thermoneutrality (36.5°C.; 97.8°F.). If the warmer is functioning properly, temperature lability caused by the warmer should not be a problem. The baby's axillary temperature should also be monitored at regular, frequent intervals as a check on the monitor.

Most radiant warmers have alarm systems that produce auditory and visual signals when the temperature is outside the preset range of 36° to 37°C. (96.8° to 98.6°F.). It is easy to turn off the alarm and forget to turn it on again, a potentially serious error.

A complication of hyperthermia, especially for the small preterm baby, is an increase in insensible water loss (see below), which can lead to dehydration. A number of studies have shown that marked increases in insensible water loss result from the use of both radiant warmers and phototherapy lights. Wu and Hodgman[65] found that insensible water loss increased from 50 to 190 per cent, depending on the size of the infant and the type of warmer. The greatest losses occurred in infants weighing less than 1500 grams.

There are advantages to the open bed of the radiant warmer. Because the baby is in an

Nursing Care Plan 23–3. Providing a Thermoneutral Environment

NURSING GOALS: To provide a thermoneutral environment for the infant to minimize metabolic need for oxygen and calories.
To prevent cold stress.

OBJECTIVES: As a result of nursing action:

1. Skin temperature will be maintained close to 36.5°C. (97.6°F.), and within a range of 36.1°C–36.7° C. (97° to 98°F.). Axillary temperature is close to 36.5°C. (97.8°F.).
2. Mechanisms of heat loss will be minimized.
3. Weight gain will be optimal.
4. Cold stress will not develop.
5. Parents will understand rationale for measures to maintain thermoneutral environment.

ASSESSMENT	POTENTIAL NURSING DIAGNOSIS	NURSING INTERVENTION	COMMENTS/RATIONALE
1. Assess infant's temperature frequently. a. Initial rectal temperature b. Subsequent axillary temperature as ordered routinely and after alteration in environmental temperature due to various intervention.	At risk for cold stress related to (specific cause, e.g., prematurity, small for gestational age)	1. Provide thermoneutral environment. a. Incubator: setting various with weight and age (see Table 23–4) b. Open bed with radiant warmer and thermistor probe c. Open crib wrapped in blankets for larger babies	Cold stress is associated with hypoxia, bradycardia, acidosis, hypoglycemia, and other serious alterations in health status (see text).
2. Assess potential for heat loss (see also Table 23–5). a. Conduction: contact with cold surfaces, equipment, hands b. Evaporation: wet skin, wet diapers c. Convection: exposure to currents of cool air, including oxygen d. Radiation: surrounding environment cold; unclothed baby	At risk for heat loss related to (specific cause, e.g., prematurity, small for gestational age)	2. Minimize heat loss (see also Table 23–5) by: a. Conduction: Warm surfaces, equipment, and hands before coming in contact with infant. b. Evaporation: Keep skin dry; bathe small areas at a time; bathe only when temperature is stable. c. Convection: Avoid air currents; warm and humidify oxygen; place plastic covering over open bed; give care through incubator portholes. d. Radiation: Use cap or bonnet, clothe baby if possible; heat shield in incubator; avoid placing baby near outside walls of nursery.	
3. Weight gain	Inadequate weight gain	If weight gain is inadequate when caloric intake is sufficient, consider the need for increased environmental temperature.	The use of calories to maintain body temperature is one reason for inadequate weight gain.

Assessment	Intervention	Rationale
4. Insensible water loss (from radiant warmer) a. Observe for weight change, urine output, urine specific gravity	Increased insensible water loss	Caloric loss also causes excess oxygen consumption.
5. Signs of cold stress a. Apnea, tachypnea, or slow shallow respirations b. Mottled skin, acrocyanosis, or cyanosis c. Increased activity (older newborns) or lethargy d. Failure to feed well e. Bradycardia f. Poor cry g. Sclerema h. Oliguria i. Hypoglycemia j. Metabolic acidosis Assess temperature every 15 minutes during rewarming.	Minimize heat loss; check all equipment for providing warmth (e.g., is it plugged in, is thermistor probe attached and dry, is it at proper setting, are incubator portholes closed, is placement in room adequate?) Provide gradual warming for cold-stressed infant (air temperature 1.5°C. or 2.5°F. warmer than body temperature). Correct other problems (e.g., hypoglycemia; metabolic acidosis).	Rapid increase of body temperature may cuse apnea.
6. Parents' understanding of thermoregulation When parents are holding infant out of bed, assess infant's temperature frequently.	Provide information about infant's need for thermoregulation; provide opportunities for questions. Assist parents to touch and hold infant while maintaining infant's body temperature; show how to hold and stroke infant's head while in thermoregulatory unit. Provide positive reinforcement for their role as parents.	Infants may become chilled when held out of bed; explain to parents in advance that first out-of-bed cuddles need to be brief and will be extended as baby's ability to maintain temperature increases.
When weaning to room temperature, assess infant's environmental temperature and infant's temperature as unit temperature is lowered. Assess weight gain. Continue to assess infant's temperature and weight gain when infant is in bassinette.	Need to maintain body temperature in normal environmental temperature	Dress infant (shirt and diaper). Bed temperature is gradually lowered over a period of hours or days, depending on infant response. When infant can maintain temperature of 36.5°C. (97.7°F.) in room air temperature (72°F.–75°F.), infant is placed in bassinette.

Infant may be able to maintain body temperature but only by using calories and thus at the expense of weight gain.

Infant may be able to gain weight in room temperature prior to discharge.

Be very careful of open "portholes" in incubator; active preterm infant can fall out.

Table 23–4.   THERMONEUTRAL ENVIRONMENTAL TEMPERATURES*

Age and Weight	Starting Temperature (°C)	Temperature Range (°C)
0–6 hours		
Under 1200 gm	35.0	34.0–35.4
1200–1500 gm	34.1	33.9–34.4
1501–2500 gm	33.4	32.8–33.8
Over 2500 gm (and >36 weeks)†	32.9	32.0–33.8
6–12 hours		
Under 1200 gm	35.0	34.0–35.4
1200–1500 gm	34.0	33.5–34.4
1501–2500 gm	33.1	32.2–33.8
Over 2500 gm (and >36 weeks)†	32.8	31.4–33.8
12–24 hours		
Under 1200 gm	34.0	34.0–35.4
1200–1500 gm	33.8	33.3–34.3
1501–2500 gm	32.8	31.8–33.8
Over 2500 gm (and >36 weeks)†	32.4	31.0–33.7
24–36 hours		
Under 1200 gm	34.0	34.0–35.0
1200–1500 gm	33.6	33.1–34.2
1501–2500 gm	32.6	31.6–33.6
Over 2500 gm (and >36 weeks)†	32.1	30.7–33.5
36–48 hours		
Under 1200 gm	34.0	34.0–35.0
1200–1500 gm	33.5	33.0–34.1
1501–2500 gm	32.5	31.4–33.5
Over 2500 gm (and >36 weeks)†	31.9	30.5–33.3
48–72 hours		
Under 1200 gm	34.0	34.0–35.0
1200–1500 gm	33.5	33.0–34.0
1501–2500 gm	32.3	31.2–33.4
Over 2500 gm (and >36 weeks)†	31.7	30.1–33.2
72–96 hours		
Under 1200 gm	34.0	34.0–35.0
1200–1500 gm	33.5	33.0–34.0
1501–2500 gm	32.2	31.1–33.2
Over 2500 gm (and >36 weeks)†	31.3	29.8–32.8
4–12 days		
Under 1500 gm	33.5	33.0–34.0
1501–2500 gm	32.1	31.0–33.2
Over 2500 gm (and >36 weeks)†		
4–5 days	31.0	29.5–32.6
5–6 days	30.9	29.4–32.3
6–8 days	30.6	29.0–32.2
8–10 days	30.3	29.0–31.8
10–12 days	30.1	29.0–31.4
12–14 days		
Under 1500 gm	33.5	32.6–34.0
1501–2500 gm	32.1	31.0–33.2
Over 2500 gm (and >36 weeks)†	29.8	29.0–30.8
2–3 weeks		
Under 1500 gm	33.1	32.2–34.0
1501–2500 gm	31.7	30.5–33.0
3–4 weeks		
Under 1500 gm	32.6	31.6–33.6
1501–2500 gm	31.4	30.0–32.7
4–5 weeks		
Under 1500 gm	32.0	31.2–33.0
1501–2500 gm	30.9	29.5–32.2
5–6 weeks		
Under 1500 gm	31.4	30.6–32.3
1501–2500 gm	30.4	29.0–31.8

*Adapted from Scopes and Ahmed: *Archives of Diseases of Children* 47:417, 1966. *In* Klaus and Fanaroff: *Care of the High-Risk Neonate.* 2nd Edition. W. B. Saunders Co., 1979, p. 102. Scopes had the walls of the incubator 1 to 2° warmer than the ambient air temperatures.

Generally speaking, the smaller infants in each weight group will require a temperature in the higher portion of the temperature range. Within each time range, the younger the infant, the higher the temperature required.

†Gestational age.

Table 23–5. HEAT LOSS IN NEWBORNS*

Type of Heat Loss	Mechanism	Conditions Contributing to Heat Loss	Nursing Intervention
Conduction	Conduction to surfaces that touch skin	Cool temperature of contact surfaces Thermal conductivity of material of contact surfaces	Avoid placing infant on cold surfaces (e.g., scales, x-ray plates, examining tables); pad with a warm diaper or blanket. Warm hands, equipment before touching baby.
Evaporation	1. Insensible evaporation from skin 2. Evaporation of moisture on skin (e.g., amniotic fluid, bath water) 3. Evaporation from the mucosa of respiratory tract	Insensible evaporation accounts for 25 per cent of heat loss. Increased skin permeability leads to insensible water loss and thus evaporative heat loss. Tachypnea increases rate of heat loss from respiratory tract.	Maintain relative humidity of 50 to 80 per cent. Keep skin dry. Do not bathe baby unless his temperature is stable. Bathe and dry only small area at a time. Warm any soaks or solutions applied to skin; keep warm. Change wet diapers quickly.
Convection	1. Air moving over the skin 2. Warm air expired during respiration 3. Convection of heat to skin surface	Exposure to currents of air, including oxygen that has not been warmed and humidified Thermal sensors on face and forehead are sensitive to cold even when rest of body is warm.	Avoid currents of air moving across skin. Warm and humidify oxygen. When infant must leave nursery (e.g., for surgery), transport in prewarmed incubator.
Radiation	Transfer from infant's skin to surrounding environment	Difference between skin temperature and environment (e.g., walls of single-walled incubator) Total radiating surface of infant—the smaller the infant the greater the surface area in relation to weight and thus the greater his loss. Large surface area of infant's head exacerbates loss.	Room temperature should be no more than 7°C. below environmental temperature. Raise incubator air temperature to 36°C. Clothe infant when possible. Keep infant's bed away from outside walls and out of drafts. Use a heat shield in incubator. Swaddle infant. Put cap or bonnet on baby, (nearly doubles insulating effect of infant's own tissues).

*Modified from Moore: *Newborn, Family and Nurse,* 2nd Edition. Philadelphia, W. B. Saunders Co., 1981.

open bed, he is more easily accessible for care. Moreover, care does not interfere with thermoregulation, as it may in an incubator. Each time the "portholes" of the incubator are opened, environmental temperature within the incubator drops to some extent. If the baby requires prolonged attention (the starting of intravenous fluids, for example), he can become hypothermic.

Another advantage of an open bed with radiant heat is the removal of a barrier between the baby and his parents. The importance of early touching of the baby by his parents is widely recognized (Chapter 28). Yet many parents are hesitant to reach inside the "box" (incubator). They seem less reluctant to hold the baby's hand or to stroke him in an open bed.

There are also disadvantages to care in an open bed. One involves infection control. There is sometimes a tendency to touch the baby without the proper preliminary handwashing,

particularly for personnel who are not working in the nursery continuously. This can be overcome with proper teaching.

A second and more difficult problem involves the recognition of those times when the baby is unable to maintain his temperature. Temperature instability is often an early sign of sepsis. In an incubator with a servomechanism, the baby's temperature may remain the same, but the fluctuation in incubator temperature will indicate temperature variability. The incubator temperature should be recorded each and every time that the baby's own temperature is charted in order to assess this temperature variability.

It is sometimes difficult to keep a very small (1000 grams or less) infant warm in an open bed. An *incubator* uses the principle of convection to provide heat—currents of warm air surround the infant. Most incubators currently available are single-walled. Room temperature affects incubator wall temperature; if the in-

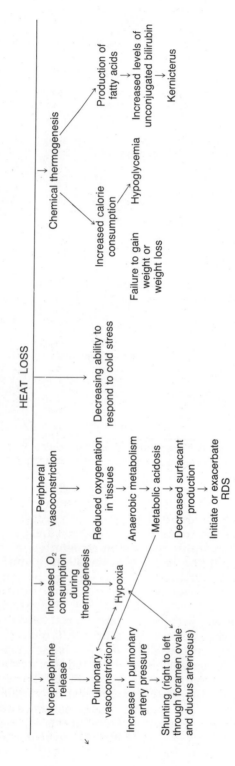

Figure 23–4. The cold stress cycle. (From Moore: *Newborn, Family and Nurse.* 2nd Edition. Philadelphia, W. B. Saunders Co., 1981.)

cubator wall is cool, the baby will suffer radiant heat loss. A plastic shield can be placed between the baby and the wall of the incubator to conserve heat. The baby will then radiate heat to the wall of the shield, which is the same temperature as the air within the incubator, rather than to the cooler wall of the incubator. One or two oxygen hoods placed over the baby can serve as a shield. Very tiny infants who have great difficulty maintaining temperature may be put on a K-pad covered with a blanket placed within the oxygen hood within the incubator.

Incubators continue to be satisfactory for many less critically ill infants. Many babies "graduate" from open beds with radiant warmers to incubators, and subsequently to open beds without radiant heat. When the baby can maintain a temperature of 97.6°F. (36.4°C.) in an 87.0°F. (30.5°C.) environment, he is ready for an open bed. If parents initially become acquainted with their baby in an open bed, the incubator may seem less of a barrier. However, we will need to both observe and talk with parents about their feelings throughout the course of their baby's hospitalization (Chapter 28).

Cold Stress. Cold stress is a danger to all newborn infants; preterm infants are particularly susceptible. A change of as little as 2°C. (3.6°F.) from a thermoneutral environment can produce profound changes in an infant. Increased production of norepinephrine along with peripheral vasoconstriction leads to the cycle shown in Figure 23–4 and ultimately to brain damage from hypoxia or death if intervention does not occur. Most of the steps in Figure 23–4 are easy to follow. Chemical thermogenesis refers to the metabolism of brown fat which, as already noted, requires oxygen.

Cold stress may occur at any time. Infants are particularly at risk during transport from one site to another within an institution or from one institution to another. Clinical signs that an infant is experiencing cold stress are summarized in Nursing Care Plan 23–3. Many of these signs are nonspecific in that they may result from problems other than cold stress. Bright red skin color can be due to the effect of low temperature on oxyhemoglobin dissociation (i.e., oxygen remains bound to hemoglobin). *Sclerema* is a hardening of the skin that can be seen in babies with sepsis and those who are moribund as well as in infants with cold stress.

It is far better to prevent cold stress than to have to treat it. Once the baby is cold, warming should occur slowly. Klaus and Fanaroff[29] suggest that the air temperature should be about 1.5°C. (2.5°F.) warmer than the abdominal skin temperature, because oxygen consumption is minimal at this temperature gradient. A rapid increase in body temperature may produce apnea.[46] During the rewarming period careful attention must be given to correcting the other problems associated with cold stress such as metabolic acidosis (due to the metabolism of brown fat) and hypoglycemia (due to the increased utilization of glycogen). Axillary temperature should be checked every 15 minutes during the rewarming period, and the environmental temperature should be adjusted accordingly until the skin temperature reaches 36.5°C. (97.8°F.).

Hyperthermia. When an infant's skin temperature exceeds 36.5°C. (97.8°F.), metabolic activity and thus oxygen and glucose consumption increase just as they do when he is cold. High environmental temperature is a major cause of hyperthermia. When either the incubator or the radiant warmer is controlled manually, hyperthermia can result. The use of phototherapy lights or extra lighting for certain procedures, or sun shining on an incubator, may produce overheating if a servomechanism is not utilized. If the servosensor probe is not taped securely to the skin or if it becomes detached, the warming unit may continue to produce heat.

Other causes of hyperthermia include dehydration and problems in central nervous system functioning resulting from injury or drugs. Infection, or sepsis, may cause hyperthermia. Changes in body temperature resulting from infection are much more variable in infants than in older children and adults.

Respiratory Distress Syndrome

The most common of all respiratory tract problems in newborns in the United States and throughout the world is *respiratory distress syndrome* (RDS), also called hyaline membrane disease (HMD). RDS occurs in approximately 0.5 to 1.0 per cent of all deliveries and in approximately 10 per cent of all preterm deliveries. In a hospital delivering 400 infants a month, from two to four infants each month could be expected to have respiratory distress. The incidence will be higher in major medical centers to which large numbers of high risk mothers are referred in premature labor. RDS is not the only respiratory disease in newborn infants, but it is the most common cause of respiratory difficulty in preterm infants. RDS generally begins within 6 to 8 hours after birth.

Pathophysiology of Respiratory Distress Syndrome

During fetal life the lungs develop more slowly than many other organ systems. The alveoli, the tiny air sacs at the terminal end of the respiratory system through which oxygen and carbon dioxide are exchanged, are not developed until 26 to 28 weeks of age. Alveolar capillaries, necessary for gas exchange between the alveolus and blood, develop at 28 weeks.

Lining the alveoli, as mentioned earlier, are type I and type II cells. In the type II cells a fatty "soaplike" substance called *surfactant* (actually a name given collectively to several compounds) is produced. Surfactant compounds enable the alveoli to remain open during exhalation, when the amount of air pressure in the lungs is decreased. Lecithin is the most abundant of these compounds, accounting for 50 to 70 per cent of surfactant. Lecithin production begins about the twenty-second to twenty-fourth week of gestation. (The monitoring of lecithin and another compound, sphingomyelin, in the fetus was described in Chapter 14.)

In RDS the production of surfactant is impaired. When the baby exhales, alveoli collapse. Each breath the baby takes must again open the alveoli, just as the first breath taken at delivery opened them. Such an effort increases the work of breathing tremendously. Moreover, there is little or no gas exchange in the collapsed alveoli. The pO_2 drops because the baby's bloodstream is unable to pick up the oxygen it needs from the collapsed alveoli. The pCO_2 begins to rise because of inadequate gas exchange in the alveoli, resulting in respiratory acidosis. As the cells of the body become hypoxic and change to anaerobic metabolism, lactic acid is produced, resulting in metabolic acidosis. The baby uses all of his accessory breathing muscles in an attempt to move air into collapsed, atelectatic alveoli. The pulmonary blood vessels respond to the lowered oxygen tension in the atelectatic alveoli by shunting blood to better oxygenated areas, resulting in local hypoperfusion. This is called an *uneven ventilation-perfusion ratio*—i.e., alveolar ventilation and alveolar blood flow are unbalanced.

Acidosis further compromises ventilation by constricting the pulmonary blood vessels, decreasing the blood supply to the lungs and leading to changes within the alveoli (Fig. 23–5). The fibrin formed within the alveoli is the hyaline membrane, one name used in describing RDS.

The baby recovers when surfactant is produced by type II cells, frequently after the third day. The goal of care is to sustain the baby during the first days by interfering with the cycle shown in Figure 23–5.

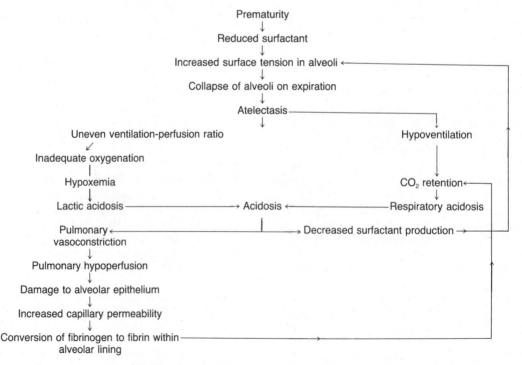

Figure 23–5.   Pathophysiology of respiratory distress syndrome.

Symptoms

The onset of RDS may occur in the delivery room or at any time within the first 6 to 8 hours following birth. Every nurse who cares for newborn infants should be thoroughly familiar with the symptoms of RDS. The principal symptoms are:

Grunting.

Retractions.

Nasal flaring.

Increased respiratory rate.

Cyanosis.

An *audible grunt* results from nature's attempt to keep alveoli from collapsing. The glottis closes to prolong expiration and thus to allow a better diffusion of the inspired oxygen across the alveolar membrane.

Marked *retractions* (intercostal, suprasternal, substernal, and sternal) demonstrate intense respiratory effort, necessary because of the collapsed alveoli.

Respiratory rates above 60 respirations per minute result from the baby's attempt to move air more rapidly through the lungs. When grunting, retracting, and tachypnea are unsuccessful in providing adequate ventilation, cyanosis and acidosis result.

Chest x-rays of babies with RDS show a characteristic "ground glass" appearance, the white areas representing collapsed, nonfunctioning alveoli.

Care

The care of a baby with RDS is basically aimed at *respiratory support* until the baby is able to produce lecithin at a rate sufficient to prevent alveolar collapse. Such care includes provision of a thermoneutral environment, maintenance of adequate respiration, initiation of alkali therapy to combat acidosis, and provision of fluids and nutrition. The baby must be closely observed and carefully cared for by nurses throughout this critical period. Nor must we forget his parents, who often feel shut out of the highly specialized world of the intensive care nursery, worried, and very much alone (see Nursing Care Plan 23–4).

We emphasize that it is difficult to care for these babies properly in a small community hospital. Their care involves skilled nursing care around the clock, 24-hour x-ray facilities, 24-hour laboratory facilities that permit close monitoring of blood gases, and specialized respiratory equipment that is usually available only in medical centers. Babies with RDS should be transferred to such a center when early signs of difficulty appear; waiting to see

if they will improve on their own may cost an infant his life or leave him severely impaired. Prompt recognition of early symptoms by nurses can be the critical difference between a healthy life and mortality or neurologic damage.

Oxygen is essential. Although neither oxygen nor any form of assisted ventilation is a cure for RDS, treatment may enable the baby to survive until he is able to begin surfactant production on his own. The amount of oxygen given to the baby (the FiO_2 or fraction of inspired oxygen) is dependent upon the arterial oxygen concentration (pO_2) of the baby. If the pO_2 is greater than 90 to 100, there is a risk of retrolental fibroplasia and/or pulmonary oxygen toxicity (see below). At pO_2 levels of less than 50, pulmonary blood vessels constrict, further hindering gas exchange in the alveoli. Brain damage may occur at pO_2 levels below 40. The level of FiO_2 necessary to maintain pO_2 levels between 50 and 90 will vary not only from baby to baby but from hour to hour within the same baby. Oxygen therapy is a risky proposition in hospitals that cannot monitor oxygen levels in the blood, preferably through an umbilical artery catheter. (Even using the umbilical artery, we are not measuring the oxygen at the level of the lungs; researchers are constantly trying to find more precise methods that are practical as well.)

Oxygen given to a baby (or to any patient) must be delivered in combination with humidity and with warmth. *Humidity* is necessary to prevent oxygen from drying out the respiratory mucosa. This leads to mucosal crusting, which impedes the normal function of the respiratory cilia and not only makes suctioning the baby difficult but increases the chance of airway obstruction. Moreover, the crusted mucus affords a medium for bacterial growth.

The need for humidity is one reason that heat is so important. Warm air holds more moisture than cold air. In order to give warm, moist oxygen to the baby, the gas must be heated to 101 or 102°F. (38.3 or 38.3°C.) at the oxygen source. Cooling occurs in the tubing carrying the oxygen to the baby, and, as a consequence, condensation occurs and water is seen in the tubing. Cold gas robs the body of water, in addition to being an additional source of chilling.

Currently the most common means of delivering oxygen to babies with respiratory distress are the head hood, continuous positive airway pressure (CPAP), and mechanical ventilation with end expiratory pressure.

Oxygen by Hood. If the baby's need is simply to breathe air with a higher concentra-

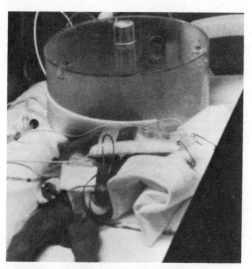

Figure 23–6. A baby receiving oxygen via hood. Note the condensation within the hood caused by the warm, moist oxygen. The opening of the hood around the baby's neck is partially covered to help maintain oxygen concentration. (From Moore: *Newborn, Family and Nurse.* 2nd Edition. Philadelphia, W. B. Saunders Co., 1981.)

tion of oxygen, FiO_2 levels of from 80 to 90 per cent can be achieved with a head hood (Fig. 23–6). The hood does not correct carbon dioxide levels, nor does it assist ventilation in any way. Oxygen concentrations in the hood should be checked and charted every 30 minutes, blood gases should be checked and charted frequently as well. Temperature within the hood should also be monitored every 30 minutes; the area can become quite warm. Constant observations of the baby's respiratory effort are essential. The symptoms described above as the initial symptoms of RDS are those with which we are particularly concerned.

Continuous Positive Airway Pressure (CPAP). Remembering that the basic problem in RDS is the tendency of the alveoli to collapse on expiration, it is logical that some form of therapy that prevents this collapse would be of value. This is the principle of CPAP. Positive pressure on both inspiration and expiration prevents alveolar collapse and enables oxygen to diffuse into the bloodstream. CPAP has no effect on the elimination of carbon dioxide. If pCO_2 levels are high (as determined by blood gas measurement), periodic bag and mask ventilation may be ordered to eliminate excess carbon dioxide.

CPAP may be administered through nasal prongs, or the baby may be intubated (Fig. 23–7). In either case the baby continues to breathe for himself. His respirations are less labored, however, because he is not working against collapsed alveoli.

CPAP is ordered both in terms of pressure

(usually from 1 to 10 mm. Hg) and of FiO_2. As already noted, the baby's respiratory effectiveness is closely monitored by determining blood gas values. If nasal CPAP is used, the prongs must be adjusted so that they do not lie on the baby's lip; the tender skin beneath can easily necrose. A cortisone ointment may be ordered for the nostrils to prevent inflammation. This is a routine order in some hospitals. As in an older patient receiving oxygen, mouth care with lemon and glycerin is helpful. A newborn's secretions are acid and should be wiped from his cheeks and neck.

Babies on both CPAP and on ventilators (see below) should be turned and suctioned every 1 to 2 hours.

Mechanical Ventilation with End Expiratory Pressure. If the baby is unable to breathe for himself, if PaO_2 is less than 50 when FiO_2 is 100 per cent, or if respiratory acidosis is severe, a mechanical ventilator may assist him (Fig. 23–8). Unlike the two modalities discussed above, mechanical ventilation controls levels of carbon dioxide as well as of oxygen. Ventilators may be pressure-cycled, volume-cycled, or time-cycled (Table 23–6). A time-cycled ventilator is frequently used in the care of newborns. Most mechanical ventilators used with newborn infants have settings for four possible breathing patterns: assist, assist-control, control, and intermittent mandatory ventilation (IMV) (see Table 23–6).

The infant who is assisted by a ventilator has an endotracheal tube that is either oral (most frequent) or nasal. Caring for this infant requires nursing skill and continual attention; if the baby is acutely ill a nurse for each baby or one nurse for every two babies is required.

Nursing care for infants on ventilators is summarized in Nursing Care Plan 23–4. Changes in management are based on blood gases, the nurse's clinical observations, and, in some instances, on transcutaneous oxygen (tc pO_2). Clinical evidence that the baby is doing well includes improved color (pink mucous membranes as well as skin), improved muscle tone, and heart rate and rhythm within normal limits (absence of either tachycardia or bradycardia). When the endotracheal tube is properly placed, breath sounds are bilateral and chest movement is symmetrical. If breath sounds are heard more clearly on one side, the endotracheal tube may be in a main stem bronchus, or a pneumothorax may have occurred. If breath sounds are heard over the stomach, the tube may be in the esophagus. Abdominal distention may also indicate esophageal placement, but abdominal distention may also occur when the endotracheal tube is

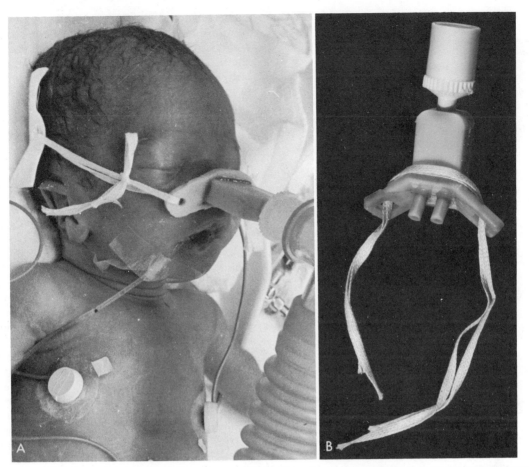

Figure 23–7. Nasal prongs for the administration of CPAP. (From Klaus and Fanaroff: *Care of the High-Risk Neonate.* 2nd Edition. Philadelphia, W. B. Saunders Co., 1979.)

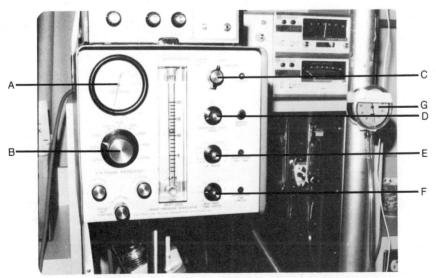

Figure 23–8. Infant ventilator. *A,* Gauge for inspiratory pressure. *B,* Dial to select O_2 concentration. *C,* Dial to select modality (CPAP, IMV). *D,* Dial to select respiratory rate. *E,* Dial to select inspiratory:expiratory ratio. *F,* Dial to select maximum inspiratory time. *G,* Pressure gauge attached to anesthesia bag (separate from ventilator) used to oxygenate baby prior to and following suction and at other times when manual ventilation may be necessary.

Table 23–6. TERMS RELATED
TO RESPIRATORY CARE

Pressure-cycled ventilator
    Delivers air until a preset pressure is
    reached; volume and time vary.
Time-cycled ventilator
    Delivers air for a preset time interval; vol-
    ume and pressure vary.
Volume-cycled ventilator
    Delivers a preset volume of air during inspi-
    ration; pressure and time vary.
Assisted ventilation
    Ventilation in which the mechanical venti-
    lator responds to the baby's respiratory ef-
    forts; the baby initiates each breath.
Assist/control ventilation
    Ventilation in which the machine assists
    spontaneous breathing but controls breath-
    ing during apnea. A ventilation machine
    with this capability is called a *guarantor.*
Controlled ventilation
    Ventilation that is entirely under the con-
    trol of a mechanical ventilator.
IMV
    Intermittent mandatory ventilation. Respi-
    rator delivers predetermined number of
    breaths per minute; baby breathes sponta-
    neously between machine breaths. Used in
    weaning baby to spontaneous breathing.
CPAP
    Continuous positive airway pressure. Main-
    tains set level of pressure in respiratory tree
    at end of exhalation to prevent alveolar col-
    lapse.
PEEP
    Positive end expiratory pressure. Maintains
    set level of pressure in respiratory tree at
    end of exhalation to prevent alveolar col-
    lapse.
FiO₂
    Fraction of inspired oxygen; the percentage
    of oxygen given to the baby. An FiO_2 of 40
    means the baby is receiving 40 per cent
    oxygen.

in the trachea. An indwelling gastric tube is frequently placed when the baby has an endotracheal tube in order to remove air from the stomach.

Mucus must be suctioned from the endotracheal tube; the frequency of suctioning varies with the amount of mucus. Careful sterile technique, including a sterile glove on the hand that holds the catheter, is essential. Preoxygenation of the baby for approximately 2 minutes with a bag and oxygen at the same FiO_2 the baby is receiving (or a slightly higher concentration) will prevent a rapid drop in pO_2 during the procedure. Sterile saline (0.2 ml.) may be placed in the tube prior to suctioning to help liquefy secretions. A sterile suction catheter should be used and replaced after each suctioning. Suction should be applied only when the catheter is withdrawn. The catheter should be inserted quickly (remember that the baby has no oxygen while the suction catheter is in the tube) and withdrawn quickly with a slight rotation. The entire process from entry to withdrawal should take no more than 5 to 10 seconds; after 15 seconds apnea and bradycardia may begin. The transcutaneous oxygen monitor is helpful during suctioning because tc pO_2 can be assessed continually (see below).

Curran and Kachoyeanos[6] have questioned the value of suctioning in relation to the apparent stress to the baby. Although their study raises some important issues that deserve further nursing research, three points must be made about their procedure: (1) they performed suctioning of the nasopharynx, which would be highly stressful to anyone; (2) the infants were not oxygenated prior to or following the procedure; and (3) no evaluation of blood gas levels was reported prior to or following the procedure. In addition, their sample included only six infants; there were no control infants.

Chest Physiotherapy. Both *position change* and *chest percussion* are aids in preventing the accumulation of secretions. Although several methods of chest physiotherapy (CPT) are utilized (a hand, a padded nipple, an electric toothbrush with a nipple attached), the electric toothbrush is a gentle method and seems more appropriate for preterm infants who are easily fatigued (Fig. 23–9). Curran and Kachoyeanos found that color, breath sounds, and pO_2 and pCO_2 (24-hour means) were higher in babies receiving CPT by electric toothbrush, but their small sample size makes it impossible to draw any conclusions. Meier[41] suggests that CPT is appropriate for infants with atelectasis, such as infants with RDS, but not for infants who have respiratory symptoms for other reasons (e.g., apnea of prematurity or heart failure). Infants may, of course, have RDS in combination with these other problems; radiographs will indicate the presence of atelectasis. The unanswered question is whether CPT, by preventing the accumulation of secretions, will prevent secondary atelectasis. Because the answer to this question is unclear, some nurses limit chest physiotherapy to areas of the chest that have proven atelectasis while others will stimulate the entire chest for 1 to 2 minutes at each site.

Meier also suggested that positioning the infant for postural drainage for 1 minute in each of the positions used for CPT (Fig. 23–10), without using CPT, is effective in aeration. Research to confirm this theory is needed.

Text continued on page 733

Nursing Care Plan 23–4.   Infants with Respiratory Distress

NURSING GOALS: To maintain exchange of oxygen and carbon dioxide in infants with respiratory distress.
To assist parents in understanding problems associated with respiratory distress and the reasons for the care given to their infant.
To assist parents in coping with their distress over their infant's illness.

OBJECTIVES:
1. During and following care, the infant will show evidence of adequate exchange of oxygen and carbon dioxide by
   a. Pink color of skin and mucous membranes
   b. Improved muscle tone
   c. Heart rate and rhythm within normal limits (120–160 beats per minute)
   d. Bilateral breath sounds
   e. Symmetrical chest movement
   f. PaO_2: 50–70 mm. Hg
      $PaCO_2$: 35–45 mm. Hg
      pH: greater than 7.2
2. Complications such as pneumothorax will be resolved.
3. Following the discontinuance of oxygen, infant's eyes will be examined for evidence of retrolental fibroplasia.
4. The parents will demonstrate:
   a. An understanding of the problems associated with respiratory distress and the reasons for the care given their infant by their behavior, comments, and questions.
   h. Evidence of coping with their distress over their infant's illness by their behavior, comments, questions.

ASSESSMENT	POTENTIAL NURSING DIAGNOSIS	NURSING INTERVENTION	COMMENTS/RATIONALE
1. Infant in a thermoneutral environment	Cold stress resulting from environment that is not thermoneutral	Provide thermoneutral environment. Warm and humidify oxygen.	Oxygen needs are minimized in a thermoneutral environment.
		Infant	
2. Respiration a. Rate b. Pattern c. Breath sounds (bilateral) d. Nasal flaring e. Grunting f. Retractions (describe)		Position infant for optimal respiratory effort: 1. Tilt mattress so head is elevated. 2. Place folded diaper under shoulders to slightly extend neck when infant on his back ("sniffing position"); avoid hyperextension and flexion.	Decrease pressure of abdominal organ on diaphragm. Provides maximum entry of air to respiratory tree and facilitates swallowing of secretions. Flexion is associated with tracheal obstruction. Hyperextension impedes air entry and swallowing; diminishes work of respiration; increases PaO_2;
Use apnea monitor as adjunct in above assessments.	Possible episodes of apnea followed by bradycardia (A's and B's)	3. Place infant on abdomen frequently. 4. Change infant's position approximately every 2 hours. 5. Provide chest physical therapy. 6. Plan care to avoid fatigue of infant.	Promote drainage of secretions with change of position and chest physical therapy.

Continued on following page

Nursing Care Plan 23–4. Infants with Respiratory Distress (Continued)

Assessment	Problem	Intervention	Rationale
3. Color (of mucous membranes as well as skin) a. Cyanosis (circumoral, acrocyanosis, general) b. Plethora c. Pallor d. Relationship of color change to activity			
4. Behavior a. Active with good muscle tone b. Lethargic with poor muscle tone			
5. Secretions (amount, character)		Suction secretions as necessary; provide humidity to prevent thickening, drying of secretions.	
6. X-ray findings a. "Ground-glass" appearance b. Areas of atelectasis			
7. Blood gas changes and acid-base balance a. $PaCO_2$ b. PaO_2 c. $NaHCO_3$ d. pH	Potential for acidosis or alkalosis	Intervene with oxygen therapy to correct imbalances (see text).	
8. Heart rate Use cardiac monitor as adjunct	Potential for tachycardia or bradycardia due to (specific reason).		Periods of apnea followed by bradycardia
9. Abdominal distention	Gastrointestinal dysfunction NEC	Insert gastric tube to compress stomach.	Distended abdomen may compromise respirations.
10. Signs of pneumothorax: restlessness, cyanosis, tachypnea, bradycardia, diminished breath sounds	Pneumothorax resulting from intensive respiratory therapy	Notify physician; transilluminate chest. Pneumothorax confirmed by x-ray; possible needle aspiration prior to chest tube insertion. (Care of infant with chest tube described below.)	
11. Eye assessment for evidence of retrolental fibroplasia (RLF)	Need for follow-up examination	Explain need for eye examination to parents; provide appropriate referral for eye examination in hospital and following discharge.	Infants less than 36 weeks gestation or less than 2000 grams at particular risk; eye examinations should occur prior to discharge and 4–6 weeks following discharge.

Parents

Assessment	Needs	Intervention	Rationale

1. Understanding of infant's problem
2. Understanding of care given infant
3. Grief reactions
  a. Denial
  b. Anger
  c. Guilt
4. Family support
5. Coping strategies
	Need for information about respiratory distress
	Need for information about procedures and protocols
		Provide information about nature of infant's problem and reason for care. Provide hope of recovery, if possible, to facilitate attachment; provide opportunities for expression of anger, guilt, etc.; provide appropriate information in response to guilt. Support coping strategies; provide privacy to allow crying, and expression of grief; facilitate group and family support.	There will be grief for the loss of the "fantasized" child as well as for the illness per se.

Modifications When Oxygen Is Administered Via Hood

Assessment		Intervention	Rationale
Assess oxygen administration in terms of: FiO_2 (frequency) Blood gases or tc pO_2 (see below) Oxygen warm and humidified Infant's condition as described above.		Measure, record FiO_2 frequently. Never use oxygen that is not humidified and warmed.	Dry oxygen causes drying of mucous membranes, accumulation of thick secretions.

Modifications When Oxygen Is Administered Via CPAP

Assessment		Intervention	Rationale
Assess oxygen administration in terms of: FiO_2 Type CPAP (nasal, endotracheal) Blood gases or tc pO_2 Oxygen warm and humidified Pressure from endotracheal tube or nasal prongs; possible skin breakdown. Signs of occluded endotracheal tube or extubation (color change, absence of breath sounds or chest movement, apnea, bradycardia, poor muscle tone)		Measure, record FiO_2 at frequent intervals. Record manometer pressure at frequent intervals. Adjust tube to prevent pressure. Provide mouth care (lemon-glycerine swabs). Orient nasal prongs properly. Suction endotracheal tube as necessary. An occluded tube must be removed and a new tube reinserted; if extubated, support with bag and mask ventilation until new tube can be inserted.	Equipment may become unattached
Assess condensation of water in tubing		Empty whenever water collects in tubing.	Water in tubing decreases diameter of tube, increases resistance and pressure in system, and decreases tidal volume.
Infant's condition as described above			

Continued on following page

Nursing Care Plan 23–4.   Infants with Respiratory Distress   *(Continued)*

Modifications When Oxygen Is Administered Via Mechanical Ventilator

Assessment	Intervention
Assess oxygen administration in terms of: F_iO_2	Ensure proper setting; record F_1O_2, rate, pressures, setting in infant's record at frequent intervals.
Ventilator rate	
Ventilator setting (IMV, assist/control, controlled)	
Peak pressure; end respiratory pressure	
Alarm on	Ensure that alarm is on in systems with alarm.
Condensed water in tubing (see CPAP above)	Suction endotracheal tube as necessary. See CPAP (above).
For signs of occluded tube or extubation, see CPAP, above.	Adjust tube to prevent pressure.
Pressure from endotracheal tube	
Sterility of all respiratory equipment	Change sterile tubing and attachments every 24 hours. Use only sterile distilled water in the system; perform all procedures, including intubation and suction, under sterile conditions.
Infant's condition as described above	

Modification Related to Measurement of Blood Gas or tc O_2

Assessment	Intervention
Assess capillary blood gas by performing heel stick.	*Obtaining sample:* Warm heel prior to sampling to increase arterial blood in sample.
Assess blood gases using umbilical artery catheter. Assess infant for:	
1. Blanching of leg (cold, white, no pulse, or mottled, pale, and dusky)	1. When blanching occurs, wrap opposite leg in warm diaper; if color does not return quickly, physician is notified; catheter is removed
2. Hemorrhage (artery or vein)	

Not sufficiently accurate for the care of acutely ill infant

Transcutaneous oxygen (tc O$_2$) monitor:
1. Temperature of electrode
2. Reddened area of skin beneath electrode
3. Effect of intervention on tc O$_2$ (note relation of activity to decreased tc O$_2$ on monitor strip)

Reddened area of skin related to use of tc O$_2$ electrode

2. When hemorrhage occurs from a. *artery:* grasp skin surrounding uambilicus; from b. *vein:* exert downward pressure on abdomen above umbilicus.

Explain use of tc monitor to parents.
Reposition electrode at least every 4 hours to prevent skin burn.
Record presence of reddened skin.
Modify nursing care when intervention causes decreased tc O$_2$ (e.g., plan care to provide longer periods of rest; decrease environment stimuli.)

Electrode temperature:
1. Too low—pO$_2$ has been underestimated
2. Too high—potential for burns

Modifications When Infant Has One or More Chest Tubes Attached to a Water-Seal Drainage System

1. Drainage
   a. Drainage receptacle lower than chest.
   b. No dependent loops or kinks in drainage tube.
   c. Fluid flows with no blood clots.
   d. Color and amount of drainage assessed and recorded.
   e. Drainage fluctuates in tube during respiration until lung re-expands.
2. Continuity of system: system must not be open at any point.
   a. Intermittent bubbling in water-seal bottle suggests air is being removed from pleural space during expiration.
   b. Continuous bubbling (during inspiration and expiration) may indicate air leak. Check catheter site and all connections.
   c. Rapid bubbling may indicate air loss.
   d. Record amount of bubbling to assess change in pattern.

At risk of inadequate respiration related to improperly functioning pleural drainage

Take particular care to maintain position of tube and receptacle when infant is moved.
Drainage tube "milked" (gently compressed toward drainage receptacle) to remove air, clots.
Place tape on drainage receptacle at drainage level.

Ensure that "rubber-shod" clamps are available at infant's bed to clamp tubing if break occurs in system.
Be sure that all connections are taped.

"Milking" chest tube:
Hold tube in one hand to stabilize; gently slide other hand down tubing away from patient.
When lung has re-expanded, fluctuation in tube stops; re-expanded lung blocks catheter openings.
System must be airtight to ensure negative pressure in pleural space. Remember that air cannot escape when tube is clamped; continuity of system must be restored quickly or air in chest may reaccumulate.

Continued on following page

Nursing Care Plan 23–4. Infants with Respiratory Distress *(Continued)*

3. Assess for potential infection.	At risk of infection related to presence of chest tube	Observe strict asepsis when changing any part of system. Use only sterile water in system.

4. Inspect site of entry of catheter into chest.
  a. Catheter should not be loose.
  b. Assess for reddened area, sign of infection.
  c. Assess for drainage around site.		

5. Check water pressure in system and maintain at desired level.		Ensure proper water pressure.	10 cm. of water is approximately the normal intrapleural pressure during inspiration.
			One-bottle water-seal system operates by gravity with no pressure; other systems (two-bottle, three-bottle, Pleur-vac) provide suction related to depth of suction control tube in water, height of column of water, or attachment to mechanical suction.
6. Assess parents' understanding of need for chest tubes.	Need for information about need for chest tubes.	Provide information: answer questions. Encourage touch and caring for baby; ensure that chest tube is secure and reassure parents that they will not harm baby by their touch.

7. Note time when lung is being re-expanded.
  a. Fluctuation in catheter stopped
  b. Drainage minimal or absent
		Anticipate removal of tube. Have petroleum gauze available to cover insertion site, prevent air entry (not always used).	Chest tube is usually removed within 24 hours after lung re-expansion if drainage is minimal.

8. Following removal of chest tube
  a. Assess for reaccumulation of air in pleural space, signs of respiratory distress (above).
  b. Assess catheter site for air leakage.
	At risk for reaccumulation of air or air leakage following removal of chest catheter.	Notify physician if signs of respiratory distress recur; may need to reinsert tube. Anticipate need for emergency needle aspiration (see text).	

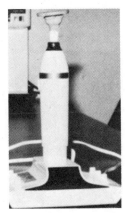

Figure 23–9. An electric toothbrush adapted with a nipple for chest physiotherapy. (From Moore: *Newborn, Family and Nurse,* 2nd Edition. Philadelphia, W. B. Saunders Co., 1981.)

The following steps are used in chest physiotherapy.

1. Perform before feeding or at least 45 minutes after feeding.

2. Observe baby carefully during physiotherapy for signs of fatigue or color change.

3. Position baby and percuss chest over each lobe using padded nipple or electric toothbrush (Fig. 23–10).

4. Suction mucus as it accumulates from mouth, nose, or endotracheal tube.

Muscle Paralysis for Infants on Ventilators. Some infants, especially larger infants, appear to "fight" mechanical ventilation yet are unable to breathe adequately without assistance. Pancuronium bromide (Pavulon) or curare may be used to paralyze muscles, allowing improved oxygenation and gas exchange. Curare relaxes not only the pulmonary vascular bed but also the blood vessels in other parts of the body and thus may cause hypotension and may decrease perfusion. Pavulon does not decrease pulmonary vascular resistance and may actually increase resistance. Careful observation of infants receiving these drugs is obviously essential.

Assessing the Adequacy of Ventilation. If ventilation is adequate, PaO_2 will be between 50 and 90, $PaCO_2$ will be between 35 and 45, and pH will be 7.2 or greater.

OXYGEN. If the pO_2 is greater than 90 to 100, there is a risk of retrolental fibroplasia or pulmonary oxygen toxicity (see below). At pO_2 levels of less than 50, pulmonary blood vessels constrict, further hindering gas exchange in the alveoli. Brain damage may occur at pO_2 levels below 40. The level of FiO_2 (fraction of inspired oxygen) necessary to maintain pO_2 levels between 50 and 90 will vary not only from baby to baby but from hour to hour in the same baby.

Adequate oxygenation in an infant may be assessed by (1) observing the color of the trunk, face, and mucous membranes of the mouth, (2) determining the pO_2 in blood samples, or (3) monitoring pO_2 continuously by catheter or transcutaneous monitor.

Color is the least valuable means of assessment and should be relied on only for short periods (e.g., during transport) when other means of assessment may not be available. Oxygen is provided at a level that just prevents visible cyanosis of the mucous membranes of the mouth. Cyanosis of the extremities is not a useful guide in newborns because acrocyanosis is not unusual in otherwise healthy infants.

Blood may be obtained from an umbilical arter catheter, the right radial artery, or a heel capillary that has been sufficiently warmed to "arterialize" the specimen (i.e., wrapping the baby's foot in a warm diaper for 5 minutes to increase blood flow). The right radial artery rather than the left is chosen because blood circulates there before reaching the ductus arteriosus; a right-to-left shunt of blood through the ductus arteriosus will affect the pO_2 in the left radial artery but not in the right. PaO_2 in the right radial artery is essentially the same as PaO_2 in the carotid arteries supplying the brain.

When the right radial artery is used for intermittent assessment, pressure is applied to prevent bleeding for 5 minutes or until the bleeding stops (whichever is longer) after withdrawing the needle. An indwelling radial artery catheter may be inserted in the right radial artery for frequent determinations; this is most commonly done when it is difficult or impossible to perform umbilical artery catheterization.

Capillary blood is of limited value in assessing oxygenation in sick newborns; it is impossible to assess the extent to which this blood is arterialized. Lower values of pO_2 are usually accepted when capillary blood is used (35 to 45 mm. Hg), but since it is not really certain what is being measured, this is potentially dangerous. Levels of pH and $PaCO_2$ should not vary in capillary and arterial blood. The amount of blood withdrawn for blood gas determinations should be recorded, and the record should be frequently assessed. In a small baby it is possible to compromise blood volume significantly by withdrawing blood frequently for specimens.

A third means of assessment that is finding increasing use in intensive care nurseries is

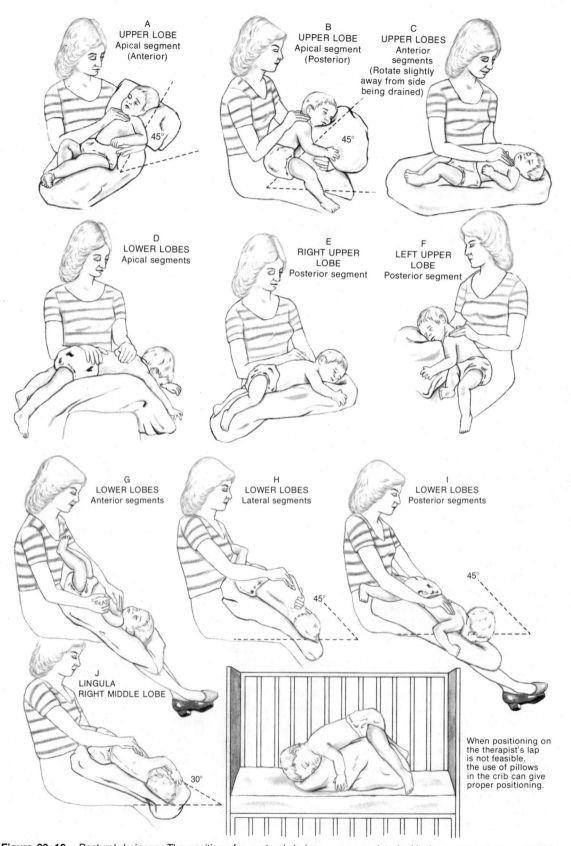

Figure 23–10. Postural drainage. The positions for postural drainage are correlated with the segment being drained. In positions *H* and *J* the child is shown on his right side; however, he must also be turned to his left side to drain both lobes. (Adapted from materials used by the Chest Physical Therapy Department, Physical Therapy Division, Department of Physical Medicine and Rehabilitation, Hospital of the University of Michigan, Ann Arbor, MI. From Tackett and Hunsberger: *Family Centered Care of Children and Adolescents: Nursing Concepts in Child Health,* 1981.)

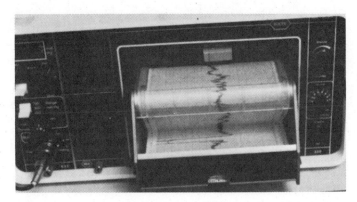

Figure 23–11. A transcutaneous monitor. Note the fluctuation in tc pO_2. (From Moore: *Newborn, Family and Nurse.* 2nd Edition. Philadelphia, W. B. Saunders Co., 1981.)

continuous measurement of oxygenation, either by intravascular oxygen electrode or by transcutaneous oxygen monitor. The transcutaneous oxygen monitor is most widely used.

Transcutaneous oxygen (tc pO_2) is oxygen that has diffused from the arterial capillaries near the surface of the skin to the skin surface. Because preterm infants have so little fatty and subcutaneous tissue, tc pO_2 measurements and arterial oxygen measurements (pO_2) have been found to correlate well.[40a] The advantage of transcutaneous monitoring is its ability to monitor oxygenation continuously in a noninvasive manner. This is particularly helpful to nurses when they care for infants with respiratory problems. The effects of position change, suctioning, chest bag ventilation, physical therapy, and many other aspects of care can be quickly assessed and care modified for the needs of each baby (Fig. 23–11).

One valuable insight that has come from the use of transcutaneous monitoring is that there is continual variation in oxygenation as measured by tc pO_2, although these changes are usually within the range of 50 to 90 mm. Hg. When the administration of nursing care causes a marked change (increase or decrease) in tc pO_2 on the printout, writing the reason for the change on the strip aids in the overall assessment of the infant's condition. When a baby has diminished peripheral blood flow because of severe hypotension, tc pO_2 is believed to correlate less closely with pO_2.

Since the electrode attached to the baby's skin is heated (Fig. 23–12), the proper temperature of the electrode is very important. If the temperature is too low, pO_2 may be underestimated; if the temperature is too high, the baby's thin skin may be burned. As further protection against burns, the electrode is repositioned every 4 hours. Even with frequent repositioning, a reddened area may appear beneath the electrode, but it will usually disappear within a few hours. This information needs to be shared with parents.

Assessment of tc pO_2 obviously is an adjunct to blood sampling, since pCO_2 and pH are not measured. However, the transcutaneous monitoring of pCO_2 is now being evaluated.

CARBON DIOXIDE ($PaCO_2$) AND ACID-BASE STATUS (pH). Carbon dioxide and pH are assessed from blood gases (from samples taken from the radial artery, umbilical artery, or capillary). The baby with RDS frequently retains carbon dioxide, leading to respiratory acidosis. Depending on the type of ventilation being used, a variety of techniques may help the baby eliminate excess carbon dioxide. Bag and mask or bag and endotracheal tube ventilation is most frequently used. Changes in ventilator pressures, volume, rate, and the ratio of inspiration to expiration time may also be considered.

Weaning from Mechanical Ventilation. It is not particularly difficult to initiate mechanical ventilation for a baby. It is often far more difficult to wean a baby from the ventilator. Historically, infants have died because they could not be weaned from respiratory assistance.

Weaning involves reduction in end expiratory pressure and in oxygen concentration. Sometimes these are decreased simultaneously; sometimes first one and then the other

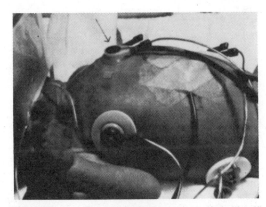

Figure 23–12. The transcutaneous electrode is identified by the arrow. Note the erythematous area lateral to the electrode where the electrode was previously placed. (From Moore: *Newborn, Family and Nurse.* 2nd Edition. Philadelphia, W. B. Saunders Co., 1981.)

is lowered. The weaning is monitored by blood gas determinations; oxygen and/or pressure is reduced, and values are checked within 30 minutes to see if the baby is able to tolerate the lower levels. Careful nursing observations to check for retractions and cyanosis are equally important.

Endotracheal tubes should not be left in place once the baby is "disconnected" from mechanical ventilation. A baby can no more breathe through an endotracheal tube without assistance than we can breathe through a straw. The resistance of the tube makes adequate air exchange impossible.

Another consideration during weaning is the way in which oxygen concentration is decreased. A very rapid drop will cause reflex constriction of the pulmonary arteries with a subsequent decrease in blood flow to the lungs, cyanosis, and other signs of respiratory distress. This behavior is sometimes termed the "flip-flop phenomenon."

Weaning usually involves a transition first from assisted ventilation to CPAP and then to the head hood.

Hazards of Oxygen Therapy

The two chief hazards of oxygen therapy, as noted previously, are retrolental fibroplasia and pulmonary oxygen toxicity (bronchopulmonary dysplasia). Overdistention and rupture of the alveoli can occur when oxygen is given under pressure (CPAP or mechanical ventilation).

Retrolental Fibroplasia. Prior to 1940 *retrolental fibroplasia* was virtually unknown. By 1950 it had become the greatest single cause of blindness in children in the United States, greater than all of the other causes combined. The fact that almost all of the cases occurred in the better-equipped medical centers while the condition was virtually unknown in small towns and rural areas was a

mystery until 1953, when it was shown that high oxygen concentrations were to blame. The large centers with the newest equipment were able to deliver oxygen much more efficiently.

As oxygen was monitored more closely, the incidence of retrolental fibroplasia dropped. There is concern that there may be a resurgence of the condition if arterial oxygen is not closely monitored, as we save more and more infants of earlier gestational age by the use of high concentrations of oxygen.

The basis of retrolental fibroplasia lies in the development of the blood supply of the retina. Until the fourth month of gestation no retinal vessels are present; vascularization of the retina is not complete until after the eighth month. A baby born at 30 weeks of gestation, for example, has no blood vessels in much of his retina (Fig. 23–13). It is the incompletely vascularized retina that is susceptible to oxygen damage. Once the vessels are completely developed, they are not damaged by oxygen.

Since newborn puppies and kittens also have incomplete retrolental vascularization, it is relatively easy to demonstrate the sequence of events when oxygen is given. The initial effect is the immediate and almost total constriction of retinal vessels. This can happen within 5 minutes after oxygen is given at concentrations of 70 to 80 per cent. It has been suggested that a careful examination of the fundus is one means of determining the level of oxygen concentration to be used; the finding of vasoconstriction indicates an immediate need to lower oxygen concentration. This is rarely done, however.

After about 10 minutes of sustained oxygen, arterioles and capillaries reopen and remain dilated for the next several hours. New blood vessels appear in the retina. Leakage of fluid and blood from these newly formed vessels and invasion by fibroblasts eventually lead to retinal detachment in the weeks that follow.

A second or cicatricial stage, during which

GESTATIONAL AGE OF FETUS

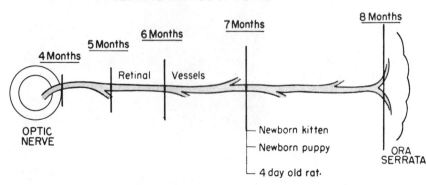

Figure 23–13. Schematic drawing showing the chronology of the development of the blood supply of the retina in the human fetus. (From Patz: *Pediatrics,* *19*:508, 1957.)

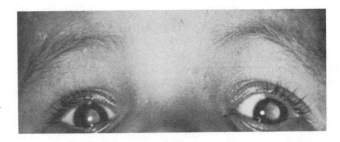

Figure 23–14. Terminal stage of retrolental fibroplasia. The child is totally blind. (From Patz: *Pediatrics,* *19*:508, 1957.)

the retrolental membrane is formed, occurs several weeks later. The extent of the damage done in the second stage depends upon the severity of the acute stage and is related to:

1. The concentration of oxygen.
2. The length of time during which oxygen is administered.
3. The degree of immaturity of the eye.

There is no cure for a fully developed case of retrolental fibroplasia (Fig. 23–14).

It is believed that by keeping pO_2 levels within the supposedly safe limits of 50 to 90 mm. Hg the danger of retrolental fibroplasia will be minimal. The danger cannot be totally eliminated, because for some babies there appears to be a danger at any oxygen level above that of room air. Long periods of oxygen therapy (3 to 10 days), even at 25 to 40 per cent oxygen, can result in retrolental fibroplasia. It is important to recognize that arterial oxygen levels in the baby can suddenly change without a change in oxygen concentration if the baby's ability to ventilate improves.

The American Academy of Pediatrics recommends the following for oxygen therapy in newborns:

1. When infants of less than 36 weeks of gestational age require supplemental oxygen, the concentration of inspired oxygen should be regulated by measuring arterial oxygen tension. If this is not possible, oxygen should be given only in a concentration sufficient to abolish cyanosis. The baby should then be moved to a hospital in which arterial blood oxygen tension can be measured.

2. Oxygen is maintained below 80 to 90 torr and usually between 50 and 70 torr.

3. The ideal sampling sites for arterial oxygen tension studies are the radial or temporal arteries. In most circumstances, however, a sample from the aorta through an indwelling umbilical arterial catheter is satisfactory.

4. Equipment for the regulation of oxygen concentration (as provided by some incubators and respirators) and devices for mixing oxygen and room air may not function properly. Therefore, when an infant is placed in an oxygen-enriched environment, the concentration of

oxygen must be measured with an oxygen analyzer at least every hour. The performance of the oxygen analyzer must be checked every 8 hours by calibration with room air and 100 per cent oxygen. Air-oxygen mixer settings should be noted every hour and calibrated every 8 hours.

5. Except in an emergency, oxygen and compressed air should be warmed and humidified before administration.

6. A person experienced in recognizing retrolental fibroplasia should examine the eyes of all infants born at less than 36 weeks' gestation or weighing less than 2000 grams (4.2 pounds) who have received oxygen therapy. This examination should be made at the time oxygen is discontinued, before the baby is discharged from the nursery and again 4 to 6 weeks after discharge.

Bronchopulmonary Dysplasia. This disorder is a second condition that may occur in newborns exposed to high concentrations of oxygen. It has been recognized even more recently than retrolental fibroplasia, being first described by Northway and associates[42a] in 1967.

Bronchopulmonary dysplasia is related to:

1. The concentration of oxygen.
2. The amount of pressure in the oxygen delivery system.
3. The length of time during which oxygen is given.
4. The presence of an endotracheal tube that disrupts normal ciliary function in the respiratory tract.

If oxygen levels above 70 per cent are given for longer than 4 to 5 days, severe pulmonary disease may result. Concentrations of 100 per cent oxygen for 36 hours can lead to pulmonary changes. The principal changes occur in the alveolar epithelium and in the endothelium of the blood vessels around the alveoli. As a result, there is progressive thickening of the blood–air barrier. In some babies these changes appear to reverse themselves over a period of 2 to 3 months. Other babies do not recover and eventually die.

Infants with bronchopulmonary dysplasia

may require oxygen therapy for a number of weeks and very slow weaning. Not only does the baby need special care, but his family will need a great deal of support to keep them from becoming discouraged.

Complications Due to the Oxygen Delivery System. When the pressure in the respiratory tract is increased, as it is when CPAP and mechanical ventilators are used, the alveoli may become overdistended and rupture, and air may escape from the respiratory tract into the surrounding tissues. If air escapes into the connective tissue adjacent to the lungs, the condition is called *pulmonary interstitial emphysema;* air may then travel to the mediastinum *(pneumomediastinum)*. Further extension of air may result in air in the pleural space *(pneumothorax)*, in the pericardial sac surrounding the heart *(pneumopericardium)*, in subcutaneous tissue *(subcutaneous emphysema)*, or in the peritoneum *(pneumoperitoneum)*.[43]

Air outside of the lungs can impede the return of venous blood to the heart, thereby decreasing cardiac output and decreasing the ability of the lung to expand.

Nurses caring for infants most frequently encounter pneumothorax. Pneumothorax may occur spontaneously in normal infants as well as in infants receiving ventilatory assistance. It is estimated that in approximately 7 per cent of all babies some degree of pneumothorax is present, but it is not always symptomatic.

The cause of pneumothorax, as noted above, is rupture of the alveoli from pressures that are too high, with escape of air into the pleural space. As more and more air escapes, breathing becomes more and more difficult. Nurses caring for babies with respiratory distress need to be alert for signs of possible pneumothorax, which often appear as *sudden* respiratory distress (cyanosis, grunting, tachypnea, restlessness, bradycardia, and a general worsening of appearance). Listening through a stethoscope for air exchange on both sides of the chest should be routine when pulse and respiration are checked.

Kuhns and associates have described the use of a high intensity transilluminating light to detect pneumothorax and pneumomediastinum.[34] After the overhead lights in the nursery are turned out, a high intensity transilluminating light is placed against the baby's chest, first in an area superior to the nipple and then inferior to the nipple on both sides.

If an area around the sternum appears translucent, or if either side of the chest transilluminates more than the other, several other spots at varying distances from the sternum on either side are transilluminated.[34]

It would seem very useful for nurses to become familiar with this rapid, noninvasive means of observation. Figure 23–15 compares the transilluminated chest of a baby with a massive pneumothorax with radiographs of the same baby's chest. The diagnosis of pneumothorax is confirmed by radiography.

Needle aspiration of air and/or placement of a chest tube is the treatment for pneumothorax. Transillumination is also being used to guide needle and tube placement.

In an emergency, needle aspiration is accomplished by attaching a syringe with a three-way stopcock to a 19- to 23-gauge scalp vein needle (Fig. 23–16). The needle is pointed toward the baby's feet and inserted into the second, third, or fourth intercostal space in the anterior axillary line (over the top of the rib), avoiding the nipple. Air is withdrawn from the pleural space and then expelled from the syringe via the stopcock. Withdrawal of air should continue until resistance occurs.

When a chest tube is inserted it is attached to underwater drainage. The precautions that are necessary with any person with a chest tube are applicable. Drainage from the chest tube is assessed and recorded, and the continuity of whatever system is used is maintained. Clamps are kept available at the baby's bedside so that the chest tube can be clamped immediately if a leak occurs in the system.

Apnea of Prematurity

In addition to RDS, preterm infants are at high risk for apnea of prematurity. Nearly all infants born at less than 30 weeks' gestation and many who are less than 32 weeks' gestation will have periods of apnea that last for more than 20 seconds and are associated with bradycardia, color change, and decreased muscle tone. Apnea may be distinguished from *periodic breathing* in that periodic breathing is cyclic (regular breathing periods of 10 to 15 seconds alternate with apneic periods of 10 to 15 seconds) and the other changes (bradycardia, color change, decreased muscle tone) are not present.

Immaturity of the respiratory centers in the central nervous system is believed to be the major reason for apnea of prematurity. Contributing factors include hypoxia, environmental temperatures outside the thermoneutral range, metabolic imbalance, sepsis, drug-related depression, and others (Table 23–7). Hypoxia and hypoxemia may occur in preterm infants because of airway congestion, poor po-

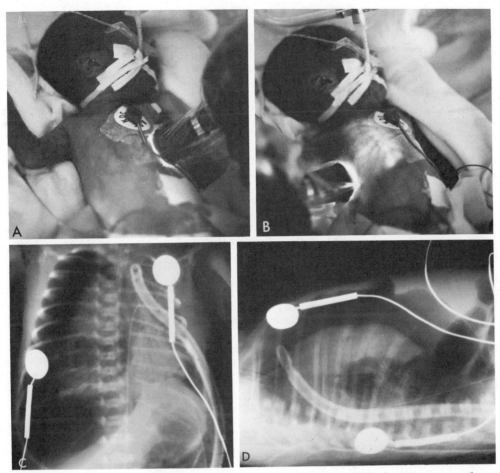

Figure 23–15. Transillumination to detect pneumothorax. *A,* Corona of light around the thorax; no pneumothorax indicated. *B,* Entire thoracic cage transilluminates; suggests large pneumothorax. *C* and *D,* Chest x-ray showing massive right pneumothorax. (From Kuhns: *Pediatrics, 56*:355, 1975.)

sitioning, or fatigue in a baby with RDS. When respiratory centers are depressed by hypoxia they are unable to respond to decreased pH or elevated $PaCO_2$. Position seems to be important in the reduction of apneic episodes. When the baby is supine a rolled diaper beneath the shoulders aids in maintaining the slight hy-

perextension that facilitates respiration. Respiration was improved in the prone position compared with the supine position in two studies.[25, 40]

The effect of environmental temperature on oxygen requirements has been noted above. Even a slight decrease in environmental tem-

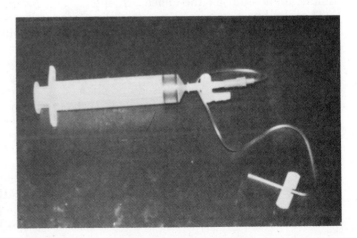

Figure 23–16. A syringe, a stopcock, and a scalp vein needle can be used to aspirate air from a pneumothorax. (From Moore: *Newborn, Family and Nurse.* 2nd Edition. Philadelphia, W. B. Saunders Co., 1981.)

Table 23–7. ASSESSMENT AND INTERVENTION IN FACTORS RELATED TO APNEA†

Factor	Assessment	Intervention
Immaturity of central nervous system	Continuous monitoring of respiratory and cardiac rates	Tactile stimulation
	Evaluation of other possible causes of apnea	Based on identified cause
		Assisted ventilation
Variation in thermoneutral environment	Frequent assessment of axillary temperature	Use of servomechanism to maintain thermoneutral environment (36.5° C [97.6° F] temperature in baby)
Hypoxia	Continuous assessment of oxygen levels: transcutaneous and/or arterial	Positioning for maximum oxygenation
	Evaluation of causes of hypoxia: airway congestion, poor positioning, tiring from respiratory efforts, patent ductus arteriosus (PDA)	Correction of underlying causes: suction
		Assisted ventilation
		Medical or surgical closure of PDA
Hypoglycemia	Dextrostix to quickly assess blood sugar level	Administration of glucose
Hypocalcemia	Assessment of serum calcium levels	Administration of calcium
Anemia	Record blood withdrawal for laboratory evaluation	Replacement of blood
	Assessment of hemoglobin and hematocrit	
Sepsis	Apnea may be early symptom of sepsis; assess other parameters	Treatment of sepsis, including supportive treatment and antibiotics
Central nervous system drug depression	Note drugs given to mother in labor	

*From Moore: *Newborn, Family and Nurse.* 2nd Edition. Philadelphia, W. B. Saunders Co.

perature can lead to apnea, as can a sudden increase in environmental temperature. Metabolic changes probably cause apnea because of their effect on the respiratory centers of the brain. Treating the underlying cause will usually result in a decrease in episodes of apnea.

Infants who might be expected to develop apnea of prematurity (including all infants under 1800 grams) should have continuous cardiac and respiratory monitoring. When apnea occurs, careful assessment of accompanying behavior is important. Does bradycardia accompany the apnea? Is there a color change? Is there a change in muscle tone? Are factors that could account for the apnea present?

Theophylline has been shown to reduce the incidence of apnea, probably because of an effect on the respiratory center in the brain. A loading dose of 5 ml. per kg. is followed by a maintenance dose of 1 to 2 ml. per kg. every 4 to 8 hours. Heart rate is assessed and charted immediately before each dose is given; tachycardia may be an early sign of theophylline toxicity. In some nurseries the dose is withheld if heart rate exceeds 180 beats per minute.

Nursing intervention during an apneic episode includes prompt tactile stimulation (rubbing the infant's back, for example). If the infant does not respond quickly, bag and mask ventilation with a low concentration of oxygen

(no greater than 30 to 40 per cent) may be necessary. When a baby continues to have constant apnea, a careful evaluation of all possible causes is essential.

Umbilical Vessel Catheterization

Catheterization of an umbilical blood vessel is an important adjunct to the care of an infant with respiratory distress. Catheterization of the *umbilical vein* for the emergency administration of drugs was described in the discussion of resuscitation earlier in this chapter. The umbilical vein catheter is inserted *just below the level of the skin,* and is removed once the baby is stabilized. The only other use of an umbilical vein catheter is in exchange transfusion in infants with hyperbilirubinemia. Umbilical vein catheters are considered more dangerous to the baby than umbilical artery catheters because the catheter tip may lodge in the portal vein, causing serious liver damage as well as other complications.

Umbilical artery catheterization, which allows frequent blood sampling as well as the administration of fluids, is a procedure that was developed in the early 1960's. An umbilical catheter can minimize the number of times a sick baby must be handled during the first week, which is decidedly to his advantage.

After the cord and surrounding area are washed with an antiseptic solution, a catheter is inserted using sterile technique into one of the umbilical arteries and fixed in place with a silk thread. The tip of the catheter should be in the abdominal aorta at the level of the diaphragm. The position of the catheter is confirmed by x-ray and the cord sutured in place. Gauze dressings are not used over umbilical artery catheters because they could delay the recognition of catheter displacement, hemorrhage, or infection.

Babies with umbilical catheters should be continuously observed for leg blanching. This could be due to arterial thrombosis that can occur shortly after the catheter is inserted or to a clot or air bubble in the leg vessels when the catheter is in place, or after the removal of the catheter. The baby's leg may appear cold and white with no pulse, or it may be mottled, pale, and dusky. Usually the catheter is removed immediately when blanching is noted. Occasionally, removal is delayed briefly if the color change is minimal; the opposite leg is wrapped in a warm diaper to see if color returns quickly to the affected leg.

Hemorrhage from an umbilical vessel is another danger in the use of umbilical catheters. Hemorrhage can result in a large amount of blood loss very quickly. Hemorrhage from the artery occurs in spurts. Downward pressure on the umbilicus is not sufficient to stop the bleeding because the arteries curve down toward the spine; the skin surrounding the umbilicus must be grasped and pinched for at least 5 minutes. Bleeding from the vein is steady. Because the vein travels toward the baby's head, pressing on the baby's abdomen above the umbilicus will control umbilical vein bleeding.[27]

Umbilical arterial catheters are removed if there is blanching of the leg or foot, as mentioned above, or as soon as supplemental oxygen is discontinued.

Problems with Acid-Base Balance. The major reason for umbilical artery catheterization is to facilitate blood gas assessment. Oxygen assessment has already been discussed. Equally important is the assessment of acid-base balance (see Table 23–8).

Emergency treatment of acidosis has been described earlier in the discussion of resuscitation. At all other times evaluation of pH and pCO_2 with the subsequent calculation of the level of bicarbonate (HCO_3) form the basis of assessment of acid-base status. Blood is obtained from an umbilical artery catheter or a radial artery catheter (or occasionally from a heel capillary).

The infant should be quiet and should have received a constant oxygen concentration for at least 10 minutes prior to the drawing of the blood specimen. If the baby has been crying or if the oxygen concentration has varied (e.g., if the hood or nasal prongs have been removed to weigh the baby), arterial gases will not correctly reflect the baby's response to the prescribed concentration of oxygen. When the blood sample is withdrawn from an indwelling line (umbilical or arterial), the blood withdrawn to clear the line must be replaced because of the infant's low blood volume. For the same reason, a careful record must be kept of blood withdrawn for specimens. Transfusion may be necessary if large amounts of blood are withdrawn for laboratory examination.

Table 23–8. ACID-BASE BALANCE IN NEWBORNS

	Common Causes	Blood Gas	Intervention
Acidosis			
Respiratory	Retention of carbon dioxide due to hypoventilation	CO_2 up pH down HCO_3 normal	Ventilation (bag and mask, mechanical)
Metabolic	Lactic acid production secondary to anaerobic metabolism Metabolic acidosis of prematurity Diarrhea Circulatory failure	CO_2 normal pH down HCO_3 down	Correction of cause Bicarbonate therapy
Alkalosis			
Respiratory	Hyperventilation (usually iatrogenic)	CO_2 down pH up HCO_3 normal	Correct cause
Metabolic	Excessive dose of $NaHCO_3$, diuretics Inadequate renal excretion, $NaHCO_3$, or excess excretion of H^+ Gastric suction, vomiting	CO_2 normal pH up HCO_3 up	Correct cause Correct fluid and electrolyte balance

Acidosis

When the pH falls below 7.3, the baby is considered acidotic. A mild acidosis (7.2) is not uncommon immediately following birth, even in newborns who are healthy, but this acidosis is generally resolved within the first 30 to 60 minutes of life as carbon dioxide levels drop to normal limits.

When the infant becomes acidotic, pulmo-

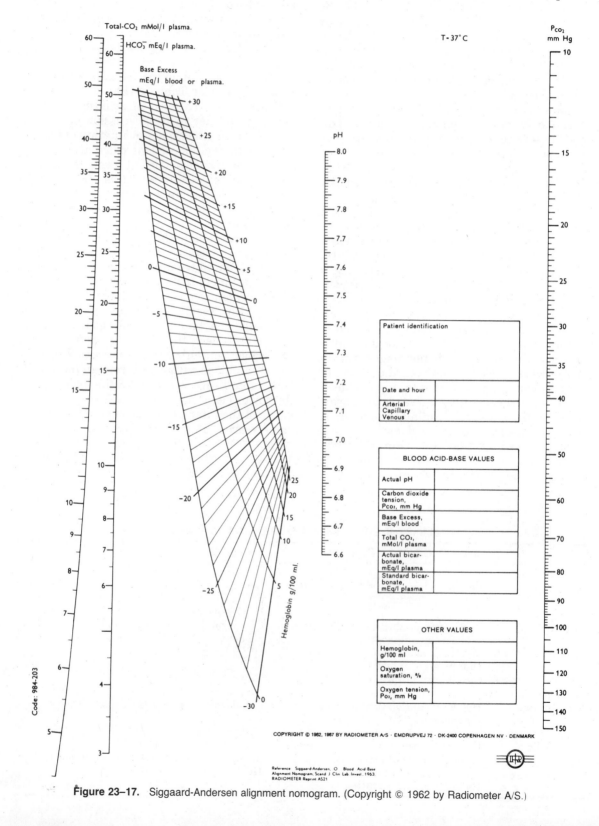

Figure 23–17.   Siggaard-Andersen alignment nomogram. (Copyright © 1962 by Radiometer A/S.)

nary vascular resistance increases, thereby decreasing the flow of blood to the lungs and subsequently leading to further increases in carbon dioxide levels. Acidosis also compromises myocardial contractility and adversely affects cell metabolism.

Respiratory Acidosis. As previously noted, infants with respiratory distress have difficulty not only in receiving enough oxygen but in getting rid of carbon dioxide, resulting in *respiratory acidosis*. Unlike the adult or older child who usually responds to respiratory acidosis by increasing acid excretion through the kidneys, the immature kidney of the preterm infant has a marked incapacity to excrete acid. Thus, preterm infants do not develop compensatory metabolic alkalosis.

Normal levels of pCO_2 in newborns are between 30 and 40 mm. Hg; a pCO_2 level of over 45 mm. Hg is considered an indication of respiratory acidosis. Acidosis that is purely respiratory in origin requires respiratory treatment; if carbon dioxide increase is mild, bag and mask ventilation may correct a transient problem. If the problem is more severe or persistent, assisted ventilation (CPAP or ventilator) may be necessary.

Metabolic Acidosis. When the baby is unable to inspire adequate oxygen to meet his metabolic needs, anaerobic metabolism results, with the subsequent production of lactic acid. In metabolic acidosis, HCO_3 is decreased. The HCO_3 level is not directly measured but is calculated from values that are directly measured. Bicarbonate levels in adults who are in acid-base balance are approximately 24 mEq. per liter. However, newborns are less able to conserve bicarbonate than adults; bicarbonate levels may be somewhat lower (20 to 21 mEq. per liter in term infants and as low as 18 to 20 mEq. per liter in preterm infants).

For practical purposes, the base deficit is calculated. One method utilizes a Siggard-Anderson nomogram (Fig. 23–17) in the following manner. After the pH and pCO_2 are determined, connect the two values with a straight line. Find the point at which this line intersects with hemoglobin concentration. The base deficit (negative number) or base excess (positive number) is read at this point. If the base deficit is 6 or more and the pH is less than 7.3, metabolic acidosis exists. The treatment for metabolic acidosis is the administration of alkali in the form of sodium bicarbonate.

Hemoglobin is important in the calculation because tissue perfusion is compromised when hemoglobin is low. If pCO_2 is 60 and pH is 7.0, base deficit is 14 with a hemoglobin of 10, but base deficit is 20 with a hemoglobin of 20. The lower hemoglobin value indicates inadequate perfusion, which is corrected by administration of blood products.

The formula for calculating the dose of bicarbonate was presented earlier in the discussion of resuscitation (see page 701). Any formula is, of course, only a rule of thumb; careful evaluation of the baby's behavior and appearance is also essential.

In administering sodium bicarbonate, several guidelines are important.

1. Dilute the prepared dose with equal parts of water for injection to lower the osmolarity. Sodium bicarbonate solutions are hypertonic; rapid injection of hypertonic solutions causes water to move into the plasma from the extravascular space, increasing plasma volume, venous pressure, and cerebrospinal fluid pressure. These pressures can lead to intracranial hemorrhage and resultant neurologic deficit or death.

2. Infuse the solution slowly (1 mEq. per minute) to avoid tissue damage as well as changes in osmolarity.

3. Be aware of the total dose given; under all but the most unusual circumstances the 24-hour dose should not exceed 8 mEq. per kg. Again, the concern is osmolarity.

4. Ventilate the baby if he is not breathing well by bag and mask or other means of assisted ventilation, so that the carbon dioxide that results from the dehydration of sodium bicarbonate will be eliminated. Otherwise pCO_2 will rise, pO_2 will fall, and the net result will be a worsening rather than an improvement in the infant's condition.

Mixed Metabolic and Respiratory Acidosis. When acidosis is purely respiratory, the HCO_3 will be normal and the carbon dioxide increased. The reverse is true for metabolic acidosis; HCO_2 is decreased and carbon dioxide is normal. Both respiratory and metabolic acidosis can exist concurrently. Both alkali therapy and excellent ventilation will be required to restore pH to normal limits. Reevaluation of blood gases approximately 5 minutes after treatment will serve as a guide to further treatment.

Alkalosis

Alkalosis is seen far less frequently in newborns than acidosis. Respiratory alkalosis may occur when an infant is hyperventilated by a mechanical ventilator. Carbon dioxide is low because too much is expired. Treatment consists of adjusting the ventilator settings.

Metabolic alkalosis may occur when the body loses acid, for example, in the persistent vomiting that can accompany an obstruction in the gastrointestinal tract such as pyloric

Nursing Care Plan 23–5.   Infants with Problems of Blood Volume and Blood Pressure

NURSING GOALS: Infant blood pressure will be maintained in normotensive range.

OBJECTIVES: As a result of nursing action:
1. Infants at risk of hypotension will be identified.
2. Infant blood pressure will be maintained within a range appropriate for infant's size.

ASSESSMENT	POTENTIAL NURSING DIAGNOSIS	NURSING INTERVENTION	COMMENTS/RATIONALE

1. Identify infants at risk of hypotension.
a. Decreased blood volume
  (1) Preterm infants
  (2) Bleeding (intrauterine, intrapartum, postpartum)
b. Drugs given to mother
  (1) Antihypertensive drugs
  (2) Adrenergic blocking drugs
c. Alterations in infant's health status (RDS, acidosis, sepsis, CNS insults, decreased cardiac output)
	At risk of hypotension	Frequent blood pressure assessment in infants at risk	

2. Hypotension in relation to infant birth weight 3000 grams: systolic <55 mm. Hg 2000 grams: systolic <50 mm. Hg 1000 grams: systolic <40 mm. Hg	Hypotension related to 1. Decreased blood volume 2. Specific maternal factors 3. Specific alterations in infant's health	1. Plasma expander is given per physician or standing order (blood, frozen plasma, Plasmanate, albumin, normal saline): 10–20 ml. per kg. body weight at the rate of 4–5 ml. per minute 2. Follow treatment of protocols for underlying cause (e.g., sepsis)	
3. Hematocrit (normal range: 45–65 per cent) High: >70 Low: <35	Alteration in hematocrit	If hematocrit is high: replace fluid loss with albumin. If hematocrit is low: replace blood loss.	High hematocrit and edema or large cephalhematoma may indicate plasma shift to extravascular space. Low hematocrit may indicate anemia.
4. Record amount of blood withdrawn for lab tests.	Decreased blood volume related to iatrogenic blood loss	Anticipate need for blood replacement.	Frequent blood testing significantly depletes blood volume.

stenosis. Usually the alkalosis per se is not treated; measures that inhibit vomiting (NPO) and correct fluid and electrolyte deficits usually restore blood pH.

Problems Related to Blood Volume and Blood Pressure

Both preterm and term infants may have problems arising from diminished blood volume or blood pressure, or both; the problem is particularly serious in preterm infants because total blood volume is initially small, the risk of blood loss is increased, and the risk of other conditions that may compromise blood pressure is also increased. Blood volume in the term newborn averages approximately 85 ml. per kg., with slightly higher values (89 to 105 ml. per kg.) in preterm infants (90 ml. per kg. is equal to 40 ml. per pound). Thus, the total blood volume of a 3000-gram infant will fill little more than an 8-ounce glass, and the blood volume of an infant weighing 1000 grams is approximately 3 ounces.

A loss of 25 per cent of blood volume will result in shock. Thus, for a 1000-gram preterm infant with a total blood volume of 90 ml., a blood loss of as little as 23 ml. will cause shock.

Blood volume may be reduced by prenatal factors (e.g., fetal bleeding or a twin-to-twin transfusion), bleeding during labor or birth (e.g., accidents of the placenta), or hemorrhage after birth. When a baby has a large cephalhematoma or significant edema, as many small preterm infants do, plasma shifts from the intravascular space into the tissues, depleting plasma volume. This condition can be recognized by a hematocrit that is higher than normal (normal is 55 to 65 per cent in term infants; slightly lower in preterm infants).

In addition to low blood volume, several other factors can contribute to hypotension in preterm (and term) infants (see Nursing Care Plan 23–5). Antihypertensive drugs given to the mother, beta-adrenergic blocking agents (given to stop premature labor, Chapter 19), RDS, acidosis, sepsis, central nervous system insults, and diminished cardiac output are major causes. A sick preterm infant may be affected by several of these factors simultaneously.

Blood pressure may be assessed in infants using several techniques; the use of a Doppler ultrasound technique is common. In the Doppler technique the sensor is placed over an artery (most commonly the brachial or the popliteal artery). In small preterm infants, blood pressure is best measured in the leg because of the relation of the size of the cuff to the limb. (In many term infants, the arm is a better choice.) If the infant is crying when the cuff is applied, soothing him before checking the pressure will result in a more accurate reading. Mean blood pressures are summarized in Table 23–9.

Haddock[23] suggests the following general guidelines as criteria for hypotension:

1. A systolic blood pressure of less than 55 mg. Hg in term infants.

2. A systolic blood pressure of less than 50 mm. Hg in preterm infants.

3. A systolic blood pressure of less than 40 mm. Hg in small preterm infants.

Systolic blood pressure below 30 mm. Hg is an indication of shock, no matter how small the infant. If not corrected quickly, hypotension results in:

1. Decreased blood supply to skin and muscles, resulting in both hypoxia and accumulation of metabolic acid waste in these areas, with increased acidosis from anaerobic metabolism.

2. Reduced red blood cell volume and thus reduced oxygen-carrying capacity when hypotension is due to hypovolemia.

3. Increased right-to-left shunting through the ductus arteriosus, further compromising oxygenation (see Patent Ductus Arteriosus, below).

Hypotension is treated by giving intravenous fluids (see below) to expand blood volume. Common solutions include blood, frozen plasma, Plasmanate, 5 per cent albumin, and normal saline. Initial doses are 10 to 20 ml. per kg. of body weight at a rate of 4 to 5 ml. per minute. Blood pressure is assessed every 10 minutes. If blood pressure does not stabilize

Table 23–9. APPROXIMATE BLOOD PRESSURES IN NEWBORN INFANTS

Weight (Grams)	Approximate Blood Pressure (Systolic/Diastolic)
800	46–48/20–22
1000	50/25
2000	60/36
3000	70/35

in an appropriate range, additional doses may be required. (See also Intravenous Fluids, below.)

Intraventricular Hemorrhage

Intraventricular hemorrhage (IVH) occurs in 40 to 60 per cent of small preterm infants, probably because of hypoxia, which damages the walls of fragile blood vessels and also causes congestion in cerebral veins. Hyperosmolar intravenous solutions such as sodium bicarbonate may also be a factor; the data are conflicting. Many of these infants will subsequently develop hydrocephalus (if they survive the initial insult) as the flow of cerebral spinal fluid is obstructed.

A tense fontanel may be the initial sign of IVH. In infants of less than 32 weeks' gestation lack of visual tracking, a diminished popliteal angle, and uncontrollable "roving" eye movements have been associated with IVH. Infants over 32 weeks' gestation are hypotonic and lethargic.[10] In infants with severe hemorrhagic shock, a bulging fontanel and an abrupt fall in hematocrit are the first signs.

The diagnosis is confirmed by a lumbar puncture in which the spinal fluid is bloody. Continued nursing assessment includes daily measurement of head size to detect possible hydrocephalus. Computerized tomography (CT scan) and cranial ultrasound are additional assessment tools. Daily lumbar punctures have been used to reduce intracranial pressure and prevent the deleterious effects of hydrocephalus, although this course of management is not practiced everywhere.[20, 44] A shunting procedure for hydrocephalus may be necessary (Chapter 24).

Cardiac Problems in Preterm Infants

Preterm infants may have any of the congenital heart defects described in Chapter 24. One condition, patent ductus arteriosus (PDA), is particularly common in small preterm infants. As many as 70 per cent of preterm infants weighing less than 1500 grams with RDS and 30 per cent without RDS may have PDA. During fetal life, the ductus arteriosus allows blood to be shunted from the pulmonary artery to the aorta. Normally, it closes functionally at birth (Chapter 20). The ductus arteriosus is more likely to remain open in preterm infants because there is less muscle in the ductus. In addition, preterm infants with respiratory distress frequently have hypoxia and acidosis, which cause the ductus to remain open. Because there is decreased pulmonary vascular resistance in preterm infants and because cardiac output is already high, heart failure may occur rapidly.

A murmur may be present in conjunction with a PDA but it may be intermittent. If the baby is breathing with the aid of a ventilator, it may be necessary to disconnect the apparatus briefly to auscultate heart sounds. A widened pulse pressure is common, as are bounding femoral and posterior pedis pulses.

Indomethacin, a drug that inhibits prostaglandin synthesis, has been used to close the PDA medically.[18, 42] The dosage should not exceed 0.2 mg. per kg. of body weight times three doses. The long-term effects of indomethacin are not known at this time: one potential short-term danger is renal shutdown due to decreased renal blood flow. Therefore, urine output must be carefully measured in infants receiving indomethacin therapy. Because of a change in platelet quality, bleeding may occur. Bleeding and problems of bilirubin metabolism as well as compromised renal function are contraindications to indomethacin.

Indomethacin therapy is most successful during the first 10 days of life and in infants who are not extremely premature. When medical closure is unsuccessful, surgical ligation may be necessary. Some physicians consider surgical ligation the treatment of choice.

If a large amount of blood is shunted through the PDA to the lungs, the baby may develop signs of heart failure toward the end of the first week. These signs are due to the following sequence:

Pulmonary vascular bed dilates
↓
Pulmonary vascular resistance decreases
↓
Blood flow to lungs increases markedly

Early signs of congestive heart failure are a deterioration in the baby's respiratory status, or an inability to wean the baby from respiratory support. Other important signs are tachycardia, tachypnea, hepatomegaly, and cardiomegaly. Digoxin and Lasix are given to infants with congestive heart failure before surgery or indomethacin is tried. Digitalizing doses of digoxin for newborns are 0.05 to 0.07 mg. per kg. of body weight orally or 0.04 to 0.05 mg. per kg. of body weight IM for term infants, and 0.03 mg. per kg. of body weight orally for premature infants. One-half of the total dose is administered immediately, and the remaining half is divided into two doses to be administered in the next 12 to 18 hours. The average maintenance dose of digoxin for newborns is 0.01 mg. per kg. Toxicity to digitalis is revealed by changes in heart rate and rhythm on the electrocardiogram (EKG). Both term and preterm infants tend to be intolerant of digitalis preparations and must be carefully monitored.

Furosemide (Lasix) is the diuretic most commonly used in infants; the dosage is 1 mg. per kg. per day intravenously (2 to 3 mg. per kg. per day orally). Careful records of urine output are kept by weighing diapers (weigh dry and again following voiding). Serum electrolytes must be carefully evaluated when diuretics are used.

Problems Associated with Water and Electrolytes

The basic needs of all infants for water have been discussed in Chapter 22. In healthy term infants this need, as well as the need for glucose and electrolytes, is met by breast or formula feeding. In preterm infants (and in sick infants) these needs must be met through parenteral fluids in the first days of life. Intravenous fluids provide water, electrolytes, and glucose. The intravenous fluid system is used to give medication and also protein and fat solutions (see Nutrition, below).

As noted in Chapter 22, fluid needs for term infants are approximately 150 ml. per kg. per day. Somewhat less fluid is provided in the first 24 hours (approximately 80 to 100 ml. per kg.), and intake is then increased to reach the maximum on the third day. One marked exception is the baby who has been asphyxiated; because of the possibility of kidney damage in such an infant, fluids may be limited to 35 ml. per kg. per day plus urine output.

Fluid loss occurs principally through urine and insensible water loss. During the first 48 hours after birth urine output may be limited to 30 to 60 ml. After the third day of life, output normally amounts to 40 ml. per kg. per 24 hours (1 to 2 ml. per kg. per hour).

Accurate urine output records are important in sick and small preterm infants. Accurate output may be assessed in two ways. A newborn urine bag may be used; the urine is withdrawn from the bag with a syringe and measured. An advantage of this method is the ease of obtaining urine for urinalysis and specific gravity, sugar, and protein checks as well as for measurement. The major disadvantage is the effect of the adhesive material of the urine bag on the skin of some newborns, especially small preterm infants. An alternative is to weigh diapers before they are placed beneath the baby, marking the weight on the diaper (each one will be different), and then weigh them again immediately after the baby voids. A sensitive scale that measures in grams is used, and a nonabsorbent diaper (e.g., a diaper wrapped in plastic wrap) is placed beneath the diaper that is to be weighed. The difference in weight between the dry and wet diaper is recorded as the output. If the baby wets an area other than the weighed diaper, the record will be incorrect, of course. With small preterm infants this is not often a problem because of the small amounts of urine voided at one time. For larger preterm infants who are not severely ill, a check on the number of wet diapers is generally sufficient.

Specific gravity of urine is assessed at each voiding, or every 2 to 4 hours in many preterm infants. A syringe (without a needle attached) can usually be used to aspirate urine from a wet diaper if the diaper is placed on a firm surface. Urine can also be collected in an infant urine bag and aspirated through a feeding tube inserted in the bag if the bag does not have tubing attached. Some small preterm infants cannot tolerate the adhesive of urine collecting bags. Only a few drops of urine are needed to determine specific gravity. The normal range for specific gravity is 1.008 to 1.012 (some accept a range of normal from 1.002 to 1.015). When urine is very dilute (low specific gravity), the baby is getting excess fluid. When urine is very concentrated (high specific gravity), the baby is not getting sufficient fluid.

Insensible water loss is fluid that is excreted through routes other than the urinary tract (e.g., the skin and respiratory tract) In term newborns insensible water loss is approximately 35 ml. per kg. per day.

Insensible water loss is particularly high in the small preterm infant because the skin is more permeable and has a higher water content and the epidermis is thinner than in term infants or older children. Insensible water loss may be increased by as much as 100 per cent in these infants. Moreover, it is the small preterm infant who is more likely to be under a radiant warmer, to be receiving phototherapy, or to have a labile body temperature, all of which contribute to insensible water loss. Phototherapy increases insensible water loss by 40 per cent, while the radiant warmer may account for an additional 100 per cent increase. Other important factors include diarrhea, vomiting, and losses through drainage from gastrostomy, chest, or other drainage tubes.

Weighing the baby is the most common method of determining insensible water loss. Usually it is sufficient to weigh the baby every 12 or 24 hours. Normal weight gain is approximately 30 grams in 24 hours. Inadequate or excessive weight gain may be related to water

Table 23–10.   ELECTROLYTE IMBALANCE: SODIUM, POTASSIUM, CALCIUM

Electrolyte	Range of Normal Values* (mEq. per liter) Preterm	Term	Basis for Imbalance	Factors Influencing Deficit	Factors Influencing Excess	Signs of Deficit	Signs of Excess	Intervention
Sodium (Na)	128–148	134–144	Hypernatremia: water deficit or sodium excess Hyponatremia: water excess or sodium deficit	Preterm infant cannot conserve Na well Furosemide, theophylline contribute to loss Diarrhea; RDS—cerebral anoxia, inappropriate ADH secretion Hypoxia—altered renal function	Heart failure Fluid loss excessive, greater than loss of Na Hypertonic IV solution	Lethargy, muscle weakness, clammy skin, decreased urine specific gravity, CNS disturbance (secondary to cerebral edema)	Irritability, muscle rigidity, dry skin, increased urine specific gravity, CNS disturbance (secondary to cerebral desiccation)	Intake of water and sodium balanced in relation to needs
Potassium (K)	Slightly lower than term infant	5.6–6.4	Hyperkalemia: increased intake, inadequate excretion cause shift from intracellular to extracellular compartment Hypokalemia: inadequate intake, excessive loss cause shift from extracellular to intracellular fluid	Diarrhea, vomiting, nasogastric drainage, IV fluids without added K	Excessive administration of K Renal failure	Lethargy, loss of muscle tone, abdominal distention, hyporeflexia, shallow breathing, tachycardia, cardiac arrhythmia; EKG: flat T wave, prolonged S-T segment	Malaise, muscle weakness, intestinal colic, diarrhea, hyporeflexia, cardiac muscle failure; EKG: T-wave elevation, depressed S-T segment, flat P wave	Hypokalemia: potassium chloride
Calcium (Ca)	7–11	8–11	Hypercalcemia: excessive Ca or vitamin D Hypocalcemia: oxytocin (antidiuretic) given to mother Formula with high ratio of phosphorus to calcium Infants of dibetic mothers; mothers with PIH Administration of citrated blood	Low Ca stores in preterm infant, depressed parathyroid secretion, stress (hypoxic, sepsis, etc.) causes steroid production—hypocalcemia frequently accompanies hypoglycemia in newborns	Usually iatrogenic Hyperparathyroidism (rare in newborns) Diuretics given to mother before birth	Apnea Twitching Jitteriness Seizures	Lack of muscle tone Cardiac arrest	Hypocalcemia: calcium gluconate (see text)

*Values for range of normal vary slightly from one laboratory to another.

balance or to inadequate calories. Changes in urine specific gravity and hematocrit will help to determine if fluid status is a factor. Hematocrit, normally in the range of 45 to 53 per cent, is increased in dehydration.

Electrolytes

As might be expected because of the rapid exchange of water and the ease with which water balance is upset, electrolytes are also exchanged rapidly and electrolyte balance is relatively unstable. Changes in sodium and potassium balance are especially likely to occur. Any loss of fluids and secretions caused by vomiting, diarrhea, or gastric suction also results in the loss of sodium, chloride, and potassium.

Table 23–10 summarizes information about three major electrolytes: sodium, potassium, and calcium. Babies with hypocalcemia may also have *hypomagnesemia* (magnesium level less than 1.2 mg. per 100 ml.); if magnesium is low, hypocalcemia will not respond to calcium treatment. Hypomagnesemia is treated with 50 per cent magnesium sulfate (0.2 ml. per kg. IM every 12 hours).

Hypocalcemia is treated with 10 per cent calcium gluconate; because of the frequency of administration and the serious side effects, nurses must be thoroughly familiar with this drug. The dosage for newborns is 2 ml. per kg. of the 10 per cent solution, mixed with an equal volume of water and given slowly. The maximum dose is 5 ml. in preterm infants and 10 ml. in term infants. The baby should be monitored with a cardiac monitor or by electrocardiogram. Rapid infusion can cause bradycardia. Calcium is given by slow push, mixed with intravenous fluids, or, in a baby who can take oral fluids, it is given orally.

When given intravenously, calcium is never mixed with a solution containing sodium bicarbonate; a salt, calcium carbonate, will form in the solution. Great care should be taken to avoid infiltrating tissues with fluids containing calcium because severe tissue necrosis can result. Calcium given through an umbilical venous catheter may cause liver necrosis; pushing calcium through an umbilical arterial catheter is considered a possible factor in necrotizing enterocolitis.[3]

Potassium needs are estimated at 2 mEq. per kg. per day; in the baby who is NPO these needs are met by adding potassium chloride to intravenous fluids or parenteral nutrition (hyperalimentation) solutions. Sodium is also provided intravenously; sodium needs are 2 to 3 mEq. per kg. per day.

Providing Fluid and Electrolytes

Electrolytes and fluids are commonly provided to preterm infants intravenously in the first days of life; small preterm infants may require intravenous fluids for a number of weeks until they are able to meet all of their needs orally. Protein, fat, and carbohydrates can also be provided intravenously (see below and Nursing Care Plan 23–6).

The type of solution and the total amount to be given, as well as the amount of solution to be given each hour, should be a part of the physician's order. Once the fluids are started, their maintenance at the proper rate becomes a nursing responsibility that involves the monitoring of both baby and intravenous equipment at the minimum of once every hour. If too small an amount of fluid is given, the baby will become increasingly dehydrated, and circulating fluid volume will be decreased. If the proper fluid level is not restored, he will die in a relatively short period of time. On the other hand, too much fluid in too brief a period of time will lead to pulmonary edema and water intoxication, and again, if uncorrected, to death. The margin for error is narrow in a newborn baby.

A first requirement for ensuring accurate intake is an intravenous set designed specifically for pediatric patients. A small amount of fluid can be transferred from the main fluid bottle to the burette—not more than the baby is to receive in a 3-hour period. In this way, even if by some accident the fluid should begin to run at a faster rate than ordered, the baby will be protected against an overwhelming fluid intake. From 5 to 10 ml. of fluid should remain in the burette at all times as a buffer, so that if an emergency does arise and fluid intake cannot be checked exactly on the hour, all of the fluid will not be gone, and the needle will not be clogged with blood.

The amount of fluid the baby receives should be checked and charted each hour. Readings are made at the fluid level at the bottom of the meniscus. The chart should be a type that can be kept at the baby's bedside and quickly checked to see the kind of fluid he is receiving, the amount he has received, and the rate of flow.

The fluid site is one area to be observed in the baby. A scalp vein, an umbilical artery, and veins in the hands and feet are frequent sites for the administration of intravenous fluids in newborns. If it is suspected that the baby will need to receive fluids for a number of days, a "cut-down" to deeper vessels may be done. The site needs to be checked for swelling

Text continued on page 755

Nursing Care Plan 23–6. Care of Infants Who Need Alternate Methods of Feeding

NURSING GOALS: To provide nourishment for the infant who is unable to have breast or bottle feedings.
To meet emotional needs commonly associated with feeding.
To assist parents in learning to feed their infant via alternative routes.

OBJECTIVES:
1. Identify infant who needs alternative feeding route.
2. Explain plan of care to parents.
3. Prevent complications associated with chosen route.
4. Provide psychosocial support normally associated with feeding.
5. Assist parents in feeding via alternative route when appropriate (e.g., infant who is to receive gastrostomy feeding at home).

ASSESSMENT	POTENTIAL NURSING DIAGNOSIS	NURSING INTERVENTION	COMMENTS/RATIONALE
1. Identify infant needing alternative feeding route: a. Less than 34 weeks' gestational age b. Illness (e.g., respiratory distress with assisted ventilation, necrotizing enterocolitis) c. Congenital anomaly of gastrointestinal tract d. Inadequate nutritional intake	At risk for inadequate fluid intake related to (specific reason) At risk for inadequate nutritional intake related to (specific reason) At risk for psychosocial deprivation related to absence of stimulation during breast or bottle feeding	Provide alternative nutrition (see specific routes, below). Provide pacifier during feeding when possible. Provide cuddling, stroking at regular intervals.	Average fluid needs: 150 ml per kg per 24 hours after 24–48 hours. 65–90 ml. per kg. per 24 hours in first 24 hours; 100–125 ml. per kg. in second 24 hours. Average caloric needs: 100–110 calories per kg. in 24 hours. Because child will not be held during feeding, regular stimulation will be necessary.
2. Assess parents' understanding of reason for alternative feeding route.	Parents' need for information (e.g., purpose of alternative feeding, appearance of infant, duration of therapy)	Encourage parents to participate in care by touching, stroking, etc. Provide appropriate information. Encourage and assist parents to hold infant with IV, gastrostomy, etc.	
3. Assess condition of infant's mouth.	Need for oral hygiene	Provide mouth care; glycerine-lemon swabs are effective.	
4. Identify indications of adequate nutrition. a. Daily weight gain of approximately 30 grams b. Weekly measurement of head circumference, progressive head growth c. Urine output and specific gravity (1) Keep strict record of output in critically ill baby by weighing diapers. (2) Check on number of wet diapers in stable		Infant should be weighed on same scale at same time of day without clothes. Note presence of any equipment (arm board, chest tube, etc.) that will affect weight on infant's record.	

Intravenous Feeding

1. Identify appropriate site (scalp, foot, hand, forearm).

   1. Secure or prepare correct solution.
   2. Label the type and amount of any medication added (e.g., potassium chloride, calcium).
   3. Restrain active infant during insertion. Use small padded board for sites other than scalp. Comfort infant following insertion. Protect insertion site (collodian, paper cup, careful taping are useful methods).
   4. Clear lines of air.
   5. Use infusion pump or pediatric IV chamber to avoid accidental fluid overload.
   6. If fluid is absorbed more slowly than ordered, do not attempt "catch-up" owing to risk of fluid overload.
   7. If fluid is blocked, do not attempt to irrigate; clot may be present and may be dislodged.
   8. Label bottle with date and time hung. Intravenous solutions and lines are changed every 24 hours.

2. Each hour during administration:
   a. Assess site and dependent areas for signs of infiltration. Note assymetry of head of scalp vein.

      At risk for tissue damage related to fluid infiltration

      Infiltration is particularly dangerous with total parenteral nutrition and solutions containing medication; skin may slough and skin graft may be required. Infusion pump will continue to push fluid into infiltrated site.

   b. Identify signs of infection (redness, edema) at site.
   c. Record fluid absorbed, rate of flow.

      At risk for underhydration or overhydration

   d. Assess lines for kinks, disconnections, air in line.
   e. Count drops per minute and check "drop" settings on infusion pump.
   f. Assess any restrained extremity for circulation.

3. Total parenteral nutrition (TPN, hyperalimination, intravenous alimentation)

   a. Peripheral administration: Assess intravenous administration as above.

      Refrigerate hyperalimentation solution until ready to use. Infusion pump, filter always used.

      Hyperalimentation solution contains glucose, protein, and other nutrients in amounts calculated to meet individual infant needs.

   b. Central administration: Inspect incisions when dressings are changed (every 24–48 hours, depending on policy, and whenever wet). Note redness, edema, drainage, condition of sutures.

      At risk of infection (local and general)

      Do not use TPN line for medications, blood withdrawal, CVP line. Start a second IV if necessary. Use sterile technique when changing dressing. Cleanse from incision line outward; date dressing change on tape. Clamp central catheter with padded hemostat when dressing is changed.

      At risk for air embolus

Continued on following page

Nursing Care Plan 23–6.   Care of Infants Who Need Alternate Methods of Feeding   *Continued*

ASSESSMENT	POTENTIAL NURSING DIAGNOSIS	NURSING INTERVENTION	COMMENTS/RATIONALE
c. With either route, assess: (1) Blood sugar (e.g., Dextrostix)	At risk of hyperglycemia, hypoglycemia At risk of osmotic diuresis secondary to hyperglycemia; at risk of brain damage secondary to osmotic diuresis		
(2) Urine sugar, protein, ketones, pH	At risk of glycosuria		
(3) Urine specific gravity			
(4) Fluid intake and output			
(5) Growth (a) Daily weight (b) Daily head circumference (c) Weekly length			
(6) Laboratory data: (a) Serum lipids (b) Serum electrolytes (see Table 23–10)	At risk for electrolyte imbalance		
4. Intravenous fat (Intralipid)		Refrigerate fat solution until ready to use. Join fat solution to TPN solution with Y connector immediately prior to entry into vein. Never infuse lipid solution through a filter.	Fat emulsion is isotonic; by infusing with hyperalimentation solution, total osmolality is decreased. Lipid solutions are delicate and easily broken down. Fat solutions may be administered through central or peripheral lines.
a. Assess signs of allergic reaction: (1) Respiratory distress (2) Cyanosis (3) Generalized rash (4) Vomiting (5) Local skin irritation (6) Fever	At risk for allergic reaction to intravenous lipid solution	Administer slowly; never faster than 3 ml. per kg. per hour. Medications are never added to fat solution.	
b. Identify signs of fatty acid deficiency: dry, scaly, or exematous skin.			
c. Identify infant with hyperglycemia.	At risk for kernicterus secondary to hyperlipidemia	Do not administer Intralipid when serum bilirubin is above 8 mg. per 100 ml. (5 mg. per 100 ml. in small preterm infant).	Large quantities of nonesterified fatty acids may displace bilirubin from albumin-binding sites.

Feeding by Orogastric or Nasogastric Tube

Need for orogastric or nasogastric feeding

1. Identify infant's need for orogastric or nasogastric feeding.

1. Select feeding tube of proper size (size 5–10), depending on infant size) calibrated syringe.
   Select proper formula.
2. Restrain active infant with diaper or blanket.
3. Position infant with head slightly extended to open oropharynx.
4. Measure distance from bridge of nose to lobe of ear to xiphoid process; mark on tube with tape.
5. Lubricate nasal catheter with sterile water; oral catheters do not require lubrication.
6. Pass catheter into infant's stomach.

Catheter in trachea

2. Observe infant for signs of dyspnea following insertion of catheter.

3. Assess residual. Large amounts of residual may be associated with NEC, intestinal obstruction.

4. Assess blood glucose (Dextrostix) prior to feeding if this assessment is necessary.

7. Aspirate stomach contents; measure residual and return to stomach. Presence of residual indicates tube placement in stomach. If no residual, infant's behavior (absence of dyspnea, agitation, etc.) indicates proper placement.
8. Provide pacifier if infant is able to suck during feeding.
9. Allow formula to flow by gravity.
10. If tube is to be removed, pinch and withdraw quickly.
11. Burp baby by placing in sitting position and gently rubbing back.
12. Turn infant to abdomen or right side to prevent aspiration.
13. Record time, amount of formula, route, addition of vitamins or other oral medications, amount of residual, infant response to feeding.
14. Transition to nipple feedings should be made gradually over a period of several days (see text)

If residual is large in relation to amount of formula, feeding may be omitted (see text).

Residual is returned to stomach to avoid loss of electrolytes.

If catheter is to remain the nasogastric route used, it is changed every 48–72 hours; alternate nares are used.

Continued on following page

Nursing Care Plan 23–6. Care of Infants Who Need Alternate Methods of Feeding *Continued*

ASSESSMENT	POTENTIAL NURSING DIAGNOSIS	NURSING INTERVENTION	COMMENTS/RATIONALE
		Feeding by Gastrostomy or Esophagostomy	
1. Inspect gastrostomy site: skin, dry, no redness or irritation.	Irritation from gastrostomy tube	A nipple, cut in half, with small part of the tip cut off, can be taped around gastrostomy tube next to skin to protect skin from irritation.	
2. Assess parents' understanding of procedure.	Parents' need for information	Technique of gastrostomy feeding:	
		1. Explain purpose and technique of feeding to family.	
		2. Prepare formula.	
		3. Provide pacifier to meet sucking needs. Hold infant if condition allows.	
		4. Attach syringe to top of tubing.	
		5. Aspirate stomach contents; measure and return aspirate.	
		6. Allow formula to flow by gravity.	
		7. Elevate tubing and syringe following (through top of incubator or attached to open bed or IV pole) to allow for gastric reflex. Explain to parents that gastric reflex is normal.	When oral feedings begin, elevate tube but leave unclamped for several days. After this period, tube will be clamped but will remain in place, frequently for several weeks.
	Need for parents to learn to feed via gastrostomy	8. Encourage parents to participate in gastrostomy feeding. If infant is to receive gastrostomy feedings at home, assist parents to become competent and comfortable with the procedure.	

at least every hour. Occasionally, in adults, the continued position of a needle in a vein is ascertained by lowering the fluid bottle to see if blood returns in the tubing. This should not be done in newborns because of the small gauge of the needle; the back-up blood may easily clog the needle, and the fluids will have to be restarted at another site. Swelling at the fluid site may indicate infiltration of fluids or merely that the tape holding the needle in place is too tight.

Even small babies have to be restrained while they are receiving fluids. Like older people with restraints, they need to have their position changed frequently and the restraints checked often. The skin under the restraint, which is so very delicate and can easily be injured, should also be checked often. If a baby is to receive oral fluids while he is restrained, his head should be lifted for feeding, and after feeding he should be turned on his side or abdomen, depending upon the fluid site. Each time the baby is turned or moved, the site and flow must be rechecked.

If the medications are added to the fluids, they must also be included in the record, just as any other medications would be.

Nutrition for Preterm Infants

In writing about nutrition for the preterm infant and other newborns who require intensive care, Rickard and Gresham say:

There is perhaps no other time when nutrition will be as important in influencing the quality of the infant's subsequent life . . . an acceptable nutritional program (is) an essential part of the comprehensive medical care these infants require.[50]

Major nutritional problems of preterm babies are summarized in Table 23–11. Because nurses have such a central role in meeting the nutritional needs of infants, we need to examine each of these problems in some detail.

Early Provision of Adequate Calories

Calories are needed both for energy and for growth. Failure to provide adequate calories results not only in inadequate growth but in starvation and in increased incidence of hypoglycemia and hyperbilirubinemia.

Energy is stored by the human body as glycogen and fat. The preterm baby has very little fat, and glycogen stores are practically nonexistent. Moreover, because of a higher metabolic rate in relation to body weight (in comparison to even the term newborn as well as to older children and adults), the energy needs of the preterm baby are relatively higher. Any metabolic or surgical stress (including the very common respiratory distress syndrome discussed above) still further increases energy needs.

How many calories does the preterm baby need for energy and growth? Recent studies suggest that the pattern of weight loss that follows the birth of a term baby, with no apparent resultant problems, may not be appropriate for a preterm baby, particularly one who is very small and/or very young in gestational age. It is felt that preterm babies should not lose more than 5 to 8 per cent of their birth weight, with smaller babies losing no more than 5 per cent. When you consider that 5 per cent of 1500 grams is 75 grams (approximately 2½ ounces) and 5 per cent of 1000 grams is 50 grams (less than 2 ounces), this is a very tiny weight loss.

Table 23–11. NUTRITION FOR THE PRETERM INFANT

Problems	Needs
Small energy stores; relatively higher energy needs	Early provision of adequate calories
Glucose intolerance: Hypoglycemia Hyperglycemia	Careful monitoring of blood glucose and glucose intake
Immature gastrointestinal system: Impaired lactose tolerance Relative inability to digest fats Increased nitrogen catabolism with respiratory distress syndrome	Feedings adjusted to the special needs of the preterm baby
Immature sucking and swallowing reflexes	Alternate routes of feeding

Lubchenco's studies show that a fetus in utero gains approximately 18 grams of weight per day from 28 to 32 weeks' gestation and 38 grams per day from 32 to 36 weeks' gestation.[35a] It has been suggested that similar gains may be appropriate for the baby of the same gestational age. Average weight gain in preterm infants is approximately 30 grams per day, although many variables affect this average.

Approximately 120 calories per kg. per day is the rough estimate currently in use, although the requirements of some preterm babies may be considerably higher. Weight gain is an important clue to the adequacy of caloric intake. For very small preterm babies, the best type of feeding remains somewhat controversial.

Hypoglycemia

It has been recognized since the 1960's that hypoglycemia is a major danger to preterm babies because of inadequate glycogen storage and the increased demands upon the body for energy, as mentioned above. Infants who are sick or stressed use glucose more rapidly than usual; glycogen stores become depleted, and hypoglycemia results. (Hypoglycemia in the infant of a diabetic mother and in the baby who is small for gestational age is discussed later in this chapter.)

Hypoglycemia is defined as a blood glucose level below 30 to 40 mg. per 100 ml. When the glucose level is below 40 mg., the baby must be carefully observed and the glucose level rechecked. When the glucose value is below 30 immediate intervention is required.

Hypoglycemia can lead to brain damage and lifelong impairment. To be consistent with a philosophy of giving parents a baby with an intact central nervous system, hypoglycemia is best noted by careful monitoring of blood glucose levels in the nursery.

Hypoglycemia is treated with glucose. Intravenous fluids containing glucose are started as soon as possible after the birth of a preterm infant.

Hyperglycemia

When babies are receiving intravenous glucose, hyperglycemia (blood sugar levels greater than 125 mg. per 100 ml.) also becomes a potential hazard. Hyperglycemia causes diuresis as the body attempts to rid itself of excess sugar, and in small babies very rapid dehydration may follow. Monitoring blood glucose levels and carefully maintaining the de-

sired rate of flow of intravenous glucose are the best ways of preventing hyperglycemia.

Immaturity of the Gastrointestinal Tract

The immature digestive system of the preterm baby makes certain dietary adjustments necessary. Not only must the type of carbohydrate, fat, and protein be adaptable to the special needs of the preterm baby but factors such as renal solute load must be considered.

Lactose is the carbohydrate of human milk and of several commercially prepared formulas. The enzyme *lactase* is necessary for lactose digestion. Since lactase enzymes do not attain maximal activity until 9 months after birth, preterm infants may have impaired lactose tolerance. Because breast milk has a higher lactose concentration than prepared formulas, some nutritionists feel that breast milk will be less well tolerated by preterm infants. (On the other hand, the possible role of breast milk in the prevention of necrotizing enterocolitis and other possible benefits of breast milk for the preterm baby are currently under investigation.)

Fats, even those digested rather easily by term infants (the fats in human milk, for example), are not believed to be well assimilated by preterm babies. Medium chain fatty acids are readily absorbed into the blood, however. Medium chain triglyceride (MCT) is an example of a fat often added to preterm infant formulas. In addition to providing essential fatty acids, added fats provide 9 calories per gram of formula in contrast to the 4 calories per gram provided by proteins and carbohydrates, making them a valuable source of energy.

Protein breakdown is very high in preterm infants with respiratory distress syndrome, occurring at a time when the body has great need for protein for brain development.

Provision of minerals is also a major problem. Lack of calcium can lead to undermineralization of the skeleton; however, it is not clear whether calcium supplementation is of any value when hypocalcemia is not present. Since iron is stored by the fetus only during the last trimester of pregnancy, preterm infants have minimal iron stores. Iron supplementation usually begins before the baby leaves the hospital, either in the form of an iron-fortified formula or iron drops. Iron is not given to babies with excessive red blood cell hemolysis (such as babies with Rh and ABO incompatibility, page 857) because the iron stores from red blood cell breakdown are not excreted.

Vitamin supplements are also frequently given to preterm babies, including vitamin E when the baby is believed to have a vitamin E–dependent anemia.

Preterm infants have a number of conditions that may contribute to a high renal solute load, including low fluid intake, high extra-renal water loss, and a decreased ability of the kidney to concentrate urine.

In view of the differences between the digestive capabilities of preterm and term infants, we may well wonder what the ideal feeding for preterm infants might be. In spite of a great deal of research, the answer to this question remains unclear. The use of human milk is again coming into favor in some preterm nurseries (below); the advantage of giving the mother an opportunity to participate in her baby's care by pumping her breasts if she so chooses is obvious. Formulas with added oil, along with added vitamins and iron, are also used. Researchers continue to search for an "ideal" preterm feeding.

Human Milk and the Preterm Infant

Historically, human milk has been considered the most appropriate food for preterm infants; in recent decades, however, the inadequacy of its protein for the rapid growth needs of the preterm baby has placed human milk in disfavor. Both the advantages and disadvantages of human milk for preterm infants are now under review.

Psychologic Advantages. A major rationale for human milk, quite apart from the nutritional significance, is the opportunity for the mother to participate in the care of her baby. As noted in Chapter 28, producing a less than perfect baby (e.g., a baby born prior to term) is a blow to a mother's self-esteem and her image of herself. If she had also planned to breast-feed and is now told she cannot (or believes she cannot), this is a second disappointment.

However, if she can provide milk for her baby, this positive step can promote both feelings of self-worth and feelings of attachment for her baby.

What if the baby is at high risk of dying? As we emphasize in Chapter 28, attachment is important to normal grieving. Mothers who have provided milk for their high risk infant have said after the baby's death, "I would do it again; giving my baby my milk made me feel that I did everything possible for him."

Immunologic Advantages and Disadvantages. The immunologic factors in human milk include secretory IgA, complement, mac-rophages, lymphocytes, neutrophils, and several others (Chapter 22). Freezing and pasteurizing human milk may eliminate many of these constitutents, but when the mother can provide fresh milk for her baby, she is also providing some protection against infection.

The immunologic disadvantages are rare when the mother is providing milk for her baby. If the mother is allergic to a medication that the baby is receiving, there is a possibility that the baby may have a reaction to that medicine. If the mother has a viral infection, the virus may be passed to her baby through breast milk. She can, however, continue to express her milk to maintain her milk supply until the infection is resolved and then again give her milk to the baby.

When human milk from a donor other than the baby's mother is used, there is a *potential* problem of an immunologic graft versus host reaction, but there is little evidence that this really does occur.

Nutritional Advantages and Disadvantages

Protein. The lower amount of protein in human milk in comparison to cow milk formulas has already been mentioned. The quality of the protein is different, however. The ratio of lactalbumin to casein, which is important in digestibility, is 60:40 in human milk and in certain commercial formulas; it is 18:82 in cow milk.

When large amounts of protein are given, the level of amino acids can be excessive, which can be a detrimental factor in brain development.

Considering total protein needs, it appears that human milk does need supplementation to provide adequate protein, but this does not contraindicate the use of human milk.

Fat. The fat content of human milk is slightly higher than that of cow milk. Moreover, the fat in human milk is better absorbed by infants, including preterm infants.

Calcium. The preterm infant's requirement for calcium is not met by human milk, but human milk is better for the baby because it also contains much less phosphate. Calcium supplementation will be necessary.

Renal Solute Load. The decreased renal solute load of human milk is an advantage for the preterm baby.

Providing Human Milk for the Preterm Baby

Because of immature sucking and swallowing reflexes (below), preterm babies will rarely be able to nurse at the mother's breast follow-

Nursing Care Plan 23–7.   Assisting the Mother in Manual Expression of Breast Milk or the Use of a Breast Pump

NURSING GOALS: To facilitate manual expression of breast milk or the use of a breast pump.

OBJECTIVES: The mother will:
1. Identify the reasons for using manual expression or a breast pump.
2. Choose the method or pump most appropriate for her needs.
3. Become skilled in the use of the technique she chooses.
4. Know how to store expressed milk properly.

ASSESSMENT	POTENTIAL NURSING DIAGNOSIS	NURSING INTERVENTION	COMMENTS/RATIONALE

1. Reasons for expressing milk by hand or pump:
a. Maternal indications: absence from infant (e.g., work, maternal hospitalization)
b. Infant indications:
   1. Infant preterm or ill, unable to nurse
   2. Infant transported to another hospital
   3. Temporary interruption in nursing due to hyperbilirubinemia
	Need to express milk due to (maternal or infant indication)	Present alternatives to mother:
		1. Hand expression
		2. Hand-held pump
		3. Electric breast pump.
		
		Allow mother to experiment with various methods (below); provide mother with information on cost and availability of various methods.
			Electric breast pump may be available in hospital but not following discharge (can be rented in some communities). Be sure that mother uses technique she can continue to use following discharge.

2. Expression of milk when infant has never nursed (e.g., preterm infant, infant ill from birth)	Need to express milk due to preterm birth	1. Begin expression of colostrum as soon as possible after birth. 2. Mother washes hands thoroughly. 3. Breast massage and nipple stimulation prior to expression stimulate oxytocin release and let-down. When a pump is used, placing the nipple slightly off center will increase nipple stimulation during pumping. 4. Encourage mother; first attempts may produce only a few drops. Explain that even these few drops are valuable for her baby and that volume will increase as expression continues.	Even a small volume of milk expressed enhances the oxytocin–prolactin cycle. Breast milk from the mother of a preterm infant changes in composition relative to infant's gestational age. When infant is preterm or ill, providing breast milk allows mother to participate in her baby's care in a very special way. Father participates by transporting milk and supporting mother.

5. Expressed milk should be stored in plastic containers; can be labeled and frozen if not used for infant immediately. Frozen milk is transported to hospital packed in ice.
6. Mother should avoid alcohol. Any medications taken by mother must be listed on label of milk.
7. Measures to encourage mother to relax encourage let-down: massage of neck and shoulder muscles by partner, warm shower, holding older sibling.

Assessment	Nursing Diagnosis	Nursing Intervention	Expected Outcome
Initial feeding at breast of preterm infant or previously ill infant. 1. Assess maternal feelings; apprehension, anxiety not unusual	Need for assistance in breast feeding	Initial feeding *at breast* of preterm or previously ill infant: 1. Explain that many infants do not "latch on" immediately. Reassure mother that first feedings are learning experiences. 2. Mother may use Lact-Aid (see text and Fig. 23–18) to supplement early breast feedings.	Expression of milk will maintain milk supply as well as provide breast milk for infant.
2. Expression of milk when breast-feeding is temporarily interrupted (e.g., infant hyperbilirubinemia, maternal or infant hospitalization)	Need to express milk due to (specific reason)	1. As above. 2. Expression will be easier after breast-feeding is established. 3. When milk is expressed because of hyperbilirubinemia, the expressed milk is usually discarded. 4. If mother is hospitalized, infant may be admitted with mother, or brought to mother for some feedings, with milk expressed at other times.	
3. Intermittent expression of milk (e.g., one or two times daily for mother returning to work) Assess a. Number of feedings to be missed b. Preferred method of expressing milk c. Possibilities for storing milk (e.g., refrigeration, packed in ice) at place of employment and for transporting milk to home	Need to express milk due to (specific reason, e.g., mother's employment)	1. Help mother develop a plan suited to her individual needs and those of her baby. 2. If milk cannot be properly stored, mother can express milk to maintain milk supply and discard, using formula for missed feedings.	

ing delivery. Often the baby may be transferred to a medical center, while the mother remains in a community hospital.

How can the nurse who cares for the mother help her succeed in providing milk for her baby?

Initial assessment begins as we ask the mother if she planned to breast-feed. So often the assumption is made, by parents, nurses, and physicians, that because she has had a preterm baby (or a baby with some other problem that necessitates care in a high risk nursery), breast-feeding is not possible for her. This isn't true. If she had planned to breast-feed, we can help her to accomplish her goal by expressing her milk until the baby is able to nurse at the breast (see Nursing Care Plan 23–7).

Expression can begin immediately after birth. The colostrum can then be given to the baby. If the mother is uncertain at first, but later decides that she wishes to breast-feed, lactation may be induced at this later time. Methods of expression are described in Chapter 26.

Milk expressed by any method is labeled with the name of the mother and the date and time of expression. If it is to be brought to the hospital that day (or if it is expressed at the hospital), the milk may be refrigerated and must then be used within 24 hours. Milk for future use is frozen. Freezing destroys many of the protective functions (e.g., macrophages) but does not appear to affect the nutritional components. If a mother lives at a great distance from the hospital and can only visit once or twice a week, freezing may enable her to provide breast milk for her baby and thus feel she is doing something for him, even when she is not with him.

Relactation and Induced Lactation

The mother of a preterm infant may not choose to breast-feed or express her milk initially but may later change her mind. A mother who was ill following delivery but subsequently recovers may also wish to breast-feed. If the baby was formula-fed but is not doing well, the mother may want to try breast-feeding. Or the mother who started breast-feeding and stopped for some reason may wish to try again. Under these circumstances *relactation* is possible.

Using a similar technique, lactation may also be induced in some women who have not been pregnant. Some adoptive mothers induce lactation in order to breast-feed their adopted infants. Although they may never totally meet their infant's nutritional needs by induced lac-

tation, mother and baby are able to share the close relationship that the mother desires.

A Plan for Relactation.   The key to lactation is nipple stimulation, which leads to the production of prolactin, which in turn stimulates milk production. Sucking by the infant every 2 hours, or 10 to 12 times in 24 hours for several weeks, is necessary to achieve lactation. Night feedings are essential. The mother must know this before she begins. Unless her motivation and her patience are high, her milk supply will not develop, and she is likely to become very discouraged.

In addition to assessment of the mother, her support systems must also be evaluated. How does the father feel about her desire to lactate? Are there other children? Will she have help in caring for them? Is there a public health nurse, a La Leche member, or a supportive neighbor available to give her counsel when she gets discouraged?

The mother's nutritional status should be good.

The personality of the baby can also be a factor in the success or failure of lactation. A very fussy baby may produce tension in the mother, which can interfere with milk production. On the other hand a very passive baby may not be sufficiently interested in frequent sucking to stimulate production.

During the lactating period the mother's milk must be supplemented by formula. After the first 48 hours, giving the supplement by dropper rather than by bottle will encourage the baby to suck from the breast, a more difficult task than sucking from the bottle. Another method of giving supplement is with a Lact-Aid (Fig. 23–18), which carries the supplement to the baby while he is nursing at the mother's breast. Adoptive mothers may use the Lact-Aid continuously.

The mother keeps a daily record, which includes:

1. The ounces of supplement given.
2. The number of times and length of time the baby nurses.

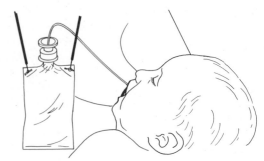

Figure 23–18.   The Lact-Aid enables this infant to nurse at his mother's breast and induce lactation while receiving supplementary feeding from the Lact-Aid bag.

3. The number of wet diapers. (There should be at least eight wet diapers a day as evidence of adequate fluid intake.)

How long will it take for the mother of a preterm baby to lactate? A general guide is 1 week for every month she has not nursed plus 1 additional week to build up a strong milk supply. For example, if it has been 2 months since her baby delivered, it should take approximately 3 weeks (2 weeks plus 1 week) for her milk supply to develop. When the baby is taking only 4 ounces of supplement in 24 hours, supplement can usually be reduced to 4 ounces in 48 to 72 hours and subsequently eliminated entirely.

Immature Sucking and Swallowing Reflexes

The sucking and swallowing reflexes of most preterm babies are insufficiently developed to enable sucking from either bottle or breast. Alternate routes of feeding include:

1. Intravenous feeding of glucose and electrolytes (see above).
2. Intravenous feeding of protein solutions (hyperalimentation).
3. Formula fed by gavage (oral or nasal).
4. Continuous intragastric drip and transpyloric feeding.

Intravenous Feeding of Protein Solutions (Total Parenteral Nutrition). Solutions for total parenteral nutrition (TPN) provide protein, vitamins, and electrolytes as well as glucose. The intravenous solution is specifically prepared for each baby under sterile conditions; hyperalimentation solutions must not be interchanged. Laboratory studies of each infant serve as a guide to determining his specific solution.

For short-term supplementation, certain hyperalimentation solutions are given in peripheral veins. More concentrated solutions for long-term hyperalimentation are administered through a catheter in the superior vena cava (Fig. 23–19).

The intravenous system for central hyperalimentation includes a millipore filter, which serves to remove particles or micro-organisms from the solution before they can reach the baby, and an infusion pump, to ensure that the solution is delivered at a constant rate throughout the 24-hour period. Both filter and pump are changed every 24 hours. The intravenous line should be labeled with the date and time of changing.

Because a number of serious complications are possible when hyperalimentation solution is administered, constant nursing attention is an absolute necessity (see also Nursing Care Plan 23–6). Septicemia is a major danger, because the glucose-protein solution is a nearly perfect medium for the growth of bacteria. The prevention of infection depends upon careful technique, not only at the time the catheter is inserted but throughout the period it is in place. The central hyperalimentation catheter should never be used for the administration of medications or for the withdrawal of blood; both procedures heighten the possibility of contamination. Babies must be observed carefully for any early signs of sepsis (see below).

In order to utilize the protein of the hyperalimentation solution for growth, the baby must also receive sufficient glucose to stimulate insulin production. The insulin, in turn, stimulates both the transport of amino acids into the cells and the synthesis of protein. If relatively large amounts of glucose are not given, the amino acids will be utilized for energy rather than for growth.

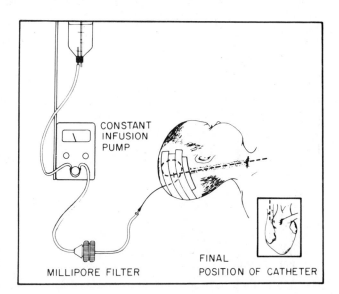

Figure 23–19. Technique of catheter insertion and delivery of fluids for total intravenous alimentation. (From Moore: *Newborn Family, and Nurse.* 2nd Edition. Philadelphia, W. B. Saunders Co., 1981.)

However, the high level of glucose, as we have already noted, can lead to rapid and severe dehydration. Urine samples are checked for glucose, and if hyperglycemia is present, either the rate of the infusion is decreased or the glucose content of the solution is decreased. Sometimes insulin is added to the solution under these circumstances. Other regimens gradually increase glucose to prevent initial glycosuria.

Hypertonic sugar solutions in combination with amino acids may, after several days of administration, lead to a hypoglycemic response within the body, whether insulin has been added or not. Therefore blood glucose levels are carefully monitored.

The baby's growth in weight, length, and head circumference is an indication of the success of total parenteral nutrition (TPN).

Intravenous Fat. Intravenous fat, in the form of Intralipid, provides a concentrated source of calories as well as essential fatty acids to infants who must be fed intravenously for more than a few days (see Nursing Care Plan 23–6). Intralipid may be given in the same peripheral vein as the hyperalimentation solution by joining the two lines with a Y-connector immediately before they enter the vein. A common line is not used prior to that point because of the delicate nature of the lipid solution. Intralipid solution is never given through a filter. The rate of administration is slow, never greater than 3 ml. per kg. per hour.

Some infants have an allergic reaction to the Intralipid solution. Intralipid therapy is contraindicated in infants with abnormal liver function.

Feeding by Gavage. Gavage feeding may be oral or nasal (see Nursing Care Plan 23–6). Nasogastric tubes are left in place between feedings; oral gastric tubes are inserted with each feeding. Because it is not difficult to insert an oral tube and because nasal tubes can cause irritation and swelling of the mucous membranes, increased mucus production and other complications, we prefer the oral tube for most babies. Babies are obligate nose breathers; occlusion of one nares with a tube when the second nares is swollen from previous tube placement can compromise breathing. Many preterm infants have a transient bradycardia or color change when the tube is first passed, which is a response to stimulation of the vagus nerve. If this response is repeatedly severe and prolonged, a nasal tube may be necessary.

Gavage tubes come in various sizes—size 5 for very tiny infants and size 8 or 10 for larger preterm babies.

The tube is measured from the bridge of the nose to the lobe of the ear to the xiphoid process. This distance is marked on the tube with tape. The catheter may be premarked, but since there are all sizes of even tiny infants, the tube should still be measured at each feeding.

Nasal catheters may be lubricated with sterile water; oral catheters do not need to be lubricated. After the catheter is passed, the baby should be observed for a moment for signs of dyspnea, an indication that the tube may be in the trachea rather than in the esophagus.

Whatever may be in the infant's stomach is gently withdrawn into a syringe attached to the feeding tube. The amount and characteristic of this *residual* is charted when the feeding is started. The residual is then replaced in the baby's stomach because it contains electrolytes. If the residual is more than 1 to 2 ml., the amount of the residual is subtracted from the feeding to be given. A large amount of residual in relation to the amount of feeding may be an early sign of necrotizing enterocolitis (below); feedings may need to be omitted when the residual is relatively large. For example, in a baby receiving 35 ml. of feeding, a residual of 5 ml. would be replaced and 30 ml. of feeding given. However, if a baby is receiving 7 ml. of feeding and has 5 ml. of residual, the 5 ml. would be replaced and the feeding probably omitted. This decision is usually made in consultation with the baby's physician.

After the residual is replaced, formula is poured into the syringe and allowed to flow into the stomach by gravity.

If the tube is not to be left in place, it is pinched and removed when every drop of formula has passed through it. A baby should be "burped" following gavage feeding, just as he is after a bottle- or breast-feeding. If he must remain in the incubator, he can be held in a sitting position and have his back gently stroked toward the neck. After feeding, the baby is placed on his abdomen or on the right side.

When a baby begins to suck on his gavage tube during feedings, he may be ready to begin the transition to bottle-feeding (Fig. 23–20). At first a few milliliters of a feeding may be offered by nipple once or twice a day *after* gavage feeding. When the baby can take one feeding per day by bottle, he can graduate to two and then three feedings. If he appears tired during bottle-feeding, the next feeding should be by gavage. It is important to chart carefully the way in which the baby takes each feeding in order to plan care for the next day.

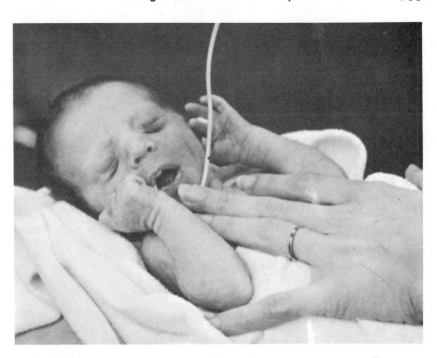

Figure 23–20. Hand-mouth gestures and a capacity to "mouth" the feeding tube are indications that this 3½ pound premature baby will soon take feedings from a nipple instead of a tube. (From O'Grady: *American J. Nursing, 71*:737, 1971.)

Patience is essential, both in increasing amounts of formula and in making the transition from gavage to bottle-feeding.

Continuous Intragastric Drip or Transpyloric Feedings. In some nurseries preterm babies are fed through a nasojejunal catheter inserted through the baby's nose and into his stomach. The baby is then turned on his right side to allow passage through the pyloric sphincter into the duodenum and ultimately into the jejunum. The position of the catheter is checked by abdominal radiograph when fluid aspirated from the catheter has reached a pH of 5.0 to 7.0.

First feedings through the catheter will be of water or dextrose, followed by half-strength and then full-strength formula. Approximately 10 to 15 ml. of formula is given by slow drip every 1½ to 2 hours.

Possible complications include occlusion of the catheter and infusion of an excess amount of formula, which may reflux into the stomach. Irrigating the tube with 1 ml. of sterile water following each feeding will help to prevent occlusion. A nasogastric tube placed in the stomach will prevent aspiration of any formula that regurgitates through the pylorus.

Necrotizing Enterocolitis

Approximately 3 to 8 per cent of preterm infants acquire necrotizing enterocolitis (NEC), a life-threatening condition. The etiology is believed to be related to hypoxia, with a resultant shunting of blood from organs that tolerate ischemia comparatively well (such as the intestines) to those areas that must be continuously oxygenated (such as the brain). Intestinal cells, damaged by hypoxia, stop secreting mucus and become damaged; they are subsequently invaded by gas-forming bacteria that produce a characteristic picture of pneumatosis cystoides intestinalis (air in the intestinal wall) on x-ray films. Intestinal perforation and death may follow if the baby's condition is not recognized. Other factors associated with NEC include sepsis, patient ductus arteriosus, exchange transfusion, umbilical vessel catheterization, low gestational age, and inappropriate oral feeding. Obviously, most babies in intensive care nurseries are potential candidates.

Nursing observations are invaluable in spotting early symptoms of NEC. A baby with abdominal distention is suspect, especially if rigidity is also present. The abdomen should be measured (Fig. 23–21) every 4 to 6 hours from the time distention is first noted; an increase of more than 1 cm. from the previous measurement should be immediately reported.

Failure to absorb feedings is another significant symptom. When a baby who has been taking feedings, either by nipple or gavage, begins to spit up formula, or when formula can be aspirated through the gavage tube at a subsequent feeding, he may have NEC. A shiny abdominal wall, absence of bowel sounds (listen with a stethoscope), and blood in the stools (check with Hemastix) are also symptoms nurses should assess.

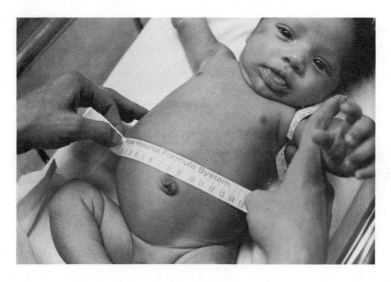

Figure 23–21. Select points on the right and the left, above or below the umbilicus, mark sites with indelible ink, and measure between them. (From Bliss: *MCN, 1*:37, 1976.)

Treatment includes the discontinuation of oral feedings for 7 to 10 days to rest the bowel and the administration of antibiotics. During this time the baby is carefully observed for signs of shock (inability to maintain temperature, decrease in blood pressure, bradycardia, and listlessness). He should be picked up as little as possible to avoid abdominal trauma, but his hands and head should be stroked for emotional satisfaction. Surgery may be necessary to remove segments of inflamed bowel. There is some evidence that the evidence of NEC is lower in babies fed breast milk, a major reason for the re-evaluation of the use of breast milk in preterm infants.

Problems Related to Bilirubin

Hyperbilirubinemia is a common problem of preterm babies for several reasons. The preterm infant has a decreased ability to conjugate bilirubin in his liver, and thus the concentration of indirect, fat-soluble bilirubin increases more rapidly than in the term infant. Bruising, more frequent in preterm babies, leads to hemolysis and increased bilirubin levels. The delay in feeding that often occurs in the sick preterm infant is another contributing factor (see also Nursing Care Plan 23–8).

Moreover, kernicterus, the brain damage that results when bilirubin enters the brain cells, can occur at bilirubin levels lower than the 18 to 20 mg. per 100 ml. in the preterm infant with acidosis or with low circulating blood volume. This is because as long as bilirubin is bound to albumin it cannot enter the intracellular fluid compartment and is therefore nontoxic to cells. The excess of hydrogen ions present in acidosis, certain other ions, and drugs such as salicylates, sulfonamides, and others compete with bilirubin for albumin-binding sites. Thus more bilirubin is able to enter the cells, even though the total amount of bilirubin in the body may be lower.

In addition, any condition that leads to lower levels of albumin in the infant, such as decreased blood volume, has the same effect of decreasing the amount of bilirubin bound to albumin.

Two modalities are principally used in the treatment of hyperbilirubinemia. They are phototherapy and exchange transfusion.

Phototherapy

It was the careful observation of a nurse at the General Hospital in Rochford, Essex, England, that led to the use of phototherapy in the treatment of hyperbilirubinemia. The nurse, whose name unfortunately is not recorded in the published report, noted that jaundice faded after babies had been in direct sunlight for a short time. Cremer and his associates[5] then began to place naked babies in direct sunlight for 15 to 20 minutes, withdrawing them for similar periods before exposing them again. During exposure the babies' eyes were protected with a plastic shield. It was discovered that although jaundice quickly disappeared from the exposed areas, it remained in the shaded areas. Subsequently, Cremer devised a source of artificial light that was found to be effective in reducing serum bilirubin levels. Phototherapy has since become a common treatment in premature and intensive care nurseries (Fig. 23–22).

Light causes bilirubin to break down into water-soluble products that are rapidly excreted in the bile, and to a lesser extent in the urine. Because of the mode of excretion, the stools of a baby who has been under the lights

Nursing Care Plan 23–8. Infants with Hyperbilirubinemia

NURSING GOALS: To identify mothers and infants at risk in prenatal period or at birth or shortly thereafter.
To recognize early signs of hyperbilirubinemia and provide supportive care and protection during therapy.
To prevent sequelae (kernicterus).

OBJECTIVES:
1. Mothers at risk of having an infant with hyperbilirubinemia will be identified in the prenatal period.
2. Infants at risk of developing hyperbilirubinemia will be identified at birth or shortly thereafter.
3. Early evidence of hyperbilirubinemia will be detected.
4. Treatment will be started early.

ASSESSMENT	POTENTIAL NURSING DIAGNOSIS	NURSING INTERVENTION	COMMENTS/RATIONALE

1. Prenatal identification: infants of mothers with
  a. Rh incompatibility
  b. ABO incompatibility
  c. Infectious illness during pregnancy
  d. Medications (sulfonamides, nitrofurantoins)
  e. Maternal diabetes mellitus or siblings with (1) cystic fibrosis, (2) liver disease, (3) metabolic error (e.g., galactosemia), (4) neonatal jaundice
	Infant at risk for hyperbilirubinemia related to (specific maternal factor)		

2. Intrapartum identification
  a. Premature labor
  b. Premature rupture of membranes
  c. Oxytocin-induced labor
  d. Vacuum extractor (Cephalhematoma)
	At risk for hyperbilirubinemia related to (specific reason)		Bruising and sepsis increase the incidence of hyperbilirubinemia.

3. Identification of infant at risk (in addition to maternal factors)
  a. Asphyxia; hypoxia
  b. Acidosis
  c. Neonatal sepsis
  d. Medications that compete with bilirubin for binding sites
  e. Large cephalhematoma (entrapped hemorrhage, RBC breakdown)
  f. Delayed passage of meconium or infrequent stools
  g. SGA
  h. Preterm
  i. Pallor (anemia)
	At risk for hyperbilirubinemia related to (specific factor)	Measures to decrease risk of hyperbilirubinemia:
		1. Supportive care
		  a. Thermoneutral environment
		  b. Appropriate respiratory support
		  c. Prevention of hypoglycemia
		  d. Prevention of sepsis
		2. Early feedings when infant's condition permits
			Supportive care reduces risk of acidosis, cold stress, which reduces binding sites for bilirubin.
			Early feeding provides stimuli, lead to early bowel emptying, decreased enterohepatic circulation of bilirubin and decreased reabsorption of bilirubin from bowel.

Nursing Care Plan 23–8.   Infants with Hyperbilirubinemia   (Continued)

ASSESSMENT	POTENTIAL NURSING DIAGNOSIS	NURSING INTERVENTION	COMMENTS/RATIONALE
j. Petechiae (intrauterine infection) k. Microcephaly (intrauterine infection) 4. Assessment of cord blood for: a. Blood type b. Rh factor c. Coombs' test d. Hemoglobin/hematocrit e. CBC			
5. Physical assessment: signs of developing hyperbilirubinemia: a. Jaundice in first 24 hours, 24–48 hours may be pathologic or physiologic (blanch skin to assess jaundice) b. Increase in bilirubin greater than 5 mg. per dl. per 24 hours c. Total bilirubin greater than 10–12 mg. per dl.	At risk for hyperbilirubinemia related to (specific reason)	Provide supportive care; anticipate need for and initiate phototherapy as ordered: 1. Infant is undressed. 2. Eyes are protected (uncover periodically to provide visual stimulation). 3. Monitor infant's temperature. 4. Assess fluid needs (output, specific gravity, weight twice daily 5. Offer water between feedings to all infants. 6. Further increase fluid intake if weight decreases by more than 2 per cent. 7. Explain reasons for phototherapy to parents, encourage and answer questions. 8. Uncover baby's eyes during part of parents' visit.	Assess jaundice in natural daylight if possible.
6. Signs of prolonged hyperbilirubinemia: clinical jaundice greater than 1 week in term infant; 2 weeks in preterm infant	Need for information about hyperbilirubinemia and phototherapy	Provide supportive care.	
7. Parents' understanding of hyperbilirubinemia and need for phototherapy, reason for eye patches, desired outcome			
8. Physical assessment: signs of serious illness a. Pallor b. Edema c. Yellow staining of cord d. Enlarged liver and spleen e. Anemia: hematocrit of less than 35 per cent f. Jaundice appearing in first 24 hours g. Rapid rise in bilirubin following birth (greater than 5 mg. per dl. per 24 hours)	At risk of kernicterus or death related to anemia, hyperbilirubinemia	Anticipate need for phototherapy (above). Anticipate need for exchange transfusion (below). Encourage parent interaction; provide appropriate information; answer questions.	Pallor, edema, enlarged liver and spleen suggest hydrops fetalis (see text).
9. Identify signs of kernicterus a. Lethargy b. Diminished reflexes		Provide supportive care. Anticipate need for phototherapy and exchange transfusion.	Many of the signs of kernicterus are also signs of other illnesses (e.g., sepsis, intracranial fluid).

d. Opisthotonus
e. Flaccidity, loss of muscle tone
f. Neuromuscular irritability

   provide appropriate information; answer questions.

Exchange Transfusion

1. Preparation phase
   a. Infant blood type
   b. Type, Rh of donor blood
   c. Freshness of blood
   d. Type of preservative

   Donor blood should be infant type or Type O and Rh negative. Blood should be as fresh as possible. Potential complications of preservatives:
1. Heparin: bleeding (may be protamine sulfate)
2. ACD or CPD: hypocalcemia, hypoglycemia, acidosis, hyperkalemia

   e. Temperature of blood

   Place blood inside incubator or in warm water (98.6°F, 37°C.)

   Cold blood will increase risk of hypothermia; overheating will damage erythrocytes, increase K level.

   f. Infant's temperature
   g. Infant's general condition

   Infant is placed under radiant warmer with servo mechanism attached.

   h. Condition of cord

   Attach cardiac monitor. If cord is dry, saline soaks 30–60 minutes prior to exchange may soften cord.

   i. Parent's understanding of reason for exchange, length of procedure, desired outcome, possible need for second exchange

Need for information about exchange transfusion

   Provide appropriate information; encourage and answer questions.

2. During exchange transfusion (1–2 hours)
   a. Assess vital signs (TPR, blood pressure).
   b. Assess infant's condition (color, respiratory status, etc.).
   c. Measure blood glucose.

   Ensure thermoneutral temperature, maintenance of intravenous fluids. Suction infant as necessary

   Keep blood mixed during exchange.
   Record transfusion (blood in, blood out, medications).

   Plasma and RBCs tend to separate; baby could get mostly plasma.

3. Following exchange transfusion:
   a. Assess vital signs.
   b. Assess infant's condition.
   c. Note bleeding from exchange site.
   d. Measure blood glucose.
   e. Perform studies for calcium, potassium, and sodium.
   f. Bilirubin assessment
      (1) Immediately following exchange
      (2) every 4–6 hours thereafter

   Continue supportive care of infant. Provide opportunity and encourage parents to be with infant.

   Rebound hyperbilirubinemia may occur.

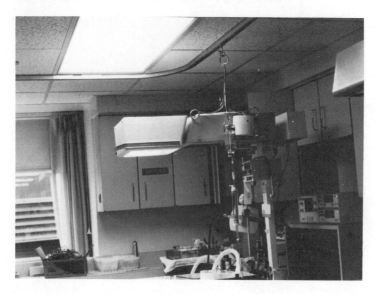

Figure 23–22.   The bilirubin light in an intensive care nursery.

are brown or dark green; the urine may be a dark golden brown.

Blue light is more effective than white light in causing bilirubin breakdown. However, it is difficult to detect changes in the baby's color, particularly changes caused by cyanosis, under blue lights. They must be turned off frequently for observation of the baby. The baby will also appear "strange" to his parents under blue lights. Even white lights are frightening and should be carefully explained. Blue lights should be flicked off so the parents can see what their baby really looks like.

Nurses caring for babies receiving phototherapy must understand several aspects of care for these babies (see Nursing Care Plan 23–8).

1. Because photodegradation of bilirubin takes place in the skin, the baby should be fully undressed while he is under the lights.

2. His temperature must be monitored; overheating with subsequent dehydration is a possibility. If a servomechanism is being used to monitor the baby's temperature, it should be covered with opaque tape.

3. Fluid intake should be increased because of increased insensible water loss, which may be increased by as much as 100 per cent in the preterm baby (and by approximately 40 per cent in the term baby). The baby should be weighed twice a day and fluid intake further increased if weight loss exceeds 2 per cent of body weight.

4. Both of the baby's eyes should be shielded completely. There is no data concerning human eye damage, but some retinal damage has been produced in experimental animals. When only one eye has been covered, permanent amblyopia (reduced vision) has been demonstrated in kittens.

5. Skin color is not an adequate guide to levels of serum bilirubin, because the skin will become less yellow during treatment. Bilirubin levels in the blood must therefore be measured.

6. Babies under the bilirubin light may have a rash from ultraviolet radiation. There should always be a Plexiglas shield between the baby and the light to filter out this radiation.

7. Stools increase in number (and change in color), adding to water loss.

8. Light emission may decay over a period of time. Specific instructions for various types of lights are contained in instruction manuals and should be reviewed periodically.

Other than the findings of the animal research studies described above, no hazards of phototherapy have been identified in the 20 years since the initial discovery of the principle, although it is recommended that lights be used only when there is a specific reason (rising bilirubin levels) and never prophylactically.

How much radiant energy does a baby receive during phototherapy? Lucey has calculated that a baby in an incubator near a window who is exposed to 6 hours of summer sunlight receives 4700 microwatts per square cm. in 24 hours.[39] A baby receiving 24 hours of phototherapy (daylight bulbs) receives 3800 microwatts per square cm.

Exchange Transfusion

A second method of treatment for hyperbilirubinemia is exchange transfusion (Nursing Care Plan 23–8). When bilirubin levels are rising rapidly, exchange transfusion is indicated rather than phototherapy. In the process of exchange transfusion bilirubin is removed.

If the exchange is done because of Rh incompatibility, sensitized red blood cells and circulating antibody are also removed.

Blood for exchange may be O negative, which has been cross-matched against maternal serum. If it is suspected before delivery that an immediate exchange will be necessary, this blood should be ready. If there is time following delivery to type the baby's blood before exchange, negative blood of the baby's type that has been cross-matched against maternal serum is used. A sample of maternal serum should be saved for future exchanges. Obtaining additional maternal blood is not a serious problem when the mother is in the same hospital as the baby. But as the transfer of very sick infants from smaller community hospitals to the intensive care units of major medical centers becomes increasingly more frequent, the nurses at both hospitals must make sure that maternal blood accompanies any baby with hemolytic anemia.

If the baby if Rh_D positive but the mother is Rh_D negative, Rh_D negative blood is used. If Rh_D positive blood is used, the antibodies already present in the infant's circulatory system will destroy the new erythrocytes, just as they are destroying his own cells; nothing will have been accomplished by exchanging one set of positive cells for another.

In addition to being the proper type, blood for exchange must be the freshest available, never more than 3 to 4 days old. Older blood is more likely to hemolyze, exactly the process that exchange transfusion is attempting to prevent. Heparinized blood is always fresh, since it must be discarded if it is not used within a 24-hour period. Babies who receive heparinized blood must be watched for bleeding following transfusion; 10 mg. of protamine sulfate may be given intravenously following an exchange with heparinized blood. Protamine sulfate counteracts the anticoagulant effects of heparin. Blood that has had acid-citrate-dextrose (ACD) or citrate phosphate dextrose (CPD) added as an anticoagulant binds calcium and lowers blood calcium levels. If the baby shows any sign of hypocalcemia (jitteriness, seizures, apnea), 2 to 4 ml. of 5 per cent calcium gluconate is administered. Calcium levels are assessed following transfusion.

The high level of glucose in ACD or CPD blood may stimulate insulin secretion and lead to hypoglycemia following exchange; assessment of blood glucose and provision of glucose to the baby is essential. Acidosis may occur if the baby's liver is unable to metabolize citrate; if the liver converts citrate to bicarbonate at a later time late metabolic acidosis may occur.

ACD or CPD blood more than 4 days old may have a potassium level that is dangerously high for infants.

The danger that the baby will be chilled during any procedure has already been discussed. In addition to the measures normally used to keep the infant warm, the blood for exchange should be warmed. An easy and safe way to do this is to place the blood in a basin of water warmed to but not exceeding 98.6°F. (37.0°C). Blood can also be warmed inside an incubator but not directly under a radiant warmer. Overheating the blood can damage erythrocytes and also increase the level of free serum potassium.

The amount of blood that will be used is figured at 85 ml. times the weight of the baby in kilograms times 2, 85 ml. per kg. being the assumed blood volume of the newborn infant. This is called a double-volume exchange. An amount equal to twice the blood volume is used because research indicates that this quantity will ensure that 85 to 90 per cent of circulating erythrocytes are effectively replaced. If the baby's hematocrit is less than 40, a partial exchange with packed red blood cells may precede the full exchange. Albumin may be given prior to the exchange; by binding bilirubin albumin increases the amount of bilirubin removed.

During the exchange itself there must be one person, doctor or nurse, who can devote full attention to the baby by monitoring pulse and respiration, observing the infant's color and general condition, and suctioning him if necessary. The amount of blood injected and withdrawn and the baby's venous pressure must also be accurately recorded. Care for the infant is summarized in Nursing Care Plan 23–8.

After the exchange is completed, the baby is observed closely both for evaluation of his general condition and for signs of hemorrhage from the exchange site. Bilirubin is assessed following the exchange transfusion; bilirubin levels may be halved. However, bilirubin levels begin to rise shortly afterward and a second exchange may be necessary.

Infection in Preterm Infants

All newborn infants are at increased risk of infection (Chapter 22). Preterm infants are particularly at risk because (1) the transfer of antibodies from mother to infant is limited by the shorter gestational period, and (2) preterm infants are more likely to be resuscitated, to need respiratory support, to have skin break-

Nursing Care Plan 23–9.   Infants with Neonatal Sepsis

NURSING GOALS: To prevent neonatal sepsis.
To identify early signs of sepsis and provide appropriate early intervention.
To avoid serious consequences of sepsis and of treatment for sepsis.

OBJECTIVES:
1. Infants at risk of sepsis will be identified from prenatal history.
2. Transmission of infection will be prevented.
3. Early signs of sepsis will be recognized.
4. Infants with infections will receive supportive care and treatment.

ASSESSMENT	POTENTIAL NURSING DIAGNOSIS	NURSING INTERVENTION	COMMENTS/RATIONALE
1. Identify risk factors in maternal history a. Rupture of membranes more than 24 hours prior to delivery b. Instrumentation or manipulation of fetus c. Maternal bleeding d. Prolonged labor e. Maternal infection (e.g., amnionitis)	At risk of sepsis		Primary sepsis (first 48 hours following birth) usually due to organisms from birth canal. Secondary sepsis (after 48 hours) usually due to nursery-acquired infection
2. Identify infants at risk a. Preterm, postterm, SGA b. Infant requiring resuscitation or ventilation c. Infant with congenital anomaly that increases exposure (e.g., myelomeningocele, gastroschisis) d. Infants requiring invasive procedures (e.g., endotracheal intubation, umbilical artery catheter, surgery)	At risk of sepsis related to (specific condition)	Gram stain of gastric aspirate frequently performed when infant is at risk; polymorphonuclear cells and bacteria suggest possible sepsis.	

	Possible sepsis	

3. Assess nursery environment for optimum technique to prevent sepsis:
  a. Careful handwashing
  b. Sterilization of equipment and supplies that contact baby
  c. Exclusion of personnel with infectious illness
		Review policies and practice of infection control frequently. Ensure systematic periodic evaluation of infection-control program.

4. Identify early signs of sepsis; physical assessment:
  a. Nonspecific change in behavior, feeding, etc., "failure to thrive," lethargy
  b. Hypotension
  c. Apnea, retractions, grunting with or without bradycardia
  d. Vomiting, abdominal distention, change in feeding pattern
  e. Pallor, mottled skin, cyanosis
  f. Temperature instability
  g. Seizures
  h. Hepatosplenomegaly
		Provide thermoneutral environment. Provide supportive care (nutrition, respiratory support, etc.)

5. Identify early signs of sepsis: laboratory assessment:
  a. Glucose intolerance: frequent Dextrostix
  b. Metabolic acidosis
  c. Hyperbilirubinemia
  d. Changes in blood count, particularly band cells (up or down); platelets (down), anemia
		Anticipate need for septic work-up:
		1. Blood culture
		2. Bladder aspiration
		3. Spinal tap
		
		Administer antibiotics (see Table 23–13).

6. Assess parents' understanding of infant's illness.		Explain each aspect of nursing intervention; provide frequent opportunities for questions; encourage visiting and participation in infant's care when possible.

down where monitors are attached, and to have intravenous lines, umbilical artery catheters, and other "invasions," each of which may potentially increase the risk of infection.

Infections affect infants in two ways. Neonatal sepsis is an acute infection in which the baby appears ill and has a blood culture that demonstrates the causative organism. About one baby in every 1000 to 2000 live term births and one in every 250 live preterm births has neonatal sepsis.

Acute infections in newborns include gonorrheal conjunctivitis (Chapter 21), urinary tract infections (which may lead to sepsis), meningitis, and infectious diarrhea.

A number of infections, several of which are acquired transplacentally, may affect the baby's long-range development but are not always obvious in the immediate newborn period. The most frequent causes of chronic infection are the organisms that are collectively known as the TORCH group (Chapter 8).

The discussion of neonatal sepsis below is applicable to any infant with neonatal sepsis; it is included in this section because of the high incidence of sepsis in preterm infants.

Signs of Neonatal Sepsis

Signs of sepsis in newborn infants, like the signs of many other problems, are more general than specific. Traditionally, clinical signs such as vomiting, failure to feed well, the baby's inability to maintain his body temperature, and gray or mottled skin color have been recognized as early evidence of sepsis. However, by the time these signs appear, the infection may be generalized. And in spite of all the antibiotics developed in recent years, there has been little change in infant mortality due to generalized sepsis.

Although we need to carefully observe and report the symptoms listed above, the current emphasis is on detecting earlier signs of infection. These signs are summarized in Nursing Care Plan 23–9.

None of these signs are routinely monitored in the apparently healthy term newborn, although these babies may become septic. However, for infants in premature and intensive care nurseries, where the risk of sepsis is even greater, these parameters are followed.

Normal white blood cell (WBC) count in newborns varies from 6000 to 25,000 WBCs and also changes from day to day, so a single value is of little help in recognizing sepsis. Any marked and sudden change, either increase or decrease, suggests sepsis. The level of band cells, a form of immature WBC, may be abnormally elevated or decreased. Band cell count in the first weeks of life normally averages from 5.5 to 9 per cent, the higher values occurring at birth.

Platelet counts decrease in septic infants; platelet counts normally exceed 80,000 to 100,000, although in preterm infants they may be as low as 60,000 in the first three days.

Either hypoglycemia or hyperglycemia may indicate sepsis. Metabolic acidosis (bicarbonate levels below 21 mEq. per liter) also suggests the possibility of an infection. Here again, a sequence of values is far more helpful than a single value in giving a clue as to what is happening to a particular baby.

Pustules or furuncles on the skin, often in the umbilical or diaper area, are a sign of staphylococcal infection. In scalded skin syndrome, an exotoxin of staphylococci causes reddening, swelling, and tenderness of the skin, and frequently desquamation as well.

Organisms Involved in Neonatal Sepsis

The types of organisms most responsible for neonatal sepsis change from time to time. Currently group B beta-hemolytic streptococci are the chief source of infection in most nurseries in the United States. Since these organisms are a part of the normal vaginal flora of many women, it is difficult to prevent their presence in neonates. Not all babies whose mothers have group B streptococci in their vaginal tract will become infected, however; only a small percentage will.

Escherichia coli, once the leading cause of neonatal sepsis, remains a major source of infection in nurseries. Other significant organisms are *Klebsiella, Staphylococcus aureus,* and *Pseudomonas.* Table 23–12 summarizes important information about common infections in newborns.

Diagnosis of Sepsis

When sepsis is suspected, a number of studies are immediately indicated. Blood cultures are drawn from a peripheral vein after disinfection of the skin with iodine. Urine for culture is obtained by suprapubic aspiration, considered less dangerous than catheterization and more reliable than a clean-catch specimen. Cerebrospinal fluid is aspirated via lumbar puncture. Any skin lesion should also be cultured.

Treatment

Good nursing care, with emphasis on careful handwashing, should effectively isolate every

Table 23–12. ORGANISMS IMPORTANT IN NEONATAL SEPSIS

Organism	Source	Form of Sepsis	Notes
Group B beta-hemolytic streptococcus	Mother: vaginal flora	Septicemia within first 12 hours of life with 50% mortality	Leading cause of neonatal sepsis
	Environment: nursery personnel and infected infants	Meningitis at 2–12 weeks of life with 20–40% mortality	
E. coli (gram-negative)	Mother (initial case in nursery); hands of nursery personnel for subsequent cases	Diarrhea Sepsis Meningitis	Until recently the leading cause of neonatal sepsis
Aerobacter (gram-negative) *Klebsiella* (gram-negative)	Intubation Surgery	Pneumonia Sepsis	
Staphylococcus	Nursery personnel, particularly hands of personnel; other infants	Meningitis Septicemia (Phage I group) Skin infection–scalded skin syndrome (Phage II group)	
Pseudomonas (gram-negative)	Respiratory equipment; bottles of distilled water and so on; sink traps	Bacteremia Pneumonia Meningitis	Difficult to treat

Table 23–13. ANTIBIOTICS FREQUENTLY GIVEN TO NEONATES WITH SEPSIS

Drug	Dosage	Route	Expiration after Mixing	Comment
Ampicillin	50–200 mg./kg./day every 6–12 hours*	IV or IM	1 hour	Against certain gram-negative organisms, along with kanamycin; initial drug used
Carbenicillin	200–400 mg./kg./day every 2–8 hours*	IV only	72 hours	Used only for *Pseudomonas* in newborn; alters platelet function
Gentamicin	3–7.5 mg./kg./day* every 8–12 hours	IM	Indefinite	Against staphylococci and resistant gram-negative organisms
Kanamycin	15 mg./kg./day* every 8–12 hours	IM	Indefinite	Against gram-negative organisms, except *Pseudomonas*, not used more than 12 days; potentially ototoxic and nephrotoxic
Nafcillin	100–200 mg./kg./day every 6–8 hours	IV or IM	48 hours	Nephrotoxic; watch for hematuria
Penicillin G	100,000–200,000 units/kg./day every 8–12 hours	IV or IM	72 hours	Against gram-positive organisms
Polymyxin	2–2.5 mg./kg./day every 6 hours	Deep IM		Most effective agent against *Pseudomonas*; nephrotoxic

*Intervals less frequent in preterm infants.

infant from every other infant in the nursery. Babies with sepsis may be isolated in separate rooms as well, but never where they cannot be closely observed, for they are usually very sick. A septic baby in a normal term nursery should be transferred to a high risk nursery to protect other healthy infants as well as to ensure him the special care he needs.

In addition to the supportive treatment that all sick newborns need, babies with sepsis receive parenteral antibiotics. Because drugs are excreted more slowly by the immature kidneys of newborns, blood levels of antibiotics remain high for a longer period of time than in older children and adults. Therefore, a 12-hour schedule is usually satisfactory. Dosage is calculated on the basis of body weight. Antibiotics commonly used in the care of newborns are listed in Table 23–13.

Four antibiotics have been found to be highly toxic to newborn infants: the sulfa drugs, tetracycline, chloramphenicol, and potassium penicillin. The sulfas compete with bilirubin for albumin-binding sites and can thus cause kernicterus and death at levels of serum bilirubin that would generally be considered safe. Tetracycline inhibits the linear growth of infants because it is deposited in the growing epiphyses and also causes permanent yellow-green staining of the enamel of the baby teeth (as does the ingestion of tetracy-

cline by the mother during late pregnancy). Chloramphenicol, because it is poorly excreted by newborns, can lead to sudden collapse and death. This is known as the "gray baby" syndrome. Potassium penicillin can cause heart block in infants.

Parents must receive careful explanations when sepsis is suspected or proved. They need to understand why their baby has been moved from the regular nursery, if this is the case, and what special care is being given to him.

Sensory Needs of Preterm Infants: The Role of Stimulation

The issue of sensory stimulation for preterm infants has been addressed in a number of studies (Table 23–14). In these studies, weight gain is present in the stimulated infant in all instances where weight is measured, although in one study[47] the difference is only slight. This finding is the converse of the finding in studies of deprivation dwarfism (i.e., infants who are not stimulated fail to thrive). Rausch[48] suggests that tactile-kinesthetic stimulation improves weight gain because of vagal stimulation, which promotes peristalsis and the subsequent expulsion of waste products, decreases gastric retention, decreases abdominal

Table 23–14. SENSORY STIMULATION IN PRETERM INFANTS

Type of Stimulation	Population	Results	Study
"Handling"	Infants weighing less than 1500 grams	More rapid regain of birth weight; improved development at 7–8 months in handled infants	Solkoff et al., 1969
"Handling"	Infants weighing 1000 to 2000 grams	Slight differences in weight gain; higher developmental scores at 2.4 and 6 months in handled infants	Powell, 1974
Rocking waterbeds; auditory stimuli	Infants less than 34 weeks' gestation	Stimulated weight infants gained more weight, increased head size and biparietal diameter	Kramer and Pierpont, 1976
Auditory	Infants 28 to 32 weeks' gestational age	Enhanced development in stimulated infants	Katz, 1971
Tactile Kinesthetic	Infants less than 36 weeks' gestational age	Less initial weight loss; improved weight gain in stimulated infants	White and Labarba, 1975
Visual Tactile Kinesthetic	Infants weighing 1300–1800 grams	Greater weight increase at 4 weeks; enhanced development at 4 weeks, 1 year in stimulated infants	Scarr-Salapatek and Williams, 1973
Tactile Kinesthetic	Infants weighing 1000–2000 grams	Increased weight gain, formula intake, and frequency of stooling in stimulated infants	Rausch, 1981

distention, and improves the baby's feeding ability. In Rausch's study, feeding intake was significantly increased in stimulated infants ($p < 0.0001$), as was stooling ($p < 0.004$). Since acceleration of growth may be associated with a variety of benefits to the infant including a shortened hospital stay with less separation of infant from parents and siblings, decreased hospital costs, and a decreased opportunity to develop nosocomial (caused by the hospital environment) infection, practices that facilitate such acceleration seem desirable.

The possibility that increased weight gain may also represent increased brain growth may be even more important, since a major long-term goal of nurses who care for preterm infants is the achievement of the infant's genetic potential in terms of intellectual development. In the study that looked at head circumference,[32] head circumference significantly increased in stimulated babies. In each of the three studies in which there was postneonatal follow-up,[47, 55, 58] differences were found in the babies who received specific stimulation when compared with controls.

Further evidence of the effect of stimulation on brain growth comes from animal studies. Rosenzweig, Bennett, and Diamond[52] reported a series of experiments, spanning more than two decades, in which they found that the cortex in rats increased in weight quite readily in response to a stimulating environment, although the weight of the rest of the brain changed very little (see Wallace[61] for a review of these studies).

In considering the advantages of sensory stimulation, it is equally important to recognize that sensory overload is also a distinct possibility (see Nursing Care Plan 23–2). Preterm infants appear to be less organized in their response to stimuli and less able to shut out stimuli. The care given to a preterm infant in itself frequently overwhelms the baby's ability to cope. The baby's physiologic response to overstimulation may include color change and even bradycardia and apnea. Continuous monitoring of tc pO_2 (see above) has shown that infants with severe RDS will have lowered PaO_2 when handled. Both the advantages and disadvantages of stimulation must be considered in relation to nursing care.

Tactile and Kinesthetic-Vestibular Stimulation

Touch, so important to the development of term infants, also appears to be significant for preterm babies. Both animal research and observations of human infants who have not been touched have shown that there are differences in the behavior of these babies when they are compared with babies who receive normal mothering. The significance of touch for both parents and babies is discussed in Chapter 28.

Preterm infants are certainly touched frequently, but what is the quality of the touch they receive? Is it only to hold them while capillary blood is extracted from a heel or an intravenous needle is placed in the hand or scalp? Is time provided for gentle stroking and caressing?

Encouraging parents to stroke their infants gently not only provides tactile stimulation but increases opportunities for closeness between parents and infants. When parents cannot be present, stroking needs must be met by the nursing staff. Combining stroking with feeding periods is one way of ensuring the stimulation of babies who are fed, because feedings in special and intensive care nurseries are usually as frequent as every 3 hours and are evenly spaced throughout the 24-hour period. Special care must be taken to meet the needs of babies who are NPO. Sammons[53] suggests that when infants are problem feeders they should have minimal social interaction during feeding and stimuli other than those directly associated with feeding should be reserved for post- or between-feeding periods. Careful observation of each infant, especially by a primary nurse who comes to know a particular baby's patterns of response, is the best guide to care for that baby.

For babies who remain in the nursery past 40 weeks' gestation, tactile stimulation can include objects of different textures, such as a washcloth, a smooth piece of material, or the smooth feel of a tongue blade.

Kinesthetic stimulation is provided by changing the baby's position frequently if he must remain in bed (e.g., the infant who has an endotracheal tube or nasal CPAP). Position changes should not be sudden.

Infants who can be removed from their beds may be rocked and carried about. In some nurseries infants who can be out of bed are carried about in cloth infant carriers, similar to those many mothers use at home. The carrier should be designed so that the infant's head is always supported.

Auditory Stimulation

In considering auditory stimulation both the negative effects of sounds that are part of the infant's environment as well as the need to provide auditory stimulation must be examined. An environmental sound of particular concern is the noise produced by the motor of the incubator. Although there are other sounds in the infant's home environment that are as loud, exposure to these sounds is almost never constant over a 24-hour period, day after day. Research is needed to assess the effect of this constant sound on infant hearing and behavior. Sudden loud noises, such as slamming the door of the incubator or dropping equipment, are probably stressful and should be avoided.

Given the evidence that preterm infants attend to voices and that their development and behavior is thereby affected, talking to infants and encouraging parents to talk to them should be a specific part of the nursing care plan (Nursing Care Plan 23–2). Sometimes parents may feel self-conscious about talking aloud to their infants in front of other people. Others feel it would be "silly" to talk to a tiny baby who may give no visible sign of response. Working class parents may express this view more frequently than middle class parents.[59] The model nurses provide by talking to each infant as they care for him and the encouragement they give to mothers and fathers can help parents overcome these barriers. Moreover, the habit of talking to their baby, begun in the intensive care nursery, may encourage more verbal behavior after discharge, behavior that many developmentalists feel is of value to long-term cognitive development.

Visual Stimulation

Although no studies have examined the effect of visual stimuli alone on the subsequent development of preterm infants, something is known about the visual preferences of term and preterm infants.

1. Infants see objects best that are 7 to 9 inches from their face.[13]
2. Preterm infants will attend to a checkerboard design placed on the side of the incubator.[13]
3. Faces promote visual attention.[35]
4. The ventro-ventral position (i.e., the position in which the baby is held to one's shoulder to burp) stimulates visual orientation.[30]

Visual stimulation may be provided by cutouts (placed in the round doors and on the inside of the top of the incubator or on the sides of an open bed) to provide an interesting environment for the baby. At the University of Virginia, where research has been conducted in preterm stimulation, cutouts of checkerboards and faces are used.[60] Because stimuli that are constantly present may cease to stimulate (due to habituation), a change in pictures seems advisable for the infant who spends a long time in the nursery.

Mobiles can be useful if they are appropriate. In general, a homemade mobile is a better visual stimulus than a commercial mobile. Most commercial mobiles are attractive to adults who view them at their own eye level and from the side. If we were to lie on our backs and look up at a commercial mobile from the bottom, we would find the view from beneath very uninteresting. Mobiles hung above the bed should be no more than 7 to 9 inches away from the baby's eyes. A mobile that the baby will view from the side should be the same distance from his eyes, but the orientation of the design should be different. Encouraging parents to construct simple mobiles of construction paper and string not only involves them in their baby's care but also reinforces the principle that they needn't buy expensive toys for their infants; the simple toys they construct are still the best.

The human face is probably the best visual stimulus of all. By letting the parents know that their faces, and their voices, are important to their baby's development involves them in his care. Nurses can assure them, "He may not look at you each time you speak to him, but he will come to know your voice and face." When a face is the visual stimulus, it should confront the baby's face. Infants appear to be very attracted to the eyes of another, and eye-to-eye contact is important for parental attachment.

Special consideration must be given to the baby who is receiving phototherapy because his eyes are covered to protect them from the light. Term babies receiving phototherapy usually have their eyes uncovered at feeding time, so there are fairly frequent opportunities for visual stimulation. Preterm babies, however, may be receiving continuous feedings and may have their eyes covered throughout the day if there is no plan for visual stimulation.

Protection from Overstimulation

Equally as important as providing stimulation is the protection of the baby from overstimulation. Some ways in which this can be achieved include the following:

1. Avoid sudden stimulation, such as loud noises, and abrupt postural change.
2. Plan care to allow for periods of sleep between periods of activity.
3. If possible, provide periods of diminished light to help the baby develop sleep-wake rhythms. This may be accomplished by covering a part of an incubator with a blanket periodically. By leaving a part of the baby uncovered and monitors attached the baby can still be closely observed.
4. Watch for signs of overstimulation. Overstimulation may be reflected by color change,

disorganized motor activity, instability in heart and respiratory rate, decreasing PaO_2, apnea, or bradycardia.

The relationship between active involvement with the baby and the time of feeding is important. Sammons[53] notes that overstimulation prior to feeding leads to poor sucking, decreased gastrointestinal motility, and vomiting or spitting. However, feeding is frequently followed by a period of sleep, and disturbing that pattern may also be distressing to the baby. Again, the responses of an individual infant may be the best indication of the pattern of intervention that best suits that baby's needs.

Planning the Preterm Infant's Discharge

As with every patient who enters the hospital, discharge planning begins at the time of admission. In the case of the preterm infant, or any high risk baby who has been separated from his parents, this is particularly important because the extent to which we are able to facilitate attachment in the days immediately following birth will be a significant factor in ensuring that the baby is welcomed at home at the time of discharge, which may be weeks or even months later. Moreover, even when initial attachment is achieved successfully, the long period of hospitalization, which may be at a medical center many miles from the parents' home, may strain the bonds. We need to keep good records of the frequency of parental visits and telephone calls, to check out the reasons when they do not occur, and to work actively to maintain bonds between parents and their babies (Chapter 28). Otherwise, the time for going home may arrive with very little attachment between parent and baby (see Nursing Care Plan 23–10).

A home visit by a public health nurse, working in close communication with the hospital, is very important before the baby is discharged. The community nurse's report to the hospital about the physical environment of the home, the preparations that have been made for the baby, and the feelings of the family is significant. If the home is found inadequate in one or more aspects, discharge may be delayed until either community or hospital nurses can help the family to better prepare for the baby. On the other hand, a baby may be discharged somewhat earlier into a home that is well prepared to care for him.

It is desirable for parents to take an increasingly greater role in the care of their baby throughout his hospitalization. In this way they will be more comfortable and confident in caring for him at home. If this is not possible throughout the period of hospitalization, perhaps because of the distance the parents live from the hospital or because of other small children in the home who cannot be left alone each day, there must be ample opportunity in the days preceding discharge for the parents to become acquainted with their baby—to feed, hold, bathe, and dress him and to understand his communication with them.

The ability of the baby to maintain his body temperature at 97.8°F. (36.5°C.) in an open bed is necessary before he can be discharged. He needs to be moved to an open bed several days before the discharge is anticipated. In addition, he must be able to gain weight while he is in the open bed. If he maintains temperature but is unable to gain weight, he is probably using too many calories for temperature control and needs to be returned to the warmer environment of the incubator somewhat longer. Usually a baby is able to maintain his temperature at about 36 to 38 weeks of gestational age and about 1800 to 2000 grams of weight.

Many parents find this waiting period difficult. Once their baby is no longer critically ill and is beginning to gain weight, they want to take him home with them right away. Sometimes it helps them to gain perspective if we ask them what their expected date of delivery was. That date may be a relatively realistic one on which they can expect to take their baby home.

As the day for discharge approaches, parents need the opportunity to discuss with nurses what the first days and weeks at home will be like. Many parents are very anxious about having the sole responsibility for a baby who has been cared for by so many persons. The baby will often respond to a change in environment by being unusually fussy, or by changes in eating and sleeping patterns. If parents know beforehand that this is not unusual they are less likely to allow these changes to further increase their anxiety and to diminish their feeling of competence as parents. As described in Chapter 22 in relation to parents of healthy term infants, a telephone link with the hospital and a telephone call from the hospital within 1 to 2 days following discharge can smooth the transition.

Parents need to know that their baby's behavior and development will vary from that of a term infant in the early months at home. Their baby even looks different, and sometimes people, even strangers, will comment thoughtlessly, "He's very small for 6 months," or "Isn't she sitting up yet?" Preparing parents for these

Nursing Care Plan 23–10. Planning Discharge of the High Risk Infant

NURSING GOALS: To ensure that both infant and parents are prepared for discharge from the hospital.

OBJECTIVE:

At the time of discharge the infant will:
1. Be gaining weight while maintaining body temperature in an environmental temperature of approximately 70°F. (22°C.)
2. Have health care needs resolved or stabilized

The parents will:
1. Be able to provide the care required by their baby, including bathing, feeding, stimulation, administration of prescribed medicines, and performance of special treatments.
2. Show evidence of attachment.
3. Anticipate variations in development.
4. Provide home environment adequate for infant's needs.
5. Have a plan for follow-up care and know how to get advice or information at any time of day or night.
6. Be aware of support groups available in community. (e.g., Parents of Prematures, Mothers of Twins, Spina Bifida Association, Ostomy Association)

ASSESSMENT	POTENTIAL NURSING DIAGNOSIS	NURSING INTERVENTION	COMMENTS/RATIONALE
		Infant	
1. Daily weight gain of approximately 30 grams	Inadequate weight gain	Delay discharge until criteria are met.	Infant may be using calories to maintain temperature, thus compromising weight gain.
2. Maintenance of body temperature at room temperature (70°F., 22°C.)	Inability to maintain temperature		
3. Apneic episodes	At risk for apnea	Delay discharge or provide apnea monitor. Instruct parents in use of monitor. Teach them infant CPR; provide emergency phone numbers.	
		Parents	
1. Assess who will provide care to infant.			In some homes a grandmother, a aunt, or other person may be the primary provider.
2. Assess caregiving by parents or by designated care-giver before discharge.	Lack of knowledge of or skill in infant care (with specific needs indicated)	Provide instruction in needed area; have parents or designated care-giver provide care while baby is in nursery until care is satisfactory and care-giver is comfortable in performance.	
a. Bathing (cord and circumcision care if applicable)			
b. Use of desired method of feeding (breast, bottle, gastrostomy)			

Assessment	Nursing Diagnosis	Intervention
c. Verbalization of desired effects and side effects of medications d. Administration of medications e. Performance of required treatments (e.g., ostomy care) f. Temperature assessment and thermometer reading 3. Assess knowledge of and need for information about: a. Safety (home and car) b. Signs and symptoms of illness c. Need for immunization and time for first immunization d. Sibling behavior, reactions	Need for specific information	Provide required information; refer to appropriate infant auto seat program if available. Discuss sibling reactions to infant, including regressive behavior, possible anger, need to feel secure about parents' love and attention. Help parents to consider ways of supporting sibling as well as new infant. Provide opportunities for siblings' visits in hospital.
4. Assess attachment behavior: a. Eye contact b. Touching and holding c. Frequency of visiting or phone calls d. Verbalizations about infant	Lag in attachment	Provide opportunities for attachment in nursery. Encourage ventilation of feelings about infant. Contact mothers who do not call or visit. Initiate public health visit before discharge.
5. Assess support system: a. Marital status b. Others in the home c. Other siblings	Lack of support system	Help parents identify sources of support appropriate to needs (e.g., public health nurse, community groups or agencies, Parents of Prematures, Mothers of Twins).
6. Assess parents' knowledge of variations in infant development that are relevant. 7. Assess parents' ability to provide appropriate stimulation.	Need for information about relevant variations in infant development Need for information about appropriate stimulation, overstimulation.	Provide appropriate information, for example: 1. Help parents recognize signs of development in their infant rather than comparing him with others. 2. Help parents recognize that there

Continued on following page

Nursing Care Plan 23–10. Planning Discharge of the High Risk Infant *(Continued)*

ASSESSMENT	POTENTIAL NURSING DIAGNOSIS	NURSING INTERVENTION	COMMENTS/RATIONALE
	Parents *(Continued)*		
8. Assess home environment.	Inadequacy of home environment; need for modification of home environment for infant's needs	will be developmental lags over the first 18 to 24 months. Hospital nurse: public health referral for assessment of environment. Public health nurse assessment: 1. Water, sanitation, refrigeration, heating, screening, etc. 2. Number of persons per number of rooms 3. Number and age of siblings and other children in home Special care will be required to meet infant's needs in overcrowded environment and home with many young children. 4. Provision for basic infant needs (e.g., sleeping, bathing, feeding) 5. Provision for special needs of infant 6. Other environmental characteristics relevant to infant care	
9. Assess plan for continuing care.	Need for continuing care	Following assessment: ensure relationship between teaching and family environment (don't assume that home has running water, heat controlled by thermostat, etc.) Provide family with information about alternatives available for continuing care; be sure that plan is made prior to discharge. Provide parents with emergency phone numbers, appointment. Provide information about community support groups. Refer to public health nurse and when appropriate to other agencies.	

possibilities can alleviate some of the distress of a difficult situation. Nurses can encourage parents to recognize their baby's signs of development—even small signs such as the growth of hair or nails—rather than to compare their baby with others. By 18 to 24 months of age most preterm infants look and behave like most other children.

All infants need a "health-care home": a nurse practitioner, physician, or clinic who will provide health care for the baby. This is particularly true of preterm infants, and some mechanisms of referral and follow-up should ensure that these babies are not "lost" from the health-care system.

Additional support is available in some communities through groups of parents of premature infants. The opportunity to share fears and concerns with parents who have had similar experiences is very meaningful to many parents.

Postterm Infants

In approximately 5 per cent of pregnancies gestation is greater than 42 weeks. Infants born after 42 weeks' gestation, however, account for 15 per cent of perinatal mortality. Signs in the newborn that indicate postmaturity are related to the length of gestation and changes in the placenta and vernix when pregnancy is prolonged.

As gestation progresses beyond term, the fetus continues to advance in development. Hair and nails grow, sometimes so long that they may curve over the tips of the fingers and toes. The baby may be very "bright-eyed" and alert. Vernix is reduced, and the protective effect of vernix is lost. At birth the baby's skin may appear wrinkled and macerated; later, as it dries, the skin is frequently cracked and peeling ("parchmentlike") (Fig. 23–23). At times the skin may appear pale and white. Skin may hang loosely because fat and muscle tissue is reduced secondary to reduced placental nutrition postterm. Placental insufficiency also reduces fetal oxygenation; as a result the baby may be meconium-stained. Yellow meconium indicates long-term staining; green meconium is of recent origin. Polycythemia occurs because reduced oxygenation in the fetus causes increased red blood cell production (see also Nursing Care Plan 23–11).

Postterm infants are at risk for a number of potential problems (Table 23–15), but the risk is not equally high with all postterm infants. Alfonso and Harris[1] note groups of mothers in

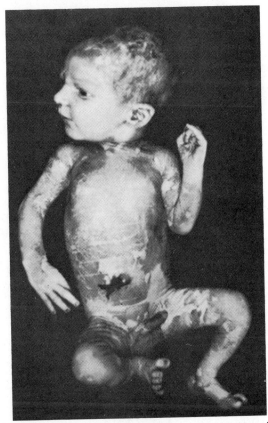

Figure 23–23. Placental dysfunction syndrome, stage III. Note long, thin infant with loose, peeling, parchment-like skin, alert expression, staining of skin and nails. (From Clifford: *Advances in Pediatrics.* Vol. 9. Chicago, Year Book Medical Publishers, Inc., 1957.)

whom the postterm pregnancy is most likely to produce adverse outcome: primigravidas (especially primigravidas over 35 years old), mothers with postterm pre-eclampsia, and mothers with prolonged labor. Risk is increased when fetal heart rate monitoring or the presence of meconium indicates fetal distress during labor.

When the baby is received into the nursery all of these factors must be assessed and noted on the record. Postterm complications are also increased when the baby is small for gestational age (SGA) or large for gestational age (LGA), or has a major congenital anomaly.

Infants Who Are Small for Gestational Age

About one-third of all low birth weight babies are preterm, term, or postterm and small for gestational age (SGA) rather than preterm and appropriate for gestational age (AGA). By

Nursing Care Plan 23–11.   Care of the Postterm Infant

NURSING GOALS: To anticipate the delivery of a postterm infant.
To meet the unique needs of the postterm infant.

OBJECTIVES: To ensure optimal growth and development of the postterm infant:

1. Infants at risk of being postterm will be identified prior to birth.
2. The fetus will be assessed during labor.
3. Signs of postmaturity will be identified.
4. Complications of postmaturity will be corrected.
5. Parents will understand the unique characteristics of their infant.
6. Parents will be supported to enhance attachment and caregiving activities and to integrate the baby into the family.

ASSESSMENT	POTENTIAL NURSING DIAGNOSIS	NURSING INTERVENTION	COMMENTS/RATIONALE
1. Identify risk factors for postmaturity in maternal history: a. Prolonged gestation assessed by maternal EDC b. Primigravida over 35 c. Postterm with pre-eclampsia (pregnancy-individual hypertension) d. Prolonged labor e. Meconium-stained amniotic fluid	At risk for neonatal complications related to prolonged gestation	Anticipate possible complications to fetus or newborn. Frequent assessment of mother and fetus prior to labor needed. Possible medical induction of labor (Nursing Care Plan 19–1)	
2. Fetal neonatal respiratory distress a. Late or variable decelerations b. Meconium staining of amniotic fluid c. Difficulty in initiating respirations	At risk for fetal or neonatal asphyxia or respiratory distress related to placental insufficiency (aspiration pneumonia), atelectasis, pneumothorax, or pneumomediastinum	Anticipate possible fetal and neonatal respiratory distress Use fetal monitor during labor (see Nursing Care Plan 18–1) Position mother for maximum oxygenation during labor. Be prepared to resuscitate newborn (adequate personnel, equipment ready; see Nursing Care Plan 23–1) Neonatal respiratory distress (see Nursing Care Plan 23–4)	Placental insufficiency is the basis of fetal and neonatal respiratory distress.

Assessment	Nursing Diagnosis	Intervention	Rationale
3. Assess gestational age. Compare gestational age with weight, length, head circumference.	Postterm infant Infant risk of complications because postterm and SGA or LGA	See Nursing Care Plans 23–13 and 23–12 for SGA and LGA infants if appropriate.	Postterm infant has a gestational age of 42 weeks or more. Risk of complications increases when the infant is postterm and SGA or LGA. Not all postterm infants have symptoms of postmaturity.
4. Physical assessment for characteristics of postmaturity: a. Long finger- and toenails b. Bright-eyed alert look c. Diminished vernix d. Wrinkled, macerated skin (shortly after delivery) e. Cracked and peeling "parchmentlike" skin f. Reduced subcutaneous tissue and muscle mass g. Congenital anomalies		Provide supportive care. Explain infant characteristics to parents; provide opportunities for questions. Trim nails or cover hands with mitts if nails are long to prevent self-inflicted scratches. Limit bathing if there are large amounts of dry skin. Protect skin (use sheepskin, position changes; avoid use of tape).	
5. Laboratory assessment for: a. Polycythemia (hematocrit over 60 per cent) b. Hyperbilirubinemia (see Nursing Care Plan 23–8 for criteria) c. Hypoglycemia (Dextrostix, biochemical evaluation) d. Hypocalcemia (less than 7 mg. per dl.) serum calcium; observe for tremors)	At risk for complications related to postmaturity	Small quantities of blood may be withdrawn and replaced with albumin by physician. See Nursing Care Plan 23–8. Initiate early oral feeding or IV fluids. Provide oral or intravenous calcium as ordered.	Many complications of postmaturity are secondary to insufficiency of postterm placenta. Hypocalcemia is secondary to bicarbonate treatment for acidosis secondary to respiratory distress.
6. Parents' response and understanding if infant is ill	Parents' need for information about infant's condition. Parents need to express fears and other feelings.	Provide parents with explanations and opportunities for questions and expression of feelings and concern.	
7. Parent–infant attachment (see Nursing Care Plan 22–1 and 28–1)	Lag in attachment	If complications limit parent–infant interaction, facilitate interaction (see Nursing Care Plan 28–1).	
8. Discharge planning (see Nursing Care Plan 23–10)	Need for infant health care Need for specialized care because of (specific factor)	Provide information about sources of health care. Help family arrange appointments if necessary. Refer to community health nurse.	Not all postterm infants have complications.

Table 23–15. POSTTERM INFANTS: NURSING PROBLEMS

Potential Problems	Physiologic Basis	Nursing Action
Fetal or neonatal asphyxia or respiratory depression	Placental insufficiency	Anticipate need for resuscitation; observe for respiratory distress
Meconium aspiration	Placental insufficiency	Anticipate need for resuscitation; careful observation for respiratory distress
Polycythemia	Placental insufficiency	Assess hematocrit; hematocrit greater than 60 per cent a concern
Hyperbilirubinemia	Polycythemia Bruising	Assess bilirubin Observe infant
Hypoglycemia	Placental insufficiency	Assess blood glucose Intravenous fluids and/or early feeding; observe for tremors
Hypocalcemia	Hypoxia; secondary to bicarbonate treatment of acidosis	Assess serum calcium; observe for tremors
Congenital anomalies		Careful assessment of infant

definition, an infant with a birth weight below the tenth percentile for age is SGA (Fig. 23–24).

Several factors appear to be related to the low birth weight of these babies, including intrauterine malnutrition, maternal smoking, infection, and congenital anomalies (see also Nursing Care Plan 23–12).

The importance of diet to a pregnant mother has already been discussed in the section on prenatal care. Nutritional deprivation seems to influence the growth of the placenta, which in turn affects the development of the fetus. There is some evidence that brain growth is

also impaired in SGA infants. Studies of infants born in Holland during the last months of World War II, a time of severe food shortages, and also in Japan, suggest that food deprivation during the last weeks of pregnancy affected the newborn's weight more significantly than did deprivation earlier in pregnancy. Maternal nutrition may be adequate or even good, but if placental transport of nutrients and oxygen is inadequate, the baby will be small for gestational age. Note in Tables 23–15 and 23–17 that many of the potential problems of the SGA infant are similar to potential problems of the postterm infant; this

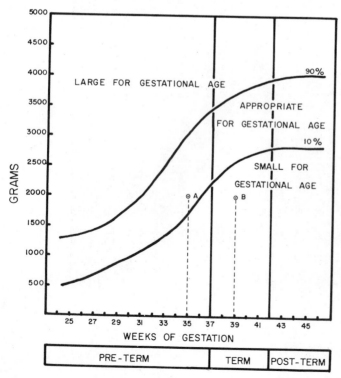

Figure 23–24. The birth weights of liveborn singleton Caucasian infants at gestational ages from 24 to 42 weeks. (From Battaglia and Lubchenco: *Journal of Pediatrics,* 71:159, 1967.)

Nursing Care Plan 23–12. Infant Small for Gestational Age (SGA)

NURSING GOALS: To identify an infant as small for gestational age. To meet the unique nursing needs of small-for-gestational-age infants.

OBJECTIVES:

To ensure optimal growth and development of SGA infants:
1. Infants at risk of being SGA will be identified prior to birth if possible.
2. Respirations will be initiated and maintained.
3. Central nervous system damage will be prevented.
4. Adequate nutrition will be provided in a manner commensurate with gestational age and health status.
5. Possible causes such as intrauterine infection/or congenital malformation will be identified.
6. Sequelae of polycythemia will be prevented.
7. Iatrogenic complications will be prevented.

Parents will:
1. Express feelings related to infant's illness.
2. Show evidence of attachment to their infant.
3. Demonstrate ability to care for their infant.
4. Integrate the baby into their family.

ASSESSMENT	POTENTIAL NURSING DIAGNOSIS	NURSING INTERVENTION	COMMENTS/RATIONALE
1. Identify risk factors from maternal health history. a. Intrauterine malnutrition secondary to pregnancy-induced hypertension, infant of diabetic mother class D or above, etc. b. Maternal smoking c. Intrauterine infection d. Prenatal suspicion of intrauterine growth retardation (1) Disparity between fundal height and gestational age (2) Disparity between fetal growth (ultrasound) and gestational age	At risk of SGA	Anticipate need for resuscitation at delivery. Early assessment of gestational age in relation to weight, length, head circumference.	Infants with weight below the 10th percentile for age are SGA.
2. Assess gestational age. Compare gestational age with weight, length, and head circumference.	SGA and preterm, term, or postterm infant At risk of complications related to SGA and those related to gestational age if infant is preterm or postterm.		Infant who is SGA may be preterm, term, or postterm.

Continued on following page

Nursing Care Plan 23–12.   Infant Small for Gestational Age (SGA)   (Continued)

3. Assess for problems common to infants who are SGA.

a. Respiratory distress (1) Hypoxia (2) Meconium (3) Pneumothorax	At risk for respiratory distress related to hypoxia, aspiration, or sequelae of resuscitation (pneumothorax)	Anticipate possibility of respiratory distress; be prepared for prompt intervention with oxygen, ventilation as required.	Chronic intrauterine hypoxia from placental insufficiency may cause birth asphyxia.
b. Environmental temperature, infant's temperature	Need for resuscitation at birth At risk of hypothermia related to ratio of large surface area to body mass and lack of subcutaneous tissue	Provide thermoneutral environment.	
c. Hypoglycemia (blood, glucose; observe for traumas)	At risk for hypoglycemia related to placental insufficiency and inadequate glycogen stores At risk of CNS damage related to hypoglycemia	Evaluate with Dextrostix. Provide early feedings and/or intravenous fluids.	
d. Hypocalcemia (Ca less 7 mg. per dl.; serum calcium; observe for tremors)	At risk for hypocalcemia related to hypoxia At risk for hypocalcemia related to bicarbonate therapy	Provide oral or intravenous calcium as ordered.	
e. Polycythemia (hematocrit more than 60 per cent)	Polycythemia related to placental insufficiency	Withdraw blood and administer albumin as ordered.	Polycythemia may result in inadequate circulation in small capillaries, including those of lungs and brain. Small quantities of blood (10 ml.) may be withdrawn and replaced with albumin by physician.
f. Intrauterine infection (TORCH titers may be assessed in mother and infant.)	Possible intrauterine infection	Provide explanation to parents. Protect pregnant personnel (Chapter 8).	Intrauterine infection is one cause of SGA.
g. Careful physical assessment for congenital malformations.	At risk for congenital malformations	Provide care appropriate to specific malformation (Chapter 24). Provide parents with opportunity to discuss malformation, grieve over "imperfect" infant.	Congenital malformation is one cause of SGA.
4. Assess nutrition. Assess feeding capability. Assess daily weight gain, weekly growth in length, head circumference.	Need for gavage feeding Need for parenteral alimentation Growth lag	Provide feedings appropriate to gestational age and health status.	

Assessment	Nursing Diagnosis	Nursing Intervention	Rationale
5. Integument Assess skin for reddened areas, skin breakdown.	At risk for skin breakdown related to diminished subcutaneous tissue and diminished muscle mass. At risk for infection in areas of broken skin	Turn infant frequently. Use soft bedding such as sheepskin. Avoid use of tape as much as possible.	
6. Central nervous system a. Muscle tone b. Tremors, pupil dilatation and reaction c. Irritability d. Reflexes (absent, symmetrical, difficult to elicit)	At risk of CNS damage secondary to hypoglycemia, birth asphyxia	Maintain respirations. Provide adequate glucose.	
7. Sepsis (see Nursing Care Plan 23–9) a. Assess nursery policies for prevention of infection. b. Identify early signs of sepsis.	At risk of sepsis because SGA At risk of sepsis because of intervention	(See Nursing Care Plan 23–9)	
8. Assess degree of sensory stimulation. a. Response to stimuli (attends, quiets, etc.). b. Signs of overstimulation vary with gestational age and infant temperament.	Need for increased stimulation Need for decreased stimulation Inappropriate stimulation Parents need information and modeling about their role in stimulation.		Sensory stimulation will vary with gestational age of infant. Preterm infant (see Nursing Care Plan 23–2) may be overstimulated. More mature infant may be able to habituate and shut out inappropriate stimuli or may show same signs as a preterm infant.
9. Parent–infant attachment (see Nursing Care Plans 22–1 and 28–1)	Lag in parent–infant attachment (see also Nursing Care Plan 28–1)	Promote attachment (see Nursing Care Plans 22–1 and 28–1).	
10. Readiness for discharge a. Infant b. Parents c. Home environment (see Nursing Care Plan 23–10).	Infant unready for discharge because of (specific cause) Parents unready for infant because of (specific cause) Home environment unready for discharge because of (specific cause)	Prepare parents for discharge (see Nursing Care Plan 23–10). Hospital nursing referral to community health nurse in advance of discharge	
11. Continuing assessment following hospital discharge based on individual needs	Need for infant health care Need for specialized care because of (specific cause)	Provide information about sources of health care. Help family arrange appointment if necessary.	

is because placental insufficiency may affect infants in both groups.

Smoking can be statistically correlated with SGA births. In experiments with rabbits it seemed that a constituent of tobacco was at fault, as smoke produced by other sources failed to cause the same effect as the tobacco smoke. Moderate smokers have twice the incidence of SGA infants as nonsmokers; infants of mothers who smoke heavily are three times as likely to be small for gestational age (Chapter 8).

Genetic factors undoubtedly account for some babies who are small for gestational age.

A woman who has delivered one SGA infant is likely to do so in a subsequent pregnancy. Therefore, the relationship between birth weight and gestational age is an important aspect of maternal history in every pregnancy.

Infections that have been demonstrated to cause SGA infants are cytomegalic inclusion disease and rubella.

Mothers who are hypertensive, who have class D through R diabetes mellitus, and who are addicted to heroin tend to produce small babies. Still other variables include certain anomalies of the sex chromosomes, high altitudes, and exposure to x-rays and some drugs.

Table 23–16. NEEDS AND CHARACTERISTICS OF LOW BIRTH WEIGHT INFANTS WITH SIMILAR WEIGHTS BUT VARYING GESTATIONAL AGES

	Preterm Infant, AGA	SGA Infant
Length of gestation	Less than 37 weeks' gestation	28–44 weeks' gestation
Duration of intensive care	Varies in relation to gestational age	Requires major care first 3 to 4 days of life
Mortality rate	Higher mortality than for growth retarded baby of same weight	—
Incidence of anomalies	—	Incidence of major congenital anomalies higher; the greater the degree of growth retardation, the greater the chance of malformation
Initial feeding	—	Susceptible to hypoglycemia; cannot tolerate prolonged fasting
Respiratory distress	Apnea, respiratory distress syndrome principal problems	Asphyxia, aspiration syndrome, pneumothorax principal problems
Maintenance of body temperature	—	Usual tables for neutral thermal environment don't apply; attempt to maintain body temperature between 96.8–97.8°F. (36.0–36.5°C.)
General appearance	Moves and cries less	Alert appearance
Weight gain	Gain is slower than would have normally been expected if had remained in utero	Loses little, if any, weight in the first 24 hours; gains more rapidly than AGA infant of same weight
Liver function	Immature; likely to have hyperbilirubinemia	Appropriate to age; hyperbilirubinemia less likely
Potential mental retardation	—	Greater chance of mental retardation in later life than AGA infant with same birth weight
Feeding	Prior to 32–34 weeks cannot suck and swallow; gastric capacity limited; small amounts of formula at frequent intervals required	Susceptible to hypoglycemia; cannot tolerate prolonged fasting; many SGA infants can nipple-feed when AGA infant of same birth weight cannot, because of being greater than 34 weeks' gestational age
Other problems	—	Polycythemia, occasionally with symptoms

Table 23-17. INFANTS SMALL FOR GESTATIONAL AGE: NURSING PROBLEMS

Potential Problems	Physiologic Basis	Nursing Action
Hypoglycemia	Placental insufficiency Low glycogen stores	Assess blood glucose level; intravenous fluids and/or early feeding; observe for tremors
Hypocalcemia	Hypoxia; bicarbonate treatment of acidosis	Assess serum calcium; observe for tremors
Polycythemia	Placental insufficiency	Assess hematocrit; hematocrit greater than 60 per cent a concern
Hypoxia Meconium aspiration	Placental insufficiency	Anticipate need for resuscitation; observe for respiratory distress
Heat loss	Large surface area, body mass; lack of subcutaneous tissue	Thermoneutral environment
Intrauterine infection	May be the cause of SGA	TORCH titers may be drawn Protection of pregnant personnel
Major malformations		Careful assessment of infant

The smaller a baby is in relation to his age, the more likely the occurrence of congenital malformations. Particularly close inspection and observations of such newborns are therefore necessary.

Table 23-16 compares SGA infants with preterm AGA infants. Table 23-17 summarizers nursing problems of SGA infants.

Infants Who Are Large for Gestational Age

Preterm, term, or postterm infants may be large for gestational age (LGA). By definition, an infant is large for gestational age if birth weight is greater than the 90th percentile (Fig. 23-24). A major problem of the preterm baby who is large for gestational age is that because of his size, his immaturity and the problems associated with it are not recognized readily (Table 23-18). He may, for example, have respiratory distress syndrome or a level of hyperbilirubinemia that might be expected for an infant of his gestational age but is not usually associated with a baby of his size. Because his sucking reflex is appropriate to his age rather than to his size, because his ability to maintain his temperature in an open bed may be poor, and because his muscle tone may be diminished (again appropriate to age but not size), he may be falsely labeled as ill (see Nursing Care Plan 23-13).

For reasons that are unknown, infants with transposition of the great vessels (Chapter 24) tend to be large for gestational age.

Infants of diabetic mothers (IDM), particularly diabetic mothers who have not been in good control during the last trimester of pregnancy, are typically large for gestational age. When delivered at 37 weeks, they may weigh

Text continued on page 794

Table 23-18. INFANTS LARGE FOR GESTATIONAL AGE: NURSING PROBLEMS

Potential Problems	Physiologic Basis	Nursing Action
Hypoglycemia	Infant of diabetic mother (IDM) (see text)	Assess blood glucose Intravenous fluids and/or early feeding Observe for tremors
Hypocalcemia	IDM	Assess serum calcium Observe for tremors
Obstetrical trauma	Delivery of large infant	Assess for bilateral movement, bilateral Moro reflex, central nervous system damage
Polycythemia	Increased RBC formation in IDM	Assess hematocrit; hematocrit greater than 60 per cent a concern
Hyperbilirubinemia	Increased in IDM	Assess bilirubin; observe infant
Respiratory distress syndrome	Delayed lung maturation in IDM	Observe respiratory effort

Nursing Care Plan 23–13.   Infant Large for Gestational Age (LGA)

NURSING GOALS: To identify an infant as large for gestational age. To meet the unique needs of the large-for-gestational-age infant.

OBJECTIVES:

To ensure optimal growth and development of LGA infants:
1. Infants at risk of being LGA will be identified prior to birth when possible.
2. A thermoneutral environment will be maintained.
3. Respirations will be initiated and maintained.
4. Sequelae of obstetrical trauma will be identified and the infant will receive appropriate care.
5. The infant of a diabetic mother will be identified and will receive appropriate care.
6. Parents will be supported to enhance attachment and caregiving activities and to integrate the baby into the family.

ASSESSMENT	POTENTIAL NURSING DIAGNOSIS	NURSING INTERVENTION	COMMENTS/RATIONALE

1. Identify risk factors from maternal history.
  a. Maternal diabetes mellitus
  b. Previous delivery of large infant
  c. Suspicion of LGA infant
    (1) Disparity in fundal height and gestational age
    (2) Disparity in fetal growth (ultrasound) and gestational age
	At risk for infant LGA	Anticipate possible cesarean birth. If cesarean birth is decided upon, provide as much information to parents as time permits.	Infants with weight above the 90th percentile for age are LGA.

2. Intrapartum risk factors associated with LGA infant:
  a. Prolonged labor with increased risk of obstetrical trauma (below), fetal hypoxia
  b. Cesarean birth with increased risk of tachypnea, possible blood loss
  c. Breech delivery with increased risk
	At risk for complications related to labor or birth factors	Anticipate possible fetal or neonatal distress; ensure that adequate personnel are present at birth to provide immediate infant care if complications occur.	

3. Assess gestational age. Compare gestational age with weight, length, and head circumference.	LGA and preterm, term, or postterm. At risk of complications related to being LGA and those related to gestational age if preterm or postterm		Infant who is LGA may be preterm, term, or postterm.

4. Obstetrical trauma
  a. Depressed skull fracture
  b. Cephalhematoma
  c. Facial paralysis
	At risk for sequelae of obstetrical trauma
	
	Injury related to infant size
		Feed infant with facial paralysis carefully in upright position. Use eye drops and patch if infant cannot close eyes.	

Assessment	Nursing Diagnosis	Intervention	Rationale
d. Phrenic nerve paralysis (1) Respiratory distress (2) Weak or hoarse cry (3) Failure of abdomen to rise on inspiration		Provide support to parents in feeding infant. Position with head elevated to minimize work of respiration. May need respiratory support (oxygen).	
e. Brachial paralysis, fractured clavicle (1) Asymmetrical movement (2) Asymmetrical Moro reflex		Position for comfort, good body alignment. Assist parents in holding and caring for infant.	
f. Trauma to soft tissue (bruising, breaks in skin)			Infants with bruising or large cephalhematoma are at risk for hyperbilirubinemia as RBCs break down and release bilirubin (see Nursing Care Plan 23–8).
g. Hemorrhage (hematocrit, hemoglobin, large cephalhematoma)			
5. Identify infants of diabetic mothers (see Nursing Care Plan 23–14).			
6. Assess infant's temperature and environmental temperature.	Hypothermia Hyperthermia At increased risk of hyperthermia due to increased amounts of fatty tissue		Hyperthermia as well as hypothermia increases metabolic needs. Not all LGA infants will have complications.
7. Parents' response if infant is ill Parent-infant attachment (see Nursing Care Plan 28–1)	Parents' need for information about infant's condition Parents need to express fears and other feelings. Lag in attachment	Provide parents with explanations and opportunities for questions and expressions of feelings and concerns. Facilitate parent–infant interaction (see Nursing Care Plan 28–1).	
8. Discharge planning (see Nursing Care Plan 23–10)	Need for infant health care Need for specialized care because of (specific factor)	Provide information about sources of health care. Help family arrange appointments if necessary.	
Continuing assessment following hospital discharge is based on individual needs (e.g., infant with facial or brachial paralysis) as well as on general infant health.			

Nursing Care Plan 23–14.   Infant of a Diabetic Mother

NURSING GOALS: To anticipate the delivery of an infant of a diabetic mother.
To meet the unique needs of the infant.
To avoid brain damage secondary to hypoglycemia and other sequelae.
To provide supportive care and education for the parents of an infant of a diabetic mother.

OBJECTIVES: As a result of neonatal care:
1. The infant of a diabetic mother will be identified in the prenatal period.
2. Early assessment of infant's glucose levels and provision of glucose by intravenous fluids or early feeding will be made.
3. Other complications will be recognized and treated.

The diabetic mother and her family will have the opportunity to:
1. Bond with the baby.
2. Participate in the baby's care.
3. Have questions about the special needs of their baby answered.

ASSESSMENT	POTENTIAL NURSING DIAGNOSIS	NURSING INTERVENTION	COMMENTS/RATIONALE
1. Maternal history for: a. Diabetes; note classification b. Pre-eclampsia—eclampsia (including any drugs given mother) c. Results of antepartum fetal testing d. Previous pregnancy outcome	Infant of diabetic mother (IDM) Parental anxiety over pregnancy outcome	Anticipate need for early feeding or IV glucose. Plan to meet physiologic needs of infant for assessment of glucose levels and provision of glucose during initial acquinatance period. Infant may need to go directly to nursery following delivery. Support parents and explain reason for separation prior to delivery. Provide opportunity for bonding as soon as possible.	A loss in a previous pregnancy (stillbirth, miscarriage) will probably influence interaction with this baby.
2. Gestational age Relationship of gestational age to weight, length, and head circumference			
3. Blood glucose levels Dextrostix Laboratory analysis Observe for tremors.	At risk of hypoglycemia related to IDM	Early feeding or intravenous fluids may be necessary.	
4. Serum calcium Observe for tremors.	At risk of hypocalcemia related to IDM	Administer calcium per physician's order (usually when calcium is less than 7 mg. per dl.).	Precautions when administering IV calcium: 1. Infant should have cardiac monitor attached. 2. Give solution slowly. 3. Possible severe tissue necrosis; careful assessment IV site; discontinue at first sign of infiltration. 4. Don't mix solution in IV line with $NaHCO_3$; it will form a precipitate calcium carbonate.

Assessment	Nursing Diagnosis	Intervention
5. Potential obstetrical trauma if LGA (see Nursing Care Plan 23–13).	At risk of obstetrical trauma related to LGA	5. Avoid umbilical vein and artery; may cause liver necrosis (umbilical vein injection) and necrosis of the bowel with possible NEC (umbilical artery injection).
6. Hematocrit greater than 60 indicates polycythemia.	At risk of polycythemia related to IDM	IDM have increased RBC formation, leading to polycythemia. Polycythemia may lead to respiratory distress, congestive heart failure, CNS symptoms, thrombosis, hyperbilirubinemia.
7. Bilirubin	At risk of hyperbilirubinemia related to IDM or polycythemia	See Nursing Care Plan 23–13. Anticipate partial exchange transfusion with fresh frozen plasma or albumin if hematocrit is above 65 per cent and infant has symptoms described here. Anticipate IV fluids. Anticipate possible need for phototherapy. If phototherapy is required, explain reasons to parents; provide opportunity for interaction with lights off and eyes uncovered.

8. Respiratory status
  a. Examine maternal record L/S ratio to indicate lung maturity.
  b. Signs of respiratory distress (see Nursing Care Plan 23–4).
	At risk of respiratory distress syndrome (RDS) related to delayed lung maturation in IDM	Anticipate possible respiratory distress (L/S less than 2–2.5).

9. Careful assessment for congenital anomalies	At risk for congenital anomalies because of maternal diabetes Parental distress or guilt if anomaly is present. Parents' need for knowledge about infant care for their infant	Specific care related to anomaly (Chapter 24) Provide opportunity for parents to express concerns, questions. Explain tests, special treatments (e.g., phototherapy, reason for IV); provide continuing opportunities for questions and expressions of feelings and concerns. Encourage parents to consider and treat baby as normal.
10. Parents' understanding of special needs of their infant in immediate postdelivery period		Mother's feelings about having diabetes may cause her to feel guilty, particularly if baby becomes ill of has congenital anomaly.
11. Parents' interaction with baby as normal infant prior to discharge		In most instances (i.e., unless there are congenital anomalies or severe respiratory distress) infant has no complications following discharge.

9 or 10 pounds. (About 10 per cent of the infants of Classes D through R diabetic mothers are small for gestational age and resemble infants with placental insufficiency). The increased size of the large IDM is due to fat (and not to edema as once believed) produced by a process described below in the discussion of glucose metabolism. Characteristically, the large IDM is fat and red-faced, lying quietly, moving very little, and crying infrequently. Not only the baby but the cord and placenta are frequently oversized (see Nursing Care Plan 23–14).

With very careful control of the mother's diabetes, especially in the last weeks of pregnancy, some diabetic mothers are delivering babies who do not have this classic appearance and who have decreased neonatal mortality as well. Although fetal and neonatal deaths are still higher for the infants of all but Class A diabetic mothers than for infants of nondiabetic mothers, neonatal mortality has decreased from 40 per cent to 10 per cent.[16]

The newborn IDM needs very careful nursing observation in the first hours and days of life. Major potential problems are hypoglycemia, hypocalcemia, hyperbilirubinemia, polycythemia, and respiratory distress syndrome. The incidence of congenital anomalies is also higher in these babies.

About 50 per cent of the infants of diabetic mothers become *hypoglycemic* during the first 6 hours after birth, probably because of the following sequence: Diabetic mothers who are not well controlled are hyperglycemic. The excess sugar, like other nutrients in maternal blood, crosses the placental barrier, causing hyperglycemia in the infant as well. To metabolize this excess sugar, the islets of Langerhans in the fetal pancreas hypertrophy in order to secrete increased amounts of insulin. The sugar is converted to glycogen and stored as excess fat, hence the large size of the baby. When the baby is born, he is removed from the source of his sugar, but his pancreas continues to work overtime for several hours. Thus he becomes hypoglycemic. The more nearly the mother's blood glucose levels can be kept within normal limits during her pregnancy, the less likely her baby is to develop hypoglycemia following delivery. The higher the maternal blood glucose level, the greater the infant's problem may be.

Most of these infants will have a transient hypoglycemia, lasting from 1 to 4 hours, after which blood glucose levels will begin to rise. In a few infants the hypoglycemia will be prolonged and severe.

Monitoring blood glucose levels was discussed earlier in this chapter. Waiting for clinical signs of hypoglycemia to appear (tremors, apnea, cyanosis, limpness, failure to feed well, convulsions) violates standards of good care. Treatment for hypoglycemia is a constant, slow infusion of 10 to 15 per cent glucose. Rapid infusion of 25 to 50 per cent glucose is contraindicated because insulin production is increased as a response, with a subsequent drop in blood glucose levels.

An increased incidence of *hypocalcemia* has been reported in infants of diabetic mothers. Tremors are the most obvious clinical sign. Polycythemia is related to increased intrauterine RBC formation. *Hyperbilirubinemia* at 48 to 72 hours occurs more frequently than in other infants of comparable weight or gestational age.

Respiratory distress syndrome is also increased in babies of Class A through Class C diabetic mothers. Apparently, high levels of insulin produced by the baby interfere with the synthesis of lecithin, which is necessary for lung maturation. In babies of Class D through Class R diabetic mothers, for whom the intrauterine environment is even less favorable, the stress resulting from poor blood supply to the uterus may lead to increased production of steroids and thus to acceleration of lung maturation.

Because infants of diabetic mothers have more fatty tissue than most babies in the nursery, their temperature must be monitored closely if they are in an incubator without a servomechanism, or they will become overheated.

Summary

Gestational age, and disparity between size and gestational age, are major causes of perinatal morbidity and mortality. By no means will every infant who is not delivered at term and is not appropriate for gestational age have all of the complications described in this chapter. The needs of a preterm infant of 34 weeks' gestation will be quite different from the needs of the 27-week-old infant. Not all infants who are postterm will have the symptoms of postmaturity described here. Some large-for-gestational-age infants are the children of large parents and will have no difficulties at all. Yet we must be aware of potential problems in each group of infants in order to protect every baby in the first hours and days of life.

In the next chapter other alterations in health are discussed. It is not uncommon for these variations to be associated with problems in gestational age and size.

REFERENCES

1. Alfonso, D., and Harris, T.: Postterm Pregnancy: Implications for Mother and Infant, Challenge for the Nurse. *JOGN Nursing*, 9(3):139, 1980.

2. Bless, V.: Nursing Care for Infants with Neonatal Necrotizing Enterocolitis. *MCN, 1*:37, 1976.

3. Book, L. Herbst, J., and Steward, D.: Hazards of Calcium Gluconate Therapy in the Newborn Infant. *Journal of Pediatrics*, 92:793, 1978.

4. Boyle, R., and Oh, W.: Respiratory Distress Syndrome. *Clinical Perinatology*, 5(2):293, 1978.

4a. Cagan, J., and Meier, P.: A Discharge Planning Tool for Use with Families of High Risk Infants. *JOGN*, 9:146, 1979.

5. Cremer, R., Perryman, P., and Richards, D.: Influence of Light on Hyperbilirubinemia of Infants. *Lancet*, 1:1094, 1958.

6. Curran, C., and Kachoyeanos, M.: The Effects on Neonates of Two Methods of Chest Physical Therapy, *MCN*, 5(5):309, 1979.

7. Dar, H., Winter, S., and Tal, Y.: Families of Children with Cleft Lips and Palates: Concerns and Counseling. *Developmental Medicine and Child Neurology*, 16:513, 1974.

8. Davis, J. A., and Dobbing, J. (eds.): *Scientific Foundations of Paediatrics*. Philadelphia, W. B. Saunders Co., 1974.

9. Drillien, C.: Abnormal Neurologic Signs in the First Year of Life in Low Birthweight Infants. *Developmental Medicine and Child Neurology*, 14:575, 1973.

10. Dubowitz, L., Levene, M., Morante, A., et al.: Neurological signs in neonatal in traventricular hemorrhage: a correlation with real time ultrasound. *Journal of Pediatrics*, 99:127, 1981.

11. Dulock, H., and Swendsen, L.: *Hypoglycemia in the Newborn*. (Module 2, The First Six Hours of Life.) National Foundation/March of Dimes, 1977.

12. Dunn, D., and Lewis, A. T.: Some Important Aspects of Neonatal Nursing Related to Pulmonary Disease and Family Involvement. *Pediatric Clinics of North America*, 20:481, 1973.

13. Fantz, R.: Pattern Vision in Newborn Infants. *Science*, 140:296, 1963.

14. Fantz, R. L., and Fagan, J. F.: Visual Attention to Size and Number of Pattern Details by Term and Preterm Infants During the First Six Months. *Child Development*, 46:3, 1975.

15. Feigun, R.: The Perinatal Group B Streptococcal Problem: More Questions than Answers. *New England Journal of Medicine*, 294:1063, 1976.

15a. Fisher, D., and Behrman, R.: Resuscitation of the Newborn Infant. *In* Klaus, M., and Fanaroff, A. (eds.): *Care of the High Risk Neonate*. Philadelphia, W. B. Saunders Co., 1973.

16. Fletcher, A. B.: The Infant of the Diabetic Mother. *In* Avery, G. B. (ed.): *Neonatology*. Philadelphia, J. B. Lippincott Co., 1975.

17. Foman, S. J.: *Infant Nutrition*. 2nd Edition. Philadelphia, W. B. Saunders Co., 1974.

18. Gersony, W.: Indomethacin Therapy for Patent Ductus Arteriosus. *Journal of Pediatrics* 91:624, 1977.

19. Gluck, L., and Kulovich, M. V.: Fetal Lung Development: Current Concepts. *Pediatrics Clinics of North America*, 20:367, 1973.

20. Goldstein, G., Chaplin, E., and Maitland, J.: Transient Hydrocephalus in Premature Infants: Treatment by Lumbar Puncture. *Lancet*, 1:512, 1976.

21. Gregory, G. A.: Respiratory Care of Newborn Infants. *Pediatric Clinics of North America*, 19:311, 1971.

22. Gregory, G., Kitterman, J., Phibbs, R., et al.: Treatment of Idiopathic Respiratory Distress Syndrome with Continuous Positive Airway Pressure. *New England Journal of Medicine*, 284:1333, 1971.

23. Haddock, N.: Blood Pressure Monitoring in Neonates. *MCN*, 5:131, 1980.

24. Hubel, D. H., and Wiesel, T. N.: The Period of Susceptibility to the Physiological Effects of Unilateral Eye Closure in Kittens. *Journal of Physiology*, 206:419, 1970.

25. Hutchinson, A., Ross, K., and Russell, G.: The Effect of Posture on Ventilation and Lung Mechanics in Preterm and Light-for-Date Infants. *Pediatrics*, 64(4):429, 1979.

26. Jacobson, S.: Long Term Parenteral Nutrition Following Massive Intestinal Resection. *Nutrition and Metabolism*, 14 (Suppl.): 150, 1972.

27. Kattwinkel, J., Cook, L., Ivey, H., et al.: *Perinatal Continuing Education Program*. Charlottesville, Va., University of Virginia Medical Center, 1979.

28. Katz, V.: Auditory Stimulus and Developmental Behavior of the Preterm Infant. *Nursing Research*, 20:196, 1971.

29. Klaus, M., and Fanaroff, A. (eds.): *Care of the High-Risk Neonate*. 2nd Edition. Philadelphia, W. B. Saunders Co., 1979.

30. Korner, A. F., and Grobstein, R.: Visual Alertness as Related to Soothing in Neonates: Implications for Maternal Stimulation and Early Deprivation. *Child Development*, 37:867, 1966.

31. Korner, A., Kraemer, H., Hoffner, E., et al.: Effects of Waterbed Flotation on Premature Infants: A Pilot Study. *Pediatrics*, 56:361, 1975.

32. Kramer, L., and Pierpont, M.: Rocking Waterbeds and Auditory Stimuli to Enhance Growth of Preterm Infants. *Journal of Pediatrics*, 88:297, 1976.

33. Krugman, S., and Gerson, A. A. (eds.): Infections of the Fetus and the Newborn Infant. *In Progress in Clinical and Biological Research*, Volume II. New York, Alan R. Liss, Inc., 1975.

34. Kuhns, L. R., Bednarek, F. J., Wyman, M. L., et al.: Diagnosis of Pneumothorax or Pneumomediastinum in the Neonate by Transillumination. *Pediatrics*, 56:355, 1975.

35. Lewis, M.: Infants' Responses to Facial Stimuli During the First Year of Life. *Developmental Psychology*, 1:75, 1969.

35a. Lubchenco, L.: The Relationship of Fetal Size to Later Physical Growth of Prematurely Born Children. *American Pediatric Society Abstracts*, 1962, p. 45.

36. Lubchenco, L. O.: *The High Risk Infant*. Philadelphia, W. B. Saunders Co., 1976.

37. Lubchenco, L. O., Delevoria-Papadopoulos, M., Butterfield, L. J., et al.: Long-term Follow-up Studies of Prematurely Born Infants. I. Relationship of Handicaps to Nursery Routines. *Journal of Pediatrics*, 80:501, 1972.

38. Lubchenco, L. O., Delevoria-Papadopoulos, M., and Searls, D.: Long-term Follow-up Studies of Prematurely Born Infants. II. Influence of Birth Weight and Gestational Age on Sequelae. *Journal of Pediatrics*, 80:509, 1972.

39. Lucey, J. F., Wolk, T., Bottogi, J., et al.: A Flux Day—Observations on Factors Influencing the Light Environment of Infants. *Pediatric Research*, 7:169, 1973.

40. Martin, R., Herrell, N., Ruben, D., et al.: Effect of Supine and Prone Positions on Arterial Oxygen Tension in the Preterm Infant. *Pediatrics*, 63:528, 1979.

40a. Martin, R., and Okken, A.: Correlation between transcutaneous and arterial oxygen tension measurements. *In* Klaus, M., and Fanaroff, A. (eds.): *Care of the High Risk Neonate.* Philadelphia, W. B. Saunders Co., 1979.

41. Meier, P.: CPT—Which Method, If Any. *MCN,* 4(5):310, 1979.

42. Moss, A.: What Every Primary Physician Should Know About the Postoperative Cardiac Patient. *Pediatrics, 63*:320, 1979.

42a. Northway, W., Rosan, R., and Porter, D.: Pulmonary Disease Following Respirator Therapy. *New England Journal of Medicine, 276*:357, 1967.

43. Oehler, J.: *Family-Centered Neonatal Nursing Care.* Philadelphia, J. B. Lippincott, 1981.

44. Papile, L., Bernstein, R., Koffler, H., et al.: Nonsurgical Treatment of Acquired Hydrocephalus: Evaluation of Serial Lumbar Puncture (abstract). *Pediatric Research, 12*:554, 1978.

45. Peacock, W., and Hirara, T.: Outcome in Low-Birth-Weight Infants (750 to 1500 Grams): A Report on 164 Cases Managed at Children's Hospital, San Francisco, California. *American Journal of Obstetrics and Gynecology, 140*:165, 1981.

46. Perlstein, P., Edwards, N., and Sutherland, J.: Apnea in Premature Infants and Incubator-Air Temperature Changes. *New England Journal of Medicine, 282*:461, 1970.

47. Powell, L. F.: The Effect of Extra Stimulation and Maternal Involvement on the Development of Low Birth Weight Infants and on Maternal Behavior. *Child Development, 45*:106, 1974.

48. Rausch, P.: Effects of Tactile and Kinesthetic Stimulation on Premature Infants. *JOGN Nursing, 10*:34, 1981.

49. Rickard, K., and Gresham, E.: Nutritional Considerations for the Newborn Requiring Intensive Care. *Journal of the American Dietetic Association, 66*:592, 1975.

50. Robert, M. F., Neff, R. K., Hubbell, J. P., et al.: The Association between Maternal Diabetes and the Respiratory Distress Syndrome. *Pediatric Research, 9*:370, 1975.

51. Robert, M. F., Raymond, K. N., Hubbell, J., et al.: Maternal Diabetes and the Respiratory Distress Syndrome. *New England Journal of Medicine, 294*:357, 1976.

52. Rosenzweig, M., Bennett, E. B., and Diamond, M.: Brain Changes in Response to Experience. *Scientific American, 226*:22, 1972.

53. Sammons, W.: Premature Behavior and the Neonatal Intensive Care Unit Environment. *In* Cloherty, J., and Stark, A. (eds.): *Manual of Neonatal Care.* Boston, Little, Brown & Co., 1980.

54. Sausville, J., Sisson, T., and Berger, D.: Blue Lamps in Phototherapy of Hyperbilirubinemia. *Journal of IES.* 112: 1972.

55. Scarr-Salapatek, S., and Williams, M.: The Effects of Early Stimulation on Low Birth Weight Infants. *Child Development, 44*:94, 1973.

56. Segal, S. (ed.): *Manual for the Transport of High Risk Newborn Infants: Principles, Policies, Equipment, Techniques.* Vancouver, Canadian Pediatric Society, 1972.

57. Smith, B. T., Giround, C., Robert, M., et al.: Insulin Antagonism of Cortisol Action on Lecithin Synthesis by Cultured Fetal Living Cells. *Journal of Pediatrics, 87*:953, 1975.

58. Solokoff, Y., Yaffe, S., Weintraub, D., et al.: Effects of Handling on Subsequent Development of Premature Infants. *Developmental Psychology, 1*:765, 1969.

59. Tulken, S., and Kagan, J.: Mother-Child Interaction in the First Year of Life. *Child Development, 43*:31, 1972.

60. Van Devender, T., Elder, W., and Hastings, S.: *The EMI-ART High-Risk Nursery Intervention Model.* Charlottesville, University of Virginia Medical Center, 1978.

61. Wallace, P.: Complex Environments: Effects on Brain Development. *Science,* 76, 1974.

62. Warrner, R. A., and Cornblath, M.: Infants of Gestational Diabetic Mothers. *American Journal of Diseases of Children, 117*:678, 1969.

63. Wennberg, R. P., Schwartz, R., and Sweet, A. X.: Early versus Delayed Feeding of Low Birth Weight Infants: Effect on Physiologic Jaundice. *Journal of Pediatrics, 68*:860, 1966.

64. White, J., and Labarba, R.: The Effects of Tactile and Kinesthetic Stimulation on Neonatal Development in the Premature Infant. *Developmental Psychology, 9*:569, 1976.

65. Wu, P., and Hodgmen, J.: Insensible Water Loss in Preterm Infants. *Pediatrics, 54*:704, 1974.

24

Care of the High Risk Newborn: Problems Related to Short- and Long-Term Alterations in Health Status

In addition to problems related to gestational age and size, newborns may have alterations in health status due to congenital anomalies, genetic errors, maternal illness, or problems of the intrapartum period. Some of these problems will be resolved during the first weeks of life; others will require special care for months and years. In this chapter the focus is on neonatal care only. Pediatric nursing texts (e.g., Tackett and Hunsberger, 1981; Marlow, 1977) provide information about infant and parental needs and nursing intervention needed past the neonatal period.

Congenital Anomalies

The embryologic basis of a number of congenital anomalies is discussed in Chapter 7. Assessment of specific anomalies is discussed in Chapter 21 in the section on newborn assessment. The needs of parents of infants with congenital anomalies are discussed in Chapter 28.

Some congenital anomalies are incompatible with or a serious threat to life itself. Others will be corrected in early infancy and will affect the infant only minimally after that time. Some anomalies are not correctable, and the task of the infant and his family becomes one of coping with the condition.

One way to differentiate congenital anomalies is to separate them into those that are reversible and those that are not. The dividing line is not always clear; some conditions are far more easily reversed than others. Some may be alleviated but not totally reversed. When surgery is necessary, it is frequently delayed for months of even years past birth, and palliative procedures are performed in the neonatal period. In addition to the direct nursing care given to a baby with a congenital anomaly and the emotional support given to parents, nurses teach parents how to care for their infant in special ways appropriate to his needs. This may include special ways of feeding, cast care, the administration of medication (digoxin, for example), or colostomy care.

Special Needs of the Newborn Infant Requiring Surgery

Many congenital anomalies require surgery in the first days of life. Some of the more common conditions that require or benefit from immediate surgical correction are (1) anomalies of the gastrointestinal tract (tracheoesophageal fistula, diaphragmatic hernia, intestinal obstruction, imperforate anus, and omphalocele), (2) skull fracture, (3) bilateral choanal atresia, (4) meningocele and encephalocele, (5) certain congenital heart defects, and (6) certain disorders of the genitourinary tract (patent urachus, obstructions). Regardless of the type of surgery, infants have some common nursing needs prior to and following surgery (see Nursing Care Plan 24–1).

Preoperative Care

The preparation of an infant for surgery involves the same principles of stabilization described in Chapter 23—thermoregulation; provision for respiratory needs and for fluid, electrolytes, and glucose; and acid-base balance. In addition, special needs related to the particular condition must be met.

Even when the surgery is to be performed quickly, the parents should have as thorough an explanation as possible of (1) the reason for surgery, (2) what they can expect the baby to look like following surgery (e.g., will there be an endotracheal tube, a ventilator, a gastrostomy tube?), and (3) whether the baby will be returning to the same nursing unit or another unit. Parents may not attend to much of what they are told initially in the stressful period before their baby's surgery, and much of what was told them initially may have to be repeated. A doll, with chest tubes, IVs, a colostomy, and other equipment attached, can help parents visualize how their baby will look.

Intraoperative Care

The baby should be transported to and from the operating room in a warmed incubator and should remain in his incubator until immediately before the procedure. Operating suites are cold; the effects of cold on newborn infants are described in Chapters 20 and 23. Other measures that may be used to keep the infant in a thermoneutral environment during surgery include:

1. Using a radiant warmer in the operating room.
2. Covering the baby's head if that is not the operative site and wrapping his arms and legs in sheet wadding or other protective covering.
3. Using nonvolatile liquids for skin preparation to reduce evaporative heat loss.
4. Warming blood for transfusion to body temperature.

Postoperative Care

Like all postoperative patients, infants require careful observation. Vital signs, bleeding, fluid intake, urine output, hypoglycemia, and hypocalcemia are assessed as well as signs related to the particular surgery (e.g., gastric drainage, chest drainage). Jaundice may be intensified by the stress of surgery or by conditions related to the surgery such as sepsis,

Nursing Care Plan 24–1. Infants Requiring Surgery

NURSING GOALS:

To prepare both infant and parents for surgery.
To protect the infant during the intraoperative period.
To support the family during the intraoperative period.
To prepare complications during the postoperative period.
To facilitate attachment.

OBJECTIVES:

1. The infant achieves physiologic homeostasis as much as possible prior to surgery.
2. Parents understand the reason for surgery and expected outcome.
3. Infant's appearance following surgery is explained (e.g., endotracheal tube, chest tube).
4. Infant is protected during the intraoperative period.
5. Family is supported during the intraoperative period.
6. Postoperative complications are prevented or quickly recognized and treated.
7. Parental attachment is facilitated.
8. A plan for continuing health care is implemented.

ASSESSMENT	POTENTIAL NURSING DIAGNOSIS	NURSING INTERVENTION	COMMENTS/RATIONALE
Preoperative period Identify infant requiring surgery.	Infant requires preoperative preparation	Provide thermoneutral environment.	Infant may require transport to regional center for surgery (See Nursing Care Plan 24–18).
Assess infant's physiologic status: 1. Vital signs 2. Blood glucose level 3. Serum electrolytes 4. Acid-base status		Initiate IV therapy. Special preparation as indicated by condition (see Nursing Care Plan for specific condition). Preparation to achieve physiologic homeostasis as far as possible.	
Assess parents' understanding of infant's condition and proposed surgery.	Parents' need for information	Explain or clarify: 1. The reason for surgery 2. How the infant will look following surgery (tubes, ventilator, dressings, etc.) 3. How the infant will behave (asleep, unable to move due to anesthesia, etc.) 4. Approximate length of surgery 5. Unit to which infant will return	Even though good explanations are provided, expect parents to ask some questions over and over; it is difficult to comprehend information in stressful state.

Continued on following page

Nursing Care Plan 24–1. Infants Requiring Surgery *(Continued)*

ASSESSMENT	POTENTIAL NURSING DIAGNOSIS	NURSING INTERVENTION	COMMENTS/RATIONALE
		Use dolls, photographs, actual pieces of equipment to explain.	
		If preoperative tests are used, explain purpose of testing.	
		Consent forms for surgery and tests should be signed only after parents understand plan of care.	
	Parents' fear of surgery for infant	Encourage parents to verbalize concerns, ask questions.	
Assess what parents have been told, or believe, about prognosis.	Lag in attachment related to fear of loss of infant (life-threatening anomaly)	Encourage parents to touch and hold infant if condition permits.	
	Lag in attachment related to infant's appearance (e.g., gastroschisis, cleft lip)	Be as positive about prognosis as condition permits.	
	Anxiety about altered body image	When anomaly involves altered body image, show pictures of infants following repair.	
Intraoperative period Assess vital signs.	At risk for hypothermia during transport to surgery and during surgery	Transport in prewarmed incubator.	
		Cover infant's head with stockinette cap and wrap arms and legs with protective covering.	
		Use nonvolatile liquids for skin preparation to avoid evaporative heat loss.	

Assess parents' status.	Parental anxiety during surgery	Allow blood for transfusion to warm to body temperature.
		Maintain contact with parents at intervals during surgery, particularly when surgery is prolonged.
		Contact clergy or hospital chaplain if desired.
Postoperative period Assess vital signs.	At risk for complications following surgery: Hypothermia Hypotension Respiratory distress Cardiac distress Bleeding Under- or overhydration Hypoglycemia Hyperbilirubinemia Sepsis	Provide thermoneutral environment.
Assess bleeding; estimate amount.		Notify surgeon if bleeding occurs at operative site or at site of arterial or central lines.
Record total intake and output hourly. Record each IV route separately, and urinary output, catheters, drains, etc. separately.		Antibiotics may be ordered; place on time schedule to achieve consistent blood levels.
Identify parents' reactions to surgery, concerns about infant.	Anxiety Fear	Allow parents to be with infant as soon as possible after surgery.
		Explain baby's condition and each piece of equipment.
		As infant's condition improves, involve parents in infant care.
Identify continuing health needs.	Parents' need for information about continuing health care	Provide information about continuing health care needs (see Nursing Care Plans for specific problems).
	Parents' need for information about community resources available to them.	Refer to community health nurse.
		Provide information about financial resources, parents' groups, as appropriate.

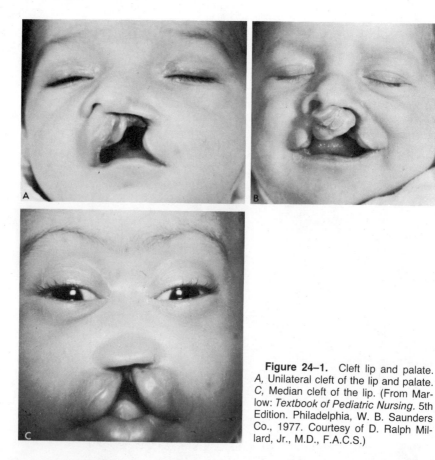

Figure 24–1. Cleft lip and palate. *A,* Unilateral cleft of the lip and palate. *C,* Median cleft of the lip. (From Marlow: *Textbook of Pediatric Nursing.* 5th Edition. Philadelphia, W. B. Saunders Co., 1977. Courtesy of D. Ralph Millard, Jr., M.D., F.A.C.S.)

the initial condition for which the baby is being treated, dehydration, or anesthesia. On the other hand, adequate hydration, antibiotics, and good general supportive care may bring about a significant fall in bilirubin level without other treatment.

Parents should have the opportunity to be with their baby as soon as possible after surgery. They will be eager, of course, to talk with the surgeon about the course of the surgery and what they can expect in the next hours and days. Nurses caring for the baby will also need to know what parents have been told.

Care Related to Specific Congenital Anomalies

Problems of the Head and Face

The most common facial anomalies are *cleft lip* and *cleft palate;* either may occur alone, or both may occur together (Fig. 24–1). Both hereditary and environmental factors have been suspected in the etiology of cleft lip and palate.

A cleft lip may be unilateral or bilateral, complete (extending into the nares) or incomplete. When parents first see their infant, they may be unable to see anything but the defect. Nurses can help parents focus on the positive aspects of their baby's appearance. Pictures of successful lip repairs may reassure parents about their baby's future appearance.

Surgery for cleft lip repair is done when the baby is approximately 1 month old. The baby will be at home with his parents during the weeks before surgery. Palate repair is commonly delayed until the second year of life.

A major concern of parents in this period is feeding (Nursing Care Plan 24–2). The cleft lip makes it difficult to maintain suction on a nipple. When the palate is also cleft, milk escapes through the nose. It is not unusual for the baby to cough and choke during feedings. Holding the baby in an upright position facilitates feeding. Because of a tendency to swallow air, the baby must be burped frequently. There are several alternative methods of feeding; experimenting may be necessary to find the most effective method for a particular baby. Some babies with a cleft lip may breast-feed. The breast may fill the defect and allow a seal around the nipple and areola. Sucking will strengthen the tongue and jaw muscles. A breast shield with a cleft-lip nipple attached may facilitate breast-feeding.[7] The ability to breast-feed an infant with a cleft palate will

Nursing Care Plan 24–2.   Infants with Cleft Lip or Cleft Palate

NURSING GOALS:
To provide immediate and long-term care for infants with cleft lip or cleft palate so that complications are prevented and good speech, hearing, and other aspects of development are enhanced.
To facilitate attachment by parents and enable them to participate in a long-range plan of care.

OBJECTIVES:
Cleft lip:
1. Parents accept their infant and are able to care for the infant both prior to and following surgery.
2. Respiratory distress is prevented.
3. Following surgery, the operative site is clean and protected from injury.
4. Parents understand and are able to participate in a long-term plan of care.
Cleft palate:
1. Cleft palate is identified.
2. Parents accept their infant and are able to care for the infant at home.
3. Multidisciplinary team is involved in care at appropriate times.
4. Parents understand and are able to participate in long-term plan of care.

ASSESSMENT	POTENTIAL NURSING DIAGNOSIS	NURSING INTERVENTION	COMMENTS/RATIONALE
Identify infant with cleft lip or cleft palate. Cleft lip is readily observable.	At risk for aspiration related to cleft lip or cleft palate.	Modify feeding: 1. Hold baby upright. 2. Burp frequently. 3. Breast-feeding may be possible for some infants; evaluate individually. Maxillary appliance may be useful.	Experimentation may be necessary to find most effective means of feeding a particular baby.

Check every infant's mouth for cleft in palate.	At risk for feeding difficulty related to cleft lip or cleft palate.	4. Alternative methods of feeding include:
		  a. Lamb's nipple
		  b. Large, soft nipple
		  c. Rubber-tipped medicine dropper or Asepto syringe (fluid placed at back of tongue)
		5. Direct flow of milk to side and back of mouth.
		6. Follow milk feeding with small water feeding.
		7. Cleanse cleft lip with water or hydrogen peroxide (one-half strength).
			Good mouth care is essential to prevent infections of middle ear.

		8. Encourage parents to feed infant. If lip surgery is delayed past neonatal period, parents will feed infant at home. Palate surgery is always delayed. 9. Infant may cough and gag during feeding. Feed more slowly. Support parent who may be frightened by this.	Cleft lip surgery may occur in the neonatal period or between 1 and 3 months. Cleft palate surgery usually begins between 12 and 18 months and may involve multiple procedures.

Continued on following page

Nursing Care Plan 24–2. Infants with Cleft Lip or Cleft Palate *(Continued)*

ASSESSMENT	POTENTIAL NURSING DIAGNOSIS	NURSING INTERVENTION	COMMENTS/RATIONALE
	Parental anxiety related to infant's appearance	Help parents accept infant (particularly with cleft lip because of altered body image). Point out infant's attractive features.	
	Lag in attachment related to infant's appearance	Provide pictures of similar infants after repair; explain infant's appearance in immediate postoperative period.	
		Explain long-range plan of care.	
		Provide opportunities for verbalization of concerns, questions.	
		Provide information about community resources.	
Postoperative care: cleft lip repair			
1. Respiratory distress	At risk for respiratory distress because of secretions, smaller airway	1. Turn infant to side (never prone), or place upright in infant seat. 2. Laryngoscope and endotracheal tube should be available at bedside. 3. A mist tent is frequently used in immediate postoperative period.	

2. Operative site
   a. Suture line clean
   b. No indication of infection
   c. No indication of trauma
	At risk for infection or injury to operative site
	
	At risk of trauma occurring secondary to injury or infection to operative site
		4. Arm restraints required to protect operative site for 2–4 weeks. Arm restraints must be removed, one at a time, at least every 4 hours and arm exercised.
		5. Site may be protected with Logan bow (curved metal appliance placed over lip and taped at each side).
		6. Suture line cleaned PRN and after each feeding. Suture line should never be rubbed.
		7. Feed with rubber-tipped dropper or syringe. Dropper is placed at the corner of the mouth; dropper should never touch suture line. Feedings are followed with sterile water to rinse mouth.
			Logan bow presents tension at suture line.
			
			Hydrogen peroxide, one-half strength, is frequently used for cleaning.

	8. Anticipate infant needs in order to decrease crying. Feed on demand. Cuddle and hold. Help parents hold infant so that operative site is not injured. Explain that holding infant now will not "spoil" infant.	Crying puts tension on suture lines.
Assess parents' ability to care for infant at home.		

Parents' need for information about infant care following discharge	1. Provide explanations, written material, and experience for parents in:
	  a. Infant feeding
	  b. Cleaning suture line
	  c. Application and removal of restraints
	  d. Need for touching, holding, stimulation
	  e. Avoidance of crying	

Parents' concern for body image	2. Explain that operative site may remain red for many months but will eventually fade. Some children will have scar revision at later age.	
Parents' need to understand long-term plan of care	3. Explain need for long-term multidisciplinary care (may include dental care, speech therapy). Refer to community health nurse for assistance in home care.	

At risk for otitis media	4. Reduce risk of middle ear infection by:
	  a. Feeding in upright position
	  b. Avoiding prolonged periods in which infant is supine
	  c. Good mouth care
	  d. Contacting health-care provider at first sign of respiratory infection
		Cleft palate associated with impaired functioning of eustacian tube; soft palate muscles normally facilitate middle ear drainage.

	5. Provide written information about signs of possible otitis media in infants:
	  a. Vomiting or diarrhea
	  b. Anorexia
	  c. Irritability, sleep disturbances
	  d. Upper respiratory symptoms: nasal congestion, cough
	  e. Fever
	  f. Red, bulging tympanic membrane
	  g. Pulling at ears
		Antibiotic therapy for 10 days is the treatment for otitis media.

depend on the extent of the defect. Appliances designed to fit the maxilla are sometimes fitted to the infant, not only to make nursing easier but also to stimulate facial development, decrease the number of ear infections, and prevent distortions of the tongue and irritation of the nasal septum.[8]

A lamb's nipple (a long nipple used for feeding lambs), a large soft nipple, a rubber-tipped medicine dropper, or an Asepto syringe with a rubber tip are other possible ways of feeding. Parents frequently show more patience and become more skilled at feeding their own infant than we are; letting them show us how they are able to care for their baby enhances their sense of competence (important to attachment) and increases our knowledge.

Caring for infants with a cleft lip or cleft palate requires team coordination—nurses in the hospital and community, physicians, and, for infants with cleft palate, speech therapists, dentists, and orthodontists. A nursing referral from a hospital to a community health nurse is important in ensuring long-term health care.

Micrognathia (hypognathia), hypoplasia of the mandible, may occur alone or in association with a cleft palate. At times the tongue may fall backward, causing respiratory obstruction; placing the baby in a prone position can prevent this from happening. During feeding, drawing the jaw forward by hooking a finger behind the angle of the jaw will enable the baby to breast- or bottle-feed. The tongue may be large in relation to the size of the mouth, requiring a small nipple. Because the human nipple fits the mouth with less bulk, breast-feeding may be easier than bottle-feeding.[7]

Respiratory Tract Anomalies

Choanal Atresia. Choanal atresia is the obstruction of one or both posterior nasal openings between the nasal cavity and the nasopharynx. The obstruction may be composed of bone or membrane; it may be unilateral or bilateral. If the obstruction is unilateral it may not be detected in the newborn period. Because infants do not breathe through their mouths, babies with bilateral choanal atresia will become cyanotic and dyspneic in the delivery room. There is increased respiratory distress when the baby's mouth is closed, and it is impossible to pass a catheter through one or both nostrils. An infant airway or, if this is not immediately available, a nipple with the end cut off is inserted in the baby's mouth to allow the baby to breathe (Nursing Care Plan 24–3). Correction is surgical; surgery can be

delayed in babies with unilateral atresia but is performed immediately when atresia is bilateral. Gavage feeding will be necessary prior to and immediately following surgery because the baby will be unable to breathe if his mouth closes around a nipple. When surgery is postponed, infants can sometimes learn to bottle-feed after an initial period of gavage feeding.

Following surgery, the infant will have a tube extending from the nares that splints the new airway. The tube will remain in place for several weeks. If it becomes obstructed, it is rinsed with saline and suctioned.[5]

Congenital Laryngeal Stridor (Laryngomalacia). When the cartilage of the larynx is unusually flaccid, the supraglottic structures may collapse into the trachea, causing a partial obstruction and stridor (noisy breathing) during inspiration. The condition improves during the first year as the baby grows and the cartilage becomes firmer. In the interim, stridor is decreased by placing the baby in a prone position, allowing the supraglottic structures to fall away from the trachea. If stridor increases during feeding, slow feedings with ample opportunities to breathe between sucking episodes may be helpful (Nursing Care Plan 24–3). Stridor is scary to parents, but cyanosis is unusual. Prompt medical intervention must be sought if the baby develops a respiratory infection because the trachea may be further narrowed by swelling.

Diaphragmatic Hernia. When the diaphragm fails to develop properly, part of the abdominal organs may herniate through the defect into the chest. If the displacement is extensive, the baby will be in acute respiratory distress from the time of birth and is likely to die without early surgery. In addition to cyanosis and retractions, infants with diaphragmatic hernia have small, scaphoid abdomens. There are no breath sounds on the affected side, which is more often the left side, and the heart beat is heard farther to the right (in left-sided displacement).

The baby must have his head elevated both pre- and postoperatively to minimize the pressure of the abdominal organs on the lungs and to allow the diaphragm to move as freely as possible (Nursing Care Plan 24–3). Postoperatively, the baby will have a chest tube connected to waterseal drainage and either a gastrostomy or nasogastric tube to keep the stomach from becoming distended. First feedings, which will begin in the second 24 hours after surgery if the baby is doing well, will be given through the tube.

Since it often takes several days for the lung on the affected side to expand fully, postoperative respiratory distress is not unusual. Po-

Nursing Care Plan 24-3. Infants with Anomalies of the Respiratory Tract (Choanal Atresia, Laryngomalacia, Diaphragmatic Hernia)

NURSING GOALS:
To provide appropriate respiratory support in addition to total physiologic support for the infant.
To assist parents in coping with the alterations in care necessitated by the infant's anomaly.

OBJECTIVES:
1. An infant with an anomaly of the respiratory tract is identified.
2. Parents are informed of their infant's health status and the proposed plan of care.
3. Gas exchange is facilitated in a manner appropriate to the individual anomaly.
4. Adequate nutrition and the protection and support of other body systems are provided.
5. Parents understand their infant's health needs and are able to care for their infant following discharge.
6. Grieving parents receive support throughout the grieving process.

ASSESSMENT	POTENTIAL NURSING DIAGNOSIS	NURSING INTERVENTION	COMMENTS/RATIONALE

1. Identify the infant with respiratory tract anomaly:
  a. Cyanosis dyspnea
  b. Cyanosis when at rest; increase in respiratory difficulty when mouth is closed (choanal atresia)
  c. Inability to pass feeding tube through one or both nares (choanal atresia)
	Respiratory difficulty secondary to anomaly of the respiratory tract
	
	Parents' need for information about infant
	
	Anxiety of parents related to congenital defect
		In all instances:
		1. Provide thermoneutral environment.
		2. Provide fluid by intravenous route or orogastric feeding appropriate to specific condition if nipple feedings are not possible.
		3. Correct alterations in pH, $PaCO_2$, PaO_2 as necessary.
		4. Provide opportunities for parents to see and touch infant.
		5. Explain infant's status to parents. Encourage parents' participation in caregiving as soon as possible.
		6. If infant requires surgery, prepare parent for infant's appearance following surgery.
		
		Choanal Atresia
		1. Insert oral airway or nipple with end cut off to provide airway.
		2. Oral feeding impossible with bilateral choanal atresia; may be difficult with unilateral atre-
			Newborn infants are obligate nose breathers; learning to breathe through the mouth requires time (usually 2–3 weeks).
			
			Continued on following page

Nursing Care Plan 24-3. Infants with Anomalies of the Respiratory Tract (Choanal Atresia, Laryngomalacia, Diaphragmatic Hernia) *(Continued)*

ASSESSMENT	POTENTIAL NURSING DIAGNOSIS	NURSING INTERVENTION	COMMENTS/RATIONALE
		Choanal Atresia *(Continued)*	
		sia. Orogastric feeding may be necessary.	
		3. If surgery is performed in the neonatal period (for cartilaginous or membranous obstruction), prepare infant and parents for surgery (Nursing Care Plan 24–1). Observe for respiratory distress in postoperative period.	
		4. If surgery is delayed (because of bony defect), support parents as they learn to feed infant, who must interrupt feeding to breathe.	
		Laryngomalacia	
d. Stridor during inspiration (laryngomalacia)	Anxiety of parents related to stridor	1. Stridor will be decreased when infant is placed in prone position.	Stridor is due to partial obstruction of trachea. Prone position allows supraglottic structures to fall away from trachea.
		2. Feed slowly if stridor increases during feedings; allow periods of breathing during sucking. Remain with parents and provide support until they are comfortable feeding infant.	
		3. Alleviate parental anxiety by providing opportunities for caretaking, encouraging verbalization of concerns, answering questions.	
		4. Explain the need to notify health-care provider immediately if infant develops respiratory infection.	Tracheal swelling during respiratory infection further narrows already partially obstructed trachea.

Diaphragmatic Hernia

In addition to cyanosis and dyspnea

e. Scaphoid abdomen
f. Dextrocardia (if left side is affected)
g. Absence of breath sounds on affected side (usually left side)

Limited gas exchange secondary to diaphragmatic hernia

Parental anxiety

1. Elevate infant's head (infant seat).
2. Provide oxygen as necessary to relieve cyanosis. If positive pressure ventilation is required, peak pressure should not exceed 20 cm. water to avoid possible pneumothorax.
3. If infant is in hospital with no thoracic surgeon, prepare parents and infant for transport to regional center (Nursing Care Plan 24–18). Provide opportunity for parents to see and touch infant prior to transport.
4. If infant is in hospital with a thoracic surgeon, prepare infant and parents for surgery (Nursing Care Plan 24–1).

Elevating the head decreases the pressure of the abdominal organs on the lungs and allows diaphragm to move more freely.

Parents' need for information.

In either instance, keep parents informed of infant status; encourage parents to see and touch infant prior to surgery.

Postoperatively

Watch for signs of respiratory distress; affected lung may require days or weeks to fully expand.

1. Infant will have chest tube connected to waterseal drainage.
2. Position baby with affected side down. Elevate head.
3. Gastrostomy tube necessary to keep stomach from distention and subsequently for initial feedings.
4. Encourage parents in caretaking. Infant may be discharged with gastrostomy tube; parents need to become comfortable caring for infant with tube in place. Infant may need to be fed slowly; parents need to become experienced at feeding their infant.
5. Provide parents with information about sources of continuing care.

Lung on affected side may take several days to expand. This position will allow maximum ventilation of unaffected lung.

If infant dies (mortality rate approximately 50 per cent) attachment through seeing, touching, caretaking facilitates grieving (Chapter 28).

Mortality related to:
1. Extent of defect
2. Condition of lungs on both affected and unaffected side

sitioning the baby with the affected side down helps the unaffected lung to expand fully in the immediate postoperative period when it is the only one functioning.

Even with superior care, not all of these babies survive. Mortality ranges from 25 per cent in hospitals where surgeons and nurses are specialists in infant care to higher than 50 per cent in general hospitals. At least part of this high mortality is due to associated anomalies of the heart, lungs, or intestines.

Congenital Heart Defects

It is suspected that 1 out of every 130 liveborn babies will have a significant congenital heart defect. In a medium-sized hospital where 30 to 35 babies are delivered each week, this means that on the average one baby each month will have a cardiac malformation. Approximately 10 per cent of all congenital defects involve the heart. Congenital heart defects are second only to prematurity as the leading cause of death in referral centers in the first month of life. Approximately one-third of all infants with congenital heart disease die within a week after birth.

Many symptoms of congenital heart defects are vague in the first days of life because certain structures of fetal circulation, such as a patent foramen ovale or ductus arteriosus, may help the baby to compensate. Since hospital stays of apparently normal mothers and babies are often limited to 4 or 5 days, clearcut symptoms of a heart defect may not appear until after the baby is discharged. Symptoms may appear in the early months of life or not for many years.

Etiology. Congenital cardiac disease may be genetic in origin, or it may be related to intrauterine infection (particularly rubella) or to other factors in the intrauterine environment such as drugs and nutrition (Nursing Care Plan 24–4). When there is a genetic predisposition, the same lesion is usually found in siblings. In most instances, however, the risk of recurrence is not considered sufficiently high to warrant the avoidance of future childbearing.

Because the heart develops mainly between the second and eighth weeks of embryologic life (Chapter 7), this is the period when teratogens will affect the heart most severely.

Types of Defects. Heart defects may exist alone or in combination, and symptoms will vary with the size of the defect and the combination of one defect with others (Table 24–1).

Shunts. Shunts are "leaks," or postnatal

openings that should not exist. There are three types of shunts: atrial septal defects, ventricular septal defects, and patent ductus arteriosus (Chapter 23). All of these conditions, when they exist alone, are acyanotic. Atrial septal defects are virtually never discovered in newborns and are seldom a problem in children of preschool age.

Of all congenital heart defects, the ventricular septal defect (VSD) occurs most frequently and is rarely symptomatic in the newborn period because the normally high pressure in the blood vessels of the lung prevents shunting from the left side of the heart to the right side through the defect (Fig. 24–2). As pulmonary pressure drops between 2 weeks and 3 months of age, blood is shunted from the left to the right side of the heart through the VSD. The lungs are flooded, and signs of congestive heart failure develop. Pulmonary artery banding is performed as a palliative procedure to alleviate the flooding of the lungs and to prevent both congestive heart failure and changes in pulmonary blood vessels. Banding itself may cause problems, chiefly necrosis of the pulmonary artery beneath the band, and an early closure of the ventricular defect with a Dacron patch may be performed (see Table 24–2).

It is important to make clear that symptoms are delayed, because parents often feel that a diagnosis was missed or that their baby was not carefully examined at birth, when in fact it was not possible to recognize the defect at that time.

Heart Blocks. There are three varieties of congenital heart blocks: aortic valvular stenosis, pulmonary valvular stenosis, and coarctation of the aorta. Aortic valvular stenosis is relatively rare, and unless it is severe it will usually not be detected in newborns but will be found at some later time during routine physical examination. The prognosis is good for children with mild to moderate stenosis but rather poor for babies who develop respiratory distress, tachycardia, and pallor in the first few weeks of life. Although these babies are initially treated with digitalis and oxygen, prompt surgery (aortic valvulotomy) is necessary to save their lives. The surgery itself carries a high risk at the present time.

Complete obstruction of the aortic valve (aortic atresia) is always fatal, generally by the time the baby is 4 to 5 days old. These babies also have an underdeveloped left ventricle and ascending aorta, the combination known as hypoplastic left heart syndrome.

Pulmonary valvular stenosis is also rare in newborns, occurring most often in infants of mothers who had rubella in early pregnancy.

Text continued on page 817

Nursing Care Plan 24—4.   Infants with Congenital Cardiovascular Disease

NURSING GOALS:
To provide physiologic and emotional support for the infant.
To enhance the coping ability of parents.
To prepare parents to care for their infant's long-term physiologic, social, and emotional needs.

OBJECTIVES:
1. The infant with congenital cardiovascular disease is identified.
2. Complications are prevented when possible, or quickly identified and treated.
3. Parents are knowledgeable about their infant's needs and comfortable in caring for their infant.
4. Parents understand the long-term plan of care.
5. Appropriate community agency referrals are made.

ASSESSMENT	POTENTIAL NURSING DIAGNOSIS	NURSING INTERVENTION	COMMENTS/RATIONALE

1. Identify infant at risk.
  a. Family member (parent or sibling) with congenital heart disease
  b. Preterm infant
  c. Maternal rubella, diabetes, viral infections, maternal drug intake, particularly in first trimester
  d. Associated with certain genetic or chromosomal disorders (e.g., Down's syndrome)
 	
2. Identify infant with cardiovascular disease.
  a. Tachypnea (respiratory rate greater than 45 breaths per minute in term infant or 60 breaths per minute in preterm infant)
  b. Failure to feed well, choking spells during feeding
  c. Tachycardia (hourly rate greater than 150 breaths per minute while infant at rest)
  d. Cyanosis (present only in specific disorders). Note color of skin and mucous membranes both at rest and during crying.
  e. Absence of femoral pulses (coarctation of aorta)
  f. Bounding femoral pulses (patent ductus arteriosus)
  g. Heart murmur
	Infant at risk for congenital heart disease
	
	Failure to feed well secondary to tachypnea and to fatigue
		1. *Prevention:*
		  a. Rubella vaccine given to all infants
		  b. Maternal rubella titer taken during prenatal period
		  c. Avoidance of nonprescription drugs during pregnancy; drugs should be prescribed by a provider who is aware of pregnancy and potential teratogenicity of drugs.
		  d. Screening for Down's syndrome in mothers over 35
		2. When cardiovascular disease is suspected, further assessment will be necessary involving one or more of the following:
		  a. X-ray
		  b. Electrocardiography
		  c. Echocardiography
		  d. Cardiac catheterization
		3. Explain or clarify explanation of procedures.
		4. Encourage parents to be with infant before and after procedure; nurse should accompany infant to testing areas outside of nursery.
		5. Provide thermoneutral environment away from nursery (chilling increases infant's oxygen needs).
		6. Provide equipment for resuscitation when infant is traveling outside of nursery.
			Incidence of congenital cardiovascular anomalies: 1 in 100 live births. Not all cardiac anomalies will be identified in the neonatal period.
			
			Assess cyanosis in natural light. Crying frequently increases cyanosis; infant cannot meet increased demands on circulatory system.

Continued on following page

Nursing Care Plan 24–4. Infants with Congenital Cardiovascular Disease (Continued)

ASSESSMENT	POTENTIAL NURSING DIAGNOSIS	NURSING INTERVENTION	COMMENTS/RATIONALE
	Cardiac Catheterization		
1. Assess infant's vital signs (temperature, apical pulse, respiration, blood pressure, acid-base balance, fluid intake).			Slow or irregular pulse may indicate interference with cardiac electrical conduction system. Reaction to dye may cause blood pressure to fall, temperature to rise.
2. Cut-down site for bleeding		If bleeding occurs: 1. Apply pressure at site of bleeding for arterial bleeding. 2. Elevate extremity for venous "oozing." 3. Notify physician.	Arterial thrombosis is a risk in infants.
3. Assess limb distal to catheter insertion for pulse, color, warmth.			Distal pulses may be initially weak but should increase in strength.
4. Dyspnea	Dyspnea secondary to possible pulmonary embolism, pneumothorax	Notify physician. Provide oxygen. Be prepared to give respiratory assistance (see Nursing Care Plan 23–1).	
	Care During the Neonatal Period		
Assess parents' understanding of reason for modifications in newborn care.	Parents' need for information about infant care	Explain rationale for care given by nurses as preparation for care at home following discharge. Encourage parents' participation in care during hospitalization.	
Assess parents' comfort in caring for infant.	Parental anxiety about infant health status, infant care	1. Provide opportunity for infant rest by giving care in blocks followed by blocks of time for rest. 2. If infant is dyspneic, position in infant seat.	

Continuing assessment of infant nutrition.
1. Growth in length, weight, head circumference
2. Condition of skin, hair

Parents' need for assistance in learning to feed infant

At risk for malnutrition because of feeding difficulty and cardiovascular disease

3. Daily bath may not be necessary if infant tires easily. Sponge and cleanse diaper area.

Feed infant with soft nipple. Burp frequently. Feed slowly.

Help parents understand that feeding at home may be time-consuming; parents may need help in incorporating infant care into daily activities. Refer to community health nurse for coordination of care.

At risk for infection and sequelae of infection

Explain or clarify explanation related to potential timing of corrective surgery (Table 24–2).

Explain to parents:
1. Protect infant from persons with infection.
2. Avoid large crowds.
3. All who care for infants should wash hands first.

Assess parents' response to long-term needs of infant with cardiovascular disease.

Parent's perception of infant as incapacitated

Increased potential for overprotection, restriction in activity

Encourage parents to:
1. Treat their infant as they would any other child.
2. Avoid concern about limiting activity. Infants will limit their own activity.
3. Set behavioral limits as infant grows older as they would for another child.

Parental anxiety and other feelings are related to presence rather than severity of disease.

Related to infant's heart disease:
Parental grief
Parental guilt
Parental anger
Parental anxiety
Parental fear

Provide information about resources available in infant development, parent-infant relationships.

Anxiety about costs of long-term care

Provide information about financial resources.

Identify signs of congestive heart failure.
1. Respiratory distress (dyspnea, retractions, nasal flaring, expiratory grunt, tachypnea, cyanosis

Plan of care in congestive heart failure:
1. Oxygen may be necessary.
2. Diuretic may be ordered to relieve edema, pulmonary congestion.

Etiology of congestive heart failure.
1. Decreased cardiac output
2. Overloading of pulmonary circulatory system → respiratory inhibition.

Continued on following page

Nursing Care Plan 24–4. Infants with Congenital Cardiovascular Disease *(Continued)*

ASSESSMENT	POTENTIAL NURSING DIAGNOSIS	NURSING INTERVENTION	COMMENTS/RATIONALE
		Care During the Neonatal Period *(Continued)*	
2. Tachycardia 3. Edema (may not have pitting edema; sudden weight gain may indicate edema; periorbital edema may be present) 4. Diaphoresis, especially in head area 5. Hepatomegaly secondary to venous congestion (liver may be 5–6 cm. below costal margin) 6. Feeding difficulty 7. Irritability, weak cry		a. Monitor electrolytes, particularly potassium and calcium; replacement therapy is frequently ordered. b. Weigh diapers to measure urine output; measure urine specific gravity. c. Weigh infant to assess loss of body fluid. d. Observe infant for signs of dehydration (loss of skin turgor, depressed fontanel).	3. Decreased blood supply to kidneys → ↓ glomerular filtration → ↑ retention of sodium and water. 4. Venous pressure increases back-up of venous blood.

Identify signs of toxicity to digoxin:
1. Laboratory: blood levels of digoxin greater than 3.5–4 ng. per ml. are toxic to neonate.
2. Clinical:
  a. Gastrointestinal: anorexia, nausea, vomiting, diarrhea
  b. Bradycardia
		3. Infant may be digitalized
		  a. *Total digitalizing dose (TDD)*: Digoxin, 0.03–0.06 mg per kg. (30–60 μg. per kg.); one-half TDD given immediately, one-half in each of next two doses.
		  b. *Maintenance dose*: usually one-half TDD in two divided doses per day.
		
		Count heart rate before each dose. Omit dose and contact physician if heart rate is less than 100 beats per minute unless another parameter has been specified.
			Digoxin strengthens cardiac contractions, has diuretic effect.

Assess parents' ability to administer digoxin.	Parents' need to learn to administer prescribed drug	Prepare parents to administer digoxin at home if infant will receive medication after hospital discharge. 1. Provide many opportunities for parents to measure and administer medication in hospital.	

2. Instruct parents not to vary prescribed dose.
3. Instruct parents: if single dose is omitted, do not be concerned. If two or more consecutive doses are missed, notify physician, clinic, or nurse.
4. Give dose 1 hour before or 2 hours after feeding.
5. If dose is vomited within 15 minutes after administration and appears lost, repeat. If more than 15 minutes has elapsed, or little appears to have been lost, do not repeat.
6. Notify physician, clinic, or nurse at first sign of any illness.
7. Store digoxin in a safe place. If it is accidentally ingested, bring victim and bottle to emergency room immediately.
8. If dosage is changed, provide additional opportunities for supervised practice in measuring dose.

Avoid loss of medication in case of vomiting.

Cardiac Surgery in the Neonate

Parents need for information about infant's surgery

Explain or clarify explanation of surgery.

Prepare parents for infant's appearance following surgery (possibility of endotracheal tube, chest tube, nasogastric tube, dressings, CVP line, etc.).

Provide thermoneutral environment for infant in transport to surgery. IV in place, NPO.

Most cardiac surgery is deferred beyond the neonatal period (see Table 24–2).

A doll model is helpful in preparing parents. Equipment used will vary with type of surgery.

O.R. should be ready for surgery immediately on infant's arrival. Infant should not have to wait in cold corridor or O.R.

Preoperative:
Identify information given to parents by others, parents' understanding of surgery.

Continued on following page

Nursing Care Plan 24–4.   Infants with Congenital Cardiovascular Disease   (Continued)

ASSESSMENT	POTENTIAL NURSING DIAGNOSIS	NURSING INTERVENTION	COMMENTS/RATIONALE
		Cardiac Surgery in the Neonate (*Continued*)	
	Parental anxiety about cardiac surgery	Encourage parents to ask questions, verbalize fears, concerns. Provide honest answers. Ensure that parents receive same information from all providers through documentation of teaching.	
Postoperative: Assess vital signs every 15 minutes during initial recovery period, then at gradually increasing intervals.		Maintain thermoneutral environment. Turn infant.	Infant may have become chilled during surgery. Hypothermia rarely used in neonatal period.
Identify: 1. Signs of respiratory distress (tachypnea, retractions, nasal flaring, expiratory grunt, cyanosis). Listen for bilateral breath sounds. 2. Tachycardia 3. Hypothermia			
Check operative site for bleeding.			
Monitor intake and output (weighed diapers, drainage from chest tube, nasogastric tube, drainage from dressing, etc.).			
Weigh daily.			
Assess parental coping.	Parental anxiety	Encourage parents to be with infant. Encourage questions, verbalization of concern. Provide realistic answers, neither overly optimistic nor overly pessimistic. Identify signs of progress.	

Table 24–1. CLASSIFICATION OF CONGENITAL HEART DEFECTS

	Acyanotic	Cyanotic
Shunts	Atrial septal defect Ventricular septal defect Patent ductus arteriosus	
Blocks	Aortic valvular stenosis Pulmonary valvular stenosis Coarctation of aorta	
Underdevelopment	Hypoplastic left ventricle	Hypoplastic right ventricle
Complex	Transposition of great vessels Tetralogy of Fallot (newborns frequently acyanotic)	

In combination with other defects, pulmonary stenosis may be an asset because it reduces excess blood flow to the lungs, just as banding of the pulmonary artery does artificially, and thus protects the baby from congestive heart failure.

Atresia of the pulmonary artery carries a very high risk; untreated patients die within 2 weeks to 2 months after birth, and mortality is very high following transarterial valvulotomy.

Because coarctation of the aorta (Fig. 24–3) usually occurs in combination with other defects, the term coarctation syndrome is often used. This syndrome is the most common malformation causing cardiac failure during the newborn period. Often the baby shows no symptoms during the few days he is in the hospital, but the absence of femoral pulses, which should be routinely assessed, gives the clue. If the defect is not discovered before the baby goes home, the classic triad of rapid breathing, feeding difficulty (due to rapid breathing), and tachycardia may follow. On the other hand, many children will have no symptoms, and the coarctation will be discovered only on routine examination. As with patent ductus arteriosus, treatment during infancy is aimed at eliminating congestive heart failure; surgery is ideally postponed until the baby is 3 to 5 years old. Surgery is performed in the newborn period only when congestive heart failure has not responded to medical treatment. To a large extent, the success of surgery depends on the nature of the related cardiac anomalies in the coarctation syndrome.

Underdevelopment. Either the right or the left ventricle may be hypoplastic (underdeveloped). Infants with a hypoplastic left ventricle have systemic circulation only through a patent ductus arteriosus. As the ductus narrows, the systemic circulation is increasingly impaired. Death commonly occurs in the first week of life. Because blood flow to the lungs is increased, the baby is usually not cyanotic.

In contrast, very little blood flows to the

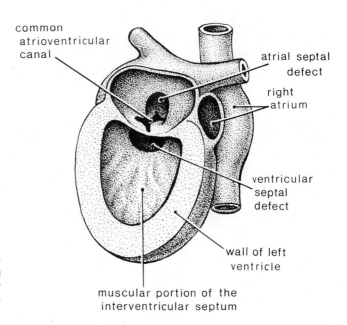

Figure 24–2. Schematic drawing of a heart illustrating various defects of the cardiac septa, including ventricular septal defect. (From Moore: *The Developing Human: Clinically Oriented Embryology.* 2nd Ed. Philadelphia, W. B. Saunders Co., 1977.)

Table 24–2. SURGICAL TREATMENT OF CONGENITAL HEART DISEASE (CHD)

Condition	Percentage of All CHD*	Surgical Intervention	Time of Surgery
Acyanotic			
Patent ductus arteriosus	5–15	Closure of ductus (ligation or division)	Preterm infant: Immediate (Chapter 23) Term infant: Varies with symptoms; usually by 12 to 18 months
Ventricular septal defect	16–20	Palliative: pulmonary artery banding Corrective: closure of defect with Dacron patch	Early total correction now favored for many infants
Coarctation of aorta	7–8	Removal of constricted segment; anastomosis	Age 3 to 5 years
Pulmonary stenosis (may cause cyanosis)	10–20	Valvulotomy	Related to symptoms
Aortic stenosis	3–5	Aortic valvulotomy (some stenosis remains)	Related to symptoms
Cyanotic	9–18	Palliative: Rashkind (balloon septostomy) or Blalock–Hanlon (surgical creation of atrial septal defect)	Palliative: following birth
Transposition of the great arteries		Corrective: Mustard (creation of new atrial septum to redirect blood flow)	Corrective: 2 to 3 years
Tetralogy of Fallot	9–15	Palliative: Blalock–Taussig (right subclavian to right pulmonary artery or left subclavian to left pulmonary artery) or Waterston (ascending aorta to right pulmonary artery) or Potts (descending aorta to left pulmonary artery)	Palliative: related to symptoms; may be in neonatal period or early infancy
		Corrective: repair VSD; repair pulmonary stenosis	Corrective: 5 to 8 years

*Defects may occur alone or in combination with other defects. Defects for which surgery is rare or for which no surgical procedure exists are not included.

lungs in infants with a hypoplastic right ventricle. When this anomaly is associated with tricuspid atresia and a ventricular septal defect, the baby will be cyanotic, but some pulmonary and systemic circulation is possible. This baby may do very well during the neonatal period. When pulmonary atresia accompanies a hypoplastic right ventricle, pulmonary blood flow depends on the ductus arteriosus, and the baby is seriously ill. Surgery linking a systemic artery to a pulmonary artery has been performed, but the risk of death is high.

Complex Malformation. The most common complex heart anomalies are transposition of the great vessels and tetralogy of Fallot. Cyanosis is the outstanding sign of transposition of the great vessels (Fig. 24–4), although even with this defect the cyanosis may not be severe in the first days until the ductus arter-

iosus closes and eliminates the mixing of blood from the two sides of the heart. After it closes, the baby has two separate circulatory systems. The aorta arises from the right ventricle rather than from the left; blood is circulated through the body and returned to the right atrium. This blood never gets to the lungs to be oxygenated. The pulmonary arteries carry blood from the left ventricle to the lungs, where it is oxygenated and returned to the left atrium. Intercommunication must be established between the two circuits or the baby will die in a few days. Treatment is the creation of an atrial septal defect that allows the blood to mix. This is commonly done through the use of a balloon cardiac catheter; an inflated balloon is drawn through the foramen ovale to enlarge the opening (Rashkind procedure) (Fig. 24–5) or through surgical creation of an atrial septal defect (Blalock-Hanlon proce-

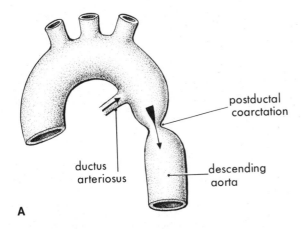

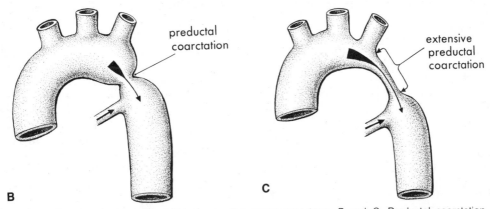

Figure 24–3. *A,* Postductal coarctation of the aorta, the commonest type. *B* and *C,* Preductal coarctation. The type illustrated in C is usually associated with major cardiac defects. (From Moore: *The Developing Human: Clinically Oriented Embryology.* 2nd Ed. Philadelphia, W. B. Saunders Co., 1977.)

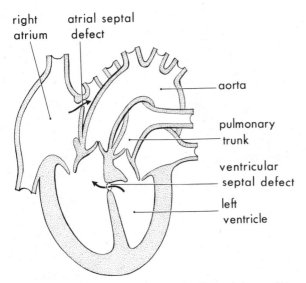

Figure 24–4. Diagram of a heart illustrating complete transposition of the great arteries. The ventricular and atrial septal defects allow mixing of the blood. (From Moore: *The Developing Human: Clinically Oriented Embryology.* 2nd Ed. Philadelphia, W. B. Saunders Co., 1977.)

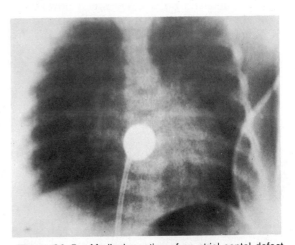

Figure 24–5. Medical creation of an atrial septal defect in transposition of the great arteries. The method of Rashkind and Miller. The anteroposterior projection of the particular cine frame shown was recorded as the balloon filled with 3 ml. contrast medium passed without deformity through the created defect. (From Rowe and Mehrizi: *The Neonate with Congenital Heart Disease.* Philadelphia, W. B. Saunders Co., 1968.)

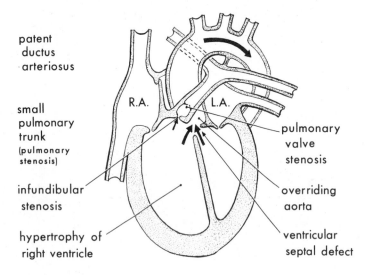

patent
ductus
arteriosus

small
pulmonary
trunk
(pulmonary
stenosis)

infundibular
stenosis

hypertrophy of
right ventricle

R.A.

L.A.

pulmonary
valve
stenosis

overriding
aorta

ventricular
septal defect

Figure 24–6. Frontal section of a heart illustrating the tetralogy of Fallot. (From Moore: *The Developing Human: Clinically Oriented Embryology.* 2nd Ed. Philadelphia, W. B. Saunders Co., 1977.)

dure). Further corrective surgery may be done when the child is older.

The four defects that comprise tetralogy of Fallot (Fig. 24–6) are (1) pulmonary stenosis (occasionally pulmonary atresia), (2) right ventricular hypertrophy, (3) ventricular septal defect, and (4) overriding aorta, which receives blood directly from both right and left ventricles.

Although tetralogy of Fallot is considered a cyanotic heart disease, cyanosis is relatively rare during the period spent in the newborn nursery, even when the pulmonary stenosis is severe. Only half of the newborns with tetralogy have a murmur, the murmur being due to the ejection of blood through the narrowed pulmonary valve. Lack of this murmur is considered a serious sign; death from anoxia will occur in a few weeks unless high risk surgery can increase the pulmonary blood flow. If the baby is having cyanotic attacks during the newborn period, one of several palliative procedures may be performed. These include (1) anastomosis of the right subclavian to the right pulmonary artery or of the left subclavian to the left pulmonary artery (Blalock-Taussig procedure), (2) anastomosis of the left pulmonary artery to the descending aorta (Pott's procedure), or (3) anastomosis of the right pulmonary artery to the ascending aorta (Waterston procedure).

Nursing Assessment of Congenital Heart Disease. A number of signs of congenital heart disease have been noted in he preceding discussion. *Tachypnea* is frequently the initial symptom. After the first 2 hours of life a respiratory rate of more than 45 breaths per minute in a term baby or 60 breaths per minute in a premature baby is usually abnormal if the baby is at rest when the observation is made. Respiratory rates are frequently not assessed in term infants, and thus failure of the baby to feed well may be the first sign noticed by the nurse. The baby is breathing so rapidly he cannot suck; he forsakes eating to continue breathing, or he may attempt to do both and choke or vomit, possibly aspirating his food and further compounding the problem. There are many other possible reasons for tachypnea in the newborn, and not all of them are of serious consequence. Yet any baby who breathes rapidly needs extra watching.

A second sign of possible congestive heart failure is tachycardia. A heart rate of more than 150 beats per minute is unusual in a healthy baby who is not crying.

Cyanosis is present only in certain defects. Both the absence of femoral *pulses* and bounding pulses are significant. The presence of a murmur should always be noted (Chapter 21).

Diagnosis of Heart Defects. Once a heart defect is suspected, diagnosis is made on the basis of (1) clinical signs that have been observed and recorded, (2) x-ray films, (3) electrocardiography, (4) echocardiography, and (5) cardiac catheterization.

The clinical signs associated with individual defects have been mentioned. The role of radiography in evaluating heart size and some outstanding anatomic changes seems obvious. It is very important that the baby be comfortably at rest and not crying when chest films are taken if they are to be detailed enough to be of any real value. If the baby is to go to the x-ray department for films he should be transported in a heated bed and should spend as little time as possible outside it. A nurse should go with him and remain with him throughout the entire procedure, wearing a protective apron to shield her from radiation while the pictures are being taken. A bottle of water or a pacifier will help to soothe the baby and keep him from crying. A bulb syringe for suctioning and a hand-operated bag resuscitator should accompany the baby; infants at times become apneic in x-ray departments and other areas of the hospital away from the nursery, and equipment for resuscitation is not always immediately available. Mouth-to-mouth resuscitation can be used in an acute emergency, of course, but there is always a risk of introducing pathogens into the respiratory tract of an already sick baby. It is much easier to be prepared.

Electrocardiograms (EKGs) of newborns differ from those of children from age 2 through adulthood, and those of premature infants often vary from the EKGs of term babies. The problems involved in the interpretation of newborn EKGs are beyond the scope of this book. As with babies who are to be radiographed, the infant should be warm and comfortable so that he will lie quietly during the procedure.

Echocardiography is a noninvasive technique that uses ultrasound to diagnose congenital heart disease. Information available from an echocardiogram includes the size and location of the chambers of the heart and the great vessels. The motion of valves can also be seen. Some conditions, such as a hypoplastic left ventricle, can be diagnosed with great accuracy; others can only be suspected. In many instances cardiac disease can be differentiated from respiratory disease. Echocardiography is proving extremely valuable because it eliminates the need for cardiac catheterization in some infants.

Cardiac catheterization (see Nursing Care Plan 24–4) presents somewhat different problems in newborns from those encountered in patients in other age groups. Although the mortality in newborns is in the neighborhood of 5 per cent, a large proportion of the babies who die have inoperable defects and would have died under any circumstances. Nevertheless, catheterization is a hazardous procedure in the newborn period for several reasons:

1. The hazards of chilling the baby during the procedure are greatest in newborns.

2. The baby is often in very serious condition before the catheterization begins; he may be cyanotic or acidotic or in congestive heart failure.

3. Needle punctures and even traction on small vessels can cause thrombosis and can impair circulation.

4. Catheterization in newborns is often combined with angiography in order to make an accurate anatomic diagnosis, thereby necessarily increasing the risk.

5. Full exploration of the heart, rather than just right-heart catheterization, may be necessary.

Measures that minimize the risk include the following:

1. Early detection of the possibility of a heart defect before the baby is critically ill.

2. Avoidance of premedication and anesthesia; local anesthesia and a cutdown are used. The umbilical artery is sometimes used for a cutdown in the first days of life.

3. Treatment of acidosis.

4. Treatment of serious arrhythmias by electrical conversion.

5. Use of a minimum amount of contrast material.

After the baby returns from catheterization, there must be careful monitoring of temperature (which often drops during the procedure), apical pulse, respiration, acid-base balance, and fluid intake. The cutdown site should be checked for bleeding, and the color and pulsation in the limb in which the cutdown was done should be observed. Thrombosis is a particular danger in tiny newborn vessels. If there is no pulse 4 hours after the study has been completed, arterial thrombosis has usually occurred. Fortunately, collateral blood supply usually prevents gangrene, but occasionally surgery will be necessary.

Caring for the Baby. In addition to the careful assessment that leads to the recognition of the infant with congenital heart disease and of changes in his condition, nurses must help parents learn to care for their infant at home (Nursing Care Plan 24–4). In many instances, this means helping them to cope with a chronic problem, offering appropriate protection but avoiding overprotection, a very fine and often difficult distinction.

Some infants with congenital heart disease have feeding problems. Nutrition may be inadequate because the baby may tire so easily that he takes an insufficient amount of formula, or he may choke and become dyspneic and the mother will discontinue feeding him. Because of an increased cardiac workload and an increased expenditure of energy, he actually needs more calories than the usual newborn. When this is the case, it may be necessary to use a formula that increases the concentration of calories within the limits of a small fluid intake. The formula should have a fairly low concentration of sodium and a low renal solute load. Parents can be helped to understand their baby's feeding problem and to be patient with his need to feed slowly.

Some babies will need to receive digoxin when they return home. Parents (or the person who will give the digoxin—sometimes it is the grandmother or another person) must have instruction and practice before the baby leaves the hospital. The following guidelines are suggested (modified from Jackson[6]).

1. Give the prescribed dosage without variation.

2. If one dose is missed, do not be concerned; do not double or increase the next dose to compensate. If two or more consecutive doses are missed, notify physician, clinic, or nurse.

3. Give doses at regular intervals as prescribed (usually every 12 hours).

4. Give doses 1 hour before or 2 hours after feedings (this facilitates passage into the bloodstream and avoids loss in case of vomiting during feedings). If dose is vomited within 15 minutes after it is administered and most of it appears to be lost, repeat dose. If vomiting occurs more than 15 minutes after administration, or if you feel that little has been lost, do not repeat the dose.

5. Notify physician, clinic, or nurse at the first sign of any illness, including colds or flu. (Loss of appetite, vomiting, and diarrhea are all signs of illness.)

6. Store digoxin in a safe place; if it is accidentally ingested by anyone, bring that person to an emergency room immediately and bring the digoxin bottle with you.

These guidelines may seem simple, but Jackson found that many parents who were giving their infants digoxin did not know these basic principles. In addition, many were unsure of how to measure the dose, particularly if the original dosage was changed. Parents need opportunities for supervised practice in the administration of digoxin not only during the initial hospitalization but whenever the dosage is changed.

Anomalies of the Gastrointestinal Tract

Anomalies may occur throughout the gastrointestinal tract. Most of these anomalies are corrected by surgery; many will require correction in the first days of life. Alternative methods of feeding (gastrostomy, parenteral alimentation) and of defecating (colostomy) are frequently necessary. Babies who are not fed orally need a pacifier for sucking needs. The baby may initially be discharged with a gastrostomy or colostomy; assisting the parents to care for their infant's special needs is an important nursing responsibility. Community health nurses, as well as hospital nurses, should be able to serve as a resource for parents.

Caring for an Infant with a Gastrostomy and Esophagostomy. When an infant first returns from surgery with a gastrostomy tube in place, the tube serves as a gravity drainage tube. Subsequently, the tube is elevated and attached to a syringe. When feedings begin, stomach contents are aspirated, measured and refed; this gastric aspirate is subtracted from the amount of the feeding, just as it is in gavage feeding (Chapter 23). Formula is poured into the syringe and allowed to flow by gravity into the baby's stomach. Between feedings the tube remains elevated; it is *not* clamped. In this way it serves as a safety valve so that fluid in the stomach will not enter the esophagus. When the baby cries, stomach contents will be seen in the tube and syringe and will not enter the esophagus.

When oral feedings are started, the gastrostomy tube at first remains open; if feedings go well, the tube is clamped but remains in place for several weeks following discharge. During the period before discharge, parents should have many opportunities to hold and feed their baby so that the gastrostomy tube is not a barrier between them. The gastrostomy site is washed with soap and water during the infant's bath.

Some infants will be discharged while receiving feedings through the gastrostomy; further corrective surgery is scheduled when the child is older. The parents need to become very comfortable feeding their baby by gastrostomy prior to discharge.

Occasionally an esophagostomy (an opening into the esophagus) is performed in infants in whom the esophagus ends in a blind pouch (esophageal atresia) and when corrective surgery is to be delayed. The esophagostomy allows secretions to drain from the esophagus and protects the baby from aspiration of secretions into the respiratory tract. Parents are taught (1) to protect the skin around the esophagostomy with ointment and frequent changes of protective dressings and (2) to give the baby oral feedings that meet sucking and swallowing needs and drain from the esophagostomy tube.

Caring for an Infant with an Ostomy. Many infants with congenital gastrointestinal defects will have temporary colostomies or ileostomies during the period between birth and the complete repair of their anomaly many months after birth. Regardless of the specific anomaly, nursing action to help parents become comfortable in caring for their infant with an ostomy begins by encouraging them to talk about their reactions to the ostomy (Nursing Care Plan 24–5). Parents are encouraged to assume gradually more of the total care of their baby so that by the time of discharge ostomy care has become a comfortable part of their daily routine.

Nursing Care Plan 24–5. Caring for an Infant with a Stoma

NURSING GOALS:
To provide immediate and long-term care for the infant with a stoma.
To prepare parents of an infant with a stoma to care for their infant.

OBJECTIVES:
1. Parents are prepared for the infant's surgery.
2. Following surgery, the incision remains clean and dry; the skin surrounding the stoma is clean, dry, and intact, and the ostomy is functional.
3. Parents accept their infant and are able to help siblings accept the infant.
4. Parents are able to care for their infant.
5. Parents are aware of community resources available to them.

ASSESSMENT	POTENTIAL NURSING DIAGNOSIS	NURSING INTERVENTION	COMMENTS/RATIONALE
Preoperative:			
1. Assess parents' knowledge about appropriate ostomy procedure.	Parents' need for information about ostomy	Provide information through use of doll, models, pictures to prepare parents for infant's appearance following surgery.	
2. Assess parents' reactions to proposed ostomy.	Anxiety about ability to care for infant with ostomy	Provide opportunities for parents to verbalize concerns, ask questions.	
	Anxiety about infant's altered body image	Explain reason for ostomy, duration (if temporary).	
Postoperative, immediate:		*Stoma care:*	
1. Condition of stoma: moist, red, lumen open	At risk for contamination of operative site	1. Wash around stoma with soap and water; dry area.	
2. Surrounding skin clean and dry	At risk for impairment in skin integrity from drainage	2. Apply Stomadhesive cut in doughnut shape to fit around stoma. Stomadhesive may remain in place for 1 to 2 weeks if skin beneath it remains dry.	Alternative skin preparations include zinc oxide ointment, silicone ointment, Karaya gum preparation.
3. Incision clean and dry, free of infection		3. Apply ostomy bag after peristalsis resumes (24–48 hours), or dressing secured with Montgomery straps. Dressing must be changed and site inspected every 2–3 hours.	Never put a single dressing over stoma and incision.
	At risk for bowel stenosis near lumen of stoma	Dilate stoma with catheter as directed by surgeon after 24 hours.	Infant may have catheter in stoma following surgery.
			Initial dilatation is done by surgeon; dilate carefully to prevent bowel perforation. Dilatation is not always necessary.

Continued on following page

Nursing Care Plan 24–5.   Caring for an Infant with a Stoma   *(Continued)*

ASSESSMENT	NURSING DIAGNOSIS	NURSING INTERVENTION	COMMENTS/RATIONALE
Postoperative, after 24 hours: 1. Continue assessment of stoma, skin, incision.			
2. Note characteristics of stool.	At risk of diarrhea related to: 1. Short bowel syndrome 2. Metabolic problems such as lactose deficiency, galactose malabsorption	Aids to maintenance of skin integrity and healing: 1. Karaya gum powder 2. Tincture of benzoin 3. Heat lamp 4. Exposure of area to air, if stool production allows	
	At risk of skin breakdown secondary to watery, diarrheal stool		
Assess parents' reactions to ostomy.	Altered body image of infant Anxiety about reactions of family and others	Encourage parents to verbalize feelings, concerns. Give them time to adjust to appearance of ostomy before involvement in ostomy care.	
	Fear of hurting infant during holding, caretaking	Assure parents they are not hurting infant by touching stoma, holding infant to shoulder, placing infant on abdomen. Encourage contact with infant to facilitate attachment.	Bowel has few nerves, thus touching stoma is not painful.
Assess parents' ability to care for infant.	Parents' need for information and practice in caring for stoma Anxiety about infant care	Develop a teaching plan: 1. Explain care given by nurse, step-by-step. 2. Let parents begin by preparing materials (Stomadhesive, dressing, etc.) and become comfortable with them before giving direct care to baby. Take one step at a time. Begin before discharge. 3. Provide written as well as verbal instructions. 4. Be sure parents have a source for necessary supplies (ostomy bags, Stomadhesive, etc.) Remind them to reorder supplies before all are used; in some communities supplies are not	Parents must know how to empty, cleanse, and change ostomy bag. Encourage both parents to participate. Responsibility often becomes solely the mother's if only the mother learns care during hospitalization.

Parents' need for information about total care of infant with stoma	immediately available. Provide information about sources of financial help for supplies.	
	Discuss total infant care with family:	
	1. Treat infant as normal.	
	2. Bathe daily; tub or sponge bath. Use lukewarm water. A long tub bath on the day Stomadhesive is changed facilitates removal.	Stomadhesive does not need to be removed during bath.
	3. Dress baby to avoid overheating. Cloth diapers are cooler than disposable ones. Plastic pants are hot, not necessary at home. Clothes with elastic waistbands may be uncomfortable.	Keeping baby cool facilitates attachment of Stomadhesive.
	4. Special formulas may be necessary, depending on reason and results of surgery.	Nutramegen, Probana, and Pregestomil are formulas for infants with disaccharidase deficiency.
	Identify resources for help in cost of special formulas.	
	Explain reason for special formula; be sure that parents understand why other formulas should not be substituted.	
	5. Instruct parents to report diarrhea to healthy-care provider immediately.	
Siblings need to understand ostomy.	Discuss with parents need to explain ostomy to siblings; show siblings stoma and bags.	
	Help parents to consider time management: extra time is needed to care for infant with ostomy and siblings also need time.	
	Babysitter will need to be familiar with ostomy and ostomy care.	
Need for continuing care following hospital discharge	Refer to community health nurse for continuing assessment and intervention in areas described above.	

Stomadhesive, a soft, pliable material, protects the skin around the stoma but allows it to "breathe." Stomadhesive is cut in a doughnut shape; it should fit closely to the walls of the stoma. The skin should be clean and dry. An ostomy bag is then attached to the Stomadhesive. The open end of the bag is folded and closed with a rubber band. To empty the bag the rubber band is removed and stool is squeezed from the bag. The ostomy bag is changed when it is soiled or when the seal between the Stomadhesive and the bag is no longer effective. Stomadhesive may remain in place for 1 to 2 weeks if the skin beneath it remains dry.

The baby can be bathed with the Stomadhesive in place, but the water should be only lukewarm for a tub bath. Water that is too warm can loosen the Stomadhesive. When it is time to change the Stomadhesive, soaking in warm water can make it easier to remove.

Not only water but clothing that is too warm can loosen the Stomadhesive. Cotton diapers are cooler than disposable diapers. Rubber pants make the baby warm and should be avoided. Clothes with elastic waistbands may be uncomfortable.

Infants with Specific Anomalies

Anomalies Associated with Maternal Polyhydramnios. Maternal polyhydramnios during pregnancy is a sign of a possible gastrointestinal anomaly. The fetus generally swallows amniotic fluid but is unable to do so if there is an obstruction in the gastrointestinal tract. Although other factors are also associated with polyhydramnios, infants whose mothers have this history should be assessed particularly carefully.

Tracheoesophageal Fistula. The signs indicating that a baby has a tracheoesophageal fistula vary somewhat with the type of anatomic anomaly involved (Fig. 24–7). In the most common type of anomaly (Fig. 24–7*A),* the esophagus ends in a blind pouch (a catheter cannot be passed through it), accounting for the almost immediate vomiting of any fluid taken orally. Because the trachea is connected to the stomach by a short fistula, the stomach quickly becomes distended as air enters with each breath. Gastric secretions can enter the tracheobronchial tree through the fistula. When the baby is not being fed there is drooling and frequent bubbly mucus—the classic symptom. Spotting and recognizing this excess mucus before the baby is fed for the first time contributes to early diagnosis and successful care of these babies.

In Figure 24–7*B,* air does not enter the stomach nor can gastric juice reach the trachea and lungs, but milk and saliva do overflow the esophagus into the respiratory tract. The fistula in Figure 24–7*C* is often not suspected in the newborn period because the esophagus does lead to the stomach and the baby can take his feedings. However, a fistula does exist, although it may be as small as a pinpoint, and its presence is suspected as the baby grows older and has repeated pneumonitis.

Fortunately, the fistulas in Figure 24–7*D* and *E* are rare. Because the upper esophagus is connected to the trachea, any feeding taken orally will be carried directly to the lungs; the baby will cough and become cyanotic, "drowning" in the fluid.

Surgery is performed as soon as the baby is stable. Often the baby must be transported from a community hospital to a medical center (below).

Caring for the Baby with a Tracheoesophageal Fistula. The greatest preoperative problem is aspiration pneumonia. Preoperative nursing care, aside from general support, is largely directed toward preventing this difficulty (Nursing Care Plan 24–6). In the most common type, the baby's head and chest are elevated to prevent the regurgitation of gastric juice into the lung. An infant seat, with rolled diapers beside the baby's head to keep the head in position, is one way of achieving this position. The baby must be kept in this semiupright position at all times.

Surgery involves ligation of the fistula and anastomosis of the esophageal segments. When

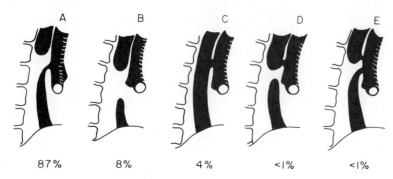

Figure 24–7. Diagrams of the five most commonly encountered forms of esophageal atresia and tracheoesophageal fistula, in order of frequency. (From Vaughan, McKay, and Behrman: *Nelson Textbook of Pediatrics.* 11th Edition. Philadelphia, W. B. Saunders Co., 1979.)

the segments are far apart, tissue from another structure, such as the colon, must be used to bridge the gap. More than one operation may be required.

The baby returns from surgery with a chest tube and a gastrostomy tube for feeding and for relieving abdominal distention. During the first postoperative hours he needs the individual attention of one nurse. Mucus may plug the respiratory tract, so frequent suctioning is necessary. He must be turned and stimulated to cry so that his lungs will fully expand. Normally there will be a minimal amount of drainage through the chest tube, and the lungs will be expanded within a few hours.

In the first days following repair, feedings are given through a gastrostomy tube. Oral feedings begin in 5 to 10 days in a baby who is doing well (but may be delayed much longer in some infants). If total repair was not possible during the initial surgery, gastrostomy feedings will continue for many months, which means that the mother will need to learn how to feed and care for her baby with the tube in place after he goes home.

Postoperatively, the biggest problem facing these babies is the healing of the esophagus. Because it has a segmental blood supply, inadequate circulation in one portion of the esophagus is not well compensated. Nor does the esophagus hold sutures well. In spite of these difficulties, surgery is generally successful when (1) the baby is full term, (2) he has no other anomalies, and (3) the esophageal segments are close together. When *esophageal atresia* exists without a fistula to the trachea, the baby will initially have a gastrostomy tube to decompress the stomach and a suction catheter in the blind pouch of the esophagus connected to a constant suction. If the proximal and distal portions of the esophagus are not close enough for anastomosis, surgery may be delayed for many months. The baby is fed through a gastrostomy tube at home, and secretions may be drained through an esophagostomy.

Postsurgical complications of tracheoesophageal fistula include pneumonia, recurrence of the fistula, and gastroesophageal reflux. Many babies will require dilatation of the esophagus in the months following surgery. Parents need to know that this may be necessary so that they will not see the need for dilatation as a setback.

Omphalocele and Gastroschisis. An omphalocele is the herniation of abdominal viscera into the umbilical cord, a failure of the intestines to return to the abdominal cavity after the tenth week of intrauterine life. The viscera are covered with a membrane; the umbilical cord extends from the membrane. Gastroschisis refers to the herniation of the bowel lateral to the midline; a covering membrane is not present. Nursing care of both anomalies is similar (see Nursing Care Plan 24–7).

If the infant is born in a community hospital he must be transported to a medical center for surgery. Prior to surgery, the goals of nursing are (1) to prevent heat and fluid loss through the exposed bowel, and (2) to protect the bowel from trauma and infection. The viscera are covered with sterile, warm saline gauze and then with plastic wrap. Fluid needs may be increased. An incubator is less likely to cause fluid loss than a radiant warmer.

Unless the amount of herniated bowel is quite small, the viscera are only partially replaced during surgery, and a Silastic envelope is created over the remainder, a little more bowel being returned to the abdomen each day to keep respiratory distress to a minimum.

Following surgery, the baby may have atelectasis or respiratory distress from the pressure of the bowel on the diaphragm. The bowel may also exert pressure on the inferior vena cava, resulting in edema of the lower extremities. A gastrostomy tube keeps the stomach decompressed and later may be used for feedings.

Nutrition is provided initially by intravenous glucose, protein, and fat (Chapter 23). Intestinal motility returns approximately 3 weeks after abdominal closure.

If the herniated bowel is necrotic and a large portion must be removed (resulting in short bowel syndrome), parenteral nutrition will be necessary for a long time, requiring a long period of hospitalization and separation from parents (Chapter 28). Babies with short bowel syndrome will need special formula (Pregestamil, Nutramigen, Probana); parents need to know where their baby's formula can be obtained in their own community so there will be no necessity to use some other type of feeding. If there are financial problems in obtaining specialized formula, contact with a WIC (Women, Infant and Children) program or local social service agencies should be made. Parents also are advised to seek medical care if their infant has even a single episode of diarrhea.[10]

Intestinal Obstruction. Intestinal obstruction may be due to atresia (absence of a lumen (passageway) or stenosis (narrowing) in some segment of the intestine, malrotation of the cecum and duodenum, or twisting of the intestine (volvulus). Meconium ileus, an early

Text continued on page 832

Nursing Care Plan 24–6.   Infants with Esophageal Anomalies

NURSING GOALS:
To encourage early signs of possible esophageal anomaly band and modify infant care.
To provide physiologic and emotional support to the infant prior to and following surgery.
To provide supportive care to parents.
To enhance parent–infant interaction.

OBJECTIVES:
1. Infant's esophageal anomaly will be recognized early.
2. Infant will be stabilized prior to surgery.
3. The physiologic, social, and emotional needs of the infant will be met in the postsurgical period.

Parents will:
1. Become attached to their infant.
2. Participate in the care of their infant.
3. Be able to care for their infant following discharge.

ASSESSMENT	POTENTIAL NURSING DIAGNOSIS	NURSING INTERVENTION	COMMENTS/RATIONALE
1. Identify factor in prenatal history that may indicate possible gastrointestinal tract anomaly: Polyhydramnios	At risk for gastrointestinal tract anomaly		
2. Postnatal assessment		Provide thermoneutral environment	
a. Excessive oral secretions ("blowing bubbles")	Respiratory distress secondary to tracheoesophageal fistula	Delay feeding.	Feeding may cause aspiration with subsequent bronchitis and pneumonia.
b. Respiratory distress			
c. Gagging, choking when feeding		Elevate infant's head (e.g., in infant seat).	Elevation of head presents gastric reflex and aspiration and facilitates respirations.
d. Inability to pass catheter into stomach		Suction	Suctioning removes excess secretions and helps to prevent aspiration; a suction tube connected to low intermittent suction may be ordered.
e. Abdominal distention			
		Provide increased humidity.	Humidity decreases viscosity of secretions.
f. Confirmation by radiography		Provide oxygen as required. Initiate intravenous fluids. Prepare infant for surgery.	
3. Postoperative assessment		*Postoperative intervention:*	
a. Airway obstruction (anxious expression on infant's face; tachypnea, apnea, retractions, cyanosis)	At risk for airway obstruction At risk for aspiration	Continue to position with head and chest elevated 20–30 degrees (e.g., in infant seat).	Avoid hyperextension of neck; will cause trauma to suture line. Respiratory distress may be due to airway obstruction or

Assessment	Intervention	Rationale
	Be prepared for rapid intervention for severe respiratory distress (laryngoscope, endotracheal tubes, oxygen and suction equipment should be immediately available).	atelectasis or pneumonia following aspiration.
	Suction carefully; have catheter marked by surgeon to indicate depth of suction to avoid area of anastomosis. Suction mouth as secretions accumulate. Chest tube in place following surgery; gastrostomy tube connected to straight drainage until gastrostomy feedings are started.	Prevent accumulation of mucus, but avoid unnecessary suctioning; suctioning increases edema.

b. Assess adequacy of nutrition
(1) Weight gain
(2) Skin turgor
(3) Urine
  (a) Volume
  (b) Specific gravity
 	
At risk of nutritional deprivation
Parental anxiety about feeding
Infant's sucking needs while NPO
	Nutrition initially provided via intravenous route (glucose, protein, fat).
	
	Gastrostomy feedings are initiated as infant's condition permits (provide pacifier to meet sucking needs prior to initiation of oral feeding).
	
	Oral feedings are begun when anastomosis is healed.
	
	Encourage parents to participate in gastrostomy and oral feeding. If infant will receive gastrostomy feedings at home, assist parents to become competent in giving them.
		(See Nursing Care Plan 23–6 for technique of gastrostomy feeding.)
		
		If repair is done in several stages, oral feedings will be delayed until repair is completed. Infant may be discharged while still receiving gastrostomy feedings.

c. After oral feedings are initiated, assess signs of stricture at the site of anastomosis (1) Difficulty in swallowing (2) Vomiting	Oral feedings: 1. Feed slowly. 2. Hold baby upright during feeding. 3. Burping frequently. 4. Explain rationale for feeding techniques to parents.	These techniques minimize the swallowing and retention of air in stomach and thus decrease the risk of regurgitation.
Lag in attachment Parental anxiety about caregiving 4. Assess parents' status with regard to: a. Attachment to infant b. Feelings in relation to anomaly (e.g., guilt, anger, etc.) c. Progress as care-givers	Encourage touching, holding, participation in care. Provide opportunities for verbalization of concern, questions. Provide positive reinforcement for caregiving behaviors. (See also Nursing Care Plan 28–1.)	
Need for continuing care 5. Identify arrangements for continuing care.	Involve parents in developing a plan for long-term care. Infant may need additional surgery, esophageal dilatation, repair of gastrostomy. Refer to community health nurse for long-term coordination of care.	

Nursing Care Plan 24–7.　Infants with Omphalocele or Gastroschisis

NURSING GOALS:
To protect the viscera and/or bowel and infant health prior to and following surgery.
To facilitate parental attachment.
To encourage parental caregiving.

OBJECTIVES:
1. Heat and fluid loss is prevented prior to surgery.
2. The bowel is protected from trauma and infection.
3. Respiratory distress is prevented.
4. Nutritional needs are met, including psychosocial needs related to feeding.
5. Parents accept their infant and are able to participate in caregiving.
6. Parents are aware of community resources available to them.

ASSESSMENT	POTENTIAL NURSING DIAGNOSIS	NURSING INTERVENTION	COMMENTS/RATIONALE
Identify anomaly.			Omphalocele: herniation of abdominal viscera into umbilical cord; membranous covering.
			Gastroschisis: herniation of bowel lateral to midline; no membranous covering.
			Infant may require transport to medical center.
Monitor vital signs.	At risk for heat loss through exposed bowel	Cover exposed bowel with warm saline sponges, then with plastic wrap to retain heat and moisture.	
	At risk of fluid loss through exposed bowel	Wear sterile gloves. Avoid pressure on abdominal contents. A sterile wall (doughnut) can be built around contents to protect during transport.	
	At risk of trauma	Incubator provides warmth with less fluid loss than radiant warmer.	
	At risk of infection	Initiate IV therapy.	
		Insert nasogastric tube to prevent distention of stomach and intestines.	
		If sac is ruptured, antibiotics are initiated in preoperative period.	

Assessment	Nursing Diagnosis	Intervention/Rationale
Identify parents' reaction to defect.	Lag in attachment; anxiety	When only a small amount of bowel has herniated through defect, Silastic envelope may not be necessary.
		Encourage parents to verbalize feelings; provide pictures of infant: 1. Immediately following surgery with Silastic envelope. 2. After closure of incision.
Assess parental attachment.	Lag in parental attachment	Encourage parents to touch infant. As Silastic envelope becomes smaller, parents become more comfortable in holding infant.
		Explain all components of the plan of care.
		Encourage questions, verbalization of concerns.
Postoperative Assess vital signs.	At risk for respiratory distress related to pressure of bowel on diaphragm	Notify surgeon; Silastic envelope (or silo) may be adjusted to relieve intraabdominal and intrathoracic pressure.
	At risk for circulatory distress related to pressure of bowel on vena cava	Prevent atelectasis by turning.
	At risk for hypothermia secondary to transport and surgery	Provide thermoneutral environment.
Inspect area where skin joins Silastic envelope for signs of infection.	At risk of infection	Cleanse area with soap and water; solutions such as half-strength Betadine may be ordered.
Assess adequacy of nutrition (daily weight, head circumference, weekly length, condition of skin).	At risk of nutritional deprivation	Early nutritional needs met by total parenteral nutrition (TNP), Intralipid; later feedings may be made via gastrostomy prior to oral feedings (see Nursing Care Plan 24–6).
		If large sections of bowel are removed, special formula maybe necessary. Explain reasons to parents.
		Help parents identify sources for formula and of financial aid for special formula.
	At risk for diarrhea related to shortened bowel	Teach parents to contact health-care provider immediately if a single episode of diarrhea occurs.

Table 24–3.   INTESTINAL OBSTRUCTIONS

Obstruction	Nursing Assessment
Atresia	
Duodenum	Vomiting soon after birth; vomitus green (if lesion is below ampulla of Vater); X-ray film shows air in upper gastrointestinal tract, no air in lower tract (double bubble)
Jejunum	Abdominal distention
Colon	Abdominal distention
Stenosis	Delayed symptoms for days or weeks; poor feeding; intermittent vomiting
Malrotation	Vomiting; may have abdominal distention; may pass meconium but fail to pass transitional or fecal stool
Volvulus	Sudden vomiting (green); sudden abdominal distention; may pass meconium but fail to pass transitional or fecal stool; bloody stool
Meconium ileus	Abdominal distention; vomiting bile; no meconium, or "puttylike" meconium
Meconium plug	Failure to pass meconium
Hirschsprung disease (megacolon	Failure to pass meconium; may not have symptoms for several weeks
Functional obstruction	
Maternal drugs (heroin)	Failure to pass meconium
Immature large bowel (e.g., preterm infants)	
Sepsis	
Hypothyroidism	
Necrotizing enterocolitis (Chapter 23)	

symptom of cystic fibrosis, can also cause obstruction in the newborn. Obstruction may be functional rather than mechanical (i.e., related to inadequate bowel function). Table 24–3 summarizes types of gastrointestinal obstructions.

Careful nursing observations of vomitus and stools are most important in recognizing an obstruction and pinpointing its location (Nursing Care Plan 24–8). Green vomitus (vomitus containing bile) is the classic symptom. Absence of stool, abdominal distention, and, occasionally, peristaltic waves from right to left are also significant observations. The lower the obstruction is located in the gastrointestinal tract, the more likely it is that symptoms will be delayed. Surgery is the treatment for mechanical obstruction (but not for meconium ileus, meconium plug, or most functional disorders). Since an obstruction is not likely to be recognized as early as other anomalies of the gastrointestinal tract, the baby may have vomited several times and lost electrolytes as well as fluid, a situation that must be corrected before he goes to the operating room.

Postoperatively as well as preoperatively, vomiting and aspiration are the chief dangers for these babies. To prevent these hazards, they should be positioned on the abdomen or side. A nasogastric tube is inserted before surgery, and either a gastrostomy tube or a nasogastric tube will be in place after surgery to prevent air and intestinal secretions from accumulating in the stomach until bowel peristalsis is restored. The return of peristalsis is indicated by normal stools and minimal gastric drainage.

Imperforate Anus.   The practice of taking an initial rectal temperature as part of the newborn assessment can detect the absence of a patent anus. If the anus is imperforate, urine is tested for the presence of meconium to determine whether or not there is a fistula to the urinary system. Rectovaginal or rectourinary fistulas are common.

Surgical repair is relatively simple when the rectum ends close to the perineum (this is more common in females) and more complicated when the end of the rectum is high and there is a fistula to the bladder or urethra. In the latter instance a temporary colostomy is created, and more extensive surgery is delayed until the baby is several months old.

Following perineal repair, specific nursing care is directed toward keeping the suture line free of feces (Nursing Care Plan 24–8). A diaper is not used so that any stool will be observed immediately and washed away. Because newborns, when they lie on their abdo-

Text continued on page 838

Nursing Care Plan 24–8. Infants with Anomalies of the Lower Gastrointestinal Tract (Intestinal Obstruction, Anorectal Malformations)

NURSING GOALS:
To recognize early signs of lower gastrointestinal obstruction.
To meet infant's physiologic, emotional, and social needs prior to and following surgery.
To assist parents in coping with infant's anomaly that may involve long-term alteration in health status.

OBJECTIVES:
1. The infant with an anomaly of the lower gastrointestinal tract is identified quickly.
2. The anomaly is repaired.
3. Parents accept their infant.
4. Parents are able to provide the care needed by their infant.

ASSESSMENT	POTENTIAL NURSING DIAGNOSIS	NURSING INTERVENTION	COMMENTS/RATIONALE
Identify factor in prenatal history that may indicate gastrointestinal tract anomaly—polyhydramnios	At risk for gastrointestinal tract anomaly.		
	Intestinal Obstruction		
Postnatal assessment		NPO	
1. Vomiting: green or not green; time of vomiting (soon after birth or delayed); projectile; blood in vomitus		Provide fluid, electrolytes via IV.	See Table 24–3 for detailed assessment.
		Explain or clarify explanation of baby's condition to parents.	
2. Abdominal distention	At risk for aspiration of stomach contents	Position infant on abdomen or side.	Position protects infant from aspiration.
3. Abnormal stool pattern: absence of meconium, "puttylike" meconium; meconium stool but no transitional or fecal stool; blood in stool (hematest)		Insert nasogastric tube; tube may be connected to low intermittent suction.	Stomach is kept empty to prevent aspiration. Irrigation of nasogastric tube with water or air may be necessary to maintain potency.
4. Aspirate gastric contents. Bile-stained fluid or gastric contents greater than 25 ml. suggests intestinal obstruction.		If infant transport is necessary prior to surgery, transport with nasogastric tube; infant in side or prone position.	
5. Radiographs will confirm clinical suspicion.		If infant must leave neonatal unit for radiography, provide thermoneutral environment, nursing observation.	
Postoperative assessment:	Parents' need to accept, care for infant with ostomy, gastrostomy	See Nursing Care Plan 24–5. Involve parents in ostomy care, one step at a time.	Not all infants will have ostomy; end-to-end anastomosis may be performed.
1. If infant has an ostomy, determine if temporary or permanent. Inspect stoma, surrounding skin.			

Continued on following page

Nursing Care Plan 24–8.   Infants with Anomalies of the Lower Gastrointestinal Tract (Intestinal Obstruction, Anorectal Malformations)   *(Continued)*

ASSESSMENT	POTENTIAL NURSING DIAGNOSIS	NURSING INTERVENTION	COMMENTS/RATIONALE
		Intestinal Obstruction *(Continued)*	
2. Assess functioning of nasogastric tube.	At risk for aspiration	Nasogastric tube is left in place until infant defecates, through ostomy or anus (usually 2–3 days). Explain to parents. Ensure potency of tube. Provide pacifier to meet sucking needs.	
3. Assess gastrostomy site.		Gastrostomy tube is initially placed low for drainage, then raised as oral feedings are initiated. Leave tube unclamped—this serves as a safety valve (Nursing Care Plan 23–6).	
4. Assess intravenous site. Central elimination line may be placed.		Long-term intravenous elimination may be necessary until healing occurs (see Nursing Care Plan 23–6).	
		Anorectal Malformations	
Identify infant with imperforate anus. 1. Inability to insert rectal thermometer 2. Absence of anal opening on observation 3. Absence of stools 4. Stooling through vagina (rectovaginal fistula) or flecks of stool in urine (rectourinary fistula) 5. Delayed abdominal distention and vomiting (at 2–3 days of life) X-ray films used to define the problem.	Parents' need for information about infant's condition	Explain or clarify condition to parents. Nursing management is coordinated with medical care plan. 1. Anal stenosis: anus dilated; parents may be taught to perform digital dilatation. Stool softener may be recommended. 2. Imperforate membrane: membrane is surgically perforated in neonatal period; observe stooling to ensure no further difficulty. 3. Anal agenesis: anoplasty in neonatal period or before 6 months. Following surgery: a. Baby is positioned on side to prevent tension on suture line.	

b. No diapers used until anoplasty heals.

c. Keep suture line clean. Remove stools with soft material and water (no gauze; may adhere to suture). Cotton-tipped applicators are useful for cleaning between sutures.

d. Ointments are sometimes used to promote healing.

e. *No rectal temperatures.* Take axillary temperature.

f. Daily dilatation of anus may be necessary for several months; explain to parents and help them become comfortable with dilatation.

g. Rectal agenesis and atresia require temporary colostomy in neonatal period, surgical correction usually between 6 and 12 months (see colostomy care, Nursing Care Plan 24–5).

All Anomalies

Provide opportunities for parents to express concerns, ask questions. Involve parents in infant's care. If infant is to be discharged with gastrostomy or ostomy, provide many opportunities for practice so that parents become comfortable in caring for infant.

Provide written material for use following discharge.

Refer to community health nurse for home follow-up.

Provide information, telephone numbers about community resources.

Assess parental attachment, parental ability and comfort in caring for infant. (Nursing Care Plan 28–1.)

Lag in attachment
Need for assistance in learning to care for infant

Nursing Care Plan 24–9.   Infants with Anomalies of the Urinary Tract

NURSING GOALS:
To identify the infant with a urinary tract anomaly.
To provide immediate and long-term care so that complications are prevented.
To facilitate attachment and infant care by parents.

OBJECTIVES:
1. The infant with a urinary tract anomaly is identified.
2. Parents understand the plan of care.
3. Attachment is facilitated.
4. Complications are prevented.
5. Parents are comfortable in caring for their infant prior to hospital discharge.
6. Referral to appropriate community resources is made prior to discharge.
7. Parents receive support during the grieving process when the infant's prognosis is poor.

ASSESSMENT	POTENTIAL NURSING DIAGNOSIS	NURSING INTERVENTION	COMMENTS/RATIONALE
Preoperative period Identify signs of possible genitourinary tract anomaly 1. Maternal oligohydramnios 2. Single umbilical artery 3. Low-set ears 4. Abdominal mass 5. Anomalies of face, limbs, lungs (Potter's syndrome) 6. Family history of urinary tract disease	Infant at risk for anomaly of urinary tract		
Identify signs of urinary tract anomaly 1. Absence of voiding after 24 hours 2. Decreased voiding (diaper is not damp every 3–4 hours) 3. Weak, dribbling urinary stream in male 4. Drainage of urine from umbilicus 5. Exposure of bladder mucosa 6. Epispadias, hypospadias 7. Absence of abdominal muscles (prune belly syndrome) 8. Distended bladder 9. General symptoms of impaired health (e.g., poor feeding, failure to thrive)		Keep accurate record of frequency of voids. When anomaly is identified, explain or clarify explanation of anomaly, plan of care.	
If surgery is indicated, assess parents' understanding of proposed surgery.	Parents' need for information	Provide or clarify explanation of proposed surgery in simple terms.	

Assessment	Intervention	Rationale/Comments
Immediate postoperative period: 1. Vital signs 2. Drainage from all catheters; drainage from each catheter should be recorded separately (amount, color). Assess drainage on hourly basis.		
Fear of attachment because of infant's illness causes lag in attachment.	Use doll, illustrations, to prepare parents for infant's appearance following surgery (catheters, drains, etc.). Encourage parents to hold infant, give care when possible.	
Absence of drainage from urinary catheter	Check for obstruction in catheter (kink, pressure, etc.). Notify physician if no external reason is discovered for absence of drainage.	
Bloody drainage	Notify physician if drainage has consistency of blood.	Normal drainage color: 0–24 hours (approx.)—red but thin, watery; 24–48 hours to 3–4 days—dark red, brown; 4–7 days—increasingly yellow, small clots.
3. Identify signs of pain: crying, restlessness Pain related to bladder spasm; bladder spasm related to surgical trauma or presence of catheter.	Inspect catheters, tubing for kinks. Administer antispasmodic medication.	Kinked tubing is a common cause for bladder spasm. Narcotics are not effective for bladder spasm.
Following stabilization: Assess parents' understanding of surgery performed. Parental anxiety	Explain or clarify surgery.	
Parents' need for information	Explain "tubes," reason for color of drainage.	Parents may interpret "red urine" as severe bleeding; explain that even small amount of blood colors urine.
Parents' need for involvement in caregiving	Assist parents to hold infant with tubes. Encourage and provide opportunities for participation in infant care.	
Parents' need for information	Provide information about continuing care.	
Assess parents' understanding of need for continuing care appropriate to infant's condition.	Refer to community health nurse and other appropriate resources.	
Parents' grief process (see Nursing Care Plan 28–2) When condition is untreatable (e.g., bilateral renal agenesis, severe bilateral hydronephrosis)	See Nursing Care Plan 28–2.	

men, have a tendency to pull their legs up under them, creating tension in the perineal area, the baby should be positioned on either side following perineal surgery and his position changed frequently. Colostomy care is described above.

Hernias. A hernia (protrusion of a part of the bowel through the abdominal wall) may be noted in the nursery or may not appear for several months. The hernia may be visible only when the baby is crying or stooling.

The most common hernias are located in the umbilical or inguinal (groin) area. Surgery is usually *not* performed in the newborn period. Most umbilical hernias will resolve by themselves.

Folk culture has suggested the use of binders, a coin, or tape to compress an umbilical hernia, but there is no evidence that these methods are effective. The belief in the effectiveness of these remedies is probably related to the high incidence of spontaneous cure. Umbilical hernias rarely incarcerate. The incidence of incarceration of inguinal hernias is high in the first months of life; parents are instructed to call their clinic or physician if there is redness or increased swelling in the area of the hernia or if they are unable to reduce the hernia.[116]

If surgery is necessary it is sometimes performed on an outpatient basis.

Anomalies of the Genitourinary Tract

Hypospadias, epispadias, and ambiguous genitalia are visible anomalies of the genitourinary tract (Chapter 21). Other anomalies are less obvious (see Nursing Care Plan 24–9). Problems frequently associated with urinary tract anomalies are a single umbilical artery, low-set ears, an abdominal mass (due to a multicystic kidney), and maternal oligohydramnios (because failure of the fetus to excrete urine decreases the amount of amniotic fluid).

A variety of abnormalities may cause obstruction in the urinary tract. The most common site is the junction of the ureter and the pelvis of the kidney. Because of the obstruction, urine collects in the pelvis of the kidney, and hydronephrosis results. The severity of the obstruction is directly related to the severity of the hydronephrosis. In addition, the oligohydramnios that results from the lack of urine production by the fetus is related to anomalies of the face, limbs, and lung (Potter's syndrome). Severe hydronephrosis results in a kidney filled with cysts that is nonfunctioning. Intrauterine surgery has, in several instances, relieved the obstruction. A catheter is placed in the fetal bladder to drain urine into the amniotic fluid.

A weak, dribbling urinary stream in male infants, accompanied by a distended bladder, indicates an obstruction in the urethra. Surgery relieves the obstruction. Following surgery, the infant may have a nephrostomy tube (draining urine from the kidney) or a ureterostomy tube (draining urine from the ureter) as well as a catheter to drain urine from the bladder. In addition, drains outside of the urinary tract to drain any extravasated urine and stents to ensure the patency of an anastomosis may be present.

The drainage from each catheter is recorded separately. Immediately following surgery the urine is bright red and watery, becoming darker after 12 to 48 hours. After 4 to 7 days the urine has become yellow and contains occasional blood clots. Frank bleeding is always abnormal. The absence of drainage may be due to kinks or compression of the tube.

It takes time to position a baby with many tubes so that his parents can hold him, but it is essential to take that time. As with any surgery for congenital defects, preparing the parents to expect the baby's postsurgical appearance will help to ease their anxiety when they first see him after surgery.

A *patent urachus*, an opening between the bladder and the umbilicus, is present when urine drains from the umbilicus. A urachal cyst may develop from the urachus in the area between the bladder and the umbilicus. Surgery is the treatment for both conditions.

Exstrophy of the bladder may take varying forms; usually the bladder is everted, and the

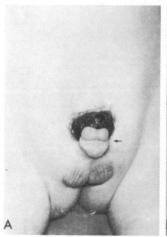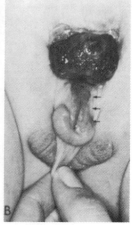

Figure 24–8. Exstrophy of the bladder. *A,* Male infant with exstrophy. *B,* Dorsal view of the short, broad epispadias. (From Vaughn, McKay, and Behrman: *Nelson Textbook of Pediatrics.* 11th Edition. Philadelphia, W. B. Saunders Co., 1979.)

mucosa is exposed. The urethra, penis, clitoris, anus, and pubic bones may be affected (Fig. 24–8).

The exposed bladder is covered with single strips of Vaseline gauze, and the diaper is changed frequently. If the defect is small, it may be closed surgically, and normal bladder capacity and urinary control can be expected. When the defect is large, a surgical procedure to divert urine, frequently into the sigmoid colon, may be performed when the infant is older.

Anomalies of the Musculoskeletal System

Common anomalies of the musculoskeletal system are far less devastating and more easily corrected than many of the other conditions described in this chapter. They are nevertheless distressing to parents. Reassurance that the baby will not be crippled following treatment helps parents to cope with the defect initially and during the many weeks of treatment (Nursing Care Plan 24–10).

Congenital Clubfoot. A clubfoot involves bones, muscles, and tendons. Clubfoot occurs approximately once in every 1000 births; it may be unilateral or bilateral and is more common in males. Of the several varieties of clubfoot, *talipes equinovarus*, in which the foot is turned medially and in plantar flexion with the heel elevated, accounts for approximately 95 per cent of all instances of clubfoot. The second most common variety is *talipes calcaneovalgus*, in which the foot deviates laterally and is dorsiflexed.

It is not difficult to recognize the presence of a clubfoot in an infant if his foot is inspected carefully. It is, however, important to differentiate true clubfoot from a foot that appears to be deformed because of the position the fetus has assumed in utero. In the latter instance, the foot can easily be positioned normally or in an overcorrected position, whereas a true clubfoot cannot.

Treatment for a true clubfoot usually begins with a cast applied before the baby leaves the hospital. The cast will be changed at frequent intervals, often weekly, for a period of several months. At each cast change the baby's foot will be manipulated to assume the corrected position more closely. Following correction, an orthopedic device such as a Denis-Browne splint (a metal bar with corrective shoes attached) will be used for a period of time.

Nurses who care for the baby in the first days after birth should teach parents basic information about cast care that will be important at each cast change. It is valuable to have the information in written form that parents can take home with them. With all that parents must learn in this period about baby care, it is easy to forget important points.

Basic information about cast care includes the following points (Nursing Care Plan 24–10).

1. Plaster casts take approximately 24 hours to dry; fiberglass casts dry much more quickly. The cast should be uncovered and handled carefully until it is dry. Turning the baby from front to back facilitates drying.

2. Check toes for swelling, coldness, and cyanosis every hour during the first 4 to 6 hours after the cast is applied and every few hours afterward during the first 24 hours. Pain and numbness, signs of cast pressure in older children, are difficult to assess in newborns.

3. Check for rough edges on the cast and any irritation on the baby's skin. "Petals" of adhesive tape can cover the cast edges to prevent irritation.

4. Keep the cast clean and dry. The baby will need sponge baths rather than tub baths. If the cast becomes wet or soft it must be replaced as soon as possible.

Parents can hold their baby with cast in place with minimal difficulty but may need encouragement at first. Positioning the baby for breast-feeding may also seem difficult. The baby can be positioned with his legs pointing toward the mother's side rather than toward her abdomen.

Congenital Hip Dysplasia. The inability to abduct one thigh is an indication of *congenital hip dysplasia*, in which there is abnormal development of the hip joint (Fig. 24–9). Dysplasia may be partial (congenital subluxation of the hip), in which the head of the femur is partially dislocated from the shallow acetabulum, or complete (congenital dislocation), in which the head of the femur is completely

Text continued on page 844

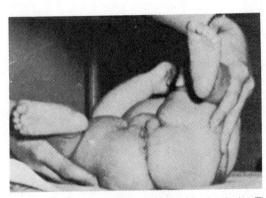

Figure 24–9. Infant with congenital hip dysplasia. The nurse is able to abduct the right thigh down to the level of the table, but not the left. (From Pray: *Pediatrics, 9:*94, 1952.)

Nursing Care Plan 24–10. Infants with Positional Foot Deformity and Congenital Clubfoot (Talipes Equinovarus, Talipes Calcanovalgus)

NURSING GOALS:
To identify the infant with congenital clubfoot and ensure initial and continuing care so that neither deformity or impairment of function occurs.
To enable parents to care for their infant.

OBJECTIVES:
1. The infant with congenital clubfoot is identified and treatment is initiated.
2. Parents accept their infant.
3. Parents understand the plan of care and are able to care for their infant.

ASSESSMENT	POTENTIAL NURSING DIAGNOSIS	NURSING INTERVENTION	COMMENTS/RATIONALE
Differentiate positional deformity from true clubfoot. 1. Positional deformity: foot can be manipulated into a normal position. 2. Clubfoot: anatomical deformity prevents foot from being manipulated into normal position. Varies in severity.	Parents' need for information about infant's status Parental anxiety about infant anomaly, ability to care for infant	Deformity is usually readily apparent. Encourage parents to verbalize concerns about infant's appearance and prognosis.	
	Need for information about plan of care	Explain or review plan of care. If *positional deformity*, parents are taught passive exercises for correction. Observe parents in performance of exercises on several occasions before discharge. Refer to community health nurse for follow-up. Provide parents with names and phone numbers of resources if questions develop following discharge. If *clubfoot*, a cast is usually applied prior to initial discharge. Cast will be changed at weekly intervals.	
Following application of cast, assess toes for: 1. Swelling 2. Color (cyanosis, pallor)	Parents' need for information about cast care	Provide parents with written information about cast care: 1. Handle casts very carefully until dry (24 hours for plaster; shorter	

3. Temperature (coldness)
4. Pedal pulses
5. Pressure areas
6. Areas of skin irritation

period for fiberglass). Turning baby facilitates drying.

2. Teach parents to assess toes following every change of cast.

3. "Petal" cast edges to prevent irritation. Teach parents to "petal" cast.

4. Sponge baths given rather than tub baths. Explain importance of keeping cast clean and dry. Baby should wear plastic pants or disposable diapers to keep urine from cast. Explain why parents must contact physician immediately if cast becomes wet or soft.

At risk for decreased parent–infant interaction secondary to casts

Help parents find comfortable ways to hold infant. Explain importance of holding, cuddling; demonstrate holding with legs pointed toward mother's side rather than abdomen. Help mother find comfortable ways to hold infant during feeding.

Need for continuing care

Explain importance of continuing care; casts must be changed as scheduled (often weekly).

Refer to appropriate community resources for help with economic or transportation problems.

Assess possible transportation, economic problems that may be a barrier to continuing care.

Explain that following correction an orthopedic device (e.g., Denis-Browne splint) will be used for a period of time.

Nursing Care Plan 24–11.   Infants with Congenital Hip Dysplasia

NURSING GOALS:
1. To identify the infant with congenital hip dysplasia in the neonatal period.
2. To ensure early correction and continuing care so that neither deformity nor impairment of function occurs.
3. To enable parents to care for their infant.

OBJECTIVES:
1. The infant with hip dysplasia is identified in the neonatal period.
2. Correction measures are initiated.
3. Parents understand the plan of care and are able to care for the infant.
4. Plans are developed for continuing health supervision of the infant.

ASSESSMENT	POTENTIAL NURSING DIAGNOSIS	NURSING INTERVENTION	COMMENTS/RATIONALE
Identify infant with congenital hip dysplasia. 1. Ortolani's maneuver: with infant supine, flex legs at right angles to trunk and adduct; adduct one thigh at a time to allow head of femur to slip over acetabulum. Listen for "click of exit" as femur slips out of acetabulum and "click of entry" when pressure is relieved, thigh is abducted, and head of femur slips back into acetabulum (subluxation).	Parents' need for information about infant care related to congenital hip dysplasia Anxiety related to outcome of hip dysplasia	Explain condition to parents; describe expected plan of care. Assist parents in initial care as prescribed by physician. 1. Use two or three diapers rather than a single diaper, or 2. Use Frejka pillow or splint, or 3. Use a spica cast, or 4. Use traction, reduction, and spica cast (dislocator).	Subluxation (more common): head of femur is partially dislocated from shallow acetabulum. Dislocation: head of femur is completely dislocated from acetabulum. Early recognition and treatment is essential for optimal outcome. Frejka pillow is applied over diaper and plastic pants. Spica cast may follow use of Frejka pillow.

2. Allis's sign: leg appears shorter on affected side when head of femur overrides acetabulum (dislocation).

At risk for skin breakdown secondary to treatment for hip dysplasia

Excellent skin care necessary with each method; keep baby dry, ensure that cast or pillow does not rub. For cast care, see Nursing Care Plan 24–10.

3. Asymmetry of gluteal folds; folds appear higher on affected side (dislocation).
4. Limited abduction of thigh on affected side (dislocation; may occur in subluxation after neonatal period)

At risk for decreased parent-infant interaction secondary to treatment for hip dysplasia

Infant is more difficult to cuddle and hold; encourage these behaviors by explaining the importance of holding, cuddling, and playing and by helping parents find comfortable ways to hold infant.

Assess possible transportation, economic problems that may be a barrier to continuing care.

Need for continuing care

Explain importance of continuing care with regular visits to health-care provider.

Refer to community health nurse to assess and help mother with caregiving at home.

Provide information about possible sources of financial assistance for long-term care.

Reassure parents that with early and continuing treatment, prognosis is usually excellent.

dislocated from the hip. Congenital subluxation is much more common.

Early recognition and treatment of congenital hip dysplasia is important in achieving good results (Nursing Care Plan 24–11). Since subluxation may not result in a limitation of abduction in the first few weeks of life, every infant should be assessed using Ortolani's maneuver. With the baby lying on his back, the legs are flexed at right angles to the trunk and abducted. One thigh is then adducted, still flexed, with pressure applied in such a way that the head of the femur slips over the posterior lip of the acetabulum. A "click of exit" is felt as the femur slips posteriorly from the acetabulum; a second "click of entry" is felt when the pressure is relieved, the hip is abducted, and the head of the femur consequently slips back into the acetabulum. Other signs that may lead to a suspicion of hip dysplasia include shortening of the leg (Allis' sign) and asymmetry of skin folds of the buttocks; both are rare in subluxation but common in dislocation.

Initial treatment may consist of using two or three diapers or a pillow covered with plastic to maintain the baby's legs in an abducted position, thereby forcing the head of the femur into the acetabulum and enlarging the socket by the constant pressure. When the hip can be easily dislocated this is not sufficient because the hip may slip from the socket at each diaper change. Casts or splints may be required. If treatment is started at birth or shortly thereafter, the hip is commonly normal by the time the baby is 3 months old. If diagnosis, and thus treatment, is delayed, more extensive treatment, including hospitalization for orthopedic traction and a hip spica cast, may be required.

Central Nervous System Anomalies

Major anomalies of the embryologic neural tube, which develops into the central nervous system, include anencephaly and hydrocephaly, and meningocele, myelomeningocele, and encephalocele. Prenatal screening for neural tube defects was described in Chapter 14. A neural tube defect is sometimes discovered during an ultrasound examination for some other purpose.

Anencephaly, an absence of the cerebral hemispheres as well as a lack of development in the skull, results in death, usually at the time of birth or within the first days of life. The birth of an anencephalic infant, who does not even look human to many parents, is a devastating experience. They will need the opportunity to talk about their feelings in professional counseling sessions not only during the immediate postpartum period but in the weeks that follow. Genetic counseling should be a part of the counseling sessions. (See Chapter 28 for a more complete discussion of family support.)

Hydrocephalus results from an imbalance between the secretion and absorption of cerebrospinal fluid within the ventricles of the brain. The etiology of hydrocephalus is summarized in Table 24–4.

Hydrocephalus may occur in utero; because of an enlarged head, vaginal delivery is not possible. In 1981 shunting procedures were used to drain cerebrospinal fluid from the fetal brain in several fetuses in whom prenatal hydrocephalus was diagnosed. A plastic tube, about 5 inches long with a one-way valve to prevent backflow of amniotic fluid, is guided through a hollow needle that has pierced first the mother's abdomen, then the uterus (as in amniocentesis), and then the fetal head. When the needle is withdrawn, approximately half of the catheter remains in the fetal brain, the remainder extending into the amniotic fluid. In preterm infants hydrocephalus is frequently a sequel to intraventricular hemorrhage (Chapter 23). In milder forms of congenital hydrocephalus the baby's head may be a normal size at birth but grows rapidly after birth.

Table 24–4.   NEONATAL HYDROCEPHALUS

Types	Etiology in Newborn
Communicating Obstruction in subarachnoid space; abnormal absorption of cerebrospinal fluid	Frequently unknown; subarachnoid hemorrhage; toxoplasmosis, CID, bacterial meningitis; Arnold-Chiari malformation—medulla and cerebellum displaced into cervical canal; compression obstructs flow of cerebrospinal fluid; secondary to myelomeningocele
Noncommunicating (obstructive) Obstruction within the ventricles; cerebrospinal fluid cannot reach subarachnoid space	Inherited sex-linked disorder; fetal viral infection; intraventricular hemorrhage

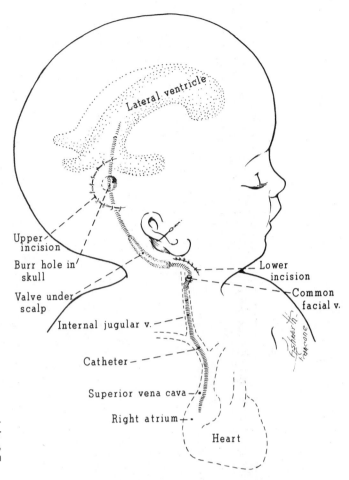

Lateral ventricle

Upper incision

Burr hole in skull

Valve under scalp

Internal jugular v.

Catheter

Superior vena cava

Right atrium

Lower incision

Common facial v.

Heart

Figure 24–10. Operative procedure for hydrocephalus in which a catheter drains the ventricular system into the right atrium. (From Jacob, Francone, and Lossow: *Structure and Function in Man.* 5th Edition. Philadelphia, W. B. Saunders Co., 1982.)

Transillumination of the head, in which a cuffed flashlight or a Chun-gun (a focused bright light) is held against the skull, will indicate abnormal fluid collection in the skull. Further studies utilize computerized axial tomography and cranial ultrasonography.

In general, the treatment of hydrocephalus is a shunting procedure in which a plastic tube with a one-way valve is inserted into the ventricle to carry excess cerebrospinal fluid to a site outside of the head such as the right atrium (Fig. 24–10) or peritoneum. Even when the long-term prognosis is not considered good, a shunting procedure may enable a family to care for their baby at home for several weeks and months, an opportunity that means a great deal to most parents. With treatment, approximately 70 per cent of infants with hydrocephalus will live beyond infancy; 40 per cent of these infants can be expected to have normal intelligence. It is frequently not possible to predict in advance which infants will have normal brain function. Some children with marked dilatation of the ventricles and a thin cerebral mantle have normal intelligence.[15]

During the preoperative period nurses can help parents become comfortable with their baby. If the baby's head is already large they will need both encouragement and assistance in holding their baby, supporting his head. Their baby may feed slowly and may need small, frequent feedings. Parents should be encouraged to feed their baby. Nurses can help parents by showing acceptance of the baby and a relaxed attitude in caring for him.

After surgery the baby will initially be kept lying down to prevent too rapid a decrease in intracranial pressure. The baby's head is positioned on the nonoperative side to prevent pressure on the shunt. Changes in position are important, however, to prevent pressure areas from developing. A piece of lamb's wool beneath the baby's head is softer than the bed (Nursing Care Plan 24–12).

Nurses observe and teach parents to observe for signs of increased intracranial pressure. In newborns, because of the open fontanels, a bulging fontanel and separation of the sutures may be noted. Irritability, fretfulness, lethargy, vomiting, dilation of scalp veins, and a shrill high-pitched cry are other signs. Intracranial pressure is increased when the shunt becomes occluded or kinked.

Infection is a serious complication; bacteria

Nursing Care Plan 24–12.   Infants with Hydrocephalus

NURSING GOALS:
To prevent sequelae of hydrocephalus through early detection and acute and long-term intervention.
To assist parents in coping with an anomaly that involves long-term alteration in health status.

OBJECTIVES:
1. Neonatal hydrocephalus is identified.
2. Infant's physiologic, social, and emotional needs are met.
3. Parents accept their infant and are to participate in the plan of care.
4. Parents are aware of community resources available for their family.

ASSESSMENT	POTENTIAL NURSING DIAGNOSIS	NURSING INTERVENTION	COMMENTS/RATIONALE
Prenatal: hydrocephalus may be detected:	Parents' need for information about hydrocephalus, available options	Provide or clarify information.	
1. During ultrasonogram for other reasons		Provide opportunities for parents' questions; encourage them to verbalize feelings.	
2. As a result of screening for neural tube defect if accompanied by open defect such as meningocele.			Hydrocephalus occurring without open neural tube defect will not be detected by neural tube screening (Chapter 14).
Postnatal: Identify infant at risk for hydrocephalus.			
1. Preterm infant	At risk for hydrocephalus secondary to intracranial hemorrhage	Measure head circumference daily; tape measure should be directly above eyebrows and across most prominent area of occiput.	
2. Infant with meningocele, myelomeningocele	At risk for hydrocephalus secondry to neural tube defect		
Identify signs of hydrocephalus.	Parents' need for information about hydrocephalus	Provide or clarify information.	
1. Rapidly growing head	Parental anxiety related to hydrocephaly	Encourage questions, verbalization of concerns.	Increasing head size is occasionally due to subdural hematoma or brain tumor.
2. Bulging, tense fontanels			
3. Widening sutures		Provide or clarify information about diagnostic procedures, which may include:	
4. Shiny, tough scalp		1. Computerized axial tomography (CAT or CT scan)	
5. Dilated scalp veins		2. Ventriculogram	
6. "Setting sun" eyes; sclera visible above iris			
7. Lethargy			
8. Irritability			
9. Vomiting			
10. Bradycardia			

Assess parents' ability to care for infant. 1. Holding 2. Feeding 3. Provision of sensory stimulation Assess parents' knowledge of 1. Signs of increased intracranial pressure 2. Care of shunt (if appropriate) 3. Signs of dehydration 4. Strategies for preventing skin breakdown If infant is to have surgical treatment:	Need for assistance in caregiving	Assist parents in holding baby if head enlarged. Support head in line with body. 1. Place baby on pillow for holding and carrying. 2. Use chair with arm support to assist in support of head. Encourage parents to feed infant. Infant may feed slowly, need small frequent feedings.	
1. Preoperative: Assess parents' understanding of shunt procedure.	Need for information about shunt procedure	Provide or clarify information about shunt procedure. Parents must understand that shunt will be revised periodically. Explain how infant will look following surgery (head shaved, sutures in scalp and at side of neck [ventriculoatrial shunt], or below sternum [ventricularperitoneal shunt], visibility of tube). Drawings are helpful.	Most common shunts: 1. Ventriculoatrial or ventriculojugular 2. Ventriculoperitoneal
2. Postoperative		Infant will usually lie flat or with head slightly elevated for 2 to 4 days. Confer with neurosurgeon for specific recommendation. Explain to parents.	If infant is held upright, ventricular size may decrease so rapidly that cortex is torn from dura, resulting in subdural hematoma.
a. Signs of increased intracranial pressure (above)	At risk for increased intracranial pressure	Shunt pumping may be prescribed (ventriculoatrial shunt): locate valve, compress carefully a specific number of times per hour or as recommended by neurosurgeon. This procedure is taught to parents prior to discharge.	

Continued on following page

Nursing Care Plan 24–12.   Infants with Hydrocephalus   (Continued)

ASSESSMENT	POTENTIAL NURSING DIAGNOSIS	NURSING INTERVENTION	COMMENTS/RATIONALE
b. Signs of infection (1) Swelling, redness, tenderness along shunt tract (2) Signs of central nervous system infection (irritability, high-pitched cry, bulging fontanel)	At risk of infection	Elevating head may also relieve pressure; consult surgeon. Shunt revision may be necessary. Explain changes in plan of care to parents: 1. Large doses of antibiotics will be prescribed. 2. Removal of the shunt may be necessary; new shunting procedure may await resolution of infection. 3. Ventricular taps may be performed to decrease intracranial pressure until new shunting procedure is done.	
c. Signs of impairment in integrity of skin: reddened areas	At risk for impairment in skin integrity	Use foam rubber or sheepskin under head. Change position frequently. Avoid lying on operative site.	
d. Feeding		Feed small amounts. Encourage parents to feed infant.	Vomiting increases intracranial pressure.
e. Stimulating		Provide age-appropriate sensory stimulation; involve parents in stimulation; explain importance of stimulation at home.	
Plans for continuing care	Parental anxiety about caring for infant at home	Refer to community health nurse. Provide phone number as resource when questions arise—e.g., is shunt functioning properly? Does the infant have infection? Provide information about community support groups.	

may colonize the shunt, and ventriculitis or septicemia may result. If infection occurs, the entire shunt may need to be replaced. The newborn infant who has a shunt will have it throughout his life; revisions are necessary as the baby grows and the distance between the brain and the heart or other shunted areas increases.

In addition to the factors mentioned above, parent education should include the development of a program of physical and sensory stimulation for the baby that will be modified as he develops. Referral to a community resource that specializes in infant development may be appropriate if it is available. Referral to a community health nurse for long-term nursing consultation is always appropriate.

Several defects can result from faulty closure of the embryonic neural tube (Nursing Care Plan 24–13). Anencephaly has been noted above. An *encephalocele* consists of a herniation of the brain and meninges through a defect in the skull, resulting in a saclike structure. The defect is repaired surgically, but the infant frequently develops hydrocephalus and is at risk for diminished intellectual function.

A *meningocele* is a saclike structure that protrudes through a defect in the vertebra (a *spina bifida*). A meningocele will transilluminate because it contains no spinal cord. Surgery is performed for excision of the sac.

In a *meningomyelocele*, the sac contains a portion of the spinal cord and terminal nerves (Fig. 24–11). The sac is not translucent. Nearly three-fourths of babies with meningomyelocele have or will have hydrocephalus. There are varying degrees of paralysis due to motor nerve involvement and loss of sensation related to sensory involvement. In the initial assessment it must be decided whether the infant can move his legs. If meconium continually oozes from the anus and urine appears to dribble from the urethra, it is likely that the baby lacks sphincter control, a significant observation in regard to neural involvement.

If the baby is born in a hospital where there is no neurosurgeon, the sac must be protected during transportation to a medical center. The area is covered with a sterile dressing and sterile plastic and is protected by a "doughnut" of foam rubber that has been wrapped in sterile gauze and secured with a binder or a gauze doughnut.

Surgery for a meningomyelocele involves the excision of the sac and the replacement of nerve tissue in the spinal canal. Wound healing takes from a week to 10 days. During this time the area must be kept scrupulously free of urine and stool, a goal that is often more difficult to achieve than with normal newborns because sphincter control is commonly lacking. To facilitate this aspect of care, the baby is kept unclothed and prone in an isolette or on a frame raised above the level of the mattress so that waste products will drain to a container below the frame. The baby is fed in the prone position and is not lifted for weighing until the wound is healed.

Parents cannot hold the baby in their arms during this period, but they can be encouraged to hold their baby's hand, to stroke his arms and legs, and to talk to him *en face* (i.e., maintaining eye contact).

After the wound has healed, the parents should participate with staff in developing a plan of care that will include physical exercises and sensory stimulation. Good skin care continues to be essential because of urinary and bowel incontinence. Parents are taught to empty the bladder using the Credé maneuver by applying firm, gentle pressure beginning at the umbilicus, progressing toward and then beneath the symphysis pubis, and then moving toward the anus (Fig. 24–12). The Credé maneuver is generally performed every 2 hours.

There are support groups of parents of children with myelomeningocele in many communities; peer support as well as the support of a team of professionals is necessary to help parents cope with the long-term needs of their baby.

Problems Related to Inborn Errors of Metabolism

Inborn errors of metabolism is a term used to describe genetic defects that disrupt normal metabolic function. Hundreds of such errors have been described. The error may affect the metabolism of carbohydrates, amino acids, lipids, vitamins, minerals, and other substances. Most are inherited as autosomal recessive characteristics (Chapter 3); some may be detected by prenatal aminocentesis once it is known that the parents are carriers (Nursing Care Plan 24–14). Many inborn errors in metabolism cause severe mental retardation unless they are recognized soon after birth. Screening for one inborn error in amino-acid metabolism, phenylketonuria (PKU), is described in Chapter 21 and in Nursing Care Plan 24–14.

Galactosemia. Like PKU, galactosemia is inherited as an autosomal recessive trait. An infant with galactosemia lacks a specific enzyme, i.e., galactose-1-phosphate uridyl transferase. Because of this he is unable to metab-

Text continued on page 857

Nursing Care Plan 24–13. Infants with Defects Related to a Failure of Neural Tube Closure (Encephalocele, Meningocele, Meningomyelocele)

NURSING GOALS:
To protect the infant from trauma and infection in the immediate postdelivery period.
To participate with parents and other health-care providers in the development of a multidisciplinary plan of care.
To assist parents in coping with an infant with an anomaly that involves long-term alterations in health status.
To ensure genetic counseling.

OBJECTIVES:
1. The defect is repaired when possible.
2. The infant is protected from sequelae (e.g., infection, hydrocephalus).
3. Parents accept their infant and are able to participate in plan of care.
4. Parents are aware of community resources available to them.

ASSESSMENT	POTENTIAL NURSING DIAGNOSIS	NURSING INTERVENTION	COMMENTS/RATIONALE
Identify infant with neural tube defect. Assess extent of involvement.	Parental anxiety related to neural tube defect	Encourage parents to see and touch infant following birth.	Attachment requires acceptance of infant as he really is.
	Lag in attachment related to defect	Do not try to hide defect. Encourage parents to see positive as well as negative aspects of child's appearance (e.g., eyes, face)	

1. Ability to move legs; flaccidity or spasticity of legs
2. Bowel and bladder dysfunction
  a. Continuous oozing of meconium
  b. Continuous dribbling of urine
	Alterations in motor function
	
	Alterations in bowel and bladder function
		Describe the immediate plan of care; infant may be transferred to another hospital for neurosurgical evaluation. During transport, protect sac with "doughnut" or gauze-wrapped foam rubber; transport in prone position.	

3. Presence of hydrocephalus. Measure head circumference at birth and daily thereafter. Assess anterior fontanel (bulging, tense) at birth and daily thereafter.		Infant is kept in prone or side-lying position. Turn carefully to avoid tension on sac. Lower extremities should never dangle. Sac must be kept free from urine and feces.	Of infants with myelomeningocele, 90 per cent will develop hydrocephalus. Early detection allows early treatment (see Nursing Care Plan 24–12).
Assess defect for: 1. Leakage of cerebrospinal fluid 2. Injury to sac 3. Skin irritation 4. Local signs of infection (red skin, purulent drainage) 5. Increase in size of sac	At risk for breakdown of incision At risk for infection from contamination of incision by urine or feces Impairment of skin integrity, potential or actual	If surgery to excise sac is performed: 1. Infant should remain prone until incision heals. Do not weigh. Placing infant on split Bradford frame allows infant to void and defecate without diaper and	Handling infant may cause tension on suture line.

Assessment	Nursing Diagnosis	Intervention	Rationale
			without contamination of incision by urine or feces. Taping sterile plastic sheet below defect protects skin from contamination. Sheepskin reduces risk of skin breakdown from pressure.
	At risk for positional deformity of feet from improper positioning	Support infant's ankles so that toes do not touch frame or mattress.	
	At risk for lag in attachment	2. Feed infant in prone position. 3. Encourage parents to feed, touch, sponge bathe infant (avoiding area of incision).	Parents will not be able to hold infant until incision heals, but attachment can be facilitated by involving parents in caretaking.
Assess infant's ability to empty bladder.	Urinary incontinence related to myelomeningocele At risk for urinary tract infection	4. Credé maneuver for bladder may be necessary if infant dribbles urine continuously; apply firm gentle pressure beginning at umbilicus and progressing toward and under symphysis pubis and across perineum toward anus. After incision heals, parents are taught to perform Credé maneuver. This procedure should be done every 2 hours during day.	Urinary stasis from bladder that is never emptied predisposes infant to urinary tract infections, nephritis.
Identify signs of infection. 1. Inspect wound for redness, drainage. 2. Assess infant for signs of central nervous system infection (irritability, lethargy, bulging tense fontanel, high-pitched cry, decreased feeding).	At risk of infection secondary to repair	Antibiotic therapy will be prescribed.	
Nutritional intake: a. Blood chemistries for electrolyte balance (particularly if cerebrospinal fluid is lost through leakage from sac)	Nutritional deficit	Oral intake may need to be supplemented by intravenous fluids to meet fluid and electrolyte needs.	
Parents' understanding of reason for passive exercise and how to perform prescribed exercises	Parents' need to learn how to provide passive exercise for infant	Teach parents how to give prescribed passive exercise. Physical therapy consultation may be appropriate.	

Continued on following page

Nursing Care Plan 24–13.   Infants with Defects Related to a Failure of Neural Tube Closure (Encephalocele, Meningocele, Meningomyelocele) *(Continued)*

ASSESSMENT	POTENTIAL NURSING DIAGNOSIS	NURSING INTERVENTION	COMMENTS/RATIONALE
Parents' understanding of need for sensory stimulation	Need for information about age-appropriate sensory stimulation	Involve parents in age-appropriate sensory stimulation prior to discharge. Explain importance of stimulation at home.	
Parents' understanding of infant's safety needs	Need for information about safety measures for infant with myelomeningocele	Explain that infant is vulnerable to injury of lower extremities because of lack of sensory information.	
		Protect infant from sharp objects, hot bath water, wrinkled clothing, wet diapers, etc.	
Parents' coping with infant's complex health needs	Anxiety related to ability to care for infant (physically, emotionally, financially)	Encourage parents to verbalize fears, concerns. Explain that fear and concern are normal reactions. Be available to talk at any time.	
	Guilt related to infant's disorder	Provide specific information about infant's needs through resource material.	
	Negative self-image related to infant's disorder		
	Ineffective individual coping	Provide information about Spina Bifida Association in local community and national address.	Spina Bifida Association of America, P.O. Box 5568, Madison, Wisconsin 53705
	Ineffective family coping	Help parents consider the care of this infant in context of total family, considering needs of siblings. Provide opportunity for sibling visiting.	
		Make positive comments about infant. Keep parents informed of even small changes.	
		Refer to community health nurse for long-term coordination of care.	
Parents' understanding of risks, testing available in future pregnancy	Need for information about prenatal testing for neural tube defects	Provide information about prenatal testing for neural tube defects (Chapter 14).	
		Refer parents to appropriate resources for genetic counseling.	

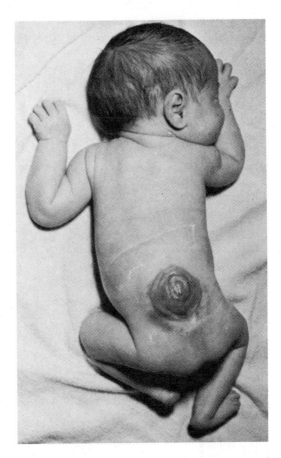

Figure 24–11. Lumbar meningomyelocele in a 3-day-old infant. There is moderate weakness of the proximal muscle groups and more extensive weakness of the distal musculature in the lower extremities. The lesion was flat at birth but began to elevate in the next 2 days. (From Schaffer, and Avery: *Disease of the Newborn.* 4th Edition. Philadelphia, W. B. Saunders Co., 1977.)

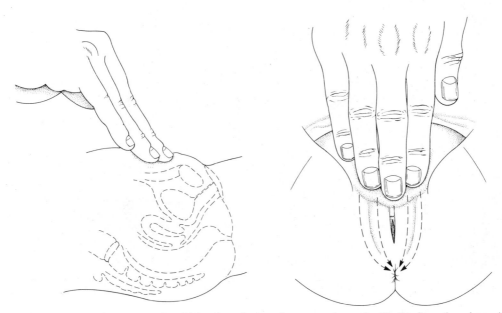

Figure 24–12. The Credé maneuver, in which external manual pressure is used, with the fingertips of one hand (for infants) pressing inward and downward over the abdomen starting over the umbilicus and moving down below the pubis as urine is eliminated. The Credé method permits manual emptying of the bladder and is an important part of the bladder training program. (From Tackett and Hunsberger: *Family-Centered Care of Children and Adolescents: Nursing Concepts in Child Health.* Philadelphia, W. B. Saunders Co., 1981.)

Nursing Care Plan 24–14.   Infants with Inborn Errors in Metabolism

NURSING GOALS:
To identify the infant with an inborn error in metabolism.
To prevent mental retardation and other sequelae by facilitating appropriate care of the infant by parents.
To refer parents for genetic counseling.

OBJECTIVES:
1. Infants at risk for inborn errors of metabolism are identified.
2. Infants with inborn errors of metabolism are identified.
3. Parents understand and are able to participate in the plan of care.
4. Mental retardation and other sequelae are prevented.
5. Genetic counseling is provided.

ASSESSMENT	POTENTIAL NURSING DIAGNOSIS	NURSING INTERVENTION	COMMENTS/RATIONALE
Identify the infant at risk of inborn error of metabolism.	At risk of inborn error of metabolism	When family history suggests possibility of inborn metabolic error, refer for possible prenatal amniocentesis.	The more quickly the diagnosis is established, the better the long-term prognosis.
1. History of unexplained neonatal deaths in family		Infant should be delivered in center where postnatal testing is immediately available. Explain to parents reason for delivery site.	
2. Symptoms are unrelieved by usual therapy and have no evidence of cause such as infection, CNS hemorrhage, etc.		Testing (electrophoresis, chromatography, spectometry) is performed on cord blood and on blood and urine at 12, 24, and 48 hours.	
a. Feeding difficulties, weight loss			
b. Vomiting			
c. Hepatomegaly			
d. Coarse facial features			
e. Seizures			
f. Jaundice			
g. Hypoglycemia			
h. Metabolic acidosis			
i. Ketosis			
j. Abnormal odor of sweat or urine (maple syrup odor, ammonia odor)			
k. Lethargy		When results of initial screening are equivocal or positive, further testing is indicated. Explain reason for further testing to parents.	
Screen all infants for PKU; in some states infants are screened for galactosemia.		When inborn error is suspected from genetic history: 1. Initial feedings of Polycose are given (contains no protein). 2. Fat added to feedings after 24 hours (Nil Prote contains glucose, fat, vitamins, minerals).	Inborn errors are autosomal recessive traits; one infant in four with positive history will have condition.

Assessment	Nursing Diagnosis	Intervention
Assess parental reactions.	Diminished self-esteem Emotional distress related to genetic disorder Difficult adaptation to genetic problem: 　Guilt 　Anxiety 　Anger	3. Protein introduced at 48 hours if testing is negative; testing repeated after 48 hours on protein (breast milk or low-protein formula). 4. If no abnormality is found, feeding proceeds with careful observation. Encourage verbalization of concerns, questions; accept negative feelings (e.g., anger). Reinforce positive coping.	
Assess parents' understanding of genetic process.	Need for genetic counseling	Explain services of genetic counselor, including prenatal testing in future pregnancies. Provide referral for genetic counseling (see also Nursing Care Plan 3–1).	

Phenylketonuria

Assessment	Nursing Diagnosis	Intervention	
Screen all newborn infants 1. Blood tests 　a. Guthrie inhibition assay: most commonly used in neonatal period; level greater than 8 mg. per dl. is considered evidence of PKU. 　b. La-Du Michael 　c. McCaman-Robbins 2. Urine tests 　a. Dintrophenylhydrazine (DNPH) test 　b. Urine tests not valid prior to 6 weeks of age 　c. Ferric chloride diaper test 　d. Phenistix test	Special nutritional needs due to inability to metabolize phenylalanine	Explain purpose of test to parents. Infant must have ingested milk for at least 24 hours prior to testing. If infant is discharged prior to this time, explain and arrange for testing (by community health nurse on home visit or ambulatory health visit). Insufficient blood on filter paper is a common reason for inadequate Guthrie test.	Screening tests are also used for monitoring PKU throughout life. Early identification through mass screening and early treatment is essential to prevent irreversible brain damage.
Assess parents' understanding of condition and plan of care.	Need for information about PKU and care of infant with PKU	Focus on neonatal needs first; add other information as parents become ready to assimilate more. Supplement teaching with written material.	

Continued on following page

Nursing Care Plan 24–14. Infants with Inborn Errors in Metabolism (Continued)

ASSESSMENT	POTENTIAL NURSING DIAGNOSIS	NURSING INTERVENTION	COMMENTS/RATIONALE
Phenylketonuria (Continued).			
Assess parents' feeding technique, formula preparation. Monitor diet by continued testing: 1. daily for 1 week 2. weekly for 7 weeks 3. bi-monthly until 1 year Goal is to maintain serum phenylalanine level between 3 and 10 mg. per dl.	Anxiety about ability to feed infant	Facilitate skill in preparing and giving special formula. Encourage participation in preparation and feeding in hospital. Refer to community health nurse for help in preparation of formula and feeding at home. Teach relaxation techniques; explain that occasional missed feeding will not be disastrous. Encourage smaller frequent feedings if infant cannot take large amounts at single feeding. Include both parents or others in home in preparation and feeding instruction.	Parents are aware of importance of formula intake and subsequent development; may try to force-feed.
Assess parents' reactions.	Sense of inadequacy related to ability to meet infant's special needs	Provide positive support related to parents' caregiving competency.	Parents must trust both themselves and health-care team if long-term needs of infant are to be met.
Galactosemia			
Identify infant with galactosemia: urine positive for reducing substance (Clinitest) but negative for glucose (glucose-oxidase dipstick). Other tests include: 1. Serum galactose-1-phosphate uridyltransferase 2. Urine galactose Physical findings: 1. Failure to gain weight or weight loss 2. Persistent jaundice 3. Subcutaneous bleeding 4. Vomiting, diarrhea 5. Cataracts 6. Lethargy 7. Hepatomegaly 8. Hypoglycemia	Special nutritional needs due to inability to metabolize lactose and galactose	Teaching related to special nutritional needs and parents' reactions to those needs (see PKU, above).	Galactosemia may be lethal in neonatal period if unrecognized and untreated.
	At risk of dehydration due to vomiting, diarrhea	Inform parents that they should notify health-care provider at first sign of diarrhea.	

olize lactose and galactose, so that galactose-1-phosphate accumulates in the red cells (hence galactosemia), and reducing sugars, for which specific tests are available, are found in the urine. Glucose, however, is not present in the urine.

The symptoms of galactosemia are not always easy to detect. Common findings are failure to gain weight and jaundice, which, unlike physiologic jaundice, persists beyond the first week. There may also be subcutaneous bleeding, vomiting, diarrhea, and subsequent dehydration. If the disease is not detected, the baby usually deteriorates progressively, developing physical and mental retardation, signs of malnutrition, cirrhosis of the liver, and cataracts (Nursing Care Plan 24–14).

The treatment is simple in theory. Since lactose occurs naturally only in milk, the newborn infant who shows signs of galactosemia is fed a formula, such as Nutramigen, that does not contain milk. Soybean formulas have also been found to be satisfactory if the baby does not have diarrhea. Problems in feeding arise as the baby grows older and needs a more varied diet, since milk and milk components such as lactose, casein, and whey are incorporated into so many commercial foods. Lactose, for example, is added to many canned and frozen fruits and vegetables during processing.

The removal of lactose from the diet changes the course of galactosemia markedly, even when the condition has gone unrecognized for several months. Appetite improves; vomiting, diarrhea, and jaundice subside; and liver function improves. In some instances, cataracts disappear.[3a]

Problems Related to Maternal Health Factors

A number of potential or actual problems in the neonatal period are related to maternal health factors. The characteristics and needs of an infant of a mother with diabetes mellitus are discussed in Chapter 23. Other maternal factors include Rh_D and ABO incompatibility, maternal pre-eclampsia, and maternal drug addiction.

Hyperbilirubinemia due to Blood Group Incompatibility

"Physiologic" jaundice is discussed in Chapter 21, and the hyperbilirubinemia of premature infants is described in Chapter 23. Jaundice may also reflect neonatal sepsis, intrauterine infection, and a number of relatively rare conditions. Hyperbilirubinemia caused by blood group incompatibility may be due to the Rhesus factor (Rh factor), to ABO incompatibility, or to minor blood group incompatibilities.

Rh_D Incompatibility

The genetic basis of Rh_D incompatibility is discussed in Chapter 3.

As soon as the baby is delivered, blood is Rh typed and a Coombs' test for the presence of antibodies is done. The Coombs' test is important, in addition to blood typing, because a baby with negative blood who has a great many antibodies may type positive. If the Coombs' test is negative, there are no antibodies present, and the baby should have no difficulty from Rh_D incompatibility. If the Coombs' test is positive, indicating that the infant's red blood cells are coated with antibodies, further blood studies are done (hemoglobin and hematocrit determinations, indirect bilirubin level, and reticulocyte count).

Some D-positive babies are in obvious distress at the time of birth. They are not immediately jaundiced, because the bilirubin produced in utero has been cleared through the placenta, although the cord may be stained yellow. Commonly they are pale and edematous and have an enlarged liver and spleen. Blood studies show marked anemia, which can lead to heart failure and metabolic acidosis. Exchange transfusion shortly after birth is usually necessary for these infants, whose condition is termed *hydrops fetalis*.

Erythroblastosis fetalis describes the condition of D-positive babies who become significantly jaundiced, usually in the first 24 to 36 hours, from the high level of bilirubin that results from the destruction of their red blood cells by maternal antibodies at a rate so rapid that the liver cannot conjugate the bilirubin.

Not all babies with erythroblastosis require exchange transfusion. The decision is based on laboratory evaluation of hemoglobin levels (which indicate the destruction of the baby's red blood cells) and levels of bilirubin (which is the breakdown product of the destroyed red blood cells, as previously described); on the presence of signs of kernicterus (which always call for exchange transfusion at any level of bilirubin); and on other parameters that affect the binding of bilirubin to albumin (discussed in Chapter 23 in relation to the hyperbilirubinemia of prematurity). The blood for exchange transfusion is Rh negative, crossmatched with the infant's blood or type O. Phototherapy is usually used in conjunction with exchange transfusion (Chapter 23).

ABO Incompatibility

ABO incompatibility exists in approximately 20 per cent of all pregnancies, but the incidence of severe hemolytic disease is very low. The mother is blood group O; the baby is blood group A or B. Antibodies to types A and B occur naturally in the plasma of type O individuals in response to A and B substances that are present in foods and in gram-negative bacteria. Why some women develop high levels of antibody and others do not is unknown. It is the type A and B infants of those women with high antibody titers who may develop ABO disease. However, because there are a limited number of sites on the fetal red blood cells that will accept the antibody, the disease is usually not severe, and the Coombs' test may be only weakly positive.

There are no preventive measures against ABO incompatibility that can be taken during pregnancy. Unlike Rh_D incompatibility, ABO incompatibility may occur in first pregnancies. Occurrence in second and subsequent pregnancies does not produce more severe disease.

A Coombs' test on cord blood should be done at the time of delivery for the infants of all type O mothers. A positive Coombs' test will alert the nursery staff to the presence of antibodies.

Phototherapy, and occasionally exchange transfusion, is the treatment for ABO incompatibility if treatment is needed. Blood for exchange transfusion is always type O, with Rh factor the same as the baby's.

It is possible, of course, for a mother–infant pair to have both Rh and ABO incompatibility, as in the case of a type O D-negative mother with a type A or B D-positive baby.

Table 24–5 summarizes major factors in Rh and ABO incompatibility.

Minor Blood Groups

In less than 5 per cent of all infants with hemolytic anemia, a blood factor other than Rh_D, A, or B is involved. E, C, and the Kell (K) factors may be responsible for severe hemolytic disease and even for hydrops fetalis. The Coombs' test is positive. Very careful cross-matching with maternal serum is necessary, so that the blood used for transfusion will not contain the antigen responsible for maternal sensitization.

Infants of Mothers with Pregnancy-Induced Hypertension

Infants of mothers with pre-eclampsia commonly have some degree of intrauterine growth retardation (IUGR) or SGA because of diminished placental perfusion and consequent diminished fetal nutrition. In addition, labor may be induced prior to term because of the mother's illness. Common problems of SGA and preterm infants are discussed in Chapter 23.

Magnesium sulfate given to the mother as treatment for pre-eclampsia or eclampsia

Table 24–5.   COMPARISON OF Rh_D AND ABO INCOMPATIBILITY*

	Rh_D	ABO
BLOOD GROUP SET-UP		
Mother	Negative	O
Infant	Positive	A or B
CLINICAL ASPECTS		
Occurs in firstborn	5%	40–50%
More severe in subsequent pregnancy	Usually	No
Stillbirth and/or hydrops	Frequent	Rare
Severe anemia	Frequent	Rare
Degree of jaundice	—	—
Hepatosplenomegaly	—	—
LABORATORY FINDINGS		
Direct Coombs' test (infant)	Positive	Not always positive
Maternal antibodies	Always	Not clear-cut
TREATMENT		
Antenatal measures	Yes	No
Exchange transfusion		
Frequency	Approximately 66%	Approximately 10%
Donor blood type	Rh_D negative; group specific	Rh as infants; group O only
Late anemia	Common	Rare

*Adapted from Oski. *In* Avery: *Neonatology.* Philadelphia, J. B. Lippincott Co., 1975.

(Chapter 13) also affects the neuromuscular junctions in the newborn, resulting in hypotonia, hypothermia, and hypocalcemia. Hypotonia may lead to respiratory failure. Vasodilation, decreased muscle flexion, and inability to shiver contribute to hypothermia, already a risk for a preterm and/or SGA baby. Magnesium is believed to inhibit the secretion of parathyroid hormone, which in turn leads to increased secretion of calcium by the kidneys.

The Infant of a Mother Addicted to Narcotics

As drug use among young women increases, as it has during recent years, the incidence of infants being born to mothers addicted to narcotics has increased. In some urban medical centers relatively large numbers of newborns addicted to morphine, heroin, and methadone are currently being seen. The problem for the nurse is to recognize these babies.

The most prominent sign of heroin withdrawal is central nervous system irritability. The baby is frantic and inconsolable, he may have tremors, and the Moro response may be incomplete. His shrill cry is not unlike that of babies with central nervous system damage. In addition, there may be a large amount of mucus or such generalized symptoms as diarrhea and vomiting. Either excessive weight loss, because of fluid loss from vomiting or diarrhea, or failure to gain weight, because of a very high expenditure of energy, prevents these babies from growing normally in the nursery.

The symptoms of withdrawal from methadone are the same as those of heroin withdrawal, but they are frequently more severe and last for a longer period of time. Although symptoms of heroin withdrawal usually appear within 24 to 48 hours following birth, withdrawal symptoms from methadone begin between 4 and 12 days of age and sometimes even later, because methadone is a longer-acting drug. Seizures are more common in infants with methadone withdrawal.

Less attention has been given to withdrawal symptoms from nonnarcotic drugs, including barbiturates, sedatives, and tranquilizers. Because these drugs are more widely used than narcotics, the possibility of neonatal addiction is also increased. Passive addiction may occur even when a therapeutic dose is used by the mother over a long period during pregnancy.[11] The onset of withdrawal symptoms may be delayed because the drug is metabolized and excreted slowly and thus remains in the infant's system. Withdrawal symptoms are frequently the opposite of the usual pharmacologic effects of the drugs and are similar to the symptoms of withdrawal from narcotic drugs, including irritability, tremors, a high-pitched cry, convulsions, gastrointestinal disturbances, tachycardia, tachypnea, and sleep disturbances (Nursing Care Plan 24–15).

Since all these symptoms are common to many other kinds of newborn problems, it is important that the nurse be alert to signs of addiction in mothers, such as scarred veins and withdrawal symptoms, in order to evaluate the symptoms in babies. Addiction should be suspected, and the possibility should be evaluated in mothers with venereal disease, hepatitis, cellulitis, and thrombophlebitis.

The diagnosis in the baby is confirmed by the discovery of narcotic breakdown products in the blood and urine. Specimens need to be collected shortly after birth because these narcotic metabolites disappear quickly.

The care of a passively addicted baby is directed toward immediate supportive care, the initiation and fostering of a bond between mother and baby, and long-term follow-up. Major elements of supportive care include a darkened environment (e.g., covering the top of an incubator with a cloth), swaddling the baby, and providing a pacifier. Some babies will respond to holding during withdrawal, but others will become more frantic when they are held. Bedding must be soft to prevent skin abrasion. Diarrhea and vomiting can lead quickly to dehydration, the major cause of mortality in addicted infants. Careful records of intake and output and weight will help in evaluating fluid balance. Sucking and swallowing may not be well coordinated, making feeding slow and difficult; gavage feeding may be necessary.

Several medications have been used to help infants with severe withdrawal (Table 24–6). Although the use of drugs may be essential in some instances, the use of nursing measures to avoid or limit their use is optimal. One important reason is that the mother, after she returns home, will probably be giving her baby a drug to solve his or her problem, just as she has used drugs to solve her own problems. In addition, a sedated baby provides limited reinforcement to the mother in response to caregiving. However, a highly irritable, unconsolable baby makes a mother feel inadequate and rejected. The mother, in turn, may reject her baby, and the forming of a bond between them becomes even more difficult. Further complicating attachment is the guilt the mother may feel because of her baby's withdrawal symptoms. Longer periods of hospitalization, often with the baby in a special care nursery, can be an additional barrier to attachment.

Plans for careful, long-term support of both

Nursing Care Plan 24–15. Care of the Infant of a Mother Addicted to Narcotics

NURSING GOALS:

To identify the infant of a drug-dependent mother.
To provide supportive care and early treatment to reduce perinatal mortality.
To encourage decision making by the mother about keeping or relinquishing her baby and about realistic plans for infant care.
To facilitate attachment and caregiving behavior in the drug-dependent mother.
To ensure care of the infant following hospital discharge.

OBJECTIVES: As a result of nursing action:

1. Infants at risk of passive addiction will be identified.
2. Signs of withdrawal will be identified.
3. The infant will be more comfortable.
4. Serious morbidity (e.g., dehydration, electrolyte imbalance) will be prevented.
5. Mortality will be prevented.
6. Parent–infant interaction will be assessed and facilitated.
7. A comprehensive plan will be initiated for continuing health care following delivery.

ASSESSMENT	POTENTIAL NURSING DIAGNOSIS	NURSING INTERVENTION	COMMENTS/RATIONALE
Identify infants at risk: maternal history	Infant at risk of passive addiction		
Signs of withdrawal in passively addicted infant:	At risk of withdrawal symptoms	Reduce environmental stimuli. Swaddle infant.	
1. CNS irritability		Plan care to provide extended periods of rest.	
a. Inconsolability			
b. Tremors (location, relation to other activities mild, moderate, severe)		Medications (Table 24–6) may be useful.	
c. Shrill cry (onset, duration)			
d. Incomplete or hyperactive Moro reflex			
e. Hypertonicity			
2. Gastrointestinal symptoms			
a. Diarrhea (frequency, water loss			
b. Vomiting (projectile, frequency, color)			
c. Poor sucking (uncoordinated)			
d. Large amounts of mucus			

Assessment	Nursing Diagnosis	Intervention	Comments

3. Respiratory symptoms
  a. Tachypnea
  b. Retractions (location, severity)
  c. Nasal flaring
  d. Skin color
  e. Sneezing; nasal stuffiness			

4. Signs of dehydration
  a. Skin turgor
  b. Weight loss
  c. Sunken fontanels
	At risk for dehydration related to (diarrhea, vomiting, poor feeding)	Record intake and output. Keep careful weight record. Feed slowly; if sucking and swallowing are very uncoordinated, feed by gavage.	

5. Electrolyte imbalance	At risk for electrolyte imbalance related to (diarrhea, vomiting, poor feeding)		
6. Pyrexia		Adjust environmental temperature to keep infant temperature in thermoneutral range.	
7. Reddened or broken areas from rubbing skin against bedding; scratches on face	At risk of skin breakdown related to activity	Provide soft bedding, such as sheepskin; pull shirt over hands to make mitts.	
Assess mother–infant attachment (see also Nursing Care plan 28–1) 1. Feeding and other caretaking behaviors 2. Naming infant 3. Positive and negative comments about infant 4. Hugs, kisses, smiles 5. Response to infant's crying	Lag in attachment behavior; infant at risk of neglect or abuse related to mother's drug-dependence	Encourage mother to participate in infant's care. Demonstrate her infant's unique characteristics. Provide information about infant development. Provide opportunity to discuss feelings about self and baby.	Unrealistic expectations are one factor in infant abuse.
Assess plans for continuing care for infant as well as mother	Lag in attachment; inability of mother to care for infant; lack of realistic plans for infant care. Lack of source of emotional support; lack of economic support for mother	Refer to public health nursing for continuing care. Refer to social worker for help with specific economic and social needs. Consider possibility of foster care for infant if maternal care is assessed as inadequate.	Symptoms of withdrawal may occur following discharge; mother's health must be closely supervised during first weeks following birth.

Table 24–6. MEDICATION USED IN TREATMENT OF PASSIVELY ADDICTED NEWBORNS*

Category	Drug	Dose	Comments
Narcotic substitute	Paregoric	0.2–0.7 ml. every 3 hours; begin at lowest level, raise by 0.05 ml. until symptoms are controlled	Stabilize in 1–3 weeks; slow withdrawal over 25–45 days; infant may be lethargic, constipated
Narcotic substitute	Methadone	0.3–0.5 mg. every 4–12 hours	Gradually decrease dose
Tranquilizer	Diazepam (Valium)	1–2 mg. every 8 hours	Dose decreased by 50 per cent, interval increased to 12 hours as symptoms are controlled. Observe for respiratory arrest diarrhea, hyperbilirubinemia
Tranquilizer	Chlorpromazine (Thorazine)	2–3 mg. per kg. per 24 hours in four doses	Treat for 2 weeks to 2 months
Sedative	Phenobarbital	5–10 mg. per kg. per 24 hours in 3–4 days	Treat for 10–40 days; taper over 1–3 weeks. Sedation may interfere with feeding, bonding

*Based on data from Harper and Edwards, 1977.

mother and baby must be made before discharge. The passively addicted baby is often difficult to care for under the best of circumstances. The mother's living conditions are less than ideal. The baby's father may also use drugs. The mother's own needs may interfere with parenting behavior. The risk of child abuse and neglect is high—abuse coming from the man in the house and allowed by the passive mother, neglect coming from the mother herself. Unless the mother has strong support from other adults in her environment who can provide responsible 24-hour care, foster care is frequently necessary.[3] Further discussion of the addicted mother is found in Chapter 13.

Persistent Fetal Circulation

Persistent fetal circulation (PFC) is a syndrome in which pulmonary artery pressure is so high that the transition from fetal to neonatal circulatory patterns does not occur (Nursing Care Plan 24–16). Other terms for this syndrome include persistence of fetocardiopulmonary circulation, persistence of pulmonary hypertension of the newborn, and several others. Although the term persistent fetal circulation is actually a misnomer because the placenta is not a part of the postnatal circulation, it appears to be the most widely used.

In patent ductus arteriosus (Chapter 23), pulmonary vascular resistance drops and blood is shunted from the left (systemic) to the right (pulmonary) circulation because that is the area of lowest pressure. In PFC, pulmonary vascular resistance is high, and blood therefore is shunted from the right (pulmonary) to the left (systemic) circulation. Because so little blood goes to the lungs to be oxygenated, the baby is cyanotic and tachypneic.

Pulmonary hypertension may be due to (1) failure of the pulmonary arterioles to relax after birth, (2) spasm of the pulmonary vessels, and (3) hypertrophy of the walls of the pulmonary arterioles. Associated problems include intrauterine hypoxia, asphyxia, primary pulmonary disease, perinatal hypoxia, acidosis, and conditions that may be related to hypoxia and acidosis. Both hypoxia and acidosis, whatever the origin, may cause spasm of the pulmonary blood vessels. Because the muscle layers of the pulmonary arterioles are frequently hypertrophied in PFC and these muscle layers develop late in gestation, PFC occurs primarily in term and postterm infants rather than in preterm infants.

Tolazoline (Priscoline), an alpha-adrenergic blocking agent, may be given to infants with PFC. Tolazoline relaxes the muscles of the pulmonary vessels, reducing pulmonary vascular resistance and increasing pulmonary blood flow. The initial IV dose of 1 to 2 mg. per kg. of body weight is followed by either continuous infusion (1 to 2 mg. per kg. per hour) or intermittent doses. In order to exert the maximum effect on the pulmonary system the drug is administered through a scalp vein.

Side effects are related to vasodilation in other areas of the body. Because profound systemic hypotension is possible, blood pressure is monitored carefully, and blood, plasma, or albumin should be readily available to prevent shock. Flushing of the skin may be seen following drug administration.

Seizures in Newborn Infants

It is not unusual for healthy newborn infants to have brief, spontaneous tremors. Infants with hypoglycemia and hypocalcemia may become "jittery"; jitteriness may be the first sign of a problem in infants who are not monitored for these conditions. Seizures are a more serious symptom; long-term prognosis is related to the underlying cause. Intracranial hemorrhage, birth asphyxia, hypoglycemia, and meningitis are the most common reasons for neonatal seizures (Nursing Care Plan 24–17).

Seizures in newborns are rarely the generalized tonic-clonic seizures seen in older children and adults, probably because of the immaturity of the cerebral cortex. Frequently the only signs of a seizure are deviation of the eyes, repetitive blinking of the eyelids, cyanosis around the mouth, chewing motions, or drooling. Nursing records that report suspected seizure activity should very specifically record the behavior observed during the seizure as well as the length of the seizure and the baby's behavior before and afterward. (See Table 24–7).

When a seizure is suspected, nursing action proceeds in the following manner:

1. Assess respiratory effort. Clear secretions and provide ventilation (bag and mask) if necessary.

2. Determine blood glucose level (with Dextrostix). Hypoglycemia is a frequent cause of neonatal seizures.

3. Observe behavior, paying special attention to behaviors in Table 24–7. If the infant is having tremors, movement can generally be stopped by flexing the involved limb. Note the state of consciousness, muscle tone, and posture.

4. Record observations specifically and notify physician.

The treatment of seizures includes correction of the underlying problem, when possible (hypoglycemia or hypocalcemia, for example), and administration of phenobarbital. The initial dose of phenobarbital is 10 mg. per kg. IM, followed by a maintenance dose of 5 mg. per kg. per day IM or orally in two to three divided doses. When phenobarbital alone does not control the seizures, phenytoin (Dilantin) is used in addition.

Transport of the High Risk Newborn

When an infant with a condition that puts him at risk of serious illness or death is born in a community hospital, he may require transport to a large medical center in order to receive the specialized care he needs. In general, in the following situations an infant should receive care at a regional center: (1) weight of less than 1500 grams; (2) emergency surgery required (e.g., for tracheoesophageal fistula, diaphragmatic hernia, gastroschisis); (3) congenital heart disease suspected; (4) major complications during delivery (e.g., meconium aspiration, birth asphyxia); and (5) poor condition due to some unknown reason.

The ideal form of transport of the high risk infant is before birth within his mother's uterus, the delivery of the baby taking place in the medical center. This is occurring with increasing frequency, but it will never be possible for all high risk babies for two basic reasons.

First, not all high risk deliveries can be anticipated. Although some mothers can be identified as likely to produce a baby needing special care even before they become pregnant (for example, the mother with diabetes or the mother who has previously delivered a child with erythroblastosis), other mothers have sudden, premature labor, or have unanticipated difficulty during labor or delivery, or have a child with a major congenital anomaly without any prior indication. Under these circumstances transport of the baby will be necessary.

Second, even when a high risk baby is expected, it will not always be possible for the mother to leave her own community to be cared for in a hospital many miles away for a period of time that may involve 1 to 2 weeks or longer. Not only the economic cost but the social cost in terms of separation from husband and family may be too high. Planning for hospitalization of such a mother will have to include planning for all the needs of the family, not just for the mother's (and later the baby's) medical problems.

Systems of Transport

There are three basic ways in which newborn transport is accomplished, regardless of the mode of transport (ambulance, helicopter, fixed wing aircraft). A team (nurse and/or physician and/or respiratory therapist) may go

Text continued on page 869

Nursing Care Plan 24–16.   Infants with Persistent Fetal Circulation (PFC)

NURSING GOALS:
To identify the infant at risk of PFC.
To prevent PFC, when possible, by adequate resuscitation of asphyxiated infants.
To provide physiologic support for the infant with PFC.
To support parents during a period of critical illness.

OBJECTIVES:
1. The infant at risk for PFC is identified.
2. All infants with intrauterine hypoxia or birth asphyxia receive immediate resuscitation, if necessary.
3. Hypoxemia and acidosis are prevented.
4. Persistent fetal circulation is resolved; side effects of treatment are prevented.
5. Parents are supportive throughout the infant's illness.

ASSESSMENT	POTENTIAL NURSING DIAGNOSIS	NURSING INTERVENTION	COMMENTS/RATIONALE
Identify infant at risk for PFC	At risk for PFC	Identify fetal hypoxia and correct (Nursing Care Plan 18–1). Have adequate personnel and equipment available for resuscitation at delivery.	Hypoxia and/or acidosis can cause spasm of pulmonary blood vessels → pulmonary hypertension → right-to-left shunting → further hypoxia and acidosis.
1. Term or postterm infant			
2. History of intrauterine hypoxia, birth asphyxia			
3. Presence of primary pulmonary disease		Assist in the provision of immediate resuscitation for newborn. Be prepared to provide adequate oxygen ventilation and to correct acidosis.	Prevention of hypoxemia and acidosis is essential for prevention of PFC.
4. Presence of hypoxemia, acidosis			
Identify infant with PFC	Inadequate oxygenation secondary to PFC	Provide neutral thermal environment.	
1. Cyanosis			
2. Tachypnea		Provide glucose and calcium as necessary.	
3. Severe hypoxemia			

Assess 1. Serum glucose levels 2. Serum calcium levels 3. Acid-base balance 4. Hematocrit for polycythemia		Correct acid-base imbalance, polycythemia. Infant will usually be ventilated mechanically (see Nursing Care Plan 23–4 for care of infant on ventilator).	A partial exchange transfusion may be used to treat polycythemia.
Infant receiving tolazoline: 1. Assess flushing of skin following administration. 2. Take blood pressure following administration and at frequent intervals.	At risk for hypotension secondary to vasodilation following administration of tolazoline.	Drug therapy: 1. Tolazoline (Priscoline), 1–2 mg. per kg. followed by 1–2 mg. per kg. per hour, IV via scalp vein. Have blood, plasma, or albumin ready for immediate use if hypotension occurs. 2. Dopamine (Intropin) 5–10 mg. per kg. per minute may be used to maintain or restore systemic blood pressure.	Tolazoline causes both pulmonary vasodilation (reason for administration) and systemic vasodilation (side effect that may cause hypotension and shock).
Assess parents' reactions.	Anxiety related to severely ill newborn	Explain plan of care to parents. Encourage parents to see and touch infant. Explain reason for each piece of equipment. Keep parents informed of changes in infant's condition. Support grieving parents if infant dies (Nursing Care Plan 28–2) or progressively involve parents in care as infant improves.	

Nursing Care Plan 24–17.   The Infant with a Seizure Disorder

NURSING GOALS:
To identify the infant with seizure activity.
To describe seizure activity and associated factors precisely.
To explain or clarify seizure activity to parents.
To assist parents in learning to care for their child.

OBJECTIVES:
1. Infant with seizure activity is identified.
2. Infant is protected during seizure.
3. Precise observation of infant's seizure activity and associated factors (relation to external stimuli, blood glucose levels, etc.) are recorded.
4. Information about neonatal seizure are explained to parents.
5. Parents are competent to care for infant; they will know what to do if seizure occurs and how to administer appropriate medication.
6. Parents are aware of community resources available to them.

ASSESSMENT	POTENTIAL NURSING DIAGNOSIS	NURSING INTERVENTION	COMMENTS/RATIONALE
Identify infant at risk for seizure.	At risk for seizure secondary to (specific condition)		
1. Perinatal complications occur in 30 to 50 per cent of neonatal seizures)			
a. Fetal distress			
b. Birth asphyxia			
c. CNS trauma in breech, difficult forceps delivery			
d. Intracranial hemorrhage			
2. Metabolic problems			
a. Hypoglycemia			
b. Hypocalcemia			
c. Hypomagnesemia			
d. Hyponatremia			
e. Hypernatremia			
3. Sepsis (delayed; usually occurs after first week)			
4. Maternal drug addiction with subsequent infant withdrawal			
5. Other causes			
Identify the newborn with a seizure.			
1. Deviation of the eyes			
2. Repetitive blinking of the eyelids			
3. Circumoral cyanosis		Clear secretions. Provide bag and mask ventilation if cyanosis persists.	
4. "Chewing" movements			
5. Drooling			
6. Apnea			
Differentiate "jitteriness" from seizure activity (Table 24–7)			

Assessment	Nursing Diagnosis	Plan/Intervention	Rationale
Assess and record: 1. Relationship of stimuli to onset 2. Areas affected 3. Cyanosis, if present 4. Rhymicity of movements 5. Effect of passive flexion of limb on movement 6. Length of time seizure lasts 7. Behavior following seizure			The cause of a neonatal seizure cannot always be identified.
Assess blood glucose level (Dextrostix, etc.)	Seizure related to hypoglycemia	Provide IV glucose to correct hypoglycemia.	
Assess blood pressure, serum electrolytes, and pH	Seizure related to (specific reason)	Underlying cause will be corrected when possible. Medication: Phenobarbital, 10–20 mg. per kg. IM or IV as loading dose; maintenance dose: 2.5–5 mg. per kg. per day IM or PO If seizure activity is not controlled, give phenytoin 5–10 mg. per kg. IV to control seizure; maintenance dose 4–7 mg. per kg. per 24 hours in two doses (IV)	Monitor pulse when giving IV phenytoin; administer slowly.
Assess parents' understanding	Parents' fear related long-term development of infant	Encourage parents to verbalize fears. Provide information about community resources. Refer to community health nurse for continuing care.	Relationship of seizure activity and normal development varies with etiology of seizure. Predictions are not made in neonatal period.
Assess information provided parents	Parents' need to learn to administer prescribed anticonvulsant medication	Phenobarbital is the primary medication given at home. Provide multiple opportunities for parents to learn to measure and administer it. Explain that: 1. Medication must be given on regular schedule. 2. Infant may be drowsy, have rash, have gastrointestinal disturbances. Parents should notify health care provider. 3. Blood levels of medication must be monitored at regular intervals. Encourage parents to use crib pad and playpen pad; avoid pillows.	

Table 24–7.   DISTINGUISHING CHARACTERISTICS OF JITTERINESS AND SEIZURE ACTVITY*

Jitteriness	Seizure Activity
Not accompanied by ocular movement	Frequently accompanied by ocular movement
Highly sensitive to stimuli	Stimuli not important in onset
Movements rhythmic, equal in rate and amplitude	Movements have fast and slow components
Flexion of affected limb can stop movement	Flexion of limb does not stop movement

*From Moore: *Newborn, Family, and Nurse.* 2nd Edition. Philadelphia, W. B. Saunders Co., 1981.

Table 24–8.   EQUIPMENT NEEDED FOR TRANSPORT OF HIGH RISK INFANTS*

Need	Equipment
Warmth	Transport incubator with servomechanism Thermometer Blankets Additional wrapping materials: plastic wrap, cotton batting, foil
Ventilation	Oxygen supply Laryngoscope with blades—#0, #1 (include spare batteries) Oral airways Endotracheal tubes (2.5–4.0 mm) Resuscitation bag and mask Stethoscope Adhesive tape Scissors Suction catheters with suction equipment Oxygen concentration monitor to monitor F_{IO_2} Flashlight CPAP† Mechanical ventilator† Equipment for in-transport monitoring of blood gases and correction of acid-base imbalance†
Prevention of hypoglycemia	Dextrostix Intravenous fluids and supplies (scalp vein needles, alcohol swabs, collodion, tape, cotton balls) Infusion pump Glucagon (if unable to start IV)
Assessment of vital signs	Thermometer (noted above) Stethoscope (noted above) Infant blood pressure monitoring equipment

Preparation for potential in-transport emergency	Drugs
	  Sodium bicarbonate
	  Calcium gluconate
	  Epinephrine 1:10,000
	  Furosemide
	  KCl
	  Saline
	  Heparin
	Syringes
	  (tuberculin, 3 cc, 10 cc, 20 cc)
	  Needle thoracocentesis
	    30 cc syringe
	    Three-way stopcock
	    Scalp vein needles (19–23)

*From Moore: *Newborn, Family and Nurse.* 2nd Edition. Philadelphia, W. B. Saunders Co., 1981.
†Additional equipment (not required)

from a medical center to the referring hospital to begin intensive care from the moment they receive the baby, often in a specially equipped vehicle that is an intensive care unit in itself. Obviously such a vehicle is very expensive and by no means universally available. A team may also go from a medical center to receive the baby with far less in terms of equipment but with special experience in caring for the baby during transport.

The referring hospital may also have specially trained nurses or teams to send with the baby and have access to a modern transport incubator in which most babies can be cared for quite well. One problem with this system is that if the community hospital sends its best trained person (who may be the only registered nurse in the neonatal area, or even in the entire obstetric area), their own coverage becomes inadequate.

A third possibility is the use of emergency medical personnel to care for the baby during transport. It is essential that these men and women be given adequate initial training and continuing education in the care of high risk babies.

In addition to a vehicle, specific equipment is necessary for infant transport to meet the baby's specific needs (Table 24–8).

Stabilization and Preparation for Transport

Stabilization prior to transport can be a significant factor in reducing mortality and morbidity (Nursing Care Plan 24–18). There is an understandable inclination to get the baby to the regional center as soon as possible However, speed should never be accomplished at the expense of stabilization. Stabilization includes:

1. Maintenance of a thermoneutral environment to keep the infant's skin temperature at 36.3 to 36.5° C. (97.5 to 97.7° F.).

2. Provision of oxygen and appropriate assistance in ventilation.

3. Provision of fluid and electrolytes. Leaving an inch of cord stump at delivery in an infant who may be expected to need blood gas evaluation will make it easier to insert an umbilical artery line in the receiving hospital.

4. Correction of acidosis and hypoglycemia.

5. Specific treatment of emergency conditions (e.g., pneumothorax).

6. Specific treatment for the baby's problem (e.g., tracheoesophageal fistula, myelomeningocele).

It is very important for the mother to *see and touch* her baby before the baby is moved to another hospital. Fathers often come with the baby or are able to see him soon after at the medical center. Mothers must remain in the community hospital for several days until the time of their own discharge. Over and over fathers tell us, "She (i.e., the mother) doesn't even feel like she has had a baby . . . it is totally unreal to her." Mothers share the same kinds of comments with us when they are able to come to the nursery several days later for the first time.

An explanation of why the baby must be transported is also essential. Parents will not understand a great deal of what we tell them at this time. They may hear nothing more than "we feel your baby should be transferred to the intensive care unit at the Medical Center." Later we will need to go back over what we have told them. But it is nevertheless important to give honest, realistic information prior to the transport of their baby. (See Chapter 28 for further discussion.)

A Polaroid picture of the baby can be quickly made before transport so that the mother will have tangible evidence of the reality of her baby. The father and other family members may be able to visit the baby at the regional center before the mother's discharge, but she can feel very left out. A picture may seem an inadequate substitute for a real baby, but mothers have said that it does help.

Prophylactic vitamin K and silver nitrate should be given and charted, so that the dose will not be repeated at the receiving hospital. A gavage tube is passed into the stomach, and the contents are gently aspirated to prevent aspiration during transport. The baby must also be properly identified.

In addition to preparing the baby, records must be available to send to the receiving hospital. These include copies of:

1. The baby's record.

2. The mother's prenatal history and labor and delivery record.

3. The mother's admission sheet, which contains valuable information such as telephone numbers and places of employment that can facilitate communication.

Two tubes of the mother's blood, one clotted and one unclotted, and of the baby's cord blood, if available, should be sent.

Finally, it seems a simple thing to be sure that the gas tank of the ambulance is full, but our experience indicates that this phase of the transport is easily overlooked.

Care en Route

Throughout transport, warmth, oxygen, glucose, and suction continue to be essential (see Nursing Care Plan 24–18).

The tremendous importance of *warmth* for

Nursing Care Plan 24–18. Infants Requiring Transport

NURSING GOALS:
To provide infant transport in a manner that protects the infant from complications and ensures arrival at the destination in the best possible physiologic state.
To facilitate attachment in mother separated from her infant.

OBJECTIVES:
1. Infants requiring transport are identified and plans for transport are initiated quickly.
2. Infant's vital signs, blood glucose level, acid-base balance are stabilized prior to transport.
3. Parents see and touch infant prior to transport.
4. Parents know how to communicate with nursery in referral hospital.
5. Infant's condition is continually assessed during transport, and appropriate intervention is initiated or continued.
6. Information about transport is provided to referring hospital and to parents.
7. Record of transport is reviewed.

ASSESSMENT	POTENTIAL NURSING DIAGNOSIS	NURSING INTERVENTION	COMMENTS/RATIONALE
Prior to transport			
Assess infant's:	Need for physiologic homeostasis prior to initiating transport	Provide thermoneutral environment.	
1. Vital signs		Provide oxygen and assisted ventilation as necessary.	
2. Blood gases (ph, PaO_2, HCO_3)		Insert orogastric or nasogastric tube.	
3. Glucose level (Dextrostix, etc.)		Provide fluids and line for medication via umbilical artery or peripheral IV.	
4. Weight		Correct acidosis.	
		Correct hypoglycemia.	
		Treat specific emergency conditions (e.g., pneumothorax).	
		Provide appropriate care as indicated for specific problem (Table 24–9).	
		Assemble equipment needed for transport (Table 24–8).	
Assess initial attachment.	Need to initiate attachment prior to separation from mother	Provide opportunity for parents to see and touch infant prior to transport.	In some instances mother may be transported with infant to avoid period of separation.
		Take picture of infant with "instant" camera to leave with mother.	
		Provide phone number and other information about referral hospital, such as pamphlet with pictures of nursery.	

During transport
1. Assess vital signs every 15–30 minutes.
2. Assess blood glucose level (Dextrostix).
3. Monitor heart rate and respiratory rate continuously, if possible.

At risk for:
Hypothermia
Hyperthermia
Repiratory distress
Cardiac distress
Hypotension
Hypoglycemia

Provide thermoneutral environment. Covering head, arms, and legs will help to provide warmth. Transport incubator should have servomechanism.

Leave with full oxygen tank. Plan for twice as much oxygen as necessary.

Provide oxygen as necessary to prevent cyanosis of mucous membranes if blood gas cannot be analyzed during transport.

Maintain intravenous fluids. Dextrose, 10–15 per cent, is a common solution (2–4 ml. per hour for preterm infant; 10 ml. per hour for term infant).

Be prepared to give emergency medications according to institutional protocol.

Record vital signs, nursing observations, medications (including oxygen) just as when infant is in nursery.

Identify signs of pneumothorax:
1. Restlessness
2. Irritability
3. Apnea
4. Bradycardia
5. Hypotension
6. Diminished breath sounds
7. Shift in heart sounds
8. Abdominal distention

At risk for pneumothorax

Be prepared for needle aspiration of pneumothorax.
1. Assemble syringe, stopcock, scalp vein needle
2. Insert needle in second, third, or fourth interspace, in anterior axillary line, pointing toward feet.
3. Withdraw air, turn stopcock, expel air.
4. Continue until resistance occurs.
5. Continue careful assessment of infant; pneumothorax may recur.

Following transport
Assess infant's:
1. Vital signs
2. Acid-base balance
3. Blood glucose

Complete record.

Inform referring hospital of infant's condition. Communicate information to parents.

Replace supplies used during transport in preparation for next transport.

If infant becomes hypothermic, hypotensive, or hypoglycemic, review transport procedures and consider possible changes in technique in future transports.

all babies, and particularly for the high risk baby, has already been discussed in detail. A transport incubator that provides warmth as well as visibility is ideal. The battery should be fully charged at all times so that warmth is continuous. Alternatives include the careful use of hot water bottles filled at 105° F. (40° C.) (not really satisfactory but better than nothing at all), wrapping aluminum foil around the baby's blanket (good insulation, but visibility, which is very important, is compromised), and wrapping the baby's arms and legs in cotton batting. This last measure, freuently used in baby surgery, is a useful adjunct to other methods and will reduce heat loss without compromising visibility.

The baby's temperature should be checked prior to transport and en route, if the trip lasts more than an hour, and recorded in the nurse's notes.

Table 24–9.   ADDITIONAL NURSING CARE FOR INFANTS WITH SPECIFIC PROBLEMS DURING TRANSPORT*

Condition	Special Points in Care
Tracheoesophageal fistula Esophageal atresia	Elevate head at a 45° angle at all times to prevent chemical pneumonia from gastric acid reflex to lungs (use an infant seat) Suction bubbly secretions in mouth and oropharynx Insert a catheter (#10 French) into blind pouch (or into stomach if tracheoesophageal fistula occurs without esophageal atresia) and connect to low intermittent suction Avoid crying by infant (air forced into stomach may cause gastric reflux to lungs)
Pneumothorax	Transport with normal side uppermost Aspirate air Watch for sudden worsening of respiration and/or shift in position of apical heart sounds
Diaphagmatic hernia	Transport with side with better lung function uppermost (usually the right side) Elevate head so abdominal organs do not compromise limited lung function Pass orogastric tube to decompress bowel Avoid positive pressure ventilation if possible, because bowel in chest will fill with air and further compromise respiration Intubate, if essential, into main stem bronchus of unaffected side Observe carefully for pneumothorax in unaffected lung
Abdominal distention (e.g., intestinal block)	Insert nasogastric tube; aspirate gently with syringe and record amount aspirated; administer low intermittent suction if possible Observe carefully for signs of shock
Exposed internal organs (e.g., gastroschisis, ectopic bladder)	Cover exposed internal organs with warm sterile saline dressing, then Vaseline gauze; an outer wrapping of plastic drape provides further insulation (infant is at high risk of heat loss because of exposed organs)
Meningocele	Transport prone Use doughnut support around meningocele Cover with sterile saline dressing or dry sterile dressing
Hypognathia, Pierre Robin syndrome	Transport face down so that tongue will fall forward; tongue falling back will lead to respiratory obstruction
Choanal atresia or stuffy nose for some reason	Baby is obligate nose breather; to assist him to breathe through mouth, insert oral airway or cut a large hole in a nipple and tape it to mouth
Eyelids open (as in severe facial palsy, occasionally in hydrocephalus)	Administer eye drops and ophthalmic ointment

*From Moore: *Newborn, Family and Nurse.* 2nd Edition. Philadelphia, W. B. Saunders Co., 1981.

Oxygen can be given by bag and mask or by bag and endotracheal tube during transport when it is needed. An extra, full cylinder of oxygen should be taken along, because any lapse in oxygenation, even of short duration, can lead to possible brain damage. Plan for twice the amount of oxygen that appears to be needed (based on flow rate and amount of time in transport). The trip may be prolonged beyond the anticipated time. During a trip of more than 30 minutes, it is ideal to monitor oxygen concentration. Some transport systems are able to provide CPAP or respirator assistance during transport.

Hypoglycemia during transport is a major concern. How often a baby arrives at a medical center with an initial Dextrostix of 0 and no indication of how long his blood glucose has been that low. As noted above, glucose may be given through an umbilical artery catheter or through a peripheral line. Ten or 15 per cent is the common solution, given at approximately 10 ml. per hour for term infants and 3 to 4 ml. per hour for preterm babies. A battery-run infusion pump will assure a constant rate. Spare sterile supplies, both fluids and peripheral intravenous equipment, should be taken on the trip.

If it is not possible to get an intravenous line started, some physicians suggest that a small amount of glucose may be gavaged into the stomach. If this is done, the baby must be transported on his abdomen with his head up to minimize the danger of aspiration.

A number of special points of care for specific conditions are summarized in Table 24–9.

A record of nursing care during transport is just as important as records kept in a hospital or health agency. The record should include:

1. Vital signs.
2. The type of fluids given, the rate, and the amount absorbed each hour.
3. The amount of oxygen given.
4. Blood glucose level, if assessed.
5. Observations of the baby's condition, including color, respirations, and seizure activity.

Summary

Many of the problems of infants described in this chapter have long-term effects on both the baby and his family. (The needs of families are discussed in Chapter 28.) Because infants and families will have a long association with the health-care system, it is imperative that the care they receive during this period be of excellent quality so that future interaction with health-care providers will not be compromised, and the long-term developmental needs of both family and baby will be enhanced.

REFERENCES

1. Bishop, W., and Head, J.: Care of the Infant with a Stoma. *MCN, 1*:315, 1976.
2. Christian, E., and Clark, J.: Potential Stresses during Infancy: Irreversible Alterations in Health Status. *In* Tackett, J., and Hunsberger, M. (eds.): *Family-Centered Care of Children and Adolescents.* Philadelphia, W. B. Saunders Co., 1981.
3. Carr, J.: Psychological Aspects of Pregnancy, Childbirth, and Parenting in Drug-Dependent Women. *In* Rementeria, J. (ed.): *Drug Abuse in Pregnancy and Neonatal Effects.* St. Louis, C. V. Mosby Co., 1977.
3a. Cornblath, M., and Swartz, R.: *Disorders of Carbohydrate Metabolism in Infancy.* 2nd Edition. Philadelphia, W. B. Saunders Co., 1976.
4. Harper, R., and Edwards, G.: Management of the Neonatal Narcotic Withdrawal Syndrome. *In* Rementeria, J. (ed.): *Drug Abuse in Pregnancy and Neonatal Effects.* St. Louis, C. V. Mosby Co., 1977.
5. Hunsberger, M.: Congenital anomalies of the Respiratory Tract. *In* Tackett, J., and Hunsberger, M. (eds.): *Family-Centered Care of Children and Adolescents.* Philadelphia, W. B. Saunders Co., 1981.
6. Jackson, P.: Digoxin Therapy at Home: Keeping the Child Safe. *American Journal of Maternal Child Nursing, 4*:105, 1979.
7. Lawrence, R.: *Breastfeeding: A Guide for the Medical Profession.* St. Louis, C. V. Mosby Co., 1980.
8. Lubet, E.: Cleft Palate Orthodontics: Why, When, How. *American Journal of Orthodontics, 69*:562, 1976.
9. Marlow, D.: *Textbook of Pediatric Nursing.* 5th Edition. Philadelphia, W. B. Saunders Co., 1977.
10. Oehler, J.: *Family-Centered Neonatal Nursing Care.* Philadelphia, J. B. Lippincott Co., 1981.
11. Ostrea, E., Ting, E., and Cohen, S.: Neonatal Withdrawal from Non-narcotic Drugs. *In* Rementeria, J. (ed.): *Drug Abuse in Pregnancy and Neonatal Effects.* St. Louis, C. V. Mosby Co., 1977.
11a. Sarahan, T., and Hunsberger, M.: Gastrointestinal Tract Anomalies. *In* Tackett, J., and Hunsberger, M. (eds.): *Family-Centered Care of Children and Adolescents.* Philadelphia, W. B. Saunders Co., 1981.
12. Saucier, P.: Persistent Fetal Circulation. *JOGN Nursing, 9*(1):50, 1980.
13. Schaffer, A., and Avery, M.: *Diseases of the Newborn.* Philadelphia, W. B. Saunders Co., 1977.
14. Tackett, J., and Hunsberger, M.: *Family-Centered Care of Children and Adolescents.* Philadelphia, W. B. Saunders Co., 1981.
15. Vaughan, V., McKay, R., and Behrman, R.: *Nelson Textbook of Pediatrics.* 11th Edition. Philadelphia, W. B. Saunders Co., 1979.

The Puerperium

25

Normal Physiologic and Psychologic Variations During the Puerperium: The Basis of Nursing Care

By Ora Strickland, R.N., Ph.D.

OBJECTIVES

1. Define:
   a. puerperium
   b. parturient
   c. involution
   d. lochia rubra
   e. lochia serosa
   f. lochia alba
   g. prolactin
   h. engorgement
   i. "taking-in"
   j. "taking-hold"
2. Describe the physiologic changes of the uterus, cervix, vagina, and perineum that occur during the puerperium.
3. Describe the physiologic changes that take place in other body systems: urinary tract, gastrointestinal tract, circulatory system, and skin.
4. Describe the process by which milk is secreted. Indicate the basis of nursing action to relieve the discomfort associated with engorgement and to promote breast care.
5. Identify maternal behavior during the taking-in and taking-hold phases. Indicate how nurses can meet the needs of mothers in each of these phases.
6. Describe nursing intervention for mothers with "postpartum blues."

When labor is completed and the infant, placenta, and membrane have been delivered, the *puerperium*, also called the *puerperal period* or the *postpartum period*, has begun. The term puerperium usually refers to the 6 weeks of physical restoration that occur after parturition, wherein the reproductive organs are restored to their normal nonpregnant state. Rubin has extended the definition of puerperium to include the psychologic processes that occur after delivery.[16] She defines the puerperium as "a complex state of the childbearing experience, during which the physical and psychological work of gestation and delivery becomes final." The mother who has recently delivered an infant is often referred to as the *puerpera* or *parturient*.

The puerperal period is marked by rapid retrogressive and progressive changes in the mother's body. Retrogressive changes occur in the uterus, vagina, and genitalia as these organs return to their nonpregnant state. Progressive changes occur in the breasts as they are prepared for lactation. Psychologic and behavioral changes occur, as the mother adapts to the rapid physical changes common to the puerperal period and as she takes on her new role as mother. The puerperal period is an interval of physical and psychologic transition, and nursing care is based on the variations that occur during the puerperium.

Anatomic and Physiologic Changes

The Process of Involution

The term *involution* refers to the process by which the reproductive organs return to their normal size and functioning during the 6-week puerperium. However, not all of the changes of pregnancy are completely reversible. During pregnancy, physical modifications occurred gradually, but the process of involution is more rapid, with the most profound and distinctive changes occurring in the first 3 or 4 days of the postpartum period. As profound and rapid as these changes are, the process of involution is a normal physiologic process, and the normal postpartum period is not a period of illness. Because the physiologic changes associated with involution closely resemble pathologic problems, it is vital that the nurse understand the normal physiologic changes that occur during the puerperium and be able to quickly distinguish variations from the norm. Furthermore, these physiologic changes dictate and serve as the basis for a great deal of the nursing care provided to the postpartum woman.

Involution of the Uterus

Immediately after labor and delivery, the uterus is a large, flattened organ that weighs about 2 pounds and is about the size of a grapefruit. Its mucous surface is denuded, and the placental site is one large wound with exposed veins containing superficial thrombi. During the puerperium, remarkable retrogressive and restorative changes take place in the uterus, and by the end of the puerperal period the uterus is a much smaller organ that weighs approximately 60 to 80 grams. Its endometrial surface is epithelialized and ready for normal reproductive functioning again. These involutional changes in the uterus are caused by three main processes: (1) contraction of the uterus, (2) autolysis of some of the protein substances of the cells of the uterine wall, and (3) regeneration of the endometrium.

During pregnancy the walls of the uterus are thinned and stretched in order to accommodate the growing fetus and other products of conception. Immediately after placental expulsion, the uterine musculature contracts so that the walls of the uterus are thick and the anterior and posterior walls lie in close opposition. The fundus or corpus of the contracted uterus can be easily palpated through the abdominal wall as a solid mass of tissue between the umbilicus and the symphysis pubis. The contracted state of the uterus is one of nature's ways of preventing postpartum hemorrhage and reducing the bulk of the enlarged organ. Uterine contraction controls bleeding by compressing and sealing off the blood vessels that enter the area left denuded by the placenta. Therefore, as long as the uterus remains sufficiently contracted, the danger of excessive bleeding from the uterine cavity is reduced. The size and bulk of the uterus are also reduced as the uterus contracts because the muscle fibers become shorter.

Although the main mechanism responsible for the diminution in the size of the uterus is contraction, its reduction in size is also aided by the process of autolysis. In this process some of the protein materials in the cells of the uterus are reduced into simpler elements that are then absorbed by the bloodstream and are cast off, mainly in the urine. Thus, the nitrogen content of the urine greatly increases for several days because of the excretion of the components of broken-down protein. During the process of autolysis the uterine muscle cells become much smaller; however, the total number of muscle cells does not decrease greatly.

The approximate rate of the decrease in size of the uterus is estimated by noting the height of the uterine fundus in relation to the umbilicus. The fundus is usually located below the level of the umbilicus immediately after delivery. It soon rises to the umbilical level, and about 12 hours after delivery the fundus is likely to be palpated a little above the umbilicus. The uterus then begins to decrease steadily in size and gradually descends into the pelvis as involution progresses. The diminution in the size of the uterus is reflected by the descent of the height of the fundus at a rate of about 1 fingerbreadth (2 cm.) each succeeding day (Fig. 25–1). Therefore, on the first day after delivery the fundus of the uterus is palpable at 1 fingerbreadth below the umbilicus, on the second day postpartum at 2 fingerbreadths below the umbilical level, and so on. By the tenth to twelfth day it can no longer be felt through the abdominal wall.

Involution of the uterus tends to occur more rapidly in primiparas and in women who breast-feed their babies. In primiparas the rapidity of uterine involution is probably due to greater contractility of the uterine muscle because the women's uterine muscle fibers are likely to be more elastic when only one full-term pregnancy has been experienced.

Secretion of oxytocin during breast-feedings, producing uterine contractions, is one explanation for the more rapid involution of the uterus during lactation. The diminished estrogen secretion during lactation may also be responsible for the more rapid uterine involution, since estrogens tend to enlarge the uterus.[8]

Methylergonovine maleate (Methergine) may be prescribed for some women for the first 3 to 5 days postpartum to encourage uterine contraction in an attempt to promote uterine involution. Adams and Flowers[1] found that methylergonovine administration had no appreciable effect on the amount of lochia flow nor on the fundal heights of women who had received the medication in comparison with those who did not receive it. Therefore, the administration of the drug seems to have minimal effect on the progress of involution. In addition, those who received methylergonovine complained of much more discomfort resulting from uterine cramping.

Nursing Care. Observation of the consistency and height of the fundus is an important aspect in the nursing care of the postpartum mother. These observations should be made at least every 15 minutes during the first hour after delivery and then at least every 4 hours for the next 23 hours. Daily observations are necessary on subsequent days. The uterus should feel firm upon palpation. A mother with a "flabby" uterus is likely to bleed heavily or hemorrhage. A well-contracted uterus seals off the open blood vessels at the former placental site and decreases blood loss.

As noted in Chapter 17, when palpating for the fundus, the nurse should first support the lower portion of the uterus with one hand, which is placed just above the symphysis pubis. The other hand is then used to palpate for the fundus. (See Chapter 17, Figs. 17–9 and 17–10.) The consistency and height of the fundus are then noted. If the uterus is not firmly contracted and the fundus feels soft or flabby, the nurse should gently massage the uterine fundus with one hand until it is firm, while keeping her other hand in the position as described above to support the uterus. Care should be taken not to overmassage the fundus because overstimulation can cause overcontraction of the fundus and subsequent muscle fatigue. If blood and clots have been retained in the uterine cavity, they should be gently

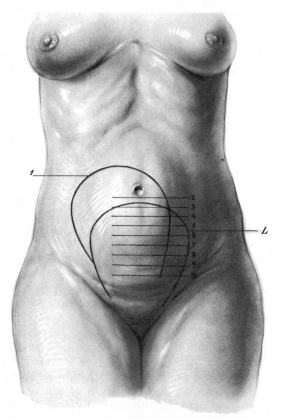

Figure 25–1. Frontal view of the abdomen indicating progressive changes in the height of the uterus postpartum with the bladder empty. *L,* Immediately after labor; *1* to *10,* fundal height on each successively numbered day. (From Greenhill and Friedman: *Biological Principles and Modern Practice of Obstetrics.* Philadelphia, W. B. Saunders Co., 1974.)

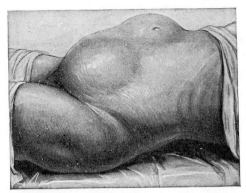

Figure 25–2. The uterus pushed up by a full bladder. (From Davis and Rubin: *De Lee's Obstetrics for Nurses.* 18th Ed. Philadelphia, W. B. Saunders Co., 1966.)

expressed from the uterus with one hand while the other hand supports the lower portion of the uterus. Force should not be used while expressing clots from the uterus. Gentle pressure is all that is required.

Usually the fundus will be palpated at the midline of the abdomen rather than at either side. However, the ligaments that support the uterus are stretched and loose after delivery, and the uterus easily becomes displaced within the abdomen until these ligaments recover their tone. Therefore, observations of the fundal height should be made after the bladder is emptied, since a full bladder will displace the uterus and invalidate the measurement. A full bladder may push the uterus upward several centimeters, usually to the right side of the abdomen (Fig. 25–2). A distended colon can also cause a similar effect.

Observation of the rate of uterine involution by measurement of fundal height is important, and any marked delay should be reported to the physician. Failure of the uterus to decrease progressively in size is an indication that involution is not proceeding satisfactorily. Failure of the uterus to return progressively to its normal size and condition within 6 weeks after delivery is called *subinvolution.* Retained placental fragments and infection are conditions that slow down the progress of involution and are among the most common causes of subinvolution.

Regeneration of the Endometrium

Just as the endometrium must undergo certain specific changes to prepare for pregnancy (Chapter 7), after delivery it must prepare to resume nonpregnant functioning. At the time of delivery both the placenta and the membranes separate from the spongy layer of the decidua, leaving a portion of the decidua in the uterus. The denuded placental site is a raw, open surface that is infiltrated with blood. If we can imagine this jagged, bloody wound surface, it is not difficult to understand why so many new mothers died from infection in generations past and why protection from infection is still a vital part of care in the puerperium.

Within 2 or 3 days, the portion of the decidua that remained in the uterus after delivery becomes differentiated into two layers as healing begins. Leukocytes invade the remaining decidua, and a layer of granulation tissue is formed, which separates the necrosing, sloughing decidua on the surface from the deeper, healthier layer. This granulation tissue serves somewhat as a protective barrier against infection. The superficial layer of the decidua then is cast off in the discharge from the uterus, referred to as the lochia (see below), leaving an inner layer adjacent to the uterine musculature. This remaining inner layer contains connective tissue and the bases of uterine glands. This is the source from which a new endometrium will regenerate. The regeneration of the endometrium is rapid except at the former placental site, which requires up to 7 weeks to heal completely. Elsewhere the endometrium is restored in about 3 weeks. The large blood vessels of the placental area that were present during pregnancy become invaded by fibroblasts, and there is recanalization of some of the vessels with smaller lumens.

The Lochia

After delivery, there is a vaginal discharge that usually persists throughout much of the puerperium, termed *lochia.* The amount and quality of lochia vary from day to day as involution progresses, providing an index of the healing process by which the endometrium of the uterus regenerates. Initially, the lochia consists of blood, along with small amounts of decidua and mucus, and occasionally it contains vernix caseosa, lanugo, and meconium. Because the appearance of the lochia varies in the days following parturition; it has been classified into three groups according to its characteristics: lochia rubra, lochia serosa, and lochia alba (Table 25–1).

The early discharge, called *lochia rubra* because of its dark red color, persists for 3 or 4 days. Since the bleeding from the placental site is more copious during the early puerperium, lochia rubra consists mainly of blood. As the blood vessels of the placental site become thrombosed, the oozing of blood from the healing surface diminishes. Then the lochia appears as a sanguine-serous discharge called

Table 25–1. LOCHIA

Type	Characteristics	Components	Duration
Lochia rubra	Consists mainly of blood	Blood Shreds of decidua Vernix (occasionally) Lanugo (occasionally) Meconium (occasionally)	3 or 4 days following delivery
Lochia serosa	Pink to red-brown Creamy consistency	Serous exudate Leukocytes Erythrocytes Shreds of degenerating decidua Cervical mucus Micro-organisms	From third or fourth day to 14 days postpartum
Lochia alba	Resembles cream	Decidual cells Leukocytes Epithelium Cells from uterus Mucus Bacteria	From tenth to fourteenth day until 6 weeks postpartum (may stop earlier)

lochia serosa, which is pink or a serous brown-red. Between the tenth and fourteenth days of the puerperium the lochia becomes thinner and greatly decreased in amount and assumes a yellowish or whitish color. These are the characteristics of *lochia alba,* which may last up to 6 weeks postpartum.

At first the lochial discharge is somewhat heavy, but it gradually diminishes over time. The presence of frank, fresh bleeding from the vagina, however, is not normal at any time. Neither should there be large clots or a persistence of bright red blood in the lochia. In the first hour after parturition the woman can be expected to saturate no more than two perineal pads. During the next 8 hours a perineal pad may be saturated within 2 to 4 hours. After the first 8 hours, the vaginal discharge is not much heavier than a regular menstrual flow. Excessive lochia may indicate a relaxed uterus. If this is the case, corrective massage of the fundus should be done immediately. Excessive loss of blood should be reported immediately.

There is great variation in the amount of lochial flow in an individual mother and among mothers. The total discharge ranges from 150 to 400 ml., but the average is about 225 ml. Multiparas tend to have more profuse lochia than primiparas. Mothers who breast-feed generally have a lesser amount of discharge, though there may be a temporary increase while the infant is nursing. During the night, when the mother is in a recumbent position, the lochial flow is less than during the day. Mothers who have had cesarean deliveries tend to have scantier lochia. The amount of discharge is increased when the mother is

more active and when she is out of bed, particularly for the first time. If the woman has not been told that this is common, she may be frightened by the increase in lochial flow when she is more active.

Because the characteristics of the lochia are indicators of the progress of involution and the restorative changes of the uterine lining during the puerperium, it is vital to judge whether the discharge is or is not normal.

First, the *lochia should not be excessive in amount.*

Second, although the odor of lochia varies, *lochia should never have an offensive odor.* The odor of the lochial discharge is determined by the kind of bacteria present in the vagina of an individual patient. A highly unpleasant odor of the lochia suggests infection, decomposing clots, or perhaps a retained sponge or packing. Investigation is imperative.

Third, *there should not be large pieces of tissue* in the lochia. The passage of distinguishable tissue in the lochia, particularly when accompanied by complaints of severe discomfort, may be indicative of retained placental fragments or membranes. If involution is to progress satisfactorily, tissues that are retained after delivery must be removed, since this predisposes the mother to hemorrhage and subinvolution. Passage of tissue in the lochia should be reported promptly.

Fourth, *lochia should not be absent* during the first 3 weeks of the puerperium. Normally, the flow of lochia does not cease until the endometrium is healed and the uterus has returned to its normal size and position in the pelvis. Suppression of lochia may indicate postpartum uterine infection.

Finally, *the characteristics of the lochia should proceed from rubra to serosa to alba.* Once a mother's lochial flow has progressed to serosa or alba, there should not be a red flow of lochia again. An exception to this is when a mother has received a prolonged course of estrogen therapy for the suppression of lactation. The lochial discharge contains more red blood and increases somewhat in amount after such therapy.

The Cervix

The cervix, which became stretched and edematous during the birth process, is a soft, flabby, collapsed structure immediately after delivery. It is very succulent and may be bruised and infiltrated with blood and fluid. However, during the puerperium the cervix rapidly regains its tone, and small lacerations sustained during labor heal.

Within 18 hours after delivery the soft, spongy cervix becomes firmer and shorter. The cervical canal becomes progressively smaller, so that although two fingers can be passed through the internal os into the uterus on the second postpartum day, by the twelfth day only one finger can reach the internal os, but the finger cannot be passed through it into the uterus. By the fourth week the external os is a small, transverse slit in contrast to the oval pregravid external os. Once a woman has undergone vaginal delivery, the external os of the cervix never regains its pregravid state. Although the internal os is closed as before, the external os remains somewhat open and has lateral indentations at the site of lacerations. These permanent changes in the external os distinguish the multiparous woman from the nulliparous woman.

The Vagina

Restorative changes in the vagina progress slowly following a vaginal delivery. The vagina is a soft, enlarged, and smooth-walled passage during the first part of the puerperium. As in the uterus, the muscles of the vagina slowly contract to diminish its diameter. About the third week of the puerperium, the vaginal rugae begin to reappear. Lacerations sustained during the delivery usually heal readily. The vagina does not completely return to its nulliparous condition, however. Residual tags of the torn hymen, called *carunculae myrtiformes*, remain and are characteristic of parous women. The vaginal introitus will remain slightly more distended than before.

Because of the amount of stretching that the vagina endures during a vaginal delivery, some parents may be concerned about the possible effects that this will have later on coitus and sexual gratification. Usually, changes in the vagina as a result of a vaginal delivery do not interfere with sexual functioning after involution is completed. Perineal or Kegel exercises, previously described, can promote the restoration of muscle tone in the vagina and perineal area. In addition, perineal exercises can help in the immediate postpartum period by helping to reduce edema and improve circulation. The exercise is performed by contracting and relaxing the perineal muscles, as if trying to stop a voiding. This exercise is more effective if it is done five times in succession three or four times each day.

The External Genitalia or Perineal Region

The appearance of the external genitalia reflects the stress that was placed on the perineal region during the vaginal delivery. The mucous surface of the vulva has a deep red, velvety appearance for several weeks following delivery. The muscles of the pelvic floor may be torn and overstretched, and the perineal tissues may be infiltrated with bloody serum. For several weeks after the delivery, the blood vessels of the perineum are fragile, and capillary oozing may complicate any perineal surgery that may be performed. Lacerations and bruises are often evident around the clitoris, vaginal introitus, and labia minora, particularly in primiparas. An episiotomy, which is an incision of the perineum frequently made during the second stage of labor to prevent perineal lacerations, may also have been performed. Edema often becomes more pronounced within 24 hours after delivery, giving a puffy appearance to the perineum.

In the absence of infection, the episiotomy and the lacerations of the perineal region heal with little inflammatory reaction. Restoration of the tonicity of the perineum is surprisingly rapid and takes about 6 weeks. Both the labia minora and the labia majora ordinarily remain flaccid in the parous woman.

Perineal Care

Special attention should be given to cleaning the perineal region and to promoting perineal comfort for each postpartum mother. Although the perineum is anatomically the area between the vagina and rectum, perineal care is more inclusive and involves cleansing of the perineum along with the vulva and rectal area. This procedure is done to prevent infection because perineal wounds and the build-up of dried lochia in the perineal region are conducive to bacterial growth. At the same time, cleansing of the perineum promotes maternal comfort because the procedure is refreshing to the perineal region. Hence, frequent perineal care is necessary to prevent infection and to promote healing and maternal comfort.

Perineal care is usually administered by the nurse in the early postpartum period and offers an opportunity for the nurse simultaneously to inspect the perineum for edema, and to check for capillary effusion of blood into the tissues of the perineum and the presence of hemorrhoids. After the mother becomes ambulatory, this aspect of care is usually attended to by the mother herself, but the nurse will still want to inspect the perineum at least once daily to assess the progress of healing and to observe any evidence of infection. Perineal care is done as part of the daily bath and after each time that the mother voids or evacuates her bowels.

Although hospitals differ as to the type of cleansing solutions and articles used to carry out perineal care, the basic principles of the procedure are the same. At one time perineal care was done as a sterile procedure in some hospitals, but now most nurses agree that it should be conducted as *clean* procedure requiring clean technique. Thus sterile water, sterile gloves, and sterile utensils are not necessary. Hand washing prior to initiation of the perineal care is required.

Some hospitals use soap or detergent solutions for cleansing of the perineum, and others use plain tap water. A pitcher or spray can, washcloths, cotton balls, or gauze sponges may be used in the procedure. As just mentioned, the hands should be washed thoroughly prior to beginning perineal care. A hip pad should be placed under the mother's buttocks to prevent soiling of the bed. The nurse should note the color, amount, and odor of the lochia as she removes the perineal pad. The perineal pad should be removed from front to back, and the cleansing of the perineal region should proceed from the pubis toward the anal area. This approach is taken to prevent the contamination of the vaginal vestibule by bacteria from the anus. It is most effective to clean the anal area first, except when disposable washcloths are used. With the mother on her side, the buttocks are gently separated, and the area is washed with cleaning solution, rinsed, and dried. The sponges used to clean the anal area are discarded immediately after use.

In hospitals in which a pitcher or spray can is employed to cleanse the perineum, the cleaning solution is poured over the perineum as the mother lies in a dorsal recumbent position.

The perineum is then rinsed with plain tap water in the same manner. The labia should not be separated during the procedure, since neither cleaning solution nor water should be allowed to seep into the vagina. Gauze sponges or cotton balls are then used to dry the area. The labia are dried, starting from the pubis, using a single downward stroke, and each gauze sponge or cotton ball should be discarded after each stroke. This is repeated with as many cotton balls or sponges as are necessary to dry the area.

When gauze sponges or cotton balls are used to cleanse the perineum, a sponge is moistened with cleaning solution, and the labia are cleaned first, proceeding from the pubis downward to the perineum. A single downward stroke is made with the sponge, and this is repeated with as many moistened sponges as are necessary to clean the area. Each sponge is discarded after use. Drying is done by using the same procedure described with dry sponges.

If disposable washcloths are used instead of gauze sponges, a similar technique is also used. The washcloth is first moistened with cleaning solution, and the labia are cleaned on one side down to the perineum. The other side is cleaned in the same manner. Then the anal area is washed last, and the washcloth is disposed of. The same technique is used to rinse and dry the perineal region; however, a second washcloth is used for rinsing the area and a third one for drying.

The perineal region is likely to be sore and tender from the trauma of delivery. Hence, perineal care should be done gently.

Once perineal care has been administered, the mother will want to put on a clean perineal pad. Contamination of the surface of the perineal pad, which will be next to the vulva, should be avoided. Therefore, the pad should be grasped on the outside when it is applied. Application of the pad should be from front to back. The sanitary belt is fastened in the front first; then the back of the pad is secured.

Perineal Care by the Mother. When the mother is ambulatory or is allowed to get up to go to the bathroom, she should be shown how to administer her own perineal care. The equipment that is to be used should be explained to her, and she should be shown where it is kept. Often it is best to give the mother simple instruction in perineal care as the nurse carries out the procedure. This can be done prior to the time the woman becomes ambulatory. When the mother ambulates for the first time, the nurse will want to review the procedure with her again. This instruction should also include the principles of perineal hygiene. Handwashing prior to initiating the procedure and cleaning the vulva from front to back should be particularly emphasized.

Measures to Promote Perineal Comfort. Complaints of perineal tenderness and pain are common among mothers who have had a vaginal delivery. Perineal discomfort is most often experienced by primiparas, who generally are more likely to have an episiotomy at delivery, and by women who have had difficult vaginal delivery.

Having the mother use a pillow or rubber ring to sit on will help relieve pressure on the perineum and decrease discomfort. A mild analgesic such as aspirin, Tylenol, or Darvon, which has been prescribed by the physician, is also helpful. However, local methods of treatment are immediately soothing and are effective in promoting perineal comfort. Local anesthetic sprays and ice packs are helpful when the mother complains of "pulling" or "tight" perineal stitches. Perineal care should be done just prior to the application of local anesthetic sprays. A few women may be allergic to such sprays. Therefore, mothers should be watched for signs of an allergic response, such as a rash or itching. If a perineal ice pack is used, it should be placed on the perineum for about 15 minutes. When a perineal ice pack is not readily available, one can be devised by placing crushed ice in a rubber glove and sealing it securely. The ice pack should then be wrapped with gauze before applying it to the perineal area.

Heat lamps and warm sitz baths are also used during the early puerperium to promote perineal comfort. In addition to being soothing to the mother, both of these treatments stimulate circulation in the perineal area, thus promoting healing of the episiotomy. Warm sitz baths are usually administered two or three times a day for 10 to 15 minutes. Generally, plain warm tap water is used for sitz baths. Care should be taken to make sure that the water is not too hot. Most sitz bath units fit easily over the bathroom commode. At many hospitals, plastic sitz bath equipment is available, which the mother may take home with her at the end of her hospital stay. If individually purchased equipment is not available, the sitz bath units should be sterilized between users.

When a heat lamp is used, the perineum is exposed to heat from a 25-watt bulb two or three times a day for a 15- to 20-minute period. Perineal cleansing should be done just prior to starting the treatment. The mother is instructed to lie in the dorsal recumbent position. The heat lamp is placed between the woman's legs about 10 to 12 inches away from the perineum, making sure that it is not so close that the heat from the bulb will be too hot. The light is adjusted so that it shines directly on the perineal area. The mother can be easily draped with the bed linen when the treatment is in progress.

Clinical Changes in Other Body Organs and Systems

Since pregnancy brings about both local and general physiologic alterations, it can be expected that puerperal changes will also involve local and general readjustments. As the new mother's reproductive system is adapted and restored to a nonpregnant state, so too are other body systems that have been changed or affected by the pregnancy or delivery. The puerperal alterations in other body systems occur in varying degrees, and in the physically healthy woman there should be no significant effects of pregnancy once the puerperium is complete.

The Urinary Tract

During pregnancy the ureters become markedly dilated and lose much of their tone. This is due in part to softening of walls of the ureters as a result of endocrine influences. During the postpartum period the ureters regain their tone and return to normal within 4 to 6 weeks.

Proteinuria is typical in the first few days following delivery. This increased nitrogen content of the urine is caused by autolysis or protein catabolism in the walls of the uterus, whereby muscle cells become smaller as protein is broken down into its components. Some of the products of protein catabolism are absorbed while others are eliminated in the urine. Proteinuria usually disappears about the third day postpartum.

Substantial amounts of sugar may also be present in the urine during the early weeks of the puerperium because of lactose absorption from the mammary glands into the bloodstream. This lactose sugar is subsequently excreted in the urine.

One of the most significant aspects of the puerperium is the large volume of urine excreted by the kidneys between the second and fifth postpartum days. This puerperal diuresis represents a reversal of the hydremia that was necessary for the nurture and support of the growing fetus during pregnancy. Since the increased extracellular fluid is unnecessary, its volume is reduced by copious urination. Sometimes the daily urine output of a postpartum mother may be as high as 3000 ml., and as much as 500 to 1000 ml. may be excreted at one voiding.

Spontaneous voiding during the first 8 hours of the puerperium may be very difficult or impossible for some puerpera. There are several reasons for this problem. The fetal head exerts a great deal of pressure on the urethra and trigone during the second stage of labor. As a result of the trauma of labor and delivery, some edema and loss of bladder tone are present for a short time after parturition. Pain from a sutured episiotomy or laceration may cause reflex spasm of the urethral muscle, making voiding very difficult. General swelling of the vulva may also inhibit voiding.

Another result of the trauma sustained during labor and delivery is a transient loss of some bladder sensation. Therefore, the puerpera is not as sensitive to a full bladder. The condition is found most often in women who have had long labors or an instrumentally assisted delivery. The mother may not void because she does not feel that her bladder is full, since there is a lack of a sensation to void. Anesthetics can have a similar effect on bladder sensitivity. A spinal anesthetic or general anesthesia given during childbirth may also interfere with bladder sensation, and, until their effects diminish, may predispose the woman to bladder distention.

Related Nursing Care. Since the newly delivered mother may not sense a full bladder, she should be encouraged to void, even though she may not feel a desire to do so. The puerpera should be offered the bedpan within the first 4 hours following childbirth. However, the nurse must not stick strictly to a timetable to determine when the patient needs to void. It is well to keep in mind that women who have received or who are receiving intravenous fluids are more likely to develop a full bladder. Assessment skills should be used to help determine when the mother has a full bladder.

The bladder may fill to such an extent that it rises and protrudes above the symphysis pubis. If markedly distended, it can easily be observed bulging between the uterus and the symphysis pubis. The uterus may be pushed upward and to the side of the abdomen. Palpation and percussion of the lower abdomen can also determine a full bladder. When palpated by the examiner's palm, the distended bladder feels like a soft fluid-filled sac, while the fundus feels solid and has a firmer tone. On percussion both the uterus and full bladder emit a dull sound; however, the full bladder is not likely to feel as firm and dense as the contracted uterus, which may protrude above or to the side of the bladder. A full or distended bladder requires immediate attention. A full

bladder can interfere with the contraction of the postpartum uterus and can render the mother susceptible to postnatal hemorrhage. A distended bladder further diminishes bladder tone and is a cause of urinary retention, which can lead to cystitis resulting from urinary stasis.

Voiding for the first time after delivery will be difficult for some mothers. However, when a mother has difficulty voiding spontaneously, several steps should be taken to encourage bladder activity. Voiding can be stimulated by exposing the mother to the sound of running water in the sink or shower, having her dabble her fingers in warm water, pouring warm water over her wrist or vulva, and having her drink a warm beverage.

Ambulation facilitates urination. Hence, the mother who is allowed to ambulate early is less likely to have difficulty voiding. If the mother is confined to bed, the nurse can facilitate urination by helping her to be more comfortable when she needs to void. Interventions that can encourage urination when the puerpera must use the bedpan include providing her with privacy, offering a warmed bedpan, and helping her to assume a comfortable upright position with body support. An upright sitting position facilitates urination because of the pressure on the urethra.

Since the mother may not have a spontaneous awareness of her need to void, it is advisable to offer the mother the bedpan at 2- to 3-hour intervals during the first 24 hours postpartum. The urine should be measured and recorded after each voiding for the first day of the puerperium until there is some certainty that the bladder is emptying completely.

Once the puerpera has voided spontaneously for the first time, she will usually not have difficulty with urination on subsequent attempts. The nurse will want to watch for signs of residual urine by noting the amount of urine voided at each attempt. At least 100 ml. should be voided to be considered sufficient. Large voidings are expected during the first few days. If, after several frequent voidings, the mother tends to excrete only small amounts of urine, residual urine may be present. It is likely that these voidings result from an overflow of a distended bladder. At this point the nurse will want to determine whether the bladder is empty by judging fundal height and position and by palpating and percussing the lower abdomen for a full bladder. If the mother is not able to empty her bladder sufficiently, catheterization for residual urine is indicated.

Catheterization. When catheterization becomes necessary, every effort should be made to prevent the introduction of bacteria into the bladder. Therefore, strict asepsis is imperative. Perineal cleansing should be done prior to beginning the catheterization procedure in order to further reduce the possibility of introducing bacteria. The nurse should keep in mind that the perineum is sore and tender and that any manipulation to expose the meatus is painful. Hence, the procedure should be carried out gently to prevent further perineal pain and discomfort. Because of edema and distortion in the perineal area, the meatus may not be easily visualized, making catheterization of a postpartum mother difficult. To facilitate the procedure, good lighting should be available and should be directed at the vulva. The nurse must gently separate the labia to prevent pulling on the perineal sutures. The solution that is used to cleanse the urinary meatus and surrounding area should be at least room temperature so that it will not feel too cold for the mother. While cleaning the area, care is taken not to allow any of the solution to flow into the vagina, to prevent inadvertent contamination of the birth canal. Lochia may be prevented from spreading upward to contaminate the meatus by placing a dry sterile cotton ball at the vaginal introitus. The catheter tip is then inserted into the meatus.

An indwelling catheter, which remains in place for 2 or 3 days, is preferred by a few physicians. This eliminates the need for frequent catheterization and permits the bladder to rest until some bladder sensation returns. Other physicians prefer catheterization as necessary, rather than an indwelling catheter, with the hope that the bladder will regain its tone more readily if it is permitted to empty and fill with some regularity. Because an indwelling catheter is likely to result in an ascending infection, preventative precautions include encouraging an increased fluid intake, keeping the urine receptacle below the level of the bladder, and ensuring good perineal cleansing.

The Gastrointestinal System

The enlarging pregnant uterus causes considerable displacement of the gastrointestinal organs, and the rise in the progesterone level during pregnancy causes the motility of the gastrointestinal tract to become more sluggish and less efficient. During the puerperium the normal motility of the gastrointestinal tract is restored, and gastrointestinal displacement is corrected. Pressure on the pelvic floor during delivery causes decreased tone of the anal sphincter. Therefore, the mother should be told that she may not have complete anal sphincter control for several days after childbirth.

Most mothers are able to eat and drink an hour after delivery if general anesthesia was not used and if there are no complications. However, a few mothers may feel nauseated and may vomit immediately after delivery. In general, the alert mother will usually have a good appetite after giving birth and may be ready to eat immediately.

Intestinal Elimination. The puerpera may experience some difficulty evacuating her bowels during the first week of the postpartum period, and constipation may result. This sluggishness is mainly caused by a tendency of the bowels to remain somewhat relaxed during the early puerperium, along with the relaxed condition of the abdominal walls. Once the products of conception have been delivered, the abdominal walls, which have been stretched during pregnancy, do not exert enough pressure to readily cause a bowel movement. Hemorrhoids and perineal stitches may further contribute to constipation because the mother may be reluctant to try to defecate owing to fear of pain.

Some women worry, probably more than is necessary, because they are having difficulty moving their bowels. If the woman had an enema during labor, there is probably little solid waste to be eliminated for the first several days.

Early ambulation after delivery will aid in preventing and correcting constipation. Some new mothers will need laxatives in order to produce spontaneous bowel evacuations early in the puerperium. To prevent constipation, many physicians routinely order a stool softener to be given each night after delivery. A laxative, suppository, or cleansing enema may be ordered if the mother has not defecated by the third postpartum day. If a suppository or an enema is given, these should be administered gently, as the anal sphincter may be tender and sore.

The new mother should be requested to employ measures that will encourage natural evacuation of the bowels. Roughage in the diet; adequate intake of fluids, especially of fruit juices; and exercise are effective in preventing constipation. If a mother is breast-feeding, she should be advised to consult her physician and follow his prescription if laxatives are required. Certain laxatives that are excreted in breast milk will affect the nursing infant.

Flatus. Flatus is also a common complaint during the early postpartum period, particularly in women who have had a cesarean birth. Although the displacement and replacement of the gastrointestinal tract during the childbearing experience contribute to flatus, the retention of waste products in the bowel produces flatus and resultant distention. Mothers can suffer great discomfort because of "gas pains." Drinking an effervescent beverage such as ginger ale will help provide some relief. Ambulation and bowel eliminations usually help to reduce flatus. Insertion of a rectal tube may be indicated.

Hemorrhoids. Hemorrhoids are a common problem for some women during the puerperium, as they are during pregnancy. They result from the entrapment and stasis of blood in the rectal veins. Pressure exerted on the pelvic floor by the presenting part and straining during labor and delivery may have precipitated the development of hemorrhoids or caused aggravation of the condition, if hemorrhoids were present previously. Usually, hemorrhoids are most painful during the first 2 or 3 days after delivery. They tend to reduce in size and become less painful as the puerperium progresses.

Hemorrhoids can cause much discomfort for the postpartum mother. Painful hemorrhoids are relieved by anesthetic sprays, sitz baths, and cool astringent compresses. Cold witch hazel compresses are ordered by some physicians, and they are very effective in abating discomfort and in reducing hemorrhoids.

Further irritation and pressure on hemorrhoids should be prevented. The perineal pad should be loosened or detached to relieve irritation of the rectum. The assumption of the Sims position by the mother while she is in bed relieves some of the pressure and congestion of the rectal veins.

Hemorrhoids that were not present prior to pregnancy will probably disappear during the latter half of the puerperium. Hemorrhoids that were present prior to pregnancy are likely to return to their prepregnancy condition.

The Circulatory System

During the early puerperium, the total blood volume remains high. However, as the excess fluid that was necessary during pregnancy is excreted after childbirth, the blood volume decreases and returns to normal. The total blood volume returns nearly to its prepregnant level by the end of the first week postpartum. A high fibrinogen level that was pregnancy-induced persists during the same period. Consequently, an elevated sedimentation rate is found during the immediate puerperium. The leukocytosis that occurs during the labor and delivery process is reflected in the puerpera's leukocyte count for the first few days after delivery.

The hemoglobin and hematocrit levels and red blood cell count tend to be variable from woman to woman. If the mother is not well hydrated after a long labor, these values may be somewhat elevated for about 3 days postpartum because of hemoconcentration. On the other hand, if the woman has lost a considerable amount of blood, hemoglobin and hematocrit levels and red blood cell count may be low, with subsequent fluid redistribution. If a mother tended to be anemic during pregnancy, then anemia will likely persist in the puerperium. It is imperative to note hemoglobin and hematocrit levels, since women with low levels need rest and are liable to experience weakness and faintness. Iron preparations, and possibly transfusions, may be ordered by the physician to help correct low hemoglobin and hematocrit levels. Dietary counseling with a focus on iron-rich foods is also indicated.

As during pregnancy, women with superficial varicosities will continue to require special attention. Usually, there is some improvement in varicose veins as the blood volume decreases after childbirth. Constricting garters or other clothing that causes pressure and interference with the flow of blood, particularly from the lower extremities, should not be worn. Although elevation of the legs may help varicosities of the lower extremities, the patient should not elevate her legs above the level of the buttocks while her head is also elevated, since this causes pooling of the blood in the pelvic region and engorgement of pelvic veins. Elastic stockings should be worn to give support to the weak walls of the veins.

Vital Signs

Pulse. The pulse rate is slower during the early puerperium than at other times. Puerperal bradycardia is a good prognostic sign and is a transient phenomenon. The pulse rate averages between 60 and 70 beats per minute, but sometimes is as low as 40 or 50 beats per minute on the first or second day postpartum. The heart rate returns to normal by the seventh to tenth day after delivery. Although the cause of the phenomenon is not known, it has been suggested that it results from a reduction in cardiac output without a reduction in stroke volume. A decrease in the pulse rate is a compensatory mechanism that results in a decrease in cardiac output, which may be related to the markedly lower flow of blood through the placental site.[9]

A rapid pulse rate in the early puerperium may be an indication of marked blood loss, cardiac disease, or nervousness.

Temperature. The mother's temperature may increase slightly after delivery without an apparent cause. In the normal puerpera,

temperature elevations should not exceed
100.4°F. (38°C.) in any two consecutive 24-
hour periods, excluding the first 24 hours postpartum. A woman who has endured a long and
difficult labor is likely to have a temperature
that is slightly elevated in the first 24 hours
after giving birth, but it rarely exceeds
100.4°F.

Any mother with a temperature exceeding
100.4°F. should have her temperature and
pulse taken every 4 hours throughout the day
and evening. The pulse rate is a helpful guide
in judging the significance of an elevated temperature during the puerperium. A mother
with a slightly elevated temperature and a
slow pulse rate is not likely to have a complication. However, an elevated temperature during the puerperium suggests the possibility of
an infection of the genitourinary tract. The
mother with an elevated temperature should
be assessed for other signs of infection, such
as general discomfort, chills, and local pain
and tenderness.

The establishment of lactation on the third
or fourth postpartum day was formerly believed to cause a natural elevation of temperature. This so-called milk-fever was regarded
as a normal accompaniment of the early phase
of lactation. However, today, milk-fever is not
a recognized process and is considered a fal-
lacy. Although extreme lymphatic and vascular engorgement of the breasts can on rare
occasions cause a sharp elevation in temperature, this rise *should not last* longer than 12
hours.

The Skin

Most of the pigmentary changes that developed during pregnancy either disappear or
regress during the postpartum period. Facial
deposits of pigment (chloasma) usually disappear completely. The increased pigmentation
of the breasts and abdomen becomes less pronounced. Spider nevi that developed during
pregnancy disappear, and striae gravidarum
become lighter in color.

In addition to the regression of skin changes,
there is an increase in the activity of the sweat
glands in the immediate puerperium. Diaphoresis occurs during the first few days of the
postpartum period, as the body rids itself of
the excess water retained during pregnancy.
Perspiration is usually most profuse at night
and may be accompanied by desquamation of
the skin. By the end of the first week postpartum, diaphoresis gradually subsides.

The postpartum mother should be reassured
that profuse sweating during the puerperium
is normal and is a process that aids the body

in returning to its prepregnant state. Wearing
of hospital gowns may be preferable at night,
when perspiration is most profuse. Protection
of the mother from chilling is important during
periods of diaphoresis.

Bathing. A bath or shower is refreshing
and stimulating for the postpartum mother,
particularly during periods of diaphoresis.
Most mothers find a bed bath administered by
the nurse in the recovery room a source of
comfort. This is best done after the woman has
rested and settled down somewhat from the
labor and delivery experience. Mothers usually
enjoy having the nurse give the first bath after
delivery, and it provides an opportunity for the
woman to talk to the nurse about the childbirth experience. It also is an excellent time
for the nurse to introduce the mother to basic
postpartum care, such as perineal care, breast
care, elimination, and hospital routines. However, the discussion and teaching activities
should be guided by the mother's readiness to
learn. The new mother can only retain so much
information during this early phase of the
puerperium, and much of the information may
need to be reviewed at another time. In the
first few hours after delivery, most women are
excited and caught up in their labor and delivery experience and have a need to talk with
someone about it and about the new baby.
Therefore, teaching and demonstration of basic
postpartum care may need to be postponed
until later.

Showers are usually permitted when the
mother becomes ambulatory. The first few
times that the mother takes a shower, it is
particularly important that she be accompanied by a nurse or attendant, who should
remain close by for safety. Some women become faint and light-headed while in the
shower and need assistance. The patient who
has had a cesarean delivery will need to keep
her incision dry until healing is well under
way. Thus she may not be allowed to take a
shower although she is ambulatory.

Tub baths are not allowed by some physicians following delivery. The danger of introducing infection through the vagina from the
bath water is the major rationale for prohibiting tub baths in the early puerperium.

The Abdominal Wall

The return of the prepregnancy "figure" is
one of the concerns of many postpartum mothers. A minimum of 6 weeks is required for the
abdominal wall to regain its muscle tone. Immediately after delivery, the abdomen is flat,
soft, and flabby. The abdominal wall never
regains its tone in some women, remaining

soft and covered by loose, wrinkled skin. The return of abdominal tone is influenced by the degree of distention of the abdominal muscles and by the mother's individual constitution. Women who have generally poor muscle tone, who have pregnancies that follow each other in close succession, or who have had excessively distended abdomens because of multiple pregnancy or hydramnios are more likely to have difficulty regaining their original abdominal muscle tone.

If the abdominal wall is so weakened that the rectus muscles separate at the midline (diastasis recti), this will be recognizable as a dark groove down the middle of the abdomen. The width of the diastasis recti should be noted and recorded. With active exercise, the width of the separation will narrow. A good diet, proper posture, and rest will further aid in the restoration of abdominal muscle tone.

At one time tight abdominal binders or girdles were used by postpartum mothers in the hope that this would restore the mother's figure and aid involution. Today, the general consensus is that abdominal binding is not necessary for the postpartum mother. However, an abdominal binder or an ordinary girdle may help the puerpera feel more comfortable if her abdomen is flabby and pendulous.

Weight Loss

Weight loss after delivery is a special concern for most mothers who desire to return to their prepregnancy weight as soon as possible. One of the first acts of some new mothers after they become ambulatory is to weigh themselves. These mothers may anxiously anticipate the day that they can again wear the clothes that they wore prior to pregnancy, and may be disappointed after delivery because they do not quickly return to their prepregnancy weight and size.

The average weight loss at delivery is approximately 12 pounds. This initial weight loss is mainly due to the delivery of the products of conception, which include the fetus, placenta, membranes, and amniotic fluid. An additional 5 pounds is lost during the first 2 weeks after delivery. This loss in weight is largely due to the elimination of excess fluid in the tissues through urination and perspiration.

In his study of 200 mothers during the first 8 days following normal delivery, Sheikh found that weight loss occurred in some mothers and weight gain in others during the first 3 postpartum days.[18] Of the mothers included in his study, 28 per cent showed a weight gain during the first 3 days postpartum, 40 per cent showed

a weight loss, and the other mothers' weight remained stable. However, from the fourth day onward most of the mothers began to lose weight. Primiparas and breast-feeding mothers were more likely to lose weight in the early puerperium. Mothers given lactosuppressants tended to have stable weights with little weight loss or gain. This was probably a result of the water and salt retention effect of estrogens given to suppress lactation.

The nurse should discuss weight loss with the mother after delivery and should point out that it usually takes the full 6 weeks of the postpartum period for her to return to her prepregnancy weight. Except for the additional weight of the lactating breasts in the mother who is breast-feeding, excess weight at the end of the postpartum period represents additional fat. If the woman has had previous problems controlling her weight, the nutritionist should talk with her about her diet habits prior to pregnancy and should provide some suggestions that may be of help to her. If a nutritionist is not available prior to the mother's return home, the nurse should review her diet history and offer assistance to her.

Afterpains

As pointed out previously, contraction of the uterus is a major process by which the uterus returns to its nonpregnant size during the puerperium. Uterine contractions after childbirth cause cramping sensations in some women similar to those accompanying a menstrual period. These are called "afterpains." Multiparas experience afterpains more frequently than primiparas. The uterus tends to remain tonically contracted in primiparas, while it often contracts and relaxes at intervals in multiparas. Painful sensations may occur with contractions, which sometimes are severe enough to require an analgesic.

Afterpains are also more likely to be a complaint when the uterus has been greatly distended during pregnancy, such as following multiple births, a large baby, or hydramnios. Women who are breast-feeding will notice that afterpains tend to occur when the infant is put to breast. The release of oxytocin from the posterior pituitary during the infant's suckling increases contractions of the uterus and gives rise to afterpains. As the puerperium progresses, afterpains decrease in intensity and frequency. By 48 hours following the delivery, they are usually mild. Usually the administration of a mild analgesic will abate or alleviate afterpains and help the woman feel more comfortable.

The Breasts

Breast development begins at puberty and is stimulated by the estrogens of the monthly sexual cycles. These estrogens stimulate growth of the ductile system and stroma. With pregnancy, additional growth of the breasts occurs, as the glandular tissue of the breast becomes completely developed for the final goal of milk production after parturition. Estrogen, progesterone, and chorionic somatomammotropin (human placental lactogen), which are secreted by the placenta, are responsible for accelerated breast development during pregnancy. There is growth and branching of the ductile system, further fat deposition, growth of lobules, and budding of the alveoli of the breasts. Development of the secretory characteristics of the *acini cells*, or the milk-producing cells of the alveoli, also occurs. Thus by the end of pregnancy, the mother's breasts have become fully developed for actual milk production, and colostrum, a thin, yellowish milk precursor, is secreted in small amounts. The actual production of milk does not occur until after the baby is born.

After parturition, no change in the condition of the breasts will be noted until about 2 days postpartum. Colostrum continues to be secreted in small amounts until lactation begins. Milk secretion begins by the third or fourth day postpartum. The onset of lacteal secretion is accompanied by larger, firmer, and more tender breasts. The veins become more prominent, and the breasts feel heavier to the mother. Some women may complain of a burning or prickling sensation in the breasts. This early breast tenderness and congestion are referred to as *primary engorgement*. At about the same time, the secretion from the nipples changes from yellow, the color that is characteristic of colostrum, to bluish-white, the color of normal breast milk.

Secretion of Milk. After childbirth, milk is produced in response to the hormone prolactin (also called luteotropin, LTH, or the lactogenic or mammogenic hormone), which is secreted by the anterior pituitary. High levels of prolactin secreted after delivery of the placenta are responsible for the initiation of lactation. The high blood levels of progesterone and estrogens during pregnancy are believed to have an inhibitory effect on the secretion of prolactins by the pituitary gland, and thus on milk secretion by the breasts. The reduction of estrogen and progesterone secretion after the placenta is delivered allows production of prolactin by the anterior pituitary because of the removal of the inhibitory effects of these two hormones (Fig. 25–3). Prolactin secretion stim-

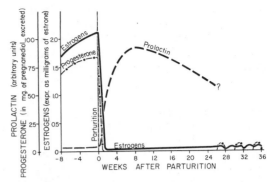

Figure 25–3. Changes in rates of secretion of estrogens, progesterone, and prolactin at parturition and during the succeeding weeks after parturition, showing especially the rapid increase in prolactin secretion immediately after parturition. (From Guyton: *Textbook of Medical Physiology.* 6th Edition. Philadelphia, W. B. Saunders Co., 1981.)

ulates the synthesis of fat, lactose, and casein by the acini cells in large quantities, and milk is produced.

The quantity of milk produced varies from woman to woman and from day to day in the same woman. Frequent and complete emptying of the breasts is necessary for the secretion of milk to continue. Milk production is inhibited by full breasts, and the amount of milk produced is generally dependent on the quantity of milk removed. Thus the infant's requirements for milk directly affect the quantity of milk produced. This is nature's way of ensuring an adequate amount of milk for the infant. As more and more milk is suckled from the breasts, the production of larger quantities of milk occurs. Usually less than an ounce is withdrawn from the breasts at each feeding on the first day after delivery. Thereafter the baby's consumption increases steadily, and by the end of the first postpartal week he removes about 2 to 3 ounces of milk from the breasts at each feeding. At the height of lacteal secretion 1.5 liters of milk may be produced each day.

If the breasts are not emptied regularly, secretion of prolactin is not stimulated, and milk production decreases and eventually ceases. When milk is not continually withdrawn, lactation will cease in 1 to 2 weeks. Milk secretion continues for as long as the breasts are emptied frequently and sufficiently. Secretion of milk normally decreases by 7 to 9 months, but this mainly depends on the amount that is withdrawn continually. The suckling of the breasts seems to be the stimulus that fosters continued prolactin secretion and milk production. Lactation can continue for several years if the mother's breasts are suckled frequently.

Other factors that influence the amount and quality of milk produced are the mother's diet and fluid intake, her activity level, and the amount of rest that she gets. An increased caloric intake is vital for the nursing mother, along with increased amounts of protein, iron, calcium, vitamins, and fluids. The mother who is breast-feeding needs to stay well rested and prevent fatigue. A midday rest period may be necessary in addition to a good night's sleep of at least 8 hours. Although moderate exercise is beneficial, the woman should not overexert herself, because fatigue has an adverse effect on lacteal secretion.

Some mothers may be concerned that their breasts are not large enough for sufficient milk production. These mothers' concerns can be alleviated by the understanding that the quality and quantity of milk produced are not related to the size of the breasts but to the amount of glandular tissue in the breasts. Breast size is related to the amount of fatty tissue in the breasts and not to the amount of glandular tissue. Since the milk is produced from the secretory mammary glands of the breasts, the amount of fat in the breasts has no influence on lactation.

Nursing care of the breast-feeding mother is discussed in detail in Chapter 26.

Engorgement.   Several days after delivery the mother may experience breast discomfort due to engorgement. Engorgement is local congestion and distention of the breasts and is related to the initiation of lactation. This condition has been attributed to an increase in the venous and lymphatic circulation in the breasts and to the filling of the lobules of the breasts with milk. *Primary or initial breast engorgement* occurs about the third or fourth day postpartum and is caused mainly by lymphatic and venous distention as lactation is being established. Engorgement that occurs after lactation has been established is referred to as *secondary or late engorgement* and is primarily due to the filling and distention of the lobules with milk.

When lactation is initiated, the breasts become heavier, larger, firmer, and more sensitive. The skin covering the breasts becomes tight and shiny. On palpation the breasts feel warm and tense. The individual lobules that are distended can be felt as hard lumps, and milk ducts can be felt as hard strings. There may be a darker or bluish coloration to the surface of the breasts, but rarely do they become reddened.

The degree of engorgement varies in severity. Varying degrees of discomfort are felt by the mother; however, engorgement is frequently quite painful. Primiparas usually suffer more discomfort from breast engorgement than multiparas. In addition to breast discomfort, the mother may complain of lassitude and headache. At one time, engorgement was believed to cause the mother to become febrile. Today engorgement is not accepted as a cause of fever in the postpartum mother. A mother's temperature may rise slightly (less than 1°F.) with engorgement, but if the mother's temperature exceeds 100.4°F. or 38°C., some other cause should be suspected.

Engorgement is a transitory condition that is usually present for 24 to 48 hours; however, it requires prompt attention. If the puerpera is nursing her infant, engorgement can interfere with the ease of nursing. If the condition is not corrected early in the nursing mother, emptying of the breasts becomes very difficult. Lactation will be terminated if the milk is not removed.

In the nursing mother, engorgement can be prevented, or at least decreased, by rooming-in. When rooming-in is practiced, the mother and infant are together constantly, and the mother can nurse according to the infant's demand and when her breasts feel full. Nursing can thus be initiated as necessary to maintain maternal and infant comfort. If the breast-feeding mother is not rooming-in, nursing staff need to make the infant available to her as often as is necessary to meet the infant's needs and to empty her full breasts.

Relief of the discomforts of engorged breasts is prompted by breast support, analgesics for pain relief, and application of heat or ice bags to the breasts. In the nursing mother removal of milk from the breasts can provide relief. A firm supportive bra will uplift and help alleviate pain and tenderness in heavy engorged breasts. Bra straps should be wide enough to prevent cutting into the shoulders. Fifteen- to 20-minute application of hot packs (for the breast-feeding mother) or ice bags (for the nonbreast-feeding mother) to the breasts can be comforting to mothers with engorgement. Relief can also be provided by applying hot or cold wet compresses or by using a towel that has been wrung in hot or cold water. Some women find that warm water from a shower that falls on the breasts is soothing.

Analgesics need to be administered as necessary for headache and local pain that may result from engorgement. If the mother is nursing, analgesics should be administered early enough prior to nursing so that the effects can provide relative comfort during the nursing period.

Removal of milk from the breasts of nursing mothers can provide some relief. This may be accomplished by manual expression of the milk or by use of a breast pump. A nipple shield may be indicated when engorgement interferes with the infant's ability to grasp the nipple. If a mother is not breast-feeding, removal of milk from the breasts is not an appropriate treatment, since this encourages further milk production.

Suppression of Lactation. When a mother chooses not to breast-feed, milk will still be produced by her breasts unless lactation is suppressed. The nonnursing mother should wear a well-fitting bra or breast binder to support and prevent manipulation of the breasts. The woman should be told not to remove any breast milk, as this encourages further milk secretion. If engorgement is present, it generally subsides in several days, since accumulation of milk in the breasts prevents milk production. At one time it was believed that restriction of fluids and the administration of diuretics would aid in the suppression of lactation; however, such treatment has not been found to be effective.[19]

When women choose not to breastfeed, the physician will usually prescribe hormones to suppress lactation. An estrogen-androgen combination or oral progestins, estrogens, or androgens alone have also been used.[20] These hormones are believed to interfere with or suppress the release of prolactin in the nonnursing mother. Diethylstilbestrol, quinestrol, and chlorotrianisene (TACE) are hormone medications that are usually prescribed for oral administration over 2 or 3 days during the early puerperium to suppress the secretion of milk. Deladumone, a long-acting estrogen-androgen combination, is administered intramuscularly. It is given in a single injection during the second stage of labor or immediately after delivery.

Estrogen-androgen combinations have been found to be most effective in preventing lactation.[20] Administration of hormones does not always effectively suppress lactation, however. Some women who have received lactosuppressants may experience filling of the breasts a few days postpartally, or as late as several weeks after delivery. Women who receive hormones for the purpose of lactosuppression should be told that filling of the breasts may occur, but this usually disappears spontaneously if milk is not removed from the breasts.

Side effects sometimes occur with the administration of lactosuppressant hormones. The administration of estrogenic hormones has been associated with heavier lochial discharge and with a greater proportion of bright red blood in the lochia, particularly after the treatment is discontinued. Thromboembolic diseases have been found to occur rarely after the use of estrogen for postpartum milk suppression. A delay in the onset of menstruation and the development of virilizing effects may be observed following the administration of androgens.

Lactation also may be suppressed by bromocriptine mesylate (Parlodel), which is a dopamine receptor agonist. It act directly on the dopamine receptor sites of prolactin-secreting cells in the anterior lobe of the pituitary gland to inhibit secretion of prolactin, thereby interfering with lactogenesis. Among the side effects of bromocriptine mesylate are headaches, dizziness, nausea, and hypotension. Because of the potential of a hypotensive reaction to the drug, the nurse should not administer bromocriptine mesylate until the mother's vital signs have been stabilized and not sooner than 4 hours after delivery. Bromocriptine mesylate is usually prescribed for oral administration over a 2- to 3-week period.

Breast Care. The importance of proper breast care for the postpartum mother cannot be overemphasized. Care of the breasts during the puerperium is aimed at providing good breast support and maintaining hygienic care. A supportive bra with wide straps is necessary. The bra should provide upward support for the breasts, but at the same time it should not be too tight. A bra should be worn during the night as well as during the day. Some women, particularly breast-feeding mothers, may be concerned that their breasts will begin to sag after childbirth. If adequate support is given, pendulous, sagging breasts are not likely to result.

The mother should be instructed to wash the breasts daily with soap and water as she showers. In nursing mothers, soap and other drying agents should not be used to cleanse the nipples because such preparations may remove the natural protective oils and leave the nipples more prone to damage during suckling. In the breast-feeding mother, nipples should be cleaned with plain water before and after suckling. Dry nipples are less likely to become macerated than nipples that stay wet and damp. Therefore, nursing mothers should leave the bra flaps that cover the nipples down for a few minutes after nursing, so that the nipples will air and dry.

Massage of the breasts between breast-feedings in nursing mothers can be helpful, by keeping the lacteal ducts open.[19] Breast massage can also aid in preventing engorgement once lactation is established.

Fissures of the nipples are portals through which infection may be introduced into the breasts. When cracks and fissures of the breasts are present, the nurse should be alert for signs of mastitis or breast infection, which include local redness, swelling, pain and tenderness, general malaise, and a high fever. If breast infection occurs in a nursing mother, termination of breast-feeding may be recommended by the physician.

Menstruation and Ovulation

Prior to returning home, mothers will want to know when they can expect their menstrual flow to appear again and when ovulation is likely to occur. The menstrual flow usually returns within 6 to 8 weeks after delivery if the woman does not breast-feed her infant. Variations are observed in the recurrence of menstruation and in the return of ovulation.

Generally, menstruation does not occur while the woman is breast-feeding. This phenomenon is called *lactation amenorrhea*. Although the most common time for the reappearance of menstruation in the lactating mother is during the third to fourth month postdelivery,[9] El-Minawi and Foda[5] noted that the duration of postpartum lactation amenorrhea ranged between 6 weeks and 26 months. They also found that lactation amenorrhea persists for a longer period of time if breast-feeding is not supplemented.

A substantial degree of infertility occurs jointly with lactation, as long as lactation amenorrhea persists. However, the mother may ovulate while she is breast-feeding, even though the menstrual flow has not reappeared. Therefore, all breast-feeding mothers should be informed of the potential occurrence of a pregnancy. Some type of birth control method should still be used while breast-feeding if the woman wants to prevent a pregnancy at that time.

Psychologic and Behavioral Reactions of the Puerperium

After delivery there is a period of psychologic adjustment for the postpartum mother. This psychologic or emotional adjustment is directly related to the physical or bodily changes she is experiencing and to her role and relationship to her new baby.

Just as the woman had to adjust to a new body image during her pregnancy, a similar adjustment is required after delivery. Once again the mother's body image changes, and she may feel a void and emptiness where the baby once was. The change in her body shape tells her that her infant is an individual, sep-

arate and real. The mother must begin to feel whole and not empty before she can reconcile herself completely to the actual birth of her baby. Initially there may be a feeling of bewilderment in the mother as she has difficulty feeling that the baby is really hers and because the sight of the newborn does not evoke an overwhelming feeling of maternal love.[13] However, as time passes she will become relieved as she begins to identify her infant as a separate individual to whom she has a binding emotional tie.

If the mother has experienced discomforts or difficulties related to the pregnancy or to the labor and delivery process, she may be anxious and fear that her body's level of functioning will never be quite the same again. When the mother has anticipated the return of her figure to the prepregnant state, she will be disappointed and frustrated during the early puerperium to see that she is still larger than she was prior to her pregnancy. It is imperative that the mother understands that these physical changes are normal, so that her anxieties and fears will be alleviated. Thus, the nurse should tell the mother about these normal alterations and should give her simple explanations about the cause of her discomforts and about their usual course before they end.

Phases of the Process of Regeneration and Restoration

Predictable psychologic and behavioral reactions occur during the course of the puerperium as physical healing and restoration progress. Rubin has described the common reactions that occur in the hospitalized mother and has distinguished two phases of puerperal adjustment—the "taking-in" phase and the "taking-hold" phase.[16] How well these phases apply to the mother who delivers at home is not known, since these maternal reactions may be influenced by the mother's hospital confinement. However, we can safely assume that the common physical changes that occur in the postpartum mother will affect her behavioral and psychologic processes similarly, whether she delivers her infant in the hospital or at home.

The Taking-in Phase. The first 2 or 3 days after the delivery the mother is in the taking-in phase of the puerperium. Characteristic of this phase is the importance of sleep and food to the mother. She tends to be passive and dependent during this period, and her psychic and physical energies are usually centered more around herself and the events of the immediate past.

Sleep and rest are necessary during the

taking-in phase of the puerperium. Uninterrupted sleep is vital for the mother as she recovers from the labor and delivery experience. In the first hours after delivery the mother feels exhausted and will fall into a deep sleep. If she is not allowed to get the sleep that she requires, a "sleep hunger" may result, and the restorative processes of the puerperium may be prolonged. As a consequence the mother may become irritable and feel fatigued for several days. Therefore, the nurse will want to ensure that the mother is allowed adequate periods of rest and sleep.

The mother's desire to ingest food is apparent during the taking-in phase. When she is not eating, she may talk about food until she eats and her hunger is satisfied. This reaction is probably partly physical and partly psychologic. Labor and delivery require hard work of the mother and a lot of energy. In addition, most mothers have gone for a long period of time without food during the labor and delivery process. Thus, the body requires food to aid in the restorative process. Food also has a great psychologic benefit for the mother, since the taking in of food may be emotionally satisfying and may signify an early step in the recovery process. Recognizing the mother's need for nourishment, the nurse should foster the woman's intake of nutritious food in the early puerperium.

Since dependence and passivity are characteristic of the mother during the taking-in phase, she does not actively initiate self-care activities. As the receiver of care, she accepts the care given to her without much input, and she does what she is told without much autonomy. The nurse will want to respect this seemingly natural response during the early puerperium by meeting the woman's dependency needs. The mother should not be forced to carry out physical activities that she is not ready to do and that seem to fatigue her. The nurse will need to have a major role in providing physical care for the mother during the first 24 hours after childbirth and should be available to assist and guide her in any self-care activities that she may initiate. The nurse will also notice that the woman's expressed needs tend to center on herself more than on her infant. The mother requires help from the nurse while she is learning to meet her own puerperal needs before she can sufficiently reach out beyond herself to meet the needs of her infant.

During the taking-in phase the mother responds psychologically to the childbirth experience by reviewing the details of labor and delivery. The woman has a need to talk about the birth events repeatedly, so that she can comprehend and grasp the reality of the whole event and of her motherhood. She needs to pull the whole event together by discussing every detail. The mother may discuss her labor and delivery over and over with several different people, so that she can better realize the completeness of birth experience. The nurse should lend a receptive ear to the mother and expedite this assimilative work, so that the mother can move on to the realities of the immediate present.

The Taking-hold Phase. In the taking-hold phase the mother reaches out more beyond herself and begins to focus on the order of things in the immediate present. This phase is marked by increasing independence and autonomy, as the mother becomes the initiator and producer of self-care and infant-care activities. The mother generally arrives at the taking-hold phase about the third postpartal day.

The mother seemingly was resting and recuperating after the events of labor and delivery in the taking-in phase. However, she now begins to move forward to deal with the events of the present in the taking-hold phase with an urgency, an immediacy that was not characteristic of her in the previous stage. Her focus is on the reality of "right now," and she presses forward to become involved and to get things organized. Her ability to carry out self-care activities becomes paramount initially, as she tries to take control of her own bodily functions. There is an element of anxiety about this, and she becomes less tolerant of delays and indications of her own inadequacies.

At this time she is concerned about her ability to evacuate her bowels and her bladder. If she is breast-feeding, she wants to know when the milk will "come in" or if she will be able to produce enough milk for her baby. As she becomes more confident of her own bodily functions, the woman begins to take hold of some of her mothering tasks with greater ease. It is as if the woman's involvement and concern with her bodily functioning are extended to her infant once she has successfully coped with the changes that occurred in her own body.

As her mothering tasks become paramount, the woman focuses on her ability to care for her infant. She has high ideals about how she should perform as a mother and feels inadequate and frustrated when she has not performed at the level that she expects. If she is having difficulty getting her baby to eat for her or if she feels awkward in providing his care, she may feel that she is failing in her mothering tasks. Her confidence is very delicate at this time, and she needs constant reassurance that she is performing well.

The woman may be overwhelmed by the

dependence of the small, helpless infant. She is curious about the infant-care tasks and is concerned about her infant's bodily functions. Most new mothers want to know the details of infant care—if the infant is getting enough to eat or if he is evacuating his bowels satisfactorily. The mother's anxiety will increase if there appears to be any defect in the infant's functioning or appearance (e.g., forcep marks, caput succedaneum, or jaundice), since she may feel that these reflect on the adequacy of her functioning during the gestation period or during labor and delivery. Thus, the nurse should discuss infant behavior and any variations from the expected with the mother. When explanations are given, they should be simple and easy for the mother to understand.

Because the woman is interested and curious during the taking-hold phase, it is a stage when receptiveness and readiness for learning are heightened. The nurse will want to take advantage of the mother's readiness for learning by providing instruction in infant care, self-care, and personal hygiene. She also can be of much assistance by giving anticipatory guidance to the mother about what to expect in the coming weeks after her return home and how to deal with these changes.

When the woman has begun to cope successfully with her mothering tasks in relation to her baby, her energies begin to extend beyond herself and her infant to encompass her role responsibilities as they affect other family members. Much of the taking-hold phase will take place at home, since this stage lasts about 10 days. Thus, prior to the mother's return home, the nurse will want to help her establish realistic expectations for herself. New mothers may involve themselves with too much activity during this phase and exhaust themselves in their drive for excellence.

Psychologic Reactions After a Cesarean Birth

From 10 to 30 per cent of women deliver their babies by cesarean birth. In many instances the woman has not been expected to have a cesarean delivery and she and her partner may have gone through prepared childbirth in anticipation of a vaginal delivery. It is not unusual for a couple to face a cesarean delivery with little or no preparation for such an event. For some there may have been little time to prepare themselves for the impact of surgery.

The loss of the opportunity to deliver their babies vaginally may precipitate feelings of failure and lack of achievement for some mothers. A labor that leads to a cesarean delivery

may be difficult to integrate and may threaten the woman's self-image. Some women who have had a cesarean birth feel disappointed and cheated because they believe they have missed an important experience related to childbirth and womanhood. One mother who had all four of her children by cesarean delivery described her feelings this way:

"I know that all of my children are mine but I don't feel like I really had them myself. I wish I could have gone through labor and had a baby like women are supposed to at least one time."

The nurse should keep in mind that mothers need to feel that their labor performance was acceptable. Cesarean mothers may be highly critical of their performance and, therefore, need reassurance.[11] As with all mothers, cesarean mothers should be encouraged to talk about their delivery experience so that they can be cognitively integrated and emotionally dealt with after delivery. It is important to fill in gaps in her memory about the events surrounding the birth and to explain details that she did not understand. The woman's labor partner can be helpful to her as she reviews and integrates the events surrounding the birth.[3, 11]

Some women view their cesarean delivery and the resulting discomforts as an experience undergone for the welfare and benefit of their babies. This moral, masochistic way of viewing the childbirth experience might be interpreted as a positive sign. Moral masochism is an essential quality of maternal behavior that is exhibited by mothers as they adapt to the increasing demands of motherhood.[11]

Although many women view their cesarean deliveries with disappointment, others do not seem greatly concerned about the method of delivery. Still others may perceive a cesarean birth as a means whereby they have escaped the discomforts of labor and vaginal delivery, particularly if surgery was performed prior to the onset of labor.

Cesarean mothers also must cope with the physiologic stress of surgery, and often have delayed contact with their infants. Because of the discomforts of surgery, cesarean mothers may display evidence of greater ego constriction in the early puerperium than those who have vaginal deliveries.[11] Women who have had a cesarean delivery may be more self-centered for a longer period of time and may tend to focus on the pain and discomfort of surgery. This may make it difficult for them to extend their psychic and physical energy from themselves to others, making it difficult for them to reach out to "mother" their babies. When cesarean delivery has been compounded by delayed maternal–infant contact, this also may delay the progression of maternal–infant attachment.

The nurse should exercise patience with cesarean mothers and view them in the context of women involved in adjusting to the consequences of major surgery in addition to the changes associated with the puerperium. Nursing care should be planned to meet cesarean mothers' physical and emotional needs with these two factors in mind.

Postpartum Blues

One of the emotional aftermaths of childbirth that some women experience is a depression or "blue" feeling for which the mother may not be able to determine an apparent cause. Postpartum blues, as it is called, usually appears between the third and tenth day postpartum but may occur earlier or later. The incidence of this phenomenon has been shown to range from 50 to 80 per cent. Mild depression, anxiety, and a feeling of being a bit slow or "not quite with it" are most characteristic of the phenomenon.[14] The mother may also have periods of weepiness and irritability. All of these symptoms are transitory and usually last from 1 or 2 hours to several days.

Several psychologic and social factors interact to influence the mood of women during the puerperium. Even though this is the case, the transient depression of postpartum blues is believed to result from the impact of the additional responsibilities of motherhood on the woman. Another explanation that has been offered is that the reaction is precipitated by a drop in hormonal levels after childbirth. Fatigue and anxiety about the baby and about her adequacy in carrying out the maternal role may also contribute to the condition.

The nurse can be of assistance to the mother by recognizing postpartum blues from the mother's behavior and by discussing the phenomenon with her. The mother will be relieved to know that her feelings are not unusual and that her crying is acceptable to the health-care team. Since a large number of mothers are likely to experience postpartum blues after they return home, women and their mates should be warned of the possible occurrence of this condition after they leave the hospital. If the condition persists for several days or if the mother becomes deeply depressed, her physician should be contacted. Infrequently, a postpartum mother may develop a more serious depressive reaction for which she will need close psychiatric supervision.

Summary

In general, the emotional state of the postpartum mother during the early puerperium tends to be somewhat labile and is affected by the mother's physical state and well-being. She is required to make adjustments to the rapid changes that have occurred and that continue to occur in her body. She is in a transitory period and is faced with stress and strain as she adapts to the new responsibilities of her maternal role. Although commonalities have been emphasized in this review of the mother's physical, psychologic, and behavioral reactions during the puerperium, the nurse must be aware of the great range of variability among postpartum mothers. Therefore, nursing care during the postpartum period must not be considered to be "routine," but each mother's individual situation and condition must be considered in planning and providing care.

REFERENCES

1. Adams, H., and Flowers, C. E.: Oral Oxytocic Drugs in the Puerperium. *Obstetrics and Gynecology,* 15:280, 1960.
2. Barnes, J.: The Aftermath of Childbirth: Physical Aspects. *Proceedings of the Royal Society of Medicine,* 68:223, 1975.
3. Boyd, S. T., and Mahon, P.: The Family-Centered Cesarean Delivery. *MCN, The American Journal of Maternal Child Nursing,* 5:176, 1980.
4. Dessouky, D. A.: Myometrial Changes in Postpartum Uterine Involution. *American Journal of Obstetrics and Gynecology,* 110:318, 1971.
5. El-Minawi, M. G., and Foda, M. S.: Postpartum Lactation Amenorrhea: Endometrial Pattern and Reproductive Ability. *American Journal of Obstetrics and Gynecology,* 111:17, 1971.
6. Eppink, H.: Catheterizing the Maternity Patient. *American Journal of Nursing,* 75:829, 1975.
7. Greenhill, J. P., and Friedman, E. A.: *Biological Principles and Modern Practice of Obstetrics.* Philadelphia, W. B. Saunders Co., 1974.
8. Guyton, A. C.: *Textbook of Medical Physiology.* 5th Edition. Philadelphia, W. B. Saunders Co., 1976.
9. Hellman, L. M., and Pritchard, J. A.: *Williams Obstetrics.* 14th Edition. New York, Appleton-Century-Crofts, Meredith Corporation, 1971.
10. MacDonald, H. N., Good, W., and Stone, J.: Changes in Common Plasma Solute Levels during Labor and the Puerperium. *Journal of Obstetrics and Gynecology of the British Commonwealth,* 81:888, 1974.
11. Marut, J. S.: The Special Needs of the Cesarean Mother. *MCN, The American Journal of Maternal Child Nursing,* 3:202, 1978.
12. Nott, P. N., Franklin, M., Armitage, C., et al.: Hormonal Changes and Mood in the Puerperium. *British Journal of Psychiatry,* 128:379, 1976.
13. Pines, D.: Pregnancy and Motherhood: Interaction

Between Fantasy and Reality. *British Journal of Medical Psychology, 45*:333, 1972.

14. Pitt, B.: Aftermath of Childbirth: Psychological Reactions to Childbirth. *Proceedings of the Royal Society of Medicine, 68*:223, 1975.

15. Rubin, R.: Basic Maternal Behavior. *Nursing Outlook, 9*:683, 1961.

16. Rubin, R.: Puerperal Change. *Nursing Outlook, 9*:753, 1961.

17. Salazar, H., Tabon, H., and Josimovich, J. B.: Developmental, Gestational and Post-gestational Modifications of the Human Breast. *Clinical Obstetrics and Gynecology, 18*:113, 1975.

18. Sheikh, G. H.: Observations of Maternal Weight Behavior during the Puerperium. *American Journal of Obstetrics and Gynecology, 111*:244, 1971.

19. Stone, S. C., and Dickey, R. P.: Management of Nursing and Nonnursing Mothers. *Clinical Obstetrics and Gynecology, 18*:139, 1975.

20. Vorherr, H.: Suppression of Postpartum Lactation. *Postgraduate Medicine, 52*:145, 1972.

26

Nursing Approach to the Postpartum Family

By Ora Strickland, R.N., Ph.D.

OBJECTIVES

1. Identify the basic principles underlying postpartum care.
2. Describe physical assessment of the mother. Indicate how maternal education can be incorporated into the assessment.
3. Describe the mother's need for rest, ambulation, nutrition, and exercise. Indicate nursing intervention to ensure that these needs are met.
4. Describe nursing actions to assist the breast-feeding mother prior to feeding, during feeding, and following feeding.
5. Describe methods of expressing breast milk.
6. Indicate parental concerns related to sexual relationships during the puerperium.
7. Describe factors that contribute to family-centered maternity care.
8. Define attachment. Describe factors that contribute to attachment. Indicate how nurses can assess and contribute to attachment.
9. Identify methods by which mothers incorporate the maternal role. Describe how a nurse can facilitate the attainment of parenting roles.

The postpartum mother and her newborn are the major focus of nursing care on the postpartum unit. The parturient mother receives special attention because she is experiencing major physical changes with resultant emotional adjustments after giving birth. Special consideration is given to the newborn because he is making a delicate transition from intrauterine to extrauterine life.

In providing nursing care during the puerperium, we must remember that childbirth has implications for others beyond the mother–infant dyad. Reproduction and childbearing are a family experience that touches the lives of all family members. The mother's most intimate contacts, such as with her husband, her other children, and her own parents and siblings, will be most profoundly affected by the birth. The arrival of the newborn will require adjustments and adaptations to be made by all members of the immediate family. Family relationships will have to be modified to incorporate the new baby. The quality of care that the family receives during the postpartum period can influence the family as it reorganizes and adjusts after the birth and can be viewed as an important basis of future family health.

We must recognize the importance of the birth to all family members and must realize that each mother, baby, and family is unique and has different needs. Every effort should be made to make sure that those family members who are most important to the mother and who will be influential in the life of the newborn are incorporated into nursing care whenever possible.

In providing postpartum care, our nursing approach is based on two basic principles:

1. The mother's body is readjusting and is being restored to the nonpregnant state.

2. With each birth a "new" family begins, as new relationships are established with the newborn and former relationships are modified.

In assessing the needs of the postpartum mother and her family, factors to be considered are:

1. Maternal physical aspects of the puerperium.

2. Parent–infant interaction.

3. Teaching needs.

The specific nursing needs of the postpartum family must be determined to ensure that comprehensive nursing care is provided.

The Postpartum Mother

The postpartum period is not an entity in itself, nor does the mother start the puerperium with a blank slate. She brings with her a history that affects her needs, expectations, and responses during the postpartum period. Information regarding the mother's family, previous childbearing experiences, sociocultural background, and other maternal characteristics can be vital in assessment and in planning nursing care. The uniqueness of each mother's history, along with her current physical condition and behavioral responses, will influence the care provided to her.

Care in the Immediate Postpartum Period

During the first hours after birth, much of the nursing care will be related to the physical aspects of the puerperium to ensure that the mother's physical condition is good. The major threat to the mother during the first 24 hours after delivery is the possibility of excessive bleeding (see Nursing Care Plan 26–1). The fundus should be checked at least every 15 minutes during the first hour postpartum to determine if it is firm and contracted. The mother's lochia flow should be checked at the same time intervals to assess the amount of bleeding. After the first hour, the fundus and lochia flow should be checked at least every 4 hours for the next 23 hours.

The patient's history should be considered when making a judgment as to whether she should be assessed for excessive bleeding more frequently. If the mother had an operative delivery or lacerations of the perineum, vagina, or cervix, she will need to be observed more closely for bleeding. The older multipara who has delivered several children and the mother whose uterus has been extensively distended (e.g., because of a large infant, multiple pregnancy, or hydramnios) are more prone to uterine atony and hemorrhage and also require closer observation.

If the uterus is atonic, it should be gently massaged until it is firm again. The uterus must be supported at the suprapubic area with one hand when it is being massaged and when blood that has pooled in the uterine cavity is being expressed. To prevent inversion of the uterus with resultant hemorrhage and shock, expression of blood from the uterus should be done only when the uterus is firm and well contracted.

A distended bladder can result in a less firmly contracted uterus. Some mothers will need to void within the first hour or two after delivery. Bladder distention should be checked and the mother should be offered the bedpan within 2 to 4 hours after parturition.

The mother's pulse, respirations, and blood pressure are taken immediately after delivery

Nursing Care Plan 26-1. Ensuring Involution for the Postpartum Mother

NURSING GOALS: To promote optimal involution to ensure minimal blood loss and recovery time.
As a result of nursing actions:

OBJECTIVES:
1. Blood loss is minimal.
2. Recovery is uncomplicated.
3. The mother is in good physical shape and in control.

ASSESSMENT	POTENTIAL NURSING DIAGNOSIS	NURSING INTERVENTION	COMMENTS/RATIONALE

Review the prenatal, labor, and delivery records for factors predisposing to hemorrhage.
1. History of excessive bleeding
2. Placenta previa
3. Abruptio placentae
4. Larger than average uterus
  a. Multiple pregnancy
  b. Polyhydramnios
  c. Large baby
5. Long labor
6. Difficult delivery
7. Multiple parity
8. Anemia
9. Medication history (e.g., aspirin)
10. Excessive analgesia or anesthesia
11. History of a tendency to bleed
 	
In women at risk for hemorrhage:
1. In fourth stage assess blood pressure, pulse, and fundus *at least* every 15 minutes. Assess amount of lochia, woman's skin color.
	At risk for postpartum hemorrhage	Explain to the family the rationale for the assessments and the normalcy of the findings.
		
		Explain to the family the importance of more frequent assessments when there are factors predisposing to hemorrhage.
		
		If factors predisposing to hemorrhage are present, continue intravenous fluids until stability of the bleeding is assured.
		
		Give oxytocin drugs as ordered. maintain administration of oxytocin longer than is routine if there is a history of factors predisposing to hemorrhage.
			If one or more predisposing factors are present, make assessments more often than routine. Hemorrhage is the leading mortality. Postdelivery hemorrhage is the most common and most serious type of excessive obstetric blood loss. Control of bleeding from the placental site is accomplished by prolonged contraction and retraction of interlacing strands of myometrium. Uterine contractions control bleeding by compressing and sealing off the blood vessels that enter the area left denuded by the placenta. Failure of the uterus to decrease progressively in size is an indication that involution is not proceeding satisfactorily. A firm or contracted uterus does not bleed after delivery.
			
			Families are more relaxed, cooperative, and follow through with care more when they are aware of the reasons for the care. The rate of the IV fluid that continues from the delivery is often a nursing judgment.
			
			Continued on following page

Nursing Care Plan 26–1. Ensuring Involution for the Postpartum Mother (Continued)

ASSESSMENT	POTENTIAL NURSING DIAGNOSIS	NURSING INTERVENTION	COMMENTS/RATIONALE

2. After the recovery room period and as long as the findings are within normal limits, assess the mother every 4 hours during the next 23 hours. After the first 24 hours make the assessments at the beginning of each shift every 8 hours.
a. Fundal check and massage if necessary
  1. Firmness
  2. Position—relationship to the midline and the umbilicus
b. Lochia
  1. Amount
  2. Color
  3. Consistency
c. Blood pressure
d. Pulse
e. Color—pale, flushed, etc.
f. General feeling of well-being
			Maintaining the IV longer would facilitate an open vein for medication (e.g., oxytocin) or blood.
			
			Lochia diminishes in amount and changes color daily (rubra, 1–3 days; serosa, 4–10 days; alba, 12th day to 3rd–6th week).
			
			The pulse rate falls a short time after delivery (range of 50–70 beats per minute) and bradycardia may persist for 6–8 weeks. Elevation of pulse rate indicates hemorrhage.
			
			Blood pressure should remain the same. A drop in blood pressure could indicate hemorrhage.

Assess for a full bladder if the fundus is elevated or displaced from the midline.	Possible displacement of uterus due to a full bladder	Have the patient void before palpating the fundus. When the fundus is elevated or displaced, question the frequency and amount of voiding. Compare uterine position and consistency before and after voiding if a problem is suspected. Keep a record of intake and output for the first 24 hours.	The uterus cannot contract and descend correctly when there is a full bladder. A newly delivered mother may not sense a full bladder. A full bladder typically pushes the fundus above the umbilicus and to the right side of the abdomen. There may be a full bladder that is spilling small amounts (50–100 ml.) of urine frequently (about every hour): retention with overflow. An intake and output record can help in estimating the amount of urine that should be voided.

Observe for the occurrence of "afterpains."	Possible afterpains due to 1. Multiparity 2. Suckling of the infant 3. Receiving oxytocin medication	Inform the family of the prevalence and the etiology of afterpains. Encourage the patient to lie flat on her abdomen as often as possible. Give analgesics as needed and 30 minutes prior to suckling the infant. Also may give analgesic with oxytocin medication if desired. Teach mother to massage fundus.	The uterine tone is maintained and involution occurs by contraction and retraction of the uterine muscles. During the first 12 hours after delivery, contractions are strong and regular. Thereafter, intensity, frequency, and regularity decrease. Afterpains occur for 2–3 days and are more prevalent in multiparas than in primiparas. Lying on the abdomen alleviates some of the discomfort of afterpains. An understanding of the etiology of the pain relieves the fear and therefore the tension and pain. The release of oxytocin from the posterior pituitary during the infant's suckling increases contractions of the uterus and gives rise to afterpains.
Determine amount of activity of the patient.	Possible poor muscle tone	Encourage erect posture while sitting and standing. Encourage a balance between ambulation and rest. Encourage and demonstrate postpartum exercises to the parents.	In addition to promoting involution and a speedy convalescence, postpartum exercises aid in the restoration of the mother's figure by retoning the muscles. Increased muscle tone and good posture assist the uterus and perineum in regaining tone and position.

Contributed by Hazel N. Brown.

and every 15 minutes during the first hour or until stable. It is usually best to take the vital signs at the time when the fundus and the amount of lochia flow are evaluated during the first few hours after delivery. This is done in such a manner that the mother will not be frequently disturbed, so that she can get more rest.

Some time in the first hours after childbirth, the mother is allowed to visit with her spouse or another significant family member of her choice. In some hospitals the father is allowed to stay with the mother in the recovery room. This practice should be encouraged, since the father is important in the childbearing experience.

Parents often want to be together in the immediate puerperium. This provides the couple with an opportunity to talk about the birth and about their baby. If the infant is not having any problems, he can also remain with the parents in the recovery room, at least for a short while, so that the parents can cuddle and explore their newborn. Affectional bonding of parents to the infant is facilitated by this early parent–infant interaction. The few minutes that parents spend with each other and with their infant immediately after delivery can become a precious memory that is recalled with warmth and joy.

The mother should have a bed bath prior to the time that she is transferred from the recovery area to her room. Many newly delivered puerperae find the bath refreshing. Mothers who have not been able to relax previously may then settle down and get some sleep after the excitement of the delivery.

Postpartum Physical Assessment and Related Patient Teaching

The mother's physical condition and the progress of involution are assessed daily while she is in the hospital. At the same time that the nurse is doing the postpartum physical assessment, she can teach the patient about involution and physical care. In addition, the nurse can help the mother feel that she is being included in the assessment by sharing her findings and discussing variations that are expected as the puerperium progresses. The approach to the postpartum physical assessment should follow a logical order, proceeding from the breasts downward. If the mother's bladder is full, it should be emptied prior to the initiation of the assessment. If the mother needs to void, her perineal pad should be checked before she uses the bathroom in order to observe her lochia flow.

The assessment is begun by taking the mother's vital signs. Temperature, pulse, respirations, and blood pressure are taken and recorded. If the temperature is elevated, along with a rapid pulse rate, the nurse should be particularly alert for signs of infection.

Breasts

The mother removes her bra so that the breasts can be easily inspected and palpated. The breasts are observed for contour, symmetry, color, fullness, firmness, venous distention, nodules, warmth, and secretion from the nipples. As the breasts are palpated, the mother is asked if there is breast tenderness or tingling. The firmness or fullness of the areola of the nursing mother is particularly noted, along with characteristics of the nipples. Nipple prominence is observed, and reddened, cracked, sore, or fissured nipples are noted. Full or firm breasts and the secretion of yellowish colostrum or bluish-white milk are characteristic in the lactating mother. Breasts that are bluish or darker in color (because of venous distention) and that are hard, tender, lumpy, and tingling are engorged. Proper treatment should be instituted immediately. Breasts that are red and hot may be indicative of breast infection, particularly if the mother's temperature is also elevated. In the nursing mother, fissured, sore, or cracked nipples must be treated promptly, and breast shields may need to be used at feeding time.

Several teaching opportunities are provided during the breast examination. These include discussing the process of milk production, the characteristics of colostrum and human milk, manual expression of milk, nipple care, breast self-examination, and the importance of adequate breast support. Of course, not all of these things will be covered at one time but can be taught during the several days before the mother returns home.

Back

The mother's back is checked for acute pain or tenderness. The presence of flank pain or pain in the area of the kidneys is also checked. Flank pain and deep tenderness are a sign of kidney infection. Mothers should be told about the importance of drinking adequate fluids daily.

Abdomen

The abdomen is observed for distention and diastasis. A large abdomen, with or without diastasis, indicates poor muscle tone. If diastasis is present, its width should be measured. Abdominal tightening exercises should be explained to the mother with poor abdominal muscle tone, and she should be encouraged to carry them out throughout the 6 weeks of the puerperium. One effective exercise is that of lying flat in bed and lifting the head to touch the chin to the chest for five times at least twice daily. If the mother places her hand on her abdomen while she does the exercise, she will be able to feel her abdominal muscles become more tense as she raises her head.

During the examination of the abdomen, the fundus of the uterus is checked for firmness, tenderness, and height in relation to the umbilicus. The presence of bowel sounds and of abdominal tenderness is also checked. If a cesarean delivery was performed, the dressing is checked for drainage. The inguinal lymph nodes are also checked for enlargement. When a woman has had a cesarean delivery, the nurse may have some difficulty palpating the fundus if a bulky dressing has been applied. However, she can gently palpate around it to determine the firmness and position of the uterus. Because some mothers complain of some abdominal tenderness on palpation around the incision, palpation should not be conducted with unnecessary pressure (see Nursing Care Plan 26–2).

Descent of the uterus is an indication of involution. The presence of bowel sounds is a sign of bowel functioning. Some mothers will have fundal tenderness, which is related to the intermittent contractions of the fundus during labor. However, this usually subsides in a few days. General abdominal tenderness is a sign of infection, particularly when accompanied by enlarged inguinal lymph nodes and an elevated temperature.

As the abdominal examination is performed, the patient can be taught what the fundus feels like and how to massage the fundus properly, without overstimulating it when it is not firm. Teaching should also include a discussion of the process of involution.

Suprapubic Area

The suprapubic area is examined for bladder fullness. The bladder should be empty if the mother voided prior to the initiation of the physical assessment. If the bladder is full, the mother should be encouraged to void. If the mother has difficulty voiding, special measures should be taken to stimulate urination (Chapter 25). Inability to empty the bladder spon-

taneously indicates that catheterization may be necessary. Since a full bladder interferes with accurate assessment of fundal height, the fundal height may need to be re-evaluated.

The amount and frequency of voidings, the odor of the urine, and whether pain, urgency, and burning occur on urination are also ascertained. Malodorous urine, urinary urgency and frequency, and pain and burning on micturition often occur with cystitis. However, the mother will normally excrete large volumes of urine during the first week of the puerperium. The mother should be taught about the normal diuresis that occurs in postpartum women and should also be told to void frequently, since she may have less of a sensation to void.

Vaginal and Perineal Area

With the mother lying on her back, the nurse inspects the vaginal area and lochial flow. She also checks the perineal pad to assess the type of lochial flow (rubra, serosa, or alba) and the odor of the lochia. The amount of flow can be estimated from the number of pads soaked in 1 hour. Asking the mother if her flow is heavier than, the same as, or less than a normal menstrual flow assists in estimating the amount of lochia. The presence of clots in the lochia should also be noted. Observation of the lochial flow can help determine if involution is progressing normally or if complications such as infection, hemorrhage, or retained placental fragments are present.

The mother can be told about changes in the appearance of the lochia, the proper application of perineal pads, and when she can expect the discharge to cease. She should be told not to use tampons while the lochia is flowing. The nurse should make sure that the mother has a clear understanding of the nature of the lochia flow. Some women may think that the lochia is a menstrual period if they do not understand its basis.

The perineal area is more easily inspected if the mother turns on her side with her top leg flexed forward. Use of a pocket flashlight makes visualization of the perineum and anal area easier. The perineum is observed for bruising, hematoma, swelling, and tenderness. If an episiotomy or laceration repair was done, the site should be inspected for healing. The anal area is inspected for hemorrhoids. Information regarding the amount of sphincter control can be provided by the mother. While examining the perineum, the nurse can discuss perineal care with the mother. Exercise for perineal tightening (repeatedly tightening the

Text continued on page 910

Nursing Care Plan 26–2. Caring for the Mother Following a Cesarean Birth

NURSING GOALS: To promote complete recovery following a cesarean birth.

OBJECTIVES: As a result of nursing actions:
1. Comfort is optimal.
2. The family understands the reasons for the cesarean birth and for the procedures used.
3. Mother is able to care for herself and infant.
4. Complications are prevented.

ASSESSMENT	POTENTIAL NURSING DIAGNOSIS	NURSING INTERVENTION	COMMENTS/RATIONALE
1. Determine the history of pain and pain intervention that occurred prior to admission to the postpartum unit.	Possible severe pain due to major surgical procedure and possibly complications (e.g., long difficult labor)	Give analgesics and narcotics as ordered and needed to keep patient comfortable.	The degree of remaining anesthesia will determine, in part, the time and amount of analgesia needed.
Review chart. Receive report from the labor and recovery nurse.		Schedule patient activity (e.g., turning, coughing, deep breathing, fundal check, and infant interaction) when the patient is comfortable—for instance, 30 minutes after receiving medication, instead of when needing medication.	If the patient had analgesia in the recovery room, she may be more comfortable on admission to the postpartum unit.
Determine the time and type of anesthesia and pain medication given.			A patient who has suffered more trauma, difficult labor, and emergency cesarean birth may require more analgesia and need more rest.
2. Assess the degree of discomfort and pain on admission to the postpartum unit.			The more comfortable the mother is, the more active she will be, turning, ambulating, and caring for herself and infant.
Assess the remaining level of anesthesia (e.g., fully awake from general anesthesia; full or partial numbness of abdomen and extremities following a saddle block or epidural).			
3. Assess the family's understanding of the reasons for the cesarean birth and for the procedures used.	Potential for fear, guilt, or anger because she had a cesarean instead of a vaginal birth, especially when the cesarean birth wasn't planned	Allow the parents to describe the events of and reasons for the cesarean birth as they understand them. Encourage them to ventilate feelings and emotions. Accept their feelings of joy and disappointment. Supply information when knowledge is lacking or when there is a misunderstanding of information.	Only by listening to the parents can the nurse determine their perception of the events surrounding the cesarean birth. Information can then be given to clarify events or correct misunderstandings.
4. Assess the mother's physical and emotional readiness for giving self- and infant care.	Potential for expecting the mother to do too much self- and infant care too soon in the postpartum period	During the first 24 hours postpartum, give almost total patient care.	Mothers are not capable of caring for their own or infant's needs during the first 24 hours postpartum.
		Organize care so that patient is comfortable when being moved.	When the mother is comfortable she will move more readily.
		Give complete bed bath.	

Turn, cough, and deep breathe, and give good perineal care every 4 hours.

Teach "huff" breathing; mother exhales forcibly. May be more comfortable than coughing. Mother should support incision with hands during coughing and "huffing" for comfort.

Encourage exercise while in bed (deep breath, arch ankles, wiggle toes, flex calves, reach one arm at a time across body). Leaving side rails up will help mother to turn herself.

Allow mother to view, hold, and cuddle infant.

Mother–infant attachment should begin immediately after delivery and continue throughout the postpartum period.

According to Rubin the mother is emotionally ready to "take hold" and begin learning to care for self and infant after the third postpartum day.

5. Identify discomfort related to gas pains.

Gas pains

Take advantage of the additional days of hospitalization (cesarean birth, usually 5 days; vaginal birth, usually 3 days) for giving experience with and teaching about self- and infant care.

Help reduce the severity of gas pains through early ambulation.

Assist mother in coping by encouraging the following:

1. Lie on left side with knees drawn up against chest.
2. Massage upper abdomen from right to left.
3. Practice abdominal breathing.
4. Ambulation.
5. Avoid carbonated beverages and apple juice until gas pains no longer a problem.

Gas pains usually occur at approximately 3 days, the time when bowel function begins to return.

6. Identify discomfort during feeding.

Discomfort during infant feeding related to cesarean delivery

Help mother find comfortable position.

1. Football hold so that baby's feet are directed away from abdomen.
2. Side-lying position (help her to turn, leave side rails up for help in turning).
3. With head of bed elevated and a pillow in her lap to support baby and protect incision.

These positions are helpful for both breast- and bottle-feeding.

Continued on following page

Nursing Care Plan 26–2. Caring for the Mother Following a Cesarean Birth (Continued)

ASSESSMENT	POTENTIAL NURSING DIAGNOSIS	NURSING INTERVENTION	COMMENTS/RATIONALE
7. Assess history of any problem or potential problem. a. Emotional b. Uplanned cesarean delivery c. Hemorrhage d. Hypertension e. Obesity (1) Mobility (2) Phlebitis Review chart for prenatal and intrapartal factors predisposing to complications (e.g., complicated labor, hypertension, hemorrhage, infant morbidity or mortality).	Possibility of complications is greater with a patient who has had a cesarean birth than with a patient who has had a vaginal birth.	Constant surveillance of normalcy and impending complications. Encourage parents to discuss the pregnancy, delivery, and the infant.	Complications are easier to prevent than treat. A good history and constant assessment, combined with preventive care, assist in preventing complications. Verbalization assists parents in clarifying events and resolving negative feelings.
8. Assess progress of involution of the uterus (See Nursing Care Plan 26–1).		Palpate the fundus every 4 hours, then once each day.	The fundus is usually located below the level of the umbilicus immediately after delivery. About 12 hours after delivery the fundus is likely to be palpated a little above the umbilicus. Thereafter, the fundus descends about one fingerbreath per day. By the 10th to 12th day the uterus is not palpable through the abdominal wall. Failure of the uterus to descend in this way combined with more profuse and red lochia indicates subinvolution, possibly inadequate healing, infection, or retained placental fragments.

9. Assess lochia by observing for a change in the color, amount, or odor of lochia that deviates from normal:
   1. Lochia rubra—first 3 days
   2. Lochia serosa—day 4 to day 14
   3. Lochia alba—day 15 to third or sixth week.

Lochia is heavy immediately after delivery—saturates 2–4 perineal pads. After 8 hours lochia is similar in amount to regular menstrual flow. Lochia in a patient with cesarean delivery may be less than with vaginal delivery.

Foul odor of lochia indicates endometritis.

10. Assess for symptoms of PIH if there is a history of it, or if any one symptom of PIH has been evident.
    a. Blood pressure
    b. Edema
    c. Proteinuria
    d. Deep tendon reflexes
    e. Weight

The first 12 hours postpartum are critical for the assessment of PIH, especially when there have been previous symptoms.

11. Assess postoperative recovery related to respiratory and circulatory systems.
    a. Blood pressure
    b. Pulse
    c. Heart sounds
    d. Respirations
    e. Lung sounds
    f. Symptoms of thrombophlebitis

Turn, cough, deep breathe every 4 hours during the first 24 hours. Ambulate beginning the first postpartum day. Larger women tend to need more encouragement to ambulate.

Turning, coughing, deep breathing, and ambulation are vital for all postpartum patients, and are more important for patients with cesarean births to increase circulation and to prevent lung congestion and thrombophlebitis.

12. Assess plans and ability to perform for self- and infant care following hospital discharge.

Need for information about care following discharge

Encourage woman to resume activities slowly following discharge.

Demonstrate lifting baby and other objects by bending at the knees.

Postpartum exercises deferred for 3–4 weeks.

Encourage mother to plan for some help at home at least part of the day, particularly if there are young siblings (husband, extended family, neighbor, etc.).

Contributed by Hazel N Brown.

Nursing Care Plan 26–3. Providing Rest for the Postpartum Mother

NURSING GOALS: To help the mother to be comfortable and rested to enable her to enjoy learning how to care for herself and her infant.

OBJECTIVES: As a result of nursing actions:

1. Rest is optimal.
2. Time that the family is together is pleasant and meaningful.
3. Parents understand the importance of the mother's rest to her physical and emotional health and to successful parent–infant attachment.
4. At the time of discharge, the parents feel confident about their ability to provide for the mother's and infant's care.

ASSESSMENT	POTENTIAL NURSING DIAGNOSIS	NURSING INTERVENTION	COMMENTS/RATIONALE
1. Identify factors from mother's prenatal and labor history relevant to rest needs—e.g.: a. Type of analgesia and anesthesia b. Length of labor c. Type and difficulty of delivery d. Condition of infant	Possible exhaustion due to, e.g., long labor, difficult delivery, complication of self or infant	Establish a restful environment. 1. Establish with the family a routine for assessing physical recovery based on patient's condition and need for rest. 2. Allow for several hours (4, possibly followed by 4 more after physical assessments are made) of sleep after mother returns to her room from recovery room. 3. Allow 1 or 2 hours of uninterrupted rest during day hours. Allow minimum of 4-hour rest periods at night. 4. Give medication for discomfort, rest, or sleep as needed. Coordinate the giving of medications with other activity to allow for rest. 5. Listen to the patient to determine her anxieties and concerns. 6. Intersperse appropriate activity with rest.	Sleep and rest are necessary during the taking-in phase (first 2–3 days) of the puerperium. With inadequate rest and sleep the mother becomes irritable and tired. A combination of rest and activity is necessary for proper body functioning (circulation, elimination, lactation, etc.). Breast-feeding mothers should avoid sleep medications.

2.	Interview family to identify ethnic or cultural variations and nursing care desired in relation to rest needs.	At risk for misinterpretation of what "should or should not" constitute good postpartum care for the mother and infant	Develop with the family a plan of care, emphasizing adequate rest periods. 1. Give the family the rationale of the care needed, both now and during the next 6 weeks. 2. Consider the family's customs and beliefs in developing the plan of care.	It's easier and more meaningful to adapt a plan of care to one's cultural needs than to try to change one's cultural beliefs. Mother and infant care will be implemented only if it is in agreement with one's cultural beliefs.
3.	Determine parents' emotional status and extent of skill in self-care and infant care while carrying out other assessments and during teaching and counseling.	At risk for parent–infant attachment problems and/or inadequate learning of self-care and infant care due to emotional problems	Begin the plan of care based upon the parents' emotional status and present knowledge of and ability to perform self- and infant care. 1. Ask open-ended questions about the family, support systems, pregnancy, labor, birth, impressions, expectations, etc. 2. Give most of the physical care during the 1st 24 hours and assist with physical care during the next 24 hours.	Important to determine what the parents want and need to know. Knowledge is best received and retained when it's wanted and needed, and when it builds upon present knowledge. Dependence and passivity are characteristic of the mother during the taking-in phase (first 2–3 days). She requires help from the nurse while she is learning to meet her own puerperal needs before she can sufficiently reach out beyond herself.
4.	Determine the proper relationship of the parent–infant attachment needs of the family and the rest needs of the mother.	At risk for fatigue due to infant being constantly in the room with parents (rooming-in)	Arrange with the family and nursery personnel to have infant with parents when parents are rested and comfortable and wish to feed, care for, or enjoy their infant. 1. Have father assist in infant care. 2. Have infant taken back to nursery when mother needs to rest.	Contact and interaction between parent and child are essential parts of parenting. Contact is vital for attachment to evolve. A good parent–infant relationship is necessary to ensure that the child's needs will be met and that his development will be optimally facilitated. A balance between relaxed purposeful interaction of parents and infant with adequate rest, sleep, and care of self is critical.

Contributed by Hazel N. Brown.

perineal muscles as if stopping the flow of urine) should be encouraged.

Lower Extremities

The lower extremities are examined for edema, varicosities, symmetry, size, shape, temperature, and color. Range of motion is observed. Check to see if the mother experiences pain in her calf when her foot is flexed while her leg is extended flat on the bed (Homans' sign). If pain is experienced, this is a sign of possible thrombophlebitis.

The pulses of the lower extremities (femoral, popliteal, posterior tibial, and dorsalis pedis) are checked to determine if they are palpable. Fever, swelling, and absence of one or more of the pulses in an extremity are also signs of thrombophlebitis. The mother should be taught the signs of thrombophlebitis, since the condition usually occurs after she returns home rather than in the early days of the postpartum period. Advise the mother against leg massage and the use of constricting garters and other clothing that interferes with circulation.

Physiologic Changes

The nursing care related to the specific normal physiologic changes of the puerperium was discussed in Chapter 25.

Other Considerations

Rest and Sleep during the Puerperium

The postpartum mother needs adequate rest during the puerperium. While she is in the hospital, the mother's environment should be as conducive to rest as possible, and she should get adequate periods of uninterrupted sleep. The new mother is usually tired after labor and delivery and needs several hours of sleep. Without them, the mother may feel tired and fatigued for several days and feel that she just cannot get enough sleep. The nurse may have to vary hospital routines in order for the mother to get adequate periods of sleep (Nursing Care Plan 26–3).

The mother needs to be comfortable and relaxed after delivery. Anxiety, tension, and worry can interfere with her ability to rest. Her mate and other significant family members need to be made aware of her need for relaxation and rest. If the mother becomes overly exhausted from frequent visitors both they and the length of their stay may have to be limited.

The mother should be told about her contin-ued need for rest after she returns home. Some mothers may try to take care of a new infant along with carrying out all of their former household tasks. This will be too much for them to do. The mother should not expect to keep a thoroughly cleaned house when she has the responsibility of caring for a newborn. We must help the mother accept the idea that she will have to limit her activity at home during the puerperium. Having someone assist her during the first week or two after she returns home is beneficial. Some husbands may be willing to stay home and help their wives for a few days after they return home. It is especially important that breast-feeding mothers get adequate rest and sleep, since fatigue can adversely affect the secretion of breast milk and interfere with the let-down reflex (page 923).

Ambulation

At one time the newly delivered mother was confined to bed from 1 to 2 weeks after delivery. However, early ambulation (within the first 4 to 8 hours after childbirth) has been found to be the most advantageous practice. When the mother is allowed to ambulate early, her circulation is increased and her bowel and bladder function is stimulated. Hence, early ambulation should be encouraged to prevent thrombophlebitis, constipation, and urinary retention.

Most mothers will be able to ambulate within 4 to 8 hours after parturition. Women who have had spinal anesthesia, however, should be kept in a recumbent position for 8 to 12 hours postdelivery. Most physicians believe that spinal headaches occur because spinal fluid leakage through the puncture site in the dura causes a decrease in cerebrospinal fluid and pressure. Cerebrospinal fluid leakage is precipitated and spinal headache is more likely to occur when the head is elevated prior to the time that the puncture site seals.

A new mother may be weak and may easily become faint during the first few hours after giving birth. For this reason, the mother should begin to ambulate slowly. Rapid elevation of the head with rapid ambulation should be avoided to discourage fainting. The patient should first sit upright and "dangle" for a few minutes before she attempts to walk. Then she can be allowed to stand and walk for a short distance near the bed. If she feels faint, she can quickly be returned to bed.

After the mother has successfully ambulated for short distances, gradually longer excursions can be taken. The nurse should remain close by when the mother initially ambulates until she safely returns to bed. Standing for long periods of time should be discouraged at first, until the patient is strong enough to ambulate safely. The nurse should remain close by when the mother goes to the bathroom or showers during the first day after delivery, in case she becomes dizzy or faint.

Prior to ambulating for the first time, the mother should be told to call someone before getting up. Some mothers will try not to "burden" the nurse by attempting to get up for the first time alone. Others may feel that they are strong enough not to require assistance. We should explain to these women why it is necessary to have assistance when ambulating initially. On the other hand, some mothers may want to stay in bed rather than ambulate. The advantages of early ambulation should be discussed with these women, and they should be encouraged to get out of bed. When a mother ambulates for the first time, her reactions (whether she becomes dizzy or faint or whether she ambulates successfully) should be recorded.

Diet

The mother may begin to eat almost immediately after delivery unless she is nauseated or has received general anesthesia. Most mothers are hungry and ready to eat at this time.

The diet for the mother who is bottle-feeding her infant should be the same as that recommended for the average nonpregnant woman of her size and body build. The diet should be well-rounded, with adequate amounts of protein, iron, calcium, calories, and vitamins. Foods from the four basic food groups should be included in sufficient amounts.

The lactating mother has additional nutritional requirements. (See also Chapter 12.) Approximately 700 additional calories are needed to provide for milk production and for the calories contained in the milk. The amounts of some other nutrients required, such as calcium, iron, thiamine, ascorbic acid, and vitamin D, are similar to those needed during pregnancy. The lactating mother will need about 10 less grams of protein than she required during pregnancy. She will need about 1000 international units of additional vitamin A above the amount that she needed during pregnancy. More riboflavin and niacin are also necessary.

Since the average daily output of milk is 850 ml., a large volume of fluid intake is necessary to ensure adequate milk production. The recommended fluid intake for the lactating mother is between 2500 and 3000 ml. per day under usual circumstances. With increased physical activity and increased activity of the sweat glands, even more fluids may be necessary.

We must be sure that the breast-feeding mother is aware of how her present diet differs from her diet during pregnancy. Nursing mothers should also know that certain foods that they may eat can have adverse effects on their infant. Excessive amounts of chocolate or any food to which the infant is allergic can cause skin rash in the newborn. Foods that cause discomfort in the infant should be decreased or deleted from the mother's diet.

Postpartum Exercises

As with early ambulation, postpartum exercises can do much to prevent complications and speed the recovery of the muscles that were overstretched during pregnancy. In addition to promoting involution and a speedy convalescence, postpartum exercises aid in the restoration of the mother's figure by retoning the muscles (see Nursing Care Plan 26–4).

These exercises can be initiated on the first postpartum day. The mother should not overexercise initially. Exercises should be introduced gradually, as the puerperium progresses. As illustrated in Figure 26–1, a new exercise should be added during each succeeding day of the puerperium. Each exercise should be done four times in the morning and evening for at least the 6 weeks of the postpartum period.

Care of the Nursing Mother

The parents' decision to breast-feed or not to breast-feed their infant is affected by a wide variety of interrelated psychologic, social, and physical factors. With proper support and guidance during the antepartum period, the couple should have arrived at a decision regarding the method of infant feeding prior to delivery.

Because of modern technology and scientific knowledge, breast-feeding is not necessary for infant welfare. Adequate nutrition for infant growth can be provided by artificial means as well as by breast-feeding. Therefore, the decision whether to breast-feed or not can more readily be made by the parents, based on their own attitudes and personal situation, without fear of "short changing" the infant.

Health-care personnel, particularly nurses who work with parents, have a definite bearing on breast-feeding behavior. The nurse can influence parents in their decision to breast-feed by her actions, which imply negative or posi-

Text continued on page 916

Nursing Care Plan 26–4. Meeting the Learning Needs of the Postpartum Mother and Her Family for Self-Care

NURSING GOALS: To define, with the family, each mother's learning needs.
To assist the family in meeting learning needs.

OBJECTIVES: As a result of nursing actions:
1. A complete assessment of learning needs is made.
2. Learning readiness of the family is determined.
3. Learning needs of the family are met.
4. Evaluation of the family's learning is done.

ASSESSMENT	POTENTIAL NURSING DIAGNOSIS	NURSING INTERVENTION	COMMENTS/RATIONALE
1. Assess learning needs by reviewing the prenatal and intrapartum record, noting potential learning needs (e.g., dietary—too little or too much weight gain, low hemoglobin; understanding of pregnancy, labor, and delivery; self-care), previous children, attendance at preparation for childbirth classes, and contraceptive needs (previous spacing of pregnancies and contraceptive use).	Possibility of not identifying the family's learning needs due to inadequate review of history, inadequate direction of conversation with the parents, not listening to the parents	Teaching should be directly related to the identified needs of the family. Parents should have expressed a desire or need for knowledge, or have been convinced that knowledge of and compliance with something is necessary for the mother's health. In discussion with parents, use phrases like "tell me about" (e.g., how you will do perineal care at home).	When patients identify a learning need, they are then motivated to meet that need through acquiring information and skill. Too often the needs identified are those that the nurse assumes the family needs and wants to know more about.
Assess, through listening to the parents discuss the pregnancy, labor, and delivery, their parenting skills and their individual needs.		Assessment and teaching should begin with the first contact with the family and continue with each contact (e.g., when checking the breast for engorgement, tenderness, and condition of the nipples). Explain what is being done, why, when to expect engorgement, what can and will be done about it, and the present status of her breasts and nipples.	Open-ended statements elicit more information, thoughts, and feelings. Assessment and teaching are more meaningful when related to patient care.
		In addition to assessment and teaching during the giving of nursing care, plan 20- to 30-minute sessions to sit and talk with the parents about their learning needs.	Longer periods of time to sit with the parents establish rapport and elicit pertinent information.

2. Determine the readiness of the parents to learn based upon their physical well-being (comfort, rest); emotional well-being (relaxed, not upset about self, infant, or family); and Rubin's phases of puerperal adjustment.

Lack of readiness for learning

Care for the patients physical needs (discomfort, pain, inability to void, etc.), and their emotional needs (concern about themselves or infant's well-being) before addressing the learning needs.

Review postpartum teaching during a readiness period in the third postpartum day or later.

In the hierarchy of needs, physical and emotional needs must be met before a person is receptive to meeting learning needs.

Patients who have had a vaginal birth tend to be discharged on the 3rd postpartum day; patients who have had a cesarean birth tend to be discharged about the 5th postpartum day. In the first 2–3 days after delivery the mother is in the "taking-in" phase, characterized by dependence and passivity. The mother generally arrives at the "taking-hold" phase about the 3rd postpartum day. This phase is characterized by increasing independence and autonomy; she becomes the initiator and producer of self- and infant care. The areas and degree of concern of mothers during the puerperium are listed in order under Assessment. Mothers are concerned about infant care and behavior, but their chief concerns are about themselves.[20]

3. Assess the learning needs for:
   a. Exercise—return of figure to normal
   b. Adjusting to new role of parent
   c. Rest
   d. Emotional health—tension, time for self, feeling of being tied down
   e. Sexual relations
   f. Contraception
   g. Perineal care
   h. Breast care
   i. Constipation
   j. General activity: exercise, work, travel

Need for information about (specific area)

Exercise: begin exercises on the first postpartum day (head raises) and progress according to written directions. The patient shouldn't tire from exercises.

Adjusting to role of parent: Discuss with both parents how they can regulate the demands of the spouse, children, housework, and job, for optimal satisfaction for the whole family.

Rest: See Nursing Care Plan 26–2.

Emotional health: Discuss with parents the importance of rest, diversion (eating out, movie, etc.), good communication, and the authenticity of postpartum blues.

Continued on following page

Nursing Care Plan 26–4. Meeting the Learning Needs of the Postpartum Mother and Her Family for Self-Care (Continued)

ASSESSMENT	POTENTIAL NURSING DIAGNOSIS	NURSING INTERVENTION	COMMENTS/RATIONALE
		Sexual relations: Give information that coincides with physician information. Typical information includes: (1) resuming sexual intercourse after the cessation of lochia and when the mother is comfortable, (2) use of contraception, (3) if breast-feeding, possible dryness of vagina and expression of breast milk during climax.	
		Perineal care: Daily shower or sponge bath. Clean perineum from front to back with separate, clean washcloth. Change perineal pad 4–6 times a day (minimum) and observe for normal lochia changes.	
		Report immediately any foul odor of lochia (see Nursing Care Plan 27–2).	Foul odor indicates possible endometritis.
		Report immediately any sudden bright vaginal bleeding (see Nursing Care Plan 27–1).	Late postpartum hemorrhage is typically due to fatigue or retained placental fragments.
		Breast care: Patient should wear a good supporting bra at all times (except during sleep). Daily bathing of the breast with plain water is sufficient. For engorgement or sore nipples, see Nursing Care Plan 26–5.	Soap or other astringents aren't necessary for cleanliness and may cause dryness and cracking of nipples.

Constipation: Prevention of constipation is important. Eat foods with roughage, drink plenty of fluids, and respond promptly to defecation stimuli. Consult physician for stool softener or laxative.

Following the trauma of delivery there is lessened sensation of the urge to defecate.

General activity: Activity should be gauged according to the mother's feeling of well-being. A combination of rest and physical activity (walking, bicycling, tennis, etc.) is important. Work may typically be resumed 6 weeks after delivery, depending on how the mother feels, what she needs and desires to do, and the type of work. Travel that is not too tiring is acceptable.

The mother's general feeling of well-being is the best indicator of the proper activity.

4. Determine how well the parents have learned the appropriate care of the mother.

Parents have possibly not understood care of the mother until they have actually done self-care.

Have the mother return demonstrations of self-care and perform self-care as much as possible before discharge.

Performing a task or procedure is the best way to learn how to do it.

Give written instructions when possible and pictures (e.g., of exercises and contraceptives).

When something is in writing, especially accompanied by pictures or diagrams, it is easier to understand, and the literature serves as a reminder to do the task.

Encourage the parents to come in for the scheduled postpartum check-up. Evaluate mother's self-care at the time of check-up. Continue with teaching and clarify any questions. Topics that continue to need discussion at the time of check-up are:
1. Balance of rest and exercise
2. Figure
3. Sexuality
4. Contraception

Check-ups are a vital part of maternity care. Further assessment and teaching of learning needs should be done at that time.

Contributed by Hazel N. Brown

10 Exercises after Pregnancy

Worried about your appearance? Your problem is largely temporary—if you avoid excessive weight-gain, wear an expertly fitted bra, even during sleep, and start these re-toning exercises before you leave the hospital. Add a new exercise each day. Do each one 4 times, twice each day, morning and evening, for a month or more.

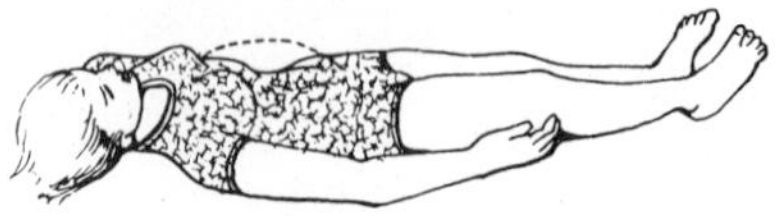

1st Day: Breathe deeply, expanding your abdomen. Hiss as you slowly exhale, then forcibly draw in your abdominal muscles.

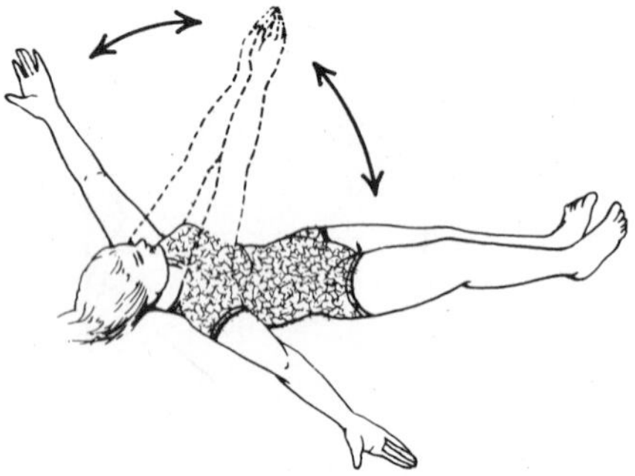

2nd Day: Lying on your back with your legs slightly parted, place your arms at right angles to your body and slowly raise them, keeping your elbows stiff. When your hands touch, lower your arms gradually.

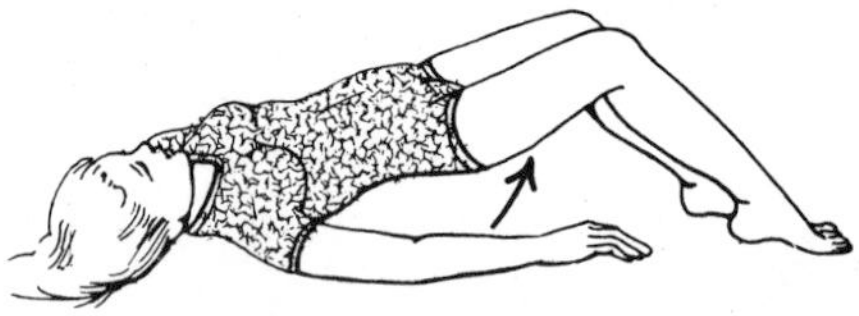

3rd Day: Lying with your arms at your sides, draw your knees up slightly, arch your back.

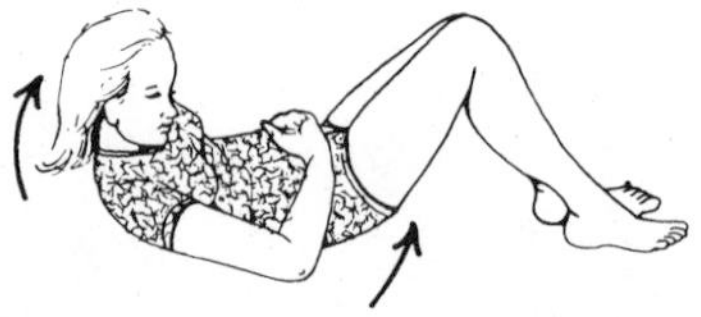

4th Day: Lying with your knees and hips flexed, tilt your pelvis inward and tightly contract your buttocks as you lift your head.

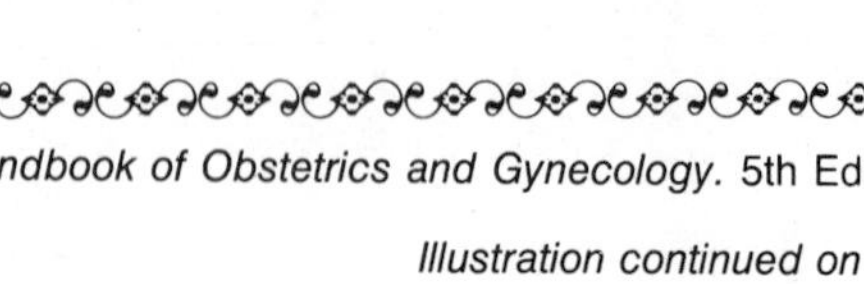

5th Day: Lying with your legs straight, raise your head and left knee slightly, then reach for (but do not touch) your left knee with your right hand. Repeat, using your right knee and left hand.

Figure 26–1.   Postpartum exercises. (From Benson, R.: *Handbook of Obstetrics and Gynecology*. 5th Edition. Los Altos, CA, Lange Medical Publishers, 1974.)

Illustration continued on opposite page

tive attitudes. She must remember that whatever decision is made by the parents regarding the method of infant feeding must be accepted and respected. Thus, the nurse should not pressure parents to make a decision for or against breast-feeding. However, she should be able to provide parents with information that they may need in order to make their own decision about which method is best for them.

Once the parents decide to breast-feed, their success will be greatly influenced by the quality of guidance and care provided by the nurse who works with them. Breast-feeding is not a totally instinctive behavior in humans. Therefore, the parents will need much assistance from the nurse (see Nursing Care Plan 26–5). The successful establishment of lactation is largely determined by the care and assistance that the mother receives during the first few postpartum days.

An environment conducive to breast-feeding must be established. In a favorable environ-

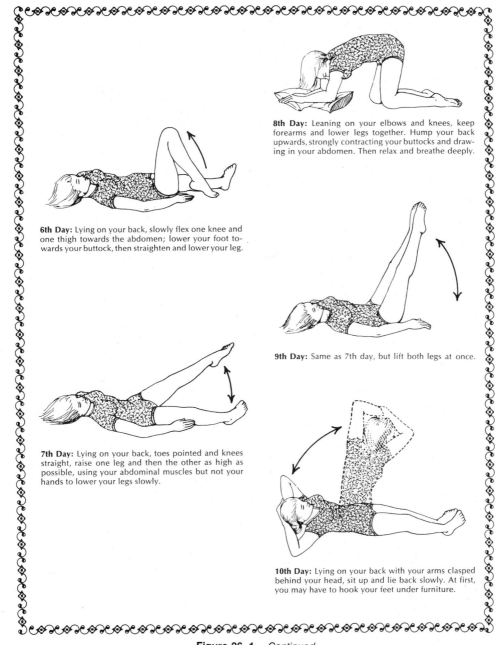

8th Day: Leaning on your elbows and knees, keep forearms and lower legs together. Hump your back upwards, strongly contracting your buttocks and drawing in your abdomen. Then relax and breathe deeply.

6th Day: Lying on your back, slowly flex one knee and one thigh towards the abdomen; lower your foot towards your buttock, then straighten and lower your leg.

9th Day: Same as 7th day, but lift both legs at once.

7th Day: Lying on your back, toes pointed and knees straight, raise one leg and then the other as high as possible, using your abdominal muscles but not your hands to lower your legs slowly.

10th Day: Lying on your back with your arms clasped behind your head, sit up and lie back slowly. At first, you may have to hook your feet under furniture.

Figure 26–1. *Continued*

ment, the mother who is insecure or ambivalent about her ability to nurse her baby may be helped to become highly successful in breast-feeding (Fig. 26–2). Under adverse circumstances, even the mother who is confident and enthusiastic about breast-feeding may become discouraged. Therefore, comfortable physical surroundings and a positive emotional climate are necessary.

All too frequently, hospital routines interfere with the mother's attempt to breast-feed her infant. Often these routines have been established for the convenience of health-care personnel rather than for the benefit of the parents. To provide the best opportunity possible for the nursing mother, we should consider whether established routines interfere with optimum care and whether these routines can be altered.

The Initiation of Breast-feeding

Breast-feeding should start as soon after delivery as possible, even though milk may
Text continued on page 923

Nursing Care Plan 26–5. Helping the Breast-Feeding Mother

NURSING GOALS: To provide the mother who chooses to breast-feed her infant with the knowledge and skills necessary to do it successfully.

OBJECTIVES:
1. Identify prior breast-feeding experience and prenatal preparation.
2. Identify mother's support system and suggest additional resources for support.
3. Assist the mother during breast-feeding.
4. Provide information about breast-feeding, including the prevention and treatment of common complications and about maternal nutrition during lactation.

ASSESSMENT	POTENTIAL NURSING DIAGNOSIS	NURSING INTERVENTION	COMMENTS/RATIONALE
1. Prior experience in breast-feeding a. Successfully breast-fed another child b. Attempted to breast-feed another child but was unsuccessful c. Mother herself and her siblings were breast-fed as infants d. Mother's peers have successfully breast-fed	Lack of experience in breast-feeding Lack of success in previous breast-feeding experience	Provide maximum support during early breast-feeding experiences when mother has had no prior experience or prior experience has been negative.	
2. Support of breast-feeding by infant's father, other family members, and friends	Lack of support for breast-feeding	Encourage mother to discuss with husband and family her desire to breast-feed. Provide information about additional sources of support in community.	Lack of support is a major barrier to *successful* breast-feeding. Support is important for adequate rest, feelings of confidence.
3. Prenatal preparation a. Assess information provided as to: (1) Content (2) Source b. Preparation techniques utilized: (1) Toughening nipples (2) Breast massage (3) Nipple rolling (4) Avoidance of drying substances (5) Specific problem identified and corrected (e.g., inverted nipples)	Lack of prenatal preparation		See Nursing Care Plan 12–2 for discussion of prenatal preparation.

Assessment	Nursing Diagnosis	Nursing Interventions	Rationale

4. Intrapartum history
  a. Complications of labor
  b. Complications of birth
	Mother at risk of fatigue from complications of labor or birth (cite specific complication)		

5. Initial breast-feeding
  a. Location
    (1) In birthing or delivery room
    (2) in recovery room
	Need for assistance in breast-feeding	Early breast-feeding with mother lying on her side, a pillow at her back for support. Plan other care to provide some periods of uninterrupted rest.
		
		Explain the benefits of first feeding (colostrum, stimulation of milk production, uterine contraction). Help mother assume comfortable position, relax (demonstrate rooting reflex; use relaxation techniques as in labor).
			For first feeding
			1. Mother should be side-lying or
			2. Head of bed should be elevated, pillow to support mother's arm as she cradles baby.
			
			Baby should not be on his back (makes swallowing difficult).
			
			Many infants do not suck well at initial feedings; explain to parents that this is perfectly normal.

b. Outcome
    (1) Mother's actions, comments
    (2) Infant's actions (infant must compress areola between tongue and palate); assess tongue action
    (3) Father's or companion's comments
    (4) Subsequent feedings
		Compress nipple and areola between two fingers prior to inserting it into infant's mouth.
		
		Allow infant to find nipple.
		
		Ensure that areola is in infant's mouth.
		
		Limit initial feeding to 3 to 5 minutes for each breast.
		
		Show mother how to break suction with finger before removing infant from breast.
		
		Demonstrate positions for burping.
		
		Allow infant to breast-feed as frequently as he desires but at least every 4 hours.
		
		Feeding time:
		Day 1: Five minutes for each breast each feeding. Alternate starting breast.
		
		Days 2–7: Increase gradually to 15–20 minutes for each breast each feeding.
			Rooming-in facilitates breast-feeding: mother knows when infant is hungry; infant can feed with minimal delay.
			
			Most breast-fed babies will nurse every 2–3 hours in first days or 6 to 12 feedings every 24 hours.
			
			To determine intervals, count from beginning of one feeding to beginning of next.
			
			By day 7 infant must nurse 15–20 minutes at each breast in order to get its hind milk, with its higher butterfat content.

c. Maternal nutrition
  (1) Food intake on "typical day"
  (2) Identify areas of need
  (3) Identify food preferences
	Need for information related to breast-feeding and nutrition	Maternal nutrition during lactation
		1. Calories should be increased by 500 per day above basic requirements.
		2. Protein should be increased by 20 grams per day.
			These requirements should be translated into maternal food preferences (e.g., peanut butter sandwich [2 tbsp peanut butter] and 1 cup whole milk will provide 500 calories and 21.5 grams protein).

Continued on following page

Nursing Care Plan 26–5. Helping the Breast-Feeding Mother *(Continued)*

ASSESSMENT	POTENTIAL NURSING DIAGNOSIS	NURSING INTERVENTION	COMMENTS/RATIONALE
		3. Calcium should be increased by milk intake (by amount of milk provided infant) or by calcium supplementation. 4. Vitamins should be increased 50 per cent above basic requirements.	Continuance of prenatal vitamin supplementation during lactation is frequently recommended.
		If food eaten by mother appears to bother infant, discontinue it. Babies are highly individual in reactions to maternal diet.	
d. Medications (1) Assess medications used by mother on a continuing basis.	Need for information related to maternal medications and breast-feeding	Explain that medications should be approved by health-care provider who knows mother is breast-feeding. Mother should consult provider before taking nonprescription medications.	
		Oral contraceptives are usually omitted in first weeks; then oral contraceptives with low estrogen content are used.	
(2) Need for supplementation for infant (3) Decreased number of wet diapers (less than 1 per feeding) (4) Inadequate weight gain (less than half an ounce a day averaged over 2–3 weeks)	Posible need to supplement breast-feeding related to (specific factor)	Supplementation is usually unnecessary. Suggest longer and more frequent feedings.	Hindmilk, obtained after first 15 minutes, has higher caloric content.
		If baby is fussy, allow to nurse rather than provide supplement. Observe breast-feeding technique.	More frequent nursing enhances milk supply.
6. Discomforts and complications a. Sore nipples (observe breast-feeding carefully to identify practices that may lead to sore nipples)	Sore nipples related to (specific cause if one can be identified)	*Prevention* 1. Support baby's head with pillows during feeding; if baby thinks head is falling he bites nipple reflexively.	Most mothers have sore nipples to some extent; soreness is worst at about 3–5 days (approximately the time of hospital discharge).

2. Place as much of areola as possible in baby's mouth.

3. Don't allow infant to "chew" nipple.

4. Break suction before removing baby from breast.

5. Allow nipples to air dry after each feeding.

6. Prevent or relieve breast engorgement (see below), which aggravates sore nipples by preventing proper grasp of areola and stretching skin around nipple.

7. Feed baby in a variety of positions to avoid constant pressure on one area.

8. Avoid use of soap, alcohol, breast creams with perfume. Use of spray deodorant and hair spray with nipples uncovered can cause sore nipples.

9. Bras should be washed before being worn the first time. Old cotton handkerchiefs inside bras are soft and absorb excess moisture.

Treatment

1. All of the measures described above are used to treat sore nipples.

2. Let infant feed first at breast that is least sore for 2 days.

3. Warm tea bags held against nipples for 30 minutes after feeding, vitamin E from a gelatin capsule, pure lanolin are helpful substances. Avoid substances that must be washed off, since these cause additional chafing.

4. In instances of severe discomfort nipple shield may be used for brief period.

Sore nipples can inhibit let-down by causing tension in mother.

Infants suck most vigorously when they are most hungry, i.e., at the beginning of each feeding.

Vitamin E and lanolin should be tested on mother's arm for skin sensitivity a day prior to using on mother's breast.

Limiting breast-feeding does not resolve the problem of sore nipples.

Continued on following page

Nursing Care Plan 26–5. Helping the Breast-Feeding Mother (Continued)

ASSESSMENT	POTENTIAL NURSING DIAGNOSIS	NURSING INTERVENTION	COMMENTS/RATIONALE
(1) Check infant for monilia infection (oral or diaper area). (2) Check mother for vaginal monilial infection.	Sore nipples related to monilial infection	Mycostatin can be applied to nipple area.	

b. Breast engorgement (swelling of breast tissue with blood and lymph)
 (1) Nipples may be flat against engorged breast.
 (2) Breasts may be hot and painful.
 (3) Maternal systemic fever
	Breast engorgement	*Prevention*
		 Empty breast frequently, at least every 3–4 hours.
		
		 Treatment
		 1. Empty breasts frequently, at least every 2–3 hours.
		 2. Hand express small amount of milk from engorged breast prior to feeding so that baby can grasp areola and will not chew on nipple.
		 3. If mother smokes, avoid smoking 15–30 minutes prior to and during feeding.
		 4. Comfort measures
		   a. Warm shower on shoulders
		   b. Immerse breasts in warm water (bend over sink) and massage.
		   c. Ice packs for congestion
			When breasts are emptied less frequently, colostrum or milk accumulates, and the resulting pressure impairs circulation and hormonal action and inhibits let-down.
			
			 Pain from nipple inhibits let-down; let-down essential for good milk flow.
			
			 Narcotics inhibit let-down.
			
			 Shower may be painful on engorged breasts but can cause release of milk.
			 With methods described engorgement can usually be controlled in 12 hours.

c. Mastitis (see Nursing Care Plan 27–2)			

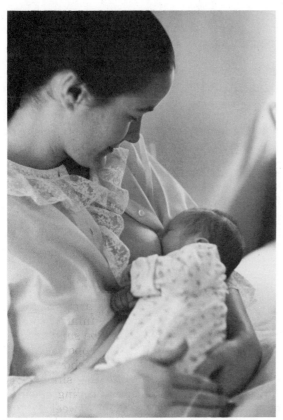

Figure 26–2. In a favorable environment, mothers are able to have highly successful breast-feeding experiences. (Photograph courtesy of Suzanne Szasz.)

not "come in" until about the third day postpartum. The infant will receive adequate nutrients from colostrum until milk is produced, as colostrum contains more protein and minerals, but less fat and sugar, than mature breast milk and is a substantial nutritional source for the infant initially.

The recommended time interval between delivery and the initiation of breast-feeding will vary according to the condition and readiness of the infant and mother and the recommendations of the pediatrician and obstetrician. Breast-feeding may begin within a few minutes after the baby's birth or as late as 12 hours following delivery.[54]

There are conflicting views about whether breast-feeding should begin immediately or several hours after birth. From the information available, there is not much support for delaying breast-feeding when the condition of the mother and infant is favorable. Initiating nursing immediately after birth has the advantage of stimulating uterine contractions and lactation in the mother. It also will fulfill the infant's need for sucking and orients the infant to the breast early. It has been conjec-

tured that the length of the interval between the baby's birth and the first breast-feeding influences his acceptance of the breast. Early initiation of breast-feeding can also affect the mother's success at nursing her infant. In a study reported by Johnson[25] women who were allowed to breast-feed their infants within 1 hour after delivery were found to be more likely to continue to breast-feed than those who waited 16 hours or more.

Some pediatricians recommend one or two feedings of water before breast-feeding begins. The ingestion of water is believed to help the infant to regurgitate any mucus or secretions that may have been swallowed during delivery. One disadvantage of initial bottle-feedings instead of initial breast-feedings is that the infant may find it difficult to accept the breast because it was easier for him to get water or milk from the bottle.

Close nursing assessment and supervision in the early hours following delivery can indicate both the mother's and infant's readiness for the initiation of breast-feeding. When the mother and infant are alert and ready, the infant may be encouraged to breast-feed. It is preferable that breast-feeding begin within an hour after delivery when possible (see Nursing Care Plan 26–5).

The "Let-Down" or "Milk-Ejection" Reflex

An important physiologic aspect of breast-feeding is the "let-down" or "milk-ejection" reflex. During lactation milk is produced and secreted continuously into the alveoli of the breasts, but milk does not flow easily into the ductile system. However, the milk must flow into the ducts before the baby can obtain it. The ejection of milk from the alveoli into the mammary ducts is stimulated by oxytocin, a hormone secreted by the posterior pituitary. This process of the "letting down" of milk from the breasts is called the milk-ejection reflex, the let-down reflex, or the expulsion mechanism.

The reflex is initially precipitated by the suckling of the breasts by the infant. The sensation of the infant's sucking is transmitted to the hypothalamus, which stimulates the secretion of oxytocin by the posterior pituitary. Oxytocin is released into the bloodstream, and when it flows to the breasts, it causes the contractile tissues that surround the alevoli, the *myoepithelial cells,* to contract and express milk from the alveoli into the mammary ducts. After milk is impelled into the lactiferous ducts, it is easily removed from the breasts by compression of the areola and suction of the nipple resulting from the infant's nursing.

The milk-ejection or let-down reflex causes milk to flow within 30 seconds to a minute after the baby begins to nurse. Suckling on one breast also causes milk to flow in the opposite breast. Hence, milk may drip from the unsuckled breast while the infant is nursing at the other breast.

In the early puerperium, the breast-feeding mother may feel painful uterine contractions while nursing her infant, as oxytocin also causes the muscle fibers of the uterus to contract. Because of the role that oxytocin plays in the let-down reflex, this hormone is sometimes administered to a nursing mother for the first few days postpartally to expedite milk flow. Oxytocin may be administered parenterally or via nasal spray just prior to nursing time. The administration of oxytocin is also effective when the let-down reflex is inhibited, such as during periods of maternal stress.

Psychogenic factors and the emotions of the mother greatly influence the let-down reflex. Such influences may be either positive or negative. For example, stimuli that are associated with nursing (e.g., the infant's crying at feeding time or actions associated with nursing) may cause milk to drip from the mother's breasts. On the other hand, pain, fear, fatigue, and emotional stress can inhibit the let-down reflex and adversely affect the flow of milk. Thus the mother needs to avoid emotional stress and strain as much as possible. The nurse can help by fostering a quiet and relaxed hospital environment, by encouraging optimum comfort for the mother, particularly at feeding time, and by maintaining a supportive attitude.

The nursing mother and her mate should be given an explanation of the let-down reflex, so that they will understand how psychogenic factors may adversely affect breast-feeding. They should be aware that a pleasant and relaxed milieu is important during periods of nursing and that various disturbances and emotional stress may interfere with breast-feeding.

Preparation and Assistance of the Breast-feeding Mother

A nurse who is knowledgeable about breast-feeding needs to be present to assist the mother and infant, particularly during their first attempt to breast-feed (see Nursing Care Plan 26–5). Even if a woman has breast-fed before, she may still need assistance and guidance. No two infants are the same; thus, a breast-feeding experience with a subsequent infant may be quite different from a previous one. Hence, the type of intervention that is necessary for each mother–infant team is assessed, based on their individual situation.

Prior to placing the infant at the breast, the mother needs to be prepared for nursing. She is given instructions about the necessity for handwashing prior to each breast-feeding. The nipples are also cleansed with plain water just prior to nursing. Ideally, the mother should wash her hands and clean her nipples immediately before she picks up the infant for feeding.

Mothers need guidance about how to hold the infant while breast-feeding, how to position themselves, and how to help the infant suckle successfully. It will take some mothers a while to determine the position that is most comfortable for them. A sitting position or a side-lying position may be equally comfortable for some women but not for others. If the side-lying position is used, the mother's arm should be raised on the side at which the infant is placed to nurse, and her head should be supported by a pillow. The infant must be supported at the breast. Some mothers need to be shown how to hold the infant at the breast, since some women feel awkward when holding a small baby. Generally, it takes about a week for the mother and infant to establish a good nursing technique.

When the infant is placed at the breast, he may not display immediate interest in feeding. Usually the infant will turn toward the nipple as he smells the milk and will begin to nurse. The rooting reflex can be used to orient the infant to the breast. If the mother gently brushes the infant's cheek on the side nearer to the breast, he will turn toward the breast and grasp the nipple. Gently directing the infant's head toward the breast will also encourage nursing.

Both the nipple and areola should be grasped by the infant while he is nursing. If the areola and nipple are not grasped, milk will not be withdrawn well. Furthermore, the mother's nipples are likely to become extremely sore and possibly damaged. Mothers should be told about the correct position of the infant's mouth on the nipple and areola. The nipple should be placed well into the infant's mouth, so that his lips are fitted well around the areola. Thus, when the infant sucks, the alternating pressure of the tongue and palate on the lactiferous ducts will encourage withdrawal of milk. The mother can make the nipple and areola more easily grasped by the newborn by compressing the tissues above the areola between two fingers while placing the nipple and areola into the infant's mouth.

Once the baby has accepted the breast, the mother should make sure that the breast does not occlude the infant's nostrils and interfere with his breathing. This can be done by holding the breast away from the infant's nose while indenting the part of the breast near the infant's nose with a finger.

Mothers consider several factors in their self-evaluation of the success of their maternal abilities. One is the reaction of the infant during feedings. If the baby does not take the nipple easily, the mother may feel rejected by the infant. A mother wants and needs to feel accepted by her infant. New mothers need to be told that it may take a day or two for the infant to be easily oriented to the breast. Once the infant learns to associate the nipple with food, he will readily grasp the nipple when it is time to feed.

The vigorousness of sucking by the infant is often important to new mothers. If the baby does not suck as soon as he takes hold of the nipple, some women may become concerned. If the infant stops nursing at any time during the feeding, it is probably because he is not hungry or has stopped to rest for a while.

The mother needs to be made aware that individual differences do exist in infants' sucking behavior. Some infants will hold the nipple in their mouth for a while before they begin to suck. Other infants will first suck and then stop at intervals during the feeding to rest. Others will suck vigorously throughout the feeding until they are full. The infant should not be prodded into a sucking pace that is not natural for him. As the mother becomes more experienced in breast-feeding, she will become familiar with her infant's sucking pattern.

Alternate Massage

To expedite early breast-feeding, alternate massage should be taught to new mothers. This procedure encourages emptying of the breasts by the nursing infant.

The mother is first taught to observe the characteristics of her infant's nursing behavior as nursing proceeds. Long, slow, and rhythmic movement of the baby's mouth indicates that the infant is compressing the milk reservoirs behind the areola (lactiferous ducts) with his palate and tongue and is withdrawing milk satisfactorily.

During the course of the feeding, the infant will rest more frequently, and the character of nursing becomes rapid and shallow. This type of nursing behavior indicates that the milk is not flowing from the breasts as freely. When the baby's mouth movements become shallow and he seems to be sleeping, the mother begins alternating breast massage with infant nursing. The baby should not be removed from the breast, but the mother should slip her hand "to the back and middle portion of the breast near the armpit and gently massage the breast several times."[24] At the same time the baby usually stops nursing; then he begins to nurse again with long, slow strokes. Only two or three strokes may be taken, since the infant quickly withdraws the milk that has flowed from the alveoli to the milk reservoirs after the massage. The massage is then repeated and the baby permitted to nurse again.

Mothers often feel the breasts softening beneath their fingers during the massage. When one area has softened, the mother should move her fingers to a new position and resume alternate breast massage, along with the infant's nursing, until the entire breast softens.

The mother is taught not to use alternate massage "until the character of the baby's nursing has changed from long, slow mouth movements to sleeping for the most part or to rapid shallow nursing. If massage is used before this time, the milk flows too fast for the baby to manage."[24]

Occasionally some mothers will have flat or inverted nipples, which the infant has difficulty grasping. Flat or inverted nipples are tested for protractility by pinching or compressing the areola between the thumb and forefinger. If the nipple elongates, this is an indication that the nipples can be pulled out manually with the fingers or with the suction from a manual breast pump just prior to placing the infant at the breast. A breast shield can also be used for the first few minutes of nursing to draw the nipples out for the infant to grasp. Usually flat or inverted nipples become more erect when the infant sucks.

Time Interval for Nursing

During the first 2 or 3 days of the puerperium, the length of the nursing period is limited to 5 minutes on each breast. This includes actual nursing time and does not include the time spent getting the infant started. As the mother's nipples become tougher and are able to tolerate longer intervals of nursing, the time interval at each breast is gradually increased.

In the first days before milk production is established, the colostrum in the breasts can usually be withdrawn during 5 minutes of nursing time on each breast. Prolonged nursing after colostrum has been removed creates undue negative pressure, which causes sore nipples.[24] The nursing period is increased up to 20 minutes as lactation becomes well established. Of course the length of the nursing period will vary according to the individual infant's need. If the infant nurses for long intervals, the mother should not be greatly concerned, as long as he is sucking intermittently and her nipples can tolerate the length of the nursing period without becoming sore. However, long intervals of nursing may be an indication that the infant's hunger is not satisfied because there is not enough milk present. If the amount of milk is adequate, the infant's own pace of nursing should not be rushed.

The mother can nurse her infant on one or both breasts at each feeding once lactation is well established. What is most important is that the mother alternate the side that is emptied at the next feeding and that at least one breast be emptied at each feeding. Remember that thorough emptying of the breast stimulates the natural production of larger volumes of milk. Less milk will be produced if the breast is not emptied well.

Removing the Infant from the Breast

The suction created by some infants while nursing is so strong that it is not an easy task for some inexperienced mothers to remove the infant from the breast. To break the suction, the mother can place a finger at the corner of the baby's mouth or apply gentle downward pressure on the infant's chin (Fig. 26–3).

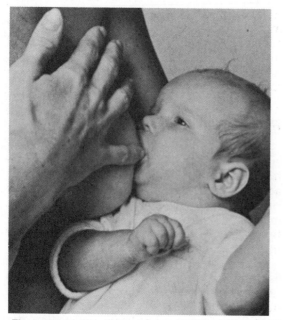

Figure 26–3. Breaking suction by placing a finger at the corner of the baby's mouth before pulling him away will help prevent sore nipples. (From Applebaum: *Pediatric Clinics of North America* 17:211, 1970.)

Burping

Infants who breast-feed do not usually swallow as much air as bottle-fed babies; however, this does not exclude breast-fed infants from the need to be bubbled or burped. Breast-fed babies are usually burped midway through the nursing period or before the mother changes the infant to the other breast, and again when the feeding period is completed. For most infants the most effective position for burping is one in which he is held in an upright position. This is done by having the mother place the infant with his head at her shoulder and his body against her chest. Some mothers find it easier to hold the infant in a sitting position in her lap, with the infant's torso supported by her forearm and with his head supported by positioning her thumb and index finger on each side of his mandible. The other arm is left free to rub the infant's back gently.

Supplementary Feedings

The use of supplementary, complementary, or prelacteal bottle-feedings for the breast-fed infant is a controversial issue. Some physicians and nurses point out that this practice reduces the success of breast-feeding by decreasing the sucking stimulation received by the breasts and thus causes less milk to be secreted. This is based on the belief that bottle-feeding causes the infant to develop a weaker sucking reflex resulting from the easy flow of milk from the bottle as opposed to removing milk from the breast. Hence, supplementary feedings are believed to cause the infant to suck less vigorously when he is placed at the breast.[36] When supplemental feedings are given, plain water, glucose water, or formula may be used.

The mother who is to use supplemental feedings at home must understand their proper function. The nurse should discuss the kind, amount, preparation, and indication for supplemental feedings with the parents before they return home. Supplemental feedings are needed when the infant remains hungry after he has nursed at the breast. When used for this reason, supplemental feedings should be given to the infant immediately following breast-feeding, when he has obtained as much breast milk as possible.

Care of the Nipples

In the early puerperium, sore nipples are a frequent complaint of breast-feeding mothers. Mothers should be encouraged to report any nipple discomfort, so that immediate intervention will be taken. When the mother's nipples are sensitive, applications of plain unmedicated hydrous lanolin after each feeding will help toughen them. Commercially prepared compounds, such as vitamin A and D ointment, may also be used.

Sore nipples should be examined for cracks, blisters, or erosion, since cracked and raw nipples are potential portals of entry for bacteria that may cause infection of the breast. Nipple or breast shields can be used during nursing periods when nipples are sore to prevent further irritation until the soreness subsides. If the mother prefers not to use a breast shield and can still withstand suckling, more frequent feedings of a shorter duration can be instituted to prevent prolonged sucking. This approach will also prevent overfilling of the breasts and engorgement, which can make the nipple difficult for the infant to grasp. Once she returns home, the breast-feeding mother can treat sore nipples by removing her bra and exposing her breasts to sunlight or room light for half-hour periods two or three times a day.

Expression of Milk

There are some situations in which the infant cannot be put to the breast to nurse or in which milk needs to be removed from the breasts because they have not been emptied sufficiently by the infant. With either of these situations, artificial means are instituted to remove milk from the breasts. *Manual expression* or a *breast pump* may be used.

Manual expression of milk can be done by the nurse or by the mother. Preferably, the nursing mother will practice manual expression of milk in the hospital, with the nurse's supervision, before she goes home so that she will know the proper procedure.

Prior to beginning manual expression, the woman should wash her hands and cleanse her nipples with plain water. The breast is gently massaged just prior to expression to stimulate the flow of milk. During breast massage one hand is placed beneath the breast while the other is placed on top. Gentle but firm pressure is exerted, with a gliding motion from the upper portion of the breast downward. Manual expression is then initiated (Fig. 26–4). One hand is used to hold the sterile receptacle for the breast milk. The fingers and palm of the other hand are placed underneath the breast for support, and the thumb of the same hand is placed above the upper edge of the areola. The thumb and forefinger are then used to gently and rhythmically compress and release the breast area just above the areola. Milk is then forced out of the breast into the receptacle.

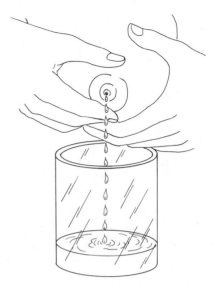

Figure 26–4. Hand expression of milk from the breast.

The fingers and thumb should not touch the areola and nipple, but they should be gradually moved around the area above the areola during the "milking" procedure to empty the breast. Manual expression should not be carried out any longer than 15 minutes at each breast.

When the breast pump is used, intermittent suction is employed to withdraw milk from the breast. Because suction is necessary to remove milk, breast pumps can cause some trauma to the breast if used improperly. Therefore, the mother is always supervised by the nurse when a breast pump is required in the hospital.

When expression of milk is implemented by an electric breast pump, low, gentle pressure can remove milk with little danger of irritation. If more suction is needed to withdraw the milk, suction must be gradually increased to prevent nipple trauma and pain.

The suction apparatus of the pump is attached to a funnel that collects the milk. This sterile glass or plastic funnel is placed over the areola so that it does not touch the nipple. As intermittent suction is applied by the pump, milk flows through the funnel to a larger sterile container. The woman is told to inform the nurse if she feels chest pain or back pain. These signs are indications that the breast has been emptied and that pumping should cease immediately. A breast pump should not be used for more than 10 minutes on one breast. If milk stops flowing during the procedure, the pumping should be promptly discontinued.

The electric pump must be cleaned well after use, since it will be used by more than one mother. The funnel, milk container, and rubber tubing should be washed thoroughly and autoclaved.

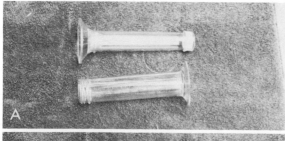
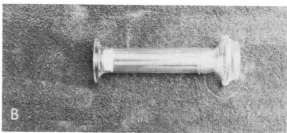
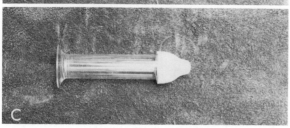

Figure 26–5. One type of hand breast pump. *A,* Separated for cleaning and sterilizing. *B,* Assembled and ready for use. *C,* With nipple attached for supplementary feeding.

A hand pump may also be used to empty the breasts (Fig. 26–5). This is a funnel-like receptacle that fits over the areola. A trap to catch the milk is located at the end of the receptacle, and a bulb syringe is attached to the container. The bulb is compressed and released intermittently to withdraw the milk. The principles that underlie the use of the electric breast pump also apply to the hand pump. The hand pump is also washed immediately after use. If more than one mother will be using the same apparatus, it should be autoclaved.

Whenever breast milk is expressed in the hospital, the amount obtained is recorded. The record should also indicate the method used to express the milk and whether one or both breasts were emptied. When only one breast is emptied, it is important to note which one it was, so that the other breast will be emptied the next time. When the milk is obtained, it should be placed in a sterile container and labeled with the mother's name and/or infant's name, the date, and the time it was collected. If the milk is not fed to the infant immediately, it must be sterilized prior to feeding. Breast milk can be frozen and used for feedings when the mother returns to work.

Excretion of Drugs in Breast Milk

The mother must understand that almost all products ingested by her are excreted in some form in her milk. Therefore, any medication that is taken by a nursing mother may be inadvertently administered to her infant.

Because a newborn has an immature enzyme system, along with incompletely developed kidney function, he is susceptible to accumulation of toxic levels of drugs. Though only small amounts of a particular drug may be in the breast milk, the cumulative amount in the milk ingested by a small infant during a 24 hour period could result in a full therapeutic dose.[37] Irritant-type laxatives taken by the nursing mother can cause abdominal pain, diarrhea, colic, and nausea in the nursing infant.

Breast-feeding mothers must not take any medication without the physician's knowledge. The mother should remind her physician that she is breast-feeding if medications are ordered for her while she is still nursing her infant.

Further Guidance and Instruction for the Nursing Mother

Although breast-feeding is a rewarding experience for most mothers, it can be frustrating when the woman has not received adequate guidance about concerns that she may have when she returns home. It is often after the mother leaves the hospital or is no longer under the direct care of the nurse that she has questions or concerns that she had not considered previously. We can help to moderate or eliminate factors that may interfere with the success of breast-feeding by anticipating these concerns.

Prior to returning home, the nursing mother needs to be given information about painful and fissured nipples. The treatment of painful nipples should be discussed. A demonstration of the use of a breast or nipple shield will also be helpful.

Leakage of milk from the breasts is often a problem for breast-feeding mothers, as lactation becomes well established and increasing amounts of milk are produced. Some mothers become distressed and embarrassed because their blouse may become soiled by leakage of milk. The nursing mother needs to be told about this before she returns home. She should be advised that wearing bra pads will prevent soiling of clothes.

Nurses need to be supportive of mothers who breast-feed their infants. Positive feedback regarding their ability in their maternal role and reassurance that their infant is nursing properly are needed. Even after the mother and baby return home, telephone calls or home visits are indicated for breast-feeding mothers until they are secure in their ability to successfully nurse their infant.[25]

As the infant grows older and the parents feel more comfortable about leaving the baby with a babysitter, some nursing mothers may feel that they cannot be away from their infant for more than a few hours. Such mothers should know that breast-feeding does not have to tie the woman down to her infant or her home. Breast milk can be expressed by the mother and left for the babysitter to feed to the infant. The mother should be reminded that breast milk should be stored in a sterilized bottle and refrigerated until the time that it is used.

Weaning

The duration of breast-feeding and weaning is an issue that should be discussed with parents. The mother needs to know that there is no set length of time to breast-feed her infant. Some infants may stop nursing as early as 3 or 4 months after birth, while others may still be breast-feeding at over 12 months of age.

In the United States, weaning from the breast usually occurs between 4 and 9 months of age. Ideally, the baby's willingness to wean rather than the mother's decision to stop breast-feeding will be the major determinant of the time for weaning. Once begun, weaning should be a slow process for mother and baby. The mother should be aware that weaning may proceed from the breast to the cup, or from the breast to the bottle and then to the cup, depending upon the infant's sucking needs.

Problems that May Complicate Breast-feeding

Breast-feeding may be complicated by problems that occur in the infant or in the mother. Oral defects in the infant may make sucking difficult. Although a cleft palate can interfere with the ability of an infant to suck, occasionally such an infant can be fitted with a prosthesis by a dentist to enable him to breast-feed.[38] Infants with facial deformities, macroglossia, or trauma or fractures to the jaw may also have dysphagia with breast-feeding. The effect of these conditions on the infant's suck-

ing ability should be evaluated in each case before a definite decision about permanent or temporary discontinuance of breast-feeding is made.

As noted in Chapter 23, prematurity and low birth weight are not contraindications if the mother wants to breast-feed her infant. If the premature baby is able to suck well, prematurity presents no special problem, except that more frequent nursing around the clock may be necessary for adequate infant intake. When small babies and premature infants have a weak sucking ability, the mother can express her breast milk into sterile containers for feeding by dropper or by a nasojejunal tube until the infant is able to nurse at the breast.

Deficient secretion of milk and illness of the mother are maternal conditions that may interfere with breast-feeding. Some bacteria and possibly some viruses can be passed to the infant through the breast milk. Active tuberculosis is one absolute contraindication to breast-feeding. In some instances mothers with an infectious disease may be allowed to breast-feed, depending on the nature of the infection.

When a mother has a fever of undetermined origin, febrile respiratory infection, gastroenteritis, or any communicable infection, she should not have contact with her infant until she is receiving appropriate treatment and is no longer contagious. During the interim when the mother is unable to breast-feed, the infant may receive donor human milk or a suitable proprietary formula. The mother's breast milk should be expressed at frequent intervals to maintain lactation until the infant can be put to breast again.

When the mother is not able to continue breast-feeding because of hypogalactia (insufficient milk secretion) or agalactia (failure of the secretion of milk), she may feel frustrated or guilty if she believes that she is not getting her infant off to the best start. This mother needs reassurance that artificial means of feeding can be just as nutritious for the infant as breast-feeding.

Sexuality in the Puerperium

Sexual Relationships

Most couples usually have some concern about when it is safe to resume sexual intercourse after pregnancy. The recommendations of physicians regarding the time to resume sexual intercourse vary widely. Some may not restrict intercourse at all as long as there is no bleeding, while others may recommend abstinence for as long as 6 weeks or more postpartum.

Abstaining from intercourse should be suggested until lochia serosa ceases because of the possibility of introducing infection to the placental site.[15] The physical discomfort that results from perineal wounds and the episiotomy is also a factor that the couple will want to consider when resuming coitus. If sexual intercourse is very painful for the woman, the couple will want to refrain from coitus for a while longer. Perineal wounds have usually healed sufficiently for the resumption of intercourse within 2 to 4 weeks postpartum.[34] Many women will suffer some discomfort from the episiotomy scar for 10 days to 2 weeks postpartum, while others may have slight discomfort for as long as 3 weeks. Clark and Hale[15] suggest that a change in position for intercourse, so that the penile shaft does not press directly on the posterior area, will reduce physical discomfort in the early puerperium. Usually, continuing sexual intercourse is beneficial because it tends to soften the episiotomy scar and thus decreases problems.[15]

Many changes in the sexual relationship of couples are likely during the postpartum period. Falicov[18] reports that a great deal of anxiety surrounds the resumption of coitus after the birth of the baby. Additionally, the ability to relax during intercourse may be affected by tension and fatigue from caring for the infant. Falicov also found that a large portion of the women in her study reported that sexual intercourse at 7 months postpartum was considerably less frequent than before pregnancy. The husbands' manifestations of eagerness and affection seem to play an important role in facilitating sexual adjustment in the puerperium. The level of prepregnancy sexual investment was associated with sexual adjustment during pregnancy and in the late postpartum period.

Landis and associates[30] reported that the general level of sexual desire of husbands and wives in their study was lower after the birth compared with prepregnancy levels. However, several factors were related to postchildbirth sexual adjustment. When wives had confidence in the contraceptive being used, the couple experienced better sexual adjustment following childbirth. Good sexual adjustment after childbirth was hindered by fear of another pregnancy.

In their investigation of the transition to parenthood, Meyerowitz and Feldman[35] found that the area of sexual adjustment was the major cause of complaint between new parents. Wives were frequently confused about what they should do regarding sexual intercourse. Psychic trauma was created for the wives when intercourse was resumed against the recommendations of the obstetrician. The mother was also found to be less interested in sexual relations than her husband at 1 month postdelivery, when she was still defining and adjusting to the maternal role.

It has become increasingly clear that healthcare providers should not ignore the sexual life of new parents following delivery. Individual needs, desires, and circumstances affect sexual adjustment in the puerperium and must be considered. The personalities of the husband and wife will play a major role in molding sexual behavior during the puerperium. The new baby can also affect the sexual relationship of new parents, particularly as adjustments are made to his presence and the additional demands that he may place on the parents. A sickly baby or an infant with deformities may place such an additional strain on the emotional lives of the parents that their coital relationship may be disrupted. Discussion of puerperal sexuality should therefore be included in the plan of care for the parents.

Sexuality and Breast-feeding

Some breast-feeding mothers find that sexual arousal occurs when their infant is nursing at the breast. This reaction may be guilt-provoking or distressing if the mother does not understand that this is a normal and frequent response. The possibility of sexual arousal during periods of breast-feeding should be discussed with the mother so that she will be aware that this reaction may occur.

Another common reaction that breast-feeding mothers may experience is the flowing of milk from their breasts when they are sexually stimulated, just as it does when they are stimulated by their baby's cry or even by the thought of their baby. This may also be distressing to some women and is another important piece of information for nurses to share with mothers while they are still in the hospital.

Just as coitus and labor and delivery have many similarities, breast-feeding and sexual intercourse can also be compared (Table 26–1). The similar physiologic responses during breast-feeding and sexual excitement are due to the release of the pituitary hormone oxytocin. The breast is an erogenous zone for most women. Sexual arousal occurs with stimulation of the breasts, regardless of the type, because of the nerve pathways to the hypothalamus from the nipples.

Table 26–1. COMPARISON OF BREAST-FEEDING AND SEXUAL INTERCOURSE

Breast-feeding	Sexual Intercourse
1. Uterus contracts	1. Uterus contracts
2. Nipples become erect; breasts are stimulated	2. Nipples become erect; breasts are stimulated
3. Skin changes; body temperature raised in submammary and mammary areas	3. Skin changes; body temperature raised in submammary and mammary areas

The New Family: Accommodating a New Member

The Family-Centered Approach to Postpartum Care

Several decades ago, childbirth was a family affair that was almost totally controlled by the parents. Because the parturient woman was attended at home, she was surrounded by family members from the time she began labor throughout the puerperium. Since the mother was confined in her own home, the father and siblings had the freedom to spend an almost unlimited amount of time with the mother and new baby. Family contact with the newborn and newly delivered mother often began within a few moments after childbirth, and the father was often present at birth.

Today, the hospital has become the major setting for childbirth. The transition of childbirth from the home to the hospital has major implications for the family. Although childbirth occurred in the family's own territory during home deliveries, movement of the event into the hospital made the family members intruders on foreign grounds.[33] When moved out of the home setting, care connected with childbirth became primarily centered on the mother and newborn infant. Even the mother and infant were separated from each other, with the mother in her own room and the infant in a separate nursery.

In some hospitals the father is allowed to visit for only short intervals, and young siblings are totally excluded from visitation. The father and siblings do not have much of a choice about what their level of participation will be because the mother and infant are confined on others' territory. The major reason given for such restrictions is that the mother and newborn must be protected from harmful infectious organisms that family members may harbor. Although there is no real justification for the practice, many hospitals still place barriers to mother–infant interaction and to the participation of fathers and siblings on postpartum units.

The family-centered approach to nursing care recognizes the need and right of fathers and other family members to be actively included in the childbearing experience. Childbirth is viewed as an experience that belongs to the family as a whole. The family on the maternity unit is viewed as a complete unit. The family-centered approach to nursing care recognizes that each family has "lines of attachment" to one another. Therefore the birth of a new family member requires readjustment by all members of the family unit. The quality of postpartum care that the family receives influences family relationships, as adjustments are made to the arrival of the newborn. Thus fathers and other family members are allowed to share in the postpartum experience to whatever extent is desirable.

In the postpartum hospital suite, the family is cared for as a unit. The father is not considered a visitor and is recognized as a vital and inseparable family member. He is considered in the nursing care plan and his needs are of paramount importance. Fathers are included in parenting classes and are allowed to come and go at will.

Rooming-in

Many more nurses and health care personnel have become aware of the importance of early and continuous contact between parents and their infant after birth. Through rooming-in, parents have increased levels of contact with the infant during the early puerperium, and parent-infant bonding is facilitated. In the rooming-in arrangement, the newborn is kept in a cot at his mother's bedside and receives most of his care from the mother. However, each mother's individual situation must be considered. Mothers who have had complicated deliveries or who are inexperienced with babies cannot be expected to care for the infants by themselves for the first few days. All mothers will require assistance from the nurse when rooming-in is practiced during the first day or so.

Fathers are also afforded greater contact with the infant when rooming-in is practiced and are likely to be more actively involved in infant care. Mothers and fathers can be taught infant care skills more easily when the infant is kept at the mother's bedside.

In some hospitals, infants are returned to the nursery at night or whenever the mother needs rest. This keeps the mother from becoming overly tired and encourages her to get adequate rest and sleep. When the mother seems not to be getting the rest that she needs, the infant should be returned to the nursery for a while. When rooming-in is practiced on units where other mothers are not utilizing such services, rooming-in infants are placed in a separate nursery.

The nurse on a rooming-in unit is in a better position to assess parenting skills and to do much more teaching. The nature of parent-infant interaction can also be more easily ascertained.

The chances of cross-infection are minimal on a rooming-in unit. Parents should be reminded, however, that they should practice frequent handwashing. Parents should wash their hands prior to handling their infant, and visitors should wash their hands upon entering the unit. Special gowns are usually worn by the father and visitors to cover their street clothes while they are with the mother and infant.

Sibling Visitation

Sibling visitation is another dimension of the family-centered approach that is practiced at some hospitals. Other children in the family should not be excluded from the childbearing experience. Visitation by siblings is beneficial for the visiting child and for the mother.

Young children are often heartbroken and feel rejected for the 3 or 4 days that their mother is away from them in the hospital. Toddlers and other young children who cannot fully understand the mother's temporary absence suffer the most adverse effects from this separation. Often these children may exhibit detachment from the mother and regress after the separation. This lack of contact between the older child and the hospitalized mother can be a major contributor to sibling rivalry when the new baby is brought home. Mothers are often also heartbroken when they have left a young child at home, particularly if the separation is the first one.

When siblings are allowed to visit, they can see their mother and their new brother or sister prior to the time that he or she is brought home. This helps the older child feel that he is also part of the birth experience (Fig. 26–6).

Of course children (and adults) who are sick or who have infectious diseases are not allowed to visit. Whenever this is the case, the nurse should encourage the mother to maintain contact with the child at home by daily telephone calls. The father and other family members who visit should be encouraged to share their visits with the child at home. Both parents should talk with the older child about the newborn, thus helping to prepare him for the infant and mother's return home.

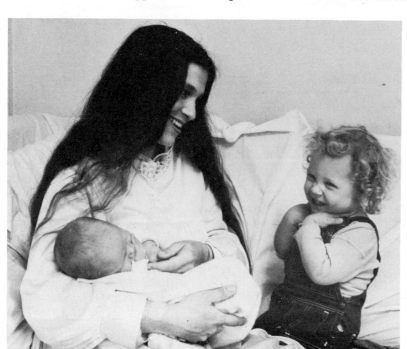

Figure 26–6. During visitation a sibling becomes acquainted with the newborn. (Photograph courtesy of Suzanne Szasz.)

Parent–Infant Attachment

When the newborn enters the world, he is in a totally dependent state. The infant is helpless and is incapable of surviving without the care of an adult. The caring adult(s), usually the mother and/or father, compensates for the newborn's incapabilities because of their attachment to him. The relationship of parents to their infant is one of the most important emotional ties that exist. This bond is vital because it promotes the survival of the infant and the species by ensuring that the helpless infant's needs will be met.

The literature concerning attachment of parents to their infant has great significance for nurses who care for infants and their families. Many of the "routine" practices of hospitals in the United States interfere with the kind of activities that seem to foster attachment. In some hospitals fathers are still excluded from delivery rooms and from direct contact with their babies. Even many mothers are only allowed to see their newborns for short periods of time during each 24-hour period, and this is usually for short periods at each feeding. Rarely are concepts such as attachment discussed with parents, either prenatally or postpartally. Even when practices such as rooming-in exist, they may be structured so they are more punitive than helpful to parents and infants.

The Nature of Attachment

Attachment involves affects and is an affectional bond between two persons or a dyad. Therefore, attachment is specific and discriminating, as it is a special tie that binds one individual to another. Because positive feelings usually predominate, attachment usually implies affection or love.[1] Attachment is a bond that is enduring over time. Once formed, this affectional tie is amazingly persistent; however, contact and interaction between two individuals are necessary for attachment to continue over time.

Behavior that promotes contact, proximity, and communication with a specific individual is characteristic of attachment. Among the common attachment behaviors are those that are signals to another (crying, talking, and vocalizing), those that include actual physical contact behavior (embracing, clinging, and touching; Fig. 26–7), and those that orient the individual to the person to whom he is attached (looking, following, or approaching). Such behaviors are indicative of attachment when they are directed specifically toward an individual to maintain a long-term affectional tie or relationship.[1]

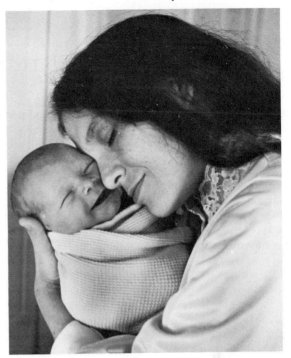

Figure 26–7. A mother embracing her infant.

The nature of parent–infant attachment is a unique kind of bond because at least some degree of parental attachment has begun to evolve prior to the infant's birth. Many factors interact to influence the degree of parental attachment to the child. Among the factors that may influence the prenatal and postnatal attachment of parents to their infant are the quality of the relationship between the parents, experiences with previous pregnancies, the parents' attitude about the addition of a new member to the family, and specific events that may occur during the pregnancy or during the labor and delivery.

Parents who have a good relationship with each other are more likely to have positive feelings toward their unborn child. When a pregnancy is welcomed and anticipated, parents will usually have positive feelings toward the child who is the product of that pregnancy. If prior experiences with pregnancy and with labor and delivery were positive and the events that surround the course of the present pregnancy are positive, a positive affect toward the baby will most likely develop.

Any information about the parents' attitude toward the pregnancy should be evaluated when it is available. Mothers and fathers who had negative feelings toward the pregnancy may have some difficulty attaching to their infant and moving into their parental roles during the puerperium. Nursing support of parents who are ambivalant toward their newborns can aid the progression of parent–infant attachment by providing appropriate guidance and by facilitating parent–infant contact.

The Attachment of Parents to Their Infant

Contact and interaction between parent and child are essential parts of parenting. Contact is vital for attachment to evolve. Mother–infant contact has generally been accepted as a requisite for the evolution of maternal attachment to the newborn. However, little emphasis has been placed on the need for early father–infant contact. Biller and Meredith[5] and Lynn[31] have pointed out that frequent contact with the infant encourages love, attachment, and nurturing behaviors in the father. Parents need frequent contact with their infant so that the evolution of a strong parent–infant bond will not be hindered.

There seems to be an innate potential for parents to become attached to their newborn, and this potential for attachment is released by early contact with the infant. Hess[22] states that Lorenz has postulated that the characteristic baby features of an infant stimulate a biologically based affection for the infant by the adult. Thus, contact by the adult with an infant encourages the adult to respond positively and to become attached to the infant.

The findings of several studies support Lorenz's contention. Hess[22] reported the results of a study by Cann that gauge the positive responsiveness of men and women to pictures of both infants and adults of several different animal species. Findings indicated that women preferred the "baby" pictures over adult pictures and that men's responses to the "baby" pictures increased as a function of marriage and parenthood. Hess[21] used enlargement in pupil size as an indication of positive response to drawings of faces progressively stylized toward greater babyishness. He found that greater babyishness of the faces elicited correspondingly greater pupil sizes. Hence, these studies not only lend support to Lorenz's thesis but also imply that positive affect and interest can even be aroused in adults by "baby" pictures.

Not only is parent–infant contact necessary for attachment to evolve but contact should occur early and frequently. Studies of parents who have been separated from their infants during the early puerperium suggest that the degree of contact and parent–infant interaction during the early days following childbirth affects later bonding to the infant and possibly affects infant development.

A study to determine whether limited maternal contact with the newborn would affect maternal behavior revealed that mothers who had extended contact with their infants in the immediate postpartum period were more attached to their infants at 1 month of age.[3] These mothers reported that they picked up their babies more in response to infant crying and that they were more likely to stay home with their babies than were those mothers who had limited contact with their infants. The mothers who had extended contact with their infants were observed to fondle their infants more, to have increased eye-to-eye contact while feeding the infants, and to comfort their babies more during doctor's office visits.

In a follow-up study a year later, there were still distinct differences in reported attachment and in observed attachment behaviors between the two groups.[27] After 2 years the mothers' patterns of speech revealed "that those who had been given extra contact with their infants during the neonatal period used significantly more questions, adjectives, words per proposition, and fewer commands and content words" than did the group of mothers who had limited contact.[42]

Fathers begin to develop a bond to their infant when they are allowed contact with their baby early in the puerperium (Fig. 26–8). Greenberg and Morris[19] found that fathers begin to develop an attachment to their infant by 3 days after birth or sooner when they have early contact with their newborn. The fathers in this study reported that they felt preoccu-

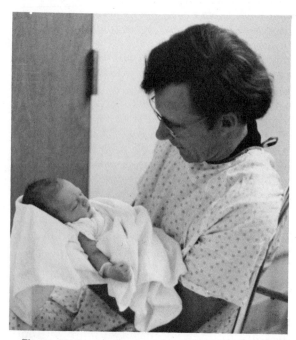

Figure 26–8. A father begins to develop a bond to his infant when they are allowed contact in the early puerperium. Bob's attachment to 2-day-old Alice seems evident.

pied, absorbed, and interested in their newborn. These fathers found that their newborn's face, activity, and eye movements held tremendous importance for them. The men often interpreted any infant activity that occurred in their presence as their infant's response to them. A new self-perception was recognized by these fathers, who described themselves as bigger, older, and more mature after seeing their newborn initially.

Parents should be helped to become acquainted with their infant by frequent and early contact. They should be encouraged to unswaddle and explore their infant. When parents can feel their infant's warm skin and cuddle the infant, bonding is further facilitated.

For the baby contact provides a source of essential security, warmth, and comfort. The infant's sense of kinesthesia is highly developed at birth and is a dominant mode of adjustment for him.[46] Therefore, touch is a major mode of stimulation and communication for the newborn. Parents should be aware of the infant's need for stimulation through touch, as well as his need for auditory stimulation from a warm and loving voice.

The attachment of parents to their infant is also affected by infant behaviors. A one-way relationship is often difficult to maintain. The parent–infant relationship is tenuous until the infant is able to actively participate and contribute to the relationship. Some mothers and fathers may have difficulty establishing a strong bond to the infant until he responds meaningfully. It is postulated that reciprocal and spontaneous infant attachment behaviors (such as crying, smiling, clinging, sucking, and rooting) are genetically determined biologic safeguards to sustain parental attachment and care of the infant.[1]

Assessing Parent–Infant Interaction and Attachment

A good parent–infant relationship is necessary to ensure that the child's needs will be met and that his development will be optimally facilitated. It is therefore vital that the nurse assess the parent–infant relationship to evaluate the future relationship and its ability to withstand stress. The immediate neonatal period presents a unique opportunity for the nurse to evaluate this relationship. If there are indications that the relationship between the infant and his parents is not progressing satisfactorily, the nurse should refer the family to the public health nurse for follow-up visits.

The parents' attitude about themselves in the maternal or paternal role is important. A parent s self-concept can be a help or hindrance to his or her bonding ability.[14] The parent's ideal self-image interacts with the actual self-image to contribute to her or his attitude in regard to the mothering or fathering role. Those traits, characteristics, abilities, and attitudes that are deemed desirable for the parental role combine to form the ideal image. How the parent views himself or herself currently constitutes the self-image. The comparison of one's self-image with the ideal image will have an impact on the developing parent–child relationship. Parents who have a positive self-image are likely to establish a positive relationship with their infant and vice versa.

Both parents' attitudes toward the newborn must also be assessed. Positive attitudes toward the infant facilitate bonding and movement of the mother and father into their parental roles. Negative attitudes will delay bonding. Assessing parental attitudes toward the infant includes consideration of whether the parents are happy about the infant's sex, whether they talk positively or negatively about the infant, and whether they move immediately to meet the newborn's needs.

The characteristics of the parents' touch can also provide information about the parents' progress in bonding to the infant. In the beginning parental relationship, there is a definite progression in the nature and amount of contact when parents touch their newborn. Movement is made from very small areas of contact to more extensive contact. Rubin[46] indicates that at first only the fingertips are used in touching, then the hands, and later the whole arms are brought in contact with the newborn. The direction of contact areas is from the periphery of the body during early stages of bonding. Then there is progression inward, centripetally, as bonding continues to evolve and the parent feels more confident in the maternal or paternal role (Fig. 26–9).

The characteristics of the parents' communication with the infant also give an indication of the ensuing parent–infant relationship. Whether the parent talks to the infant and whether the voice is warm and loving should be noted. The expression on the parent's face should be observed to determine if this is positive when interacting with the infant. Eye-to-eye contact with the infant by the parent is a positive sign of parental bonding. Whether parents call their infant by name should also be noted. Parents who do not name their infant or do not call their newborn by name may be experiencing difficulty recognizing or accepting him as a separate, whole individual, which will interfere with the parent–infant relationship.

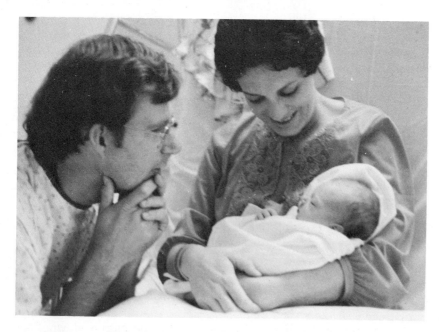

Figure 26–9. The newborn is incorporated into the family.

Finally, how the parent stimulates the infant should be noted when evaluating the parent–infant relationship. Observe if the parent attempts to elicit responses from the infant or if the mother or father is passive, with little contact with the infant. Overstimulation of the infant by slapping, pinching, hitting, poking, and the like are negative signs for the ensuing parent–infant relationship.

Incorporation of the Newborn into the Family

When the newborn is added to the family there are changes in family relationships and in the roles of the individual family members. The newborn is not quickly assimilated into the family without an internal change occurring in the family system. The newborn is an additional person with individual needs and demands that have to be considered in relation to the desires and needs of the other family members. Thus, the family must accommodate the new arrival.

Each family member's role within the context of the family changes with the new addition, and each obtains a new status. Rubin points out that "one becomes a mother or father, another a brother or sister, an aunt or uncle, a grandfather or a grandmother, simply by virtue of someone else's birth."[47] In any case, the arrival of the newborn introduces an additional person to whom the family members, particularly the immediate family members, must relate and adjust. In essence, with the newborn's arrival a new family is born.

The postpartum period is a phase accompanied by the incorporation of the infant into the family unit and by the incorporation of new roles and identities by family members. The taking on of a new role consequently brings about a new identity. The period during which the parents take on their new roles and identities is a critical time for mothers and fathers. Many parents need some assistance in order to feel comfortable about their new role. The infant is not completely incorporated into the family until each member is comfortable about his or her unique dyadic relationship with the newborn. Hence, parents must feel reasonably competent and comfortable about their parenting ability in relation to the newborn.

The postpartum nurse is in a unique position because she is an active participant in the care of families when the parents are in the early stages of their relationship with the newborn. She is accessible to the new parents as they begin to take on their parenting roles and can intervene to assist them when needed.

The Attainment of Parenting Roles

A first step in the attainment of the role of mother or father is the identification of the infant as a whole, separate individual. Part of this process involves obtaining relevant information about the newborn—sex, condition, and size.[47] Once the parents have received this information they each must weigh it in relation to their own fantasies and ideals regarding what the infant would be like. It is only after they have satisfactorily accepted and dealt with this basic information that the identification process can continue onward in an easy, eager manner.

When parents have a less-than-perfect baby or are disappointed about the basic characteristics of the infant, the identification process is delayed while disappointments are coped with. This point is of particular significance to the postpartum nurse, since these parents are likely to have difficulty in carrying out their roles. The initial step in assisting such parents is to help them accept their infant by encouraging contact with the newborn and by discussing the realities of the infant's condition with them.

Once parents have realistically dealt with their disappointments and have accepted their infant, a realignment of their anticipated relationship with the newborn can be made and the identification process can continue. Until the parents are able to accept their infant, they grieve about their disappointment. Each of their specific disappointments must be reviewed and mourned, so that their attachment to the previously desired relationship can be loosened.[47]

The identification process is fostered by direct contact and interaction with the infant. Through such contact and interaction, parents begin to differentiate the identity of the newborn. Both the infant and their parenthood become more real to them. Once parents identify their infants as separate individuals, they can more effectively proceed to carry out their roles of mother or father.

Although much of the attainment of parental roles occurs after delivery, there is evidence that a great deal of role anticipation occurs during childhood and again during the prenatal period, as parents prepare to move into their roles.[48, 49] However, Rossi[44] points out that most individuals do not receive any realistic training for parenthood in our society.

In her study of the attainment of the maternal role, Rubin found several operations by which mothers incorporated their roles.[48] Although fathers were not considered in the investigation, it is likely that similar operations influence the attainment of the paternal role. Six operations were identified: mimicry, role play, fantasy, introjection-projection-rejection, identity, and grief work.

1. In mimicry the parent adopts simple behavioral manifestations that are recognizable symbols of parenthood, such as speech, affects, or gestures.

2. Role play involves the acting out of what a parent does in a specific situation.

3. In fantasy, the daydreams, wishes, and fears of the person proliferate to help her get an idea of what the parenting role that she fantasizes will actually be like.

4. In introjection-projection-rejection the parent finds a model to emulate whose own behavior seemed to work toward resolving a specific event that the parent is presently experiencing. If the "fit" is workable, then the behavior is reinforced; however, if it is unsatisfactory, the behavior is rejected.

5. Identity is the end process in the attainment of the parenting role. When the parent reaches a sense of confidence and comfort about the role, then parental identity is reached and role attainment is complete.

6. However, final grief work occurs as the parent lets go of the former identity in some previous roles that are incompatible with the assumption of the new parenting role. It involves the review and mourning of the attachments to a former role that had to be dropped during the attainment of the new parenting role. Thus the incorporation of the parenting role and of the infant into the family requires some degree of loss of former life patterns that must be mourned and resolved. Resolutions may involve reduction of social roles or career pursuits.[20]

Rubin[49] also found that mothers most often selected their own mother or mother substitute as their role model, as they incorporated their maternal role. However, peers were also extensively used. It is also likely that fathers use peers as models to a great degree. In her study of expectant fathers, Marquart[33] found that expectant fathers reported that they sought out and spent more time with other expectant fathers or with actual fathers. These findings point to applicability of parent group discussions on the postpartum unit as a means of peer teaching.

The nurse is also used as a model by parents as they begin to carry out their parenting roles. Thus, as she interacts with the infant, parents observe her and may adopt certain aspects of her approach. This is why it is important for nurses to relate to the infant on an individual basis. She should cuddle, talk to, and smile at the infant during her contact with him, since these behaviors will hopefully be modeled by the parents. The nurse can also serve as a role model by communicating her knowledge about parenting to new mothers and fathers.

Postpartum Teaching—Helping Parents to Incorporate Their Roles

Learning to be a good parent is difficult, and few people are truly prepared for parenthood. Now that the nuclear family has replaced the extended one, parents, grandparents, cousins, aunts, and uncles are often not available to young couples to offer advice and assistance. Teaching parenting skills to new mothers and fathers is of paramount importance and should be a part of postpartum nursing care. New parents need assistance and instruction in the areas of infant care, infant behavior and characteristics, and infant development. Parents must also be knowledgeable about other areas of family life, such as sexuality, contraception, and family dynamics, in order to function well in their parenting role. Hence, the postpartum teaching needs of parents may touch on many facets of family life.

Individual Parent Teaching.   Not all parents have the same parenting capabilities. Individual instruction is a recognition of the differences in the background and experience of parents that result in specific capabilities and individual learning needs.

Certain factors must be considered when assessing the parents' individual learning needs. The most important factor is what the parents feel they need to know. People learn best what they are ready to learn and what they want to learn. The parent's own perceived need is important to her or him and is a strong motivator for learning. Most often it is best to give consideration to what the parents want to learn when they express this, so that they can then move on to accept other needed teaching.

Other factors that should be considered when assessing the learning needs of parents are the specific characteristics of the parents' individual situation, which determine the need for specific knowledge. For example, parents who have an infant with a cleft palate, hypospadias, or even a cephalhematoma require additional information regarding their infant. Individual teaching allows the nurse to relate information to the parents' particular situation at a time when the situation presents an optimum opportunity for teaching. For example, it may be more effective to explain and demonstrate perineal care to a mother as it is being done by the nurse, rather than waiting to teach it in a formalized group session. Often individualized instruction, when a teachable situation presents itself, can be used to reinforce information that was given in a group session.

Information that should be shared with all postpartum parents, that is, information that all postpartum parents can generally benefit from, is usually given in group classes.

Group Postpartum Teaching.   Group teaching is an effective method of postpartum instruction because many people can have their need for similar knowledge met at the same time. Group teaching can also ensure that a large number of parents get certain information that all parents need but are not likely to know. Information that all parents generally need to know during the puerperium includes infant care skills, infant development, normal newborn behavior, and contraceptive methods. A well coordinated program of group classes can be very effective in teaching a broad range of parenting skills, particularly when a topic requires a longer interval of time to be covered well. More parents are likely to be reached and taught a topic that requires 45 minutes than if each individual is taught separately.

In selecting topics and planning group classes for parents, the nurse should ask herself several questions: "What common information do a number of parents need to know? Is this information best taught in a group situation or on an individual basis? If this information is not taught in a group session, are parents who need to be reached likely to be taught this individually, based on the number of qualified staff who could provide the information?"

Once the topics to be included in the program of group classes have been selected, the instructor must determine what resources and approaches to teaching will be most effective. Films and other audiovisual aids, demonstrations, discussion groups, or lecture-discussions are teaching approaches and methods that can be used for group classes. Mothers may also bring their infants with them to the group class, so that they can practice what they were taught while the instructor is available to guide them.

The instructors of the classes may be staff nurses only or may also include nutritionists, public health nurses, physicians, and social workers. No matter who is included in the classes as instructors, *nurses must remember that it is their responsibility to initiate, plan, and implement an organized postpartum group teaching program.*

An often unrecognized benefit of group teaching is the peer teaching that often occurs when parents begin to discuss topics in a group. Often multiparas and experienced fathers share valuable information with their peers based on their previous experience. As previously mentioned, parents often use their peers as models as they attain their parenting roles. Parents may informally share problems and teach each other as they gather around a table for tea or recreation. A parent who is returning to older children can exchange notes

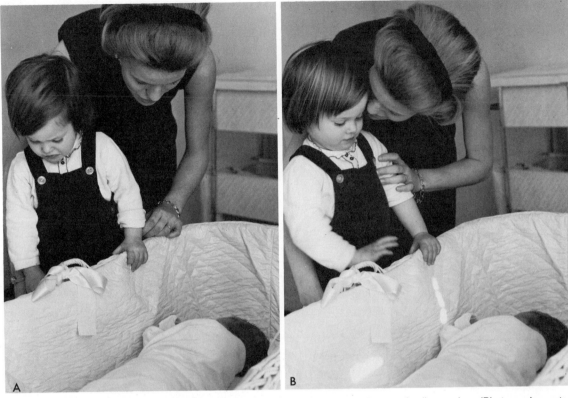

Figure 26–10. *A,* Sometimes a child needs a parent's guidance to accept the new family member. (Photograph courtesy of Suzanne Szasz.) *B,* With loving encouragement, brother and sister become friends. (Photograph courtesy of Suzanne Szasz.)

with an inexperienced parent (Fig. 26–10*A, B*). This informal interaction can also be facilitated by insuring that parents have a place to gather informally.

All of the group class sessions may not be needed by all parents. Some maternity units establish special sessions for smaller groups of parents with common special concerns. Examples are classes for breast-feeding mothers, for parents of infants requiring intensive care services, or for parents with premature infants. Of course the type of special group sessions offered will depend on the number of clients on the unit with common special concerns.

Outpatient Teaching. Once parents leave the hospital, they may be cut off from needed supportive and teaching services. Studies by Sumner and Fritsch[55] and by Gruis[20] show that parents still have teaching needs and parental concerns when they return home. Once faced with the care of the infant in their home without assistance, the parents find that questions and concerns arise that had not surfaced previously. In many communities postpartal parent groups have been established to assist those who need further instruction and support. Usually some of the purposes of these groups are to increase parents' knowledge of childrearing and child development and to pro-

vide a supportive atmosphere while parents incorporate their roles.

Parents may receive a similar type of assistance during the postpartum period from the public health nurse, a community liaison nurse from the hospital postpartum unit, or through the private sector. A telephone service whereby parents can share their concerns with nurses and have their questions answered can be beneficial, particularly for those parents who may not be able to attend group classes outside their home.

Discharge from the Hospital

At the time that the mother and infant are discharged from the hospital (Fig. 26–11), the nurse or the mother's obstetrician usually gives her special discharge instructions. One of the things discussed is a short review of self-care between the time of her release from the hospital and the time of the postpartum check-up. Usually the mother is advised to return to her usual activities gradually. She is advised against heavy work and lifting. Stair climbing is also limited until after the second week postpartum. The mother is told not to douche until after her postpartum check-up. She is encouraged to get adequate rest and sleep to

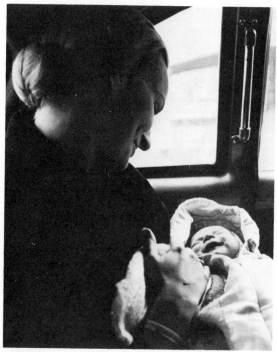

Figure 26–11. A mother returns home with her baby. (Photograph courtesy of Suzanne Szasz.)

prevent fatigue. The mother should be aware that she can take tub baths and showers and wash her hair when she returns home. The resumption of sexual activity by the couple is also included in the discharge discussion.

Special instructions regarding infant care may be given by the pediatrician. If the infant is bottle-feeding, the type of formula to be used is reviewed with the parents, and they may be given other special instructions about their infant's care.

Even though the major points above are reviewed at the time of discharge, the family is constantly being prepared for discharge while they are at the hospital. Therefore, a more in-depth discussion of this information should be led by the nurse at some time prior to the discharge.

The family's need for support systems should be assessed before they return home. Mothers or infants with special problems or conditions should be followed at home by a visiting nurse or a public health nurse. Appropriate referrals should be made to other health-care providers when needed.

In some hospitals and birthing centers, mothers who have had normal vaginal deliveries are allowed to return home as early as 24 hours after delivery. This does not allow much time for the nurse to provide the depth of instruction and guidance that mothers may

need to readily take on their maternal role and to understand their own care after giving birth. In such instances, follow-up by a nurse is important and the services of a visiting nurse or public health nurse take on special significance. Follow-up telephone calls from the postpartum nurse or a telephone line that mothers can use to call to the postpartum unit for assistance could be a valued service, particularly when the mother has been discharged very early after delivery.

Care Following Discharge

The care of childbearing families does not end with discharge from the hospital or a birthing center. Families need to know what kinds of resources are available to them in the weeks following delivery. They need to know very specifically where to find answers to questions such as whether they should call the hospital or birthing center nurse, the health department nurse, or the nurse in their private physician's office. In some perinatal care delivery systems nurses call or visit new parents within the first few days following hospital discharge to assess both their physiologic and their psychosocial status.

The traditional 6-week postpartum check-up now may occur at 4 weeks; in many communities nurse practitioners, nurse midwives, and other health-care providers are seeing women and their families within 2 weeks after birth in order to identify possible physiologic or psychosocial problems that require intervention and to provide appropriate nursing intervention or referral.

The follow-up visit must include assessment of problems identified in the prenatal or intrapartum phases of pregnancy to ensure their resolution or appropriate intervention. For example, a woman who has had a urinary tract infection during pregnancy should have a careful urinary tract assessment following the puerperium.

For women who plan to have more children, the period between pregnancies is a time in which health can be improved. For example, a woman's specific nutritional needs may be addressed. If she is overweight, plans for weight loss that would have been inappropriate during pregnancy can be developed in consultation with her. Anemia, low weight, and hypertension are other examples of health problems that, if addressed during this period, can influence future pregnancies.

Good health can be stressed for all women.
Text continued on page 945

Nursing Care Plan 26–6. Caring for the Mother During the Puerperium: Weeks 4 to 6

NURSING GOALS: To evaluate physiologic restitution during the puerperium.
To evaluate incorporation of the new infant into the family.

OBJECTIVES:
1. Vital signs (temperature, pulse, respiration, and blood pressure) are within normal limits for nonpregnant women.
2. Weight is within normal limits for the woman's age and height.
3. Hemoglobin and hematocrit are within normal limits for nonpregnant women.
4. Bowels are functioning without difficulty.
5. No evidence of urinary tract disease is present.
6. Abdominal muscle tone is improved, approximating prepregnant tone. Postpartum exercises are taught or reinforced.
7. Breasts in nonlactating mother are soft and nontender and have no reddened areas or palpable masses. Woman is taught breast self-examination.
8. Lactating woman does not have sore, cracked nipples or signs of mastitis. Appropriate counseling about continued lactation is provided.
9. Lochia is absent by 6 weeks after delivery.
10. Uterus has returned to approximate prepregnant size by 6 weeks after delivery. External os is closed. Pelvic floor has good muscle tone; importance of continuing pelvic floor exercises is reinforced. Vulva and perineum are intact.
11. Papanicolaou test is completed.
12. Family planning needs are identified, and appropriate counseling is provided.
13. Family reports satisfaction with parenting roles, attachment to infant, absence of severe sibling rivalry, absence of family discord.

ASSESSMENT	POTENTIAL NURSING DIAGNOSIS	NURSING INTERVENTION	COMMENTS/RATIONALE
1. Vital signs should be at pre-pregnancy level by 4 to 6 weeks		Temperature elevation: further assessment and referral for possible infection	
If client appears excited or anxious, provide period for relaxation before assessing vital signs.		Tachycardia, irregular pulse: further assessment and possible referral to identify basis	
		Tachypnea: further assessment and possible referral to identify basis	
		Hypertension: refer for further assessment	
2. Weight should be at prepregnancy level by 6 weeks.	Inadequate weight loss Excessive weight loss Need for information related to nutrition	Compare weight with desirable weight for height. Provide dietary counsel to help woman achieve ideal weight during interpartum period.	
		Evaluate woman with inadequate weight loss for edema.	

Continued on following page

Nursing Care Plan 26–6.   Caring for the Mother During the Puerperium: Weeks 4 to 6 *(Continued)*

ASSESSMENT	POTENTIAL NURSING DIAGNOSIS	NURSING INTERVENTION	COMMENTS/RATIONALE
3. Hematocrit: 37 per cent ± 5 per cent Hemoglobin: 12 g. per 100 ml.	Need for nutritional assessment related to low hemoglobin, hematocrit	Assess daily food intake and activity level. Provide or refer for diet counseling. Evaluate dietary intake in woman with excessive weight loss; provide or refer for diet counseling.	
	Need for referral to identify causes of anemia other than iron deficiency	Supplemental iron may be indicated. If hemoglobin is less than 9, anemia may be related to factors other than iron deficiency; refer for further evaluation.	
4. Bowel function: return to prepregnancy function by 6 weeks.	Constipation	Evaluate diet if constipation is present; counsel to increase intake of whole grains, fruits, vegetables, and fluids; exercise.	
Identify rectocele, if present.	Fecal incontinence secondary to rectocele		
Identify hemorrhoids.		If hemorrhoids are present, stool softeners may be helpful.	
5. Bladder function a. Identify cystocele.	Urinary incontinence secondary to cystocele	Refer woman with cystocele to physician.	Woman who had urinary tract infections during pregnancy should have a careful evaluation of the urinary tract 2 to 3 months following delivery.
b. Assess presence of (1) Frequency (2) Urgency (3) Burning on urination	Urinary incontinence secondary to trauma to urethra	Teach or reinforce teaching of pelvic floor exercise (see Chapter 11).	
	Urinary frequency and/or burning secondary to urinary tract infection	Refer for treatment of urinary tract infection.	
c. Obtain clean-catch urine specimen; no evidence of infection should be present in lactating mother.			
6. Abdomen a. Muscle tone approaching prepregnancy status by 6 weeks. No diastasis recti (separation of rectus muscles at midline)	Need for information about exercise to strengthen abdominal muscles	Teach or encourage continuation of postpartum exercises.	
	Need for encouragement to continue postpartum exercises		

Physical Assessment/Normal Findings	Alterations	Nursing Intervention
b. Linea nigra fading; striae may still be red		Explain that linea nigra will continue to fade; striae will gradually become silvery in appearance.
c. Incision is healed in woman following cesarean birth.		
7. Breasts		
a. Nonlactating mother: by 6 weeks should approximate prepregnant size, be soft, no tenderness, no redness	Need for information about breast self-examination	Teach or reinforce teaching of breast self-examination.
	Possible breast infection (red, tender breast)	If mass is present in breast, refer for further evaluation.
		If infection (mastitis) is present, see Nursing Care Plan 27-2.
b. Lactating mother: breasts full; identify signs of complications: (1) Sore, cracked nipples (2) Infection (mastitis)	Need for information about identified complications	See Nursing Care Plan 26–5 for care of sore nipples; Nursing Care Plan 27–2 for care in mastitis.
Identify mother's plans for breast-feeding or weaning if she is returning to work.	Need for information about breast-feeding in relation to working schedule	Review options with mother: 1. Use of breast pump while away from infant; milk saved for infant 2. Use of breast pump to maintain milk supply; milk discarded and formula substituted 3. Gradual weaning. Help mother identify plan best suited for her; refer to community health nurse or provide resource for continuing consultation.
8. Reproductive tract		
a. Lochia: absent by 6 weeks	Persistence of lochia after 6 weeks	Assess for subinvolution or infection in mother with persistent lochia; culture lochia. Refer for additional evaluation and treatment.
b. Menstrual period (1) Absent in breast-feeding mother; first period may be delayed for several months. (2) Resumption of menses at approximately 4 to 6 weeks in nonlactating mother	Persistence of lochia rubra after 2 weeks	Remind mother that ovulation precedes menses; counsel about contraceptive use (Nursing Care Plan 6–1).
c. Pelvic examination (1) Uterus returned to approximate prepregnant size by 6 weeks (2) Cervix: external os closed; appears as transverse slit	Subinvolution (uterus larger than appropriate; os open)	Refer for further evaluation of subinvolution or infection. Dilatation and curettage may be necesary for subinvolution.

Continued on following page

Nursing Care Plan 26–6.   Caring for the Mother During the Puerperium: Weeks 4 to 6 (Continued)

ASSESSMENT	POTENTIAL NURSING DIAGNOSIS	NURSING INTERVENTION	COMMENTS/RATIONALE
(3) Pelvic floor: good muscle tone	Poor muscle tone in pelvic floor muscles	Teach or reinforce teaching of pelvic floor exercise (see Chapter 11).	
(4) Vulva and perineum: episiotomy or laceration healed			
(5) Introitus: allows intercourse without discomfort			
d. Papanicolaou test		If abnormal cells (Class 3, 4, 5) are identified, contact client and refer for further evaluation and treatment.	
9. Assess plans for family planning (Nursing Care Plan 6–1).	Need for information about family planning	Provide information appropriate to individual. Refer for appropriate intervention (e.g., prescription for oral contraceptives, insertion of IUD, etc.). See Nursing Care Plan 6–1.	
10. Assess family interaction. a. Reports of satisfaction with parental role: mother does not feel totally overwhelmed with infant care; reports assistance from significant others.	Inadequate coping with parental role	Mother may initially report general feelings; take adequate time to help her identify specific problems. Home visit by community health nurse may be helpful. Develop specific plan; e.g., help with one feeding each day, help with bath every other day. See Nursing Plan 22–1.	
b. Signs of attachment (see Nursing Care Plan 22–1) Strong signs of attachment should be present by 4 to 6 weeks. If attachment seems weak, identify possible causes in order to develop specific intervention.	Lag in attachment related to specific cause (e.g., maternal illness, characteristics of infant, family problems, etc.)	If attachment is not present at this time, refer to community health nurse for continuing assessment and intervention to facilitate attachment.	
c. Sibling acceptance of newborn (See Nursing Care Plan 22–1.)	Sibling difficulty in coping with newborn infant	Provide opportunity for parents to verbalize concerns about sibling rivalry; identify specific problems. Home visit by community health nurse may be essential for full assessment and intervention. Continuing or severe problems in sibling adjustment may need to be referred for counseling to appropriate resource (e.g., Family Service Agency, Mental Health, etc.).	The appropriate agency will vary from one community to another. Nurses are responsible for being aware of services available in their community.

The advantages of health in terms of vitality and appearance as well as the prevention of future health problems are stressed. Health teaching, including breast self-examination and the need for periodic examinations including a Papanicolaou test, is emphasized.

In addition, adequate time should be provided during this visit to talk with the mother, and ideally, with other members of her family about her (and their) adjustment to the new infant's presence. By 4 weeks, most families will have integrated infant care into their pattern of living. Mothers may still be fatigued, particularly if there are other small children, but most will have developed their own style of coping. Activities such as bathing and feeding will no longer be overwhelming.

When comments by the mother or another family member indicate that they continue to be overwhelmed by the new baby, further identification of specific problems and appropriate intervention are needed. Perhaps there is a feeling of isolation that could be alleviated by participation in a new mother's group. Perhaps homemaker services, available in some communities, would help. Further assessment and intervention from a community health nurse may be essential. Evidence of lack of copying should never be dismissed with the "hope" that the situation will automatically improve with further experience. The components of postpartum evaluation at 4 to 6 weeks following birth are described in Nursing Care Plan 26–6.

REFERENCES

1. Ainsworth, M. D. S.: The Development of Infant-Mother Attachment. *In* Caldwell, B. M., and Ricciuti, H. R. (eds.): *Review of Child Development Research.* Vol. 3. Chicago, The University of Chicago Press, 1973.
2. Atkinson, L. D.: Is Family-centered Care a Myth? *American Journal of Maternal Child Nursing,* 1:256, 1976.
3. Barnett, C. R., Leiderman, P. A., Grobstein, R., et al.: Neonatal Separation: The Maternal Side of Interactional Deprivation. *Pediatrics,* 45:197, 1970.
4. Benson R. C.: *Handbook of Obstetrics and Gynecology.* 5th Edition. Los Altos, Cal., Lange Medical Publications, 1974.
5. Biller, H. G., and Meredith, D.: *Father Power.* New York, David McKay Co., Inc., 1975.
6. Bishop, B.: A Guide to Assessing Parenting Capabilities. *American Journal of Nursing,* 76:1784, 1976.
7. Bowlby, J.: *Attachment and Loss.* Vol. 1. New York, Basic Books, 1969.
8. Brazelton, T. B.: The Parent-Infant Attachment. *Clinical Obstetrics and Gynecology,* 19:373, 1976.
9. Cahill, A. S.: Dual-purpose Tool for Assessing Maternal Needs and Nursing Care. *JOGN Nursing.* 4(1):28, 1975.
10. Childbirth and Postnatal Care a Family Experience Shared by the Father. *Nation's Hospitals,* 2:40, 1972.
11. Clark, A. L.: The Adaption Problems and Patterns of an Expanding Family: The Neonatal Period. *Nursing Forum,* 5:93, 1966.
12. Clark, A. L.: Introducing Mother and Baby. *American Journal of Nursing,* 74:1483, 1974.
13. Clark, A. L.: Recognizing Discord between Mother and Child and Changing it to Harmony. *American Journal of Maternal Child Nursing,* 1:100, 1976.
14. Clark, A. L., and Affonso, D. D.: Infant Behavior and Maternal Attachment: Two sides to the Coin. *American Journal of Maternal Child Nursing,* 1:95, 1976.
15. Clark, A. L., and Hale, R. W.: Sex during and after Pregnancy. *American Journal of Nursing,* 74:1430, 1974.
16. Cox, B. S.: Rooming-In. *Nursing Times,* Aug. 8, 1974, p. 1246.
17. Eckes, S.: The Significance of Increased Early Contact between Mother and Newborn Infant. *JOGN Nursing,* 3(4):42, 1974.
18. Falicov, C. J.: Sexual Adjustment during First Pregnancy and Post Partum. *American Journal of Obstetrics and Gynecology,* 117:991, 1973.
19. Greenberg, M., and Morris, N.: Engrossment: The Newborn's Impact upon the Father. *American Journal of Orthopsychiatry,* 44:520, 1974.
20. Gruis, M.: Beyond Maternity: Postpartum Concerns of Mothers. *American Journal of Maternal Child Nursing,* 2:182, 1977.
21. Hess, E. H.: Ethology. *In* Freedman, A. M., and Kaplan, H. I. (eds.): *Comprehensive Textbook of Psychiatry.* Baltimore, The Williams & Wilkins Co., 1967.
22. Hess, E. H.: Ethology and Developmental Psychology. *In* Mussen, P. H. (ed.): *Carmichael's Manual of Child Psychology.* 3rd Edition. New York, John Wiley and Sons, Inc., 1970.
23. Hogan, A. I.: The Role of the Nurse in Meeting the Needs of the New Mother. *Nursing Clinics of North America,* 3:337, 1968.
24. Iffrig, Sis. M. C.: Nursing Care and Success in Breast Feeding. *Nursing Clinics of North America,* 3:345, 1968.
25. Johnson, N. W.: Breast-feeding at One Hour of Age. *American Journal of Maternal Child Nursing,* 1:12, 1976.
26. Jones, W. L.: The Emotional Needs of the New Family. *Nursing Mirror,* Oct., 1975, p. 49.
27. Kennell, J. H., Jerauld, R., Wolfe, H., et al.: Maternal Behavior One Year after Early and Extended Post-partum Contact. *Developmental Medicine and Child Neurology,* 16:172, 1974.
28. Klaus, M. H., Jerauld, R., Kreger, N. C., et al.: Maternal Attachment. *New England Journal of Medicine,* 286:460, 1972.
29. Knafl, K.: Conflicting Perspectives on Breast Feeding. *American Journal of Nursing,* 74:1848, 1974.
30. Landis, J. T., Poffenberger, R., and Poffenberger, S.: The Effects of First Pregnancy upon the Sexual Adjustment of 212 Couples. *American Sociological Review,* 15:766, 1950.
31. Lynn, D. B.: The Father: His Role in Child Development, Monterey, Cal., Brooks/Cole Publishing Co., 1974.

32. *The Mammary Glands and Breastfeeding*. Ross Laboratories, 1972.

33. Marquart, R. K.: Expectant Fathers: What Are Their Needs? *American Journal of Maternal Child Nursing, 1*:32, 1976.

34. Masters, W. H., and Johnson, V. E.: *Human Sexual Response*. Boston, Little, Brown and Co., 1966.

35. Meyerowitz, J. H., and Feldman, H.: Transition to Parenthood. *Psychiatric Research Report 20*, Washington, D. C. American Psychiatric Association, Feb. 1966, p. 78.

36. Newton, N., and Newton, M.: Lactation—Its Psychologic Components. *In* Howells, J. H. (ed.): *Modern Perspectives in PsychoObstetrics*. New York, Brunner/Mazel Publishers, 1972.

37. O'Brien, T. E.: Excretion of Drugs in Human Milk. *American Journal of Hospital Pharmacy, 31*:844, 1974.

38. Oseid, B. J.: Breast-feeding and Infant Health. *Clinical Obstetrics and Gynecology, 18*:149, 1975.

39. Otte, M. J.: Correcting Inverted Nipples—An Aid to Breast Feeding. *American Journal of Nursing, 75*:454, 1975.

40. Penfold, K.: Supporting Mother Love. *American Journal of Nursing, 74*:464, 1974.

41. Rich, O. J.: Hospital Routines as Rites of Passage in Developing Maternal Identity. *Nursing Clinics of North America, 4*:101, 1969.

42. Ringler, N. M., Kennell, J. H., Jarvella, R., et al.: Mother-to-Child Speech at 2 Years—Effects of Early Postnatal Contact. *The Journal of Pediatrics, 86*:141, 1975.

43. Rising, S. S.: The Fourth Stage of Labor: Family Integration. *American Journal of Nursing, 74*:870, 1974.

44. Rossi, A. S.: Transition to Parenthood. *Journal of Marriage and the Family, 30*:26, 1968.

45. Rubin, R.: Basic Maternal Behavior. *Nursing Outlook, 9*:683, 1961.

46. Rubin, R.: Maternal Touch. *Nursing Outlook, 11*:828, 1963.

47. Rubin, R.: The Family-Child Relationship and Nursing Care. *Nursing Outlook, 12*:36, 1964.

48. Rubin, R.: Attainment of the Maternal Role: Part I. Processes. *Nursing Research, 16*:237, 1967.

49. Rubin, R.: Attainment of the Maternal Role. Part II. Models and Referrants. *Nursing Research, 16*:342, 1967.

50. Rubin, R.: Maternity Nursing Stops too Soon. *American Journal of Nursing, 75*:1680, 1975.

51. Schroeder, M. A.: Is the Immediate Postpartum Period Crucial to the Mother-Child Relationship? *JOGN Nursing, 6*(3):37, 1977.

52. Shaw, N. R.: Teaching Young Mothers Their Role. *Nursing Outlook, 22*:695, 1974.

53. Sonstegard, L. J., and Egan, E.: Family-centered Nursing Makes a Difference. *American Journal of Maternal Child Nursing, 1*:249, 1976.

54. Stone, S. C., and Dickey, R. P.: Management of Nursing and Nonnursing Mothers. *Clinical Obstetrics and Gynecology, 18*:139, 1975.

55. Sumner, G., and Fritsch, J.: Postnatal Parental Concerns: The First Six Weeks of Life. *JOGN Nursing, 6*(3):27, 1977.

27

Physiologic and Psychologic Variations in the Puerperium

OBJECTIVES

1. Define:
   a. early hemorrhage
   b. late hemorrhage
   c. puerperal infection
   d. subinvolution
   e. mastitis
2. Describe common causes, nursing assessment, and nursing action relevant to early and late postpartum hemorrhage.
3. Identify women at risk for puerperal infection. Indicate nursing actions to prevent infection.
4. Describe signs of postpartum infection and nursing action in the treatment of infection.
5. Describe common breast complications, indicating appropriate nursing assessment and action.
6. Identify common reasons for subinvolution. Indicate factors in assessment that suggest subinvolution.
7. Describe the signs of upper and lower urinary tract infection. Indicate nursing for mother and infant.
8. Differentiate the signs of superficial and deep thromboembolic disease. Describe nursing actions for each problem. Indicate potential complications.
9. Describe emotional complications of the puerperium.

For most women the puerperium is a time of physiologic restitution and of individual and family integration. For some women and families, these goals are more difficult to achieve. Two major barriers are complications in the mother and illness in the infant. In this chapter both physiologic and psychologic variations in the puerperium are discussed. The effect of these alterations on maternal–infant attachment is discussed in Chapter 28.

Physiologic Complications During the Puerperium

Postpartum Hemorrhage

Normal blood loss following separation and expulsion of the placenta is 200 to 400 ml. Postpartum bleeding of more than 500 ml. is considered excessive and is defined as *postpartum hemorrhage*. When the bleeding occurs within the first 24 hours following delivery, it is considered *early* or *immediate* postpartum hemorrhage. *Late* or *delayed* postpartum hemorrhage occurs from 24 hours to the end of the puerperium. Characteristics of each type of hemorrhage are summarized in Table 27–1.

Although the potential for postpartum hemorrhage exists in all women, certain prenatal and intrapartal factors increase the risk (Table 27–2). Nursing assessment and intervention can frequently prevent postpartum hemorrhage or lead to its early recognition.

Uterine atony is by far the most common reason for early postpartum hemorrhage—i.e., hemorrhage in the first 24 hours following birth. Early hemorrhage occurs in 2 to 5 per cent of postpartum women.

Following the delivery of the placenta, the

Table 27–1. POSTPARTUM HEMORRHAGE

Type	Cause	Intervention
Early	Vaginal laceration Cervical laceration	Direct suture of laceration
	Tears of vaginal varicose veins	Packing of vagina
	Uterine atony	Massage of fundus Oxytocic drugs Packing uterus (if above inadequate) Hysterectomy (if above inadequate)
	Retained placenta	Removal Curettage
	Placenta accreta (placenta firmly adherent to myometrium) Placenta increta (placental tissues infiltrate myometrium)	Hysterectomy
	Laceration or rupture of uterus	Hysterectomy (Chapter 14)
	Inversion of uterus	Manual replacement and oxytocic drugs Laparotomy to reposition uterus (if above inadequate) Prophylactic antibiotics
	Coagulation defects	Treatment of cause Heparin Fibrinogen (see Fibrinogenopenia, Chapter 10)
Late	Retained placenta or membranes	Curettage
	Subinvolution of the uterus	Depends on cause (see text) Curettage Antibiotic drugs Oxytocic drugs
	Endometritis	Penicillin therapy Curettage (if no response to above)

Table 27–2. WOMEN AT INCREASED RISK OF POSTPARTUM HEMORRHAGE: RISK FACTORS

Reproductive History
    Previous postpartum hemorrhage
    Grand multiparity
    Uterine fibroids
General Health History
    Idiopathic thrombocytopenia purpura
    Chronic anemia
Current Pregnancy (prenatal or intrapartal factors)
    Abruptio placentae
    Placenta previa
    Uterine overdistention
    Prolonged precipitate or traumatic labor
    Chorioamnionitis
    Cesarean delivery
    General anesthesia
    Oxytocin induction
    Coagulation defect

uterus should be hard and globular as a result of the contraction of the interlacing myometrial fibers. These contracted fibers compress the blood vessels, thus providing hemostasis. The firmness of the fundus is assessed every 15 minutes; if the fundus is not firm it is massaged with one hand while the other hand is kept on the symphysis pubis to prevent inversion of the uterus (Chapter 17). The height of the fundus must also be noted; an increase in height may indicate the accumulation of blood or clots in the uterus. Because a full bladder is associated with uterine atony, bladder fullness is assessed, and the mother is encouraged to void.

Oxytocic drugs (Table 27–3) are routinely given in some delivery services to prevent hemorrhage. The same effect is provided naturally by the mother's own body when the baby is put to breast to nurse immediately after birth; endogenous oxytocin is released into the mother's circulation and the uterus contracts.

Bleeding is also assessed every 15 minutes (see Nursing Care Plan 27–1). An accurate assessment of blood loss is facilitated by weighing perineal pads; each gram of increase in weight is equivalent to 1 ml. of blood loss (see the section on weighing of diapers in high risk newborns to estimate urine output in Chapter 23). A count of the number of pads used is more commonly used, although it is less precise. Evaluation of blood pressure and pulse and the recording of fluid intake and output will also help to identify changes that are characteristic of hemorrhage and the resulting hypovolemia (i.e., decreasing blood pressure, increasing pulse, decreased urine output (see Nursing Care Plan 27–1).

When any of these signs are recognized, massage of the fundus may be all the intervention that is necessary. If massage is not successful, bimanual compression, in addition to stimulating uterine contraction, will exert pressure on the uterine veins and slow or stop bleeding. In severe hemorrhage, compression of the aorta just above the bifurcation between one's fist (or heel of the hand) and the vertebrae may slow bleeding. Because of the diastasis of the rectus abdominis muscle, this is easily achieved in the postpartum mother.

When hemorrhage is suspected, an IV is started immediately if it is not already in place. Those who argue for the use of an intravenous line in all laboring women believe that one reason this is important is the possibility of postpartum hemorrhage and the very rapid need for an IV in this instance. Those opposed believe that an IV is unnecessary for all women when only 2 to 5 per cent will have a postpartum hemorrhage, and many of these women will have risk factors that can be identified in advance.

If oxytocic drugs have not been given prophylactically, they are given when hemorrhage is suspected. Additional doses are usually given even when preventive medication was administered. Note in Table 27–3 that synthetic oxytocin lasts for a short time; ergot derivatives have longer action but the onset of action is slower than that of synthetic oxytocin.

If these measures do not stop the bleeding, further assessment of the cause by a physician is necessary. Bleeding in the presence of a firm uterus frequently indicates a laceration, the second most common reason for early postpartum hemorrhage. Other causes and interventions are summarized in Nursing Care Plan 27–1.

Continuing nursing assessment may detect signs of hypovolemic shock. Initially, the mother may be alert and anxious with the signs of hypovolemia described above and in Nursing Care Plan 27–1. If shock continues to progress she will become confused, pale, and cold, blood pressure will worsen, and tachycardia and tachypnea will occur. In late shock she may not respond to volume expansion.

When a mother suffers from shock she will need a level of intensive care equal to that given other shock victims, including oxygen, fluid therapy, and continuing assessment. Depending on individual hospital facilities, she may receive care in an intensive care unit. Special care must be taken to meet her needs as a new mother as well as her physiologic needs.

Late postpartum hemorrhage may occur as late as 6 to 8 weeks after birth. Late hemor-

Text continued on page 955

Table 27–3. MEDICATIONS TO PREVENT OR CONTROL UTERINE RELAXATION

Drug	Route	Dose	Onset of Action	Duration of action	Contraindications	Potential Side Effects	Comments
Synthetic oxytocin							
Pitocin	IV*	10–40 U (1–4 ml.)*	2–3 minutes	Sustained: 5–10 minutes	Hypertension	Nausea/vomiting (rare)	Uterus may fail to respond in woman with calcium deficiency
Syntocin	IM	10 U (1 ml.)		Intermittent: 30–45 minutes			
Ergot derivatives Ergonovine (Ergotrate)	Oral	0.2 mg.	5–10 minutes	1½–3 hours	Hypertension		
	IM	0.2 mg.	2–5 minutes		Breast-feeding	Hypertension Overdose: vomiting, diarrhea, dizziness, increased or decreased blood pressure	
Methylergonovine (Methergine)	Oral	0.2 mg.	5–10 minutes	1½–3 hours	Precautions: Sepsis	Nausea/vomiting Transient hypertension	
	IM	0.2 mg.	2–5 minutes		Heart disease Hepatic disease		
	IV†	0.2 mg.†	Immediate		Renal disease	Dizziness, headache, dyspnea	

*When Pitocin is given IV it is added to 500 to 1000 ml. of intravenous solution to dilute it; not to do so can lead to profound hypotension in the mother.

†Methergine is given IV only as an essential life-saving measure; it may cause sudden hypertension and cerebral vascular accident. If given IV it is given over a period of no less than 1 minute with continuous blood pressure monitoring.

Nursing Care Plan 27–1. Caring for the Mother with Postpartum Hemorrhage*

NURSING GOAL: To prevent postpartum hemorrhage.
To promote optimal recovery from postpartum hemorrhage.

OBJECTIVES: As a result of nursing actions:
1. Predisposing factors to hemorrhage are noted early.
2. Appropriate nursing measures are taken when hemorrhage occurs.
3. The parents understand the causes and treatment of hemorrhage.
4. The parents are allowed to ventilate their feelings.
5. Further complications are prevented.

ASSESSMENT	POTENTIAL NURSING DIAGNOSIS	NURSING INTERVENTION	COMMENTS/RATIONALE

1. Review the prenatal, labor, and delivery record for predisposing factors to hemorrhage.
a. History of excessive bleeding
b. Placenta previa
c. Abruptio placentae
d. Larger than average uterus
  1. Multiple pregnancy
  2. Polyhydramnios
  3. Large baby
e. Long labor
f. Difficult delivery
g. Multiple parity
h. Anemia
i. Medication history (e.g., aspirin)
j. Excessive analgesia or anesthesia
k. History of a tendency to bleed
	At risk for postpartum hemorrhage	Explain to the family the rationale for the assessments and the normality of the findings.
		
		Explain to the family the importance of more frequent assessments when there are factors predisposing to hemorrhage.
		
		If factors predisposing to hemorrhage are present, continue intravenous fluids until stability of the bleeding is ensured.
		
		Give oxytocic drugs as ordered. Maintain oxytocin longer than is routine if there is a history of factors predisposing to hemorrhage.
		
		When predisposing factors are present, the recovery room period will probably be longer. During the first 8 hours on the postpartum unit assess the patient at 1 hour, then every 4 hours during the next 15 hours.
			If one or more predisposing factors are present, make assessments more often than is routine. Hemorrhage is the leading cause of maternal mortality. Postdelivery hemorrhage is the most common and most serious type of excessive obstetric blood loss. Control of bleeding from the placental site is accomplished by prolonged contraction and retraction of interlacing strands of myometrium. Uterine contractions control bleeding by compressing and sealing off the blood vessels that enter the area left denuded by the placenta. Failure of the placenta to decrease progressively in size is an indication that involution is not proceeding satisfactorily. A contracted uterus does not bleed after delivery.

2. Assess and identify the first sign or symptom of excessive bleeding.	Potential for serious hemorrhage and complications if hemorrhage is not assessed and treated at immediate onset.	Keep accurate record of blood loss and report to physician: 1. Pad count—how often changed and how completely the pad is saturated 2. Record the characteristics of the bleeding: Color—bright or dark; consistency—thick or thin; clots—note size and number. 3. Determine cause of bleeding.	Pad count is the only accurate way to determine blood loss. Bright bleeding indicates current bleeding. Dark blood indicates blood that has collected in the uterus. Thin blood means current bleeding with poor clotting potential. Thick blood has more clotting potential.

Table continued on following page

Nursing Care Plan 27–1. Caring for the Mother with Postpartum Hemorrhage* Continued

ASSESSMENT	POTENTIAL NURSING DIAGNOSIS	NURSING INTERVENTION	COMMENTS/RATIONALE
3. Assess for cause of bleeding: a. Uterine atony b. Laceration c. Hypofibrinogenemia d. Retained placental fragments		a. Uterine atony—gentle massage of fundus, give or increase oxytocin medication. If massage fails to contract uterus, hold uterus tight with fist until other measures are available.	Oxytocin facilitates uterine contractions.
		b. Laceration—notify physician so that suturing may be done. Meanwhile, apply firm pressure and ice to laceration when possible.	Pressure tampons bleeding vessels. Ice constricts vessels to slow down or stop bleeding.
		c. Hypofibrinogenemia—in addition to other measures, give fibrinogen. (See Nursing Care Plan 13–10.)	Treatment for hypofibrinogenemia is fibrinogen replacement.
		d. Retained placental fragments—usually the cause of late hemorrhage. When early hemorrhage and other causes are ruled out, suspect retained placental fragments. Notify physician and institute all of the measures prescribed above and below for hemorrhage.	Bleeding from retained placental fragments may be immediate or sometime between the first and third weeks postpartum.
4. Ongoing assessment every 5 minutes until hemorrhage lessens: a. Fundal check b. Assess lochia, pad count, color, and consistency c. Blood pressure d. Pulse e. Skin color		4. General nursing measures for any type of hemorrhage. a. Massage if not firm; note the position of uterus in relation to umbilicus. Be alert to changes in position and changes in consistency of uterus.	Overmassage of uterus may cause uterine atony; therefore, massage only when uterus is atonic. A drop in blood pressure indicates hemorrhage. A rise of pulse rate or a weak, thready pulse indicates hemorrhage. Pale color, associated with other symptoms of hemorrhage, is significant.

Assessment	Intervention	Rationale
	b. Keep physician informed.	Physician should be informed, if not present, every 15–30 minutes when hemorrhage is critical or worsening. Notifications of physician should be recorded.
	c. Keep IV line open.	
	d. Administer oxytocin continuously.	
	e. See that blood is typed and cross-matched.	Because of time necessary to perform type and cross-matching, this should be done at the earliest sign of hemorrhage so that blood will be ready when needed.
	f. Keep bladder relatively empty.	A full bladder may keep the uterus from contracting, therefore causing more bleeding.
	g. Administer oxygen as indicated.	Since the red blood cell carries oxygen through the system, depletion of the blood supply depletes maternal oxygen. Administering oxygen can assist in compensating for oxygen loss through blood loss.
	h. Trendelenburg position as indicated.	Trendelenburg position causes maternal blood supply to gravitate toward the vital centers—head and heart.
5. Determine the parents' level of understanding of hemorrhage and its treatment. Possibility of lack of knowledge or misinterpretation of events.	During the emergency when the staff are busy with procedures, make time to give clear, simple, honest explanations to *both* parents of what is happening and what is being done. Encourage and answer questions. As soon as possible, listen to the parents and give and clarify information.	Parents cooperate with and tolerate emergency procedures much better when they understand the reasons for them. Explanations relieve some of the fear of the unknown.
	After the crisis is over, encourage and allow the parents to discuss their feelings and interpretation of events. Support the parents in their right to have the feelings they have. Make referrals to counselors, social workers as needed.	Parents need to have their immediate informational needs met, but later they need to discuss the events of the crisis with a nurse who will *listen,* clarify information, and support their opinions and feelings.

Table continued on following page

Nursing Care Plan 27–1.   Caring for the Mother with Postpartum Hemorrhage* *Continued*

ASSESSMENT	POTENTIAL NURSING DIAGNOSIS	NURSING INTERVENTION	COMMENTS/RATIONALE
6. Be alert to signs and symptoms of complications that may follow hemorrhage (e.g., infection, emotional disturbances, general debilitation). a. Change in vital signs (temperature, pulse, respirations, blood pressure) b. Lochia characteristics—color, odor	Possible further complications due to hemorrhage	1. All nursing measures should observe good medical asepsis: a. Handwashing b. Good perineal care. Always cleanse from front to back. c. Place untouched side of perineal pad to perineum.	Hemorrhage is the leading cause of maternal mortality. Infection is the number 2 cause. Many times infection is preceded by the debilitating effects of hemorrhage.
		2. Encourage good nutrition. a. Determine the patient's likes and dislikes. b. Encourage high protein and iron diet. c. Encourage plenty of fluids.	Protein and iron are needed for tissue regeneration and building hemoglobin. Increase in fluids will assist in preventing infection by increasing circulatory volume. Any two temperature readings of 100.4°F. or higher after the first 24 postpartum indicate infection.
		3. Encourage activity. a. Turning, coughing, and deep breathing while in bed. b. Early ambulation interspersed with adequate rest.	An increase in pulse and respiration could be symptomatic of infection. Early and continued activity is the best way to prevent postpartum infection.
7. Assess for any sign of emotional maladjustment. Particularly note mother–infant attachment.			When there are complications for the mother, she needs additional time and support to deal with her comfort and health before she can reach out to care for others such as infant or husband and other children when at home.

*Contributed by Hazel N. Brown

rhage is less frequent than early hemorrhage, occurring in 0.1 to 1.0 per cent of postpartum women. The most common cause is the retention of a fragment of placental membrane tissue. The retained tissue degenerates, interferes with involution, and becomes a culture medium for bacterial growth. A second cause, subinvolution (below) frequently occurs at the placental site. An underlying infection, which leads to sloughing of previously thrombosed blood vessels, is frequently associated with late postpartum hemorrhage.

If late postpartum hemorrhage occurs while the mother is hospitalized following delivery, treatment will generally include oxytocin, IV fluids, and curettage. Any evidence of infection will also be treated. Women with severe bleeding, as in early hemorrhage, require intensive assessment and nursing care.

If the mother has returned home and the bleeding is minimal, bed rest at home and an oral oxytocic (methylergonovine [Methergine]) may resolve the bleeding. Antibiotics are given if there is any evidence of endometritis (below). If bleeding following discharge is more than minimal, the mother is readmitted to the hospital. Plans for continued mother–infant interaction are essential if this should occur. Separation is very distressing, and every effort is made to maintain family interaction within the context of the mother's physical needs. Every hospital should have a plan of care that focuses on the mother–infant pair as well as the physiologic needs of the mother. Following readmission, physiologic intervention is the same as it was prior to discharge; IV fluid, oxytocin, curettage, and antibiotics if there are signs of infection. Blood loss and hypovolemia are assessed as described in Nursing Care Plan 27–1.

Puerperal Infection

Puerperal infection is a term that encompasses all bacteria-caused infections of the reproductive organs during labor or the puerperium. Synonyms include *puerperal sepsis, puerperal fever,* and *childbed fever.*

Prior to the twentieth century, puerperal sepsis was the major cause of maternal death. Many of our current practices that are now being questioned—the rigid separation of mothers and babies from other family members, for example—developed in the attempt to control puerperal sepsis.

Historical Perspective. Allegemeines Krankenhaus in Vienna was the largest maternity hospital in the late eighteenth and early nineteenth centuries. In 1840 the maternity service was divided. In one section, in-struction was given to medical students and care was given by them; in the other, midwives were taught and they gave the care. Although the medical students used cadavers in their studies, the midwives only used mannequins. By 1846, four times as many women on the wards where mothers were delivered by medical staff were dying as on the wards where midwives cared for mothers. The maternal mortality for the medical students' ward was 9.9 per 100 mothers, although two and three decades earlier the maternal mortality rate for the entire hospital had been only 1.3 per 100 mothers.

In 1846, Ignaz Philipp Semmelweis became assistant director of the medical students' clinic and began to search for the cause of the high rates of maternal mortality. He found that (1) infections were far more common in women with labors lasting more than 24 hours, and (2) sepsis was rare in women who delivered at home.

While Semmelweis pondered the possible significance of these facts, a friend cut his finger during an autopsy and subsequently died after a course of illness very similar to puerperal sepsis. Semmelweis was then able to recognize infection carried from the dissecting rooms to the mothers as the source of puerperal sepsis.

In 1847 Semmelweis asked medical students to scrub their hands with chloride of lime before they examined women who were pregnant. By 1848 the maternal mortality rate (which had risen to 11.4 per cent in 1846) was 1.27 per cent, lower even than that of the midwives (1.33 per cent in 1848). Nevertheless, Semmelweis and his ideas were ridiculed by most of his colleagues, and Semmelweis became embittered, and mentally ill before his death in 1865.

A generation later, in 1879, Pasteur demonstrated the relationship between bacteria (the existence of which was unknown until 1863) and puerperal sepsis.

Meanwhile in the United States in 1843 Oliver Wendell Holmes was also suggesting that physicians might be a causative factor in puerperal fever, an idea no more welcome to the American medical community than that of Semmelweis to his European colleagues. Holmes, however, became the Dean of the Harvard Medical School and in a publication in 1855 titled *Puerperal Fever as a Private Pestilence* was able to win his point. Maternal mortality improved significantly, but the isolation of mother and baby from the contaminated outside world (including fathers) also became an increasingly frequent practice.

Etiology. The anatomic and physiologic

Table 27–4.   GENERAL CLASSIFICATION OF PUERPERAL INFECTIONS

Type	Source	Predisposing Factors	Comments
Endogenous infection	Bacteria in the genital tract Septicemia Sepsis in adjacent organ	Excess bruising of tissue due to prolonged labor Traumatic delivery Instruments used in labor or in delivery Retained placenta, membranes, or clots of blood Exhaustion superimposed on trauma Hemorrhage superimposed on trauma Severe anemia Malnutrition	Usually mild; rarely fatal
Exogenous infection	Organisms from nurses, physicians, and other caretakers Environment Marital partner (gonorrhea and syphilis) Patient's hands	Same as for endogenous infection	Most common type of infection

changes of pregnancy and of delivery leave the reproductive tract of the woman recently delivered particularly susceptible to infection. In addition, certain women are at increased risk, including:

1. Women with untreated local infections during pregnancy.
2. Women with prolonged labor (more than 24 hours) or difficult labor and/or delivery.
3. Women with anemia.
4. Women in whom lacerations of the reproductive tract occur.
5. Women who require uterine exploration following delivery (for example, exploration for a retained placenta).
6. Women who have had a cesarean delivery.

Infection may develop from organisms already present in the reproductive tract (endogenous or autoinfection) or, more commonly, from organisms introduced from other individuals or the environment (Table 27–4).

Infections are also classified by site. Common sites include the vulva *(vulvitis)*, the vagina *(vaginitis)*, the endometrium *(endometritis)*, connective tissue in the pelvis *(pelvic cellulitis)*, and the pelvic cavity *(peritonitis)*. Local infections may lead to septicemia, bacterial invasion of the bloodstream, and thrombophlebitis (inflammation of the veins of the pelvis and legs).

Common causative organisms include streptococci (particularly beta-hemolytic streptococci), *Escherichia coli*, staphylococci (particularly *S. aureus* and *S. albus*), and *Bacteroides*.

Symptoms. A temperature of 100.4°F. (38°C.) after the first 24 hours following delivery that remains elevated for more than 24 hours strongly suggests the possibility of puerperal sepsis. Other signs, more specific to the varying types of sepsis, are summarized in Table 27–5.

Treatment: General Principles. The treatment of puerperal sepsis is similar to that of all infections. Antibiotics specific to the causative organisms, once the results of cultures are known, have made a remarkable difference in treatment.

Nursing measures remain important, nevertheless (Nursing Care Plan 27–2). A high fluid intake is encouraged, usually from 3000 to 4000 ml. per day. If the mother is unable to take adequate fluids orally, parenteral fluids are given.

Rest is a major component of care. A semi-Fowler's position may be recommended to promote the flow of lochia; keeping the mother comfortable in this position is part of the nursing challenge.

Keeping the uterine muscle contracted by fundal massage and administration of oxytocics will slow the spread of bacteria through

Text continued on page 962

Nursing Care Plan 27–2. Caring for the Mother with Postpartum Infection*

NURSING GOALS: To prevent infection of the postpartum mother.
To provide optimal care for the postpartum mother with infection.

OBJECTIVES: As a result of nursing actions:
1. Predisposing factors to infection are noted early.
2. Appropriate care is provided for the mother with infection.
3. The parents understand the causes and treatment of the infection.
4. Mother–infant attachment is facilitated as much as possible.
5. Further complications are prevented.

ASSESSMENT	POTENTIAL NURSING DIAGNOSIS	NURSING INTERVENTION	COMMENTS/RATIONALE
1. Review the prenatal, labor, delivery, and postpartum record to date for predisposing factors to infection. a. Untreated local infections during pregnancy or labor b. Prolonged or difficult labor c. Premature or prolonged rupture of membranes d. Anemia e. Lacerations of the reproductive tract during delivery f. Uterine exploration following delivery g. Sore or cracked nipples or bruised breast tissue h. Varicose veins or tenderness or soreness of legs i. Poor ambulation j. Hemorrhagic complication	At risk for postpartum infection	1. When any predisposing factors are present, meticulous attention should be directed toward the prevention of postpartum infection. General nursing care for the prevention of infection: a. Handwashing—for nursing staff and patient before caring for patient, especially breast and perineal care. b. Cleanse perineum from front to back. Keep perineum as clean and dry as possible. c. Place untouched side of perineal pad to the perineum. d. Encourage good nutrition, especially protein, iron, and fluids—3000 to 4000 ml. per day. e. Encourage activity—turn, cough, and deep breathing while in bed. Early ambulation.	Most microorganisms are transported by unclean hands. Wiping from front to back prevents organisms from the rectum from entering the vagina. Protein and iron are needed for tissue regeneration and for building hemoglobin. An increase in fluids assists in the prevention of infection by increasing the circulating volume. Early and continued activity prevents infection by increasing circulation.

Table continued on following page

Nursing Care Plan 27–2. Caring for the Mother with Postpartum Infection* (Continued)

ASSESSMENT	POTENTIAL NURSING DIAGNOSIS	NURSING INTERVENTION	COMMENTS/RATIONALE
2. Assess for changes in vital signs, general status, lochia. a. Temperature, pulse, respirations b. Pain—breast, abdominal, perineal, leg c. Lochia—character, color d. Signs and symptoms of infection—chills, loss of appetite, general malaise		f. Ensure adequate rest.	Rest is important for tissue healing and for general well-being. Any two temperature readings of 100.4°F. or higher after the first 24 hours postpartum indicate infection. Increases in pulse and respiration rates are symptomatic of infection.
3. Determine the appropriate nursing care for the specific infection.	Potential for further complications if appropriate nursing care is not given	2. *Puerperal sepsis†* a. General nursing care (no. 1, above) b. Antibiotics specific to the causative organism c. Semi-Fowler's position while in bed d. Keep uterine muscles contracted by fundal massage and oxytocin. e. Isolation procedures †Usually becomes manifest on the third or fourth postpartum day. 3. *Thrombophlebitis‡* a. General nursing care (no. 1 above) b. Be alert to early signs and symptoms. (1) May be preceded by endometritis (2) Positive Homan's sign (3) An area of leg (usually calf) is white with a drained appearance, and the area below the affected part is edematous.	A culture is done to determine the specific causative organism. The specific antibiotic for the organism can be given. Semi-Fowler's position promotes lochia flow and uterine drainage. A contracted uterus slows the spread of bacteria through the walls of the uterus and aids in the expulsion of clots or retained membranes or placental fragments that facilitate infection. Isolation procedures prevent the transfer of organisms to nurse, other staff, and other patients. If early signs and symptoms are detected, treatment may prevent critical problems. Infection in the vein is accompanied by arterial spasm that diminishes arterial circulation. This decreased circulation and edema give the leg the white, drained appearance.

(4) Decrease in breast milk (amount)	Breast milk decreases due to the increase in temperature and the body's attempt to conserve fluid.
c. Report immediately early signs and symptoms and later symptoms. 　(1) Chills 　(2) Stiffness, pain, and redness in the affected part. d. Antibiotics specific to the causative organism	
e. Bed rest with affected leg elevated and protected with a cradle	The leg is elevated to facilitate circulation. The cradle keeps the pressure of bedclothes off the affected leg to decrease sensitivity of the leg and to improve circulation.
f. Never rub or massage the affected leg. g. Early ambulation is the best prevention of thrombophlebitis.	Ambulation or rubbing the leg could dislodge the thrombus, which would then become an embolus.
h. Anticoagulants.	Anticoagulant therapy may be started to prevent further formation of clots and to dissolve the present one.
‡Thrombophlebitis becomes manifest around the tenth postpartum day.	
3. *Mastitis* a. General nursing care (no. 1, above). b. Be alert to early predisposing factors: 　(1) Cracked or fissured nipples	When the patient can prevent sore, cracked nipples (see Nursing Care Plan 26–5), the chances of having mastitis are greatly lessened.
(2) Clogged milk duct 　(3) Infant colonized with staphylococci in the hospital nursery.	Mastitis may occur as early as seventh postpartum day or when the infant is weeks or months old. Therefore, the mother needs careful instruction in early detection of signs and symptoms of mastitis.
c. Teach mother to report early the presence of predisposing factors, and the importance of preventing sore, cracked nipples.	

Table continued on following page

Nursing Care Plan 27–2. Caring for the Mother with Postpartum Infection* *(Continued)*

ASSESSMENT	POTENTIAL NURSING DIAGNOSIS	NURSING INTERVENTION	COMMENTS/RATIONALE
		d. Be alert to symptoms and report immediately.	
		(1) General: headache, malaise, chilling, "flulike" symptoms, rapid pulse	
		(2) Specific: breast— engorged, red, hard, hot to touch, tender, and painful	
		e. Specific treatment:	
		(1) Rest	Rest is important to conserve maternal energy to respond to the infection.
		(2) Local heat to breast	Heat increases circulation to the area. The increased circulation brings more nutrients for healing.
		(3) Keep breast as empty as possible.	Breast needs to be empty to reduce congestion and allow healing.
		(4) Wear supporting bra.	Supporting bra facilitates good circulation in the breast.
		(5) Take analgesic medication before nursing.	Neither the infection nor the antibiotic affects the infant.
		(6) Antibiotic specific to the causative organism	Endometritis may present while the patient is hospitalized or later. Thrombophlebitis and mastitis tend to present after the patient is discharged from the hospital. Therefore, it is imperative that parents know how to prevent the condition and how to recognize early signs and symptoms of infection.
4. Determine the parents' understanding of the infectious process and the treatment being given.	At risk of being noncompliant if they do not understand what is happening with the mother	Teach parents the early signs and symptoms of infection and how to prevent infection.	
		Keep parents informed continuously.	
		Listen to their concerns and questions.	

5. Determine the quality of the mother–infant attachment.

Possible inadequate mother–infant attachment due to the illness of the mother

Unless the mother has an infection that is contagious and the infant might contract it if exposed to the mother, take the infant to the mother every 4 hours for viewing and holding, even though the mother is on bed rest.

If mother is breast-feeding, continue to feed unless infection is contagious (puerperal sepsis).

Explain to parents that a delay in the mother's "mothering feelings" is normal when mother is ill.

Encourage the father to try to compensate with father–infant attachment.

Note and compliment good attachment.

Make arrangements to follow through with evaluation of mother–infant attachment:
1. At time of check-up
2. Public health nurse

Rubin has noted that even well mothers have a need for normal body function before they begin to "mother." This behavior is appropriate when there is a maternal complication, but it is a barrier to mothering.

Mothers with mastitis and mothers with thrombophlebitis may continue breast-feeding, even though they are unable to perform infant or self-care.

Milk supply may be diminished due to elevated temperature. The supply should resume if the baby nurses well after temperature becomes normal.

Missed opportunity for initial attachment may affect later attachment. Therefore, attachment should be followed up.

6. Determine the extent of further complications from the infection.

At risk for further complications from the infection

Give the best nursing care possible to promote maximum recovery and prevent further complications.

Complications that may follow infections are:
1. Puerperal sepsis → peritonitis, septicemia, septic shock, and death.
2. Mastitis → breast abscess, incision and drainage → septicemia and death.
3. Thrombophlebitis → thromboembolus, pulmonary embolism, heart attack, cerebral vascular accident, and death.

Infection is the second leading cause of maternal mortality. With prevention and early detection and treatment most complications can be prevented.

*Contributed by Hazel N. Brown.

Table 27–5.   PUERPERAL SEPSIS IN VARIOUS SITES

Infection	Cause	Symptoms	Treatment
Vulvitis; vaginitis	Trauma Infection during labor	Inability to urinate Local pain from swelling	Removal of sutures to effect drainage Sitz baths Perineal heat lamp Antibiotics
Endometritis		Slight chills Temperature above 100.4°F. (38°C.) Rapid pulse Uterus relaxed and tender Foul-smelling or profuse lochia Malaise Vomiting and diarrhea (as infection progresses)	Appropriate antibiotics for organism involved
Pelvic cellulitis	Lacerations of the cervix, lower uterine segment, or vagina	Tender unilateral swelling of cervix that spreads laterally Temperature above 100.4°F. (38°C.) for more than 24 hours; may be several degrees higher	Bed rest Antibiotics Maintain hydration Blood transfusion if hemoglobin level drops
Pelvic peritonitis	Spread of infection from genital organs	Acute local pain Temperature above 100.4°F. (38°C.) for more than 24 hours Rapid pulse Frequent vomiting Abdominal distention (usually subsequent to above symptoms) Rapid and tender abdomen during acute attack	Same as for cellulitis
Septicemia	Septic invasion of the bloodstream	Acute onset during first 3 postpartum days Rapid pulse in absence of blood loss High temperature Scant or absent lochia in overwhelming septicemia	Antibiotics Fluids Bed rest

the walls of the uterus and aid in the expulsion of clots or membranes that facilitate infection.

Ideally, the nurse who cares for mothers with an infection should not care for other mothers. This is not practical in every setting. Scrupulous handwashing along with other isolation precautions can protect other mothers, however.

The policies of most hospitals will not allow mothers with sepsis to hold and care for their babies. Many of the organisms that cause infection in the mother, beta-hemolytic strepto-

Table 27–6.   SUPERFICIAL AND DEEP THOMBOPHLEBITIS

	Clinical Signs	Time of Onset	Treatment	Complications
Superficial	Slight temperature elevation Slight tachycardia Leg pain, tenderness Localized redness, heat	3–4 days postpartum	Bed rest Warm soaks Elevation of affected leg Elastic bandages or stockings Bed cradle to keep covers away from leg Analgesics or anti-inflammatory drugs; aspirin, phenylbutazone	Spread to deep vein
Deep	Marked temperature elevation, chills Tachycardia Severe leg pain Tenderness along course of affected vessel Positive Homan's sign* Edema of ankle, leg, thigh Extremity may be cold and pale (arterial spasm)	6–10 days postpartum	All of above Anticoagulant therapy—heparin or coumarin Antibiotics	Pulmonary embolism

*Homan's signs: With the mother's leg extended on the bed, place one hand on her knee, applying gentle pressure. With the other hand dorsiflex the foot. Calf pain is a positive Homan's sign.

cocci, for example, are highly dangerous for newborns (Chapter 23) and can be a cause of death. It becomes our responsibility to talk with the mother about her baby and in as many ways as possible to facilitate bonding during the time mother and baby must be separated (above). Lawrence[16] has stated that once a therapeutic level of antibiotics has been established for 12 hours, infants can be permitted to breast-feed. Bottle-fed infants are usually separated from their mothers for a longer period of time because they are not receiving the protective advantages of breast-feeding. Table 27–6 summarizes the specifics of treatment.

Septicemia and Septic Shock

Localized infection, if not recognized early and treated vigorously, may become systemic (septicemia) and in a few instances may result in septic shock.

Signs of septicemia include tachypnea, respiratory alkalosis, and later, fever and chills, tachycardia, and oliguria. The mother frequently appears confused and restless. Initially, cardiac output is increased, and vasodilatation occurs as the body responds to increased metabolic demands of the cells. Hyperventilation, another coping response, leads to respiratory alkalosis. Blood pressure may be low in spite of increased cardiac output because of peripheral vasodilatation.

If the mother is already hypovolemic, cardiac output will be low, with low central venous pressure and hypotension. As shock deepens, metabolic acidosis occurs. Acid accumulates in the cells, the capillary arteriolar sphincters relax, blood pools in the capillary beds, arterial blood pressure decreases, the myocardium becomes depressed, and heart failure ensues. (For a more detailed explanation see Kenner.[15]) The mother is critically ill and requires an intensive level of continuing assessment and care including intravenous fluids, oxygen, antibiotics, and vasoactive drugs. Drainage of infected areas, dilatation and curettage, and occasionally hysterectomy may be necessary in order to remove the source of infection. (See Kenner[15] and other critical care nursing texts for a discussion of septic shock.) Nurses who care for postpartum mothers should be alert to the early signs of infection (above) to prevent these serious sequelae.

Breast Complications

Breast complications occur on a continuum. The least serious complications are the most frequent; the most serious are relatively rare. Moreover, proper attention to the less serious consequences will often prevent more serious problems.

Potential breast complications are sore nipples (Chapter 26), cracked or bleeding nipples, engorgement (Chapter 26), a clogged milk duct, mastitis, and breast abscess.

A part of the nursing care plan for mothers who are breast-feeding is teaching them to recognize early signs of these complications so that they can be promptly treated, and less severe complications will not become more severe.

Clogged Milk Duct. When one section of the breast is tender, with a small, sometimes reddened area, it is possible that the milk duct in that area has become clogged. Untreated, a clogged milk duct may become infected.

The principle of treatment of a clogged duct is keeping the breast as nearly empty as possible and the milk flowing. The baby is nursed frequently (every 2 to 3 hours) and always on the affected side first, so that that breast will be more completely emptied. After each feeding, any milk remaining in the affected breast is expressed by hand. The mother should make sure that her bra is not too binding or too tight in any area, since this may place pressure on a part of the duct system. She can also be sure that any dried secretions covering the nipple are rinsed away (they may need prior soaking to loosen them) so that the milk flows freely.

Mastitis. There are several potential routes by which a mother may develop mastitis. If her baby has become colonized with staphylococci in a hospital nursery, he may transmit the organism to her breasts. The mother's own hands or the hands of hospital personnel may introduce the organism. If nipples are cracked or fissured, if breast tissue is bruised, or if a duct is clogged, the potential for infection is higher. Therefore early recognition of these predisposing factors is important.

Symptoms. Initial symptoms of mastitis may be one or more of the following: headache, an elevated temperature with or without chilling, malaise, aching and other "flulike" symptoms, and a rapid pulse rate. The breast may be engorged, reddened, very hard and hot to the touch, and tender and/or painful.

Treatment. The treatment of mastitis includes rest for the mother, local heat to the affected breast, and keeping the breast as empty as possible. Specific suggestions to the mother include the following:

1. Rest in bed as much as possible; a prone (face down) position is preferable.

2. Apply warm, lightweight, wet compresses to the affected breast. Clean washcloths are fine. Cover the compresses with plastic wrap to hold the moisture. Change every 2 hours.

3. Nurse the baby frequently; every 2 to 3 hours. Nurse on the affected side first to empty that breast more completely. (At one time the mother with mastitis was told to discontinue nursing or to discard the milk from the affected breast. This is no longer believed to be necessary because the causative organism is probably already in the baby's nose and mouth. Nor will the antibiotics that may be prescribed for the mother harm the baby.)

4. A firm bra will support the mother's breasts and make her more comfortable.

5. One aspirin-phenacetin-caffeine (A.P.C.) tablet may be taken prior to nursing.

If the mother has a fever, penicillin may be prescribed (penicillin G, 250,000 units, every 4 hours is a usual recommendation).

Early treatment usually resolves mastitis in a short time, often in 2 to 3 days, and the mother is able to continue breast-feeding as long as she desires. In the rare instance when a mother has repeated mastitis, we must help her examine handwashing practices, her methods of laundry, and so on.

Breast Abscess. A breast abscess is a localized complication of a more generalized infection (mastitis), in which pus accumulates in a local area. The treatment for an abscess is an antibiotic and may also include surgical incision and drainage of the abscess.

When an abscess occurs, the mother should discontinue nursing on the affected side; she should express milk by hand from that breast and discard it until the abscess heals. Meanwhile, she can continue to nurse on the unaffected breast.

When a staphylococcal *epidemic* occurs in the nursery, mothers may develop a staphylococcal breast abscess 2 weeks to 8 months following birth.

Shinefeld[23] has suggested that colonized infants should not be breast-fed when there is an epidemic. The organism may pass from the infant's nasopharynx to the mother's breast and back to the infant. However, infant colonization is usually not recognized until after breast-feeding begins. Symptoms occurring in the mother are a spiking fever, chills, tachycardia, malaise, headache, and a localized red, tender, swollen area on the breast. Breast-feeding is stopped when symptoms appear, and antibiotic treatment is started. The abscess may require draining. There is no consensus on whether to resume breast-feeding.

Subinvolution

Subinvolution is the term that describes the failure of the uterus to return to postnatal size and consistency within the usual period of time. Two common reasons are retention of placental fragments or fragments of the fetal membranes or infection of the endometrium (endometritis).

In checking the height of the fundus each day and the color and amount of the lochia, the nurse may suspect subinvolution. The fundus will be higher than expected and the lochia more profuse and red.

The treatment will depend upon the cause; it may include curettage to remove retained fragments, antibiotics for infection, and an oxytocic preparation to stimulate contraction of the uterine muscle.

Complications of the Urinary Tract

The effect of labor and delivery on the bladder was described in Chapter 25. When measures are not taken to ensure adequate voiding, *cystitis,* due to residual urine and/or bladder trauma, may result. The mother may complain of frequent, painful voiding or of suprapubic or perineal pain. She may recognize the fact that she has not emptied her bladder completely. She may have a slight temperature elevation (100° to 101°F. or 37.8° to 38.3°C.). Urine examination reveals bacteria, pus, and frequently red blood cells.

Upper urinary tract infection (e.g., pyelitis, pyelonephritis) is suspected when there is flank tenderness (i.e., tenderness in the area of one or both kidneys). Other symptoms include frequency of urination, an elevated temperature that may be accompanied by chills, and nausea and vomiting. As in any infection, malaise may be present. Bacteria and pus are found in the urine.

Treatment of both lower and upper urinary tract infections includes specific antibiotic therapy, 3000 to 4000 ml. of fluid per day, and emptying of the bladder. The mother usually remains in bed.

Urinary tract infections are not a hazard to the infant unless the causative organism is a beta-hemolytic *Streptococcus* (which is uncommon). Mothers should wash their hands carefully before touching their babies.

If the mother is breast-feeding, sulfa medications should not be used during the first month following birth because they interfere with the binding of bilirubin to albumin. Ampicillin is given, and, although it is excreted in breast milk, is not considered harmful to the baby.

Thromboembolic Disease

Thrombophlebitis was at one time so closely associated with the puerperium that the condition was called milk leg. Today thrombophlebitis occurs in 1 per cent of vaginal deliveries and 2 to 5 per cent of cesarean births.

The effect of progesterone on the walls of the veins, resulting in venous stasis, predisposes women to thrombophlebitis and embolism. Women with varicosities are particularly at risk. Immobilization from anesthesia, prolonged bed rest, and the prolonged use of stirrups during the intrapartum period may also contribute to thrombophlebitis. Thrombophlebitis may occur in either the superficial or deep veins. Sites include veins in the tibial, popliteal, femoral, and pelvic areas. The symptoms of superficial phlebitis are usually milder than those that occur when the deep veins are involved (Table 27–6). However, clinical signs are present only 40 to 50 per cent of the time.

The treatment of thromboembolic disease is summarized in Table 27–7 and Nursing Care Plan 27–2. Heparin, because it is a large molecule, does not cross into breast milk; coumarin will be secreted in breast milk.

The most serious complication of thrombophlebitis (almost always deep thrombophlebitis), is *pulmonary embolism.* In 50 to 80 per cent of instances of pulmonary embolism there are no prior signs.[10] The mother experiences sudden apprehension, sharp chest pain, dyspnea, tachypnea, and hemoptysis. Auscultation reveals rales and a friction rub.

Intensive care is necessary when a pulmonary embolism occurs. Although mortality is 1 per cent in treated women it is as high as 10 to 20 per cent in untreated women. Because pulmonary embolism commonly occurs at the end of the first week, the mother may have returned home before symptoms occur. Prompt recognition of the seriousness of the symptoms, whether they are first encountered in a telephone call or in person, may be life-saving.

Treatment usually includes:

1. Hospitalization.
2. Oxygen.
3. Narcotics for the relief of pain and apprehension.
4. $NaHCO_3$ for metabolic acidosis.
5. Aminophylline for bronchospasm.
6. Heparin.
7. Streptokinase that activates the fibrino-

Table 27–7. COMMON SYMPTOMS OF POSTPARTUM NEUROSES

Symptom	Characteristics	Comments
Depression	Varies from mild and transitory to deep and long-lasting	Most common symptom Prenatal depression lasting several months may recur postpartum
Neurasthenia	Extreme fatigue Sleeplessness Emotional lability Irritability	May last from several months to a year May be incapacitating
Anxiety	Pronounced Mother may feel abandoned by short absences of husband	May become chronic if not appropriately cared for at early stage
Phobias	Fear of infanticide Fear of insanity	Often a single episode; except in schizophrenia (a psychosis), the risk of infanticide is not present
Sexual difficulties	Decreased libido Incapacity for orgasm	More pronounced than during pregnancy
Psychosomatic complaints	Frequent and varied complaints of physical symptoms	Distinguish carefully from physical symptoms

lytic enzyme in the serum in order to rapidly dissolve clots and the fibrinous portion of exudates.

Nurses who care for mothers with pulmonary embolism should be thoroughly familiar with both the condition and the side effects of the medications used. Frequently, the mother will be in an intensive care unit, which is better equipped to meet her physiologic needs than the maternity unit. As soon as the mother is physically able, her needs as a new mother must be incorporated into her plan of care.

Foot Drop

Postpartum foot drop, a sudden loss of sensation along the anterolateral aspect of the leg and foot combined with a loss of ankle dorsiflexion, occurs in 1 of 2500 deliveries. Compression and stretching of the lumbosacral nerve trunk or peripheral peroneal nerves is the basis of foot drop; compression may be caused by retractors or hematomas in a cesarean birth, by the fetal head during a prolonged labor, or by forceps. At times, foot drop occurs after an apparently uncomplicated vaginal delivery.

The mother will limp on the affected side and experience numbness. Generally, improvement occurs within a week, although total recovery may take as long as 3 months. A foot pushboard and splinting will prevent contractions. Occasionally complete recovery does not occur.

It is not hard to imagine a mother's distress at having her mobility compromised at a time when the needs of her new baby make mobility especially important. Reassurance that the problem resolves spontaneously in a few weeks in most instances can help. Parents may need help in planning for infant care and other activities during these weeks.

Separation of the Symphysis Pubis

Relaxation of the symphysis pubis and the sacroiliac joints occurs in many women during the prenatal period. In some women pubic ligaments rupture, and the symphysis separates from 1 to 8 cm., often in association with such factors as abnormal presentation, shoulder dystocia, use of forceps, precipitous delivery of a large infant—all situations in which tension is placed on the pubic ligaments.

The mother experiences suprapubic pain; it is difficult for her to turn in bed or to get out of bed. If she is able to walk she has a waddling gait; her feet and legs rotate externally. The area over the symphysis is swollen and very tender. A gaping defect may be palpated.

The goal of therapy is immobilization of the joint; this is accomplished by bed rest and a pelvic binder. Bed rest at home is very difficult for a new mother. Parents will need help in planning for infant care as well as in meeting their own needs. Some families may need the help of a homemaker service (available in some communities) or other assistance. A referral to a community health nurse will help to ensure continuity of nursing care.

Emotional Complications During the Puerperium

Just as physiologic problems during the puerperium can interfere with family integration, maternal emotional problems can restrict mothering and affect every member of the family.

Considerable ambiguity clouds discussion of emotional complications during the puerperium. There is often no clear distinction made between disorders precipitated by childbirth and disorders occurring in the postpartum period but not critically related to childbirth. Some postpartum reactions may begin during pregnancy; others occur after delivery.

Some reactions appear to be caused by immediate difficulties of motherhood; others seem to be based on deep-seated conflicts concerning femininity, motherhood, or sexual and reproductive roles. Nevertheless, there seem to be basic areas of agreement that can be helpful both in clinical nursing practice and in developing nursing research.

Like all emotional illness, emotional complications of the puerperium can be divided into psychoses and neuroses. Psychotic illness is far less frequent, estimated to occur in 1 or 2 women per 1000 deliveries. Neurotic illness, chiefly depression, is estimated to occur in 1 to 3 of every 100 postpartum women, or approximately 10 times more frequently. In addition, less marked symptoms occur in a larger number of women; some estimate this incidence to be as high as one out of four women in the postpartum year. (Estimates vary considerably, depending upon the definition of illness.)

Postpartum Neuroses

Neurosis is the term often used to describe all mental illness of a nonpsychotic nature. Neuroses, which restrict the individual's functioning and disturb her well-being, include anxiety states, phobias, obsessions, hypochondriasis, and depression. In the postpartum period, depression has repeatedly been found to be the most common neurosis.

Postpartum neuroses cannot be viewed as a specific entity but rather as part of the health–illness continuum. At one end of the continuum are mothers who exhibit symptoms of postpartum blues (Chapter 25), which are considered a part of normal emotion lability in the first days following pregnancy. At the opposite end of the continuum are women with symptoms sufficiently severe to require hospitalization or intensive treatment. This group represents from 1 to 3 per cent of women who have delivered.

Between these two extremes are a large number of women who exhibit some symptoms, such as despondency, tearfulness, feelings of inadequacy or inability to cope, hypochondria, irritability, undue fatigue, decrease in appetite, difficulties in sleeping, decreased libido, and fears for the baby's health.

Since these symptoms are very general and since many of them may, and usually do, occur at one time or other in most new mothers, the recognition of illness is obviously a matter of degree. For example, all mothers have periods of fatigue (lack of sleep is a frequent hazard of new parents), but chronic fatigue that is unrelieved by rest may indicate illness. There are days when each new mother may feel inadequate to cope—days when the baby seems to cry incessantly, for example—but the mother who has a constant feeling of inadequacy needs professional counseling.

Characteristics of Mothers Who Develop Postpartum Neuroses. Is it possible to predict which mothers will have postpartum neuroses and thereby to give them special attention and perhaps even to prevent their symptoms or alleviate their severity? In a very specific sense the answer is no, although certain factors in common do appear in the research literature.

In both prospective and retrospective studies,[18, 19] a past history of neurosis was found to be the single most important factor in predicting neurotic reactions during or after pregnancy.

Bardon[2] found unconscious conflicts about assuming the roles and responsibilities of mothering to be the most frequent and most important stress factor. He suggests that real or fantasized difficulties between a child and her parents—an unhappy relationship or unmet dependency needs, for example—are transferred to her own child. As the child of the mother becomes the mother of the child, she sees herself in her child and her mother in herself. Kaij and Nilsson[14] suggest that women with poor or unsatisfactory relations with their mothers during infancy and adolescence; women insufficiently informed about sexual matters, especially menarche; and women with early sexual experience and more than one sexual partner are more likely to have a negative attitude toward pregnancy and to develop postpartum neurosis.

Tod, in a prospective study of 700 consecutive pregnancies, found 20 mothers (2.9 per cent) with postpartum depression (1958 to 1963).[26] He described all of them as having "inadequate personalities" (introverted and with symptoms of neuroses). Other characteristics included: abnormal psychiatric history: 55 per cent; abnormal marital history: 55 per cent; abnormal obstetric history: 60 per cent; anemia: 40 per cent; previous medical problems: 20 per cent; and previous stillbirth or baby with a congenital defect: 25 per cent. Tod found that neither social class nor age was significant.

The presence or absence of "postpartum blues" does not appear to be indicative of future emotional problems. Behavior during the brief period of hospitalization that may indicate abnormality includes a lack of interest in the child (failure to name him or call him by name, disinterest in feeding and holding him, and so on) and a marked concern about the problems to be faced by the mother when she returns home.

Barglow and associates[3] found that 25 per cent of women with postpartum mental illness had a recurrence in a subsequent pregnancy.

Contributing Factors. In addition to factors within the mother's personality, other variables have been suggested as possible contributors to postpartum neuroses.

Hormonal factors, particularly the postnatal fall in progesterone, have been postulated as contributing to neurosis.

Tod has questioned the role of folic acid as a causative factor. From 1958 to 1963, he found an incidence of depression of 2.9 per cent in 700 women.[26] In a retrospective study of 700 women who delivered between 1965 and 1970, only 0.9 per cent of the second group were depressed. He suggests that the fall may be related to the routine administration of folic acid during pregnancy during the second time span. Folic acid has been shown to be related to mental disturbance in some other conditions, including tropical sprue, prenicious anemia, and postgastrectomy anemia.[24, 25]

Cone found the incidence of depression to be lower in mothers who delivered at home than in mothers who delivered in hospital.[7] Her study, done in Cadiff, Wales, where home deliveries are common, may reflect differences in mothers who choose home versus mothers who choose hospital (mothers were matched for parity and mode of delivery) or may suggest factors in the hospital environment, an idea worth exploring further.

Other areas that have been investigated, with no conclusive findings, include age, social status, parity, and specific genetic factors.

Symptoms. The most common symptoms of postpartum neuroses are summarized in Table 27–7.

Treatment. The treatment will vary with the specific diagnosis. Antidepressive drugs, psychotherapy, and allowing the mother to express her distress and incompletely acknowledged hostilities are major principles of treatment.

Bardon[2] suggests that when hospital admission is necessary, admitting both mother and infant will enable them to have good experiences together, rather than confirming the mother's existing doubts and feelings of inadequacy.

Untreated, symptoms may persist for a year or more, with potentially devastating consequences for the entire family.

Postpartum Psychoses

As noted above, psychoses are far less common than neuroses, but the impact of a psychotic mother on her family can be monumental.

Symptoms of puerperal psychosis include mixed or rapidly changing affects; a clouding of consciousness; hypochondriacal delusions; hallucinations; erroneous beliefs that the child is dead, malformed, or severely ill; and general anxiety.

The duration of illness may range from a few days to a year to a chronic state lasting many years. Kaij and Nilsson[14] report about 20 per cent of the women recovering within 1 month; 40 per cent having a course of illness lasting 6 months or longer, and 15 per cent becoming chronically ill. When the illness is chronic, there is some question as to whether it is a true postpartum psychosis or a preexisting condition that becomes more evident when the mother is faced with new responsibilities.

Although for many women the postpartum psychosis represents a single, discrete event, as many as 30 per cent may have further psychotic episodes. The ratio of risk of a subsequent postpartum psychosis occurring has been estimated to be as high as 1:7, although some researchers suggest only a slightly increased risk.

Treatment is directed toward the specific psychotic symptoms.

Fourth Trimester Care

Two generations ago, when mothers remained in the hospital from 10 days to 3 weeks, assessment of potential complications was not difficult. Today, however, with mothers returning home from 1 to 3 days after delivery, the opportunity for close assessment no longer exists. We have already noted that many mothers leave the health care system when they are discharged. Few will fail to seek medical attention for a dramatic symptom, such as marked hemorrhage or a high fever. But without follow-up, many women, particularly those without a private physician, may not seek care for less obvious problems, either physical or emotional.

One of the immediate challenges to our system of nursing care is a *systematic* way to provide care during the "fourth trimester." Donaldson[8] describes a follow-up program at Hoag Memorial Hospital-Presbyterian in California that includes:

1. Initial telephone contact with families after they return home.
2. Assessment of needs.
3. Reinforcement of teaching.
4. Repeated calls, home visits, and referral to other agencies when necessary.
5. Communication with appropriate staff and agencies.

Mothers know, and are reminded during the telephone calls, that they may call the maternity unit at any time, 24 hours a day.

In many communities in England, home visits by community health nurses are frequent for several weeks after delivery for all patients.

Nurses everywhere need to evaluate the fourth trimester care in their communities to better meet the needs of childbearing families.

REFERENCES

1. Assali, N., and Brinkman, C. (eds.): *Pathophysiology of Gestation.* Vol. 1, Maternal Disorders. New York, Academic Press, 1972.
2. Bardon, D.: Puerperal Depression. *In* Morris, N. (ed.): *Psychosomatic Medicine in Obstetrics and Gynecology.* Basel, S. Karger, 1972.
3. Barglow, P., Wilson, J., and Shipman, W.: The Nature of Post Partum Mental Illness. *In* Morris, N. (ed.): *Psychosomatic Medicine in Obstetrics and Gynecology.* Basel, S., Karger, 1972.
4. Barnard, M.: Supportive Nursing Care for the Mother and Newborn Who are Separated from Each Other. *MCN,* 1(2):107, 1976.
5. Brown, W.: A Prospective Study of Post Partum Psychiatric Disorders. *In* Morris, N. (ed.): *Psychosomatic Medicine in Obstetrics and Gynecology.* Basel, S. Karger, 1972.
6. Charles, D., and Klein, T.: Postpartum Infection. *In* Charles, D., and Finland, M. (eds.): *Obstetrics and Perinatal Infections.* Philadelphia, Lea & Febiger, 1973.
7. Cone, B.: Puerperal Depression. *In* Morris, N. (ed.): *Psychosomatic Medicine in Obstetrics and Gynecology.* Basel, S. Karger, 1972.
8. Donaldson, W.: Fourth Trimester Follow-up. *American Journal of Nursing,* 77:1176, 1977.
9. Eiger, M., and Olds, S.: *The Complete Book of Breastfeeding.* New York, Bantam Books, 1972.
10. Frisoli, G.: Physiology and Pathology of the Puerperium. *In* Iffy, L., and Kaminetzky, H. (eds.): *Principles and Practice of Obstetrics and Perinatology.* New York, John Wiley, 1981.
11. Grossman, E.: Helping Mothers to Nurse Their Babies. *GP,* 31(4):78, 1965.
12. Holmes, O. W.: Contagiousness of Puerperal Fever. *New England Quarterly Journal of Medicine and Surgery,* 1:503, 1842–1843.
13. Holmes, O. W.: *Puerperal Fever as a Private Pestilence.* Boston, Ticknor and Fields, 1855.
14. Kaij, L., and Nilsson, A.: Emotional and Psychotic Illness Following Childbirth. *In* Howells, J. (ed.): *Modern Perspectives in Psycho-Obstetrics.* New York, Brunner/Mazel, 1972.
15. Kenner, C.: Multisystem Failure. *In* Kenner, C., Guggetta, C., and Dossey, R. (eds.): *Critical Care Nursing.* Boston, Little, Brown & Co., 1981.
16. Lawrence, R.: *Breastfeeding: A Guide for the Medical Profession.* St. Louis, C. V. Mosby Co., 1980.
17. Newton, M., and Newton, N.: The Normal Course and Management of Lactation. *Child and Family,* 9(2):102, 1970.
18. Nilsson, A.: Para-natal Emotional Adjustment. *Acta Psychiatrica Scandinavica,* Suppl.:220, 1970.
19. Nilsson, A., Kaij, L., and Jacobson, L.: Postpartum Mental Disorder in an Unselected Sample. The Importance of Unplanned Pregnancy. *Journal of Psychosomatic Research,* 10:341, 1967.
20. Pitt, B.: Psychiatric Illness Following Childbirth. *Hospital Medicine,* 2:815, 1968.
21. Pitt, B.: Neurotic (or Atypical) Depression Following Childbirth. *In* Morris, N. (ed.): *Psychosomatic Medicine in Obstetrics and Gynaecology.* Basel, S. Karger, 1972.
22. Schwarz, R.: *Handbook of Obstetric Emergencies.* Flushing, N.Y., Medical Examination Publishing Co., 1973.
23. Shinefeld, H.: Staphyloccal Infections. *In* Remington, J., and Klein, J.. (eds.): *Infectious Disease of the Fetus and Newborn Infant.* Philadelphia, W. B. Saunders Co., 1976.
24. Smith, A.: Megaloblastic Madness. *British Medical Journal,* 2:1840, 1960.
25. Strachan, R., and Henderson, J.: Psychiatric Syndromes Due to Avitaminosis B_{12} with Normal Blood and Marrow. *Quarterly Journal of Medicine,* 34:303, 1965.
26. Tod, E.: Puerperal Depression. *In* Morris, N. (ed.): *Psychosomatic Medicine in Obstetrics and Gynecology.* Basel, S. Karger, 1972.
27. Varney, H.: *Nurse-Midwifery.* Boston, Blackwell Scientific Publications, 1980.
28. The Womanly Art of Breastfeeding. Franklin Park, Ill., La Leche League, 1963.

28

Alterations in the Process of Attachment

OBJECTIVES

1. Define crisis. Identify factors that may influence reaction to crisis.
2. Describe common reactions of parents to the birth of a baby who is ill or has a congenital anomaly.
3. Identify criteria for the assessment of attachment.
4. Describe nursing actions that facilitate attachment in parents of high risk infants.
5. Describe ways in which nurses can help parents meet the needs of the siblings of newborns who are ill or dying.
6. Describe special attachment problems in multiple births.
7. Define the vulnerable child syndrome. Discuss its implications for nursing.
8. Identify the special needs of parents and siblings of a dying infant. Discuss the implications for nursing in this situation.
9. Identify the manifestations of grieving in nurses. Suggest strategies that are supportive to nurses.
10. Identify alterations in attachment related to maternal illness. Discuss implications for nursing.
11. Identify mothers who are at risk for alterations in attachment for reasons other than maternal illness. Indicate the implications of their problems.
12. Describe ways in which nurses can assess slow progression in attachment.

Attachment between parents and their infant is not a single event but a process that occurs over time and results in a bond that endures over time. The development of attachment is discussed in this book in relation to the prenatal period (Chapter 9), the intrapartum period (Chapter 20), and the puerperium (Chapter 26).

Attachment is reciprocal; it is influenced by parental and infant characteristics as well as by the circumstances surrounding birth. The process of attachment may be altered because of maternal or infant illness or because of social and emotional factors.

In this chapter alterations in attachment will be explored. In most instances these alterations are due to a crisis at the time of birth or in the immediate postpartum period. In Chapter 9 the view of some that childbearing per se is a crisis is discussed.

A crisis may be defined as a situation that cannot be easily handled by an individual's or a family's usual problem-solving mechanisms. Reaction to a crisis may be, "I've never faced anything like this before; I just don't know what to do." Certainly, then, it is possible for the birth of a healthy infant to a healthy mother to be considered a crisis under certain circumstances. When the infant is ill or has a congenital anomaly (Chapters 23 and 24) or when the mother is ill (Chapter 27), the definition of crisis will almost always apply. Parents are faced with a need to cope with overwhelming stimuli (see Roy's adaptation theory, Chapter 2). The extent of the crisis (the seriousness of the illness or anomaly) and the coping ability of the individual parents will be important in the ability of each family to adapt. Some families may have more difficulty in adapting to what may seem to nurses to be a relatively minor alteration in health (congenital hip dysplasia, for example), while other families will appear to adapt easily to what we perceive as a more serious problem (the birth of an infant at 32 weeks' gestation, for example).

Alterations due to Infant Illness or Anomaly

The appearance of an infant is thought to be a powerful stimulus to attachment. Adults have demonstrated a preference for pictures of young animals and humans over pictures of adults of the same species.[7] When a baby does not have the characteristics of "babyishness" because of prematurity or a congenital anomaly, that stimulus is lacking or diminished.

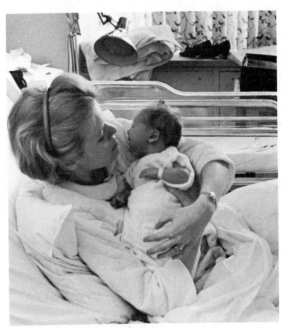

Figure 28–1.   The baby's response to cuddling stimulates attachment. (Photograph courtesy of Suzanne Szasz.)

A second stimulus to attachment is infant behavior. The quiet alert look and responses to cuddling and feeding are examples of ways in which infants facilitate the bonding process between themselves and their parents to them (Fig. 28–1). When the infant does not respond to parents because of marked prematurity or illness this stimulus is lacking.

Attachment requires personal interaction. When parents are separated from their infants during the first hours and days of life, the attachment process is delayed, and attachment may only be achieved after several weeks (see Nursing Care Plan 28–1).

Reactions of Parents

Although every parent will have individual emotions when a child who in some way appears less than perfect is born, there seem to be patterns of reactions of parents. These emotions, which are the emotions of the grief process associated with death and dying, occur even when the defect is one that to us may appear relatively minor and repairable (a cleft lip, for example), as well as when the problem is major, life-threatening, or terminal. The grief process is not only common; it seems to be essential for the parents to grieve for the lost baby of their imagination before they can accept their baby as he really is.

Mrs. Andrews' third child was a full-term healthy newborn with a unilateral cleft lip that extended

Text continued on page 976

Nursing Care Plan 28–1. Alterations in Attachment Due to Infant Illness or Anomaly

NURSING GOAL: To facilitate attachment and effective family coping when an infant is ill or has a congenital anomaly.

OBJECTIVES:
1. Parents accept their infant's condition.
2. Parents resolve feelings of anger, guilt, diminished self-esteem, denial, oversolicitude.
3. Parents demonstrate positive signs of attachment to their infant.
4. Family coping is effective.
5. Siblings accept the infant and are secure about their place in the family.
6. Parents are comfortable in caring for their infant in hospital and following discharge.
7. Parents utilize appropriate community resources.
8. The infant receives appropriate continuing health supervision.

ASSESSMENT	POTENTIAL NURSING DIAGNOSIS	NURSING INTERVENTION	COMMENTS/RATIONALE
Identify the reaction of parents to their infant and the alteration(s) in their infant's health status.		Keep both parents fully informed of infant's condition, plan of care, reason for each piece of equipment, tests, etc. Encourage questions.	Any or all of the reactions described may occur at different times. Continuous assessment is essential.
1. Shock, disbelief, denial	Denial		
2. Shame, embarrassment	Shame		
3. Loss of self-esteem	Loss of self-esteem		
4. Guilt	Guilt		
5. Anxiety	Anxiety		
6. Sadness	Sadness	Realize the need to repeat information given parents. Accept parental feelings. Provide privacy for times of crying.	
7. Anger	Anger		
8. Hostility	Hostility		
9. Oversolicitude	Oversolicitude		
10. Acceptance of infant's condition	(Each of the above is secondary to birth of infant who is ill or has a congenital anomaly)	Show sympathy and caring for infant and family. Indicate acceptance of the infant regardless of appearance. Point out positive attributes of infant.	
11. Acceptance of self without guilt or diminished self-esteem.			
Identify signs of ineffective family coping.	Ineffective family coping secondary to infant illness	Encourage parents to verbalize their perception of the effect of infant's illness on family.	The community health nurse making a home visit will frequently identify signs of family disruption not readily apparent to hospital staff or to parents themselves.
1. Quarreling			
2. Reports of psychosomatic illness in one or more family members, including siblings		Refer to community health nurse for home assessment.	

3. Reports of school problems, interpersonal problems, regression in behavior of siblings

Provide information about appropriate support groups in community (Parents of Prematures, Spina Bifida Association, etc.). Referral for family counseling will be necessary in some instances.

Sibling anxiety, guilt, other reactions

Provide opportunities for sibling visiting.

Counsel parents on discussions with siblings that are age-appropriate.

Use (or demonstrate for parents to use) doll play to help young children to express feelings about infant.

Provide opportunities for older siblings to participate in care.

Encourage parents to find some special time to spend with siblings (e.g., family picnic).

Lag in attachment

If parents do not initiate contact, hospital and community health nurses must maintain lines of communication with parents: telephone calls, home visits, pictures of infant, "letter" from infant. Share information that makes infant seem like a "real baby."

Identify behaviors that indicate growing attachment.

1. Parents try to be with infant as frequently as possible.
2. When parents cannot be present, they call or write.
3. Parents touch, caress infant, talk or sing to infant, use positive terms in commenting on infant.

Model positive behavior to infant. Call infant by name.

4. Parents try to establish eye contact with infant.
5. Parents attempt to soothe crying or fussy infant; stop behaviors that appear to disturb infant.

Help parents differentiate soothing and irritating behaviors (e.g., "John seems to enjoy hearing your voice").

6. Parents see family characteristics in infant (e.g., his father's eyes).

Encourage and support parental caregiving. Allow parents to assume increasing responsibility for activities of daily living.

Table continued on following page

Nursing Care Plan 28–1.   Alterations in Attachment Due to Infant Illness or Anomaly *(Continued)*

ASSESSMENT	POTENTIAL NURSING DIAGNOSIS	NURSING INTERVENTION	COMMENTS/RATIONALE
7. Parents participate in caregiving (e.g., notice that infant's diaper is wet and either change diaper or ask nurse to change diaper).			
8. Parents ask frequent and specific questions about infant's condition.		Answer questions gladly, even when information has been previously provided. Refer to appropriate sources for information nurse is unable to provide.	
9. Parents are able to express negative feelings.			
10. Anxiety is appropriate to infant's condition.			
Identify signs that indicate slow progress in attachment.	Lag in attachment		
1. Infrequent visiting, calls			
2. Visits to infant brief; limited interaction with infant. Do not touch, ask questions, etc.		Refer to community health nurse for home assessment and attempt to discover cause of infrequent visiting.	When parents do not visit hospital, this opportunity is provided by community health nurse.
3. Expressed feelings of inadequacy in relation to infant's care		Provide opportunities for verbalization of feelings.	
4. Frustration in relation to infant's crying; inability to comfort			
5. Negative comments about infant (note affect as well as words)			
6. Lack of preparation for infant's homecoming		If lack of transportation, family situation, etc., is limiting visiting, seek help from appropriate source (social services, hospital chaplain, etc.).	

Identify family readiness for discharge. 1. Acceptance of infant's condition 2. Acceptance of self without guilt or diminished self-esteem 3. Realistic understanding of infant's need for protection without overprotection 4. Provision for infant care at home (e.g., supplies for infant) 5. Comfort in caring for infant: recognize infant's needs and respond appropriately 6. Ability to meet special need (e.g., ostomy care, chest physical therapy, special feeding, etc.) 7. Expressed satisfaction in parenting activities 8. Identification of support system (e.g., who will babysit) 9. Plans for appropriate continuing care (well-child care, care appropriate to infant's problem).	Ineffective family coping patterns Lack of support system Lack of preparation for infant care at home Lack of knowledge about infant needs Fear, anxiety related to care of infant at home	Begin preparing family for home care early in hospitalization: participation in care, discussion. Refer for one or more community health nursing visits prior to discharge: 1. To establish relationship 2. To assess readiness 3. To identify potential problems 4. To provide support and counsel Encourage verbalization of anxiety related to infant care at home. Make positive comments about infant normality. Provide phone numbers (hospital unit, community health nurse, other appropriate resources).	Sources of nursing intervention may be community health nurse, nurse in ambulatory clinic, nursery nurse through follow-up phone calls.
Assess family coping following discharge. Utilize parameters as in family readiness for discharge; identify family's ability to act on parameters. Observe infant care at home. Is the parent comfortable in feeding, holding infant? What does she report about infant sleep patterns? Where does infant sleep? Have parents utilized babysitter? Are appointments for continuing care made and kept? What do parents report about sibling reaction to baby?	Ineffective family coping patterns Lack of support system Lack of knowledge about infant needs	Reinforce positive parenting behaviors. Encourage verbalization of concerns. Provide information as needed. Refer to appropriate support services as needed or desired (parent groups, homemaker service, etc.).	

into the nares. The first night after the baby was born, Mrs. Andrews cried frequently and was obviously very sad. However, on subsequent days she learned to feed him and seemed very comfortable with him, cuddling him and talking to him. She wanted her 19-year-old daughter to see the baby prior to the lip repair, which was done when the baby was 5 days old, so that her daughter too would accept him as he was.

Her behavior on the morning of surgery, when she came to the nursery early to hold him before he went to the operating room, indicated to us that she had formed a strong bond with her son, even prior to a successful surgical repair. She told us, "At first all I could do was cry, but now he seems no different from my other children."

Shock and disbelief are usual first reactions—"Why me?"—"Why us?" they ask. Denial is one way of coping with the shock. "I don't believe it . . . I can't believe it . . . I won't believe it." Sometimes denial leads to behavior by parents that nurses view as very inappropriate. Their baby is critically ill, yet they seem unconcerned; they may even be laughing. Only gradually does the full impact of their baby's problem become real for them.

A second group of feelings, normal to this situation, are those of *shame, embarrassment, loss of self-esteem,* and *feelings of personal inadequacy.* "What caused this?" they ask, which may often be translated, "What is wrong with us that we couldn't have a normal child?"

A seemingly routine request may thus bring a sharp response. As noted in Chapter 3, it is customary to karyotype the chromosomes of both the mother and father of a baby suspected of having Down's syndrome in order to determine the type of chromosomal problem and assess the risk of recurrence. When this was explained to one father, he angrily answered, "There's never been anything like that on my side of the family." His wife was not present when he made the statement. Had she been, he might not have said what he did, but he most certainly would have thought it. We need to be ready to accept such feelings and to let parents know that other parents also feel this way under similar circumstances.

Guilt about the origin of an anomaly or prematurity is another frequent response to abnormality. Is it something we did? Our long-standing beliefs about sin and punishment, a part of our heritage for many centuries, leave the nagging fear that this is a punishment for some deed or for some thought. Perhaps the pregnancy was originally undesired—many are, even when the baby is later accepted. Maybe an abortion was contemplated or even attempted; the feeling of guilt here can be

almost overwhelming. Guilt feelings, unresolved, may lead to depression.

Parents are *anxious* for many reasons. What will become of this child? How will we care for him—physically, emotionally, financially? Can we love him as we love our other children? Will this child hurt our other children? A particularly important question is—will future children run the risk of a similar defect?

Anger, also common, is probably the hardest of all the grief-related emotions for us to deal with, because so often we, the nurses, are the target of that anger, and it seems so unjustified. We wonder, what did *we* do to deserve this? It isn't *our* fault that the baby is ill or malformed. Of course it isn't. But anger is a part of the grief process. If we can accept this idea, the anger, even when directed at us, should not really upset us.

Why are parents angry? They are angry that this happened to them. Even though they know it is irrational, they are often angry at the baby. They may be angry at each other. And they feel guilty because they are angry. The anger will come out in many ways. The bath water is too hot, the bed is too hard, or the food is terrible.

Family Disruption

Since we know that the birth of a normal, healthy infant brings changes to a family's style of life, it is reasonable to expect that the birth of a high risk baby will be even more disruptive. In addition, the strong individual emotions that accompany a high risk birth—anger, guilt, and the like—may further cause family disruption.

The Shutt family, both mother and father, traveled over 100 miles every day from the time of the baby's birth until his death 7 months later, to visit their infant son in the hospital. During all this time, a 7-year-old-daughter was at home with her grandmother.

If the baby is obviously sick at the time of birth or during the first days afterward, family problems may appear early. When the disorder is not diagnosed until later, disruption may be evident from the time of diagnosis.

A first example is of a family that had apparently been well adjusted prior to the diagnosis of cystic fibrosis in their baby, who was 9 months old. The same types of behavior, however, may be evident in families of children with neonatal problems.

Quarrels between parents concerning interpersonal psychosexual behavior and genetic prognosis had ensued almost immediately thereafter. Both parents had turned to their own parents to air their grievances.[6a]

Tips also noted that the three older children had been informed by classmates of the complex family situation. The behavior and social and academic standing of the children had deteriorated as a consequence.[24]

A second example describes a family with two unaffected children and a third and fourth child with congenital spastic paraplegia of genetic origin.

Immediately after receiving the adverse and distasteful genetic prognosis, the parents had become concerned about their interpersonal relationships. Nocturnal arguments had ensued and the mother had developed severe dyspareunia. She had become overly concerned with the management of the affected children and had neglected the older children who developed behavioral disturbances and began failing in school. The father, previously dominant, had withdrawn and assumed a passive role in the family circle . . .

During the consultation, the parents refused to communicate with one another, but both were excessively free in the discussion of family problems with all team members. As the family history was discussed, both parents overtly degraded the other's family. Each parent also strongly suspected the other of extramarital affairs.[24]

In both instances counseling enabled the parents to identify their concerns, to talk about them more realistically, and ultimately to resolve them.

Acceptance is the final step in the grief process. We need to realize that it may be many months, even a year or more, before that acceptance comes. Nurses who care for the infant and his family at the time of birth do not often see parents at this point. We must not expect acceptance in the 3- to 5-day period that mothers remain on the obstetric unit, or even in the weeks that the baby is in the nursery.

Attachment Between Parents and Their High Risk Baby

The steps by which parents form attachments to their healthy newborn babies were discussed in Chapter 26. Attachment is equally important for the parents of the high risk baby. Studies indicate that approximately one-third of all infants who are battered or "fail to thrive" in the absence of physiologic disease were either preterm babies or babies who were ill in the period following birth. The common denominator was separation from their parents during the early days when attachments are formed (Fig. 28–2). Facilitating the attachment of high risk babies and their parents is obviously very important.

Attachment is equally important if the baby is expected to die. Parents will grieve, regardless of whether or not they have formed an attachment. It is far healthier for them to grieve for a specific, tangible baby than for a vague entity they have never known. Normal grief can be resolved. Undefined grief may linger—as anger or sadness or in some other form—for a very long time.

It is not surprising that parents are reluctant to form attachments to their sick or malformed baby. They fear the pain they will suffer if the baby dies. Their problem is then compounded by the guilt they experience about not feeling love for their baby.

Assessment of Attachment

The assessment of attachment behavior when the infant is ill must take into account

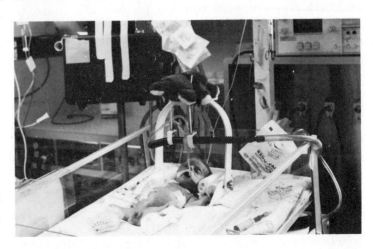

Figure 28–2. The complex and technical nature of the care of the high risk infant contributes to the difficulties in attachment, separation being a major problem.

the stage of the grief cycle. A single assessment on a single day is of little value. A series of observations noted in the infant's record (and the mother's record while she is hospitalized or in interaction with a community health nurse) is essential. The following questions will guide nursing assessment during the attachment process. Although the initial evaluation of parents may indicate a negative, unhealthy response, the response will frequently become positive as the parents have increased opportunities to interact with their baby and to mobilize their coping strategies.

1. Do parents seek opportunities to be with their baby, to touch him, and to hold him if that is possible? When they cannot be present, do they call or write the nursery? (Some parents cannot afford to call long distance.)

2. Do parents seek information about their baby's condition, asking frequent and specific questions?

3. Can parents express their negative feelings—fear, anger, disappointment—or do they deny having negative feelings?

4. Is parental anxiety generally appropriate to the seriousness of the baby's condition? Do parents deny the seriousness of a life-threatening condition and refuse to discuss it?

5. Is support available from grandparents or other family members? Do the parents support one another or are they angry with one another or blame each other for the baby's problem? (See also Indications of Slow Progression of Attachment, below.)

Nursing Action to Facilitate Attachment and Assist Coping

Initial Communication With Parents. The moment at which parents are first told that their infant is dead or critically ill or has a birth defect is a very difficult one for parents, nurses, physicians, and other health team members. The situation raises a number of questions. Who should tell the parents? Who should be told—the father first, the mother, both parents together? What if the father is not available? How should the parents be told? What should they be told? These questions have concerned us for many years, but changes in other aspects of maternity care have caused us to think again about the way we answer them.

Several decades ago, when many mothers were asleep at the time their infants were delivered and for some time afterward, and when fathers were kept in distant waiting rooms, "telling" was often postponed. Today, in a growing number of hospitals, the mother is watching the delivery with her husband beside her. Such postponement is not possible under these circumstances. Occasionally, a father may be asked to leave the delivery room when a complication is suspected. We have to consider whether such a practice offers psychologic protection to the delivery room personnel rather than to the father. If there is a serious problem to be faced, it might be that the support the mother and father could offer to one another would be of real value. There are probably individual exceptions to this concept, but they should be exceptions and not the rule.

A second traditional practice that is fortunately on the decline (but hardly eradicated) is explaining the baby's condition to the father or some other member of the family but withholding part or all of the truth from the mother. The assumption here is that the father is better able to cope with reality and to make decisions than the mother who has recently delivered. Aside from the fact that this assumption is, at best, questionable and that is places a tremendous burden on a new father, the delay not only doesn't fool the mother but adds to her anxiety. Her energy is drained in wondering what is wrong, why she hasn't seen her baby, why the nurses and perhaps her husband are avoiding her, and why no one answers her questions. Moreover, if we are less than honest with either parent in the hours after a problem is first recognized, they may easily doubt what we tell them later, wondering if we are still "putting them off."

What is initially said to parents will depend, of course, on the baby's condition. In every instance it is important to be honest. However, even when the baby is quite ill, honesty can often be combined with a note of optimism, such as "many babies as sick as your baby do get well." Some optimism is helpful in encouraging parents to develop an attachment to their baby.

At this time parents need some idea of the tests and procedures that may be carried out; we must get their written permission for those procedures. Talking with both parents together, as soon as the baby's problem is recognized, is nearly always the most helpful course. In this way, the same information is given to both parents. The physician or midwife who delivered the baby should be present; he or she may be the only member of the team who has known the parents, and is known to them, prior to delivery. A nurse who will be caring for the mother in the first days following delivery should also be present, not only for support but so that she too will know what the parents have been told. Nursing records should include the basic information given to the family, so that everyone who subsequently

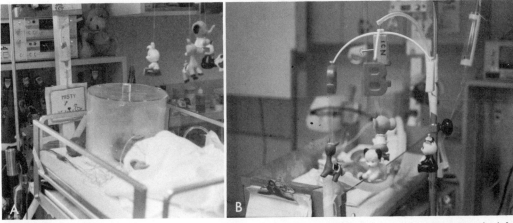

Figure 28–3. *A* and *B*, The opportunity to provide toys and personalized items helps parents accept the infant.

cares for this family will be better able to support them.

After the parents have been told about their baby's condition, the nurse needs to be available to them for support and to answer questions that may arise. Many of us feel at a loss for words, but words are not always necessary; touch can also convey concern. "Hit and run," in which the parents are "hit" with distressing information about their baby and then we "run" away, leaving them to deal with what has been told them in solitude should be unthinkable.

The initial shock of their baby's condition will block out much that is told them at this time. Some written information about the nursery in which their baby will receive care should be given to them; they will turn to it in the hours and days that follow, and it will help to remind them of what we have said in these first minutes.

Most important, this early time of communication should give parents the feeling that we are concerned about them and about their baby and that we will be available to answer their questions or just to listen whenever they wish us to do so. We want them to know we will be honest and open in trying to answer their questions.

If the baby is to be transferred to another hospital (e.g., from a community hospital to a medical center with an intensive care nursery), the reasons should be explained to the parents in a way they can understand. Parents should *see and touch* their baby before the transfer. This is particularly true of the mother who, because of her own hospitalization, may not be able to see her baby for several days—critically important days in terms of maternal attachment.

If the baby is to remain in the same hospital, the parents should have early and frequent opportunities to visit him in the nursery. Helping the parents to cope during these visits is discussed later in this chapter.

This initial period of communication is not a time to discuss every complication that may occur. For example, the preterm baby may develop hyperbilirubinemia in 2 to 3 days, but this can be dealt with later. To bring out too much initially will raise a barrier to attachment.

Interaction with Parents When the Baby Is in the Nursery. During the days, perhaps weeks, that a sick baby may be hospitalized, nurses can continue to foster attachment in a number of specific ways.

Showing Acceptance. The importance of our own attitude toward the baby has already been mentioned. The baby, despite any defect that he may have, should not be hidden in a corner of the nursery. The baby can be talked to, and about, as a baby. The parents should be encouraged to name the infant, his name should be placed on his bed, and the baby should always be called by name (Fig. 28–3).

Explaining Equipment. How did you feel when you walked into the intensive care nursery for the first time? If you were in a medical center, with monitors, respirators, alarms, intravenous lines, and the like, you may have thought, "I could never work in a place like this." If nurses who are familiar with hospitals feel this way (and many registered nurses do), consider how parents must feel in an intensive care nursery for the first time, with *their* baby as a patient (Fig. 28–4).

How can we help them cope with such an overwhelming experience? Even before they enter the doors for the first time, we can describe what they will see—the reason for each piece of equipment, about the way it is helping their baby—and also tell them something about the way their baby will look. Then

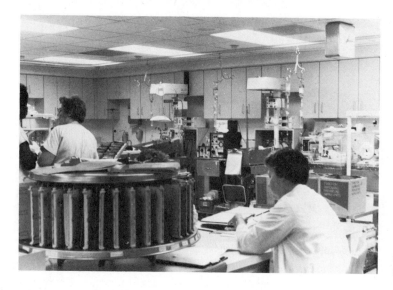

Figure 28–4. The highly technological environment of the intensive care nursery can be threatening to parents.

we can accompany them to their baby's bed, again explaining everything carefully, for much of what we have previously said will not be comprehended. Continuing explanations are necessary as the baby's condition changes.

Continuing Communication. Parents need to feel welcome each time they telephone or come to the nursery. Increasingly, parents are allowed to visit intensive care nurseries as frequently and as long as they desire (as we become more knowledgeable about the importance of attachment in infant care), although they may be asked to leave briefly during certain procedures involving their own or other babies.

Many questions about their baby and his care will be asked more than once; answers may not have been understood or may have been forgotten in the stress surrounding the family. These questions should be answered with patience and care each time.

Good communication among nurses, physicians, and other workers in the nursery is also essential to good communication with parents. Nothing can be more confusing or distressing to parents than to hear different stories from different people. Major information communicated to parents should be documented and easily accessible to everyone caring for the baby. A check sheet can be one aid in this area, as well as being a help in assessing attachment (below).

Equally as important as knowing what parents have been told is knowing what they understand about what they have heard. We need to listen for clues about their understanding or lack of it. For example, when the father of a baby with serious brain damage talks about his son as a future Little Leaguer, communication has certainly been ineffective for

some reason. It may be that this father is not psychologically ready to accept what he has heard. Or we may have been unclear about what we said to him. An important question to ask about each family each day is "Where are they in their understanding of their baby's condition?"

In addition to picking up clues in conversation, we can ask them what they have been told. For example, if a mother says, "How much longer will my baby need to have that needle in his head (intravenous line)?" we might first ask her what information she has already been given. Many parents will ask a question of several nurses and physicians, just to see if they will get the same answer. It is a way of looking for assurance, but it can certainly be very hard on staff if our own communication is not good.

Encouraging Parents to Participate in Their Baby's Care. As with healthy term babies, attachment formation with high risk babies involves seeing, touching, and caretaking. Many parents who will eagerly caress a term baby may shrink from a preterm infant or a child with a defect (Fig. 28–5). This is one more reason why we need to be with them the first times they visit, and we should always remain close by. We may have to encourage their touch. "Would you like to hold your baby's hand?" we can say. Sometimes if we hold his hand or stroke his head or leg while we are talking, we can encourage parents to be less fearful. Fathers often need a great deal of encouragement to handle tiny babies, although in some families the father may be less reluctant than the mother.

It is more difficult to involve parents in caretaking with a very sick baby than with the term baby. At first parents may not be

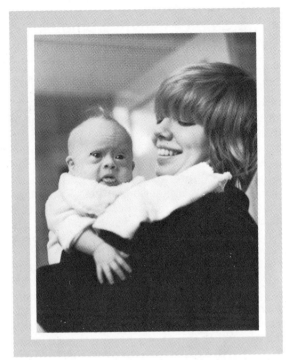

Figure 28–5. This mother is learning to care for her child who has Down syndrome. (From Smith and Wilson: *The Child with Down's syndrome.* Philadelphia, W. B. Saunders Co., 1973.)

able to feed their baby or bathe or diaper him, but we can assure them that their gentle stroking and talking to him play a real role in his care (Fig. 28–6). We can also use our ingenuity to involve the parents in as many ways as possible. For example, if the baby is to have a gavage feeding, we might insert the tube and be sure of its position; the mother might then pour the premeasured formula into the syringe. As the baby's condition improves, the parents can assume a more active role in his care.

Encouraging Attachment When Parents Are Separated from Their Baby. The centralization of high risk newborns in medical centers, although obviously offering significant advantages from the standpoint of physiologic care, presents some real barriers to attachment. Parents may live 50 or 100 miles from the hospital in which their baby receives care; they may even live in a different state. Many times they lack transportation to travel back and forth except on weekends. Often there are other children at home who also need care. How do we foster attachment on a long-distance basis? No one has final answers to this question, but attempts are being made to deal with the problem.

The telephone is an important means of communication for parents. It gives us a chance to tell them how much their baby has gained, how he is eating, and little personal bits of information such as, "He opened his eyes while I was bathing him," that not only mean a lot to most parents but contribute to their feelings of attachment. An ideal situation is a telephone number that can be called long distance at no charge to the family. Many parents cannot afford long distance calls each day; some have no access to telephones at all.

Letters and photos from the hospital can be helpful if the mother and father are unable to come for several weeks at a time.

Contact through public health nurses in the parents' home area, if for some reason it is difficult to reach the parents themselves, is another avenue of communication. Certainly the public health nurse should be contacted before the baby is discharged so that she may come to know the family and be available to them for teaching and counsel.

The concept of "back-transfer," that is, sending the baby back to the hospital nearer to his home community for intermediate level care before discharge, is growing in popularity. Not only is the baby nearer his family, which facilitates their visiting and their learning to care for him, but local care is often less expensive.

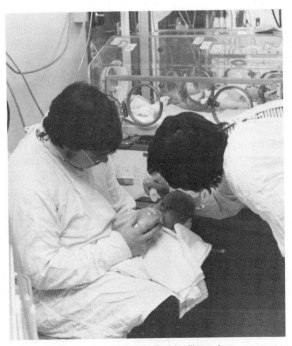

Figure 28–6. Even though Todd still requires some oxygen, his father can feed him while his mother holds the tubing carrying oxygen close to his face.

Reactions of Siblings

In caring for parents and their sick or anomalous infant it is very easy to overlook the brothers and sisters of that infant, whom nurses may never have seen. It is very easy for parents to be so caught up in their own feelings about the baby (which are a normal part of grieving) that they are unaware of the needs of the other children, who perhaps have been sent to stay with a grandmother or friends or other relatives. Even when parents are aware of the needs of their other children, they may find it difficult to answer their questions or may feel inadequate to give them support.

Preschool-age children, with their limited understanding of cause and effect and a focus that is primarily self-centered, may feel that in some way they are responsible for the baby's illness. For example, a child may have said or thought "I don't want a baby brother" and may now feel that he is thereby responsible for the baby's illness. For a preschool child the separation from his parents that accompanies the new baby's illness can be devastating. Regression of preschool-aged children is not unusual even when the childbirth is normal; it should not be surprising, therefore, when either the infant of the mother is ill.

Nursing assessment should include checking with the parents about what siblings have said or what the parents may have observed in sibling behavior changes. A nurse could say, "Brothers and sisters often have worries about their baby brother (sister). Has Johnny asked about the baby?"

When the baby must remain in the hospital for days or weeks after birth, sibling visiting should be arranged. The small child, held up by his parents to view the baby in an incubator or an open bed, will often give the baby the briefest attention. Older children may have many questions. Many children bring the baby a present—a picture they have colored, for example.

When the baby looks different (a baby with a cleft lip, for example) explanations and perhaps pictures that are suitable to the siblings' age are helpful. Doll play can be used with young children to help them understand more about their baby brother or sister and also to help them express their feelings about the baby. Older children may be able to participate in the baby's care if they wish. If the baby's problem is going to be of long duration, most families will need a source of continued counseling and group support to help them meet the needs of siblings as well as other needs in the months and years ahead.

Vulnerable Child Syndrome: A Reaction to Neonatal Illness

When a newborn is severely ill and expected to die but survives, the relationship between parents and their baby may be affected by reactions that have been collectively described as a *vulnerable child syndrome*. Parents believe that their baby is vulnerable to accident or serious illness and is destined to die during childhood. (Vulnerable child syndrome can also occur following serious illness in an older infant or child.) Serious maternal illness that is life-threatening may also be a factor; the mother may displace her own fear of dying to the infant.

When the child is seen as vulnerable, parent–infant interaction is affected. Mothers fear any separation. The baby will frequently sleep in the parents' bedroom; they will awake several times during the night to check on him and also check frequently during the day when he is asleep. Parents may report that the baby does not sleep well; in fact, they may unconsciously keep the baby awake at night because of a fear that if he falls asleep he may die.

Babysitters are rarely used by these parents. As the infant grows older, parents are unable to set limits on their child's behavior. Feeding problems are common, and school phobia or underachievement occurs in later years. The consequences are far reaching.

Nursing intervention may prevent extreme overconcern in some parents. In planning for discharge, a nurse can explain that many parents are fearful of assuming total responsibility for a baby who has been so ill. Parents can be encouraged to verbalize their own fears and to consider whom they might choose as a babysitter so they can have some time away from the baby. Reassurance that their baby is now healthy is important. Some preterm babies who are at increased risk of apnea may have an apnea monitor for use at home.

As the baby recovers, comments should focus on his increasing normality (e.g., weight gain, increased oral intake, visual tracking, listening to a music box) rather than on how ill he has been in the past (e.g., "He almost didn't make it").

Signs of possible vulnerable child syndrome can frequently be assessed within a few weeks following the baby's discharge from the hospital by a community health nurse during a home visit or during a follow-up conference at the hospital. Assessment should include the areas described, such as sleeping patterns and periods of separation. The infant's health-care provider should be aware of potential signs of difficulty so that parents can be reassured when their baby is examined and found to be healthy.

When parental behavior indicates undue concern, they can be helped to recognize the basis of that concern and to modify their behavior gradually. For example, a mother could be encouraged to find a trusted babysitter and then to leave her baby with that person for a brief period. Plans could then be made for a second, slightly longer separation. Similar gradual modification of behavior may help the mother who must awaken to check on her infant frequently during the night or who is reluctant to allow him to sleep.

Attachment in Multiple Births

When twins or triplets are born, parents must become attached to each infant separately. Because infants in multiple births are frequently preterm, the problems associated with separation and infant illness are added to the already complex attachment needs. Twins will be used as the example in this discussion but the principles of care apply to all infants in multiple births.

Nurses can facilitate attachment by helping parents identify the unique characteristics of each baby.[5] The use of items from the Brazelton Assessment Scale (Chapter 21) is helpful. Parents may see that one baby is particularly responsive to an auditory stimulus, such as the sound of the mother's or father's voice, while the twin is more interested in visual stimuli. Each baby may respond differently to position changes, to being held, to feedings. Nurses caring for the babies will be able to share their observations of each baby's uniqueness. Calling each baby by name, rather than Twin A or the Jones twins, further emphasizes their uniqueness.

One problem area is discharge planning for twins. It is not unusual for one baby to be ready for discharge earlier than the other. There is concern that if one twin returns home before the other, especially if a difference of several weeks is involved, parental attachment to that twin may be enhanced at the expense of the other. Not only will there be a marked difference in the amount of interaction between the parents and the two infants, but spending time with the hospitalized twin may be more difficult when there is an infant at home. On the other hand, keeping an infant who is ready for discharge in the hospital to await a sibling's discharge is very difficult; costs and allocation of space alone would prohibit such a practice if more than one or two days is involved.

Mothers of many singly born newborns are often overwhelmed by the care of their baby; for mothers of more than one infant the task may seem impossible. Prior to discharge, hospital nurses and community health nurses need to assess the mother's feelings about infant care and the resources available to her. In many communities peer support from groups such as Mothers-of-Twins is available. When a great deal of infant care is provided by others—a grandmother, a neighbor, or someone employed to help the mother—attachment may be hindered because providing care is part of the attachment process. Nurses might suggest that helping persons help with noninfant care tasks, and that mothers and fathers provide at least part of the care for each baby each day.

In assessing parental attachment to twins, all of the behaviors assessed in relation to singly-born infants are relevant, although attachment may proceed more slowly. Attachment to individual twins is indicated when parents refer to each baby by name rather than to the twins collectively as "they".

When one twin is more seriously ill than the other, or when one twin dies, attachment to the living or more healthy twin is affected by grief for the other baby. Parents may deny their feelings of grief and need reassurance that it is "all right" to grieve for their dead baby. They may withdraw or be reluctant to become attached to the living twin, afraid of the pain of still another loss. Attachment in such a case is likely to proceed slowly and to require significant nursing support.

The Dying Infant

As we have already noted, one of the most difficult aspects of the care of high risk infants is facing the reality that many of our patients will not recover. Duff and Campbell[6] suggest that two philosophies underlie the way in which we care for these babies and their families:

1. A "disease-oriented" philosophy, which sees death only in a highly negative context of failure.

2. A "person-oriented" philosophy, which recognizes that under some circumstances death is not only inevitable but is not necessarily the worst of fates.

The way in which we have traditionally treated the dying newborn and his family is not much different from the way in which the American culture in general, and the nursing and medical subcultures that preside over our dying, have dealt with death at any age. With a few exceptions (the baby with anencephaly or the baby of less than 25 weeks' gestation, for example), we make heroic efforts to save the baby. However, if we fail, we then feel we have done all we can and frequently withdraw from the baby and family, emotionally if not physically.

Some newborns die in spite of anything we can do. For others, life may be prolonged, but not necessarily saved, by a variety of means. The intensity and duration of care given to a particular baby must take into account not only medical factors but family feelings as well. We find great satisfaction working in a nursery in which the understanding and feelings of parents are discussed along with laboratory values and respiratory status on daily rounds.

Consider the difference that the feelings of parents made in the care of two infants who happened to be in the same intensive care nursery at the same time. Baby A was able to breathe only in 100 per cent oxygen; Baby B required a tracheostomy and continual ventilation. During week after week of intensive care, repeated attempts were made to help both babies become able to breathe normally in room air. Careful studies were undertaken to discover the underlying cause of each baby's problem. Both mothers and fathers visited every day; their attachment was evident. Baby A was entered in her church's "beautiful baby contest" via photographs. Baby B had his sister's picture taped to his isolette along with mobiles and music boxes.

Gradually, it became evident to the staff that neither baby was likely ever to breathe independently, and the information was shared with the parents. Over the next few days the parents of Baby A decided, along with staff, that their baby would receive no more oxygen. We could continue to feed her and care for her in every other way for as long as she was able to live. They continued to visit her each day and brought her 2-year-old sister so that she too, might see her. In a few days, Baby A died.

Baby B's parents continued to believe that he would recover until the time of his death. Because of their wishes, the baby was ventilated via a respirator throughout his life.

Different families deal with death in different ways; in these instances including the parents in the decision-making resulted in two different courses of action. What is helpful for one family may not be so for a second.

One aspect worth noting in the behavior of both of these families, and in the family described below as well, is the involvement of siblings. Because small children are often jealous of a brother or sister, particularly one who

separates them from their parents for the long periods of time that hospital visits require, they may wish that the baby dies, so that their parents will become available to them once again. Since for a small child wishing something to happen is hard to differentiate from causing it to happen, there may be a great deal of guilt when the baby does in fact die. Often parents, wrapped up in their own grief and their concern for the baby, need some help in realizing that their other children need support through this difficult period. A question such as, "What does your child (children) say about the baby?" will remind parents to be sensitive to their other sons and daughters.

Can we make the death of an infant, despite the inevitable sorrow, a positive experience for families? We submit the following as evidence that we can:

A premature infant was believed to have a hopeless prognosis. The parents and doctor, with the agreement of the medical and nursing staff, decided to stop all heroic measures. The parents informed their healthy 3-year-old daughter that her brother probably could not live, and, on her request, she was brought to see the baby.

Later, after contemplating autopsy and plans for disposition of the baby's body (both discussed at their request), the parents were asked which they preferred–to leave; to be beside their baby's incubator; or to have the baby, with all his tubes and apparatus removed, brought to them in a private room. Immediately, they chose the last. In the company of the doctor, they held their infant for 55 minutes while he died. During this time, they wept, talked to their daughter about him, found humor in some incongruities, or were silent. The mother cradled the baby to her bosom most of the time, while the father stroked his wife and baby.

He told us that the scene of mother and dying child was one of sublime beauty despite its occurrence in the midst of tragedy. He later said he believed that the time interval spent in intimacy with their baby was about 2 hours, not 55 minutes. She told us, "We had to say hello to him before we could say goodbye."

They came to think of this experience as a fitting funeral from which they gained greater strength for living. They helped each other. They also helped their daughter over the ensuing weeks as she overcame her abnormal fears of dying and openly dealt with her guilt for feeling that her bad wishes had killed her brother.[6]

Nursing Interaction with Families During the Time of Dying

When an infant is clearly dying, nurses can initiate positive action to help families cope with the event (see Nursing Care Plan 28–2). One of the most difficult problems in some nurseries is the provision of privacy so that families can be alone with their baby. Unlike units for adults, nurseries are not usually designed with private rooms or even curtains to screen one patient from another. Each nursery must designate a place where families can comfortably spend private time with their infant, holding the baby if they wish.

Although some time for the family to be together by themselves may be desired, a nurse should be with the family or immediately available most of the time. She may sit quietly, saying little or nothing, but her presence indicates that support is available. Other professionals—hospital chaplain, the family clergyman, nursery social worker, physician—may also provide support. No family should feel alone and abandoned during this difficult time.

Many families have religious beliefs and practices that are important at the time of death. For example, Roman Catholic and Episcopal families will desire infant baptism. Some families will have a brief prayer service at the infant's bedside, in which they affirm their belief that their baby is returning to God. Particularly, when families are away from their home community because the baby has been transferred to a regional center, nurses need to assess the parents religious desires and be able to help the family contact their own clergyman or a clergyman of their denomination if they wish to do so.

Group meetings of parents of infants who are dying or have died are very helpful to some families, whereas other families may not feel that they will be helpful to them. Informal support of one family by parents of other babies in the nursery may also occur. Each family will deal with grief in a manner unique to them; thus nurses must assess family needs individually, provide information about the resources available, and allow families to decide if a particular resource will be helpful.

Nursing Interaction Following Infant Death

The responsibility of nurses and their professional colleagues to the family does not end with the death of their infant. Continued support of the family in the period immediately following death is easier when the mother is still hospitalized from childbirth. When the infant dies several days or weeks after birth, the parents will generally leave the hospital shortly after the baby's death. Each nursery needs a plan to provide further support to these parents.

Consider first the mother who is herself in hospital at the time of the baby's death. Many mothers find it difficult to remain in a maternity unit filled with happy parents and their healthy babies following the death of their own baby. The option of care in another unit or perhaps an early discharge if the mother's health permits should be available to them. If the mother is transferred to another unit, nurses in the area to which she is moved should be knowledgeable in caring for mothers who have lost an infant in death. In some units the father may remain with the mother overnight.

Sedation of the mother is not generally considered helpful. Expressions of grief, such as intense crying, are important to the process of grief resolution and are only impeded, never resolved, by chemicals.

Some mothers report that "everyone" avoids talk of their dead infant "as if he never had existed." It is painful for the staff to talk about the baby because they perceive that it is painful for the parents. Both nurses and parents must recognize that pain is an inevitable and necessary part of the resolution of grief. Nurses must sit with parents and help them express their grief. One might begin by acknowledging the sorrow: "I know it is very difficult (very painful) to talk about your baby, but other parents have found this helpful." Mothers often review their pregnancy, looking for a reason for their baby's death. Fathers also search for possible causes. Nurses can help parents accept the fact that they are not responsible for the death of their infant by answering their questions as clearly as possible.

Many parents, especially fathers, need reassurance that it is "all right to cry" and that crying is not only appropriate but a normal part of grieving that will help them make progress toward eventual grief resolution.

Parents face one very practical decision very soon after the baby's death: Should there be a funeral? If death has occurred over a period of days, the family may have considered the issue. When death is sudden and unexpected, parents feel completely unprepared to make any decision. Parents usually have several options:

1. The hospital disposes of the body without charge; no funeral or memorial service is held.
2. The hospital disposes of the body but the family holds a memorial service.
3. The body is sent to a funeral home and a funeral is held.

Parents frequently ask nurses for help in making this decision. A memorial service or a funeral provides public recognition of the reality of the baby's death, a socially acceptable mechanism for expressing grief, and the op-

Nursing Care Plan 28-2.   Caring for the Family when Fetal or Neonatal Death Occurs

NURSING GOAL: To facilitate grieving in parents and siblings when fetal or neonatal death occurs.

OBJECTIVES:
1. Parents grieve for and eventually accept the death of their fetus or newborn.
2. Family dysfunction is avoided.
3. Appropriate counseling related to genetic disease, family planning, and family crisis is provided.

ASSESSMENT	POTENTIAL NURSING DIAGNOSIS	NURSING INTERVENTION	COMMENTS/RATIONALE
Identify parents' reactions to their dying infant, stillborn infant, or aborted fetus. 1. Shock, disbelief, denial 2. Loss of self-esteem 3. Guilt 4. Anxiety 5. Sadness 6. Anger, hostility 7. Acceptance	Anticipatory grieving Denial Loss of self-esteem Guilt Anxiety Sadness Anger Hostility	When infant is clearly dying but is still alive: Provide opportunities for parents to see, touch, and hold infant. Dress infant in clothes. When the infant has died or is stillborn, or when a fetus is aborted: Allow parents to hold fetus, wrapped in blanket or dressed. Point out attractive features; help parents to see family resemblance. Support family during this procedure. Take picture of infant for family. In either instance: Encourage verbalization and other expressions of feelings. Assure that it is "all right to cry." Encourage parents to verbalize to one another. Provide privacy but do not abandon family. Assure them that support is available to them. Be available to talk whenever parents desire. Provide picture of infant for family. Avoid statements that minimize significance of infant's dying (e.g., "You can always have another baby.") Explain that the resolution of grief is a slow process, proceeding gradually over a period of weeks.	Each family will deal with grief in a unique way. Grief for a "real person" can eventually be resolved; grief for an "unknown object" is far more difficult to resolve. Even if family does not want picture at the time, file it for later. Most families will eventually cherish the picture.

Identify parents' desire for specific religious observance (e.g., baptism).	Desire for support from clergy Desire for specific religious observance	Contact family clergy, hospital chaplain, or clergy of appropriate denomination. If baptism is desired and clergyman is not available, follow hospital policy.	Every hospital should have a written plan for emergency baptism.
Identify sibling reactions.	Sibling grief Sibling guilt Alterations in sibling behavior (e.g., regression, fear of separation from parents)	Help parents consider ways to express their own grief to siblings and reassure siblings of continued parental support. Role play may be helpful. Books (Table 28–1) may help some parents explain death to their other children in age-appropriate ways. Help parents interpret alterations in sibling behavior. If alterations do not resolve over time, parents may need suggestions about sources of help.	Sibling reactions to infant's death will vary with age of sibling (see text).
Identify parents' wishes about funeral, memorial service, etc.	Parents' need for information about alternatives available to them	Explain alternatives available in individual community. Provide referral to appropriate resources (e.g., clergy).	Alternatives commonly available: 1. Hospital disposal of body; no service 2. Hospital disposal of body; memorial service 3. Funeral
Identify continuing needs.	Dysfunctional grieving Inadequate family coping Need for specific counseling (e.g., genetic)	Provide opportunity for follow-up conference: 1. Continuing support for family 2. Results of autopsy if performed 3. Referral for genetic counseling if appropriate 4. Other referrals as appropriate (e.g., family counseling) 5. Discussion of family planning	

portunity for friends and family to support the family.[1, 16] The disposal of the infant's body with no public recognition of the infant's existence may make both birth and death seem unreal, especially if the infant's life was brief, and may complicate the resolution of grief.

Parents need to be prepared for difficult days at home after their infant's death. The clothes and furnishings that may have been prepared for the baby must be packed away. Well-meaning friends may make statements such as "You can always have another baby," or "It was God's will" that devastate parents. A phone number that will put them in touch with someone (such as nurse, clergyman, or parents' group) who will listen to their feelings is valuable.

When the mother is no longer in the hospital herself at the time of the baby's death, maintaining contact with the family over the first hours and days is more difficult. A nursing plan for this family should include short-term follow-up care, either from the hospital where the baby died or through the use of community health nurses. The same issues discussed with the mother in the hospital need to be explored with the mother at home.

Resolution of grief takes time and proceeds at varying rates for different individuals. The time period may be as long as 6 to 8 months. Parents need to know that they will not "feel better" in a few days or even a few weeks, although the intensity of their grieving will gradually diminish. It is believed that the couple should not become pregnant during this period of grief resolution because the new infant may be considered a "replacement" for the dead infant, complicating the relationship between parents and that infant.[9]

Because grief proceeds at different rates in different persons and because individuals react to grief in different ways, a mother and father may be in different stages of grieving or behaving in ways that seem inappropriate to the other. If this possibility is not explained to and accepted by a couple, it can lead to difficulties in their relationship.

Within a few weeks after the baby's death there may be a planned conference with parents, nurses (often the baby's primary nurse), physicians, and social workers. The purpose of this conference is to assess the parents' progress through the grieving process and to identify needs for additional help. Parents have the opportunity to ask questions that may still be a source of concern to them. If there has been an autopsy, the findings are explained to the parents. Referrals for help with specific needs (marital counseling or genetic counseling, for example) or additional conferences with the nursery staff may be planned.

Helping Parents to Cope with the Reaction of the Infant's Siblings

The need to consider siblings and their feelings and reactions to a new baby who is ill is discussed earlier in this chapter. When an expected baby dies, the needs of siblings are for solace, comforting, and help in understanding the death. The way in which these needs will be met will vary with the age of the child. A very small child may not understand about the baby's death at all but will be affected by his parents' grief. Death is not real to a child under the age of 3, but separation, particularly separation from parents, is a major source of anxiety. Children between the ages of 3 and 5 may have some ideas about death, but still do not view death as permanent. Gradually, after the age of 6, children begin to understand the permanancy of death. Children between the ages of 5 and 8 seem to be more afraid of death than younger or older children.

Parents who are grieving themselves often have great difficulty talking about the baby's death with their other children. There are a number of books about death written for children that may help both parents and children verbalize their feelings of sadness (Table 28-1). Parents can be helped to acknowledge their feelings and to reassure their other children with statements such as "Mommy is sad because our baby died, but she is happy that you are here."

Parents frequently ask if siblings should attend the baby's funeral. There is no single answer to this question. Many variables, including the child's age and his wish to attend or not, must be considered. Some children would feel very isolated if they were not a part of this ritual. If children do attend a funeral, a family friend or relative should assume the responsibility for their care. If children are unable to sit throughout the service, they should be able to leave with the adults who are caring for them.

Reactions of Nurses

Not only families of infants but also nurses and their professional colleagues may have difficulty in coping with their feelings about newborn infants who are ill or dying or have major congenital anomalies. Before nurses can be helpful to parents they must be able to recognize and cope with their own feelings.

Table 28–1. BOOKS FOR CHILDREN AND THEIR PARENTS ABOUT DYING

Preschool-Age Children
  Someone Small, by Barbara Borack. New York, Harper & Row, 1969.
  The Dead Bird, by Margaret Wise Brown. Reading, Mass., Addison-Wesley, 1958.
  My Grandpa Died Today, by Joan Fassler, New York, Human Sciences Press, 1971.
  Why Did He Die? by Audrey Harris. Minneapolis, Lerner Productions, 1965.
  When Violet Died, by Mildren Kantrowitz. New York, Parents' Magazine Press, 1973.

School-Age Children (ages 6–9)
  Nana Upstairs, Nana Downstairs, by Thomas De Paola. New York, G. P. Putnam's Sons, 1973.
  Confessions of an Only Child, by Norman Klein. New York, Pantheon, 1974. (Describes the feelings of a 9-year-old when the new baby dies.)
  Death Is Natural, by Lawrence Pringle. New York, Scholastic Book Service, 1977.

Preadolescent Children (ages 10–12)
  Life and Death, by H. Zim and Sonia Bleeker, New York, William Morrow, 1970.

Parents
  About Dying: An Open Book for Parents and Children, by Sara Stein. New York, Walker & Company, 1974.
  Helping Your Child to Understand Death, by Anna Wolf. New York, Child Study Association of America, 1973.

Consider this situation: You are working in the nursery when a baby, newly delivered, arrives. His father will be coming to the nursery shortly to see his first-born son. Normally this is a joyful occasion; you get a great deal of satisfaction from "showing" babies to their parents for the first time. But in the middle of this baby's back is a large meningocele. How do you feel about showing this baby to his father? Threatened? Anxious? Helpless? Sad? Would you like to position the baby so that the father will not see the defect? Are you angry about being placed in the position of having to show the baby?

None of these feelings is unusual. They are shared not only by student nurses but by many other members of the health team. To recognize that we sometimes feel this way is the beginning of developing an ability to cope with the reality of a high risk baby and his parents.

The Sources of Our Feelings

Our own experiences, both professional and personal, influence the way we will view the problems of a particular baby and his family.

For example, if we have seen very good results in the repair of cleft lips in babies, we find we can talk quite comfortably with parents, giving this realistic assurance. Moreover, and perhaps even more important, we can handle the baby easily and affectionately. Parents are quick to perceive our reactions to their baby; our positive feelings toward them and their baby will help them to react in a positive way as well.

Nurses and other health team members may also have negative feelings toward babies who are critically ill or handicapped. One student nurse, for example, whose brother had been brain damaged at the time of birth and eventually placed in an institution, found it particularly difficult to care for babies and families who appeared to have similar problems.

Just as parents detect positive attitudes, they may even more quickly perceive negative feelings toward themselves and their baby. How do we hold their baby? Do we hide him in the corner of the nursery? Do we avoid spending time with the mother and father? Because of their own feelings of guilt and anger and disappointment, they are usually supersensitive to any indication that we reject their baby. Even a chance remark overheard in a corridor may be taken as evidence of our rejection.

Learning to explore and deal with our feelings about sick or handicapped babies can be painful. Nurses sometimes choose maternity and newborn nursing as an area of practice because they feel it involves happy people — joyful parents and healthy babies—in contrast to many other areas of health care. Because joy is the expectation, coping with sadness is even more difficult than it might be under different circumstances. To be an effective nurse for pregnant families, we must have the resources to help parents cope with unexpected grief as well as with happier moments.

Somewhat different kinds of feelings may surface in the nursery concerning decisions about how much treatment is given to a particular baby. We may feel angry about the aggressive treatment given to one infant who we feel has little chance of survival ("Why don't they let him die in peace?"). On the other hand, we may feel just as hostile about failure to treat a baby who we believe would have a good chance of surviving. Part of the frustration for nurses comes from the feeling that we have no choice in the decisions that are made; we need to recognize this. Part of the *result* of that frustration may involve subtle (and usually unconscious) manipulation of parents to one's point of view. Needless to say, this is

Table 28–2. MANIFESTATIONS OF THE GRIEF PROCESS IN NURSES AND FAMILIES*

Emotion	Nurses	Families
Shock and disbelief	Particularly acute when baby who appeared to be doing well worsens—Why this baby?	Why me? Why us? Why our baby?
Shame, loss of self-esteem	Inability to prevent death seen as threat to self-esteem	Why could we not produce a healthy child?
Guilt	Guilt about care given or not given	Guilt about preterm birth or anomaly Guilt about not wanting to attach to baby
Anxiety	Fear of helplessness Coping with anxiety by remaining detached, enforcing "rules"	Fear of attaching to baby, growing to love baby Fear of loss of baby
Denial	Denial of severity of illness to self and parents	Denial of severity of infant's illness
Anger	Anger at baby Anger at parents Anger at other team members Blaming parents and team members	Anger at baby Anger at staff Anger at other family members
Bargaining	Promises to God and others	Promises to God and others
Acceptance	Need opportunities to express feelings and ask questions Require acceptance of colleagues' expressions in nonjudgmental fashion	Need opportunities to express feelings and ask questions

*(From Moore: *Newborn, Family and Nurse.* 2nd Edition. Philadelphia, W. B. Saunders Co., 1981.)

very destructive behavior. Parents of newborns who are ill have to cope with multiple problems and feelings; our care must be supportive.

These feelings of nurses are very much like those of parents who are experiencing grief. Nurses do experience grief as they care for high risk infants and may demonstrate grief in their behavior. Table 28–2 compares the grief process of nurses with that of parents. Until we can recognize the basis of our own behavior we will be limited in our ability to help parents cope.

What can be done to help staff (nurses, physicians, and other professional workers) deal with these kinds of feelings? Frequently, opportunities for all nursery staff to meet together in multidisciplinary conferences are helpful. The opportunity for each person to share his or her ideas can enhance care tremendously. Such sessions are of little value, of course, if they are authoritarian or defensive.

Careful leadership is important in these conferences to avoid their disintegration into "gripe sessions," which can be more destructive than constructive. A discussion of group dynamics is beyond the scope of this book, but help is available within most hospital settings or from other agencies in most communities in the form of individuals who can assist nurses in developing these skills or who can share their leadership with a nursing unit.

Nursing peer support needs to be immediately available on a 24-hour basis. Nurses who care for sick or seriously handicapped babies may come to the point of tears of anger and frustration at the end of a shift. They need to talk about those feelings at that moment; otherwise they may become exhausted from trying to cope with their own grief and the grief of the parents as well as the continued physical and emotional needs of the other infants in the nursery.

With support, experiences with sick infants or infants with serious congenital anomalies and with their families can lead to emotional equanimity, which enables nurses to give compassionate care without devastating their colleagues or being devastated themselves. Without support, grief experiences may lead to an emotional detachment that prevents nurses from being responsive to the special needs of these infants and their families.

The Mother Who Is Ill During the Puerperium

The immediate postpartum period has been described as a "sensitive period," during which attachment is facilitated by the parents' opportunity to see, touch, hold, and care for their baby. What happens when the mother is unable to be with her baby because of infection, for example, or because she is too ill to care for him? Does this missed opportunity affect her initial attachment to her baby? Does it affect her long-term relationship?

A mother who is ill herself necessarily focuses on her own needs. She may have reduced self-esteem and a sense of failure because she did not have the kind of labor and birth experience she expected and because she is not able to participate in the care of her infant in the way she desires. Her illness may make breast-feeding difficult or impossible in the immediate postpartum period, although she may be able later to breast-feed using techniques of relactation (Chapter 23). She may feel powerless to cope with the needs of her new infant. Because caring for her infant is part of the attachment process, attachment may be delayed.

Mercer[13] describes a mother with idiopathic thrombocytopenic purpura who went into shock a few hours after delivery and subsequently underwent surgery for a retroperitoneal hematoma. Postoperatively she spent 4 days in an intensive care unit and was then transferred to a surgical unit. During this time she had no contact with her baby. Mercer's conversations with the mother indicate the mother's focus of attention on her own physical problems.

Rubin[20] has noted that even well mothers have a need for normal body function before they begin to "mother." This behavior on the part of the mother, while appropriate to the circumstances, is a barrier to mothering.

An additional barrier to attachment is the physical separation of mother from baby. Rules should be bent whenever possible to minimize the time of physical separation. In the interim, pictures of the baby that the mother can keep with her and frequent discussions with the mother that emphasize her baby's individuality can help to facilitate her attachment.

As the mother recovers physically she will be able to assume more mothering tasks, although it may be some time after hospital discharge before she is able to take major responsibility for her infant's care. Hospital nurses can help her set priorities for her activities at home (baby care has priority over house care, for example) and plan for a gradual increase in activities. Planning should include the identification of others who will be able to help and what those others will do. Community health nurses provide continuity in furthering or modifying the plan of care in consultation with the mother.

Nursing records should indicate the mother's progress toward attachment. When does she refer to the baby by his sex, calling the infant "him," for example, rather than "the baby"? When does she call him by name? Is she concerned about infant care in a specific way for her baby? Does she identify the unique needs and characteristics of her baby?

Mercer[13] reports on a follow-up visit to the mother described earlier when her baby was 9 months old. Even then, she never referred to her son by name. She talked much about herself but had to be questioned about her son. Although generalizations cannot be drawn from a single incident, the experience of even one family indicates the need for nurses to be aware of the potential implications of postpartum complications.

Alterations in Attachment or Caregiving due to Maternal Personality Characteristics

In addition to maternal or infant illness, other factors may influence attachment. Characteristics of the mother's personality may make attachment difficult.

Polansky[18] classified mothers who were unable to provide an adequate level of care to their infants in several groups: apathetic–futile, impulse ridden, mentally retarded, reactive depressive, and psychotic (see Nursing Care Plan 28–3). Another group of mothers who are likely to have difficulty providing care is composed of those addicted to drugs or alcohol.

Apathetic–futile mothers are characterized by emotional numbness. They feel that nothing is worth doing. They have few if any interpersonal relationships with others, a characteristic noted by other researchers as well.[8] Low competence level, a fear of failure, passive defiance of authority, negativism, and an inability to express feelings were also evident. Infants of apathetic–futile mothers were found to become withdrawn and lethargic and, be-

Nursing Care Plan 28–3. Alterations in Attachment and Infant Care Related to Maternal Illness or Personality Variables

NURSING GOAL: To facilitate attachment and effective family coping when the mother is ill or has a personality characteristic that interferes with attachment or with infant.

OBJECTIVES:
1. Mother's dependency needs are met.
2. Attachment is facilitated in a manner appropriate to the mother's problem.
3. Appropriate infant care is ensured through support services if mother is unable to care for infant.

ASSESSMENT	POTENTIAL NURSING DIAGNOSIS	NURSING INTERVENTION	COMMENTS/RATIONALE
Identify the mother at risk of difficulty in attachment.		Meet mother's prolonged dependency needs. Provide opportunities to verbalize concerns about self.	Mother will not be able to attend to infant until her own needs are met.
1. Maternal illness in the puerperium	Decreased maternal self-esteem	Mother may be limited in ability to care for infant initially. Provide opportunities for mother to see baby and touch as condition allows. At first nurse may need to hold infant so mother can see, or place infant on mother's bed beside her. Provide pictures of infant for mother between baby visits.	
2. Unexpected complications of labor or birth	Lag in attachment related to maternal illness		
		As mother recovers, encourage her to assume responsibility for infant very gradually.	
		Discuss infant care at home following discharge; help mother set priorities that allow adequate maternal rest. Guide mother to identify support persons who will assist with home and infant care.	
Identify signs of attachment or lag in attachment (see Nursing Care Plan 28–1).	Lag in attachment	Refer to community health nurse to provide intervention following discharge.	
		Provide mother with information about community resources such as Homemaker Service.	
Identify maternal characteristics that may alter attachment. *Apathetic-futile personality* 1. Nothing is worth doing 2. Emotional numbness 3. Lack of interpersonal relationships 4. Passive defiance of authority	Maternal apathetic-futile personality	Focus on small gains at a time. Don't be overambitious; don't expect too much at once. Attempt to increase mother's ability to talk about her feelings.	Potential effect on infant or child: 1. Withdrawn 2. Lethargic 3. Eventual lower intelligence (owing to lack of intellectual stimulation).

Characteristics	Intervention	Potential effect on infant or child
(continued) 5. Low competence; fear of failure 6. Stubborn negativism 7. Inability to express feelings	Provide specific training in parenting skills. Expect any change to take a long time.	
Impulse-ridden personality 1. Restless 2. Unable to tolerate stress 3. Aggressive, defiant 4. Craves excitement 5. Manipulative 6. Behavior often that of 3- to 9-year-old 7. May not keep appointments (e.g., not at home when nurse goes to visit, even though prior appointment made)	Encourage mother to place limits on behavior, first to please professional, later to please self. Encourage delayed gratification. Provide specific training in parenting skills.	Potential effect on infant or child: 1. In danger when mother succumbs to impulse to leave 2. Hostile-defiant 3. Lack of self-control
Mentally retarded mother 1. Illiterate 2. Poor sense of time 3. Finds difficulty in money management 4. Concrete, rigid understanding 5. Forgetfulness of anything if it is out of sight 6. Travels only over familiar routes 7. Finds difficulty in making adult judgments (e.g., when infant is sick) 8. Limited manual skill 9. Highly suggestible	Ensure supervision (family homemaker service, etc.) Provide specific training in parenting skills.	Potential effect on infant or child: 1. Precarious physical survival 2. Inadequate protein nutrition (irregular meals, etc.) 3. Slow language development 4. Eventual lower intelligence (lack of intellectual stimulation)
Reactive depressive mother 1. Depression in reaction to a specific external stimulus 2. Unable to care for children 3. Unable to communicate about job, excitement, love 4. Oblivious to child's signals	Encourage mother to verbalize feelings. Refer for specific treatment for depression. Provide specific training in parenting skills.	Potential effect on infant or child: 1. Withdrawn, lethargic, eventual lower intelligence (lack of intellectual stimulation)
Psychotic mother 1. Out of contact with reality 2. Social withdrawal 3. Loss of contact 4. Inappropriate mood 5. Bizarre behavior; grimaces 6. Disturbed stream of thought 7. Delusions 8. Hallucinations 9. Chronic anxiety	Refer for professional psychiatric care. Ensure infant care (mother may be unable to provide any safe care). Foster care may be necessary if no competent caregiver in home.	Potential effect on infant or child: 1. In danger due to mother's forgetfulness of feeding, hours for sleep, lack of physical care, etc. 2. Eventual lower intelligence (owing to lack of intellectual stimulation)

cause of lack of intellectual stimulation, eventually showed evidence of lower intelligence.

Impulse-ridden mothers were unable to tolerate stress. Restless, aggressive, and defiant are words that describe their behavior. They are controlled by impulses that may lead to abuse or abandonment of their baby.

Mothers who are mentally retarded often have a poor sense of time, resulting in irregular feedings and general disorganization. Out of sight may mean out of mind, so that the mother may, for example, leave home for an errand and actually forget about her baby. Language development in the baby is frequently slow because of the lack of verbal stimulation. The mentally retarded mother may have limited manual skills and will usually have difficulty in making adult judgments, such as recognizing illness in her baby.

Mothers who are depressed are frequently unable to care for their infants because they are oblivious to their child's signals. They are also unable to communicate any joy or excitement to their child.

A psychotic mother, who has lost contact with reality, may exhibit bizarre behavior, delusions, hallucinations, and inappropriate mood, and may pose a real danger to her infant.

Mothers addicted to drugs have weak commitments to interpersonal relationships, a pattern that may characterize mother–infant relationships as well as those with other persons.[22] One sign of this tenuous bond is the tendency to surrender parenting functions readily to others while in the hospital and to other persons around her after discharge. In addition, if the baby is withdrawing from narcotics (Chapter 24), the mother may receive more negative than positive reinforcement for her attempts to care for her baby.

A need common to mothers with any of the problem characteristics described above is a comprehensive plan of care that provides continuing assessment of and interaction with the family over an extended period of time. Nurses during the puerperium may identify mothers as having potential difficulties in attachment (as may nurses in the prenatal period [Chapter 10] or in the intrapartum period [Chapter 20]). Successful long-term intervention, when necessary, will require follow-up by community health nurses and other professionals. Some mothers will always need supervision in the care of their children—the mentally retarded or psychotic mother, for example. When no supervision and long-term family support is available, the issue of child custody arises. Adoption may be a necessary solution for some infants.

A second need common to these mothers is very specific help in parenting skills, and assessment of each mother's progress in attaining these skills. This process is initiated in the hospital but must be continued when the baby returns to the community.

Indications of Slow Progression of Attachment

Assessing the failure of attachment is difficult because the timing of the process varies individually, even when both mother and infant are healthy. Macfarlane[11a] reported that 27 per cent of 97 mothers said they first felt love for their babies during the first week of life, whereas 8 per cent indicated they did not have feelings of love for their baby until after the first week. Moreover, more mothers reported an increase of affection during the first 2 weeks of life than at birth. Robson and Moss[19] also found that many mothers felt that their babies were strange and unfamiliar during the first weeks of life and that their affection grew as they came to know their babies.

In assessing attachment it is essential to remember that early indications of difficulty do not necessarily indicate that there will be long-term problems. However, early assessment cannot be ignored. Once again, close communication between nurses who see mothers and infants in the period immediately following birth and community health nurses who will see them in the weeks and months that follow is essential.

Broussard[3] has been using her Neonatal Perception Inventory (NPI) for 16 years to measure a mother's perception of her baby compared with her perception of the average baby on six aspects of infant behavior: crying, spitting, feeding, elimination, sleeping, and predictability. In following infants from birth through 16 years of age, Broussard reported that those infants whose mothers perceived them as "better than average" were at low risk for developmental problems, while infants viewed less favorably were at risk for subsequent problems.

Most mothers perceive their babies as better than the average baby; in our high risk nurseries we have found that even mothers of infants who have spent a number of weeks in intensive care perceive their infants as better than average on the NPI. Therefore, when a mother perceives her baby as "less than average," especially when the baby is a month old, further interaction with her would seem to be necessary. Table 28–3 describes the NPI.

Table 28–3. NEONATAL PERCEPTION INVENTORY

1. The mothers is told, "We are interested in learning more about the experiences of mothers and their babies during the first few weeks after delivery. The more we can learn about mothers and their babies, the better we will be able to help other mothers with their babies. We would appreciate it if you would help other mothers by filling out these two forms now (first or second postpartum day) and again when your baby is 1 month old." (Forms on pages 996 and 997.)
2. The mother is given the "average baby" form. The examiner remains with the mother while she is filling out the form.
3. When the mother has completed the "average baby" form, the examiner takes it from her and gives her the "your baby" form.
4. Each behavioral item is scored on a 5-point scale ranging from "a great deal" (5 points) to "none" (1 point). (This scoring is used on both occasions of completing the forms.)
5. NPI scores are obtained by adding the numerical scores for each item and subtracting the total score of the "your baby" inventory from the total score of the "average baby" inventory. The difference between the two scores represents the NPI score. A positive score indicates a favorable perception of the infant; he has been rated as better than the average baby and is at low risk for subsequent developmental problems. A negative score indicates a less favorable perception; this infant is at risk for subsequent developmental problems.

In addition to assessing the mother's perceptions of her infant, a number of other nursing observations may indicate slow progression of attachment or potential problems in parenting. The following indications are suggested by Gray.[10]

1. The mother's hopes and expectations as well as her doubts about her own ability and the ability of the baby's father to fulfill the responsibilities of parenthood.
2. Frequency of mother's and father's interaction with baby (use of rooming-in; baby left in bassinet or held and cared for).
3. Failure of progression in skills such as diapering and feeding.
4. Mother's or father's views of the baby as too demanding, too interruptive, too messy.
5. Tendency to ignore baby.
6. Maternal or parental difficulty in handling baby's crying—"crying on purpose"—feeling helpless, feeling like crying themselves, unable to comfort.
7. The way in which parents refer to the baby, calling it by name and sex or "it," making negative remarks. Note affect, not just the words; "he eats like a little pig" could be a positive or a negative remark.
8. Establishment and maintenance of eye contact.
9. Continued disappointment about the sex of the infant.
10. Availability, or lack of it, or support for mother from father, from other kin, and from persons other than family; mother's perception of support systems as "helpful" or "not much help."

Following discharge, multiple phone calls or visits for very minor issues may indicate a lack of confidence in mothering skills; this is considered to be a high risk indicator to the mother, just as multiple calls prenatally suggest risk (Chapter 10). The mother's description of the baby as crying constantly should be verified. Is the mother perceiving constant crying correctly? If the baby is truly crying constantly there may be a physiologic basis (inadequate nutrition, abdominal pain, etc.) If the baby's behavior is "average" but the mother perceives the baby as "less than average," further evaluation of the mother–infant relationship is indicated.

Summary

There has been increasing emphasis in the late 1970's and early 1980's on the importance of the first moments after birth in forming attachment. Some researchers believe that this emphasis has been "overzealous" and that many of the studies contain serious research flaws. When immediate bonding and interaction is possible, certainly it is important and should be encouraged. But when, because of infant or maternal illness, bonding is delayed, excellent long-term attachment may still occur. The warm relationships between adoptive parents and their children support this belief. An *extreme* emphasis on the first moments of the infant's life is potentially deleterious to parents who do not have classic bonding experiences at that time; they may wonder if they will ever be able to be adequate parents.

Nurses assess and facilitate attachment in parents under a variety of circumstances, modifying the plan of care to meet the specific needs of each family.

AVERAGE BABY

Although this is your first baby, you probably have some ideas of what most little babies are like. Please check the blank you think best describes the AVERAGE baby.

How much crying do you think the average baby does?

| a great deal | a good bit | moderate amount | very little | none |

How much trouble do you think the average baby has in feeding?

| a great deal | a good bit | moderate amount | very little | none |

How much spitting up or vomiting do you think the average baby does?

| a great deal | a good bit | moderate amount | very little | none |

How much difficulty do you think the average baby has in sleeping?

| a great deal | a good bit | moderate amount | very little | none |

How much difficulty does the average baby have with bowel movements?

| a great deal | a good bit | moderate amount | very little | none |

How much trouble do you think the average baby has in settling down to a predictable pattern of eating and sleeping?

| a great deal | a good bit | moderate amount | very little | none |

YOUR BABY

While it is not possible to know for certain what your baby will be like, you probably have some ideas of what your baby will be like. Please check the blank that you think best describes what your baby will be like.

How much crying do you think your baby will do?

| a great deal | a good bit | moderate amount | very little | none |

How much trouble do you think your baby will have feeding?

| a great deal | a good bit | moderate amount | very little | none |

How much spitting up or vomiting do you think your baby will do?

| a great deal | a good bit | moderate amount | very little | none |

How much difficulty do you think your baby will have sleeping?

| a great deal | a good bit | moderate amount | very little | none |

How much difficulty do you expect your baby to have with bowel movements?

| a great deal | a good bit | moderate amount | very little | none |

How much trouble do you think that your baby will have settling down to a predictable pattern of eating and sleeping?

A | a great deal | a good bit | moderate amount | very little | none |

Figure 28–7. Neonatal perception inventories. *A,* form given on the first or second postpartum day. *B,* form given when the baby is one month old. (From Broussard: Diss Abstr 26:484, 1964–1965. Copyright 1964—Retained Elsie R. Broussard, M.D.)

Illustration continued on opposite page

AVERAGE BABY

Although this is your first baby, you probably have some ideas of what most little babies are like. Please check the blank you think best describes the AVERAGE baby.

How much crying do you think the average baby does?

| a great deal | a good bit | moderate amount | very little | none |

How much trouble do you think the average baby has in feeding?

| a great deal | a good bit | moderate amount | very little | none |

How much spitting up or vomiting do you think the average baby does?

| a great deal | a good bit | moderate amount | very little | none |

How much difficulty do you think the average baby has in sleeping?

| a great deal | a good bit | moderate amount | very little | none |

How much difficulty does the average baby have with bowel movements?

| a great deal | a good bit | moderate amount | very little | none |

How much trouble do you think the average baby has in settling down to a predictable pattern of eating and sleeping?

| a great deal | a good bit | moderate amount | very little | none |

YOUR BABY

You have had a chance to live with your baby for about a month now. Please check the blank you think best describes your baby.

How much crying has your baby done?

| a great deal | a good bit | moderate amount | very little | none |

How much trouble has your baby had feeding?

| a great deal | a good bit | moderate amount | very little | none |

How much spitting up or vomiting has your baby done?

| a great deal | a good bit | moderate amount | very little | none |

How much difficulty has your baby had in sleeping?

| a great deal | a good bit | moderate amount | very little | none |

How much difficulty has your baby had with bowel movements?

B | a great deal | a good bit | moderate amount | very little | none |

How much trouble has your baby had in settling down to a predictable pattern of eating and sleeping?

| a great deal | a good bit | moderate amount | very little | none |

Figure 28–7 *Continued*

REFERENCES

1. Barton, D.: *Dying and Death: A clinical Guide for Caregivers.* Baltimore, The Williams & Wilkins Co., 1977.
2. Broussard, E.: Psychosocial Disorders in Children: Early Assessment of Infants at Risk. *Continuing Education,* pp. 44–57, February 1978.
3. Broussard, E.: Assessment of the Adaptive Potential of the Mother-Infant System: The Neonatal Perception Inventories. *Seminars in Perinatology, 3*:91, 1979.
4. Caplan, G.: Patterns of Response to the Crisis of Premature Birth. *Psychiatry, 23*:365, 1960.
5. Dickerson, P.: Early Postpartum Separation and Maternal Attachment to Twins. *JOGN Nursing, 10*(2):120, 1981.
6. Duff, R., and Campbell, A.: On Deciding the Care of Severely Handicapped or Dying Persons: With Particular Reference to Infants. *Pediatrics, 57*:487, 1976.
6a. Dunn, D., and Lewis, A.: Some Important Aspects of Neonatal Nursing Related to Pulmonary Disease and Family Involvement. *Pediatric Clinics of North America, 20*:481, 1973.
7. Eibe-Ebesfeldt, E.: *Ethology, the Biology of Behavior.* New York, Holt, Rinehart and Winston, 1970.
8. Elmer, E.: *Fragile Families, Troubled Children.* Pittsburgh, University of Pittsburgh Press, 1977.
9. Fischoff, J., and O'Brien, N.: After the Child Dies. *Journal of Pediatrics, 80*:140, 1976.
10. Gray, J., Cutler, C., Dean, J. et al.: Perinatal Assessment of Mother-Baby Interaction. *In* Helfer, R., and Kempe, C. (eds.): Child Abuse and Neglect. Cambridge, Mass., Ballinger, 1976.
11. Green, M., and Solnit, A.: Reactions to the Threatened Loss of a Child: A Vulnerable Child Syndrome. *Pediatrics, 34*:58, 1964.
11a. Macfarlane, A.: *The Psychology of Childbirth.* Cambridge, Mass.: Harvard University Press, 1977.
12. Mercer, R.: Responses of Mothers to the Birth of an Infant with a Defect. *ANA Clinical Sessions,* 1974. New York, Appleton-Century-Crofts, 1975.
13. Mercer, R.: Postpartum: Illness and Acquaintance-Attachment Process. *American Journal of Nursing, 77*:1174, 1977.
14. Miller, C.: Working with Parents of High Risk Infants. *American Journal of Nursing, 78*:1228, 1978.
15. Moore, M: *Newborn, Family and Nurse.* Philadelphia, W. B. Saunders Co., 1983.
16. Oehler, J.: *Family Centered Neonatal Nursing Care.* Philadelphia, J. B. Lippincott, Co. 1981.
17. Opirhory, G.: Counseling the Parents of a Critically Ill Newborn. *JOGN Nursing, 8*:179, 1979.
18. Polansky, N., DeSaix, C., and Sharlin, S.: *Child Neglect: Understanding and Reaching the Parent.* New York, Child Welfare League of America, 1972.
19. Robson, K., and Moss, H.: Patterns and Determinants of Maternal Attachment. *Journal of Pediatrics, 77*:976, 1970.
20. Rubin, R.: Puerperal Change. *Nursing Outlook, 9*:753, 1961.
21. Sheer, B.: Help for Parents in a Difficult Job—broaching the Subject of Death. *MCN, 2*(5):320, 1977.
22. Singer, A.: Mothering Practices and Heroin Addiction. *American Journal of Nursing, 74*:77, 1974.
23. Stinson, R., and Stinson, P.: On the Death of a Baby. *Atlantic Monthly, 244*:64, 1979.
24. Tipe, R., Smith, G., Lynch, H., et al.: The "Whole Family" Concept in Clinical Genetics. *American Journal of Diseases of Children, 107*:67, 1964.

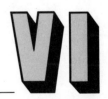

Contemporary Issues for Perinatal Nurses

29

Childbearing and Adolescence

OBJECTIVES

1. Describe trends in births to mothers under the age of 19.
2. Identify factors associated with effective adolescent contraceptive use.
3. Identify social, emotional, and health needs of adolescents who are pregnant.
4. Explain the higher rate of complications in adolescents who seek abortion.
5. Describe consequences of pregnancy for adolescent women, their infants, and society.
6. Discuss legal issues relating to the care of adolescents.
7. Describe how nurses, working with others, can address the issues of adolescent pregnancy.

Childbearing in adolescence has been a focus of attention not only of nurses and other health-care providers but also of social scientists, politicians, educators, parents of adolescents, adolescents themselves, and the general public. Much has been written and said about adolescent pregnancy. Some information is misleading, and a number of questions are still unanswered. This chapter will review adolescent childbearing in relation to the incidence, apparent causes, health and social problems of pregnancy, and the consequences for the mother, father, and infant and for the society as well.

Issues relating to adolescent pregnancy must be considered within the wider perspective of adolescent sexuality. Our concerns must encompass all adolescents, not just those already pregnant or even those already sexually active.

Incidence of Adolescent Pregnancy

The median age of first intercourse for women aged 15 to 19 in the United States who are sexually active was 16.2 years in 1976, a decrease from 16.5 years in 1971 (based on a national probability sample).[45] The median age for men was 13 years in one study.[15] Approximately 35 per cent of unmarried teenagers had experienced sexual intercourse in 1976, an increase of 30 per cent over 1971; the increase was greater among white teens than among black teens (Table 29–1).

In 1978, the last year for which complete statistics were available at the time of writing, over 10,000 infants were born to mothers who were 15 years old or younger; more than 540,000 newborns had mothers between the ages of 15 and 19.[13]

Although there is a widely held impression that there has been a significant rise in adolescent pregnancy during the last decade, a brief examination of Figure 29–1 will show that birth rates for 15- to 19-year-olds have fallen each year since 1970, and have been on a generally declining course since 1957. The birth rate reflects the number of registered live births per 1000 women in the age group. Rates for 14- and 15-year-olds peaked in 1975 and have declined since that time. The 1978 birth rate for women aged 18 and 19 was close to the lowest ever observed for this age group.[7]

A major increase has occurred, however, in the percentage of births occurring to teenaged women outside of marriage (Fig. 29–2). The term "legitimated first birth" is used to describe a first birth occurring 7 or fewer months following a first marriage. It is not possible to determine from statistical information such as that in Figure 29–2 and Table 29–2 how many marriages were a direct result of pregnancy compared with those that had been planned before conception or before the woman realized she was pregnant. Note (Table 29–2) that while in previous decades the percentage of black women marrying following premarital conception equaled or exceeded the percentage of white women marrying, there has been a marked decrease in marriage among black women and an increase among white women (see last column). Later in this chapter the advantages and disadvantages of marriage as a result of pregnancy are discussed.

The statistics on adolescent birthrates reveal only part of the extent of teenaged pregnancy. Over 300,000 adolescents terminate pregnancy through abortion each year; roughly twice as many white teens seek abortion, although the percentage of black teens is increasing annually. There appears to be a correlation between ease of obtaining abortion and the birth rate to unmarried women.[12] In addition, approximately 100,000 teenagers spontaneously abort each year.

Causes of Adolescent Pregnancy

Why do adolescents become pregnant? In examining the causes of adolescent pregnancy, the incidence and frequency of teenage sexual intercourse and their knowledge and use of contraceptives are areas to consider.

Zelnik and Kantner[45] surveyed 15- to 19-year-old women of all marital statuses to determine the prevalence of premarital intercourse as well as gathering information about other related topics. An increase of 30 per cent in incidence of premarital intercourse was found between 1971 and 1976.

One must then consider whether that intercourse was protected by the use of contraception. Contraceptive use appears to be age-related: in one study 55 per cent of 18- and 19-year-old women used a contraceptive at first

Table 29–1. SEXUAL EXPERIENCE OF UNMARRIED ADOLESCENTS (PER CENT EVER HAVING INTERCOURSE)*

	White	Black
1971	21	51
1976	31	63

*Zelnick and Kantner: *In* Furstenburg, Lincoln, and Menken (eds.): *Teenage Sexuality, Pregnancy, and Childbearing.* Philadelphia, University of Pennsylvania Press, 1981.

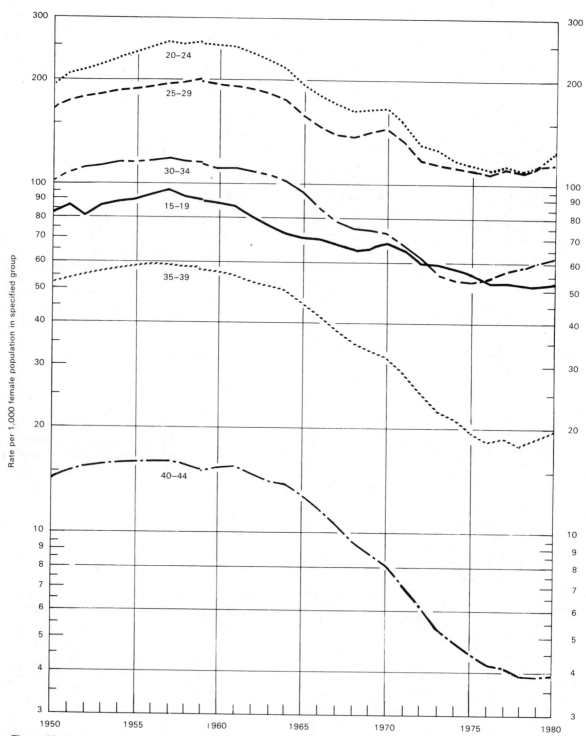

Figure 29–1. Birth rates by age of mother, United States, 1950–1980. (From National Center for Health Statistics: Advance report of final natality statistics, 1980. *Monthly Vital Statistics Report*, Vol 31, No. 8, Suppl., Nov. 1982.)

intercourse, whereas only 25 per cent of women under 15 and 41 per cent of women aged 15 to 17 did. Of those who used contraception at first intercourse, one-third do not continue to use it consistently. For many women there is a time lag approximately 1 year between the initiation of first intercourse and an initial visit to a family planning clinic. During this time, some women are using a form of contraception available in the community. However, nearly one-half of all initial teenaged pregnancies occur in the first 6 months of sexual activity.[43]

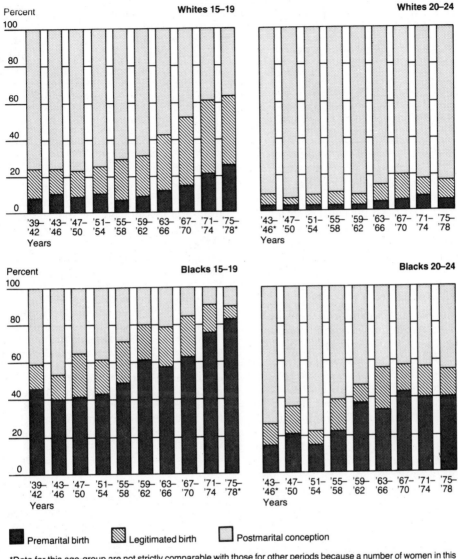

Premarital birth · Legitimated birth · Postmarital conception

*Data for this age-group are not strictly comparable with those for other periods because a number of women in this cohort are not included in the survey universe. This number is relatively small. See Tables 1 and 2.

Figure 29–2. Percentage distribution of first births to women aged 15–19 and 20–24, by legitimacy status of birth, 1939–1942 to 1975–1978. (From O'Connell and Moore: The legitimacy status of first births to U.S. women aged 15–24, 1939–1978. *Family Planning Perspectives, 12*(1):17, 1980.)

Not all pregnancies of teenagers are unintended; Zelnik and Kantner[45] report that approximately 50 per cent are desired. Twenty-three per cent occurred to women who were married prior to pregnancy, and 28 per cent occurred to nonmarried women. Of these, over 40 per cent married before the baby's birth.

Of those teenagers who did not intend pregnancy, 8 in 10 were not using any method of contraception at the time pregnancy occurred (Table 29–3).

Just as the use of contraception influences the likelihood of pregnancy, a variety of factors appear to influence the likelihood of contraception.

1. The age of the mother at the time of first intercourse has already been noted as having an inverse relation to the use of contraception; the younger the mother, the less likely it is that contraception will be employed.

2. The educational level of the teenaged woman's parents appear to be a factor in her participation in premarital intercourse, use of contraception at first intercourse, and regularity of contraceptive use. However, almost 75 per cent of sexually active teenagers used contraceptives irregularly or not at all.[16]

3. The better an individual feels about herself, the more likely she is to use contraceptives.[18, 20, 30]

4. Effective communication between sexual partners may improve contraceptive use.[22] One

Table 29–2. PREMARITAL CONCEPTION AND BIRTH FOR WOMEN AGED 15 TO 19*

	Per Cent Premarital Conceptions		Per Cent Premarital Births		Per Cent Legitimized First Birth	
	White	*Black*	*White*	*Black*	*White*	*Black*
1939–1942	25	60	10	40	15	20
1951–1954	25	60	10	40	15	20
1955–1958	29	71	7	49	22	22
1975–1978	63	90	26	83	37	7

*Data from O'Connell and Moore: *Family Planning Perspectives, 12*:16, 1980.

outcome of communication may be the acknowledgement of the possibility of intercourse and thus the need for contraception.

5. If pregnancy is perceived as rewarding (e.g., because it enables the adolescent to marry or leave home), contraception is likely to be less effective or less frequent even if pregnancy is not immediately desired.[24]

6. Adolescents who have higher educational and occupational goals are more likely to use contraceptives; frequency of contraception is related to the degree of commitment to long-term goals.[22] This is the converse of No. 5; it suggests that a difference in perceived rewards and costs makes a difference in contraceptive use (see also Exchange Theory in Chapter 2).

7. The level of cognitive development may be important. Frequently, an adolescent will state that she just didn't believe that pregnancy could happen to her,[37] a kind of magical thinking. As formal thought becomes more developed, this reasoning should be less frequent.

8. Religious affiliation and church attendance affect contraceptive use. In one study adolescents from fundamentalist religions used contraceptives least frequently, while Catholics used them most often.[45]

Adolescents Who Are Pregnant

Like the members of any other group, adolescents who are pregnant do not form a homogeneous group. Nor is every adolescent pregnancy a problem pregnancy, although many do present one or more special needs.

Mary Anne is 18 and a high school senior. Although she is not married to the man who is the father of her expected baby, the relationship is close. He hopes to be with her during labor and delivery. Both his mother and her own plan to help care for the baby next year so that Mary Anne can attend the LPN program at the community college.

Janice is 16. She lives at home with her mother and sisters; two of her sisters, 17 and 18 years old, are also pregnant. She says she feels no long-term commitment to the father of this infant and would rather have her girlfriend with her during labor.

Cara is 17 and very much alone. Her parents live in a rural community approximately 50 miles from the city where she is now living. The baby's father is from that same community; she has not seen him since she discovered that she was pregnant and does not plan to tell him. Cara has not completed high school; she worked as a waitress when she first came to the city and is now a cashier in a movie theater from 2:00 P.M. until 10:00 P.M. each evening.

When a teenaged woman becomes pregnant, she must make decisions that may be the most difficult of her life to that time. Should she continue the pregnancy or choose to have it terminated? If she continues the pregnancy, should she consider giving the baby for adoption? If she is single, should she marry? Can she continue in school or must she drop out?

Too little is known about the process by which teens make these decisions. Some decisions are undoubtedly passive. Termination of pregnancy, for example, may not be considered or decided upon until the pregnancy is so far advanced that termination is no longer an option. The baby may be kept by the mother not as a result of an active decision but because adoption was never considered.

Some data are available regarding the outcome of these decisions. Few teens choose to place the baby for adoption. Although 90 per cent of unmarried teens chose adoption a decade ago, fewer than 10 per cent now choose adoption. Approximately 30 per cent of unmarried teens seek abortions.

Table 29–3. RISK OF PREGNANCY IN SEXUALLY ACTIVE ADOLESCENT WOMEN

Method	Per Cent Risk of Becoming Pregnant
No contraception	58
Regular contraception (nonmedical method)	11
Regular contraception (medical method: pill, IUD, diaphragm)	6

Luker[24] has used a cost–reward model in her study of young women seeking abortion. The cost of continuing a pregnancy are weighed against its possible rewards. Further research within this framework may prove very useful.

To effectively help teenagers cope with pregnancy, we need to consider the developmental aspects of adolescence as well as the ways in which pregnancy interfaces with those developmental needs. In doing so, we discover that for the teenager herself, her needs and concerns are principally directed toward her adolescence rather than toward her pregnancy.

Health Needs of Adolescents Who Are Pregnant

Adolescents who are pregnant have traditionally been considered at risk for prenatal and intrapartum complications. More recent data suggest that many of the health problems of pregnant teens are related not so much to age but to a lack of prenatal care. In one survey, 7 of 10 teenagers received no prenatal care during the first trimester.[27] There are many probable reasons for delaying care. The teenager may not realize she is pregnant, may deny the pregnancy to herself, or may feel the need to conceal the pregnancy from others. She may not perceive early care as necessary, or at least sufficiently necessary to seek it out. (In the framework of rewards and costs discussed in Chapter 2, the costs may outweigh the rewards.)

When prenatal care is early and sufficient, the physical outcome of pregnancy is generally satisfactory. Nevertheless, special attention should be directed toward those aspects of care that are potential problems in adolescent gravidas (Nursing Care Plan 29–1). This kind of attention apparently reduces the risk status of pregnant adolescents to a level similar to that of all pregnant women.[35]

Identifying pregnant teens as soon as possible after conception and bringing them into a health care system that meets their special needs is obviously the first step (Fig. 29–3). Barriers to care such as lack of accessibility or an atmosphere in which teens feel unwelcome must be corrected. The requirement for parental consent before services are provided can lead to a delay of many weeks before an initial prenatal visit. Many teens are most comfortable in a service designed specifically for adolescents.

A second area of concern is the nutritional status of the pregnant adolescent. During adolescence body growth and development accelerate rapidly, being most marked in girls between the ages of 11 and 13 years and boys between the ages of 13 and 15½ years. Between the ages of 11 and 16 a girl achieves 8 per cent of her total physical development. At no other period in life after the first birthday does growth occur so rapidly.

To keep pace with this rapid development, nutritional demands both in the 11- to 14- and 15- to 18-year age groups are increased in terms of extra calories, protein, minerals, and vitamins.

The nutritional needs of pregnant women have been described in Chapter 9. There are few good studies of the specific nutritional needs of pregnant teenagers. Since growth may continue for 2 or more years following menarche, there is a possibility of conception before full physical maturity, and the younger teen is considered at highest nutritional risk. Calories, protein, calcium, the B vitamins (except vitamin B_{12}), and vitamin C are the nutrients for which teens appear to have an increased need. There is no difference in the recommended intake of vitamins A, E, B_{12}, and folacin and the minerals iron, magnesium, iodine, and zinc for adults and adolescents during pregnancy.[28]

The pregnant teen often does not prepare her own meals and frequently is uninterested in many foods that are important for her, such as vegetables and milk. Continuing diet counseling is important throughout pregnancy to help her meet her nutritional needs within bounds set by her likes and dislikes as well as by her socioeconomic status.

A mother who enters pregnancy at 10 per cent or more below standard weight is at increased risk of delivering a low birth weight infant, who is in turn at increased risk of perinatal mortality.[39] Some teenagers fall within this category. Higgens[19] reported that protein-calorie supplementation improved pregnancy outcome in underweight women; Rush[33] did not find an advantage in the use of dietary supplementation.

Although in theory only iron and folic acid require supplementation during pregnancy, the diet habits of many teenagers make the use of vitamin-mineral supplements common.

The increasing use of alcohol or other drugs by some teenagers must be considered in the assessment and planning of care for all teens. Sexually transmitted diseases are also increasing in the adolescent population.

Other health concerns cited in the literature include an increased incidence of pregnancy-induced hypertension, iron deficiency anemia, hemorrhage and miscarriage, stunted bone growth, and prolonged labor. Stunted bone

Text continued on page 1011

Nursing Care Plan 29–1. Caring for the Adolescent Woman During Childbearing

NURSING GOALS: To support the childbearing adolescent so that her physiologic, developmental, social, emotional, and educational needs are met.
To facilitate attachment between the adolescent mother and her infant.
To provide support for the adolescent mother who is relinquishing her infant for adoption.

OBJECTIVES:
1. The pregnant adolescent receives prenatal care, beginning early in pregnancy, that is designed to meet her physiologic, developmental, social, emotional, and educational needs.
2. Complications of pregnancy are prevented or identified early so that appropriate intervention is initiated.
3. Attachment is assessed and facilitated at each stage of childbearing: prenatal, intrapartal, postpartal.
4. Counseling is provided to help the adolescent mother develop plans for infant care, continuation of her own education, and family planning.
5. The mother who relinquishes her baby for adoption is supported during the grieving process.

ASSESSMENT	POTENTIAL NURSING DIAGNOSIS	NURSING INTERVENTION	COMMENTS/RATIONALE
Identify the pregnant adolescent early in pregnancy.	Pregnant adolescent	Ensure and advertise the availability and advisability of pregnancy testing; remove "barriers" to pregnancy testing and prenatal care. Through community education develop awareness in parents, teachers, and others of behavior in adolescents that may indicate pregnancy.	
		Support pregnant adolescent in "telling" parents about pregnancy—e.g., role play "telling," help her visualize reactions and consider how she will cope with different reactions.	
Identify adolescent's reaction to pregnancy. 1. Denial 2. Problem pregnancy	Denial of pregnancy Problem pregnancy	Encourage acceptance of the reality of pregnancy through nonjudgmental counseling, encouraging verbalization of reactions to the idea of pregnancy.	
Assess knowledge of alternatives to parenthood.	Need for information about alternatives to parenthood (adoption, pregnancy termination)	Provide information about alternatives to parenthood (adoption, pregnancy termination) when desired.	
	Need for problem pregnancy counseling		
	Delay in prenatal care secondary to denial of pregnancy	Develop and participate in community programs to encourage early prenatal care. Remove "barriers" that discourage early prenatal care.	

Goal	Nursing Diagnosis	Intervention	Rationale
Assess throughout pregnancy for potential physiologic complications. 1. Pregnancy-induced hypertension 2. Hemorrhage 3. Premature labor	At risk for (specific complication) secondary to pregnancy during adolescence.	See specific Nursing Care Plans 13–7, 13–10, 19–4.	
Identify nutritional needs.	Nutritional deficit secondary to pregnancy during adolescence At risk for iron deficiency anemia	Counsel to help teenager meet increased needs for calories, protein, calcium, iron, vitamins B and C within the context of foods acceptable to individual.	Teenager favorites such as hamburgers, cheeseburgers, tacos, and pizza can provide needed protein and calories. See Chapter 12 for specific dietary requirements.
	At risk for stunted bone growth in mother (particularly in adolescents less than 15 years old)	Provide continuing nutritional counseling throughout pregnancy. Allow teen to plot weight on graphic chart at each visit to encourage adequate weight gain.	Denial of pregnancy, desire to look like peers, may be factors in desire to gain less weight, look "less pregnant."
Assess weight gain and fetal growth on a continuing basis throughout pregnancy.	At risk of intrauterine growth retardation and delivery of infant who is small for gestational age (Chapter 23)	Married teens may welcome assistance in meal planning, food purchase and preparation. Assistance may be available from home extension agents, homemaker services, etc. Help teens living at home with parents plan ways to meet nutritional needs. Recognize that independence needs may interfere with nutritional needs (e.g., rejection of parent's cooking, desire to eat like peers). Explain how good nutrition enhances skin, nail, and hair appearance.	
Identify need for information about pregnancy, childbirth, and early parenting.	Knowledge deficit Need for information about pregnancy, childbirth, early parenting	Provide information through multiple channels; help the individual adolescent discover sources of information that are most helpful to her. 1. One-to-one teaching 2. Classes within school system, in community centers, in ambulatory clinics, etc. 3. Written information designed for adolescents 4. Tour of labor/birth site	

Table continued on following page

Nursing Care Plan 29–1. Caring for the Adolescent Woman During Childbearing *(Continued)*

ASSESSMENT	POTENTIAL NURSING DIAGNOSIS	NURSING INTERVENTION	COMMENTS/RATIONALE
Identify effects of pregnancy on individual's developmental, social, and emotional needs.		Provide primary nurse throughout pregnancy when possible.	
1. Need for peer acceptance 2. Need for emancipation from parents 3. Need to accept changing body image		Provide continuing opportunities for each pregnant adolescent to verbalize concerns to a nonjudgmental nurse. Interact directly with adolescent rather than with adolescent's mother.	Pregnancy may cause adolescent to be more dependent rather than less dependent on parents.
4. Need to continue education		Identify resources for continuing education in community; refer to proper resource to develop plan for continuing education during pregnancy and following delivery.	Pregnancy is the primary cause of school dropout for young women.
Identify signs of prenatal attachment.	Lag in prenatal attachment	Provide opportunities to hear fetal heart tones with a Doppler.	Some adolescents will deny pregnancy of much of the prenatal period; attachment behaviors will be delayed and may be absent.
1. Pregnancy planning 2. Early prenatal care 3. Attendance at prenatal classes 4. "Nesting" behavior		Through pictures, model, and other visual aids help mother to visualize what fetus is like at each stage of development.	
		After quickening, encourage sensitivity to fetal movement. Fetus will usually respond to "effleurage" of abdomen.	
		Suggest inexpensive ways of preparing for infant (e.g., unfinished furniture, making baby clothes, sources of inexpensive clothing, cost comparison of various sources of diapers).	
Identify prenatal complications that may affect attachment. 1. Unwanted pregnancy 2. Consideration of elective abortion			
Identify support system.	Lack of support system	Help teen identify sources of support; explore possibility of family support. Inform her about community support.	Be aware of sources of support in own community—e.g., Crittendon Homes.

Identify problems related to labor and birth. 1. Assess preparation for labor and birth. 2. Identify reaction to onset of labor.	Knowledge deficit related to labor, birth Misinformation about labor and birth Anxiety secondary to knowledge deficit, misinformation Lack of family or friend as support person during labor	Document attachment behaviors (presence or absence) to assist intrapartal and postpartal nurses in assessment and intervention. Provide primary nurse to support mother (and coach, when present). Provide information about process of labor, reason for nursing actions and actions of others. Assist in relaxation and breathing techniques, even if no prior preparation. If support person (boyfriend, girlfriend, etc.) is also very young, that person may need considerable nursing support. Labor and birth experiences influence early prenatal attachment and future birth experiences.
3. Assess coping skills during labor.		Provide positive reinforcement for coping during labor.
Identify intrapartal signs of attachment: verbal and nonverbal behaviors such as touching and holding, smiling, talking to infant.	Lag in attachment	Provide opportunity for mother (and father, if present) to see, hold, touch infant. Encourage these behaviors and provide positive reinforcement. Point out infant's attributes (quiet alert look, response to voice, etc.)
Identify complications of labor that may interfere with attachment. 1. Long, difficult labor more common in adolescence 2. Maternal complications that prevent early bonding	Lag in attachment, related to 1. Long difficult labor 2. Maternal complications 3. Neonatal complications	Provide bonding opportunities within the context of maternal and infant health and encourage maternal participation (e.g., take mother to nursery in wheelchair, provide picture if mother and infant are separated. See Nursing Care Plan 28–3.
Identify signs of attachment to newborn infant. 1. Positive verbal and nonverbal behaviors 2. Positive regard for infant's father 3. Verbalizes and exhibits joy in caring for infant 4. Verbalizes recognition of infant's unique characteristics 5. Responds appropriately to infant needs and states	Lag in attachment	Help mother (parents) discover unique characteristics of infant, infant's cues about needs. Provide positive reinforcement for caregiving efforts. Refer to community health nurse for continuing care. See Nursing Care Plan 22–1.

Continued on following page

Nursing Care Plan 29–1.   Caring for the Adolescent Woman During Childbearing *(Continued)*

ASSESSMENT	POTENTIAL NURSING DIAGNOSIS	NURSING INTERVENTION	COMMENTS/RATIONALE
Identify plans for infant care following hospitalization. 1. Self 2. Family member 3. Need for community resource	Need for information about resources available for infant care	Provide information about resources available in community. Refer to community health nurse for continuing support.	Mother's ability to return to school and complete education dependent upon family support and community resources.
Identify plans for continuing maternal education.	Need to continue education	Provide information about education alternatives available in community (e.g., self-study, learning "labs" if full-time school not possible). Refer to community health nurse for continuing support.	
Identify plans for contraception.	Need for information about contraception	Provide information about contraception. When preferred method is chosen, counsel mother in depth. Include sexual partner in discussion, when possible. Refer to community family planning resources for continuing care.	A second birth to a teenaged mother further impairs opportunities for continued education and job opportunities.
Care for the Mother Who Relinquishes Her Infant for Adoption			
Identify the mother who chooses to relinquish her infant for adoption.	Mother relinquishing infant Grief reaction	Recognize that relinquishment will cause grieving. Encourage mother to verbalize feelings, concerns. Be available as a listener. Provide opportunity for mother to see, touch, hold infant if she desires. Provide picture of infant for her. Assure her that infant is normal, if true. Inform mother about pertinent laws related to rescinding her decision. Provide information about sources of support in the community that are available for counseling after hospital discharge.	Just as grief work at death is facilitated by attachment, it appears that grief at relinquishment is also facilitated by attachment. State laws vary concerning the length of time in which mother may rescind her decision.

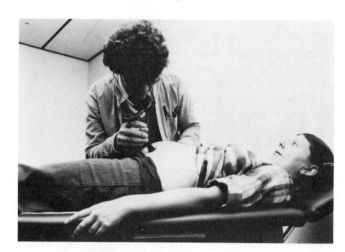

Figure 29–3. Bringing the pregnant teen into a health care system that meets her special needs helps to reduce the risks associated with labor and birth. (Photograph courtesy of Barbara Thompson.)

growth is primarily a concern when the mother is 15 or under. Many other factors may be more related to a lack of prenatal care than to age per se.

Social and Emotional Needs of Adolescents Who Are Pregnant

Need for Acceptance by Peers. Observe any group of adolescents for an hour or so, and the importance of the peer group (their fellow adolescents) becomes apparent. Teens tend to dress alike, eat the same foods, participate in the same activities, use the same vocabulary, listen to the same music, and on and on. Few teens want to be different.

An understanding of this fact has a number of ramifications for our care of the pregnant teenager. If she is a part of a group in which pregnancy is frequent and accepted, *not* being pregnant or having never been pregnant may make her different. If she is part of a group that is looking toward college or a group in which out-of-wedlock pregnancy means "bad girls," being pregnant may be highly stressful. She may choose to terminate the pregnancy early and return to "normal" as quickly as possible.

If she chooses to continue the pregnancy, she may still attempt to remain like her peers in as many ways as possible. For example, she often continues to wear the same clothes that she wore before and to eat foods that are a part of the teenaged lifestyle (soft drinks and French fries, for example) even though we suggest to her that these foods are not ideal during pregnancy.

Need for Emancipation from Parents. One of the largest of all of the tasks of the teenager is achieving independence. For many girls, pregnancy can interrupt the process of becoming independent in a very disturbing way. Our nursing behavior can facilitate her

developing independence or can be one more barrier to that independence.

Consider the following very familiar situation:

Mrs. Anderson has brought her 16-year-old unmarried, pregnant daughter Sally to the obstetric clinic. Sally is quiet, occasionally biting her lip. She does what is asked, never smiling and saying little. Her mother has a great deal to say, most of which is not very complimentary to Sally.

Both Sally and her mother have needs, and Mrs. Anderson is pressing hers upon you very hard. It's very easy to get so drawn into dialogue with in adolescent's parents that we forget that our first priority must be Sally herself—*Sally is our patient.* If we appear to be merely her mother's ally, we will not be very effective in helping Sally. The first rule is: *Remember who the patient is.*

This is not to say that her parents are not very important. A chance to express their feelings is very necessary, both for them and for their pregnant daughter. Ideally, this will come at a separate time and/or place—not during the daughter's prenatal visit. If a separate time is impossible, then a separate place to talk is needed.

Need to Express Feelings to a Nonjudgmental, Truly Interested Adult. Many pregnant adolescents have a need to express their feelings about their pregnancy. Few teenagers can share such feelings with their own parents; such discussions too often become punitive and judgmental.

For some, sharing in a group session may be easier than a face-to-face session with one individual. Here again, the support of the all-important peer group can be significant. Others may find it more difficult to express themselves in groups.

Cultural values will affect the degree to which individuals will share deeply felt emotions. When control of feelings is considered a value, sharing feelings may expose the individual to ridicule from her peers, as Lenocker and Daugherty demonstrated in their study of adolescent mothers.[23] Verbalization of feelings is largely a middle class value and a value of our profession. We need to be sensitive, however, to those groups that do not share this value and should not press our own values upon them.

One of the problems many nurses and other health professionals have in helping a teenager who is pregnant—especially the 14-, 15-, or 16-year-old—is that we also often have very ambivalent feelings about her pregnancy. Thus it is difficult to be nonjudgmental. We may feel that her pregnancy is not a good idea, so that although a part of us truly wants to help her cope with pregnancy, another part of us may want her to understand that she shouldn't be pregnant in the first place. We may fear that being too accepting of her means that we condone her behavior.

We need to recognize our own feelings and to seek guidance in coping with them if we are to be the nonjudgmental professionals that patients have a right to expect us to be.

Need for Mutual Self-disclosures. Should a nurse or other professional person share her own experiences and values about pregnancy with her teenaged patients? Traditionally, we have been told that this is inappropriate and nonprofessional. However, Lenocker and Daugherty described their work with adolescents in which they consciously chose to be open with the teenaged mothers.[23] They found that girls responded by questioning them about their attitudes toward many aspects of their (the authors') life—marriage, childbearing, men, birth control, and similar areas. The teenagers used this information not as a norm for their own life, but as a part of a process of forming perceptions about middle class white women. (The group of teens in the study were black and from low income homes.) The authors felt their openness, which included picnics at their homes, may also have demonstrated that self-revelation is an acceptable form of behavior.

Need to Be Understood Despite Language Barrier. An important characteristic of adolescent culture is a language by which teens communicate with one another. This language includes phrases that may mean something very different to the teenaged mother than they do to us. Moreover, many terms in general use are unfamiliar, especially if the teenager is from a different socioeconomic level and/or a different cultural background than the nurse.

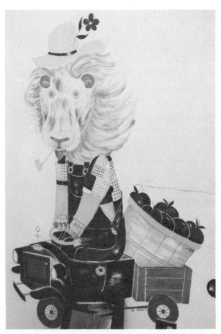

Figure 29–4. Attractive murals turn a clinic examining room into an attractive environment in which parents can learn more about interacting with their infants.

By asking for frequent feedback and by checking out what we think we hear, we can overcome these language barriers and keep communication pathways open.

Need for Information About Pregnancy, Childbirth, and Parenting. In some communities childbirth education may be, or seems to be, inaccessible to teenaged or single mothers. When the focus of prenatal classes is on husbands and wives, a 16-year-old and her girlfriend or boyfriend or mother (any one of whom may serve as her coach) may feel very uncomfortable. Yet few mothers are more in need of support from someone they know during labor than are young teens. Provision must be made, either in classes in which all parents feel comfortable or in classes designed especially for teens, for the opportunity to become well prepared for childbirth. Information about parenting can be provided initially during the prenatal period but should continue to be available after birth in attractive settings where teens feel welcome and comfortable (Fig. 29–4). A variety of programs have been developed throughout the country designed to foster attachment and help young mothers provide cognitive stimulation for their infants.

Need to Accept Changing Body. Accepting the changes in her own body is one of the developmental tasks that each teenager must achieve. The amount of time spent in front of the mirror is evidence of the importance of this task. The tremendously greater body changes that occur during pregnancy are superimposed upon this already major job.

How does she respond? Denial, exhibited by wearing a tightly buttoned coat or by refusing to wear maternity clothes, is one response. The 16-year-old in her seventh month of pregnancy, sitting in the obstetric clinic in a sweater and jeans, is not necessarily lacking funds to buy more appropriate clothing.

Need to Continue Education. One of the most serious consequences of teenaged pregnancy is the effect of that pregnancy on a young woman's education. Caring for the teenager who is pregnant will hopefully lead nurses to investigate what their community offers to meet the educational needs of adolescent gravidas. What happens to pregnant teenagers—married and unmarried—in your local school system? Do they have to drop out of school? Do they have an opportunity to learn about how to care for themselves and their babies? Is there a readily accessible person with whom they can talk?

In the past, and to this day in many parts of the United States, pregnancy has automatically meant exclusion from school, often not only during the prenatal period but for varying lengths of time after the baby is born. As a result, for most of the girls involved, pregnancy means an effective termination of their education. A survey by Gordon in 1971 documents that local practices rather than statutes or regulations are the determinants of such customs.[17] Although arguments such as concern for the health of the teenaged gravida may be advanced as the basis of such policies, one suspects that the fact that these girls have violated community norms and the fear that they might, by their presence, encourage others to do so, seems closer to the real reason.

Recent court decisions suggest that this kind of exclusion may be a violation of legal rights. Whether or not this will ultimately be shown to be true, it is certain that the beginning of pregnancy is a poor time to interrupt a girl's education. To her increasingly important need for a basic education is now added a need for knowledge of pregnancy and child care. She needs more, not less, education and counseling (Fig. 29–5).

A number of communities across the United States have dealt with the needs of the pregnant teenager in varying ways. Two of these programs are described below.

The Winston-Salem, North Carolina Program. When a teenager attending public school in Winston-Salem thinks she is pregnant, she goes to her school guidance counselor. If it is her choice to continue her pregnancy, she may transfer to the Continuing Education Center or remain in her base school.

Prior to 1964, when the continuing education concept was originated, most girls terminated their schooling when they became pregnant. Few returned, since policies dictated that they must remain at home until after their baby's first birthday, a policy that was applied uniformly to married and unmarried students alike. Beginning with eight girls and one teacher, the program now serves more than 200 girls each year with a staff that includes a full-time director, a social worker, two nurses, seven teachers, the services of a vocational rehabilitation worker, a child development specialist, and college students who volunteer to tutor students in subjects not offered by the center. In addition to basic junior and senior high school subjects, students study the processes of pregnancy, newborn care, and home economics and participate in group discussions, termed Laboratory for Effective Living, conducted by nurses, a social worker, and a child development specialist (Fig. 29–6).

The nurses follow the students physically after their initial examination by a physician until the last month of pregnancy, when they

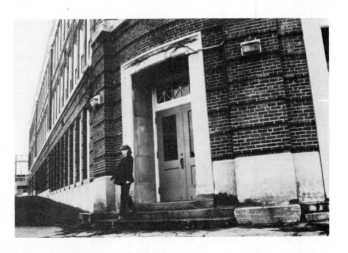

Figure 29–5. The pregnant teenager continues to have educational needs. Many communities are considering how best to meet these needs. (Photograph courtesy of Barbara Thompson.)

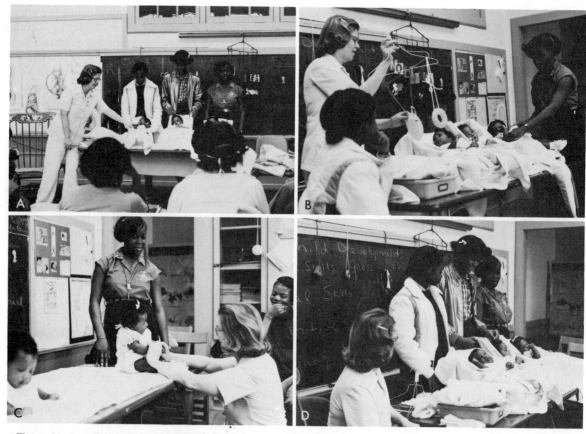

Figure 29–6. "Baby Day" in a in-school class for pregnant teens *(A)*. The nurse teaches infant stimulation using homemade mobiles and paper plates *(B)*; she models interaction *(C)* and helps to develop parenting skills in adolescents *(D)*.

return to the physician's care. The services of physicians are also available if any sign of complication arises.

After delivery, students usually return to classes within 2 weeks. They may return to regular school classes when a new semester begins or may remain at the Continuing Education Center until the end of the school year.

The Atlanta Adolescent Pregnancy Program. In Atlanta approximately 80 per cent of the pregnant students remain in their neighborhood schools throughout their pregnancy. They find this a feasible, workable, and inexpensive option. Special education classes are available, however, for the very young student in grammar school, who requires a greater degree of privacy and protection than regular school offers; for the student who does not plan to keep her baby; and for any student who feels a strong need for concealment.

Since this is a relatively new concept and one that may grow in the future, both opposing points of view and Atlanta's arguments for this type of program seem worth considering.

REASONS FOR EXCLUDING PREGNANT STUDENTS FROM REGULAR SCHOOL CLASSES.

1. Pregnant students are unable, for medical reasons, to carry out the usual school program. The Atlanta program argues that this is not true for the majority of students, just as it is untrue for most women who are employed or care for their homes.

2. Allowing the student to remain in school makes it appear that the school board favors or approves of teenaged pregnancy.

3. The teenager who is pregnant needs teachers who are sympathetic and understanding. Experience in Atlanta showed that some teachers of regular classes were quite hostile, some quite sympathetic, but that the majority did not have strong feelings either way. It was not difficult to avoid the openly hostile teachers. It is also likely that the too sympathetic instructor might not be the most helpful, since the student must get along with the varied attitudes of people in the real world.

REASONS FOR INCLUDING PREGNANT STUDENTS IN REGULAR SCHOOL CLASSES.

1. Relationships with teachers and friends are already built. At an age when peer relationships are very important, these ties are not broken by transfer to a special school.

2. Requiring a student to leave her regular school can be interpreted by the student as evidence that she is "undesirable" or "bad," creating or reinforcing a feeling of alienation. It is felt that it may be difficult for her to return to a school in which she feels she is not wanted.

3. The regular school can offer a wider range of educational and extracurricular activities. Although the small and specialized classes of a special school may seem ideal, what is the long-range gain once the student has returned to her regular classrooms?

4. Transportation problems are less likely when the student remains in her regular school.

5. The cost to the school system is less. Special facilities and teachers for small groups of students are not required.

6. School-aged pregnancy is visible, an important factor in helping communities deal realistically with the needs of teenaged gravidas.

The Adolescent Couple

Both in research and in clinical practice, nursing interaction with adolescents as *couples* appears to have been very limited (an adolescent couple is defined as an adolescent male and female who consider themselves a couple). They may be married, but more often they are not. They may be engaged, but often they are not.

Our society has generally assumed that when pregnancy has occurred outside of marriage, the relationship was not one of commitment and that there was no couple per se, only an unwed mother. And, of course, this is true in some instances. It may even be true in a majority of instances. However, in one study of 44 teenagers in Rochester, N.Y., the investigators[9] found that the pregnancy typically resulted from an extended and serious relationship with a single mate, who frequently contributed to the child's support. Only a minority of involvements were severed following the pregnancy.

Rosen,[32] in a study of 432 pregnant girls aged 18 or less, found that in adolescents who chose to keep their infants (n = 207), male partners were the major influence. Mothers were the most important influence in the issue of abortion versus adoption.

For many nurses a teenaged couple, especially an unmarried couple, presents an ethical or moral dilemma. They feel that if they support the couple as a couple, they are supporting or even encouraging teenaged sexual activity

(illegitimacy), a whole package that conflicts with some very basic values. In their hearts they feel that these teenagers should be punished, not supported. Punitive attitudes once focused on teenage mothers may now be focused on teenage couples in some instances.

From a research standpoint couples as an entity, married or single, have been even more neglected, whatever their age. To be sure, research on couples has been reported in the literature for several decades, but much of it has been based on the response of one person of a dyad to an interview or questionnaire. In decision-making research, the emphasis has been on what Olson,[29a] calls *final-say* research (i.e., research on who made a final decision rather than on the process of decision-making).

The reasons for this are largely logistical (it is easier to contact and interview one person than two, easier to analyze the data afterward, and of course the whole process is cheaper), but some of us believe that the results probably don't reflect a true understanding of the dynamics of couple interaction.

Why should we increase our focus on couples rather than concentrating solely on women or on men? For many teens, their relationship as a couple, whether married or unmarried, is an important one to them. Their relationship may not last forever, but not all marriages do either.

There are a number of studies that suggest that interpersonal relationships within the adolescent dyad may be important in decisions made by adolescents about issues such as sex and contraception.[22] The two models diagrammed on the following page demonstrate the importance of the adolescent couple's relationship in decision-making.

Scales[36] looked at couples in terms of the interpersonal power and influence of the adolescent female in a relationship vis-à-vis the male, and found that the traditional sex role pattern in which the male was more powerful and the woman more passive

1. Discouraged male contraceptive responsibility.

2. Supported male adventurousness and sexual conquest.

3. Led to different perceptions about the relationship of sexual intercourse and long-term dyadic commitment.

4. Inhibited comfortable and rational interpersonal communication about sexual relationships and contraceptive behavior.

Scales concluded that the lower the influence and interpersonal power of the female, the greater the risk of eventual exposure to pregnancy.

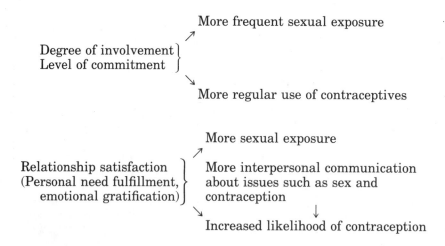

Jorgenson[22] and associates came to similar conclusions. Their research was based on interviews with the female partner only (147 12- to 18-year-olds attending family planning clinics in urban and rural Arizona). They found that the relationship within the adolescent dyad was a stronger and more consistent factor in risk of exposure to pregnancy than either peer or family relationships. Increased satisfaction in the relationship led to an increased probability of contraceptive use. Decreased female power in the dyad led to a decreased probability of contraception and increased probability of frequent sexual intercourse.

As a result of their study, Jorgenson's group concluded that the adolescent couple "is able to construct and maintain firm psychological and normative boundaries that distinguish it from other social groups. This 'couple identity' renders the teenage couple somewhat impervious to the normative and behavioral influences of peers and family members, especially parents."[22]

Considering the findings from even this limited amount of research, it is imperative to consider couples as couples and to appreciate the importance of the couple's identity as well as understanding adolescent men and women as separate individuals.

Supporting Adolescent Couples

Family Planning Programs. Family planning programs need to provide an atmosphere in which both young men and women feel comfortable; they also need to provide same basic information to both. Many teenaged men have limited opportunities to obtain factual information about contraception.

In providing information about contraceptives we need also to be aware of other factors besides knowledge and availability that are important in contraceptive risk-taking, and then help young men and women in these

areas. The literature suggests that understanding the dynamics of power in a relationship and the role of self-esteem may be just as important as knowledge of when and how to take pills. In relationships in which the male has more power, how can we expect to make a consistent impact if we leave males out of decisions about contraceptives?

If male power, as Scales and Jorgensen have indicated, discourages contraceptive responsibility, then perhaps one focus of family planning programs should be to help young women develop skills that increase their power in a relationship. Power is derived from resources, both tangible and intangible. Individuals with increased tangible resources (e.g., education, knowledge, financial support) and increased intangible resources (e.g., self-esteem) are likely to have more power in a relationship with their male partner than women who lack those resources.

Prenatal Visits. Nurses can allow teenaged couples to participate as a couple in prenatal visits if they choose and are able. During examinations the father can be at the head of the table just as he is in the delivery room. He can hear the baby's heart beat, hear the discussions with the nutritionist or nurse or physician.

There seems to be a relationship between involvement and attachment. Many of Klaus and Kennell's steps to attachment (Chapter 9) occur before birth. The other steps—hearing, seeing, touching, holding, and then caretaking—are postbirth experiences. If we don't acknowledge the couple as a couple, if we shut the father out—out of clinic or office visits, out of childbirth preparation, out of the labor and birth experience—how is optimal attachment to occur?

Prenatal Education. Couple-oriented prenatal education should be available for all couples regardless of age and sex. Often the assumption is made that "clinic patients" won't come to such classes, or we assume that the father or some other significant person won't be interested, but he may be more interested than we suspect. The success of prenatal education for anyone, and particularly for teens who can be supersensitive, is the attitude of the person involved.

Using only first names on name tags is an easy way to eliminate the obvious identity of couples as married or unmarried. Conveying the attitude of acceptance of each couple is essential regardless of how we may feel about the pregnancy. The pregnancy is a fact. If the couple is coming for childbirth education, they are usually planning to keep the baby; now we must move from that fact to helping them have a positive labor and birth experience so that they will be in the best possible position to be good parents. Because low self-esteem is a variable linked with teenaged pregnancy and also with child abuse, it would seem that whatever we can do to enhance self-esteem and to provide coping mechanisms should build feelings of self-worth and lead to better parenting.

Another facet of childbirth education is establishing an appropriate level of understanding—neither talking down to the participants nor overwhelming them. This is achieved in part by an atmosphere of openness so that everyone feels free to ask questions. For example, in discussing basic anatomy and physiology we can say to everyone—doctors, nurses, lawyers, and college professors as well as factory workers and teens—"You probably already know this. But just so you'll know what I mean when I use certain terms, let's review." Sometimes a teenager who took high school biology the year before is more knowledgeable than the mother with a Ph.D. in English.

Labor and Birth. The value of a supportive person in continuous attendance in any labor has been documented. In one study[38] women with a supportive person were found to have shorter labors (8.8 hours compared with 19.3 hours) and to engage in increased stroking, smiling, and talking to the baby than mothers without companions (women were randomized in experimental and control groups).

Who that supportive person should be is obviously up to the mother; for some adolescents it will be the baby's father, and if that is their choice, then that is the person we should support. Again, we need to evaluate our attitudes and responsibilities as professionals. If we can interact with adolescents who choose to be couples as we interact with other couples rather than treating them as wayward children or less than desirable adults, we will

enhance the coach's support of the mother and contribute to the growth of both mother and father.

Postpartum Period. Traditionally, one of the goals of the postpartum period, at least from the standpoint of nursing, has been to teach the mother how to care for her baby. We need to rethink our practices to include the father in postpartum teaching. In the 1980's the strong sex role segregation in families, in which only mothers bathe and feed and nurture babies and fathers are the providers in terms of income, no longer applies to a great many families. Remembering that caretaking is part of the attachment process, it is apparent that adolescent fathers, as well as fathers of every age, need the opportunity to begin caretaking activities in the postpartum period (Chapter 22).

Consequences of Adolescent Pregnancy

The consequences of adolescent pregnancy affect young parents, their teenaged children, and society as a whole. These consequences involve the health of the mother and the infant, and the social and economic aspects of their lives as well as the lives of all of us (Table 29–4).

It is hard to separate biologic consequences of teenaged pregnancy from social factors. For example, the increase in the delivery of low-birth-weight infants, maternal anemia, and pregnancy-induced hypertension, appears to be related to a lack of prenatal care, as discussed previously. Nevertheless, as long as many teens do not seek early prenatal care the consequences remain. For the 10,000 mothers each year under the age of 15, biologic problems (anemia, pre-eclampsia, eclampsia, cephalopelvic disproportion, difficult labor, abnormal bleeding) may occur even when prenatal care is good.[34] Mothers under 15 have a 60 per cent higher maternal mortality rate from complications of pregnancy, birth, and delivery than mothers over 20, and an infant mortality rate two to four times higher. Mothers under 15 years old are 3.5 times, and mothers 15 to 19 years old 1.5 times, more likely to die of toxemia than mothers over 20, even in studies in which race and parity are controlled.[2] Suicide is five times more common in these mothers than in teenage women who have no children.[6] Low birth weight is twice as common among teenaged mothers.

Equally important as health consequences are the social consequences of adolescent pregnancy. Many teen mothers drop out of school;

Table 29–4. CONSEQUENCES OF ADOLESCENT CHILDBEARING

	Mother	Infant	Community/Society
Health	Increased mortality and morbidity Increased rates of suicide	Increased mortality Increased prematurity and low birth weight Increased neurologic defects (white mothers under 15 years old)	Increased need for specialized health care services for mothers and children
Social	Decreased education Increased marital separation	Increased child abuse or neglect Decreased cognitive development Decreased school achievement Increased likelihood of becoming adolescent parent	Increased number of single-parent families Loss of contributions of individuals who do not achieve their potential
Economic	Increased likelihood of long-term poverty	Family poverty decreases opportunities for growing child	Increased probability of welfare assistance Increased health care costs High unemployment among individuals with limited education

white mothers and mothers who marry are more likely to drop out than black mothers and mothers who continue to live at home with their parents. The availability of infant care is an important factor; mothers who have support from adults in their families are more likely to be able to continue their education. Dropping out of school leads to limited job opportunities or none and frequently to a second pregnancy, which further damages prospects of economic self-sufficiency.[41] Welfare assistance may become necessary.

When teenaged pregnancy leads to marriage, the likelihood of separation or divorce is increased. Both premarital pregnancy and teenaged pregnancy are associated with increased marital disruption.[25]

In addition to increased mortality and morbidity in infants of teenaged mothers, lower cognitive development in these infants appears to be a risk. It is difficult to separate the effects of other characteristics such as poverty from the effects of maternal age; however, when these effects are controlled, some statistically significant difference does remain. The presence of another adult in the household who helps to care for the child, often the child's grandmother or another close relative who provides more than custodial care, is a positive influence on cognitive development.[1, 7] Card reviewed the histories of 375,000 teens and found that even when social and economic factors were controlled, children of younger mothers showed decreased cognitive development, were more likely to live in single parent homes, and were likely to bear children early themselves. Teenaged parents may be more

likely to abuse their children.[10] Baldwin and Cain[1] summarize a number of other studies related to the children of teenaged parents.

What about society as a whole? The consequences of teenaged childbearing affect not only teens themselves and their immediate families. Teenaged mothers have an increased need for health care services and frequently for social services as well. In 1975 federal and state governments disbursed 4.65 billion dollars through Aid to Families with Dependent Children (AFDC) to households in which women bore their first child as teenagers. This figure does not include administrative costs, Medicaid, food stamps, or health care.[26]

Mecklenburg County, North Carolina, estimated that a 20-year cost of nearly 17 million dollars would be generated by births to teenaged mothers in a single year (1979). Included were health (maternal, pediatric, Medicaid, and WIC) and welfare (AFDC, food stamp, school lunch, and day care) benefits.[14]

In addition, society suffers when individuals, and later their children, are caught in a cycle of early childbearing, decreased education, low income, and marital dissolution. Few persons can live up to their potential under such circumstances.

The Law and Patients Under 18 Years of Age

At one time the basic legal theory that governed relationships between nurses and other givers of health care and patients under

18 years of age was that treatment of a minor without parental consent was assault. However, the 1979 decision of the United States Supreme Court (*Bellotti v. Baird*) invalidated state laws requiring parental consent and parental notification for "mature minors" seeking abortion or medically prescribed contraceptives. "Mature" minor is not clearly defined and may be left to the provider's discretion. The *Bellotti* decision also allows services to "immature" minors if the court determines this to be in the minor's best interest. Legislation is still controversial and changing.

Many health-care providers feel that this change in the law will benefit teenage health. For example, the need to inform parents of a pregnancy before receiving care might mean a delay in health care, often well past the important first trimester of embryologic development. The inability of a minor to have an abortion without parental consent could delay the abortion until a time when a more complex procedure is necessary or when the abortion itself is not possible.

Not everyone is in favor of allowing adolescents to assume responsibility for their own health care. The major opposition has come from parents who see such efforts as one more assault on the family, by taking from the parents still another of their responsibilities.

Adolescents Who Choose to Terminate Pregnancy

It is estimated that more than 300,000 teens seek abortions annually. In some communities the number of teenagers seeking abortions is greater than the number who choose to continue pregnancy. To some observers the decision to terminate pregnancy is a responsible one, given the long-term consequences of teen-aged childbearing (below). Others, of course, feel that abortion is never a solution to the problem of pregnancy. Teens themselves tend to be conservative in their attitudes toward abortion, favoring this solution in particular circumstances but not in all situations.[11, 44, 45]

The risk of physical complications during or following abortion is related to the gestational age of the fetus, the overall rate of complications being approximately 12 per cent. Because teenaged women are more likely to defer the decision for pregnancy termination until later in gestation, risks for the group as a whole tend to be higher (see Chapter 30). There do not appear to be long-term emotional sequelae.[3, 29b]

Luker[24] has suggested that the decision by an individual to terminate a pregnancy will vary from one pregnancy to the next. At each pregnancy the costs versus the rewards are weighed. For most adolescent women, the sexual partner plays a prominent role in the decision.[8]

Community Action and Adolescent Sexuality and Pregnancy

Community action in relation to adolescent sexuality and pregnancy must involve not only health-care providers but a broad group of persons including adolescents themselves. Nurses with a holistic perspective of the issues may serve as catalysts for community organization. Table 29–5 lists nine groups in one county (Mecklenburg County, North Carolina) that worked together as the Mecklenburg Council on Adolescent Pregnancy and the initial contributions of each group.

The research described in this chapter suggests that a large part of the intervention needed to prevent undesired teenage pregnancy must occur before teenagers become sexually active. The questions that must be asked include: How can we reach these teens? What can we say or do to delay sexual involvement until an older age?

One priority is advocating comprehensive family life education, which includes communication skills for children and parents, decision-making skills for teenagers, and alternatives to sexual involvement as well as specific information about reproductive anatomy and physiology, the likelihood of pregnancy, and means of contraception (Table 29–6). Although it is probably unrealistic to expect teens who are already consistently sexually active to become "sexually inactive," younger teens and preteens may decide to delay sexual involvement as a result of such family life education.

Organized family planning programs have frequently been less than successful at reaching young persons who are sexually active before a first pregnancy; services designed specifically for teens may achieve greater success.[21] No matter how accessible these services are, they will not be sought until teens feel themselves to be sufficiently at risk for pregnancy. Thus, for both sexually active and sexually inactive teens, early education appears to be a priority.

In many communities, educational programs dealing with any aspect of reproduction remain highly controversial. Nurses acting as advocates may join with others to encourage such programs.

Table 29–5. MECKLENBURG COUNCIL ON ADOLESCENT PREGNANCY 1981 COMPLETED PROJECTS

Coalition	Project
Agency:	Identified and evaluated services and resources available, related to adolescent pregnancy.
	Organized this information into a resource directory for use by the community.
	Organized 15 agencies and organizations and presented a Family Film Festival to over 280 parents and teens at five showings in five different locations in the Charlotte–Mecklenburg Community.
Business:	Prepared a document determining the actual cost of adolescent pregnancy in 1979 in Charlotte.
Clergy:	Awareness presentations have been made to individual church groups and to the Executive Board of the Charlotte Area Clergy.
Government/Legal:	Prepared incorporation papers for the Council. Presented information/awareness program for State Legislators.
Media:	Assisted in initial information/awareness programs.
Medical:	Documented pregnancies, deliveries, abortions, miscarriages, and adoptions for period September 1, 1980 to August 31, 1981 in Charlotte–Mecklenburg.
	Mapped the geographical distribution of this data.
Parents/Community:	Identified leaders in a majority of community groups.
	Developed an awareness program presentation and prepared a list of potential group projects relating to teenage pregnancy.
	Presented a "mini awareness conference" to selected community leaders.
	Organized workshop on "Seminars for Parents on Adolescent Sexuality." Trained 18 volunteers to take this workshop into the community.
Peers:	Wrote and received a grant from the North Carolina State Youth Council.
	Conducted information/awareness meeting for peer group to begin training for staffing of Teen Hot-Line.
Schools:	Organized group to prepare information/awareness program on primary prevention for all Charlotte–Mecklenburg superintendents and principals.

Adolescents who are pregnant need access to counseling to help them make their own informed decision about the pregnancy, and they need support for the decisions they make. Support includes access to the services their decision requires. For those who choose to continue the pregnancy and to keep their infant, education for childbirth prior to delivery and after the birth of the baby needs to be available.

Table 29–6. DECISIONS AND INTERVENTION IN ADOLESCENT SEXUALITY

Status of Adolescent	Decision of Adolescent	Intervention by Providers
Not sexually active	To become sexually active or delay sexual activity	Provide information and skills in communication, decision-making, alternatives to sexual activity, reproductive physiology
Sexually active but not pregnant	Use of effective contraceptive	Provide information about reproductive cycle, contraception, consequences of teenage pregnancy
Pregnant	Termination or continuation of pregnancy; keeping baby or giving it up for adoption	Provide counseling on advantages and disadvantages of each option; support and facilitate decision (including referrals); provide opportunities to continue own education
Early parenting	Provision of child care; continuation of maternal education	Provide information on parenting, options for continuation of own education

REFERENCES

1. Baldwin, W., and Cain, V.: The Children of Teenage Parents. *In* Furstenberg, F., Lincoln, R., and Menken, J. (eds.): *Teenage Sexuality, Pregnancy and Childbearing.* Philadelphia, University of Pennsylvania Press, 1981.
2. Battaglia, F. C.: Obstetric and Pediatric Complications of Juvenile Pregnancy. *Pediatrics, 32*:902, 1963.
3. Bracken, M., Klerman, L., and Bracken, M.: Abortion, Adoption, or Motherhood: An Empirical Study of Decision Making During Pregnancy. *American Journal of Obstetrics and Gynecology, 130*:251, 1978.
4. Campbell, A.: The Role of Family Planning in the Reduction of Poverty. *Journal of Marriage and the Family, 30*:236, 1968.
5. Card, J.: *Long-Term Consequences for Children Born to Adolescent Parents.* Palo Alto, CA, American Institute for Research, 1978.
6. Chap, M.: *Better Choices for a Better Future: Teenage Pregnancy in North Carolina.* Raleigh, NC: Governor's Advocacy Council on Children and Youth, 1980.
7. Chillman, C.: Social and Psychological Research Concerning Adolescent Childbearing, 1970–1980. *Journal of Marriage and the Family, 42*:67, 1980.
8. Cobliner, W., Shulman, H., and Romney, S.: The Termination of Adolescent Out-of-Wedlock Pregnancies and the Prospects for Their Primary Prevention. *American Journal of Obstetrics and Gynecology, 115*:432, 1973.
9. De Amicus, L., Klovman, R., Hese, D., et al.: A Comparison of Unwed Pregnant Teenagers and Nulligravid Sexually Active Adolescents Seeking Contraception. *Adolescence, 16*:11, 1981.
10. Egeland, B., Phipps-Yonas, S., et al.: A Prospective Study of the Antecedents of Child Abuse. *Caring,* National Committee for Prevention of Child Abuse, Winter, 1979.
11. Evans, J., Selstad, G., and Welcher, W.: Teenagers: Fertility Control Behavior and Attitudes Before and After Abortion, Childbearing or Negative Pregnancy Test. *Family Planning Perspectives, 8*:192, 1976.
12. Field, B.: A Socio-Economic Analysis of Out-of-wedlock Births Among Teenagers. *In* Scott, K., Field, T., and Robertson, E. (eds.): *Teenage Parents and Their Offspring.* New York, Grune and Stratton, 1981.
13. Final Natality Statistics, 1978. *Monthly Vital Statistics Report, 29*(1): 1980.
14. *Financial Report on Adolescent Pregnancy*: A Business Look at a Major Issue. Charlotte, NC, Mecklenburg Council on Adolescent Pregnancy, 1980.
15. Finkel, M., and Finkel, D.: Sexual and Contraceptive Knowledge, Attitudes and Behavior of Male Adolescents. *In* Furstenberg, F., Lincoln, R., and Menken, J. (eds.): *Teenage Sexuality, Pregnancy and Childbearing.* Philadelphia, University of Pennsylvania Press, 1981.
16. Ford, K., Zelnik, M., and Kantner, J.: Differences in Contraceptive Use Among Socioeconomic Groups of Teenagers in the United States. Paper presented at the annual meeting of the American Public Health Association, New York, November 4–8, 1979.
17. Gordon, L.: National Survey of Legislation Relative to Schoolage Parents. National Alliance Concerned with Schoolage Parents. Unpublished, 1971.
18. Herold, W., Godwin, M., and Lero, D.: Self-esteem, Locus of Control and Adolescent Contraception. *Journal of Psychology, 101*:83, 1979.
19. Higgins, A.: Nutritional Status and the Outcome of Pregnancy. *Journal of the Canadian Dietetic Association, 37*:17, 1976.
20. Hornick, J., Doran, L., and Crawford, S.: Premarital Contraceptive Usage Among Male and Female Adolescents. *Family Coordinator, 28*:181, 1979.
21. House, E., and Goldsmith, S.: Planned Parenthood Services for the Young Teenager. *Family Planning Perspectives, 4*:27, 1972.
22. Jorgenson, S., King, S., and Torrey, B.: Dyadic and Social Network Influences on Adolescent Exposure to Pregnancy Risk. *Journal of Marriage and the Family, 42*:141, 1980.
23. Lenocker, J., and Dougherty, M.: Adolescent Mothers: Social and Health-Related Interests: Report of a Project for Rural Black Mothers. *JOGN Nursing, 5*:9, 1976.
24. Luker, K.: *Taking Chances: Abortion and The Decision Not to Contracept.* Berkeley, University of California Press, 1975.
25. McCarthy, J., and Menken, J.: Marriage, Remarriage, Marital Disruption and Age at First Birth. *In* Furstenberg, F., Lincoln R., and Menken, J. (eds.): *Teenage Sexuality, Pregnancy and Childbearing.* Philadelphia, University of Pennsylvania Press, 1981.
26. Moore, K., Hofferth, S., and Wertheimer, R.: Teenage Motherhood: Its Social and Economic Costs. *Children Today,* September-October, 1979.
27. National Center for Health Statistics: *Vital Statistics of the U.S., 1974.* Washington, D.C., U.S. Government Printing Office, 1976.
28. National Research Council: *Nutritional Services in Perinatal Care.* Washington, D.C., National Academy Press, 1981.
29. O'Connell, M., and Moore, M.: The Legitimacy Status of First Births to U.S. Women Aged 15–24, 1939–1978. *Family Planning Perspectives, 12*:16, 1980.
29a. Olson, B., and Cromwell, R.: Power in Families. In Olson, B., and Cromwell, R. (eds.): *Power in Families,* New York, Wiley, 1975.
30. Reiss, I., Banwart, A., and Foreman, H.: Premarital Contraceptive Usage: A Study and Some Theoretical Exploration. *Journal of Marriage and the Family, 37*:619, 1975.
31. Robertson, E.: Adolescence, Physiological Maturity, and Obstetric Outcome. *In* Scott, K., Field, T., and Robertson, E. (eds.): *Teenage Parents and Their Offspring.* New York, Grune & Stratton, 1981.
32. Rosen, R.: Adolescent Pregnancy Decision-Making; Are Parents Important? *Adolescence, 15*:43, 1980.
33. Rush, D., Stein, Z., and Susser, M.: A Randomized Controlled Trial of Prenatal Nutritonal Supplementation in New York City. *Pediatrics, 65*:683, 1980.
34. Safro, J.: Adolescent Sexuality, Pregnancy and Childbearing. *In* Smith, P., and Mumford, D. (eds.): *Adolescent Pregnancy.* Boston, G. K. Hall, 1980.
35. Sandler, H., Vietze, P., and O'Connor, S.: Obstetric and Neonatal Outcomes Following Intervention with Pregnant Teenagers. *In* Scott, K., Field, T., and Robertson, E. (eds.): *Teenage Parents and Their Offspring.* New York, Grune & Stratton, 1981.
36. Scales, P.: Males and Morals; Teenage Contraceptive Behavior Amid the Double Standard. *The Family Coordinator, 2b*:211, 1977.
37. Shah, F., Zelnik, M., and Kantner, J.: Unprotected Intercourse Among Unwed Teenagers. *Family Planning Perspectives, 7*:39, 1975.
38. Sosa, R., Kennell, J., Klaus, M., et al.: The Effect of a

Supportive Companion on Prenatal Problems, Length of Labor, and Mother-Infant Interaction. *New England Journal of Medicine, 303*:597, 1980.

39. Thompson, A., and Hylten, F.: Nutrition in Pregnancy and Lactation. *In* Beaton, G., and McHenry, E. (eds.): *Nutrition, A Comprehensive Treatise,* Vol. 3. New York, Academic Press, 1966.

40. Torres, A.: Telling Parents About Adolescents' Use of Family Planning and Abortion Services: Clinic Policies and Teenage Behavior. *Family Planning Perspectives, 12*:284, 1980.

41. Trussell, J., and Menken, J.: Early Childbearing and Subsequent Fertility. *In* Furstenberg, F., Lincoln, R., and Menken, J. (eds.): *Teenage Sexuality, Pregnancy and Childbearing.* Philadelphia, University of Pennsylvania Press, 1981.

42. Wilson, S., Keith, L., Wells, J., et al.: A Preliminary

Survey of 16,000 Teenagers Entering a Contraceptive Program. *Chicago Medical School Quarterly, 32*:26, 1973.

43. Zabin, L. S.: Pregnancy Risk to Adolescent Girls in Early Years of Intercourse. Dissertation. The Johns Hopkins University, School of Hygiene and Public Health, Baltimore, 1979.

44. Zelnik, M., and Kantner, J.: Attitudes of American Teenagers Toward Abortion. *Family Planning Perspectives, 7*:89, 1975.

45. Zelnik, M., and Kantner, J.: Sexual and Contraceptive Experience of Young Unmarried Women in the United States, 1976 and 1971. *In* Furstenberg, F., Lincoln, R., and Menken, J. (eds.): *Teenage Sexuality, Pregnancy and Childbearing.* Philadelphia, University of Pennsylvania Press, 1981.

30

Problem Pregnancy Counseling and Elective Abortion

OBJECTIVES

1. Identify the role of the counselor when women have a problem pregnancy. Describe areas that could be discussed in the counseling process.
2. Identify the reasons that a pregnancy may present a problem to an individual woman.
3. Describe the major arguments of those who oppose elective abortion and those who support the right to elective abortion.
4. Describe the responsibility of nurses in relation to abortion, the rights of nurses, and the rights of clients.
5. Identify the components of nursing assessment prior to abortion.
6. Describe the procedures used to abort, indicating the appropriate period of gestation, contraindications, and potential complications, including mortality rates.
7. Identify possible sequelae of abortion—short-term and long-term, physiologic, and psychological.
8. Describe the nursing interventions appropriate to each stage of the abortion process.
9. Identify significant legislation related to legal abortion in the United States.

Any nurse who spends even a few weeks with potential mothers and fathers will come in contact with women and men for whom pregnancy, for any one of a number of reasons, presents a problem, either physical or emotional. By no means will all nurses formally become problem-pregnancy counselors. But all of us need to know enough about the process to talk with women and men in a way that is both informed and helpful and to make the best possible referrals.

Problem-pregnancy counseling is that which the phrase implies: counseling women (and their mates when it is at all possible) who have a pregnancy that either they, or sometimes we, see as a problem. Problem-pregnancy counseling is *not* abortion counseling, although abortion may be an alternative that is discussed. It is *not* a service only for, or even primarily for, the single woman. It may include genetic counseling or a referral for genetic counseling. At some point it will probably include discussion of responsible sexuality and contraceptive information.

Counselors may be nurses, physicians, family counselors, clergymen, or lay persons with special training. In addition to a basic understanding of the counseling process, those who counsel women with troubled pregnancies must be fully aware of the resources that their own and other communities offer.

Ideally, the initial counselor for a woman or couple with a troubled pregnancy should *not* be attached to an agency to which a patient might later be referred. For example, if the counselor works in an abortion clinic, no matter how objective he or she is in dealing with the alternatives open to the woman, the counselor's own position seems to suggest that he or she thinks highly of abortion as a solution. A counselor who works with an adoption agency, highly cognizant of the current shortage of adoptable babies, may unconsciously put this solution in a favorable light. Counselors working with some groups will not even suggest abortion as an alternative.

It is difficult for any of us to be totally objective, but the more successful we are in our attempt at objectivity, the better able we will be to help each woman. Counselors have no right to force their own wishes and views on women, or even to suggest them.

Mace describes the role of the problem-pregnancy counselor as accepting and supporting each woman as she struggles to reach the decision that is right for her.[12] If we can do this well, the crisis of a problem pregnancy can become, despite the misery, a chance for personal growth.

A particular pregnancy may be a problem for varied reasons:

1. The health of the mother may be threatened. Examples are the mother with serious heart pathology, diabetes that is poorly controlled, or major kidney disease. She may be mentally ill or feel that emotionally she cannot cope with the infant.

2. Previous children or one of the parents may have a major hereditary defect that makes the prospect of another child both emotionally and financially difficult. The family with one or more children with cystic fibrosis, for example, may be very threatened by another pregnancy.

3. A couple may feel that financially they just cannot care for another child, or even for a first child.

4. A couple may feel that they do not wish to add to the world's population. Many younger couples today (and some who are not so young) take the concept of zero population growth both seriously and personally.

5. The mother may be single and may not wish to bear a child.

Options for the single woman with a problem pregnancy were discussed in Chapter 5. Genetic counseling was discussed in Chapter 3. Here we will explore the alternative of elective abortion.

Elective Abortion

Of all the realities of maternity nursing, elective abortion may be the most difficult for many nurses. In certain hospitals a nurse may be asked to give life-saving care to a 27-week preterm infant on one day and assist in the abortion of a 24-week fetus on the next.

The issue of elective abortion is multifaceted. Nurses must deal with their own feelings about the ethical considerations involved and their proper professional response. Nurses must be aware of possible reactions of women to abortion, and they must understand the various procedures that result in the termination of pregnancy.

Social and Historical Perspectives

Elective abortion has been practiced throughout recorded history. Aristotle saw abortion as a legitimate means of maintaining optimal population size.[18] Early Roman Catholic theologians were concerned with abortion once the soul had entered the body; Augustine concluded in the fourth century, however, that no soul was present prior to quickening. Nine hundred years later, Thomas Aquinas stated that the soul infused the male embryo at 40 days following conception and the female embryo at 80 days, a concept derived from Aristotle. It was another 400 years, in the seventeenth century, before the life of the embryo or fetus of any gestational age was considered to be equivalent in value to that of the mother in Roman Catholic thought.

Following the Reformation, elective abortion became widespread in Protestant areas of Europe, both as a surgical procedure and through the use of herbal abortifacients. English common law made abortion a crime only after quickening and then only a misdemeanor. Early nineteenth century abortion statutes in the United States, however, did not distinguish abortion prior to and following quickening.

In 1896 Pope Pius IX banned abortion, labeling the act as homicide and excommunicating those who performed it. Not until 1917 was the woman who had an abortion considered a "sinner" and subject to excommunication. Prior to that time the woman was considered an innocent party, the passive recipient of the actions of another.[5] Pope Pius reaffirmed the position that fetal life was sacred in 1930, a position still supported by the Catholic Church.

Historical attitudes toward abortion have not occurred in a vacuum. Resistance to abortion has frequently been high when populations were decreased (such as periods following long wars) and has been low during times or in areas of the world where overpopulation was a concern. As mortality rates declined in northwestern Europe and Japan, individuals began to limit population growth, at least partly through abortion, to ensure the well-being of themselves and the children they chose to have.

The changing aspirations, status, and roles of women in the second half of the twentieth century raised new questions in discussions of abortion. Who should decide if the woman should bear a child? The woman herself? A psychiatrist who would declare that childbearing would be dangerous to her mental health? What if the child was conceived as a result of rape? What if the child was recognized to be seriously deformed, physically or mentally, or to have a genetic disease that would probably lead to an early death?

A second group of questions was also debated. If safe, legal abortion was a component of health care and if health care was a right rather than a privilege, should abortion be available to all women, regardless of their ability to pay? Who should pay?

The changing climate of the 1960's and 1970's led to a number of significant changes in the status of abortion in the United States through actions of the Congress and the Supreme Court of the United States.

1973   *Roe v. Wade* and *Doe v. Bolton.* The Supreme Court of the United States ruled that a woman's right to decide whether she should have an abortion during the first trimester was protected by her constitutional right to privacy. As a result, all state laws restricting abortion were rendered unconstitutional. After the first trimester, the state may impose regulations that protect maternal health.

       After "viability" of the fetus occurs, the state may impose regulations to protect the life of the fetus and may prohibit abortions except when it is considered necessary to preserve the life or health of the mother. Viability is defined as the time when the fetus may sustain life outside of the womb, with or without artificial assistance.

1973   Medicaid funding becomes available for medically indigent women.

1976   Medicaid funding becomes available for medically indigent women.

1976   *Planned Parenthood v. Dunforth.* The Supreme Court of the United States ruled that the state cannot impose the requirement of consent by a third party on a woman's right to abortion. This means that neither spouse, parent, nor guardian can veto the woman's request for abortion.

1976   Hyde amendment first passed; barred the use of federal funds for most abortions. Passed annually each year since.

1980   *Harris v. McRae.* The Supreme Court of the United States upheld the constitutionality of the Hyde amendment.

1983   Debate over abortion continues in Congress.

The Ethical Problem of Abortion

For most people, lay persons as well as professionals who give health care, the issues surrounding abortion require careful thought. These issues are discussed in churches, at women's meetings, in state legislatures, in the Congress of the United States, and by the President of the United States. What are the major concerns? What are the arguments for and against abortion?

Opposition to Abortion

The Fetus as a Human Being. Most people who oppose abortion believe that a unique being with a life of its own exists from the moment of conception. They point out that the zygote has, encoded in its DNA, all the potential for full development as a person. There will never again be another being exactly like this being. Therefore, to destroy this life at any point is to kill a human being. It is suggested that allowing judgments about who should live and who should die in one area of life is no different from deciding who lives and dies under any circumstances (if abortion, why not infanticide, for example?).

A key question in this argument is when life begins. In hearings in the Senate of the United States in 1981 this question was raised, but no consensus could be reached. Leon Rosenberg, an embryologist from Yale University, stated that science could not define life or death; the definition is a matter of personal belief, i.e., of one's religious belief or world view.

Opponents of this point of view argue that although the embryo has human potential, the embryo is not yet a person. In addition, they point to the biological reality that of all eggs and sperm, only a small proportion are fertilized and that many zygotes are lost at the menstrual period following fertilization.

The Rights of the Fetus. Closely related is the issue of the right of the fetus to live. If indeed the zygote-embryo-fetus is a human being, that fetus then has basic rights, including the right to life.

Most opponents of this argument agree that the fetus does have rights, but these rights must be balanced against the rights of the mother and perhaps also of the father, other members of her family, and even the society as a whole.

Support for Abortion

Support for abortion is embodied in several arguments: population control, financial resources, the rights of women, and the hazards of illegal abortion are four reasons discussed frequently.

Population Control. The hazards of overpopulation were documented in Chapter 6. There are those who fear that without access to liberal, legal abortion, adequate population control will be impossible. Abortion is not advocated as the principal means of limiting population but as an adjunct to other methods.

Those who disagree suggest that there are better means of population control available.

Financial Resources. Some women choose abortion because they feel they cannot financially support the child. From the societal standpoint, the cost of abortion versus the cost of supporting a child whose family is unable to care for him financially is cited by some as a reason not only for abortion but for abortion supported by state or federal funding. It is argued that no state would be able to afford the cost of caring for those children who would result from pregnancies that are now aborted.

The same argument, opponents point out, could also be made for disposing of the elderly, the mentally retarded, and others in society who are supported by the society rather than contributing to the society.

Rights of Women. In recent years one of the most frequent arguments for abortion has been in terms of the right of a woman to control her own body. This freedom would include the right to decide whether she wishes to bear a child she has conceived.

Opponents argue that the zygote is not a part of her body but is a separate entity. Although the ovum was formerly part of her body, once it has been released by the ovary, it has its own independent life. The zygote is the equal contribution of man and woman. It has its own combination of genes, different from the combination of either the man or the woman. On the other hand, it cannot grow without the protection and nourishment of the mother's body. (This may be possible some day but not currently.)

Hazards of Illegal Abortion. The argument here is not for abortion per se but for *legal* abortion, It is suggested that there have always been and will always be abortions, and in order to make them as safe for women as possible, they should be legal and available to all women.

Elective Abortion and Nursing Practice

Nurses, as well as all others in society, need to carefully consider the arguments for and against abortion. In an attempt to help nurses to practice within the framework of their own decisions, the Nurses Association of the American College of Obstetricians and Gynecologists (NAACOG) approved the following statement on abortion. The statement attempts to protect both the right of the nurse to hold and practice her own ethical standards and the right of patients whose ethical decisions may differ from those of the nurse.

The Nurses Association of the American College of Obstetricians and Gynecologists recognizes that current knowledge of human behavior, population pressure and changes in medical technology challenge the position traditionally held regarding interruption of pregnancy.

We are aware of our nursing role in relation to operating with team members in meeting the health care needs of the woman seeking an abortion or sterilization. Genuine concern and compassion for this woman is strongly urged. However, there may be concern regarding nursing practice and participation in this particular area of health care. It is therefore our aim to recommend that an individual's rights must be maintained and safeguarded by written policies.

The Association recommends the following principles and guidelines:

1. Nurses have the responsibility to provide nursing care.

2. Nurses have the right to refuse to assist in the performance of abortions and/or sterilization procedures in keeping with their moral, ethical and/or religious beliefs, except in an emergency when a patient's life is clearly endangered, in which case the questioned moral issue should be disregarded. This refusal should not jeopardize the nurses' employment nor should they be subjected to harassment or embarrassment because of their refusal.

3. Nurses, in dealing with such patients, should not impose their views on the patients or personnel.

4. Nurses have the right to expect their employers to describe to them the hospital's policies and practices regarding abortions and sterilizations.

5. Nurses have the obligation to inform their employers of their attitudes and beliefs regarding abortions and sterilizations.

Just as patients need opportunities to express their feelings in a nonjudgmental milieu, so too must nurses and others who care for patients have an opportunity to share their feelings. The convictions of nurses who choose not to participate in abortions should be respected, not only for the sake of the nurse but for the sake of the patient. Hostile or disapproving attitudes have a way of surfacing in subtle ways—in failure to provide fresh water or to answer a call light, for example.

A Woman's Decision for Abortion

Luker[11] utilized a cost-reward framework (Chapter 2) to conceptualize the decision-making process by which women arrive at the decision to have an abortion. Findings from other studies of women's reasons for abortion fit well within this context. A decision-making model is useful in both individual counseling and in health education.

For example, some women take the risk of becoming pregnant through participation in unprotected intercourse because they do not perceive the probability of pregnancy as very high. Others believe that the perceived costs of contraception (e.g., inconvenience of a diaphragm, side effects of pill or IUD) are high in comparison with the perceived rewards of pregnancy (possible marriage if unmarried, increased attention from family and friends (Table 30–1).

Table 30–1. DECISION-MAKING: SEXUAL ACTIVITY, CONTRACEPTION, AND ABORTION

Decision	Decision-Making Affected by:
Sexual activity	Perceived probability of pregnancy Perceived costs/rewards of pregnancy
Use of contraceptive	Perceived costs of contraception Perceived probability of pregnancy Perceived costs/rewards of pregnancy Perceived probability of abortion
Abortion	Perceived costs/rewards of pregnancy Perceived costs/rewards of parenthood

Women who seek abortion consider the costs of continuing pregnancy to be greater than the rewards that may accrue. Costs will be different for individual women. Examples of costs in continuing pregnancy are:

1. Financial inability to care for a child.

2. Loss of personal freedom associated with the care of a child.

3. Interruption of educational or career plans.

4. Lack of support for pregnancy and child care from the male partner, both within and outside of marriage.

5. Loss of self-esteem associated with pregnancy at this stage of their life.

For some women, the costs of having an abortion will be so great that even though the cost of pregnancy may be high, the perceived costs of abortion are higher. Examples of costs in choosing abortion are:

1. A strong belief that abortion is morally wrong.

2. Alienation from a male partner who strongly desires pregnancy and infant or who believes abortion is morally wrong.

3. Fear related to the abortion procedure.

Counseling Prior to Abortion

Nurses can use a cost-reward framework during problem-pregnancy counseling and pre-abortion counseling to facilitate decision-making by helping clients to identify the rewards and costs for themselves. The rewards and costs for all alternatives can be explored. Women may discover costs or benefits (rewards) that had not occurred to them in their initial reaction to a problem pregnancy.

Mace[12] suggests that prior to any abortion each woman should be counseled in such a way that she:

1. Understands the meaning of abortion and is sure that this is what *she* desires.

2. Is not coerced by others (boyfriend, husband, parents, friends, counselor).

3. Has considered her conscience and her values.

4. Has considered alternatives (adoption, for example).

5. Is knowledgeable about effective contraception.

The counseling process itself should give each woman an opportunity to tell her story in her own words and to express her feelings. Often she may not be in touch with her true feelings at first, but self-recognition is important before a decision is made. Options are then explored (Chapter 5). As a result each woman will be able, we hope, to take the responsibility for a decision that is in accord with her own values.

The Reactions of Women to Elective Abortion

Anger, guilt, fear and sadness are emotions common to women both prior to and following induced abortion. Anger may be expressed at oneself ("I was dumb to let this [i.e., pregnancy] happen") or at the mate. If the mate is also the husband, the anger may influence many aspects of their relationship.

Some degree of guilt is not uncommon. The accompanying discomfort (there is always at least some discomfort that is somewhat equivalent to menstrual cramps) in the days that follow can reinforce feelings of guilt.

Fear may be related to fear of the procedure (see below), fear of pain, fear of after-affects, or fear that the fact of her abortion will become known.

Sadness is sometimes expressed in statements such as "I sometimes wonder what the baby might have been like."

On the more positive side, relief, gratitude that the abortion could be experienced with some degree of dignity, and a new understanding are achieved by some women. Both positive and negative emotions often coexist in the same individual. How much some of these emotions, particularly the more negative ones, are due to the influence of a culture that for so many generations has considered not only abortion but sex outside of marriage (for females at any rate) as sin is unclear at this point in history.

When a woman presents herself for the actual abortion procedure, she will have experienced, and may be continuing to feel, all of the emotions we have mentioned. Even the woman who feels very sure that this is the right thing for her to do may be anxious about the procedure itself. We can help this anxiety somewhat by a careful explanation of exactly what will happen in some detail. For example, if she is to have a saline instillation, she can be told that the solution used to prepare her abdomen will feel cold to her. One reason we as nurses need to be quite familiar with the procedures ourselves is so that we can prepare the patient for what to expect and answer her questions in an accurate and knowledgeable way.

Patients for induced abortion often have a very low tolerance for frustration. They have made their decision, and now they want the matter concluded as quickly as possible. Sometimes there must be a period of waiting, for the results of laboratory work, for example. The very least we can do in these instances is to acknowledge how difficult this must be for the woman. "I know how hard waiting must be for you; it usually takes about 30 minutes for these reports to be ready," may be helpful.

Rules, too, may be particularly hard to accept at this time. Even though rules have been explained (such as the necessity for having nothing by mouth for the patient who is to have general anesthesia), they may need to be discussed a second and third time. Patients who are preoccupied and anxious do not learn readily; explanations are easily forgotten. For this reason, too, the period before the abortion procedure is not a good one for teaching about contraception or any other material we expect the patient to retain.

The degree of formality that is a part of the relationship between the nurse and the abortion patient (or any patient) will vary considerably. Adolescent patients usually welcome a very informal relationship in which they are called by their first name and "mothered" with warmth and acceptance. This kind of approach can be offensive to a mature professional woman. Acceptance and concern for her may be more readily appreciated when it is expressed in quiet competence.

Regardless of what we attempt, some patients who come for abortion will be hostile because of their own high level of anxiety. Being able to understand and accept these feelings is a part of their nursing care.

Physical Preparation for Abortion

Physical preparation for an induced abortion includes assessing the general health history, laboratory tests, and general and gynecologic physical assessment.

Health history is one significant factor in

deciding on the type of procedure most appropriate for an individual patient and also where the procedure might best be performed. Induced abortion in an outpatient clinic is not suitable for women with a number of conditions, including cardiac, pulmonary, hematologic, or metabolic disease. Physical conditions that should be noted in the medical history include anemia; sickle cell disease; liver, kidney, or heart disease; diabetes, and epilepsy. Any intrauterine surgery, including hysterotomy or cesarean delivery, should be recorded, as should allergies to medications. A respiratory tract infection will usually contraindicate the use of general anesthesia. On the other hand, general anesthesia may be advisable for very young or very anxious patients.

Obstetric history, including the date of the last menstrual period and previous pregnancies, is part of this record.

The time during which a nurse is recording the medical history gives her an opportunity to assess undue anxiety or ambivalence, which could indicate a need for more intensive counseling.

Laboratory work commonly includes a pregnancy test, urinalysis, complete blood count, serology, blood group and type, and sickle cell screening. When indicated, the administration of immune globulin to Rh negative women following induced abortion is just as significant in the prevention of hemolytic disease of the newborn as administration following delivery.

Pap smears (and in some clinics gonococcal smears) are done at the time of the pelvic examination.

A thorough general and gynecologic examination, in most instances by a physician, completes the physical preparation.

Abortion Procedures: First Trimester

Menstrual Extraction. Menstrual extraction is the term used in a Supreme Court decision of January 1973 to describe a procedure in which a flexible polyethylene catheter, with two openings at its distal end, is inserted through the cervix into the uterus. Suction is applied, by syringe, or a hand or foot controlled pump, or electric vacuum apparatus, and the lining of the uterus that would normally be shed in menstruation is aspirated.

Although forerunners of this type of procedure, which is called by a number of names (menstrual regulation, menstrual aspiration, miniabortion, menstrual induction, and several others) date back to 1927, it has become relatively common only in the 1970's.

By strict definition menstrual extraction is not abortion, in that it is most commonly performed in the fourth to sixth week following the last menstrual period, a time during which pregnancy tests are not reliable. It is a method of establishing nonpregnancy for the woman who *may* be pregnant and does not wish to be. Some studies indicate that as many as half of the women having a menstrual extraction were not pregnant and were, therefore, undergoing an unnecessary procedure. At least one physician has suggested that delaying menstrual extraction until from 6 to 8 weeks after the last menstrual period could eliminate these unneeded procedures.

Most reports indicate that the procedure itself has many advantages over other types of pregnancy termination. In the few studies that have been done, complications were far lower than with other types of first trimester abortions. It is an outpatient procedure that is brief and requires no general anesthesia. This contributes to a far lower cost to the patient. Menstrual extraction generally fails to terminate pregnancy in less than 2 per cent of patients, although failure rates are as high as 10 per cent when the practitioner is inexperienced.[2]

It has been suggested that paramedical personnel (including nurses) could perform menstrual extraction after specialized training. Some women's groups have advocated the use of this technique by women in their own homes. No one is sure whether there might be a danger in repeated menstrual extractions in the same woman, although most agree that it should not be a substitute for contraception. Further research seems important before these issues can be resolved.

Vacuum Aspiration. During the first 12 weeks following the last menstrual period vacuum aspiration (also termed suction curettage or vacuum curettage) is considered the safest method of terminating pregnancy.

Following a paracervical block or general inhalation anesthesia, the cervix is dilated. With the vacuum off, a vacurette is inserted into the dilated internal os; the vacuum is applied, and the tube is withdrawn gently. The uterine contents, trapped in a special container, are examined by the physician and may then be sent to a pathologist.

The patient may receive intravenous Pitocin during the procedure to reduce blood loss. Often she rests for a few minutes in the operating room before returning to the recovery suite.

Variations in the procedure may include:

1. Omitting dilation very early in pregnancy when smaller bore evacuation tubes may be adequate.

2. Inserting a cylinder made from the stem

Table 30-2. ABORTION PROCEDURES

Procedure	Time Period	Site	Symptoms following Procedure	Potential Complications	Comments	Abortion-Related Deaths per 100,000 Abortions* 1972–1978
Menstrual extraction (ME)	4–8 weeks	Ambulatory	Possible mild bleeding, cramping	Low risk	Failure rate is 2–10 per cent	
				Increased risk in nulliparas (bleeding, uterine injury)	Some women who have ME are not pregnant.	
Vacuum aspiration	First 12 weeks	Ambulatory	Bleeding as in heavy menstruation, cramping	Infection, uterine perforation	Subsequent D and C may be necessary if bleeding severe	1.0 for vacuum aspiration and D and C
				Retained fetal or placental fragments		
Dilation and curettage (D and C)	First 12 weeks	Hospital	Bleeding (usually minimal)	Infection, uterine perforation	Not widely used for abortion today	1.0 for D and C and vacuum aspiration
			Cramping	Retained fetal or placental fragments		
Dilation and evacuation (D and E)	13–16 weeks	Hospital	Bleeding, cramping	Infection, uterine perforation		13–15 weeks: 5.6
				Retained fetal or placental fragments		16 weeks or later: 14.0

Method	Time	Setting	Side effects	Complications	Comments	Mortality
Prostaglandin instillation	Late first trimester, second trimester	Hospital	Nausea, vomiting, diarrhea, abdominal cramps (during and following procedure)	Cervical laceration, cost; possible delivery of live fetus	Second injection may be necessary; Contraindicated in: Asthma, Hypertension, Epilepsy, Glaucoma	Prostaglandin, Urea: 9.0
Hypertonic saline instillation	Second trimester after 16 weeks	Hospital	Feeling of fullness following instillation of saline; Discomfort of labor	Infection; Incomplete separation of placenta; Excessive bleeding; consumption coagulopathy; failure of abortion; Entry of hypertonic saline into circulatory system; Severe side effects: tachycardia, dryness in mouth, severe headache, flushing of skin	Fetal death usually occurs within an hour of injection; Labor begins in 8–40 hours and may last as long as 24 hours	Saline: 13.9
Hysterotomy	Second trimester	Hospital	As in cesarean birth or abdominal surgery	Infection, bleeding	Rarely used for abortion	42.8

*Data from Center for Disease Control, 1981.

of dry seaweed (*Laminaria digitata*) on the evening prior to the aspiration. The seaweed expands as it absorbs moisture and dilates the cervix. However, it may migrate in the cervix and become difficult to remove. *Laminaria* may possibly increase the incidence of endometritis.[5]

Abortion by aspiration is frequently done on an outpatient basis, with the woman remaining at the clinic for approximately 6 hours. This allows time for counseling and teaching, both before and after the procedure, as well as close observation of the woman.

After the twelfth week of pregnancy the technique of abortion becomes more complex.

Dilation and Curettage. Dilation and curettage (D and C) differs from vacuum aspiration in that (1) the cervix must be more fully dilated, (2) a sharp curet rather than a suction catheter is used, and (3) blood loss may be increased. D and C is used less frequently than vacuum aspiration, and usually when vacuum aspiration is not available. Occasionally a D and C is necessary following vacuum aspiration if bleeding persists, indicating the possibility of retained fragments.

Abortion Procedures: Second Trimester

Dilation and Evacuation. Dilation and evacuation (D and E) is used during the thirteenth to sixteenth weeks of gestation. At this time the products of conception are sufficiently large that they are crushed in the process of evacuation. The cervix is dilated before the procedure, usually through the insertion of *Laminaria*. Vacuum aspiration may complete the procedure. Although D and E has been performed after 16 weeks' gestation, note in Table 30–2 that the maternal mortality rate increases significantly, from 5.6 per 100,000 at 13 to 15 weeks to 14.0 per 100,000 after 16 weeks. The use of other procedures is preferred after 16 weeks.

Saline or Glucose Injection. When hypertonic saline or glucose is injected into the uterine cavity, severe damage results to both the placenta and the fetus, and fetal death occurs. Hypertonic saline is used more often than glucose in this procedure because of the increased rate of infection associated with glucose. Hypertonic saline may not be given to the mother with heart disease.

Abortion by saline instillation is performed by:

1. Antiseptic skin preparation and draping.
2. Infiltration of the abdominal wall with a local anesthetic (such as 1 per cent lidocaine).
3. Insertion of a spinal needle into the intrauterine space through a site about midway between the umbilicus and the symphysis pubis, and the subsequent withdrawal of 200 ml. of amniotic fluid.
4. Instillation of 200 ml. of 20 per cent sodium chloride (or 50 per cent glucose). The sodium chloride may be injected manually or via drip infusion.

A major maternal danger of this procedure is the risk that the hypertonic sodium chloride will enter the woman's circulation, causing death from acute hypernatremia or causing neurologic or cardiopulmonary damage. The chances of this are felt by some to be less when a drip infusion is used. The infusion bottle can be lowered to check for a clear return flow, indicating that the needle is not in a blood vessel.

Complaints of headache or thirst by the patient also suggest direct intravenous injection; the infusion should be stopped immediately.

Prostaglandins. Prostaglandins are fatty acids of a number of varieties that occur in many human tissues. Human semen alone contains 13 varieties. In obstetrics prostaglandins are being used to induce both abortion and labor, although the latter use is still largely experimental.

Intravaginal or intrauterine (via injection into the amniotic sac) administration of prostaglandins can interrupt pregnancy as early as the first week after a missed menstrual period or at any time during the first two trimesters, although these substances currently appear most effective after the sixteenth week. Prostaglandins may also be given intravenously, but larger doses are required and the incidence of side effects is increased. Prostaglandins induce abortion by stimulating contractions of the uterine smooth muscle. In most instances, expulsion of the uterine contents occurs within 24 hours.

Because these substances stimulate the smooth muscle of the gastrointestinal tract as well as of the reproductive tract, nausea, vomiting, abdominal cramps, and diarrhea are the principal undesired reactions. Prochlorperazine (Compazine) may be given for nausea and meperidine (Demerol) for pain, but aspirin should not be used because it inhibits the body's synthesis of natural prostaglandins and thus prolongs abortion time. Special care in the use of prostaglandins is necessary for women who have asthma, epilepsy, hypertension, or glaucoma because of occasional side effects: bronchospasm, convulsions, and transient blood pressure elevation.

Some early researchers using prostaglandins hoped that they could play a major role in contraception in vaginal tampon form. They would be packaged along with a pregnancy-testing kit. However, because they are not totally effective and because of the side effects, this has not yet become practical.

Mortality and Morbidity Following Elective Abortion

The major determinant of mortality following abortion is the length of gestation. Mortality is identified in Table 30–2 in relation to procedure, the next most important determinant, and in Table 30–3 in relation to weeks of gestation. To place these figures in perspective, maternal mortality in the United States from all pregnancy-related causes is 9.6 per 100,000 pregnancies; 6.4 for white women and 23.0 for all other women.[14] Mortality from other common surgical procedures, such as tonsillectomy and laparoscopic tubal sterilization, is more than 10 per 100,000 procedures.

The implication for nursing care seems clear. Problem-pregnancy counseling must be available to women early in pregnancy so that those women who choose abortion can have the safest possible procedure. Barriers to problem-pregnancy counseling and to abortion that delay a procedure must be eliminated. This includes financial barriers, which may cause a woman to delay abortion until she is able to pay for a procedure or wait for several weeks to be certified for reduced cost or free care.

Morbidity must be considered in relation to both immediate and long-term sequelae, and in relation to both physiologic and emotional consequences (Table 30–4). For statistical purposes, the Center for Disease Control considers complications to be related to the abortion procedure if they occur within 42 days after the procedure.

Infection, excessive bleeding, retained products of conception, and trauma to the uterus or cervix are some of the complications encountered.

Table 30–4. POTENTIAL MORBIDITY ASSOCIATED WITH ELECTIVE ABORTION

	Short Term (≤ 42 days)	Long Term
Physio-logic	Infection Excessive bleed-ing Physiologic uter-ine trauma Cervical trauma Retained products of conception Complications re-lated to specific method (see Nursing Care Plan 30–1)	Increased risk of midtrimester spontaneous abortion and premature labor (varies with type of proce-dure) Infertility secon-dary to pelvic inflammatory disease secon-dary to infec-tion
Psycho-logical	Anger Sadness Denial Grief Psychological emptiness	Very rare posta-bortion psy-chosis (3 per 10,000 in one study Disruption in re-lationships

countered. Nursing intervention specific to these complications is described in Nursing Care Plan 30–1. A combination of medical and nursing prevention and intervention is usually effective in dealing with complications if nurses have been successful in teaching clients the symptoms of complications that should be reported (see Nursing Care Plan 30–1).

The association between elective abortion and subsequent spontaneous abortion and premature delivery is still being debated. Reports by Klinger,[8] Liu et al.,[10] Richardson and Dixon,[17] and Keirse et al.[6] suggest a relationship. Daling and Emanual[4] and Van der Slikke and Treffers[23] found no relationship. Repeated first trimester abortion does appear to be associated with an increased risk of subsequent preterm labor,[7] as does second trimester abortion[6] and pregnancy occurring within 1 year of either an induced abortion or a pregnancy carried to term. If further research confirms these associations, this information should be available to women during problem-pregnancy and preabortion counseling.

If infection prior to or subsequent to abortion is untreated, generalized pelvic inflammatory disease and subsequent infertility may occur. Screening all women for venereal disease during preabortion assessment and prompt treat-

Table 30–3. WEEKS OF GESTATION AND MORTALITY RATE FOR LEGAL ABORTION, 1972–1975*

Weeks of Gestation	Mortality Rate per 100,000 Procedures
≤ 8	0.5
9–10	1.7
11–12	3.0
13–15	9.9
16–20	16.3
≥ 20	27.9

*Reported by Abortion Surveillance Branch of the Center for Disease Control; cited in Page, Villee, Villee: *Human Reproduction.* 3rd Edition. Philadelphia, W. B. Saunders Co., 1981, p. 220.

Text continued on page 1038

Nursing Care Plan 30–1.   The Woman Who Chooses Abortion

NURSING GOAL: To enable the woman who chooses abortion to successfully resolve a life crisis.

OBJECTIVES:
1. Preabortion counseling is provided to all women seeking abortion.
2. Prior to, during, and immediately following abortion, physiologic and emotional support is provided.
3. The woman client understands the reason for and components of self-care.
4. The woman client receives a follow-up examination 2 to 4 weeks postabortion that includes both physiologic and emotional assessment.
5. Contraceptive counseling appropriate to the client's needs is provided.

ASSESSMENT	POTENTIAL NURSING DIAGNOSIS	NURSING INTERVENTION	COMMENTS/RATIONALE
Initial assessment of the woman with problem pregnancy. 1. Pregnancy confirmed 2. Length of gestation confirmed through history and physical assessment	Need for information about all alternatives to problem pregnancy	Counsel or refer for counseling about all alternatives to problem pregnancy.	Gestational age will determine which abortion procedures are options.
Identify reason for abortion. 1. Pregnancy not desired 2. Abortion for medical reasons: a. Fetal indication: severe fetal disease b. Maternal indication: maternal health status	Proposed abortion for (specific reason)	Woman's reaction, family support, and counseling (see below) will vary with reason for abortion.	
Prior to abortion: Identify woman's feelings about proposed abortion. 1. What does abortion mean to her? How does she picture the embryo/fetus? 2. Has she considered the advantages and disadvantages (costs/rewards) of all possible alternatives to her pregnancy? Why did she choose abortion? Identify components of decision-making. Is her decision impulsive or carefully considered? 3. Is the decision her own or does she feel coerced by others? 4. What is her relationship to her sexual partner? Does he know about the pregnancy? Does he know about her desire for abortion?	Guilt Anxiety Ambivalence Denial of feelings	Encourage verbalization of feelings and fears. Maintain a nonjudgmental attitude. Correct misconceptions about abortion procedure and alternatives with appropriate information.	A counseling process in which a woman has the opportunity to verbalize feelings about pregnancy and abortion may decrease future unwanted pregnancies.

5. How does she regard others who have abortions? How does she regard herself as a result of her desire for abortion?

Identify support system.
1. No support system
2. Support from sexual partner
3. Support from family
4. Support from friends
5. Support from community agency counselor (e.g., Planned Parenthood)

Identify woman with history of severe psychiatric illness.

Identify woman's knowledge:
1. Anatomy and physiology of reproductive tract
2. Abortion procedure

Assess general health.
1. General assessment
   a. Cardiac disease
   b. Hypertension
   c. Pulmonary disease
   d. Hematologic disease (anemia, sickle cell disease)
   e. Metabolic disease (e.g., diabetes)
   f. Epilepsy
   g. Glaucoma
2. Gynecologic assessment
   a. Last menstrual period
   b. Estimated length of gestation
   c. Intrauterine surgery
   d. Gonorrhea or other infectious disease

Absence of support system

At risk of exacerbation of illness secondary to abortion

Need for information about anatomy and physiology of reproduction

Need for information about abortion procedure

Anxiety that interferes with learning

Frustration, anger, hostility related to rules and procedures

Potential need for modification of abortion procedure

At risk of bronchospasm, convulsions, or transient hypertension secondary to prostaglandin instillation

At risk of postabortion infection

Help woman to identify source of support from family or friends.

Be aware of community sources of support for referral if appropriate.

Nursing intervention will be highly individualized. Abortion may not be performed.

Using pictures, diagrams, written material, provide information as needed.

Explain reason for variation in abortion procedure in relation to gestational age (e.g., hospitalization for second trimester abortion).

Acknowledge woman's feelings about rules and procedures.

Explain reasons for specific rules and procedures.

Explain to woman reasons for modification in procedure.

Prostaglandins should not be administered to women with asthma, epilepsy, hypertension, or glaucoma.

Treat gonorrhea and other infectious diseases prior to abortion.

Commonly used procedures:
1. Prior to 8 weeks' gestation: menstrual extraction
2. Prior to 12 weeks' gestation: suction curettage
3. 12–16 weeks' gestation: dilatation with *Laminaria* and vacuum curettage
4. 16–20 weeks' gestation: prostaglandin injection, saline injection, hysterectomy (rare)

Continued on following page

Nursing Care Plan 30–1. The Woman Who Chooses Abortion *(Continued)*

ASSESSMENT	POTENTIAL NURSING DIAGNOSIS	NURSING INTERVENTION	COMMENTS/RATIONALE

3. Laboratory assessment
  a. Urinalysis
  b. Complete blood count
  c. Serology
  d. Blood group and type.
  e. Sickle cell screening
  f. Pap smear
	Need to protect woman from Rh isoimmunization	Administer Rh immune globulin (RhoGam) to all Rh negative women following abortion	

During abortion procedure:
1. First trimester abortion
2. Second trimester abortion (a labor/delivery process)
  a. Vital signs
  b. Intake and output
  c. Progress of labor
	At risk of dehydration	Encourage oral fluid intake.	IV fluids may also be administered.

	At risk of hemorrhage	When abortion occurs, remove fetus, observe for placental separation. Administer oxytocic drug following separation.	Hemorrhage is particularly likely following placental separation.
	Pain secondary to uterine contractions and cervical dilatation	Encourage relaxation and breathing techniques as in labor. Provide comfort through cleanliness.	Anxiety about abortion may lower pain threshold.
		Utilize prescribed medications for pain relief,.	
Gastrointestinal tract disturbance following prostaglandin instillation	At risk of nausea, vomiting, diarrhea, abdominal cramping secondary to prostaglandin instillation	Explain reason for symptoms to woman. Administer antinausea medication.	Prostaglandins stimulate the smooth muscle of the gastrointestinal tract as well as the reproductive tract.
Signs of hypernatremia following saline instillation: 1. Headache 2. Tachycardia 3. Dryness in mouth 4. Flushing of skin	At risk of hypernatremia secondary to entry of hypertonic saline into circulatory system	Stop infusion. Notify physician if not present. Be prepared to start IV with dextrose (5 per cent) to prevent cerebral dehydration.	

Physical assessment following abortion.
1. Bleeding
  a. Blood pressure, pulse
  b. Perineal pad
  c. Fundus in 2nd trimester procedures (saline, prostaglandin instillation, hysterectomy)
	At risk of infection
	At risk of hemorrhage
		Provide perineal hygiene.
		Report excess bleeding or change in pulse, blood pressure.
		Be prepared to start IV therapy.
		Massage fundus.
		Administer oxytocic drug as ordered.

Assess woman's understanding of self-care following abortion.	Need for information about self-care following abortion	Explain what to expect:
		1. Some bleeding and cramping for as long as 2 weeks
		2. Spotting for as long as 4 weeks
		3. Resumption of menstruation in 4–6 weeks
		
		Explain self-care:
		1. Take temperature each morning and evening for one week. Always take temperature before taking aspirin or Tylenol.
		2. Avoid for 6 weeks
		  a. Tampons
		  b. Douching
		  c. Intercourse
		3. Refer for physical and emotional evaluation 2–4 weeks following abortion procedure.
		
		Explain when to notify clinic or physician.
		1. Temperature of 100°F.
		2. Foul-smelling vaginal discharge
		3. Increased bleeding
		4. Prolonged bleeding (i.e., after 2 weeks)
		5. Severe pain
		6. Amenorrhea after 8 weeks
		7. Menstrual irregularity: dysmenorrhea, increased flow, irregularity

	Need for information about contraception	Explain that pregnancy may occur before first menstrual period. Provide appropriate contraceptive counseling (Chapter 6).
Identify feelings of woman following abortion.	Anger Guilt Sadness Ambivalence Relief Unhappiness	Provide opportunity and encourage verbalization of feelings following abortion. Provide woman with resources for discussion of feelings she may have in the weeks following abortion. Any or all of the feelings described may be present in the same woman.

ment of all infections should prevent this complication.

Psychological Consequences of Abortion. Literature on the psychological consequences of abortion in the 1960's and early 1970's focused on resultant emotional trauma.[9] More recent studies, some of which are reviewed here, indicate less serious emotional sequelae. Two possible reasons may account for the difference.

1. Until abortion became legal throughout the United States as a result of *Roe v. Wade* in 1973, many women seeking abortion were involved in an illegal act. The atmosphere of conspiracy surrounding the abortion rather than the abortion itself may have been responsible for the findings of certain emotional consequences associated with abortion. Abortion, drug use, and prostitution were considered to be similar crimes.[21]

2. Prior to 1973, one route by which abortion was sanctioned was through a psychiatric consultation in which it was stated that the pregnancy in question was detrimental to a woman's mental health. Pfeiffer[16] suggested that the law encouraged women to feign psychiatric symptoms in order to achieve a desired goal.

Now that abortion has been legal for a decade, the emotional trauma related to these factors has undoubtedly decreased, accounting for the differences in research findings.

Women have described a variety of emotions in the period immediately following an abortion. These emotions include sadness, an "empty" feeling, and grief reactions. Zimmerman[24] quotes one mother:

I started crying in the wheelchair. Then the nurse bent over me and was really concerned with physical hurting, if I was all right and nothing was wrong with me physically. I said, "No, I'm sad," and "Just leave me alone," because that feeling—if the mother can't care, who can?

Some women report the experience as seeming unreal: ". . . it just doesn't seem like it happened. It just seems like part of my life that never did happen . . . It seemed like those few hours down there never really existed, even though they did. . ."

"I kind of guess I blocked it out of my mind. I remembered what happened but . . . I guess I just didn't want to think about it and I still don't . . ."[24]

Most women reported that such feelings resolved in the weeks following the procedure. In Zimmerman's study of 40 women, 21 reported they were completely untroubled during the hours and days immediately following the abortion. Relief and even happiness were reported by Shusterman.[22]

Feelings following abortion appear to be influenced by situational factors in the woman's life. Postabortion emotional adjustment has been associated with (1) satisfaction with the decision, which the woman made herself; (2) positive support from the male partner; and (3) initial response to pregnancy that was not unduly angry or anxious.[22]

In addition to situational factors, the degree of psychological adjustment prior to the abortion, rather than the abortion per se, seems to be the important factor in postabortion psychiatric disturbances.[11] Nursing assessment at the time of postabortion follow-up should always include an evaluation of the woman's emotional status.

Abortion psychosis was found to be far less common (0.3 per 10,000 legal abortions) than postpartum psychosis (1.7 per 10,000 deliveries) in a prospective study conducted in Britain.[3]

Disruption in one or more social relationships, principally the relationship with the male partner involved in the pregnancy, was found by Zimmerman[24] in 22 of 40 women, but other women reported increased closeness to one or more persons. As with other social and emotional factors, the characteristics of the relationship prior to the abortion were important to the effect of the abortion.

The Male Partner. There are limited data on the relationship between the male partner and abortion. Rothstein,[20] following interviews with 60 men at an abortion clinic waiting room, reported that the decision for abortion was primarily a shared one. Approximately one-third of the men cited the decision as primarily that of the woman, while one-fifth said it was primarily the man's decision. Men who accompany women to an abortion clinic may be very different from men who do not, so care must be used in interpreting these results.

A second paper by Rothstein[19] suggested that the men interviewed reacted favorably to counseling in which financial alternatives, contraception, and abortion procedures were discussed.

Commercial Abortion Agencies

With the growth of legitimate abortion agencies it was probably inevitable that some commercial agencies would develop solely for profit. One example is the commercial referral agency. The agency may advertise on radio or television or in newspapers, particularly campus newspapers. The patient calls a designated phone number and is told, "Your abortion will cost $200; bring or mail $50 down payment or deposit and we will arrange an appointment for you." After the patient has made this payment she is referred to a clinic, which may be a highly reputable clinic that knows nothing of the referral group and charges a customary fee of $150.

A second possibility is that the clinic itself is in collaboration with the referral agency and receives a "kickback" from the fee charged for the abortion.

Nurses can prevent such practices. Awareness of the fees normally charged by legitimate clinics and alertness to the possibility of such referral services are two ways of doing this. Referral through family planning clinics and other health agencies can be made available and then publicized. When patients come for abortion referral, we can be sure that they are treated in such a way that alternative referrals

will not seem more desirable. For example, the college student who fears that her request for abortion through campus health facilities will be a difficult, uncomfortable procedure may seek an alternate route. Questionable referrals are most likely to continue when they fulfill a woman's need for sympathy and individualized concern.

Summary

Elective abortion remains a controversial issue in the United States. Nurses have a responsibility to support individual clients and to participate in the public debate that will determine future policies.

REFERENCES

1. Belsey, E., Greer, H., Lal, S., et al.: Predictive Factors in Emotional Responses to Abortion. *Social Science and Medicine, 11*:71, 1977.
2. Brenner, W., and Edelman, D.: Menstrual Regulation: Risks and Abuses. *International Journal of Gynecology and Obstetrics, 15*:177, 1977.
3. Brewer, C.: Incidence of Post-abortion Psychosis: A Prospective Study. *British Medical Journal, 1*:476, 1977.
4. Daling, J., and Emanuel, I.: Induced Abortion and Subsequent Outcome of Pregnancy. A Matched Cohort Study. *Lancet, 2*:170, 1975.
5. Fogel, C.: Abortion. *In* Woods, N., and Fogel, C.: Health Care of Women: A Nursing Perspective. St. Louis, C. V. Mosby Co., 1981.
6. Keirse M., Rush, R., Anderson, A., et al.: Risk of Preterm Delivery in Patients with Previous Preterm Delivery and/or Abortion. *British Journal of Obstetrics and Gynecology, 85*:81, 1978.
7. Keirse M.: Epidemiology of Preterm Labor. *In* Keirse M., et al. (eds.): *Human Parturition.* Boston, Nijhoff Publishers, 1979.
8. Klinger A.: Demographic Consequences of the Legalization of Induced Abortion in Eastern Europe. *International Journal of Gynaecology and Obstetrics, 8*:680, 1970.
9. Kummer, J.: Post Abortion Psychiatric Illness—A Myth? *American Journal of Psychiatry, 119*:980, 1963.
10. Liu, D., Melville H., and Martin, T.: Subsequent gestational Morbidity after Various Types of Abortion. *Lancet, 2*:431, 1972.
11. Luker, K.: *Taking Chances: Abortion and the Decision Not to Contracept.* Berkeley, University of California Press, 1975.
12. Mace, D.: *Abortion: The Agonizing Decision.* Nashville, Abingdon Press, 1972.
13. Nurses Association of the American College of Obste-

tricians and Gynecologists: Statement on Abortions and Sterilizations. *JOGN Nursing, 1*:57, 1972.
14. Page, E., Villee, C., and Villee, D.: Human Reproduction. 3rd Edition. Philadelphia, W. B. Saunders Co., 1981.
15. Papevangelou, G., Vrettos, A., Papdatos, C., et al.: The Effect of Spontaneous and Induced Abortion on Prematurity and Birth Weights. *Journal of Obstetrics and Gynaecology of the British Commonwealth, 80*:418, 1973.
16. Pfeiffer, E.: Psychiatric Indications or Psychiatric Justification of Therapeutic Abortion? *Archives of General Psychiatry, 23*:402, 1970.
17. Richardson, J. A., and Dixon, G.: Effects of Legal Termination on Subsequent Pregnancy. *British Medical Journal 1*:1303, 1976.
18. Rodman, H., Sarvis, B., and Bonar, J.: *The Abortion Controversy.* 3rd Edition. New York, Columbia University Press, in press.
19. Rothstein, A.: Abortion: A Dyadic Perspective. *American Journal of Orthopsychiatry, 47*:(1):111, 1977.
20. Rothstein, A.: Mens Reactions to Their Partner's Elective Abortion. *American Journal of Obstetrics and Gynecology, 128*:831, 1977.
21. Sarvis, B., and Rodman, H.: *The Abortion Controversy.* New York, Columbia University Press, 1974.
22. Shusterman, L.: Predicting the Psychological Consequences of Abortion. *Social Science and Medicine, 13A*:683, 1979.
23. Van der Slikke, J., and Treffers, P.: Influence of Induced Abortion on Gestational Duration in Subsequent Pregnancies. *British Medical Journal, 1*:270, 1978.
24. Zimmerman, M.: *Passage Through Abortion. The Personal and Social Reality of Women's Experiences.* New York, Praeger, 1977.

31

Contemporary Issues for Perinatal Nurses

OBJECTIVES

1. Identify issues of concern to perinatal nurses and childbearing families.
2. Identify sources of ethical and legal dilemmas for perinatal nurses.
3. Describe theories of ethical decision-making.
4. Identify resources for ethical and legal decision-making.
5. Describe specialized practices in perinatal nursing—the nurse-midwife, the clinical nurse-specialist, nurse practitioner, childbirth educator, nurse clinician.
6. Explain the relationship of certification and perinatal nursing practice.
7. Define maternal, fetal, neonatal, perinatal, and infant mortality. Describe uses of mortality statistics to improve perinatal care.
8. Discuss the rationale for regionalization of perinatal health care. Indicate the advantages and problems associated with regionalization.

Because childbearing, along with childrearing, is essential to the ongoing of society, vital issues surround the nursing practice of care for childbearing families. Many of these issues have been explored in this text. Some issues that produced major debates just a few years ago (for example, the presence of fathers in labor and delivery rooms) have been resolved for many families.

Society, however, continues, and will always continue, in a state of change. New issues arise as old issues are moved toward resolution.

Nurses who desire to improve the care of childbearing families have always recognized the need to do more than provide excellent care to individuals. One nurse, Margaret Sanger, led a fight for the right of women to plan their families at a time when that issue was as controversial as pregnancy termination is today. Mary Breckinridge, a nurse-midwife, not only developed the Frontier Nursing Service (FNS) to bring care to mothers and infants in the Kentucky mountains, but also gathered baseline and ongoing statistics to demonstrate the value of the services provided. She was able to show, for example, that even in primitive environments the maternal mortality in families delivered by FNS was 1.2 per 1000 (in the period 1925–1951); national maternal mortality for the same period was 3.4 per 1000. Many other nurses, less well known, have worked in the past and continue to work for changes that are necessary to continued improvement in the health of mothers and infants.

Issues of significance to nurses may involve law, ethics, social policy, or health care policy. Frequently these areas overlap or vary according to one's perspective. For example, termination of pregnancy is primarily an ethical issue for some persons, a legal issue for others, and a matter of social or health care policy for still others.

Because of varying perspectives, nurses do not always agree on issues related to childbearing. Nevertheless, nurses have the responsibility to become active advocates for present and future clients in those arenas where decisions are made that affect the well-being of those clients.

Power: A Key Concept

Many of the issues important to the health care of childbearing families involve questions of power and control.

Where shall babies be born? In many communities those who would provide options other than hospital delivery have met with a variety of sanctions. Within hospitals, the rights of childbearing families vary widely.

Who will care for childbearing mothers? Care by nurse-midwives is an option in some communities, but in others midwives have been denied the opportunity to practice or have had to practice under less than desirable circumstances.

Who receives care? Issues include funding for health care, funding for nutritional services such as the WIC (Women, Infants and Children) nutritional program, and the availability and accessibility of family planning services.

Power may be defined as the "ability of one party to cause another to change behavior in an intended direction."[38] A major basis of power is the possession of "resources," which may be tangible (the possession of wealth, for example) or intangible (e.g., the possession of "prestige"). Although some nurses have successfully "fought the system" to bring about changes they perceived as important, others have felt "power-less" and as much the victims of the "power-full" as the clients for whom they would be advocates. One reason is a perceived lack of resources. With limited funds for court battles, legislative lobbying, or contributions to political campaigns, nurses often do not feel able to bring about change. However, nurses possess an important resource in that they form the largest by far of all the health care professions. In addition, many of the concerns of nurses for childbearing families are shared by consumers, with whom nurses can form coalitions, thus increasing their resources and their power. Nurses mobilize their strength through professional nursing organizations, such as their state associations and the American Nurses' Association, through which they can become more knowledgeable about the political process and can work for important legislation as individuals and as a group.

Decisions that affect the care of childbearing families are made in a variety of settings. The examples below are by no means all-inclusive but do suggest why nurses must be politically active at all levels of government.

Where Shall Babies Be Born? An increasing although still relatively small number of parents are choosing home or an alternative birthing center outside of the hospital as the site for birth. Opposition to this practice has been intense in many communities. Individual practitioners who have participated in out-of-hospital births have suffered varying reprisals, including loss of malpractice insurance, loss of hospital privileges, and loss of license to practice. Alternative Birth Centers must be licensed, and opposition to such licensure has also frequently been intense. Although opponents believe that their opposition will promote safer care for mothers and infants, supporters argue that parents will not seek hospital care but may choose home delivery without any professional (either nurse-midwife or physician) in attendance (see also Chapter 16).

Who Will Care for Childbearing Mothers? Decisions concerning the licensing of professionals, including the parameters of practice for nurses, nurse practitioners, and nurse-midwives, are made in state legislatures and thus vary from one state to another. In addition, individual institutions may decide the parameters of practice within the framework of state law. State law may, for example, allow nurses to perform certain acts but a particular institution may not. Many state legislatures are considering or have passed legislation concerning the role of midwifery in the care of childbearing families. In at least one state, lay midwives have been permitted to attend home births, but nurse-midwives have not been allowed to practice in homes. In another state the state nurses' association is suing both the Medical Board and the Medical Society, alleging that those groups are engaged in pursuing a conspiracy to restrain trade in the provision of health care services by nurse practitioners and nurse-midwives.

The restraint of nurse-midwives and nurse practitioners in many communities not only limits choice but may mean that services will be unavailable, inaccessible, or too costly for many clients. The practice of nurse-midwifery and other perinatal nursing specialists is described in this chapter.

Who Receives Care? What Services Will Be Available? The ability to provide perinatal care is related, at least in part, to the availability of funding. When clients have limited funds, there must be other sources of funding to ensure care. Federal and state taxes are major sources of revenue. Foundations, such as the National Foundation—March of Dimes, have provided funding for professional education, equipment, and research.

Nurses can question candidates for national and state office on their views about perinatal health care. Will they support reimbursement for providers of health care, such as nurse-midwives and nurse practitioners? Will they support legislation that allows consumers a choice of birthing environments? Will they support funding for programs such as WIC, family planning, and prenatal care? Will they support daycare or Aid to Families with Dependent Children (AFDC)? Nurses can and must actively support candidates who share their views on the importance of perinatal health.

Nurses may also choose to run for public office themselves. In Maryland in 1982 three nurses were members of the state legislature. One of those nurses, the Honorable Marilyn Goldwater, introduced legislation that allows direct third-party payment ot nurse-midwives and nurse practitioners without the need for physician support or referral, the first legislation of its kind passed in the United States.

Nurses can also actively work to educate the general public on the value of dollars spent for the care of pregnant women and children, so that there is a broad base of support for good perinatal health care. In addition, nurses can and must testify at hearings where issues related to health care are discussed. The forum may be a school board meeting where the topic is family-life education or programs for pregnant teens within the school system, a meeting of county commissioners who are debating a health department budget, the state legislature where the practice of nurses in extended roles is the subject of a proposed bill, or the Congress of the United States where decisions are made about federal health care funds and policy. Nurses can overlook none of these local and government organizations. Although nurses may participate personally at local and perhaps state levels, national participation is frequently accomplished through professional organizations such as the American Nurses' Association, which maintains an office in Washington to lobby for issues important to nurses.

In addition to interaction with elected bodies, nurses can influence perinatal care through participation in voluntary organizations. The boards of these organizations make decisions that can be important to perinatal health care. Nurses should seek to be represented on these boards to increase the likelihood that boards that fund research activities can consider nursing research and projects for care as well as those of other groups. Some states have perinatal advisory committees, which are voluntary but are appointed by and advisory to elected officials and may be influential in determining perinatal policy.

Nurses must enter political discussions from a position of experience and expertise. Statements made at hearings and in letters to officials must be factual. For example, in a recent hearing on nurse-midwives and home birth, non-nurses presented data that compared mortality in home births of past decades with hospital births today. Nurses and nurse-midwives who were present were able to challenge those data effectively and to present more relevant statistics. The legislative committee ultimately accepted the argument of the nurses and nurse-midwives. Had nurses not been well prepared, it is unlikely that they could have presented convincing arguments.

In the pages that follow a number of issues in contemporary childbearing are discussed. Other issues have been described throughout this text. As nurses move to effect change in relation to these issues, it is necessary to remember that the political route, at some level, is the way in which change is accomplished. To effectively travel that route, nurses must

1. Be aware of problems
2. Know where decisions that will affect those problems are made (within the institution or by a community board, the state legislature, or federal government)
3. Form coalitions with other groups who support their proposals
4. Demonstrate knowledge and expertise in relation to the solutions they propose (i.e., to use a popular phrase, show that they have done their homework).

Earlier generations of nurses have demonstrated that informed and articulate arguments can change perinatal health care. Contemporary nurses can do so as well.

Ethical and Legal Issues in Perinatal Nursing

The practice of nursing involves continuous decision-making. Many of the decisions described in previous chapters are based on a knowledge of scientific fact or theory. Using nursing processes, a problem is identified, a nursing diagnosis is made, appropriate intervention is instituted, the outcome is evaluated, and the plan is then continued or modified.

Scientific facts or theories, however, are not the only variables that affect decision-making. The values of clients, their families, the community, and health-care providers are increasingly recognized as major variables in decisions about health care. Some values become laws and others remain part of moral codes and belief systems. Both laws and belief systems may have a major impact on nursing interactions with childbearing families.

Ethical issues are those that involve values and moral responsibility. Values that comprise ethics are expressed in ethical behavior. The study of ethics is concerned with the way things "ought to be." A code of ethics may

define ethical behavior; for example, the ANA Code of Ethics for nurses defines how nurses are expected to behave in general terms.

CODE FOR NURSES*

1. The nurse provides services with respect for human dignity and the uniqueness of the client unrestricted by considerations of social or economic status, personal attributes, or the nature of health problems.
2. The nurse safeguards the client's right to privacy by judiciously protecting information of a confidential nature.
3. The nurse acts to safeguard the client and the public when health care and safety are affected by the incompetent, unethical, or illegal practice of any person.
4. The nurse assumes responsibility and accountability for individual nursing judgments and actions.
5. The nurse maintains competence in nursing.
6. The nurse exercises informed judgment and uses individual competence and qualifications as criteria in seeking consultation, accepting responsibilities, and delegating nursing activities to others.
7. The nurse participates in activities that contribute to the ongoing development of the profession's body of knowledge.
8. The nurse participates in the profession's efforts to implement and improve standards of nursing.
9. The nurse participates in the profession's efforts to establish and maintain conditions of employment conducive to high quality nursing care.
10. The nurse participates in the profession's effort to protect the public from misinformation and misrepresentation and to maintain the integrity of nursing.
11. The nurse collaborates with members of the health professions and other citizens in promoting community and national efforts to meet the health needs of the public.

*Published by the American Nurses' Association, 1976, and reprinted with permission. The Code with Interpretative Statements is available from the American Nurses' Association, 2420 Pershing Road, Kansas City, MO 64108.

Legal issues are those related to a body of law. Laws such as the nurse practice acts of each state define the legal practice of nursing, usually in broad, rather general terms. Broad terminology is used so that nurse practice acts will not have to be changed constantly as new technology develops. This general language, however, may leave room for much interpretation by courts. Frequently it is difficult to determine what is ethical in a particular situation and at times it may be difficult to determine the proper action under the law.

Legal and ethical issues are frequently intertwined. In a particular instance an act or behavior may be legal but not ethical, ethical but not legal, neither ethical nor legal, or both ethical and legal. Consider the following examples in perinatal nursing:

Termination of pregnancy by abortion in the United States is legal in 1982 and has been for 9 years (Chapter 30). Yet for some persons, abortion per se, and therefore assisting with abortion, is unethical. This difference in perspective is an important characteristic of the ethical basis of actions. The values of one person or group of persons frequently differ from those of others. The values of a client or patient may be different from those of a nurse. The values of nurses and physicians may vary. Nurses may differ from one another in relation to values.

The structure of our health-care system, in which nurses have much responsibility but limited authority, at times places nurses in the position of behaving in a manner that may not be legal but that is believed to be ethical. For example, both ethically and legally nurses have a general responsibility to fulfill the medical orders of a physician. But what if a nurse, in the role of patient advocate, believes those medical orders or the physician's behavior are not in the best interest of the client or patient? For example, a physician might decide to withhold information from the parents of an infant who is ill or to withhold feedings from a mentally retarded infant to hasten the dying process.

Cushing[10] describes an instance in which nurses were not only ethically but legally liable when they failed to stop a surgeon from accidentally removing a portion of bowel during surgery to remove a dead fetus.

The woman's attorney argued that the nurses should have intervened and stopped the surgeon before the extensive damage had been done. (The events had occurred over a 10-minute period.)

The nurses unsuccessfully argued that they frequently defer to a doctor's judgment even if they feel something is wrong. Their attorney said that the court decision was unfair because it held that the nurses should have countermanded the physician who had more training and expertise than any of the nurses. However, expert witnesses for the woman testified that professional ethics and hospital procedures mandate that nurses countermand a doctor's action if they feel it is incorrect.

The case is currently being appealed.

What Is the Nurse's Ethical and Legal Responsibility?

Dilemmas are situations in which no solution is ideal. For example, an unwanted pregnancy is a dilemma because no solution approaches the ideal of a wanted pregnancy. Ethical and legal dilemmas confront nurses (and other health-care providers) in all practice settings. The dilemmas of perinatal nursing are particularly difficult for several reasons.

During the prenatal and intrapartum phases of pregnancy some people believe that there are not one but two clients, the embryo–fetus and the pregnant woman. Others argue that the pregnant woman and her fetus form an "organic whole."[17] Dilemmas arise when the needs of mother and fetus differ. In decades past, the question occurred primarily when the well-being of the fetus threatened the life of the mother and one was faced with a decision: Should the mother's or the infant's life be saved? Today, with far more sophisticated techniques of fetal assessment and intervention, legal precedents are being established by which the fetus, particularly after 20 to 24 weeks, acquires the "right" to medical intervention. Courts have recently ruled, for example, that when a vaginal delivery is deemed hazardous to the fetus, a cesarean birth is required even if the gravida denies permission.[3]

The legal process may be the same as that previously used when parents have refused certain types of treatment for infants or children, such as the refusal of blood products by parents who belong to the religious denomination Jehovah's Witnesses. The court may award the custody of the fetus to an administrator of the hospital, or it may directly order a cesarean, as did a Denver court when a particular mother refused a cesarean delivery recommended because of meconium staining and signs of fetal distress on a fetal monitor tracing. The judge from the juvenile court ruled that the fetus was a dependent and neglected child.[3]

As technology makes other types of fetal intervention increasingly possible, such as intervention when infants have congenital hydrocephalus or urinary tract obstruction (Chapter 24), discussion of fetal rights will probably become more common. Nurses, in their role of patient advocate, may have to consider the question—advocate for which patient, the mother or the fetus?

A second dilemma is not unique to perinatal nursing but arises frequently because a newborn infant is unable to make decisions. When an adult is critically ill and there is no hope of recovery, previous discussions with that person, perhaps even a "living will," may provide some insight into his or her desires. Infants, however, cannot participate in decisions about their lives. As modern technology enables us to maintain life for small preterm, malformed, or seriously ill infants for days and weeks, a choice between the prolonged life, no matter how limited, and death must at times be made. Although nurses may not be directly involved in this decision-making process, the close relationship between nurses, infants, and families and the advocacy role of nurses make it essential for them to deal with the issue. (See below and also Chapter 28.)

A young adolescent who is pregnant may also, in some circumstances, be denied participation in decisions about sexuality and childbearing. She may be denied access to contraception if her parents do not give permission, denied access to pregnancy termination, or, conversely, be pressured to have an abortion.

A third factor that has influenced ethical and legal decision-making related to perinatal nursing is the rapid and continuing explosion of knowledge that has taken place during the past decade. Change requires a confrontation with values, whether that change is social or technological. When there was no possibility of diagnosing a genetic disorder while the fetus was in utero, there was no ethical dilemma about fetal treatment or abortion of a fetus with a congenital problem such as Down's syndrome or myelomeningocele. Today, the combination of contraception and abortion allows many couples or women to decide how many children they will bear and to avoid the birth of children with certain genetic defects. This possibility "has obvious and enormous ramifications for traditional sex roles, family life, composition of the work force, and patterns of child-rearing."[5]

When there were no infant respirators for ventilatory support, there were few decisions to make about the care of very tiny, very premature infants. They usually died soon after birth. Now such an infant may live for weeks or months; some will still die, others will have significant disability, and still others will become healthy children. Although statistics tell us that a certain percentage of infants of a particular birth weight and gestational age may be expected to die or have significant morbidity (and those statistics change frequently), they are of no value in predicting the outcome and thus the appropriate course of action for a particular infant.

Theories of Ethical Decision-Making

Ethical decision-making may be approached from a number of theoretical perspectives. These theories can be described only briefly in this chapter. An ethical decision may utilize more than one theoretical perspective.

In deontologic theory ethical decisions are derived from rules of conduct. For example, the basis of a decision made according to a code such as the ANA Code for Nurses or the Ten Commandments is deontologic. In a teleologic approach, the "rightness" of an action is determined by the results or consequences of the action. As Lumpp[24] states, the desired result may vary significantly. In Roman Catholic natural law, a teleologic theory, the desired end is ultimate union with God in heaven. In utilitarianism, also a teleologic theory, the desired end is happiness for the individual concerned or, in social issues, "the greatest good for the greatest number of persons."

Immanuel Kant, an eighteenth century philosopher whose thought is still a major influence in ethical decision-making, emphasizes respect for individual autonomy and universalizability as the major principles on which decisions ought to be based. Respect for individual autonomy implies the right of persons to make decisions about their own lives and to have these decisions respected. Unfortunately, it doesn't answer the questions involved in ethical decision-making when the person (such as an infant) cannot make those decisions.

Universalizability is a principle that states, "Act only on that maxim which you can at the same time will that it should become a universal law" (Kant, cited in Carroll and Humphrey[6]). Universalizability is comparable to the Golden Rule (Do unto others as you would they do unto you). It requires asking whether this decision would be appropriate for all persons in similar circumstances and whether, in similar circumstances, each person would wish the same decision to be made in relation to himself.

Curran[8] has drawn on the work of twentieth century philosopher Richard Neibuhr, who states that ethics must be based on a response to human needs rather than on a rigid system of rules. The moral ethical person is a responsible person who relates to and responds to others. Curran therefore calls his theory a Relationality–Responsibility Theory that recognizes that relationships and responsibilities must be examined within the perspective of both time and culture. The questions that arise in nursing concern the relationship of a nurse to the various actors, including herself, in a particular situation and the responsibility of a nurse to each of these actors. Lumpp states that the primary relationship is that of nurse to client and that the nurse–client relationship is one of advocacy. "To be an advocate means that one has reference for the other, and that one can establish a covenant of fidelity with the other."[24] The "covenant of fidelity"[32] involves a reciprocal agreement in which both client and caregiver agree as to what each can expect from the other and trust that the agreement will be carried out. For example, a nurse establishes an advocate relationship with a particular patient, develops a relationship of trust with her, provides information so that she is able to make necessary decisions, respects her autonomy and therefore respects the decision that is made, and then, as advocate, supports that decision actively. If a nurse finds that, to be true to herself she is unable to support the client's decision, she would be ethically required to withdraw from the situation.

Although the principal relationship in ethical decision-making for nurses is the nurse–client relationship, ethical dilemmas may be due to nurse–physician and nurse–nurse relationships, as the examples later in this chapter will demonstrate.

Professional Ethics and Individual Moral Values

It is necessary to distinguish between professional ethics and one's personal moral and religious values. This distinction is not always easy, particularly when dearly held views are in question. For example, most professional nurses respect the ethic of a person's right to make a decision for self. But what if the results of that decision are in conflict with the nurse's individual moral values? What if the mother refuses RhoGam because it is a blood product; this action is a moral decision for the mother but may violate nurses' notions of moral good because nurses believe she is seriously endangering the children of future pregnancies. What if parents elect abortion and the nurse

believes that abortion is morally wrong? What if parents refuse transfusion or surgery for their critically ill infant? Do nurses respect the parents' autonomy or treat the child anyway as the child's advocate?

Ethical decisions involve rational thought, a process described in the pages that follow. Professional ethical judgments are the product of rational thought of one or more nurses. Some state nurses' associations and some individual practice settings have ethics committees or ethics rounds that can help an individual nurse use ethical theory and decision-making processes to help determine an ethical response to a problem. This type of committee, which addresses the process of ethical decision-making, is different from committees within institutions, which determine the outcome in particular ethical dilemmas, especially those involving the withdrawal of life support.

Lestz[23] presents arguments for and against ethical decisions by committee. Advantages include the elimination of personal bias, reduction in the agony of prolonged human suffering, relieving family and individual provider of the responsibility for the decision, and relieving society of a questionable benefit by eliminating organisms that do not possess "humanhood." For Lestz, however, the disadvantages of such a committee outweigh the advantages. Disadvantages include the loss of human rights, individualism, and self-determination and a radical alteration in the relationship between the health-care provider (she focuses on the physician) and the client.

Lestz suggests ongoing education of the public and professionals to help all of us become more aware of alternatives in ethical decision-making. This kind of education in ethics should be helpful for the individual nurse as she seeks to recognize the difference between her own personal values and her ethical responsibility as a professional nurse.

The Process of Ethical Decision-Making

Ethical decision-making, like other kinds of decision-making, requires a data base. That data base includes answers to the following questions.

1. *Who are the actors involved?* Actors include a client or clients, health-care providers, family members, and perhaps others (clergy, social agencies, and so on).

2. *What is the proposed action?*

3. *What is the setting or context of the proposed action?* Is the context one in which a

decision must be made quickly (e.g., the decision to incubate an infant weighing 800 grams and use a ventilator to maintain respiration) or is there time to consider the decision (e.g., the decision to discontinue ventilator support or to terminate pregnancy when the fetus has a large meningomyelocele)?

4. *What is the intention or purpose of the proposed action?* Is the purpose to spare the family from suffering (e.g., termination of pregnancy when an infant has a genetic defect) or to protect an individual (such as an infant who would continue to undergo painful procedures with little or no hope of recovery or meaningful life)?

5. *What are the probable implications or consequences?* Here one might consider not only implications or consequences for the individuals involved but also, using the principle of universalizability, the implications or consequences if the action were always followed under similar circumstances.

6. *Are there alternatives or choices?* Clients may not always be aware of all possible choices; nurses must be sure all alternatives are presented. For example, we see clients who feel that abortion is the only choice they have in response to a problem pregnancy. For some of these clients the presentation of other alternatives (Chapter 5) allows them a choice that is more ethically comfortable for them.

Legal Decisions

Although legal decisions related to perinatal nursing may seem more clearly defined than ethical decisions, they are by no means always straightforward. The rapid changes taking place in perinatal health care raise legal issues that were not a consideration a few years ago. For example, with the widespread use of fetal monitoring, failure to seek appropriate intervention when the monitor strip indicates late decelerations is a potential legal issue today that did not exist only a few years ago.

Perinatal nurses must be knowledgeable about law in three areas—(1) the legally defined duties of all nurses to clients, (2) specific issues with legal ramifications, and (3) laws that are applicable to childbearing families.

Legally Defined Duties

Nurses have two legally defined duties to clients—"(a) a duty to possess the required knowledge and skill as possessed by the average member of the profession and (b) a duty to exercise ordinary and reasonable care in the application of such professional knowledge and skill."[10] The criterion by which a nursing action may be legally judged is whether the action was that which a "prudent" or "reasonable" nurse would have taken under the "same or similar circumstances." The law thus requires that nurses be knowledgeable, skillful, and possessed of good judgment.

When a nurse finds herself in a situation for which she feels she is not prepared, she is legally obligated to ask for assistance. If that situation is one for which her colleagues were prepared, she should seek to be at least equally well prepared. For example, a nurse who normally cares for mothers in labor in most settings can be expected to be capable of evaluating variations in fetal heart rate pattern as indicated on the fetal heart rate monitor and of intervening appropriately. This would be considered the "required knowledge and skill possessed by the average member of the profession." If she is unable to do this she should seek assistance from her colleagues in caring for a woman who is being monitored during labor, or not care for such a woman until she has the appropriate knowledge and skills. Although institutions have a responsibility to provide education, the responsibility of the individual nurse to acquire additional education remains.

"Ordinary and reasonable care" is a matter of judgment. Cushing[10] cites the following court case (*Murphy v. Rowland,* 609 S.W. 2nd 292, Texas 1980) in which a nurse lost her license because her actions were not deemed prudent and reasonable.

A woman, eight months pregnant, awoke in great pain and was driven to a lay midwife. The midwife told the family to take the woman to a hospital because she was not in labor and had a serious problem. After being examined in a hospital emergency room in Aransas Pass, Texas, by two nurses who consulted via telephone with a physician, she was referred to a second hospital several blocks away. At the second hospital, the woman remained in the car while her sister-in-law went inside and explained the situation to the nurse on duty. The nurse went out to the car, checked the pregnant woman's pulse and contractions, and examined her for bleeding.

She instructed the family to take her to another hospital, about 20 miles away in Corpus Christi, as quickly as possible. She did not consult with or notify the physician on emergency call.

When the family requested an ambulance, the nurse informed them that the only one available was from a funeral home and that their response time was slow. The family declined the nurse's offer to call for a police escort. After leaving the emergency room, the family tried to take the woman home. En route the woman died of a ruptured uterus.

The Board of Nurse Examiners stated that "the nurse's actions in failing to telephone the physician and failure to initiate appropriate nursing intervention to stabilize the patient's condition before referring her constituted unprofessional conduct." A Texas court affirmed the decision.

In this instance, the issue was not what the nurse did but what she failed to do. Nurses may be legally liable if they (1) perform an act that they are not authorized to perform, (2) perform an act improperly, or (3) fail to act when action is indicated and would be performed by a reasonable and prudent nurse.

Specific Legal Issues

It is not possible to discuss every legal issue that may be pertinent to perinatal nursing in this text; readers should refer to texts concerning nursing and the law (e.g., Creighton, 1981[7]). However, three issues that occur almost daily in varied practice settings have particular implications for perinatal nursing.

Informed Consent. *Informed consent* requires that clients are given information about risks, benefits, alternatives, and consequences of treatment. When the procedure is a medical one (such as surgery), the ultimate responsibility for obtaining informed consent is the physician's, but nurses who are caring for the client must confirm that consent has been obtained.

When the client is a pregnant woman, the effects of the proposed treatment on the fetus as well as the mother must be described. Often the effects on the fetus are unknown; this information must be shared. Issues of informed consent are a major topic in the Pregnant Patient's Bill of Rights (Appendix J), which, although it is not a legal document, is a useful guide to areas of client concern. Many clients do not realize that they have the right to refuse certain medications and treatments. Women in prenatal classes frequently fear they will be given medication during labor they don't desire. In other than true emergencies (when consent is implied) they need to know that any questions they have about a treatment for themselves of for their infant must be answered to their satisfaction before legal consent is given. When therapy is refused, clients are usually asked to sign a statement to that effect.

When the perinatal client is not legally an adult, can she give consent or must her parent or guardian sign for her? The answer to this question is generally determined by state law; nurses must know the law of their own state and the policy of the agency in which they work. In some states, if the minor is pregnant she is considered an "emancipated minor" and may consent to treatment as an adult. Recent federal rulings require that parents be informed of certain kinds of care received by minors.

Standing Medical Orders. Standing medical orders are frequently utilized in the care of healthy mothers and infants because some basic components of care are similar. For example, there may be a standing order for the administration of vitamin K to newborn infants or for certain laboratory tests for pregnant women. The nurse indicates in the nursing record when the action has been completed. Some standing orders are based on a specific contingency; for instance, if serum bilirubin exceeds 10 mg. per 100 ml., the infant is placed under phototherapy lights and the physician is notified.

Standing orders require the same obligation from nurses as any other medical order, i.e., they must use judgment and discuss with the physician factors in the client's health status that may require modification of the order.

Confidentiality. Information about clients is privileged; in general, it cannot be shared without the consent of the client. At times both legal and ethical issues impinge on confidentiality. If a minor is treated for venereal disease or seeks contraception or abortion, should parents be informed? If an individual is the carrier of a deleterious genetic trait and does not wish other family members who may be affected to be informed, what is the health-care providers' responsibility?

Laws Applicable to Childbearing Families

Nurses who care for childbearing families constantly interact with institutional, municipal, state, and federal policies and laws. Because these laws and policies vary widely, nurses must identify those laws and policies applicable to their practice. The list below suggests general issues; many are of ethical as well as legal concern.

1. Contraception, particularly in relation to minors.
2. Sterilization for all persons and for persons who are mentally retarded.
3. Treatment for venereal disease.
4. Artificial insemination and in vitro fertilization.
5. Abortion.
6. Adoption.

7. Laws affecting newborn care, including prevention of ophthalmia neonatorum and screening for specific conditions (PKU, hypothyroidism).

8. Legal requirements of birth certificates, particularly in relation to the infant's father when he is not married.

9. Orders not to resuscitate, and the removal of infants (and occasionally mothers) from life support systems.

10. Research involving fetus, newborn, and gravida.

11. Laws governing nurse-midwives, nurse practitioners, and nurses who provide neonatal and maternal transport, thus performing what may be construed as a "medical act."

12. Relationship of state nurse practice act, agency policy, and new technology.

Statute of Limitations

The "statute of limitations" is a term that refers to the number of years after an injury during which the injured party may seek legal compensation. However, when the injury occurs to a minor the period of time does not begin until the individual is no longer a minor. Thus more than two decades may elapse between the time an infant sustains an injury and the time that person may seek legal redress for injury.

Two implications for perinatal nurses are particularly important. First, all care must be carefully documented in the nursing record. For example, if an infant requires resuscitation, the resuscitation procedure, the persons involved, and the drugs given (including dosage, route, and time) must be accurately recorded. This is frequently not easy if adequate personnel are not available to assist with resuscitation, but it must be done. Should the infant suffer brain damage secondary to anoxia, it may be necessary to show in court 25 years later that the proper course of action was followed.

A second implication relates to the type of professional liability insurance needed by a perinatal nurse. The policy should cover any incident occurring during the time the policy is in effect, no matter when legal action is brought. Such a policy is called an occurrence policy. With an occurrence policy in effect in 1983 a nurse would be protected in the year 2002 should suit be brought, even if she had retired and no longer carried insurance, or even if she had died and her estate or heirs were being sued.

To summarize, the factors affecting the legal and ethical issues surrounding childbearing include the presence of two clients, the patient–client who is unable to provide consent, the explosion of knowledge and technology relevant to the fetus and newborn, and the prolonged statute of limitations in effect for minors.

Ethical and Legal Dilemmas: Some Examples

Many of the examples that follow were collected during a study by the author that is still in progress. Respondents were asked to describe situations that were stressful. For many persons, ethical and legal dilemmas were described as a source of stress. Other examples are derived from personal communications and published reports. These examples are offered for consideration and discussion.

No solutions are provided. Instead, the reader is encouraged to apply the legal and ethical principles described in this chapter.

Ethical and Legal Dilemmas in Nurse–Client Relationships

A major source of ethical dilemmas in nurse–client relationships has been noted already—there are frequently two clients. When a mother elects to have a legal abortion, but the fetus survives even briefly, for whom is the nurse the advocate? When the nurse questions the ability of parents to care for their infant, for whom is she the advocate? If the infant were separated from the parents, would the infant's life be improved?

When the client is a young adolescent, the ethical concern of involving her parents in decision-making may be a legal concern as well, because laws that permit the treatment of minors in certain circumstances without parental consent change. A conflict between legal obligations and a perceived ethical obligation to a client may prove to be a substantial dilemma for many perinatal nurses in the 1980's.

A nurse from the postpartum-gyn floor ran into the nursery stating, "We have a live saline" (a live infant following a saline abortion). I went out to the floor. The infant was gasping, heartbeat present, color pale pink. The other nurse said, "What should we do?" I stated, "We have to save the baby." The infant was given cardiac massage and placed on a ventilator. The infant subsequently died of DIC (disseminated intravascular coagulation).

A premature baby girl (3 pounds, 6 ounces) was born to a teen-aged mother who was married but lived with a boyfriend; the baby's father was in the service. The baby stayed in our nursery until she weighed 4 pounds, 12 ounces. The baby returned in three weeks with pneumonia; abuse and neglect were suspected.

An alcoholic mother is drunk when she comes to feed her premature infant.

A patient I had worked with for months was totally inadequate as a mother. She let the baby fall to the floor and became very upset over her ineptness but would not give the baby up for adoption.

An infant with multiple anomalies was sent to the medical center for evaluation of problems. After two weeks the baby was sent back to us with the understanding that another evaluation would be done in a year. The parents decided to take the baby home despite the known risks. Nursing staff felt helpless because it seemed a potentially dangerous situation. Nursing concerns were relayed to the attending physician, and referral was made to a public health nurse. Two weeks after discharge the baby suffered a cardiac arrest at home and died.

Ethical and Legal Dilemmas in Nurse–Physician Relationships

For nurses, the nurse–client relationship is primary; advocacy for the client's rights and well-being is the focus of professional nursing practice. Nurses are, however, generally expected to support and cooperate with the physician's plan of care. When this is difficult, nurses face a potential dilemma of undermining the client's confidence in the health-care system. They also may place themselves at risk of losing their jobs and, in some instances, their licenses if they pursue their advocacy too vigorously. In these situations, nurses may feel that both they and their clients are powerless.

A physician in town gives notoriously bad prenatal and intrapartal care. It is most frustrating to provide good prenatal care in the health department and then have the client or baby have complications because of gross mismanagement. This physician apparently has a huge file of incident reports at the hospital, but the administration is unwilling to do anything. The county health director is unwilling to make waves because of the power the physician has in the community. I have considered approaching the media about the problem but am unable to provide enough proof or take the risk of being "black-balled."

Nurses in the health department clinic in a rural county noticed irregular fetal heart tones and a decreased fetal heart rate in a mother at 42 weeks' gestation. The physician was notified but would neither see the woman nor refer her to the tertiary center in the adjacent county.

The nurses contacted the nursing consultant from the referral center who was also unable to effect referral. Subsequently, the fetus died in utero. Nurses in the local health department fear they may lose their jobs if they pursue the issue; the nurse–consultant was also told to let the issue drop.

A newborn with symptoms of sepsis was being cared for by a group of four physicians who had not discussed management of such babies and had not arrived at a consensus. Medicines were changed three times. Parents were told several different things. Nurses were caught in the middle.

Physicians in our hospital are resistant to implementation of an informed consent procedure prior to circumcision.

The physician was called when a sick infant arrived from the delivery room. He replied, "I'm not coming in for a dead baby." This was the second time this happened in a month.

I was involved in a delivery of a full-term child who had a tumor protruding from its abdomen at birth as big as an adult's head. The obstetrician delivered the child, who cried weakly at birth. He said that this child would never survive because all of its abdominal organs were probably in that sac or tumor and he would die. So he threw the baby up on the instrument table to die. The mother was asleep during the delivery and thus was not consulted. I was very upset at his decision. Because it was standard procedure to call the pediatrician immediately after the delivery despite the fact that the obstetrician said not to, I called the children's clinic, and a pediatrician said she would be right up. She examined the child, got very upset with the obstetrician, and called in a surgeon. They did immediate surgery on the child and found that the tumor or sac was just benign tissue. The tissue was removed, and the child lived. Two months later I saw the child in the children's clinic for a routine visit, and he was a very healthy and normal baby.[6]

A young expectant mother came into the hospital in premature labor. Her labor had progressed to the point where the physician could not delay an early delivery. She delivered a baby that weighed approximately 2 pounds. The baby was perfectly formed and began breathing on his own but with some difficulty. The physician would not allow us (the nurses) to render any life-saving measures and instructed us not to take the baby to the nursery. He felt that it would not live and if it did survive because life-saving measures were taken, it would probably be mentally retarded.

Although the baby was still alive when the delivery procedure was complete, the physician still refused to allow us to take the baby to the nursery. Since the mother had been given a general anesthetic during the delivery, she was not fully alert when brought to her room, and the physician left without telling her the condition of her baby or the decision that he had made.

When the physician left, we made the decision to disobey the physician's orders and take the baby to the nursery. The baby did survive and was normal in every respect.[6]

In some instances, nurses may find allies in the community through advocacy groups that are concerned about standards of care and increase community awareness of good (and bad) maternal and infant care. This is not an instant solution, but one needs only to consider the changes that advocacy groups have been able to bring about in the past decade to realize that joint action and public education can be effective.

Ethical and Legal Issues Related to Maternal Rights

Although the Pregnant Patient's Bill of Rights (Appendix J) is not a legal document, it is a code that suggests standards of ethical conduct in relation to perinatal care. Many of the statements in this code are far less controversial today than they were when the code was first proposed. Along with other codes and the utilization of ethical decision-making processes, the Pregnant Patient's Bill of Rights can help nurses evaluate specific practices within their agency and their community.

Ethical and Legal Dilemma: The Critically Ill Newborn

Few ethical dilemmas are more difficult for perinatal nurses than those involving decisions about the care of a critically ill newborn. Whether a decision is made to withhold care, perhaps even feedings, from an infant who appears to be severely impaired or, conversely, to be very aggressive in the care of a very tiny infant, perhaps even against the wishes of the parents, there are no easy answers. As the potential for both saving lives and reducing the sequelae of prematurity increases, even for infants with birthweights of less than 1000 grams, decisions become increasingly difficult for both parents and professionals.

A number of arguments have been suggested as a basis for decision-making. Treatment has been both withheld and prolonged in deference to parental wishes, placing the burden of decision-making on the parent rather than on the professional. This decision may occasionally be related to fear of a lawsuit if the parents' wishes are violated, but more often it arises from a philosophy of allowing parents to participate in decisions about their infant.

Fost[12] reviews three models of parent–child relationships—the long-standing but no longer acceptable view that the parent "owns" the child, a view that allowed infanticide until the nineteenth century; the view of the parent as a "trustee" with broad but not unlimited authority; and the concept of "equal rights" of the parent and the child. From the equal rights perspective, an infant would not be allowed to die simply because his existence would be a burden to his family. McCormick[25] suggests the criterion of "the potential for human relationships" as a standard for decisions; although this standard may be helpful in extreme instances, such as the withholding of care for an anencephalic newborn, it is frequently difficult to judge the newborn's potential for future interaction.

Decisions about very sick newborn infants are likely to be affected in the future by two additional variables: the cost of such care and possible judicial decisions. In the debate over the rapidly rising costs of health care, a question that is being raised with increasing frequency is the cost of neonatal intensive care. Many question whether there will be enough health care dollars, either from tax sources or from private insurance, to care for small premature infants. A very rough estimate of cost in an intensive care nursery is $8000 per infant. However, the cost for infants weighing less than 1000 grams (2.2 pounds) has been estimated at greater than $80,000 per infant. Moreover, some of these infants will require expensive health care for many years.

Few nurses want health care decisions to be based on costs. Yet resources are finite, and needs at times appear infinite. In seeking an answer to this dilemma, nurses can provide active support to programs designed to prevent prematurity. Herron, Katz and Creasy[16] report a decrease in premature births from 6.75 per cent to 2.43 per cent in one year. If prematurity rates can be reduced by one half, the dollar savings can be significant. In the 19 counties comprising the Northwest Perinatal Region in North Carolina, 7.5 per cent of the approximately 21,000 births are premature (a figure that has not changed in the last 5 years); this represents 1575 premature infants, or an average care cost of $12,600,000. If prematurity could be reduced from 7.5 per cent to 3.75 per cent, over 6 million dollars per year could be saved, and the ethical dilemma of scarce resources would be considerably diminished. In addition, some births that might still be premature (i.e., births of less than 37 weeks' gestation) might be prolonged sufficiently to allow the birth of an infant at 34 or 35 weeks' gestation rather than at 26 to 28 weeks, thus decreasing the average cost of care per infant. There seems little doubt that if nurses are not active in developing programs to prevent prematurity (see Nursing Care Plan 19–4), appropriate care may not be available for all infants.

Judicial decisions concerning fetal rights have already been discussed. In one legal case an initial court decision in 1979 that upheld parental autonomy when the parents decided against open heart surgery for a child with Down's syndrome was subsequently followed by a decision in 1981 that faulted the parents for treating the child as "permanently defective and without expectations." The child had been placed in an institution as a newborn infant in 1966 because of Down's syndrome, and little parental contact was maintained. In 1981 another family who had become interested in the child, named Phillip Becker, was awarded custody in terms of a limited guardianship because their expectation for the child gave him a chance to secure a "life worth living." (See Cushing[9] for further discussion.) It seems reasonable to expect, on the basis of decisions about fetal rights and child rights, that the judicial process may become more important as a factor in perinatal care in the coming decades.

Ethical and Legal Issues Related to Sterilization

For the woman who is not a minor and is mentally "competent," the ethical and legal responsibility prior to a voluntary sterilization includes a thorough explanation of sterilization—the risks, including psychological risks, and the benefits. The laws of many states require a waiting period between the time of initial consideration of sterilization and the procedure itself to allow each client to avoid making a decision at the time of stress. It is essential that the client understand that the procedure is irreversible.

Both ethically and legally, sterilization in a person who is judged incompetent to make a decision for himself is a more difficult problem. In general, parents are not allowed to make decisions for a mentally incompetent child; that decision is left to the court. State laws vary in regard to sterilization of persons who are mentally retarded. Nurses must be informed about the relevant laws in their own state.

Ethical and Legal Issues Related to Abortion

The ethical and legal issues related to abortion are discussed in Chapter 30.

Ethical and Legal Dilemmas in Perinatal Nursing Research

Nurses may be involved in both perinatal and neonatal nursing research and in medical research with perinatal clients. Nurses also care for clients on research protocols when they are not involved in the research itself. There are number of codes relating to human experimentation and research. They include the Nuremberg Code, developed in reaction to human experimentation by Nazi Germany in World War II; statements concerning the Protection of Human Subjects and Research on the Fetus from the U.S. Department of Health, Education and Welfare; and Ethical Principles in the Conduct of Research with Human Participants promulgated by the American Psychological Association.

The Code for Nurses of the American Nurses' Association states that "The nurse participates in research activities when assured that the rights of individual subjects are protected." Protection of the rights of subjects involves

1. Assurance that the subjects have agreed willingly to participate, understand the nature of the investigation, including costs and benefits, and understand what use will be made of the data.

2. Respect for confidentiality.

3. Permission to withdraw from the study at any time.

Research involving the fetus must also

1. Be preceded by animal studies and studies in which nonpregnant humans participated.

2. Seek knowledge that is important and that is unobtainable by reasonable alternatives.

3. Be undertaken only after description of the risks and benefits to both mother and fetus.[26]

In all research, subjects should be selected so that the risks and benefits will not fall inequitably on persons in particular economic, racial, ethnic, or social classes.

Perinatal Nursing: Specialized Roles

Perinatal nursing provides a number of opportunities for specialized practice. Several of these expanded roles are described below

The Certified Nurse-Midwife

Midwife is derived from the Middle English *mid-wif,* meaning "with woman." Even in the 1980's the word midwife brings to some persons an image of a toothless granny delivering a baby in a dark cabin. The certified nurse-midwife resembles that image about as closely as the present-day graduate of an American medical school resembles the barber-surgeon of the fourteenth century.

The earliest birth attendants in the United States were undoubtedly midwives who arrived with the colonists. Between 1750 and 1860, upper-income women in Boston and Philadelphia began increasingly to choose male birth attendants, is spite of claims that male attendants engaged in harmful, meddlesome practices.[11] Anesthesia became more widely used during childbirth following the use of chloroform in 1853 by James Simpson, who attended Queen Victoria's labor. The importance of asepsis was also more widely recognized by the end of the nineteenth century. These two factors, combined with the attitude that women were unsuited to medical practice as well as the competition presented to physicians by midwives, crystallized the attitudes of the medical profession toward midwives. Most physicians believed that midwives were uneducable and should be eliminated by law. Others accepted midwives as a necessary evil to care for poor clients.

The midwives of the eighteenth, nineteenth, and early twentieth centuries were lay midwives, often called granny midwives. A further discussion of lay midwives is found in the next section (see page 1054). Nurse-midwives first practiced in the United States in 1925 in the Frontier Nursing Service (FNS), which was organized in Kentucky by Mary Breckenridge, a nurse who continued as the active director of the FNS until her death in 1965. Because there was no school of midwifery in the United States, British nurse-midwives or American nurses educated in England or Scotland served as midwives in rural Kentucky.

When the Second World War began in Europe in 1939, this transatlantic exchange was no longer possible, and the Frontier Graduate School of Midwifery was started that year.

It was not, however, the first school for nurse-midwives in the United States. That distinction belongs to the Maternity Center Association in New York City, where the first program was established between 1931 and 1933.

A third school opened at Tuskegee Institute in Alabama in 1941, but because neither professionals nor the community was ready for nurse-midwives, it closed in 1946. During those few years, however, fetal mortality in that area of Alabama dropped from 45.9 per 1000 live births to 14.0 per 1000 live births.

Catholic University was the first university to grant a degree in midwifery, and in 1955, the American College of Nurse-Midwives was founded.

In many areas of the world, care for pregnant mothers and infants who have no complications is conducted almost totally by nurse-midwives. Several of these countries, such as the Netherlands and Norway, have rates of infant mortality below the rates of the United States. Although there are other variables, it appears obvious that nurse-midwives can be a valuable part of the team caring for childbearing families.

Studies in the United States have also proved the value of the nurse-midwife. Levy and his associates compared rates of prematurity and neonatal mortality and prenatal care in a rural California county before, during, and after a 3-year demonstration program in rural California. During the program, prenatal care increased, and prematurity and neonatal mortality decreased. After the demonstration project ended, prenatal care decreased while prematurity rose from 6.6 to 9.8 per cent and neonatal mortality rose from 10.3 to 32.1 per 1000 live births. After searching for any other factors that may have influenced these changes, it was concluded that nurse-midwives were the major factor in the change.

In Mississippi the infant death rate in 1965 was 41.5 per 1000 live births (compared with a national rate of 24.7), and maternal mortality was double the national rate. In less than 3 years (1968 to 1971) in one large county in Mississippi the Midwifery Program of the University of Mississippi Medical Center was able to reduce infant mortality to 21.3 per 1000 live births.

Preparation of the Nurse-Midwife. There are two routes by which nurse-midwives are prepared. One type of program, which leads to certification as a nurse-midwife upon satisfactory completion of the course and a national certification examination, is open to any registered nurse; such a program lasts from 8 months to a year. Other programs, which lead to a master's degree, require the registered nurses who enter to have a bachelor of science degree; these programs last from 1 to 2 years.

A current list of programs is available from The American College of Nurse Midwives, 1000 Vermont Ave., N.W., Washington, D.C. 20005. The American College also publishes *Statements of Standards, Functions, and Qualifications for the Practice of Nurse Midwifery;* a journal, *Journal of Nurse Midwifery;* and other information about nurse-midwifery.

Curricula include both theory and practice in prenatal, intrapartum, and postpartum care and in family planning. A master's program may also include courses in statistics, research, group dynamics, teaching, administration, and curriculum development. Nurse-midwives prepared at the master's level may themselves become teachers of nurse-midwifery.

Practice of the Nurse-Midwife. The nurse-midwife assumes responsibility for low risk maternity patients during the antepartum, intrapartum, postpartum, and often interpartum periods. She delivers the infant and evaluates him, as well as his mother, during their stay in the hospital. Teaching, counseling, and provision for family planning are a part of her care, as is the return postpartum examination.

Nurse-midwives have a relationship with a physician, to whom problems beyond the scope of midwifery are referred. For example, a woman who develops gestational diabetes would be referred during the prenatal period. When labor is not progressing satisfactorily, physician consultation is sought. The legal relationship between the nurse-midwife and the physician varies in state laws. In some states approval of a nurse-midwife to practice is contingent upon her association with a particular physician or group of physicians. In other states, the approval to practice is not related to association with a particular physician. The nurse-midwife establishes referral patterns just as any professional health-care provider does.

Legislation allowing direct reimbursement of nurse-midwives by third-party providers (government and private health-care insurers) was a part of the Omnibus Reconciliation Act of 1981. The nurse-midwife need not be practicing in association or consultation with a physician unless state law requires physician supervision. Because nurse-midwife services cost less than physician services, this regulation is expected to save 2.2 million dollars in health care costs in fiscal 1983 and 2.8 million dollars in fiscal 1985.[25a]

In 1982, the National Association of Blue Cross–Blue Shield agreed to reimburse federal employees with high option policies throughout the United States for 100 per cent of the cost of home birth and 80 per cent of the cost of hospital birth attended by a certified nurse-midwife. The regulation for this coverage states, "Benefits are provided for the services of a nurse-midwife for pre- and postpartum care and delivery." Nurse-midwives are new providers for the Federal Employment Program for 1982.

The higher reimbursement for home deliveries reflects a policy of Blue Cross–Blue Shield to encourage outpatient surgery when feasible. To Blue Cross–Blue Shield birth is a surgical procedure, a perspective with which many nurses would disagree.

Changes such as these, along with actions in state legislatures (e.g., the Goldwater bill passed in the Maryland legislature [page 1042]) testify to a new awareness of the value of nurse-midwives and at the same time allow many clients a choice of birthing attendant without penalizing that choice economically by withholding reimbursement.

Lay Midwives

Lay midwives are men or women (primarily women) who assist women in giving birth. There are lay midwives in every society. Some lay midwives have been practicing for many years; the term "granny midwives" is sometimes used to describe them. Dougherty[11] describes the typical granny midwife as rural, middle-aged or older, black, committed to women, and possessing limited formal education. Well into the twentieth century there were large numbers of lay midwives who delivered hundreds of thousands of infants, particularly in the South, where many hospitals would not admit black women for delivery. For example, in 1930 there were 4000 lay midwives in North Carolina alone. However, no new permits for midwives have been issued in North Carolina since 1964, and the number of midwives "permitted" under the old system had dropped to 10 by 1980. A similar decrease has been evident throughout the South.

Today, an increasing number of younger, often better educated, women are becoming lay midwives throughout the United States. A number of states have developed legislation that permits lay midwifery when established criteria are met. Lay midwives attend home births. Since both home births and lay midwifery are opposed by many physicians, legislative battles are frequently heated.

In 1981, an initial meeting of nurse-midwives and non-nurse midwives led to the formation in 1982 of the Midwives Alliance of North America, an umbrella organization to facilitate cooperation between midwives and to promote midwifery as a means of improving health care for women and their families.[11a]

The Clinical Nurse Specialist

The clinical nurse specialist has a master's degree in nursing; if she cares for childbearing families, her master's degree will be in maternal and child health nursing. The role of the clinical specialist will vary from one practice setting to another, but she usually is involved in patient care, in staff development, and in research. The clinical specialist is likely to have a flexible schedule to meet the needs of patients and staff.

Some activities of the clinical specialist include:

1. Developing nursing care plans.
2. Developing and evaluating literature for patients.
3. Conducting nursing research.
4. Initiating or revising patient classes.
5. Evaluating patient teaching.
6. Implementing staff development in formal and informal ways.
7. Serving as a role model for patient care.
8. Acting as a change agent to improve care.

Nurse-Practitioner Programs and Roles

Several types of nurse-practitioner programs prepare registered nurses to function in expanded roles. These programs commonly involve several months of intensive training followed by a preceptorship, i.e., a specified period of practice under the direct supervision of a preceptor, who is usually a physician.

Other nurse-practitioner programs are part of advanced degree nursing programs. States vary in mandating the laws that govern the practice of nurse-practitioners.

The Maternal-Child Nurse Practitioner. During pregnancy, a maternal-child nurse practitioner functions in much the same way as the nurse-midwife, with the exception of delivering the infant. However, the maternal-child nurse practitioner may continue to care for mother and child during the childbearing years (and care for the mother should she again become pregnant). Thus a continuity of care is provided that is lacking not only for women and children in public clinics but for many patients in the private sector as well, who must seek an obstetrician or obstetric clinic for maternity care and a pediatrician or pediatric clinic for child care.

Nurse practitioners may work in a rural health clinic, a public health agency, an outpatient clinic, or a private obstetric-pediatric clinic. They may follow the mother from the clinic into the hospital, where they offer support and teaching and counseling during labor, delivery, and the immediate postpartum period, and then follow her again into the community setting.

The Obstetric-Gynecologic Nurse Practitioner. The obstetric-gynecologic nurse practitioner functions in an expanded role in ambulatory settings, giving care to women in prepregnancy, pregnancy, and postpartum periods and giving gynecologic health maintenence care.

Curricula of practitioner programs include the development of clinical skills (e.g., pelvic and vaginal examinations); an understanding of the scientific and theoretical bases of maternity and gynecologic nursing care and principles of care; discussions of referrals, techniques of counseling and guidance; and evaluation of social and family systems.

A Pediatric Nurse Practitioner in a Hospital Setting. Most nurse-practitioner programs prepare nurses to function in ambulatory settings or in combinations of ambulatory and in-hospital settings, as they follow their patients from one environment to another.

Schuman describes another role, that of the pediatric nurse practitioner in a hospital setting, who has primary responsibility for physical examination and day-to-day follow-up of "well" infants and for communication with parents.[24] During her day the pediatric nurse practitioner may:

1. Discuss the importance of follow-up visits with a postpartum mother.
2. Perform newborn physical examinations.
3. Encourage the mother with a preterm or sick baby to see and touch her baby and, if the baby's condition permits, to hold and feed him.
4. Explain the reason for detention in the nursery for babies who will not be discharged with their mothers.
5. Serve as a liaison with other departments, such as the prenatal clinic or social services.
6. Teach parents and staff in formal and informal ways.
7. Write medical orders as determined by the nurse practitioner and the chief of the department, commonly for laboratory work, X-rays, discharge, and so forth.

Childbirth Educator

The term childbirth educator is used by many people—nurses, other health professionals, such as physical therapists, and lay persons—to describe themselves in a variety of roles that prepare parents for the experience of birth, and sometimes for parenting as well. Childbirth education has been described in Chapter 11.

For many nurses (nurses employed in prenatal clinics, for example) childbirth education is a part of regular practice. Other nurses contract with couples to teach psychoprophylactic preparation or the Bradley method. These nurses may undertake specialized training leading to certification. For example, the American Society for Psychoprophylaxis in Obstetrics (ASPO) has a national certification program. Candidates attend seminars, observe certified teachers, have a period of student teaching, prepare a bibliography and syllabus, and take a national examination. Postpartum reports written by mothers taught by the candidate (who is usually an R.N. or a physical therapist) are also submitted as part of the accreditation process. ASPO also conducts continuing education programs for members.

The American Academy of Husband-Coached Childbirth certifies persons in the Bradley method of childbirth. The International Childbirth Education Association (ICEA) is developing a national certification program for childbirth educators. ICEA has provided certification in some regions of the country for a number of years. (Addresses for these organizations are found in Appendix I.)

Nurse Clinician

The term nurse clinician is frequently used to describe a nurse with expertise in nursing practice. However, the term is not used uniformly in all practice settings. In some institutions, nurse clinician is the title given to a position several steps along a career ladder, while other facilities use designations such as Clinician I, II, III, and IV to indicate various steps in a career ladder.[18] Still other facilities do not use the term at all. In some institutions that designate nurse clinicians, certification in a specialty area is one criterion that may be used as a partial requirement (see Certification, below).

Standards for Nurses in Expanded Roles

With the exception of the certified nurse-midwife, for whom there are standards and a national examination for certification, there are no national standards for nurses practicing in an expanded role. Nurses with similar titles and similar functions may have varying degrees of preparation and responsibility.

We believe that one of nursing's tasks in the coming decade will be to establish some standards for nurses in new roles. Such standards will not only serve the public interest but will enable nurses to evaluate programs before they commit time and money to enrollment.

Certification

Within the nursing profession certification in a specialty has had varied meanings. Some certification provides entry into specialty practice; an example of this type of certification process is the examination taken by graduates of nurse-midwifery programs to become certi-

fied nurse-midwives. Other programs certify for expertise considered to be important to nursing practice in an area of specialization. The certification process may have specific requirements relating to clinical practice, continuing education, or educational preparation required for certification examination. Certified nurses are identified by a variety of designations; examples are RNC (registered nurse, certified), CNM (certified nurse-midwife), CPNP (certified pediatric nurse practitioner).

Eleven nursing organizations offer certification. Perinatal nurses are primarily certified by the Maternal and Child Health Division of the American Nurses' Association (Maternal and Child Health Nurse and High Risk Perinatal Nurse) and by the NAACOG Certification Corporation (Inpatient Obstetric Nurse, Ob/Gyn Nurse Practitioner, Neonatal Nurse Clinician Practitioner, and Neonatal Intensive Care Nurse). Nurse-midwives are certified by the American College of Nurse-Midwives. The certification of childbirth educators has been discussed previously (a certified childbirth educator need not be a nurse).

In general, the certification process consists of application, submission of the required credentials, and a written examination. Costs in 1982 varied from 75 dollars for ANA members taking ANA examinations (125 dollars for nonmembers) to 250 dollars for NAACOG examinations.

Maintenance or recertification programs ensure that nurses, once certified, will continue to increase their knowledge in their specialty. Re-examination or documentation of prescribed amounts of continuing education within a specified period of time are the usual procedures for maintaining recertification.

For specific information about certification programs, write to the specific nursing organization involved (Appendix I).

Mortality

Mortality rates are frequently used as one index of perinatal health care. The marked decline in maternal mortality in the past several decades has been a major achievement in the health care of women. The recognition in the 1960's that infant mortality in the United States was significantly higher than in many other developed nations resulted in increased emphasis on neonatal care including research, the allocation of resources, continuing education for health-care providers, and changes in patterns of health-care delivery, including regionalization of perinatal care.

Table 31–1. MATERNAL MORTALITY, UNITED STATES: 1970, 1974, 1978

	1970	1974	1978
National Center for Health Statistics: deaths per 100,000 births	21.5	12.8	9.9
Professional Activities Study, Commission on Professional and Hospital Activities: deaths per 100,000 births*	25.7	19.6	14.3
Professional Activities Study: Maternal deaths*	273	246	172
Maternal mortality, vaginal deliveries: deaths per 100,000 births*	20.4	15.2	9.8
Maternal mortality, cesarean deliveries: deaths per 100,000 births*	113.8	62.9	40.9

*Petitte et al.: Obstetrics and Gynecology 59:6, 1982.

Maternal Mortality

Maternal mortality is reported as maternal deaths per 100,000 births. There is concern that maternal deaths are under-reported;[29] note the difference in data from two sources in Table 31–1.

This same concern is voiced in relation to vital statistics for infants and other statistical data. Kleinman[22] noted, as did Shapiro,[35] that in spite of inadequacies, mortality statistics remain "a unique source of readily available health status indicators which provide information for clinical, epidemiologic, and health policy purposes."

Two conclusions can be drawn from Table 31–1. First, maternal mortality continued to decrease during the 1970's, both for vaginal births and for cesarean births. Improvements in anesthesia, antibiotics, and the availability of blood in labor/delivery rooms are considered major reasons.[31]

Second, the mortality rate is much higher in cesarean delivery. With a marked increase in cesarean rates (Chapter 19), the potential for maternal mortality is also increased. Maternal mortality associated with *repeat* cesarean delivery is 18 per 100,000 deliveries, low in comparison with all cesarean births but higher than that for vaginal delivery. Nurses can help in educating the public about the safety of vaginal birth after cesarean delivery when the

uterine incision from the previous delivery is in the lower uterine segment. Shy,[36] in a review of all of the English language literature, found no instance of maternal mortality directly attributable to rupture of a low segment scar.

Vaginal delivery after cesarean birth is not possible in all hospitals. Prerequisites include the capability if performing an immediate cesarean delivery should this be necessary, availability of anesthesia, 24-hour blood bank services, and maternal and fetal intensive care services. Parents have the right to be informed if a hospital cannot offer this option and where such care is available.

When a mother dies during the intrapartum period, nurses and physicians must carefully review the circumstances to identify any possible changes in practice that may be indicated.

Mortality: Fetus and Newborn Infant

Several terms describe the death of a fetus or newborn infant. *Fetal death* is a death prior to delivery of a product of human conception. In computing fetal death rates, fetal deaths resulting from pregnancies of greater than 20 weeks' gestation that are not the result of therapeutic abortion are counted. The *fetal death rate* (fetal mortality rate) is the

$$\frac{\text{number of fetal deaths}}{\substack{\text{number of live births} \\ \text{plus number of fetal deaths}}} \times 1000$$

Neonatal death is the death of an infant born alive (i.e., shows any evidence of life even briefly, such as breathing, a heartbeat, voluntary muscle movement, or pulsation of the umbilical cord) who dies under 28 days of age. Neonatal death rate is the

$$\frac{\text{number of neonatal deaths}}{\text{number of live births}} \times 1000$$

Perinatal death rates are the sum of fetal and neonatal death rates. Perinatal death rates are not always reported in vital statistics data but can be easily calculated if fetal and neonatal mortality figures are available. The perinatal death rate is considered a sensitive indicator of perinatal care because it reflects both fetal and neonatal deaths. It is theoretically possible, for example, for one population to have a lower neonatal mortality rate than another but to have higher perinatal mortality because of a high incidence of intrauterine fetal death. In general, neonatal death rates are slightly higher than fetal death rates. In

Table 31–2. INFANT, MATERNAL, AND NEONATAL MORTALITY RATES, AND FETAL MORTALITY RATIOS, BY RACE: 1940 TO 1978

[**Deaths per 1000 live births, except as noted.** Prior to 1960, excludes Alaska and Hawaii. Beginning 1970, excludes deaths of nonresidents of U.S.]

Item	1940	1950	1960	1965	1970	1972[a]	1973	1974	1975	1976	1977	1978
Infant deaths[b]....	47.0	29.2	26.0	24.7	20.0	18.5	17.7	16.7	16.1	15.2	14.1	13.8
White	43.2	26.8	22.9	21.5	17.8	16.4	15.8	14.8	14.2	13.3	12.3	12.0
Black and other	73.8	44.5	43.2	40.3	30.9	27.7	26.2	24.9	24.2	23.5	21.7	21.1
Black........	72.9	43.9	44.3	41.7	32.6	29.6	28.1	26.8	26.2	25.5	23.6	23.1
Maternal deaths[c]	376.0	83.3	37.1	31.6	21.5	18.8	15.2	14.6	12.8	12.3	11.2	9.6
White	319.8	61.1	26.0	21.0	14.4	14.3	10.7	10.0	9.1	9.0	7.7	6.4
Black and other	773.5	221.6	97.9	83.7	55.9	38.5	34.6	35.1	29.0	26.5	26.0	23.0
Black........	781.7	223.0	103.6	88.3	59.8	40.7	38.4	38.3	31.3	29.5	29.2	25.0
Fetal deaths[d]	(NA)	19.2	16.1	16.2	14.2	12.7	12.2	11.5	10.7	10.5	9.9	9.7
White	(NA)	17.1	14.1	13.9	12.4	11.2	10.8	10.2	9.5	9.3	8.7	8.5
Black and other	(NA)	32.5	26.8	27.2	22.6	19.5	18.6	17.0	16.0	15.2	14.6	14.7
Neonatal deaths[e]	28.8	20.5	18.7	17.7	15.1	13.6	13.0	12.3	11.6	10.9	9.9	9.5
White	27.2	19.4	17.2	16.1	13.8	12.4	11.8	11.1	10.4	9.7	8.7	8.4
Black and other	39.7	27.5	26.9	25.4	21.4	19.2	17.9	17.2	16.8	16.3	14.7	14.0
Black........	39.9	27.8	27.8	26.5	22.8	20.7	19.3	18.7	18.3	17.9	16.1	15.5

Statistical Abstracts of the United States, 1981.
NA Not available.
[a]Based on a 50-percent sample of deaths.
[b]Represents deaths of infants under 1 year old, exclusive of fetal deaths.
[c]Per 100,000 live births from deliveries and complications of pregnancy, childbirth, and the puerperium. For 1970–1978, deaths are classified according to eighth revision of *International Classification of Diseases. Adapted for Use in the United States;* in prior years classified according to the revision of the International Classification of Diseases in use at the time.
[d]Beginning 1970, includes only those deaths with stated or presumed period of gestation of 20 weeks or more, for prior years, includes gestational age not stated.
[e]Represents deaths of infants under 28 days old, exclusive of fetal deaths.

recent years, as neonatal mortality has improved in the United States, this has not always been true. Note in Table 31–2 that both rates were identical in 1977 and that the fetal death rate both for all races and for whites and nonwhites analyzed separately was higher than the neonatal mortality rate.

Infant mortality refers to the death of a liveborn infant before the first birthday. Infant mortality rates are frequently used in comparing populations because they are more likely to be available than some other types of data. Because neonatal deaths are the largest component of infant mortality rates, these rates do tell a great deal about newborns although not quite as precisely as other indices. Infant death rate is computed as the

$$\frac{\text{number of infant deaths}}{\text{number of live births}} \times 1000$$

Mortality rates, properly interpreted, are helpful in recognizing the need for health care and in identifying populations with particular needs, and are frequently used to help allocate scarce resources to those populations. Information linking mortality rates to particular causes of death are also valuable in health care planning. For example, preterm births are the largest single cause of neonatal mor-

tality; therefore, if one wishes to lower neonatal mortality one might address both the causes of prematurity and the care of the preterm infant following delivery.

Many factors influence mortality rates—social, economic, demographic, and cultural as well as health care. In comparing two populations all of these factors must be considered.

Infant gestational age and birth weight are highly important. Perinatal nurses need to examine data that extend beyond general mortality to gestational age-specific and weight-specific data, particularly for their own community and state. Data may be available from the agency that compiles vital statistics for the state. Mortality statistics may be used to identify the causes of death among infants born in various types of hospitals (e.g., small community hospitals, regional centers), as Hein and Brown[15] did. Those authors found, for example, that birth asphyxia, a potentially preventable cause of death, accounted for 23.5 per cent of deaths in level I hospitals, 12.6 per cent in level II hospitals, and 3 per cent in level III hospitals, even though many of the mothers at the level III hospitals had health-care problems that placed them at risk. This type of analysis suggests areas in which continuing education for nurses and other health-care providers is indicated.

Table 31–3. INFANT MORTALITY RATES—STATES: 1960 TO 1978

[**Deaths per 1000 live births, by place of residence.** Represents deaths under 1 year old, exclusive of fetal deaths. Beginning 1970, excludes deaths of nonresidents of the United States.]

Division and State	White 1960	White 1970	White 1978	Black 1960	Black 1970	Black 1978	Division and State	White 1960	White 1970	White 1978	Black 1960	Black 1970	Black 1978
U.S.	**22.9**	**17.8**	**12.0**	**44.3**	**32.6**	**23.1**	**So. Atl.—Con.**						
N. Eng.	**21.7**	**16.8**	**10.7**	**37.2**	**33.9**	**22.6**	W. Va.	24.8	22.8	14.9	38.1	30.1	21.6
Maine	25.7	21.0	10.5	ª5.7	ª38.5	ª11.0	N.C.	22.3	19.3	13.0	53.3	36.7	24.9
N.H.	23.7	18.0	10.5	ª1.39	ª28.6	—	S.C.	23.9	18.2	13.3	48.6	31.3	26.5
Vt.	24.2	17.6	13.5	—	—	ª80.0	Ga.	24.6	17.2	11.8	48.3	33.2	22.1
Mass.	21.1	16.0	10.5	37.4	36.0	20.1	Fla.	23.6	17.8	11.8	46.2	33.7	20.8
R.I.	22.4	19.3	12.2	43.2	34.1	35.2							
Conn.	20.0	15.5	10.0	37.9	32.3	23.5	**E. So. Cent.**	**25.6**	**18.7**	**12.3**	**48.5**	**35.6**	**23.7**
							Ky.	26.0	18.8	12.0	49.0	28.6	19.9
Mid. Atl.	**22.0**	**17.3**	**11.8**	**42.3**	**32.7**	**22.2**	Tenn.	25.3	18.8	13.1	43.7	30.7	21.2
N.Y.	21.5	16.9	11.9	42.8	31.6	21.9	Ala.	24.9	18.6	12.1	45.1	36.4	23.7
N.J.	21.9	16.9	10.5	42.5	33.0	22.8	Miss.	26.6	18.7	11.5	54.3	39.6	25.4
Pa.	22.6	18.2	12.5	41.2	35.2	22.1							
							W. So. Cent.	**24.9**	**19.6**	**13.0**	**44.8**	**32.4**	**23.3**
E. No. Cent.	**22.1**	**17.8**	**12.0**	**39.8**	**32.0**	**24.2**	Ark.	22.5	18.3	14.3	38.9	31.3	22.6
Ohio	22.2	17.2	12.1	39.8	29.7	21.5	La.	22.6	19.8	12.7	46.9	32.3	24.6
Ind.	22.6	18.5	11.9	38.3	28.6	23.4	Okla.	22.7	20.3	13.4	48.2	34.5	21.5
Ill.	22.2	18.3	12.8	39.9	34.8	26.7	Tex.	26.3	19.6	12.9	44.3	32.5	22.6
Mich.	22.1	18.6	11.8	40.7	31.0	24.6							
Wis.	21.2	16.0	10.9	37.2	32.1	15.2	**Mt.**	**25.7**	**18.1**	**11.8**	**42.5**	**30.2**	**19.0**
							Mont.	24.2	21.2	10.4	ª39.5	ª20.6	—
W. No. Cent.	**21.7**	**17.3**	**12.0**	**42.5**	**33.3**	**27.3**	Idaho	22.7	17.3	11.8	ª19.2	—	ª37.0
Minn.	21.6	17.3	11.6	33.3	20.7	26.7	Wyo.	27.5	19.6	13.4	ª52.6	ª76.9	ª23.0
Iowa	21.7	18.3	12.3	36.8	35.9	22.5	Colo.	26.9	19.7	11.0	42.6	24.5	17.1
Mo.	21.4	17.0	12.2	45.6	34.5	29.2	N. Mex.	30.9	19.5	13.4	39.4	42.3	ª22.1
N. Dak.	24.1	14.3	13.4	ª43.5	—	ª11.9	Ariz.	26.6	16.0	12.4	45.8	25.0	18.7
S. Dak.	24.2	16.7	12.1	ª80.0	ª83.3	ª16.7	Utah	18.8	14.9	11.3	ª58.8	ª10.3	ª23.0
Nebr.	21.3	18.5	12.1	33.3	33.3	28.1	Nev.	29.6	22.2	11.9	34.1	45.2	19.3
Kans.	21.3	16.7	11.7	35.5	30.8	22.0	**Pac.**	**22.6**	**16.7**	**11.6**	**35.6**	**27.4**	**19.8**
							Wash.	22.7	18.1	12.3	33.4	33.8	21.2
So. Atl.	**23.6**	**18.0**	**12.3**	**47.6**	**33.1**	**23.3**	Oreg.	23.0	16.0	12.9	36.3	ª20.1	ª16.9
Del.	17.8	16.3	9.9	51.2	31.5	23.4	Calif.	22.5	16.5	11.2	35.7	27.1	19.9
Md.	22.3	16.4	11.7	45.1	30.0	22.5	Alaska	27.9	20.3	13.5	ª29.6	ª48.5	ª15.3
D.C.	29.4	26.3	13.4	39.8	30.0	30.2	Hawaii	21.5	17.8	10.2	ª35.7	ª17.5	ª12.2
Va.	24.6	17.0	11.5	45.8	34.1	21.7							

Statistical Abstracts of the United States, 1981.

—Represents zero.

ªBased on a frequency of less than 20 deaths.

It is also necessary in interpreting mortality rates to consider the size of the population being described. A population (the population of a county, for example) that is small may have a rate that is excessively high or low because when the population base is small a difference of one or two deaths can affect rates far more than it does when the population base is large. In Table 31–3, notice, for example, the wide differences in mortality in black in-fants in individual New England states where there is a relatively small number of births to black women. When populations are small, combining mortality rates for more than 1 year (5-year periods are often reported) or for several similar populations (the New England states as a region, for example) will give a clearer picture than the vital statistics of a single year.

In examining Tables 31–2, 31–3, and 31–4,

Table 31–4. PERINATAL MORTALITY RATES BY RACE: 1940–1978ª
(Deaths per 1000 live births)

	1950	1960	1965	1970	1975	1976	1977	1978
Race								
White	36.5	31.3	30.0	26.2	19.9	19.0	17.4	16.9
Black and other	60.0	53.7	52.6	44.0	32.8	31.5	29.3	28.7
Total perinatal mortality	39.7	34.9	33.9	29.3	22.3	21.4	19.8	19.2

ªCalculated from Table 31–2.

two conclusions are obvious. First, over the past four decades, all indices of fetal and newborn health have improved. The most marked improvement occurred between 1940 and 1950, with steady improvement from that time on.

Second, there is marked disparity in the survival of white and nonwhite infants. The perinatal death rate for nonwhites in 1978 was higher than the perinatal death rate for whites in 1970.

There are also differences in mortality rates from one area of the country to another. Comparing regional rates with the national rate in 1978, the New England, Middle Atlantic, and Mountain-Pacific regions have lower infant mortality rates than those of the nation as a whole.

An obvious difference in every state is the continued high black infant mortality, which is frequently close to double the white infant

Table 31–5. VITAL STATISTICS OF SELECTED COUNTRIES

	Estimated Population mid-1981	Birthrate per 1000 Population[a]	Infant Mortality[b]	Life Expectancy at Birth	Urban Population (%)	Density[c]
World.............	4,492,000,000	28	97	62	41	98
Afghanistan........	16,400,000	48	185	42	15	28
Albania............	2,800,000	29	—	69	37	226
Algeria	19,300,000	46	127	56	61	44
Angola.............	6,700,000	48	192	41	21	22
Argentina.........	28,200,000	25	41	69	82	16
Australia..........	14,800,000	16	12	73	86	3
Austria	7,500,000	11	15	72	54	202
Bangladesh........	92,800,000	46	139	47	11	954
Belgium............	9,900,000	13	12	73	95	682
Bolivia.............	5,500,000	44	168	51	33	18
Brazil..............	121,400,000	32	84	64	61	58
Burma	35,200,000	39	140	53	27	340
Cambodia	5,500,000	33	150	45	14	152
Cameroon	8,700,000	42	157	45	35	55
Canada	24,100,000	15	12	74	76	35
Cen. Afr. Republic ..	2,400,000	42	190	46	41	40
Chile	11,200,000	22	38	67	81	63
China..............	985,000,000	18	56	68	25	309
Colombia..........	27,800,000	29	77	62	60	120
Cuba..............	9,800,000	15	19	72	65	185
Cyprus............	600,000	21	16	73	53	121
Czechoslovakia	15,400,000	18	19	70	67	222
Denmark..........	5,100,000	12	9	74	84	175
Ecuador...........	8,200,000	42	70	60	43	159
Egypt..............	43,500,000	41	90	55	45	1,533
El Salvador	4,900,000	39	53	63	41	383
Ethiopia	33,500,000	50	178	39	13	43
Finland	4,800,000	13	8	72	62	185
France	53,900,000	14	10	73	78	169
Germany, East	16,700,000	14	13	72	77	267
Germany, West.....	61,300,000	10	15	72	92	465
Ghana	12,000,000	48	115	48	31	90
Greece	9,600,000	16	19	73	65	105
Guatemala	7,500,000	43	69	58	36	282
Haiti...............	6,000,000	42	130	51	25	425
Hungary	10,700,000	15	24	70	54	160
India..............	688,600,000	36	134	52	22	381
Indonesia	148,800,000	35	91	50	20	524
Iran	39,800,000	44	112	58	50	66
Iraq...............	13,600,000	47	92	55	72	145
Ireland............	3,400,000	20	15	73	58	60
Israel	3,900,000	25	16	74	89	321
Italy	57,200,000	12	15	73	69	326
Japan..............	117,800,000	14	8	76	76	2,145
Jordan	3,300,000	46	97	56	42	223
Kenya	16,500,000	53	83	53	14	273
Korea, North	18,300,000	33	70	62	60	808
Korea, South	38,900,000	23	37	66	48	1,719

mortality rate. The United States Department of Human Services has a goal of reaching an infant mortality rate of 9 per 1000 live births by the year 1990, with no county and no racial or ethnic group having an excess of 12 infant deaths per 1000 live births.

Table 31–5 lists infant mortality rates for a number of world nations. Eleven of these nations have infant mortality rates lower than those of the United States. In Sweden, the neonatal mortality in 1978 was 7, the lowest in the world and almost half the rate of 13.8 in the United States for the same year. Although some have ascribed low mortality to a relatively homogeneous population, Hein[14] noted that from 1973 to 1976 even lower mortality occurred among immigrants to Sweden in spite of the fact that those immigrants were in general less advantaged in regard to income, occupation, and living quarters. Hein believes

Table 31–5. VITAL STATISTICS OF SELECTED COUNTRIES (*Continued*)

	Estimated Population mid-1981	Birthrate per 1000 Population[a]	Infant Mortality[b]	Life Expectancy at Birth	Urban Population (%)	Density[c]
Laos	3,600,000	44	175	42	13	217
Lebanon	3,200,000	34	45	65	76	904
Liberia	1,900,000	50	148	48	33	315
Libya	3,100,000	47	130	55	52	33
Malaysia	14,300,000	31	44	61	29	220
Mexico	69,300,000	33	70	65	67	71
Morocco	21,800,000	43	133	55	40	107
Netherlands	14,200,000	12	8	75	88	694
New Zealand	3,100,000	17	14	73	85	22
Niger	5,700,000	51	200	42	13	46
Nigeria	79,700,000	50	157	48	20	178
Norway	4,100,000	13	9	75	44	455
Pakistan	88,900,000	44	142	52	28	356
Panama	1,900,000	28	47	70	51	109
Paraguay	3,300,000	34	58	64	40	20
Peru	18,100,000	39	92	56	67	59
Philippines	48,900,000	34	65	61	36	538
Poland	36,000,000	20	22	71	57	189
Portugal	10,000,000	15	39	70	30	244
Rumania	22,400,000	18	30	70	48	150
Saudi Arabia	10,400,000	49	118	48	67	12
South Africa	29,000,000	36	97	60	50	30
Spain	37,800,000	16	13	73	74	120
Sweden	8,300,000	12	7	75	83	223
Syria	9,300,000	42	81	62	50	66
Taiwan	18,200,000	25	25	72	77	—
Tanzania	19,200,000	46	125	50	12	38
Thailand	48,600,000	28	68	61	14	273
Tunisia	6,600,000	33	123	57	52	87
Turkey	46,200,000	32	125	61	47	83
Uganda	14,100,000	45	120	52	12	132
USSR	268,000,000	18	36	69	65	44
United Kingdom	55,900,000	13	13	73	76	304
United States	229,800,000	16	13	74	74	53
Uruguay	2,900,000	20	48	71	84	19
Venezuela	15,500,000	36	45	66	75	70
Vietnam	54,900,000	37	115	62	19	512
Yugoslavia	22,500,000	17	32	69	42	158
Zaire	30,100,000	46	171	46	30	97
Zambia	6,000,000	49	144	48	39	17
Zimbabwe	7,600,000	47	129	53	20	104

1981 World Population Data Sheet, Population Reference Bureau, Inc., Washington, D.C.
[a]1978–79 data.
[b]Deaths under age one per 1000 live births.
[c]Persons per km² of arable land.

that there is a direct relationship between the three following factors and this low mortality.

1. Provision of accurate information to all Swedish schoolchildren about reproductive biology, responsible parenthood, family planning, and the value of prenatal care.

2. Prenatal care for 99 per cent of the population, probably reflecting both this educational emphasis and the care that clients feel meet their needs.

3. Plentiful, accessible, prenatal care.

Most prenatal and intrapartum care in Sweden is provided by nurse-midwives, who not only assess prenatal health but provide prenatal education and are available for questions and counseling at times other than those regularly scheduled for visits. Women identified at risk are cared for by obstetrical specialists.

In the Netherlands, where infant mortality is also very low (8 per 1000 live births), midwives also provide most prenatal and intrapartum care. In contrast to Sweden, where the majority of births occur in hospital, over half of the births in the Netherlands are at home. Intervention is minimized in the Netherlands. Women, in general, neither expect nor receive medication for pain, nor are other types of intervention common. "There is in Dutch birth participants a deep-seated conviction that the woman's body knows best and that, given enough time, nature will take its course."[21] Many Americans find this philosophy difficult to accept; for the Dutch, however, the philosophy results in an infant mortality rate that has not been achieved by any state within the United States.

Regionalization of Perinatal Care

When the capacity for providing care for high risk infants that was both highly sophisticated and expensive developed in the late 1960's and early 1970's, it was recognized that not every hospital could provide care for every high risk infant. Subsequently, the concept of regionalization has come to include regionalized care for the high risk mother.

A region is a geographical area within which one or more hospitals would provide complex care to high risk mothers and infants. These hospitals were designated as regional, tertiary, or Level III centers. Other hospitals within the region might be designated as Level II or Level I centers. A Level I center would care primarily for healthy mothers and infants, whereas a Level II center might provide care for certain sick infants but not an infant who was critically ill. Some leaders in perinatal health care have suggested that the use of numbers to designate levels of care was unfortunate and should be discontinued. They argue that there are no consistent definitions of Level I and Level II care and that several hospitals with varying capabilities may all be designated the same level. The terms regional center and community hospital would be used.

In addition to complex care, regional centers provide educational services to the area they serve. These services may include seminars, workshops, and opportunities for nurses, respiratory therapists, physicians, and other providers of perinatal health care to participate in guided clinical practice. Nursing consultants may be available to community hospitals and health agencies to provide clinical and classroom instruction within the community setting. Guides for self study and audiovisual materials are also available from many regional centers.

In a number of areas, state and regional perinatal advisory counsels provide active direction for perinatal care. The councils are usually multidisciplinary and may include consumers as well as providers of care. Councils are usually voluntary; activities vary and may include:

1. Providing a forum for the discussion of perinatal issues and communication of information.

2. Involving providers in the design of educational activities so that education will truly meet the needs of those providers in community hospitals.

3. Education of the general public and legislators and others concerning perinatal health care issues.

Nurses need to know whether councils exist in their region and become familiar with their role. Meetings are frequently open to anyone who wishes to observe.

There seems little doubt that regionalization, particularly when both maternal and neonatal care are involved, has contributed to improved perinatal outcome. Regionalization has not been without problems, however. The separation of infants from families for many weeks and sometimes over great distances is one obvious disadvantage.

Although regionalization was designed to make cost-efficient use of both nurses, physicians, and others with specialty education and equipment, the frequent tendency to leave infants in regional centers during convalescence is costly both economically and in relation to family bonding. Providing care for convalescing infants at community hospitals, which are generally both less expensive and more convenient for families, is a solution that has worked well in some regions.

Postlogue

You have finished this course, but you have only started to learn about childbearing families. There has never been a single day in our professional lives in which there was not an opportunity to learn—from a woman or a family, from a newborn or preterm infant, from a colleague, from a student, from a friend, and from our personal experiences in childbearing.

Perinatal nurses practice in many settings, from highly technical intensive care nurseries and maternal intensive care units to isolated rural health centers to living rooms where they may teach prenatal classes. Some of our clients glow with healthy pregnancy. A few are very ill. Childbearing brings joy to many families but the potential for grief is also present.

Each family and each of our colleagues brings the uniqueness of their personhood to our interaction with them. If we are willing to share ourselves and accept and value them, perinatal nursing will bring an excitement and joy that are possible in few other professions.

REFERENCES

1. Annas, G.: The Case of Phillip Becker: A Legal Travesty. *Nursing Law and Ethics* 1:4, 1980.
2. Bean, M.: The Nurse Midwife at Work. *American Journal of Nursing* 71:949, 1971.
3. Bowes, W. P., and Selgestad, B.: Fetal Versus Maternal Rights: Medical and Legal Perspectives. *Obstetrics and Gynecology* 58:209, 1981.
4. Brown, M., O'Meara, C., and Krowley, S.: The Maternal-Child Nurse Practitioner. *American Journal of Nursing* 75:1298, 1975.
5. Callahan, D.: Health and Society: Some Ethical Imperatives. *Daedalus* Winter, 1977.
6. Carroll, M., and Humphrey, R.: *Moral Problems in Nursing: Case Studies.* Washington, D.C., University Press of America, 1979.
7. Creighton, H.: *Law Every Nurse Should Know,* 4th Ed. Philadelphia, W. B. Saunders Co., 1981.
8. Curran, C.: *New Perspectives in Moral Theology.* Notre Dame, Indiana, University of Notre Dame Press, 1974.
9. Cushing, M.: Whose Best Interest? Parent vs. Child Rights. *American Journal of Nursing* 82:313, 1982.
10. Cushing, M.: A Matter of Judgment. *American Journal of Nursing* 82:990, 1982.
11. Dougherty, M.: Southern Midwifery and Organized Health Care: Systems in Conflict. *Medical Anthropology* 6:113, 1982.
11a. *Federal Monitor,* 1982, v (4), p. 5.
12. Fost, N.: Ethical Issues in the Treatment of Critically Ill Newborns. *Pediatric Annals* 10:16, 1981.
13. Greenlaw, J.: To Whom Is the Nurse Accountable? *Nursing Law and Ethics* 1:3, 1980.
14. Hein, H.: Secrets from Sweden. *JAMA* 247:985, 1982.
15. Hein, H., and Brown, C.: Neonatal Mortality Review: A Basis for Improving Care. *Pediatrics* 68:504, 1981.
16. Herron, M., Katz, M., and Creasy, R.: Evaluation of a Preterm Birth Prevention Program: Preliminary Report. *Obstetrics and Gynecology* 59:452, 1982.
17. Hubbard, R.: The Fetus as Patient. *Ms.* 11(4):28, 1982.
18. Huey, F.: Looking at Ladders. *American Journal of Nursing* 82:1520, 1982.
19. Hogan, A.: A Tribute to the Pioneers. *Journal of Nurse-Midwifery* Summer, 1975.
20. Jonsen, A., and Garland, M.: *Ethics of Newborn Intensive Care.* San Francisco, Health Policy Program, School of Medicine, University of California, and Berkeley, Institute of Governmental Studies, University of California, 1976.
21. Jordan, B.: *Birth in Four Cultures.* Montreal, Eden Press, 1980.
22. Kleinman, J.: The Continued Vitality of Vital Statistics. *American Journal of Public Health* 72:125, 1982.
23. Lestz, P.: A Committee to Decide the Quality of Life. *American Journal of Nursing* 77:862, 1977.
24. Lumpp, F.: The Role of the Nurse in the Bioethical Decision-Making Process. *Nursing Clinics of North America* 14(1):13, 1979.
25. McCormick, R.: To Save or Let Die: The Dilemma of Modern Medicine. *Journal of the American Medical Association* 229:172, 1974.
25a. NAACOG: *Newsletter* 9(4):5, 1982.
26. The National Commission for the Protection of Human Subjects of Biomedical and Behavioral Research. *Report and Recommendations: Research on the Fetus,* Washington, D.C., Department of Health, Education and Welfare Publication No. (05)76–127, 1975.
27. Nunnally, D., and Bird, J.: The Clinical Specialist—Link between Theory and Practice, *JOGN Nursing* 4(2):40, 1975.
28. Olrig, A.: A Nurse-Midwife in Practice. *American Journal of Nursing* 71:953, 1971.
29. Petitte, D., Cefalo, R., Shapiro, S., and Whalley, P.: In-hospital Maternal Mortality in the United States: Time Trends and Relation to Method of Delivery. *Obstetrics and Gynecology* 59:6, 1982.
30. *Promoting Health/Preventing Disease: Objectives for the Nation.* Washington, D.C.: United States Department of Health and Human Services, 1981.
31. Quilligan, E., and Keegan, K.: Cesarean Section: Some Important Considerations. *Perinatal Press* 5:111, 1981.
32. Ramsey, P.: *The Patient as a Person.* New Haven, Yale University Press, 1970.
33. Romanell, P.: Ethics, Moral Conflicts, and Choice. *American Journal of Nursing* 77:850, 1977.
34. Schuman, H.: A Pediatric Nurse Practitioner in the Neonatal Unit. *JOGN Nursing* 2(6):42, 1973.
35. Shapiro, S.: A Tool for Health Planners. *American Journal of Public Health* 67:816, 1977.
36. Shy, K.: Evaluation of Elective Cesarean Section as a Standard of Care: An Application of Decision. *American Journal of Obstetrics and Gynecology* 139:123, 1981.
37. *Statistical Abstracts of the United States, 1981.* Washington, D.C., U.S. Department of Commerce, Bureau of the Census, 1981.
38. Zartman, W.: *The 50 Per Cent Solution.* New York, Anchor Books, 1976.

Appendix A

HEMOGLOBIN, HEMATOCRIT, AND LEUKOCYTE VALUES DURING THE FIRST
6 WEEKS OF POSTPARTUM LIFE (TERM INFANT)*

Age	Hemoglobin† (Grams %)	Hematocrit† (%)	Leukocytes‡
Birth			
Mean	19.0	61	18,000
Range	16.8–21.2	53.6–68.4	9,000–30,000
7 Days			
Mean	17.9	56	12,000
Range	15.4–20.4	46.6–65.4	5,000–21,000
14 Days			
Mean	17.3	54	12,000
Range	15.0–19.6	45.7–62.3	5,000–21,000
6 Weeks			
Mean	11.9	36	—
Range	10.4–13.4	31.2–40.8	—
3 Months			
Mean	11.3	33	12,000
Range	10.4–12.2	29.7–36.3	6,000–18,000

*Standards will vary slightly from one laboratory to another.
†Range represents 1 standard deviation in study by Matoth: *Acta Paediatrica Scand., 60*:317, 1971.
‡After Oski and Naiman: *Hematologic Problems in the Newborn*. 2nd Edition. Philadelphia, W. B. Saunders Co., 1972.

ENGLISH–METRIC CONVERSION: POUNDS AND OUNCES TO GRAMS

Pounds	Ounces 0	1	2	3	4	5	6	7	8	9	10	11	12	13	14	15
0	—	28	57	85	113	142	170	198	227	255	283	312	340	369	397	425
1	454	482	510	539	567	595	624	652	680	709	737	765	794	822	850	879
2	907	936	964	992	1021	1049	1077	1106	1134	1162	1191	1219	1247	1276	1304	1332
3	1361	1389	1417	1446	1474	1503	1531	1559	1588	1616	1644	1673	1701	1729	1758	1786
4	1814	1843	1871	1899	1928	1956	1984	2013	2041	2070	2098	2126	2155	2183	2211	2240
5	2268	2296	2325	2353	2381	2410	2438	2466	2495	2523	2551	2580	2608	2637	2665	2693
6	2722	2750	2778	2807	2835	2863	2892	2920	2948	2977	3005	3033	3062	3090	3118	3147
7	3175	3203	3232	3260	3289	3317	3345	3374	3402	3430	3459	3487	3515	3544	3572	3600
8	3629	3657	3685	3714	3742	3770	3799	3827	3856	3884	3912	3941	3969	3997	4026	4054
9	4082	4111	4139	4167	4196	4224	4252	4281	4309	4337	4366	4394	4423	4451	4479	4508
10	4536	4564	4593	4621	4649	4678	4706	4734	4763	4791	4819	4848	4876	4904	4933	4961
11	4990	5018	5046	5075	5103	5131	5160	5188	5216	5245	5273	5301	5330	5358	5386	5415
12	5443	5471	5500	5528	5557	5585	5613	5642	5670	5698	5727	5755	5783	5812	5840	5868
13	5897	5925	5953	5982	6010	6038	6067	6095	6123	6152	6180	6209	6237	6265	6294	6322
14	6350	6379	6407	6435	6464	6492	6520	6549	6577	6605	6634	6662	6690	6719	6747	6776
15	6804	6832	6860	6889	6917	6945	6973	7002	7030	7059	7087	7115	7144	7172	7201	7228
16	7257	7286	7313	7342	7371	7399	7427	7456	7484	7512	7541	7569	7597	7626	7654	7682
17	7711	7739	7768	7796	7824	7853	7881	7909	7938	7966	7994	8023	8051	8079	8108	8136
18	8165	8192	8221	8249	8278	8306	8335	8363	8391	8420	8448	8476	8504	8533	8561	8590
19	8618	8646	8675	8703	8731	8760	8788	8816	8845	8873	8902	8930	8958	8987	9015	9043
20	9072	9100	9128	9157	9185	9213	9242	9270	9298	9327	9355	9383	9412	9440	9469	9497
21	9525	9554	9582	9610	9639	9667	9695	9724	9752	9780	9809	9837	9865	9894	9922	9950
22	9979	10007	10036	10064	10092	10120	10149	10177	10206	10234	10262	10291	10319	10347	10376	10404

Appendix C

TABLE OF FAHRENHEIT AND CELSIUS (CENTIGRADE) TEMPERATURE
EQUIVALENTS*

94.0–34.4	97.0–36.1	100.0–37.8
94.2–34.6	97.2–36.2	100.2–37.9
94.4–34.7	97.4–36.3	100.4–38.0
94.6–34.8	97.6–36.4	100.6–38.1
94.8–34.9	97.8–36.5	100.8–38.2
95.0–35.0	98.0–36.6	101.0–38.3
95.2–35.1	98.2–36.8	101.2–38.4
95.4–35.2	98.4–36.9	101.4–38.5
95.6–35.3	98.6–37.0	101.6–38.6
95.8–35.4	98.8–37.1	101.8–38.7
96.0–35.5	99.0–37.2	102.0–38.8
96.2–35.6	99.2–37.3	102.2–39.0
96.4–35.7	99.4–37.4	102.4–39.1
96.6–35.8	99.6–37.5	102.6–39.2
96.8–36.0	99.8–37.6	102.8–39.3

*To convert Fahrenheit to Celsius (Centigrade), subtract 32 from the Fahrenheit reading and multiply by $5/9$.

Appendix D

AMERICAN NURSES' ASSOCIATION—STANDARDS OF MATERNAL–CHILD HEALTH NURSING PRACTICE*

The development of standards of practice is important in every profession. The following *Standards of Maternal-Child Health Nursing Practice* was developed by the Executive Committee and the Standards Committee of the Division on Maternal-Child Health Nursing Practice of the American Nurses' Association in 1973. These standards are process standards.

A booklet discussing maternal-child health standards in more detail is available from the American Nurses' Association, 2420 Pershing Road, Kansas City, Missouri, 64108.

Maternal and Child Health Nursing Practice is based on the following premises:

1. Survival and the level of health of society is inextricably bound to Maternal and Child Health Nursing Practice.
2. Maternal and Child Health Nursing Practice respects the human dignity and rights of individuals.
3. Maternal and Child Health Nursing Practice is family-centered.
4. Maternal and Child Health Nursing Practice focuses on the childbearing, childrearing phases of the life cycle which include the development of sexuality, family planning, interconceptual care and child

*Reprinted by permission of the American Nurses' Association, Inc., 2420 Pershing Road, Kansas City, Missouri 64108

health from conception through adolescence.
5. Maternal and Child Health Nursing makes a significant difference to society in achieving its health goals.
6. Man is a total human being. His psychosocial and biophysical self are interrelated.
7. Human behavior shapes and is shaped by environmental forces and as such sets into motion a multitude of reciprocal responses.
8. Through his own process of self-regulation the human being attempts to maintain equilibrium amidst constant change.
9. All behavior has meaning and is influenced by past experiences, the individual's perception of those experiences, and forces impinging upon the present.
10. Growth and development is ordered and evolves in sequential stages.
11. Substantive knowledge of the principles of human growth and development, including normative data, is essential to effective Maternal and Child Health Nursing Practice.
12. Periods of developmental and traumatic crises during the life cycle pose internal and external stresses and have a positive or negative effect.
13. Maternal and Child Health Nursing Practice provides for continuity of care and is not bound by artificial barriers and exclusive categories which tend to restrict and delimit practice.

14. *All* people have a right to receive the benefit of optimal health services.

Maternal and Child Health Nursing Practice is aimed at:
1. Promoting and maintaining optimal health of each individual and the family unit.
2. Improving or supporting family solidarity.
3. Early identification and treatment of vulnerable families.
4. Preventing environmental conditions which block attainment of optimal health.
5. Prevention and early detection of deviations from health.
6. Reducing stresses which interfere with optimal functioning.
7. Assisting the family to understand or cope with the developmental and traumatic situations which occur during childbearing and childrearing.
8. Facilitating survival, recovery and growth when the individual is ill or needs health care.
9. Reducing reproductive wastage occurring at any point on the continuum.
10. Continuously improving the quality of care in Maternal and Child Health Nursing Practice.
11. Reducing inequalities in the delivery of health care services.

Standard I

Maternal and child health nursing practice is characterized by the continual questioning of the assumptions upon which practice is based, retaining those which are valid and searching for and using new knowledge.

Rationale: Since knowledge is not static, all assumptions are subject to change. Assumptions are derived from knowledge of findings of research which are subject to additional testing and revision. They are carefully selected and tested and reflect utilization of present and new knowledge. Effective utilization of these knowledges stimulates more astute observations and provides new insights into the effects of nursing upon the individual and family. To question assumptions implies that nursing practice is not based on stereotyped or ritualistic procedures or methods of intervention; rather, practice exemplifies an objective, systematic and logical investigation of a phenomenon or problem.

Standard II

Maternal and child health nursing practice is based upon knowledge of the biophysical and psychosocial development of individuals from conception through the childrearing phase of development and upon knowledge of the basic needs for optimum development.

Rationale: A knowledge and understanding of the principles and normal ranges in human growth, development and behavior are essential to Maternal and Child Health Nursing Practice. Concomitant with this knowledge is the recognition and consideration of the psychosocial, environmental, nutritional, spiritual and cognitive factors that enhance or deter the biophysical and psychological maturation of the individual and his family.

Standard III

The collection of data about the health status of the client/patient is systematic and continuous. The data are accessible, communicated and recorded.

Rationale: Comprehensive care requires complete and ongoing collection of data about the client/patient to determine the nursing care needs and other health care needs of the client/patient. All health status data about the client/patient must be available for all members of the health care team.

Standard IV

Nursing diagnoses are derived from data about the health status of the client/patient.

Rationale: The health status of the client/patient is the basis for determining the nursing care needs. The data are analyzed and compared to norms.

Standard V

Maternal and child health nursing practice recognizes deviations from expected patterns of physiologic activity and anatomic and psychosocial development.

Rationale: Early detection of deviations and therapeutic intervention are essential to the prevention of illness, to facilitating growth and developmental potential, and to the promotion of optimal health for the individual and the family.

Standard VI

The plan of nursing care includes goals derived from the nursing diagnoses.

Rationale: The determination of the desired results from nursing actions is an essential part of planning care.

Standard VII

The plan of nursing care includes priorities and the prescribed nursing approaches or measures to achieve the goals derived from the nursing diagnoses.

Rationale: Nursing actions are planned to promote, maintain and restore the client/patient's well-being.

Standard VIII

Nursing actions provide for client/patient participation in health promotion, maintenance and restoration.

Ratonale: The client/patient and family are provided the opportunity to participate in the nursing care. Such provision is made based upon theoretical and experiential evidence that participation of client/patient and family may foster growth.

Standard IX

Maternal and child health nursing practice provides for the use and coordination of all services that assist individuals to prepare for responsible sexual roles.

Rationale: People are prepared for sexual roles through a process of socialization that takes place from birth to adulthood. This process of socialization, to a large extent, is carried out within the family structure. Social control over child care increases in importance as humans become increasingly dependent on the culture rather than upon the family unit. The culture of any society is maintained by the transmission of its specific values, attitudes and behaviors from generation to generation. Attitudes and values concerning male and female roles develop as part of the socialization process. Attitudes toward self, the opposite sex and parents will influence the roles each individual assumes in adulthood and the responsibilities accepted.

Standard X

Nursing actions assist the client/patient to maximize his health capabilities.

Rationale: Nursing actions are designed to promote, maintain and restore health. A knowledge and understanding of the principles and normal ranges in human growth, development and behavior are essential to Maternal and Child Heath Nursing Practice.

Standard XI

The client's/patient's progress or lack of progress toward goal achievement is determined by the client/patient and the nurse.

Rationale: The quality of nursing care depends upon comprehensive and intelligent determination of the impact of nursing upon the health status of the client/patient. The client/patient is an essential part of this determination.

Standard XII

The client's/patient's progress or lack of progress toward goal achievement directs reassessment, reordering of priorities, new goal setting and revision of the plan of nursing care.

Rationale: The nursing process remains the same, but the input of new information may dictate new or revised approaches.

Standard XIII

Maternal and child health nursing practice evidences active participation with others in evaluating the availability, accessibility and acceptability of services for parents and children and cooperating and/or taking leadership in extending and developing needed services in the community.

Rationale: Knowledge of services presently offered parents and children is the first step in determining the effectiveness of health care to all in the community. When it is recognized that needed services are not available, accessible or acceptable, the nurse takes leadership in working with consumers, other health disciplines, the community and governmental agencies in extending and/or developing these services. Services must be continually evaluated, expanded and changed if they are to improve the health and well-being of all parents and children within our society.

Appendix E

THE NURSES ASSOCIATION OF THE AMERICAN COLLEGE OF OBSTETRICIANS AND GYNECOLOGISTS— STANDARDS FOR OBSTETRIC, GYNECOLOGIC, AND NEONATAL NURSING*

The following statements are taken from the second edition of *Standards for Obstetric, Gynecologic, and Neonatal Nursing* (1981). Specific standards for each area of practice, along with these general standards, are found in this book, which is available from NAACOG, 600 Maryland Avenue, S.W., Suite 300, Washington, D.C. 20024.

Nursing Care

Comprehensive obstetric, gynecologic, and neonatal (OGN) nursing care shall be provided to the patient and her family and shall utilize all components of the nursing process, including assessment, nursing diagnosis, planning, implementation, and evaluation; it shall reflect informed consent and respect for the rights of the patient and her family.

Professional Responsibility and Accountability

The nurse is responsible for maintaining the knowledge and clinical skills required for OGN nursing.

Health Education

Health care education for the patient and her family should be an integral part of OGN nursing practice.

Policies, Protocols, and Procedures

Development, review, and revision of OGN nursing policies, protocols, and procedures should be the responsibility of the OGN nursing division, and should be correlated within a multidisciplinary framework.

Personnel

Obstetric, gynecologic, and neonatal nursing staff requirements shall be developed to meet patient care needs.

Environment

The OGN nursing division should assist in providing a safe, comfortable, and therapeutic environment by collaborating with other disciplines and services in promoting family-centered care, planning facilities, evaluating and selecting equipment and supplies, and establishing protocols for their use and maintenance.

*Reprinted by permission of the Nurses Association of the American College of Obstetricians and Gynecologists.

Appendix F

ARIZONA NURSES' ASSOCIATION—PERINATAL NURSING STANDARDS*

The following standards were developed by the Committee for Preparation of Standards of Perinatal Nursing Practice, Arizona Nurses Association, in 1977. The objective of these Perinatal Nursing Standards is to give structure, direction, and a more formal recognition to the maternal-fetal and neonatal nursing practice, education, and evaluation. Perinatal nursing integrates the interdependent normal and high risk segments of maternal-fetal neonatal health care and includes the care of all pregnant women and neonates and their families.

A complete copy of these standards, including assessment factors, is available from the Arizona Nurses Association, 4525 North 12th Street, Phoenix, Arizona, 85014.

Standard I

Perinatal nursing practice is characterized by the continual questioning of the assumptions upon which practice is based, retaining those which are valid and searching for and using new knowledge.

Standard II

Perinatal nursing practice is based upon knowledge of the normal and abnormal biophysical and psychosocial development of the pregnant woman, her fetus/newborn and her family.

Standard III

Nursing diagnoses are based upon the collection of data about the health status of the mother/fetus/newborn.

Standard IV

The plan of nursing care includes priorities and the prescribed nursing approaches or measures to achieve the goals derived from the nursing diagnosis.

Standard V

The plan of nursing care contains a nursing history. The care plan expresses assessment of the patient/family, defines health care goals and nursing actions. This process is recorded, communicated and accessible.

Standard VI

Perinatal nursing practice provides for the use and coordination of all perinatal health care services within the region.

*Reprinted by permission of the Arizona Nurses' Association, 4525 North 12th Street, Phoenix, Arizona 85014.

Appendix G

JOURNALS USEFUL TO NURSES WHO CARE FOR CHILDBEARING FAMILIES

American Journal of Diseases of Children, American Medical Association, 535 North Dearborn Street, Chicago, Illinois, 60610.

American Journal of Nursing, American Journal of Nursing Company, 10 Columbus Circle, New York, New York, 10019.

American Journal of Obstetrics and Gynecology, C. V. Mosby Company, 11830 Westline Industrial Drive, St. Louis, Missouri, 63141.

American Journal of Orthopsychiatry, 49 Sheridan Avenue, Albany, New York, 12210.

American Journal of Public Health, 1015 Eighteenth Street, N.W., Washington, D.C., 20036.

APRS Federal Monitor, Box 6358, Alexandria, Virginia 22306.

Archives of Disease in Childhood, British Medical Association, Tavislock Square, London, England.

*Birth and Family Journal, 110 El Camino Real, Berkeley, California, 94705.

*Briefs, Maternity Center Association, Publication Office, 6900 Grove Road, Thorofare, New Jersey, 08086.

The Canadian Nurse, 50 The Driveway, Ottawa, Ontario, Canada.

Child and Family, P. O. Box 508, Oak Park, Illinois, 60303.

Children Today, Superintendent of Documents, U.S. Government Printing Office, Washington, D.C., 20402.

*ICEA News, International Childbirth Education Association, P.O. Box 20048, Minneapolis, Minnesota, 55420.

International Journal of Nursing Studies, Headington Hill Hall, Oxford, OX3 OBU, England.

*JOGN, Journal of Obstetric, Gynecologic and Neonatal Nursing, Nurses Association of the American College of Obstetricians and Gynecologists, Harper and Row, Publishers, 2350 Virginia Avenue, Hagerstown, Maryland, 21740.

Journal of the American Dietetic Association, 430 North Michigan Avenue, Chicago, Illinois, 60611.

*Journal of Nurse Midwifery, 1000 Vermont Avenue, N.W., Washington, D.C., 20005.

Journal of Pediatrics, C.V. Mosby Company, 11830 Westline Industrial Drive, St. Louis, Missouri, 63141.

*Maternal-Child Nursing Journal, 3505 Fifth Avenue, Pittsburgh, Pennsylvania, 15213.

*MCN: The American Journal of Maternal Child Nursing, American Journal of Nursing Company, 10 Columbus Circle, New York, New York, 10019.

Nursing, (77) (78), etc., Intermed Communications, 132 Welsh Road, Horsham, Pennsylvania, 19044.

Nursing Clinics of North America, W. B. Saunders Company, West Washington Square, Philadelphia, Pennsylvania, 19105.

Nursing Digest, 12 Lakeside Park, 607 North Avenue, Wakefield, Massachusetts, 01880.

Nursing Mirror, Surrey House, 1 Throwley Way, Sutton, Surrey, SM1 400, England.

Nursing Outlook, American Journal of Nursing Company, 10 Columbus Circle, New York, New York, 10019.

Nursing Research, American Journal of Nursing Company, 10 Columbus Circle, New York, New York, 10019.

Nursing Times, Little Essex Street, London, WC 2R 3LF, England.

Nutrition Reviews, 665 Huntington Avenue, Boston, Massachusetts, 02115.

Obstetrics and Gynecology, Journal of the American College of Obstetrics and Gynecology, 2350 Virginia Avenue, Hagerstown, Maryland, 21740.

Pediatrics, American Academy of Pediatrics, Evanston, Illinois, 60204.

---

*These journals are primarily devoted to childbearing topics.

Appendix H

AUDIOVISUAL RESOURCES RELATED TO CHILDBEARING

Unless otherwise indicated, resource is a 16 mm. film. Asterisk* indicates appropriate for parents or other lay-groups as well as for professional nurses. The addresses of companies supplying these audiovisual resources follow this listing.

Abortion: A Rational Approach, Audio Visual Narrative Arts, Inc. Two filmstrips with audiocassette tapes or 33⅓ RPM records discussing abortion and the Supreme Court decision of 1973.

About Conception and Contraception, Canadian Film Institute. Describes reproductive physiology, sexual intercourse, conception, and contraception.

Adapting to Parenthood, 1975, Polymorph Films. New parents discuss their initial adjustments.

The Amazing Newborn, Ross Laboratories.

Anemia in the First Week of Life, 1973, National Medical Audiovisual Center. Slides, audiocassette, and guide.

Are You Ready for the Postpartum Experience? 1975, Parenting Pictures. Includes discussion of husband-wife relationships, sleep deprivation, breast- and bottle-feeding, depression, and satisfaction.

Birth Atlas Slide Series, Maternity Center Association. A series of 22 slides, adapted from the *Birth Atlas,* and guide.

Breast Feeding: Prenatal and Postpartum Preparation, Health Sciences Communication Center, Case Western Reserve University.

The Beat of a Different Drummer, 1976, Nurse Midwife Program, College of Nursing, Medical University of South Carolina. Black adolescents share their feelings about marriage, abortion, birth control, and the experience of labor and delivery.

The Biological Aspects of Sexuality, Harper and Row. 35 mm. slides and audiotape cassette.

Birth in the Squatting Position. Polymorph Films. A Brazilian film; shows five unassisted, spontaneous births.

Birth without Violence, 1976, New Yorker Films. The Leboyer method of infant delivery.

Blueprint for Life, Milner-Fenwick, Inc. Describes chromosomes, meiosis, mitosis, fertilization, and genetic counseling.

The Bonding Birth Experience, 1977, Parenting Pictures. Includes coping techniques during labor, fetal monitoring, the father's role, bonding, family adjustment, and breast-feeding.

Bottle Babies, International Film Center. Discusses the implications of the use of commercial baby food in underdeveloped nations.

Brazelton Neonatal Behavioral Assessment Scale, Educational Development Center, Inc. A series of three films that describe the assessment of neonatal behavior; the third film is a self-scoring examination.

The Breastfeeding Experience, Parenting Pictures.

Caring and Coping: The New Parent Experience, Parenting Pictures. Six families (urban, rural, teen, working, first born, sibling adjustment) adjust to a new infant.

The Case against Rubella, National Foundation—March of Dimes. Describes the effects of maternal rubella infection during pregnancy and the development of rubella vaccine.

The Cesarean Birth Experience, 1977, Parenting Pictures. Experiences of cesarean delivery.

Changing Concepts: The Nursing Care of the Newborn, Health Media Corporation. A series of slides, audiocassette tapes, and guides: (1) Introduction of Newborn Nursing, (2) The First 12 Hours of Life, (3) Fetal Circulation, (4) Transitional Circulation, (5) Assessing Cardiac Status, (6) Forces of Labor, (7) Fetal Heart Rate Monitoring, and (8) Forces of Labor and Fetal Heart Rate Monitoring.

Contraception: A Matter of Choice, Audio Visual Narrative Arts, Inc. Two filmstrips with audiocassette tapes or 33⅓ RPM records discussing the history of fertility control, state laws, and medically-accepted means of contraception.

The Crisis of Loss, The American Journal of Nursing Company. Filmstrip with audiotape cassette or 33⅓ RPM record. Examines loss and mourning within the framework of crisis theory. Not specifically concerned with infant death but concepts applicable.

*Daughters of Time, New Day Films. Describes nurse-midwives.

Death of a Newborn, Ross Laboratories. Parents and physician discuss feelings 2 months after the death of their child.

*Diagnosis Before Birth, National Foundation—March of Dimes. Discusses the prenatal and postnatal diagnosis of birth defects and genetic counseling.

The Distressed Newborn, Network for Continuing Medical Education. Videotape.

Early Complications of Pregnancy, Medcom Press. Slides, audiocassette, and guide.

*Essential Exercises for the Childbearing Year, Polymorph Films.

Facilitating Self-Disclosure, The American Journal of Nursing Company. Filmstrip with audiocassette tape or 33⅓ RPM record. Examines skills that facilitate a patient's or parent's expression of feelings in both psychiatric and nonpsychiatric clinical settings.

*Family Planning, Trainex Corporation: 35 mm. filmstrip with audiotape cassette or 33⅓ RPM record in English or Spanish for patient teaching; discusses six methods of contraception and problems when contraception is not used.

Fetal Growth and Development, Mead Johnson Laboratories. 16 mm. film or videotape with study guide.

First Breath, Childbirth Education Films, Inc. For health professionals; describes the benefits of prepared childbirth through interviews with psychiatrists, pediatricians, and obstetricians.

*From Generation to Generation: Genetic Counseling. National Foundation—March of Dimes. Filmstrip or slides with audiocassette or record discussing genetics in easily understood terms.

*Help! I'm a New Parent, Churchill Films. The reality of changes a baby makes in parents' lives.

Hospital Maternity Care: Family Centered, The American Journal of Nursing Company. Describes family-centered care for childbearing families.

*How Babies Begin, The American Journal of Nursing Company. Filmstrip describing reproduction and contraception in simple terms; for use in patient teaching.

*How Many Children Do You Want? The American Journal of Nursing Company. A series of three filmstrips with audiotape cassettes or 33⅓ RPM record for patient teaching: (1) How Babies Begin, (2) Drugstore Methods and Least Effective Methods of Birth Control, and (3) Doctor Methods of Birth Control.

Human Embryology, W. B. Saunders. Slides of illustrations from the book *Human Embryology* by Keith L. Moore, published by W. B. Saunders Company.

*Hunger in America, Parts I and II, CBS Reports Program, Carousel Films. Emphasizes the effects of malnutrition and starvation on mothers, babies, and children in varied areas of the United States.

Hydatidiform Mole, Oxford Tape-Slide Series. Slides, audiocassette, and guide.

Hypoglycemia, National Foundation—March of Dimes. Slides, audiocassette tape, and guide.

I'm Seventeen, Pregnant and Don't Know What To Do, Children's Home Society of California.

*Inside My Mom, National Foundation—Supply Division. Filmstrip or slide set with audiocassette or record describing nutrition as basic to life in cartoon style.

Introduction to Congenital Heart Disease, National Medical Audiovisual Center. Series of slides, audiocassette tapes, and guides: (1) Perinatal Circulation, (2) General Background, (3) Common Acyanotic Lesions, (4) Common Cyanotic Lesions, and (5) The Large USD in Infancy.

Jaundice in the Newborn, 1973, National Medical Audiovisual Center. Slides, audiocassette, and guide.

Maternity Nursing, The American Journal of Nursing Company. A series of 15 classes, 44 minutes each, available as 16 mm. film, videotape, or audiotape cassettes.

*More Than Love, National Foundation—March of Dimes. Filmstrip, record, and guide discussing prenatal care and birth defects.

*Nan's Class, ASPO. Prenatal and intrapartal experiences of couples in a Lamaze class.

Neonatal Infections: Diagnosis and Prevention,

Mead Johnson Laboratories. 16 mm. film or videotape with study guide.

Neurological Evaluation, Health Sciences Communication Center, Case Western Reserve University. Describes and demonstrates neurological examination of the newborn.

The Neurologically Suspect Infant, 1973, National Medical Audiovisual Center. Slides, audiocassette, and guide.

*Newborn, 1972, West Glen Films. Focuses on the experience of a mother and father and their first child.

*Nicholas and the Baby, Centre Productions, Inc. For children 3 to 12 and their parents.

Normal Puerperium, Oxford Tape Slide Series. Slides, audiocassette, and guide.

Nutrition in Pregnancy, Jay Hathaway Productions, Inc.

Nutritional Support of the Premature, Mead Johnson Laboratories. 16 mm. film or videotape with study guide.

*The Only Kid on the Block, National Foundation—March of Dimes. Describes the impact of a serious birth defect on a boy, his family, and neighbors.

The Perinatal Assessment of Maturation, 1973, National Medical Audiovisual Center. Slides, audiocassette, and guide.

Physical Examination of the Newborn, Medcom Press. Slides, audiocassette, and guide.

Postpartum Haemorrhage, 1976, Parts I and II, Oxford Tape-Slide Series in Obstetrics and Gynecology. Slides, audiocassette, and guide.

*Poverty in Rural America, United States Department of Agriculture. A graphic presentation of lifestyles in mountain hollows and along dirt roads.

*Pregnant Fathers, Joseph T. Anzalone Foundation.

*Purposes of Family Planning, Canadian Film Institute. Describes the positive purposes of family planning for consumers of all ages and income levels.

Respiratory Distress Syndrome, 1973, National Medical Audiovisual Center. Slides, audiocassette, and guide.

Respiratory Distress Syndrome, Mead Johnson Laboratories, 16 mm. film or videotape with study guide.

Resuscitation of the Newborn, Mead Johnson Laboratories. 16 mm. film or videotape with study guide.

Resuscitation of the Newborn, 1977, ACOG Film and Video Service. Discusses resuscitation from the perspectives of prenatal assessment, intrapartum monitoring, and recognition and care of the depressed baby.

*A Shared Beginning, Judy Christiansen.

*A Shared Cesarean Beginning, Judy Christiansen.

*The Teenage Pregnancy Experience, Parenting Pictures. Two school-age mothers are followed from pregnancy through postpartum.

Thermal Regulation of the Neonate, Mead Johnson Laboratories. 16 mm. film or videotape with study guide.

*The Story of Eric, Centre Films, Inc. Describes preparation for labor and labor and delivery using the Lamaze method in a conventional delivery room.

*Together, With Love, Centre Films, Inc. A birthing room delivery and a family-centered cesarean delivery.

*Tomorrow Happens Today, National Foundation—March of Dimes. Filmstrip with record or cassette and guide discussing prenatal care and protection of the unborn child.

The Use of Nasal CPAP, 1976, Health Sciences Communication Center, Case Western Reserve University. Principles of CPAP, techniques and administration, characteristics of the infant with RDS, and related therapies are included.

*Wednesday's Child, Human Betterment League, N.C., Inc. Describes biologic, emotional and social aspects of genetic disease and genetic counseling.

*Welcome, Emily, Diane Gent. Slides and cassette; birth in a homelike setting.

Addresses for Films

ACOG Film and Video Service, P. O. Box 299, Wheaton, Illinois, 60187.

The American Journal of Nursing Company, Educational Services Division, 10 Columbus Circle, New York, New York, 10019.

ASPO (American Society for Psychoprophylaxis in Obstetrics, 1840 Wilson Blvd., Suite 204, Arlington, Virginia, 22201.

Audio Visual Narrative Arts, Inc., P. O. Box 398, Pleasantville, New York, 10570.

Canadian Film Institute, 303 Richmond Road, Ottawa, Ontario, Canada.

Carousel Films, 1501 Broadway, Suite 1503, New York, New York, 10036.

Centre Films, Inc., 1103 North El Centro Ave., Hollywood, California, 90038.

Centre Productions, Inc., 1327 Spruce St. #3, Boulder, Colorado, 80302.

Childbirth Education Films, Inc., 648 Riverside Road, North Palm Beach, Florida, 33408.

Children's Home Society of California, 3100 West Adams Boulevard, Los Angeles, California 90018.

Churchill Films, 662 N. Robertson Blvd., Los Angeles, California, 90069.

Diane Gent, 445 South Green Rd., South Euclid, Ohio, 44121.

Educational Development Center, Inc., Distribution Center, 39 Chapel Street, Newton, Massachusetts, 02160.

Harper and Row, Media Department, 10 East 53rd Street, New York, New York, 10022.

Health Media Corporation, P. O. Box 167, Tulsa, Oklahoma, 74101.

Health Sciences Communication Center, Case Western Reserve, University Circle, Cleveland, Ohio, 44106.

Human Betterment League of North Carolina, Inc., P. O. Box 3036, Winston-Salem, North Carolina, 27102.

International Film Center, 33 Sixth Ave., New York, New York, 10014.

Jay Hathaway Productions, Inc., 4349 Tujunga Avenue, North Hollywood, California, 91604.

Joseph T. Anzalone Foundation, P. O. Box 5206, Santa Cruz, California, 95063.

Judy Christiansen, 2068 Cynthia Way, Los Altos, California, 94022.

Maternity Center Association, 48 East 92nd Street, New York, New York, 10028.

Mead Johnson Laboratories, Evansville, Indiana, 47721.

Medcom Press, 2 Hammarskjold Plaza, New York, New York, 10017.

Milner-Fenwick, Inc., 3800 Liberty Heights Avenue, Baltimore, Maryland, 21215.

National Foundation—March of Dimes, Supply Division, Box 2000, White Plains, New York, 10602.

National Medical Audiovisual Center, Washington, D.C., 20409.

New Day Films, P. O. Box 315, Franklin Lakes, New Jersey, 07417.

Network for Continuing Medical Education, 15 Columbus Circle, New York, New York, 10023.

New Yorker Films, 43 West 61st Street, New York, New York, 10023.

Oxford Tape-Slide Series in Obstetrics and Gynecology, Pretest Service, Inc., 71 South Turnpike, Wallingford, Connecticut, 06492.

Parenting Pictures, 121 N.W. Crystal Street, Crystal River, Florida, 32629.

Polymorph Films, 118 South Street, Boston, Massachusetts, 02111.

Ross Laboratories, 585 Cleveland Avenue, Columbus, Ohio, 43216.

Trainex Corporation, Subsidiary Medcom, Inc., P. O. Box 116, Garden Grove, California, 92642.

United States Department of Agriculture, Washington, D.C., 20250.

W. B. Saunders Company, West Washington Square, Philadelphia, Pennsylvania, 19105.

West Glen Films, West Glen Communications, Inc., 565 Fifth Avenue, New York, New York, 10017.

APPENDIX I

Organizations Concerned with Childbearing

American Academy of Husband-Coached Childbirth, P. O. Box 5224, Sherman Oaks, California, 91413.

American Academy of Pediatrics, P. O. Box 1034, Evanston, Illinois, 60204.

American College of Home Obstetrics, c/o Gregory White, M.D., 2821 Rose Street, Franklin Park, Illinois, 60131.

American College of Nurse Midwifery, 330 West 58th Street, New York, New York, 10019.

American Diabetes Association, Inc., 1 West 48th Street, New York, New York, 10020.

American National Red Cross, 17 and D Street, N.W., Washington, D.C., 20006.

The American Nurses' Association, 2420 Pershing Road, Kansas City, Missouri, 64108.

American Society for Psychoprophylaxis in Obstetrics, 1840 Wilson Blvd., Suite 204, Arlington, Virginia, 22201.

Child Study Association of America, 9 East 89th Street, New York, New York, 10028.

C/Sec, Inc., 66 Christopher Road, Waltham, Massachusetts, 02154.

The Couple to Couple League, P. O. Box 11084, Cincinnati, Ohio, 42511 (natural family planning).

International Childbirth Education Association, P. O. Box 20048, Minneapolis, Minnesota, 55420.

La Leche League International, Inc., 9616 Minneapolis Avenue, Franklin Park, Illinois 60131.

Maternity Center Association, 48 East 92nd Street, New York, New York, 10028.

National Family Planning Federation of America, Inc., 1221 Massachusetts Avenue, N.W., Washington, D.C., 20005.

The National Foundation—March of Dimes, 1707 H Street, N.W., Washington, D.C., 20006.

National League for Nursing, 10 Columbus Circle, New York, New York, 10019.

National Organization of Mothers of Twins Clubs, 5402 Amberwood Lane, Rockville, Maryland, 20853.

Nurses Association, American College of Obstetrics and Gynecology, 600 Maryland Ave. SW, Suite 200 East, Washington, D.C., 20024.

Parents of Prematures, 7838 Hummingbird, Houston, Texas, 77071.

Parents Without Partners, 7901 Woodmont Avenue, Bethesda, Maryland, 20014.

Planned Parenthood Federation of America, Inc., 810 Seventh Avenue, New York, New York, 10019.

The Pregnant Patient's Bill of Rights*

The American Hospital Association has developed a Patient's Bill of Rights that is increasingly recognized as a standard of care.

Because the woman who is pregnant represents two patients, herself and her fetus, she should be recognized as having additional rights. The following Pregnant Patient's Bill of Rights has been suggested by Doris Haire and was published in the *Journal of Nurse Midwifery, 20*:29, 1975.

1. *The Pregnant Patient has the right,* prior to the administration of any drug or procedure, to be informed by the health professional caring for her of any potential direct or indirect effects, risks or hazards to herself or newborn infant which may result from the use of a drug or procedure prescribed for or administered to her during pregnancy, labor, birth or lactation.

2. *The Pregnant Patient has the right,* prior to the proposed therapy, to be informed, not only of the benefits, risks and hazards of the proposed therapy but also of known alternative therapy, such as available childbirth education classes which could help to prepare the Pregnant Patient physically and mentally to cope with the discomfort or stress of pregnancy and the experience of childbirth, thereby reducing or eliminating her need for drugs and obstetric intervention. She should be offered such information early in her pregnancy in order that she may make a reasoned decision.

3. *The Pregnant Patient has the right,* prior to the administration of any drug, to be informed by the health professional who is prescribing or administering the drug to her that any drug which she receives during pregnancy, labor and birth, no matter how or when the drug is taken or administered, may adversely affect her unborn baby, directly or indirectly, and that there is no drug or chemical which has been proven safe for the unborn child.

4. *The Pregnant Patient has the right,* if cesarean section is anticipated, to be informed prior to the administration of any drug, and preferably prior to her hospitalization, that minimizing her and, in turn, her baby's intake of nonessential preoperative medicine, will benefit her baby.

5. *The Pregnant Patient has the right,* prior to the administration of a drug or procedure, to be informed if there is *no* properly controlled follow-up research which has established the safety of the drug or procedure with regard to its direct and/or indirect effects on the physiological, mental and neurological development of the child exposed, via the mother, to the drug or procedure during pregnancy, labor, birth or lactation — (this would apply to virtually all drugs and the vast majority of obstetric procedures).

6. *The Pregnant Patient has the right,* prior to the administration of any drug, to be informed of the brand name and generic name of the drug in order that she may advise the health professional of any past adverse reaction to the drug.

7. *The Pregnant Patient has the right* to determine for herself, without pressure from her attendant, whether she will accept the risks inherent in the proposed therapy or refuse a drug or procedure.

8. *The Pregnant Patient has the right* to know the name and qualifications of the individual administering a medication or procedure to her during labor or birth.

9. *The Pregnant Patient has the right* to be

*Reprinted by permission of the *Journal of Nurse-Midwifery.*

informed, prior to the administration of any procedure, whether that procedure is being administered to her for her or her baby's benefit (medically indicated) or as an elective procedure (for convenience or teaching purposes).

10. *The Pregnant Patient has the right* to be accompanied during the stress of labor and birth by someone she cares for, and to whom she looks for emotional comfort and encouragement.

11. *The Pregnant Patient has the right* after appropriate medical consultation to choose a position for labor and for birth which is least stressful to her baby and to herself.

12. *The Obstetric Patient has the right* to have her baby cared for at her bedside if her baby is normal, and to feed her baby according to her baby's needs rather than according to the hospital regimen.

13. *The Obstetric Patient has the right* to be informed in writing of the name of the person who actually delivered her baby and the professional qualifications of that person. This information should also be on the birth certificate.

14. *The Obstetric Patient has the right* to be informed if there is any known or indicated aspect of her or her baby's care or condition which may cause her or her baby later difficulty or problems.

15. *The Obstetric Patient has the right* to have her and her baby's hospital medical records complete, accurate and legible and to have their records, including Nurses' Notes, retained by the hospital until the child reaches at least the age of majority, or, alternatively, to have the records offered to her before they are destroyed.

16. *The Obstetric Patient*, both during and after her hospital stay, has the right to have access to her complete hospital records, including Nurses' Notes, and to receive a copy upon payment of a reasonable fee and without incurring the expense of retaining an attorney.

It is the obstetric patient and her baby, not the health professional, who must sustain any trauma or injury resulting from the use of a drug or obstetric procedure. The observation of the rights listed above will not only permit the obstetric patient to participate in the decisions involving her and her baby's health care, but will help to protect the health professional and the hospital against litigation arising from resentment or misunderstanding on the part of the mother.

Appendix K

PREPARED CHILDBIRTH: A COURSE OUTLINE

Class I

Goals

1. Make each couple feel comfortable about being in the class.
2. Explain what prepared childbirth means.
3. Dispel myths about prepared childbirth.
4. Review the anatomy and physiology of reproduction.
5. Overview development of embryo and fetus.
6. Discuss pain during labor.
7. Introduce the topic of relaxation and teach passive relaxation.
8. Review basic concepts of prenatal care.
9. Encourage attendance at hospital tour.

Objectives

At the completion of this class the couple will be able to:

1. Describe the basic concept of the Lamaze method of prepared childbirth.
2. Give two examples of ways in which a prepared mother differs from an unprepared mother.
3. Correctly identify the terms uterus, fundus, cervix, vagina, and perineum.
4. Cite two sources of pain during labor and three strategies for coping with labor pain.
5. Give two examples of the way in which relaxation aids in labor.
6. Give one example of the value of relaxation techniques and of benefit other than during pregnancy and labor.
7. Demonstrate passive relaxation (mother relaxes, coach checks).
8. Tell the ideal weight gain during pregnancy.
9. Name foods that should be eaten during a single day.
10. Describe the position for resting and the amount of rest and sleep needed during the third trimester.
11. Describe one value of exercise during pregnancy.
12. Indicate when sexual intercourse is permissible during pregnancy and when it is not.
13. List at least seven danger signs during pregnancy.
14. Indicate what to do if danger sign is present.
15. Tell when hospital tours are available.

Outline

I. Before class
   A. Registration
   B. Book browsing (a variety of books and other materials available).
II. Introductions
   A. Self
   B. Couples
III. Couples' reasons for coming to class (discussion)
IV. What is the Lamaze method of prepared childbirth?
   A. Definition
   B. Brief history
   C. Advantages
   D. What we do not promise
V. Review of anatomy and physiology
VI. Embryo-fetal development
VII. Relaxation
   A. Role of relaxation

B. Carryover value
C. Types of relaxation
D. Teach passive relaxation
VIII. Basic concepts of prenatal care
   A. Diet and weight gain
   B. Rest
   C. Exercise
   D. Clothing
   E. Bathing
   F. Feelings—emotional changes
   G. Sex
   H. "Minor" discomforts
   I. Importance of keeping appointments
   J. Symptoms that should be reported immediately
IX. Tell about times for hospital tours; encourage to go during the next 2 to 3 weeks.

Class II

Goals

1. To teach touch relaxation, reinforcing again the role of relaxation.
2. To re-emphasize the importance of body building (mentioned in Class I) and to teach specific body-building exercises.
3. To overview the stages and phases of labor.
4. To describe the contractions of early labor in more detail.
5. To teach slow chest breathing.
6. To discuss infant feeding.

Objectives

At the completion of this class, the couple will be able to:

1. Demonstrate touch relaxation.
2. Check for relaxation.
3. Describe two effects of body-building exercises.
4. Demonstrate pelvic rock, bent leg lifts, tailor sitting, and tailor press.
5. Describe two values of the Kegel exercise.
6. Describe the Kegel exercise.
7. Name the stages of labor, telling when each begins and ends.
8. Name and differentiate the phases of the first stage of labor.
9. Correctly define duration and frequency and describe duration and frequency in first phase.
10. Tell when slow chest breathing is used.
11. Define cleansing breath, effleurage, and focal point, and tell how each is used in psychoprophylaxis.

12. Demonstrate slow chest breathing.
13. Describe advantages and disadvantages of methods of infant feeding.

Outline

   I. Review
  II. Touch relaxation
 III. Physical fitness exercises
   A. Why physical fitness
   B. Exercises
     1. Kegel
     2. Pelvic rock
     3. Bent-leg lift
     4. Tailor sitting
     5. Tailor press
 IV. Stages and phases of labor
  V. The contractions of early labor in more detail
   A. Characteristics
   B. Duration
   C. Frequency
 VI. Slow chest breathing
   A. When
   B. Cleansing breath
   C. Demonstrate slow breath
   D. Effleurage
   E. Focal point
   F. Relaxation
VII. Infant feeding
   A. Breast-feeding
     1. Advantages
     2. Prenatal preparation
     3. Basic approach to breast-feeding
     4. Community resources
   B. Bottle-feeding
     1. Comparison of methods and costs of various ways of preparing formulas.
     2. Importance of holding baby during feeding.
     3. Potential complications: "bottle-mouth," otitis media.
VIII. Remind about hospital tours

Class III

Goals

1. To review the stages and phases of labor and slow chest breathing.
2. To describe the active phase of labor in detail.
3. To teach shallow breathing.
4. To discuss hyperventilation.
5. To discuss the signs of labor and the differentiation between true and false labor.

6. To discuss what to take to the hospital.
7. To discuss fetal monitoring so that the monitor will not be a source of anxiety.
8. To review relaxation and teach concentration relaxation.

Objectives

At the completion of this class the couple will be able to:

1. Describe actual labor in terms of frequency and duration of contractions, length of the phase, reactions of the mother, and role of the coach.
2. Demonstrate shallow breathing and tell when it is used.
3. Define hyperventilation, tell the cause, at least three signs, and list three treatments.
4. List three signs of labor.
5. Differentiate true labor from false labor in at least three ways.
6. Name five items to pack in the suitcase and five items from the Lamaze bag.
7. Tell one reason fetal monitoring is used.
8. Describe at least one aspect of external fetal monitoring and one aspect of internal fetal monitoring.
9. Demonstrate concentration, relaxation.
10. Cite one aspect of the film, *Nan's Class,* which was meaningful to them.

Outline

   I. Review stages and phases: slow chest breathing
  II. Second phase/first stage
    A. When
    B. Contractions
    C. Reactions of mother
    D. Coaching
 III. Shallow breathing
    A. When
    B. How
 IV. Hyperventilation
    A. What is hyperventilation
    B. Signs of hyperventilation
    C. Reasons
    D. Treatment
  V. Discussion
    A. Signs of labor
    B. True vs. false labor
    C. What to take to the hospital
 VI. Fetal monitoring
    A. External and internal monitoring
    B. Demonstration of external monitor
    C. Reasons for use of monitor; advantages and disadvantages

    D. Using monitor to help prepared mother
 VII. Relaxation
    A. Review passive and touch relaxation
    B. Teach concentration relaxation
VIII. *Nan's Class*: Film and discussion

Class IV

Goals

1. To discuss the transition phase of labor and couples' response to transition.
2. To review relaxation, slow and shallow breathing.
3. To discuss obstetric intervention: episiotomy, forceps, and types of anesthesia.
4. To describe back labor and ways of coping with back labor.
5. To describe and discuss breech and cesarean birth.

Objectives

At the completion of this class the couple will be able to:

1. Cite five signs of transition.
2. Describe the contractions of transition.
3. Demonstrate coping with the contractions of transition.
4. Cite one reason for an episiotomy.
5. Describe two ways a mother can facilitate episiotomy healing.
6. Briefly describe in lay terminology each of the following types of anesthesia and analgesia, in relation to route of administration, time of administration, and action.
7. Cite two potential causes of back labor.
8. Describe two ways the coach can help alleviate the discomfort of back labor.
9. Define breech labor and identify one problem.
10. Describe two possible reasons for cesarean delivery.
11. Describe ways in which fathers may participate in cesarean birth.
12. Identify special maternal needs following cesarean birth.

Outline

  I. Transition
    A. What is transition
    B. Signs of transition
    C. The contractions of transition
    D. Coping with transition

E. Breathing patterns
F. Premature urge to push
II. Review
  A. Relaxation
  B. Slow chest and shallow breathing
III. Obstetric interventions
  A. Episiotomy
  B. Forceps
  C. Anesthesia
IV. Back labor
  A. Definition
  B. Major causes
  C. Characteristics
  D. Coping with back labor
V. Breech birth
VI. Cesarean birth (including film: *Cesarean Birth Experience* and discussion)

Class V

Goals

1. To review previously taught breathing patterns, checking for relaxation, use of focal point, effleurage, cleansing breath before and after.
2. To discuss "pushing": when not to push, how not to push, when and how to push.
3. To discuss the immediate postpartum period in the hospital.
4. To discuss the needs of newborn infants.
5. To discuss the needs of the parents of newborn infants.
6. To discuss the needs of siblings of newborn infants.

Objectives

At the completion of this class the couple will be able to:

1. Demonstrate previously taught breathing patterns (slow-chest, shallow and transition breathing).
2. Cite two examples of when and why not to push.
3. Demonstrate two techniques for not pushing during a practice contraction.
4. Tell when pushing is appropriate.
5. Demonstrate the technique for effective pushing.
6. Describe one advantage of rooming-in.
7. Describe classes available in hospital for mothers following delivery; encourage attendance.
8. Identify at least two needs of parents, newborn infants, and children.

Outline

I. Reverse role review of relaxation and breathing
II. Pushing
  A. When not to push
  B. How not to push
  C. When to push
  D. How to push
III. Beginning focus on postpartum
  A. Immediately following delivery
  B. Recovery room
  C. Rooming-in
  D. Father's visiting hour
  E. Classes available in hospital
  F. Feeding your baby
IV. Needs of parents and babies
  A. Needs of parents
  B. Characteristics and needs of babies
    1. Physical characteristics and needs
    2. Sensory characteristics and needs
    3. Social characteristics and needs
  C. Needs of siblings

Class VI

Goals

1. To help couples integrate all they have learned through a rehearsal of the labor experience, posing hypothetical situations and reviewing major steps.
2. To further discuss the postpartum period with particular attention to the needs of each family member, postpartum exercises, sexuality, contraception, fatigue, and a review of infant feeding.
3. To invite a recently delivered couple to share their experience of childbirth with the class.
4. To allow those couples who desire to listen to the baby's heartbeat with a fetoscope or stethoscope.

Objectives

At the completion of this class the couple will be able to:

1. Show by their answers and through demonstration that they understand the Lamaze method of preparation for childbearing.
2. Describe or demonstrate at least two postpartum exercises in addition to the Kegel exercise.
3. Tell when sexual intercourse may be resumed following delivery.

4. Name three methods of contraception.
5. Describe two ways in which a mother can prevent fatigue after she returns home.

Outline

I. Rehearsal for delivery
  A. Situation
  B. Second situation
  C. Review signs of labor
  D. Review: what to do when you believe you're in labor
  E. Review hospital admission procedure
  F. Review coping with early labor
  G. Dealing with interruptions
  H. Shallow breathing
  I. Transition
  J. Premature urge to push
  K. Pushing
  L. Baby arrives—Hooray
  M. Third stage
II. Continued discussion of postpartum (including film and discussion of postpartum experiences)
  A. Postpartum exercises
  B. Sexuality
  C. Contraception
  D. Fatigue
III. Listen to baby's heartbeat with fetoscopes and stethoscopes
IV. Discussion with recently delivered couple
V. Plans for class "reunion" after all infants are born.

Class Preparation for Cesarean Birth
(for women and their families expecting cesarean birth)

Outline

I. Prenatal preparation common to all mothers
II. Reasons for cesarean delivery, including opportunities to share reasons for feelings about previous cesarean birth
III. Relaxation exercises—useful during Braxton-Hicks contractions, pelvic examinations
IV. Prenatal tests: a way of communicating with baby
V. Hospital policies
  A. Tours
  B. Predelivery preparation
  C. Anesthesia
  D. Cesarean birth process
  E. Father participation
  F. Recovery room
  G. Infant care immediately following delivery
VI. Special needs of infant born by cesarean birth, including special concerns about bonding
VII. Postpartum period
  A. Physiologic dimensions
  B. Emotional dimensions, feelings
VIII. First weeks at home

Glossary _____

abortion, elective: interruption of pregnancy at the choice of the woman for reasons other than her own physical safety.

abortion, habitual: three or more consecutive spontaneous abortions.

abortion, incomplete: spontaneous abortion in which only part of the products of conception are expelled.

abortion, induced: deliberate interruption of pregnancy.

abortion, inevitable: spontaneous abortion with bleeding, uterine contractions, and progressive cervical dilatation.

abortion, missed: abortion in which the fetus dies but is retained in the uterus for 8 weeks or longer following death.

abortion, septic: abortion in which infection occurs in the endometrium and the products of conception.

abortion, spontaneous: the process by which a nonviable fetus is expelled from the uterus.

abortion, threatened: transcervical bleeding in a gravida when the fetus is less than 20 weeks' gestational age.

abortus: fetus of less than 20 weeks' gestation or 500 grams.

abruptio placentae: premature separation of a normally implanted placenta; may be complete or partial.

acini cells: milk-producing cells of the alveoli in the breast.

acme: highest point (as in the acme of a contraction).

acrocyanosis: peripheral cyanosis of the hands and feet, common in newborns.

adaptation level: state of coping (Roy's Adaptation Theory).

adaptive modes: intervening variables between basic needs and behavior; the four adaptive modes are physiologic, self-concept, role-function, and interdependence (Roy's Adaptation Theory).

afterbirth: term used by laymen to describe placenta and membranes expelled following delivery.

AGA: appropriate for gestational age; babies with birth weights between the tenth and ninetieth percentiles.

agalactia: failure of the secretion of milk.

agenesis: failure of an organ to develop; e.g., renal agenesis—failure of the kidneys to develop.

alae nasi: the nostrils.

albuminuria: detectable amounts of albumin present in the urine.

allantois: embryonic structure; a tubular diverticulum from the posterior yolk sac; allantoic blood vessels develop into the umbilical vein and arteries.

alleles: contrasting forms or states of a gene.

alpha-fetoprotein (AFP): the major circulating protein of the early human fetus; highly elevated levels of AFP in amniotic fluid are associated with neural tube defects (e.g., spina bifida, hydrocephalus).

amenorrhea: the absence of menstruation.

amniocentesis: process by which amniotic fluid is withdrawn from the amniotic sac through a needle inserted through the abdominal and uterine walls.

amnion: inner of two fetal membranes forming the amniotic sac.

amnionitis: infected amniotic fluid.

amniotic fluid: fluid surrounding the fetus within the amniotic sac.

amniotomy: the artificial rupture of the membranes.

anaerobic metabolism: metabolism occurring in the absence of oxygen; utilizes body compounds to produce energy.

analgesia: a substance that relieves pain.

android pelvis: narrow "male-type" of pelvis.

anencephalus: absence of the cranial vault, due to a failure of the anterior end of the neural tube to close.

anesthetic: a substance that causes loss of sensation, with or without the loss of consciousness.

anomaly: malformation.

anoxia: absence of oxygen.

antenatal: before birth.

antepartal: before labor.

anthropoid pelvis: pelvis in which the anteroposterior diameter equals or is greater than the transverse diameter.

antibody: a substance produced by the body that is antagonistic to a specific antigen.

antigen: any substance capable of causing the

production of an antibody; may be an invading organism, a foreign protein, and so forth.

Apgar scoring: a method of rapid assessment of the newborn in the delivery room, originally suggested by Virginia Apgar, M.D.

apnea: temporary absence of respiration.

areola: pigmented area surrounding the nipple.

artificial insemination: instrumental injection of semen into the vagina for the purpose of fertilization.

Aschheim-Zondek test: a pregnancy test involving the injection of urine from a woman into a mouse. After 5 days the mouse is sacrificed; if the mouse's ovaries are enlarged, the test is positive. Used less frequently today than in past decades.

asphyxia: a condition of an organism in which oxygen is decreased or carbon dioxide is increased.

atelectasis: a condition of the lungs in which many of the alveoli are collapsed.

atresia: absence of a passage normally present in the body; e.g., esophageal atresia.

auscultation: assessment by listening to sounds within the body.

autosomes: all of the chromosomes except the sex chromosomes.

axis: a real or imaginary line that runs through the center of a body, e.g., pelvic axis.

bag of waters: amniotic sac (lay term).

ballottement: a sign elicited by the examiner when two fingers are placed in the vagina; the fetus is felt to "bounce."

Bandl's ring: thickened muscle tissue between the upper and lower segments of the uterus.

Barr body: a chromatin mass derived from one of the X chromosomes. The number of Barr bodies is one less than the number of X chromosomes.

Bartholin's glands: two small glands near the vaginal orifice with ducts opening between the edge of the hymen and the labia minora.

bicornuate uterus: an anomaly of the uterus.

bilirubin: a product formed by the breakdown of red blood cells.

biopsy: removal of a small segment of tissue for examination.

---blast: a suffix designating a developing cell; e.g., neuroblast, a developing nerve cell.

blastocyst: an early stage of embryologic development.

Braxton Hicks contractions: intermittent uterine contractions occurring during pregnancy.

Brazelton assessment: a set of criteria assessing the interactional behavior of a newborn.

breech presentation: buttocks or feet as presenting part. Complete breech: buttocks and feet present. Footling breech: one or both feet present. Frank breech: buttocks present; hips flexed.

bregma: the area of the anterior fontanel.

bronchopulmonary dysplasia (BPD): a lung disorder secondary to oxygen therapy in newborns.

brown fat: source of energy for heat production in newborns.

bruit, uterine: the sound of the passage of blood through the uterine blood vessels; sometimes mistaken for fetal heart rate.

Candida vaginitis: a vaginal infection accompanied by intense burning and itching.

caput: occiput of the fetal head presenting at the vaginal opening prior to birth.

caput succedaneum: edema of the superficial tissues that overlie the bone of the part of the head presenting first at delivery.

caul: fetal membranes covering the head during delivery.

centromere: the point at which the strands of a chromosome are joined.

cephalhematoma: collection of blood between a cranial bone and the overlying periosteum.

cephalic presentation: when the head is the presenting part.

cephalopelvic disproportion (CPD): when the size or shape of the fetal head is too large to pass through the maternal pelvis.

cervix: the segment of the uterus between the corpus and the external os.

cesarean section: an operative procedure by which an infant is delivered through an incision in the abdominal and uterine walls.

Chadwick's sign: a bluish-violet color of the vagina during pregnancy due to increased vascularity.

chloasma: pigmentation of the face during pregnancy; "the mask of pregnancy."

choanal atresia: a congenital defect in which there is a bony or membranous obstruction of the posterior nares.

chorioamnionitis: infection in the amniotic membranes.

chorion: the outer layer of fetal membranes.

chorion frondosum: becomes the fetal component of the placenta.

chromosomes: rod-shaped bodies within a cell, on which genes are located (visible under the microscope).

circumcision: surgical excision of the foreskin (prepuce) of the penis.

cleft lip: congenital fissure of lip, called hare-lip by laymen.

cleft palate: failure of the palate to fuse during embryonic life; may involve hard and/or soft palate.

climacteric: a period of time, usually several years, during which ovarian function becomes less and less responsive to the stimulation of the gonadotropic hormones.

clitoris: erectile tissue at the anterior end of the vulva; homologous to the male penis.

coccyx: last four bones of the spinal column.

coitus: sexual intercourse.

colostrum: yellowish fluid secreted from the breasts prior to the secretion of milk.

complement: a natural property of food that is a factor in the destruction of bacteria.

concept: term that represents some aspect of reality.

conceptus: the embryo or fetus, the fetal membranes, the amniotic fluid, and the fetal portion of the placenta.

confinement: the period of birth and the early puerperium.

congenital: occurring during intrauterine life.

conjugate, diagonal: distance from the sacral promontory to the point at which the lower margin of the symphysis pubis rests on finger inserted in the vagina.

conjugate, true: anteroposterior diameter of the pelvic inlet; cannot be measured directly but is derived by subtracting 1.5 to 2.0 cm. from the diagonal conjugate.

conjunctiva: mucous membrane lining the eyelid, which is reflected onto the eyeball.

conjunctivitis: inflammation of the conjunctiva.

contextual stimulus: any stimulus, external or internal, other than a focal stimulus, which affects a situation, can be measured or is reported by an individual (Roy's Adaptation Theory).

contraception: prevention of conception.

contraction stress test (CST): a test to evaluate fetal well-being by observing the response of fetal heart rate to spontaneous or oxytocin-induced contractions.

copulation: sexual intercourse.

corona radiata: follicular cells bordering the ovum.

corpora cavernosa: (1) two cylinders of spongy tissue within the penis, (2) tissue within the clitoris.

corpus albicans: the term for the corpus luteum during the final portion of the regressive phase.

corpus luteum: the follicle after the ovum has been extruded; so called because the follicle is filled with a yellow material.

corpus spongiosum: a cylinder of spongy tissue within the penis.

cotyledon: one lobule of the placenta.

Couvelaire uterus: "boardlike" uterus due to hemorrhage within the myometrium following abruptio placentae.

CPAP: continuous positive airway pressure; one method of treating respiratory distress syndrome.

craniotabes: softening of localized areas in the cranial bones.

creatinine: a body chemical found particularly in blood and muscle; measurements of creatinine in mother's urine correlate with the amount of fetal muscle mass and thus with fetal size.

Credé prophylaxis: instillation of silver nitrate ophthalmic solution in the newborn infant's eyes to prevent ophthalmia neonatorum.

crowning: the appearance of the presenting part at the entrance of the vagina.

cul-de-sac of Douglas: peritoneal pouch between the anterior wall of the rectum and the posterior wall of the uterus.

cultural imposition: the attempt to impose one's cultural values on those with differing cultural values.

culture: the knowledge, beliefs, customs, laws, attitudes, values and behavior of members of a society.

culture shock: a reaction that occurs to persons in unfamiliar situations as a result of multiple environmental stresses.

curettage: scraping of the uterine endometrium with a curette.

cyesis: pregnancy.

cystocele: herniation of the bladder into the vagina.

decidua: the endometrium during pregnancy.

decidua basalis: maternal side of the placenta.

decidua capsularis: the decidua surrounding the chorionic sac.

decidua vera: the decidua other than that of the placenta.

decrement: decline or decrease, as in a contraction.

deletion: a piece of one chromosome that breaks off and is lost.

ΔOD_{450} (read delta OD_{450}): a measurement of the optical density of amniotic fluid in the evaluation of Rh_D sensitized mothers.

developmental task: a problem in social development that must be resolved during a particular stage of development for future development to proceed normally.

dextrocardia: having the heart on the right side of the body.

DHEA (dehydroepiandrosterone): an estrogen precursor; significant in the measurement of estrogens as a test of fetal well-being.

diaphoresis: profuse perspiration.

diaphragmatic hernia: congenital anomaly in which the diaphragm does not form completely, allowing abdominal organs to be displaced into the thoracic cavity.

diastasis rectus: condition in which the abdominal rectus muscles separate at the midline.

dilatation: the process by which the cervix dilates to 10 cm. in diameter.

dissonance: a characteristic of culture conflict; values and behaviors of one group do not "fit" with values and behaviors of another group.

dizygotic: from two zygotes, as dizygotic twins.

DNA (deoxyribonucleic acid): protein that contains genetic information.

dominant inheritance: inheritance requiring a gene from one parent only.

Down's syndrome: a condition in which there are three number 21 chromosomes (trisomy 21).

Dubowitz assessment: set of criteria used in the assessment of gestational age of the newborn infant.

ductus arteriosus: an anatomic connection between the pulmonary artery and the aorta, normally patent during fetal life but closing shortly after birth.

ductus venosus: an anatomic connection between the umbilical vein and the inferior vena cava, allowing most blood to bypass the liver during fetal life but closing shortly after birth.

Duncan's mechanism: delivery of the placenta with the maternal surface outermost.

dura (dura mater): the outer covering of the brain and spinal cord.

dysmenorrhea: difficult menstruation.
dyspareunia: difficult or painful intercourse.
dystocia: difficult labor.

ecchymosis: bruising.
eclampsia: occurrence of one or more convulsions, not attributable to other cerebral conditions, in a woman with pre-eclampsia.
ectoderm: outer layer of embryo from which skin, hair, nails, and so forth develop.
ectopic: in an abnormal position.
ectopic pregnancy: implantation of the fertilized ovum outside of the uterine cavity.
EDC: estimated date of confinement; the date the baby is expected to be born.
effacement: the process by which the cervical canal becomes shorter and thinner.
effleurage: light massage with the fingertips.
ejaculation: expulsion of semen from the urethra.
embryo: the developing conceptus from 2 to 8 weeks following fertilization.
embryologic age: the age of the embryo-fetus dated from the time of conception.
endometriosis: condition occurring when patches of endometrium are found outside the uterus.
endometrium: mucous membrane lining the inner surface of the uterus.
engagement: the status of the fetus when the largest part of the presenting part has passed the pelvic inlet and entered the true pelvis.
engorgement: vascular congestion, resulting in distention, as in breast engorgement.
entoderm: inner layer of the embryo from which internal organs develop.
epicanthus: fold of skin extending from the nose to the median aspect of the eye, covering the inner canthus; characteristic of Oriental persons; may occur in persons with Down's syndrome.
episiotomy: an incision made in the perineum, using blunt scissors.
epispadias: opening of the urethra on the dorsal aspect of the penis.
epithelial pearls (Epstein's pearls; Bohn's nodules): raised white areas of epithelial cells on the hard palate or gums.
Erb-Duchenne paralysis: paralysis of the upper arm resulting from injury to the fifth and sixth cervical nerves during delivery.
erythema toxicum: a rash of unknown etiology occurring in the newborn; resolves spontaneously.
erythroblastosis fetalis: hemolytic disease of the newborn due to incompatibility between the blood group of the mother and the blood group of the fetus.
estradiol: an estrogen.
estriol: the oxidized end product of estradiol and estrone; formed in the liver.
estrogens: hormones secreted by the cells of the ovarian follicle, the corpus luteum, and, during pregnancy, by the placenta.
estrone: an estrogen.
estrus: period of sexual activity in mammals other than primates.

ethnocentrism: the belief that one's own culture is superior to that of other groups.
exchange transfusion: replacement of 75 to 80 per cent of recipient's blood with donor blood by withdrawing and replacing small amounts at a time.
extension: the stretching-out of a limb or part; the opposite of flexion.

fallopian tubes (uterine tubes): tubes extending laterally from each side of the uterus to the area of the ovary.
ferning: the branching pattern that cervical mucus exhibits just prior to ovulation when it is allowed to dry on a glass slide.
fertilization: penetration of the ovum by a sperm.
fetal death: death of a fetus weighing 500 grams or less or of 20 weeks' gestation or less.
fetal heart rate, baseline fetal heart rate: the rate between contractions. Baseline fetal heart rate variability: fluctuations normally present in baseline fetal heart rate.
fetal mortality rate: number of fetal deaths per 1000 births.
fetoscopy: an experimental procedure in which a fetoscope is introduced into the amniotic cavity through the abdominal wall for the purpose of blood or skin sampling or visualization of the fetus.
fetus: the term given to the conceptus from 8 weeks after fertilization until birth.
fibrin: an elastic substance, deposited in fine threads, that causes the blood to clot.
fibrinogen: a protein that is changed to fibrin during the process of clot formation by the action of thrombin.
fibrinogenopenia: a deficiency of fibrin and fibrinogen.
fibroid: a tumor consisting of fibrous and muscular tissue.
fimbria: any fringelike structure; e.g., the fringelike extension at the distal end of the fallopian tube.
FiO$_2$ (fraction of inspired oxygen): the amount of oxygen an individual is receiving.
fissure: a groove.
fistula: an abnormal tubelike passage; e.g., tracheoesophageal fistula, an abnormal passage between the trachea and esophagus.
flexion: bending or being bent; the opposite of extension.
focal stimulus: environmental change in a given situation (Roy's Adaptation Theory).
follicle: a small excretory duct or tubular gland (see also graafian follicle).
follicle-stimulating hormone (FSH): hormone that stimulates the maturation of the graafian follicle; produced by the anterior pituitary gland during the first half of the ovarian cycle.
fontanel: space at the intersection of the sutures on the fetal head.
fontanel, anterior (bregma): diamond-shaped space at the junction of frontal, sagittal, and coronal sutures.

fontanel, posterior: triangular space at the junction of the sagittal and lambdoid sutures.

foramen ovale: opening in the septa between the atria of the heart during fetal life; normally closes shortly after birth.

foreskin (prepuce): fold of skin covering the glans penis.

fornices of the vagina: anterior and posterior spaces formed by the protrusion of the cervix into the vagina.

fornix: an arched structure (plural, fornices).

fossa: a shallow depression.

fourchette: a band or fold of mucous membrane connecting the posterior ends of the labia minora.

fraternal twins (dizygotic twins): twins that result when two ova are fertilized.

frenulum: a membranous fold connecting parts or restricting their separation.

frenulum clitoridis: frenulum joining the inner labia minora on the undersurface of the clitoris.

frenulum linguae: frenulum from the lower gum to the root of the tongue.

frontum: forehead.

fundus: upper portion of the uterus between the point of attachment of the uterine tubes.

galactorrhea: excessive secretion or flow of milk.

galactosemia: a condition in which the infant cannot metabolize lactose and galactose due to lack of a specific enzyme; inherited as an autosomal recessive trait.

gametes: sex cells.

gastroschisis: a defect in the abdominal wall lateral to the midline.

gastrostomy: a surgically created fistula through the skin into the stomach; provides an alternative pathway for gastric reflux and for feeding.

gavage: feeding through a tube passed into the stomach.

genes: determiners of hereditary traits.

genotype: genetic composition of an individual; e.g., possessing a gene for cystic fibrosis.

gestation: pregnancy, the period of pregnancy.

gestational age: the age of the embryo-fetus dated from the time of the last menstrual period.

gestational diabetes: diabetes that occurs only during the period of pregnancy.

glabella: smooth area above the nose between the eyebrows.

glans penis: smooth, round head of the penis.

glycosuria: presence of glucose in the urine.

gonad: sex gland; the ovary or testis.

Goodell's sign: softening of the cervix in the second month of gestation.

graafian follicle (vesicular follicle): mature ovarian cyst containing the fully developed ovum that will be released at ovulation.

gravid: pregnant.

gravida: a pregnant woman.

grunt: sound made by the closing of the glottis to prolong expiration and thus keep the alveoli from collapsing.

gynecoid pelvis: the typical female pelvis in which the inlet is round.

gynecology: the study of the diseases of the female reproductive tract and associated structures.

harlequin sign: momentary variance in color between right and left sides of body; of no pathologic significance.

Hegar's sign: softening of the lower uterine segment during the second and third months of pregnancy.

hematocrit: the volume of red blood cells per unit of circulating blood.

hematoma: a collection of blood in tissue.

hemoglobin: a component of blood consisting of globin, a protein, and hematin, an organic compound of iron.

hemorrhagic disease of the newborn: bleeding disorder in the first days of life related to a deficiency of vitamin K.

hermaphrodite: possessing genital and sexual characteristics of both sexes.

heterozygous: having different alleles for a trait on each gene of a pair; e.g., a genotype Dd.

histogenesis: the process by which tissues differentiate.

homoiotherm: an animal that can maintain its internal temperature at a specific level regardless of the environmental temperature.

homozygous: having the same alleles for a trait on each gene of a pair; e.g., a genotype DD.

human chorionic gonadotropin: a hormone produced by the trophoblast; the basis of testing for pregnancy.

human chorionic somatomammotropin (HCS): a hormone produced by the placenta; basis of one test of fetal well-being. Also called human placental lactogen (HPL).

human placental lactogen (HPL): human chorionic somatomammotropin.

hyaline membrane disease (HMD): a disease primarily of preterm newborns, characterized by a lack of surfactant in the alveoli of the lungs; also termed respiratory distress syndrome (RDS).

hydatidiform mole: a developmental anomaly of the placenta in which some or all of the chorionic villi degenerate into transparent vesicles.

hydramnios: amniotic fluid in excess of 2000 ml.

hydrocele: serous fluid in a saclike cavity, such as the cavity that surrounds the testicle.

hydrocephalus: a condition in which excessive cerebrospinal fluid leads to rapid head growth.

hydrops fetalis: describes the fetus of a sensitized Rh_d (negative) mother with intrauterine anemia and congestive heart failure.

hymen: a pinkish membrane of elastic and collagenous tissue at the entrance of the vagina. An *imperforate hymen* has no opening.

hymenal tag: hymenal tissue protruding from the floor of the vagina.

hymenotomy: surgical incision of the hymen.

hyperbilirubinemia: excess of unconjugated bilirubin in the blood.

hypercapnia: excessive carbon dioxide in arterial blood.

hyperemesis gravidarum: prolonged, severe nausea during pregnancy.

hypermagnesemia: excessive serum magnesium; may occur following the administration of magnesium sulfate.

hyperplasia: increase in the number of cells.

hypertensive states of pregnancy: hypertensive disease occurring during pregnancy, including pre-eclampsia and eclampsia.

hypertrophy: increase in the size of cells.

hypofibrinogenemia: deficiency of fibrinogen; may occur following a missed abortion or abruptio placentae.

hypogalactia: insufficient milk secretion.

hypogastric plexus: a large plexus of motor fibers formed above the promontory of the sacrum near the bifurcation of the aorta.

hypoglycemia: in the newborn, blood glucose level below 40 mg. per 100 ml. after 72 hours; blood glucose level below 30 mg. per 100 ml. prior to 72 hours.

hypomagnesemia: low serum magnesium; may occur following blood transfusion.

hypoplasia: the underdevelopment of an organ.

hypospadias: a condition in which the urethra opens on the ventral surface of the penis.

hypoxemia: inadequate level of oxygen in the blood.

hypoxia: inadequate level of oxygen in the body.

hysterectomy: surgical removal of the uterus.

hysterectomy, abdominal: removal of the uterus through an abdominal incision.

hysterectomy, pan---: removal of the entire uterus, the ovaries, and tubes.

hysterectomy, subtotal: surgical removal of the fundus and body of the uterus, but not the cervix.

hysterectomy, total: removal of the entire uterus, but not the ovaries and tubes.

hysterectomy, vaginal: removal of the uterus through the vagina.

hysterotomy: surgical incision into the uterus.

iatrogenic: medically caused; e.g., an iatrogenic condition would be caused by the treatment, such as blindness in a preterm infant due to high levels of arterial oxygen concentration.

icterus: jaundice.

idiopathic: of unknown cause.

idiopathic respiratory distress syndrome: see respiratory distress syndrome or hyaline membrane disease.

IDM: infant of a diabetic mother.

IgA: primary immunoglobulin of colostrum.

IgG: immunoglobulin that crosses the placenta and confers passive immunity to those infections to which the mother is immune (e.g., diphtheria, measles, and so forth).

IgM: first immunoglobulin made by infant after birth (or before birth if there is intrauterine infection).

impetigo contagiosa: a contagious staphylococcal infection of the skin.

implantation: attachment of the fertilized ovum, normally occurring in the uterine mucosa.

impotence: inability to participate in sexual intercourse; term usually refers to male partner.

inborn error of metabolism: hereditary deficiency of a specific enzyme resulting in a problem in metabolism; e.g., galactosemia, phenylketonuria.

incompetent cervix: inability of cervix to remain closed throughout pregnancy, resulting in spontaneous abortion or preterm delivery.

increment: increase, as in the increment of a contraction until the acme is reached.

induction: (1) intervention to cause labor to begin, (2) in embryology, the process by which one tissue transmits a stimulus that leads to the development of neighboring tissues.

inertia: inactivity; e.g., the absence of uterine contractions during labor.

infant mortality rate: number of deaths in the first year of life per 1000 live births.

innominate bone: hip bone.

interstitial cell-stimulating hormone (ICSH): stimulates the production of testosterone by the interstitial cells of Leydig in the testes; corresponds to luteinizing hormone (LH) in the female.

intertuberous diameter: distance between ischial tuberosities; measures the plane of the pelvic outlet.

intervillous space: areas filled with maternal blood in the maternal portion of the placenta, where maternal-fetal exchange takes place.

intrathecal: within the subarachnoid space.

introitus: entrance; e.g., of the vagina.

intromission: insertion of one object into another; e.g., insertion of the penis into the vagina.

inversion of the uterus: when the uterus is turned inside out; may be caused by pulling on the umbilical cord before the placenta has detached.

inverted nipple: a condition in which the nipple does not protrude from the breast.

involution: the process by which the reproductive organs return to their normal size and function.

ischium: posterior and inferior part of the lower portion of the innominate bone.

IUD (intrauterine device): devices placed within the uterus as a means of contraception.

IUGR (intrauterine growth retardation): failure of the fetus to grow properly, because of intrauterine infection, placental pathologic processes, and so forth.

jaundice (icterus): yellow discoloration of tissues, due to the deposition of unconjugated bilirubin.

jaundice, breast milk: jaundice that occurs when pregnanediol in mother's milk inhibits the conjugation of bilirubin by interfering with the enzyme glucuronyl transferase.

jaundice, pathologic: any jaundice that is not physiologic.

jaundice, physiologic: jaundice occurring in an

otherwise healthy newborn more than 24 to 36 hours of age.

karyotype: systematic arrangement of photographed chromosomes in order to demonstrate structure and number.

Kegel exercise: exercise for the muscles surrounding the vagina.

kernicterus: brain damage due to the deposit of unconjugated bilirubin in brain cells.

ketosis: the accumulation of ketone bodies (e.g., acetone) in the body as a result of incomplete metabolism of fatty acids.

kinesthetic: the sense that perceives movement, position, weight and resistance; proprioceptive.

labia: lips or liplike.

labia majora: the large, outer lips of the vulva.

labia minora: the thin, pink, hairless inner lips of the vulva.

laceration: a cut or tear.

lactase: the enzyme necessary for lactose digestion.

lactation: refers to (1) the secretion of milk or (2) the period during which milk is secreted.

lactiferous ducts: ducts through which milk travels from the lactiferous sinus to the nipple.

lactiferous sinus: located beneath the edge of the areola of the breast, the sinus holds milk and must be compressed by the baby's lips to send milk through the lactiferous duct to the nipple opening.

lactogenic hormone: hormone produced by the anterior pituitary; stimulates the growth of breast tissue and the process of lactation (also called prolactin, luteotropin).

lactose: the sugar in human milk.

lambdoidal suture: the suture between the occipital and parietal bones.

laminaria tent: a cone of *Laminaria* (dried seaweed), which swells when it becomes moist; may be used to dilate the cervix in an induced abortion.

lanugo: fine, downy hair covering the fetus from 20 weeks until birth.

laparotomy: abdominal incision.

let-down reflex: response to oxytocin that allows milk in the alveoli of the breast to flow into the milk ducts.

leukorrhea: white or yellow-white mucus discharged from the cervix or vagina; may be physiologic or pathologic.

levator ani: a broad muscle helping to form the floor of the pelvis.

LGA: large for gestational age; babies with birth weights greater than the ninetieth percentile.

libido: sexual drive.

lie: the relationship between the long axis of the fetus and the long axis of the mother.

lightening: the descent of the uterus when the baby's presenting part becomes fixed in the pelvis.

linea nigra: pigmented line seen from the umbilicus to the pubes in some women during pregnancy.

linea terminalis: divides the upper or false pelvis from the lower or true pelvis.

lithotomy position: lying on one's back with thighs flexed upon the abdomen and lower legs flexed upon the thighs.

lochia: vaginal discharge during the puerperium.

lochia alba: yellowish or whitish lochia after the second postpartum week.

lochia rubra: dark red vaginal discharge during the first 3 to 4 days following delivery.

lochia serosa: pink or serous brown-red lochia, usually occurring from 4 to 10 days following delivery.

low forceps delivery (outlet forceps): forceps are applied after the fetal head is crowning.

L/S ratio (lecithin/sphingomyelin ratio): a test to assess lung maturity in the fetus by measuring the phospholipids in amniotic fluid; a ratio of 2.0 or better usually indicates mature lungs.

luteinizing hormone (LH): hormone that stimulates ovulation and the development of the corpus luteum; produced by the anterior pituitary gland.

luteotropic hormone (LTH): hormone believed responsible for the maturation of the corpus luteum; produced by the anterior pituitary gland (see also lactogenic hormone).

macerated: softened by steeping in fluid; e.g., a macerated fetus.

macroglossia: enlarged tongue.

macrophages: monocytes in tissues and human milk; important in resistance to infection.

macrosomic: of large body size, as in some infants of diabetic mothers.

malpresentation: abnormal fetal presentation.

mastectomy: surgical removal of part or all of a breast.

mastitis: infection of breast tissue.

meconium: odorless, viscid first stools after birth; from dark green to black in color.

meconium ileus: paralysis of the lower gastrointestinal tract due to thick, putty-like meconium; a neonatal sign of cystic fibrosis.

meconium staining: condition of a newborn with hypoxia in utero.

mediastinum: the folds of the pleura and intervening space between the right and left lung.

meiosis: the process by which ova and sperm divide.

---melia: refers to a limb; e.g., phocomelia, absence of part of a limb.

menarche: first menstruation.

meningocele: congenital malformation of the spine in which the meninges protrude through a defect in the vertebrae.

menopause: the cessation of menstruation.

menorrhagia: profuse or excessive menstrual flow.

menses (menstruation): periodic vaginal discharge.

mentum: chin.

mesoderm: middle layer of embryo from which muscle, bone, and connective tissue develop.

metritis: inflammation of the uterus.

metrorrhagia: bleeding between menstrual periods.

microcephalus: a small head resulting from failure of the skull and brain to grow.

micrognathia: abnormally small jaw.

midforceps delivery: forceps are applied when the head is engaged but has not yet reached the perineal floor.

midwife: a person who delivers infants.

midwife, certified nurse (CNM): a registered nurse who has graduated from a nurse-midwifery program and passed a national certification examination.

midwife, "granny": a woman with no formal training who delivers infants, usually in a rural area.

midwife, lay: a person, usually a woman, who delivers infants but is not a nurse-midwife or a physician.

milia: tiny white papules seen on the face of newborns that disappear spontaneously.

miscarriage: lay term for spontaneous abortion.

mitosis: the process by which all cells divide, except the sex cells, after the stage of the primary oocyte and primary spermatocyte.

molding: the process by which the shape of the fetal head changes to fit the pelvis during labor.

Mongolian spot: pigmentation in the area of the lower back and buttocks, usually seen in nonwhite infants, which fades as the child grows older.

moniliasis: fungal infection of skin or mucous membrane.

monocytes: white blood cells important in resistance to infection.

monozygotic: originating from a single fertilized ovum; e.g., monozygotic twins.

mons pubis (mons veneris): fatty tissue covering the bony pubic symphysis.

monstrosity: major congenital abnormality (derived from the Latin *monstrare* [to show] because of the ancient belief that the birth of deformed infants was a sign from the gods).

montrice: an individual trained in psychoprophylactic methods who supports women during labor.

morbidity: disease or abnormal condition.

Moro reflex: reflex normally present in term newborn involving extension and then embracing movements of arms and flexion of knees and thighs.

morphogenesis: the process by which organs of the body and the body itself take shape.

mortality: death.

mortality, fetal: death of a fetus weighing 500 grams or more or of 20 weeks' gestation or more.

mortality, infant: death in the first year of life.

mortality, maternal: death of a woman during pregnancy and for a varying period following delivery.

mortality, neonatal: death of a newborn who has shown any sign of life within 28 days following birth.

mortality, perinatal: fetal mortality plus neonatal mortality; i.e., death from 20 weeks' gestation (or 500 grams weight) until 28 days after birth.

mortality rate: number of deaths per a specific population; e.g., deaths per 1000 births.

mortality rate, fetal: number of fetal deaths per 1000 births (or live births).

mortality rate, infant: number of deaths in the first year of life per 1000 births.

mortality rate, maternal: the number of maternal deaths per 100,000 births.

mortality rate, neonatal: number of neonatal deaths per 1000 births (or live births).

mortality rate, perinatal: the sum of the fetal mortality rate plus the neonatal mortality rate.

morula: a ball of cells in the very early development of the embryo.

mosaicism: condition in which there are different chromosomal patterns within the cells of a single organism.

mucous membrane: specialized mucus-secreting tissue lining many body structures.

mucus: fluid secreted by mucous membranes.

multigravida: a woman pregnant for the second or subsequent time.

multipara: a woman who has delivered two or more viable infants.

multiple pregnancy: pregnancy involving more than one fetus; e.g., twin pregnancy.

mutation: change in a gene.

myelomeningocele: congenital malformation of the spine in which the meninges and spinal cord protrude through a defect in the vertebrae.

myoepithelial cells: contractile cells surrounding the alveoli in the breast, which contract and express milk from the alveoli into the mammary ducts.

Nägele's rule: method of estimating the expected date of confinement (EDC). Count back 3 months from the first day of the last menstrual period and add 7 days.

navel: umbilicus.

necrotizing enterocolitis: a condition believed to result from lack of oxygenation to the bowel and infection, resulting in necrosis of the bowel wall.

neonatal death: see mortality, neonatal.

neonatal death rate: see mortality rate, neonatal.

neonate: an infant from birth to 28 days of age.

neonatologist: a physician with special training in the care of the newborn.

neonatology: the study of the neonate.

nephrostomy: a surgically created fistula into the kidney pelvis.

nevus: a congenital area of pigmentation in the skin (mole).

nevus flammeus: port wine stain; an area of discoloration of the face and neck.

nevus vasculosus (strawberry hemangioma): elevated area consisting of immature capillaries and endothelial cells; slowly regresses over a period of several years.

nidation: implantation of the fertilized ovum in the endometrium.

nonshivering thermogenesis: the process by which newborns produce heat by increasing their metabolic rate.

nucleotide: single segment of the helical strand of DNA.

nulligravida: a woman who has never been pregnant.

nullipara: a woman who has never delivered a viable infant (20 weeks' gestation or more).

nurse-practitioner: a registered nurse with additional education who practices in an expanded role.

occiput: back part of the head.

oligohydramnios: abnormally small amount of amniotic fluid; may indicate a defect of the fetal urinary tract.

oliguria: diminished secretion of urine.

omphalitis: infection of the umbilical stump.

omphalocele: congenital defect in which the abdominal wall fails to close and the abdominal contents herniate through the navel.

oogenesis: the process by which oogonia develop into mature ova.

oogonia: the forerunners of the mature ova.

oophorectomy: surgical removal of an ovary.

ophthalmia neonatorum: gonococcal infection of the newborn's eyes.

opisthotonos: an arched, hyperextended position of the body.

orgasmic platform: the congested walls of the lower vagina during intercourse.

orifice: opening, as in vaginal orifice.

os: mouth, as in uterine os.

ovary: gland that contains ova (in many stages of development) and that also produces estrogen and progesterone.

ovulation: discharge of the ovum from the ovary.

ovulation method of family planning: a method based on observation of changes in cervical mucus and abstinence during the days surrounding ovulation.

ovum: egg; female germ cell.

oxytocic: a pharmacologic agent that stimulates uterine contractions.

oxytocin: hormone from the posterior pituitary gland; stimulates uterine contractions and the let-down reflex during breast-feeding.

oxytocin challenge test: a test of fetal well-being in which the mother is given a small dose of oxytocin to stimulate contractions, and the fetal heart rate is monitored; also called contraction stress test (CST).

Paco$_2$: the partial pressure of carbon dioxide in arterial blood.

palliative: relieving symptoms but not curative.

palpation: physical examination using the fingers or palms.

Pao$_2$: amount of oxygen that has diffused through the alveoli into the arterial blood.

Papanicolaou test: a test for cervical cancer that involves "scraping" the ectocervix, the endocervix, and the vaginal pool.

para: a term describing the number of pregnancies in which an infant of more than 20 weeks' gestation was delivered (whether alive or dead).

paracervical nerve block: administration of a local anesthetic into the pelvic plexus.

parametritis: inflammation of the parametrium.

parametrium: smooth muscle, fatty tissue, and connective tissue extending laterally from the uterus between the layers of the broad ligaments.

parenteral: any route other than oral through which medications or nutrients are administered.

parity: number of live or stillborn infants of more than 20 weeks' gestation that a woman has delivered.

parturient: woman in labor.

parturition: process of giving birth.

patent: open.

pathogen: a substance or organism capable of producing disease.

pathogenic: productive of disease.

pathognomonic: characteristic symptom of a disease that helps to differentiate that disease from others.

peak experience: an experience that provides a deep sense of inner satisfaction and joy and enables a person to see self as a changed person with enhanced potential for further development.

pedigree: a diagram of the genetic history of a particular trait.

PEEP: positive end expiratory pressure; a modality used in conjunction with a ventilator in the treatment of respiratory distress.

pelvic inlet: upper margin of the pelvic cavity.

pelvic outlet: inferior margin of the pelvic cavity.

pelvimeter: instrument used in measuring pelvic diameters.

pelvimetry: process of measuring pelvic diameters to assess capacity for vaginal delivery.

pelvis, false: that portion of the pelvis above the linea terminalis and the symphysis pubis.

pelvis, true: that portion of the pelvis below the linea terminalis.

peridural anesthesia: the injection of an anesthetic into the extradural space; anesthetic does not penetrate the dura or the spinal cord.

perinatal mortality: see mortality, perinatal.

perinatal mortality rate: see mortality rate, perinatal.

perinatologist: an obstetrician with special interest in the perinatal period, with particular interest in high risk mothers and infants.

perineum: area between the vulva and the anus, made up of skin, muscle, and fascia.

periodic breathing: brief periods of apnea without cyanosis common in the respiration of preterm infants.

pessary: supportive device placed inside the uterus.

petechiae: minute hemorrhages.

pH: the chemical symbol for hydrogen ion concentration; the greater the number of hydrogen ions, the more acidic the solution and the lower the pH.

phagocyte: a white blood cell that destroys micro-organisms.

phagocytosis: ingestion and digestion of bacteria and particles by phagocytes.

phenomenologic: a psychological perspective that emphasizes the systematic investigation of conscious phenomena (experiences).

phenotype: genetically expressed characteristics of an individual; e.g., hair color, presence of hemophilia.

phenylketonuria (PKU): an inborn error in metabolism; the infant cannot metabolize phenylalanine, an essential amino acid.

phimosis: tightness of the foreskin of the penis, so that the foreskin cannot be pushed back over the glans penis.

phlebitis: inflammation of a vein.

phlegmasia alba dolens: "milk leg"; thrombophlebitis resulting in blanching, swelling, and pain in the thigh and leg.

phototherapy: the use of light as a treatment for hyperbilirubinemia.

pica: nonfood substances that are eaten.

pinna: cartilage of the ear.

placenta: organ through which fetal-maternal exchange of gases (oxygen and carbon dioxide), nutrients, and wastes occurs.

placenta accreta: invasion of the uterine muscle by the placenta; separation of the placenta thus becomes impossible in most situations.

placenta, battledore: insertion of the umbilical cord into the margin of the placenta.

placenta circumvallata: a raised white ring at the edge of the placenta.

placenta previa: abnormal implantation of the placenta in the lower uterine segment.

placenta, retained: condition in which part or all of the placenta remains in the uterus following delivery.

placenta succenturiata: an accessory placenta.

placentae, abruptio: see abruptio placentae.

placental infarct: hard, whitish area on the fetal or maternal side of the placenta.

platypelloid pelvis: oval pelvis with a shortened anteroposterior diameter.

plethoric: of a deep, beefy red color.

pneumomediastinum: accumulation of air in the mediastinum.

pneumopericardium: air in the pericardial sac.

pneumothorax: air in the thoracic cavity.

podalic version: shifting the position of the fetus to bring the feet to the pelvic outlet.

polycythemia: increased erythrocytes.

polydactyly: an extra finger or toe.

polygenic inheritance: traits controlled by more than one gene.

polyhydramnios: see hydramnios.

polymorphonuclear leukocytes (polys): white blood cells important in the resistance to infection.

polyuria: excessive secretion of urine.

position: relationship between the presenting part and the mother's pelvis.

post-term infant: an infant with a gestational age of more than 42 weeks; also termed postmature.

precipitate delivery: rapid labor and delivery.

pre-eclampsia: hypertension with proteinuria, edema, or both, occurring after the twentieth week of pregnancy.

prepuce (foreskin): fold of skin covering the glans penis.

presenting part: the part of the fetus that first enters the vagina.

preterm infant: an infant with a gestational age of less than 38 weeks; also termed premature.

primigravida: a woman during her first pregnancy.

primipara: a woman who has delivered one viable infant.

prodromal: early symptoms of a disease.

progesterone: hormone secreted by the corpus luteum and, during pregnancy, by the placenta.

projectile vomiting: expulsive vomiting.

prolactin: see lactogenic hormone.

prolapse of the umbilical cord: condition in which the umbilical cord is at or below the level of the presenting part.

proliferative phase of the menstrual cycle: precedes ovulation.

prophylaxis: prevention.

proposition: a statement that states a relationship between variables.

prospective study: a study of events that are expected to occur after the study is initiated.

prostaglandin: a biologic substance present within the body that plays a role in many body processes, including contraction of the uterus.

proteinuria: protein in the urine; one symptom of pre-eclampsia.

pruritus: itching.

pseudocyesis: a condition in which a woman believes she is pregnant but is not (false pregnancy).

psychoprophylaxis: a method of preparation for labor.

ptyalism: excessive salivation.

puberty: the period of life during which the reproductive organs mature.

pudendal nerve block: administration of a local anesthetic into the pudendal nerves on the right and left of the perineum.

puerperal sepsis: infection of the pelvic organs during the puerperium.

puerperium: the period of time from the completion of the third stage of labor until the complete involution of the uterus, usually occurring 6 weeks later.

pulmonary oxygen toxicity (POT): a condition that occurs in some infants who have received too much oxygen at too much pressure for too long a period of time; also termed bronchopulmonary dysplasia, chronic lung disease.

pulse pressure: the difference between systolic and diastolic blood pressure.

pyelonephritis: inflammation of the kidney and its pelvis.

quickening: fetal movement perceived by the mother.

radioimmunoassay: a test for pregnancy that measures an antigen-antibody reaction by a radioisotope technique.

rales: sounds heard as air passes through fluid in the bronchi and alveoli; classified as dry or moist.

recessive inheritance: inheritance requiring genes from both parents.

rectocele: herniation of the rectum into the vagina.

rectovaginal fistula: an opening between the rectum and vagina.

residual stimulus: any characteristic of an individual that is relevant to a specific situation (Roy's Adaptation Theory).

residual urine: urine remaining in the bladder after voiding.

respiratory distress syndrome (RDS): a disease primarily of preterm newborns, characterized by a lack of surfactant in the alveoli of the lungs; also termed hyaline membrane disease (HMD).

restitution: at delivery, the rotation of the presenting part of the fetus after it emerges from the vagina.

retroflexion of the uterus: condition in which the body of the uterus is tipped posteriorly but the position of the cervix remains unchanged.

retrolental fibroplasia: a condition caused by oxygen given in too high concentration to the immature infant, resulting in blindness.

retrospective study: a study of events that occurred before the study was initiated.

retroversion of the uterus: condition in which the body of the uterus is tipped posteriorly with the cervix pointing anteriorly; uterine displacement.

Rh$_D$ factor: a factor in blood that is a possible antigen when the mother lacks the factor (Rh$_D$ negative) but the fetus has the factor (Rh$_D$ positive).

rhythm method: a method of contraception in which the couple abstains from intercourse on days prior to and following ovulation.

Ritgen maneuver: method of controlling the delivery of the fetal head.

RNA: ribonucleic acid; a protein within each cell.

role: the carrying out of rights and responsibilities associated with a particular status (e.g., the parent role).

Rubin test: a test for patency of the uterine tubes by the insufflation of carbon dioxide.

rugae: folds or creases (e.g., rugae of the vagina).

sacrum: bone comprised of five fused vertebrae located between the fifth lumbar vertebra and the coccyx.

saddle block: injection of medication into the conus of the dural sac; anesthetizes the area that would come in contact with a saddle while riding a horse.

sagittal suture: membranous space between the parietal bones from the anterior fontanel to the posterior fontanel.

scaphoid abdomen: "sunken" abdomen; e.g., the abdomen of a newborn infant with diaphragmatic hernia.

scapula: shoulder blade.

Schultze's mechanism: delivery of the placenta with the fetal surface outermost.

sclerema: hardening of the skin and subcutaneous tissue.

secretory phase of the menstrual cycle: follows ovulation.

semen: secretion from the male urethra in which sperm are transported.

SGA: small for gestational age; babies with birth weights below the tenth percentile.

Shake test: a test to assess lung maturity in the fetus by measuring the phospholipids in amniotic fluid; more rapid and less complex than the L/S ratio.

significant other(s): individual(s) who have a close, meaningful relationship with a particular person.

simian crease: a single abnormal transverse crease in the palm of the hand.

Skene's ducts: paraurethral ducts, found on each side of the urethral meatus.

smegma: cheeselike secretion around the labia minora.

souffle: soft blowing sound heard on auscultation.

souffle, funic: sound produced by fetal blood rushing through the umbilical vessels; synchronous with fetal heart rate.

souffle, placental: sound produced by blood flow in placenta; synchronous with maternal pulse rate.

souffle, uterine: sound produced by blood in the arteries of pregnant uterus; synchronous with maternal pulse rate.

spermatic cord: cord from which the testis is suspended; contains blood vessels, nerves, muscle fibers, and the vas deferens.

spermatogenesis: the process by which spermatogonia develop into sperm.

spermatogonia: forerunner of mature sperm.

spina bifida occulta: congenital malformation of the spine in which the posterior portions of the vertebrae fail to close.

spinnbarkeit: a property of cervical mucus that enables it to make a thread when placed between two glass slides.

station: the level of the presenting part in relation to the pelvis.

station zero: when the presenting part is at the level of the ischial spines (engaged).

strabismus: crossed eyes.

striae gravidarum: red, slightly depressed streak marks on the abdomen, and occasionally on the breasts, during pregnancy; "stretch marks."

stridor: harsh, high-pitched respiratory sound.

subinvolution: failure of the uterus to return to normal size and state following pregnancy.

subluxation: incomplete dislocation; e.g., congenital subluxation of the hip.

supernumerary nipples: excessive number of nipples, usually located along an embryologic nipple-line.

supine hypotensive syndrome: hypotension caused by the interference with the flow of blood returning to the heart via the inferior vena cava; due to the weight of the uterus on the inferior vena cava when the mother is supine.

suppuration: formation of pus.

surfactant: a substance formed by Type II cells in the alveoli of the lungs that reduces surface tension and prevents the alveoli from collapsing.

sutures: membranous spaces between the bones of the cranium in a fetus or newborn infant.

symbolic interaction: a social-psychological perspective in which the focus is the interaction between persons.

symphysis pubis: area where pubic bones join at the midline.

syndactyly: webbing of the fingers or toes.

tachypnea: rapid respiration (in newborn, a respiratory rate greater than 60 per minute).

talipes calcaneovalgus: a congenital condition in which the foot is flexed and deviates laterally.

talipes equinovarus: a congenital condition in which the foot is extended and deviates medially.

teratogen: any environmental factor, chemical or physical, that affects the embryo-fetus adversely.

term infant: an infant with a gestational age from 38 weeks to 42 weeks.

testicle: a gland in the male scrotum that produces sperm and the hormone testosterone.

testosterone: hormone secreted by the interstitial cells of the testes.

tetanic contraction: a contraction that exceeds 90 seconds in duration.

tetany: a state of excessive muscle tone.

theory: set of interrelated concepts and propositional statements.

thermoneutral environment: environment that allows a baby to maintain a body temperature of 36.5°C. (97.7°F.) with a minimum use of energy.

thromboembolus: obstruction of a blood vessel by a clot that has migrated from the site of formation.

thrombophlebitis: inflammation of a vein with subsequent formation of a clot.

thrombus: blood clot obstructing a blood vessel.

thrush: an infection caused by the fungus *Candida albicans*.

tine test: screening test for tubercular infection.

toco---: a prefix referring to labor or birth.

tocolytic: refers to the inhibition of uterine contractions, as in premature labor; derived from *toco-* (labor, birth) and *lysis* (gradual decline in the signs of a condition).

tonic: prolonged muscular contraction.

TORCH organisms: refers to toxoplasmosis, other (syphilis), rubella, cytomegalovirus, and herpes simplex, organisms that may injure the embryo-fetus in utero.

toxemia: term previously used to describe hypertensive states of pregnancy, including pre-eclampsia and eclampsia.

tracheoesophageal fistula: congenital anomaly in which there is a connection between the trachea and esophagus.

traditional societies: societies in which cultural change occurs slowly, so that there is minimal change from one generation to the next.

transient tachypnea of the newborn: rapid respiratory rate for several days following birth due to fluid in lungs that clears spontaneously as fluid is absorbed.

transition: the last phase of the first stage of labor, from the time the cervix is approximately 8 cm. dilated until complete dilatation.

translocation: refers to a piece of one chromosome that breaks off and subsequently attaches itself to another.

trauma: physical or psychologic injury.

Trichomonas vaginalis: a protozoan causing a vaginal infection, Trichomonas vaginitis.

trimester: three month period.

trisomy: the presence of three chromosomes rather than the usual two. Example: trisomy 21 (i.e., three of the number 21 chromosome) results in Down's syndrome.

trophoblast: outer layer of cells of the developing blastocyst.

tubercles of Montgomery: small papillae that appear on the surface of the nipples and the areolae; secrete a lipoid substance that lubricates the nipples.

tunica albuginea: tight fibrous sheath enclosing each testis.

ultrasonography: a technique by which high frequency sound waves are beamed into the body.

umbilical cord: the structure linking fetus and placenta, normally containing two umbilical arteries and one umbilical vein.

umbilical hernia: protrusion of the bowel at the umbilicus through a defect in the abdominal wall.

umbilicus: navel.

urachus: an epithelial tube connecting the fetal urinary bladder with the allantois; normally closes and forms the umbilical ligament following birth; occasionally remains patent.

ureterostomy: a surgically created external ureteral fistula.

urinary frequency: a frequent need to void.

uterine tubes (fallopian tubes): tubes extending laterally from each side of the uterus to the area of the ovary.

vagina: tube between the uterus and the vaginal orifice.

vaginismus: intense spasm of the muscles surrounding the vagina.

variables: concepts that vary along a dimension (e.g., age: from young to old).

varices: varicose veins; distended veins.

vas deferens: tubelike structures through which spermatozoa leave the testes.

vasectomy: a surgical procedure in which the vas deferens is severed and tied, blocking the passage of sperm.

vernix caseosa: a fatty secretion of fetal sebaceous glands and dead epidermal cells that covers fetal skin during the second half of pregnancy.

version: an attempt to "turn" the baby in a transverse "lie" to a longitudinal "lie." Version may be *external* or *internal podalic*.

vertex: top of head.

vertex presentation: presentation in which the head is the presenting part.

viable: capable of living, as a viable fetus, a fetus of 28 weeks' gestation or more.

villi: small vascular protrusions on a membranous surface; e.g., chorionic villi.

vulva: the collective term for the external female genitalia.

vulvectomy: surgical removal of the external female genitalia.

Wharton's jelly: a jelly-like substance surrounding the umbilical arteries and vein within the umbilical cord.

womb: uterus.

X-linked inheritance: inheritance through genes located on the X chromosome.

zona pellucida: the covering of the discharged ovum.

zygote: fertilized ovum.

Index

Note: Page numbers in *italics* refer to illustrations. Page numbers followed by the letter *p* refer to nursing plans. Page numbers followed by the letter *t* refer to tables.